Advanced Medical Statistics

2nd Edition

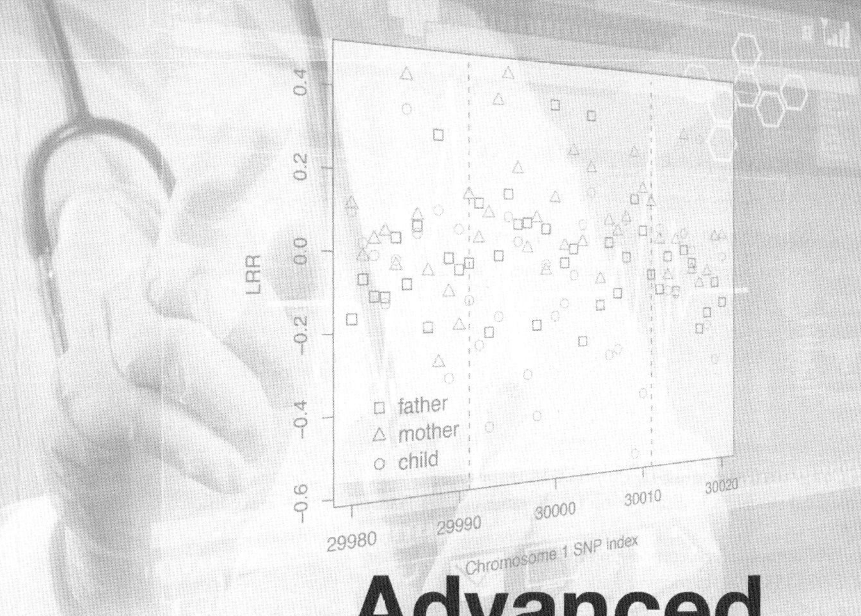

Advanced Medical Statistics

2nd Edition

Editors

Ying Lu
Stanford University, USA

Jiqian Fang
Sun Yat-Sen University, China

Lu Tian
Stanford University, USA

Hua Jin
South China Normal University, China

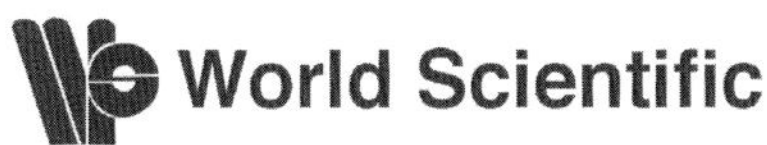

NEW JERSEY • LONDON • SINGAPORE • BEIJING • SHANGHAI • HONG KONG • TAIPEI • CHENNAI

Published by

World Scientific Publishing Co. Pte. Ltd.
5 Toh Tuck Link, Singapore 596224
USA office: 27 Warren Street, Suite 401-402, Hackensack, NJ 07601
UK office: 57 Shelton Street, Covent Garden, London WC2H 9HE

Library of Congress Cataloging-in-Publication Data
Advanced medical statistics / editors, Ying Lu, Jiqian Fang, Lu Tian, Hua Jin. -- 2nd edition.
p. ; cm.
Includes bibliographical references and index.
ISBN 978-9814583299 (hardcover : alk. paper)
I. Lu, Ying, 1960– , editor. II. Fang, Ji-Qian, 1939– , editor. III. Tian, Lu, editor. IV. Jin, Hua, 1967– , editor.
[DNLM: 1. Statistics as Topic--methods. 2. Biomedical Research--methods. WA 950]
R853.S7
610.7'27--dc23
2014048409

British Library Cataloguing-in-Publication Data
A catalogue record for this book is available from the British Library.

Typeset by Stallion Press
Email: enquiries@stallionpress.com

Printed in Singapore

PREFACE TO THE SECOND EDITION

Since the publication of the first edition, there have been tremendous advances in biostatistics and bioinformatics. The new edition tries to cover as many important emerging areas and reflect as much progress as possible. Many distinguished scholars, who greatly advanced their research areas in statistical methodology as well as practical applications, also have made invaluable contributions to the new edition by revising some chapters with relevant updates and writing new ones from scratch.

The new edition has been divided into four sections: Statistical Methods in Medicine and Epidemiology, Statistical Methods in Clinical Trials, Statistical Genetics, and General Methods. The first section includes new chapters on covariate-specific predictive value of prognostic biomarkers with survival outcome and personalized medicine: both discuss the newest development in statistical methods for predicting future clinical outcome or treatment response based on potential comprehensive baseline profiling of genomic and/or biomarker information. The following book chapters in this section are also substantially revised to reflect new advances in the field: Describing Data, Modeling Variation, and Statistical Practice, Meta-analysis, and Capture and Recapture Methods in Epidemiological Surveillance. The second section includes new chapters on Surrogates for Qualitative Evaluation of Treatment Effect, Adaptive Trial Design in Clinical Research, and Statistics in the Research of Traditional Chinese medicine. These introduce new methodological developments in either the design or analysis of clinical trials under different settings. We also include four revised book chapters: Statistics in biopharmaceutical research and development, Statistics in pharmacology and preclinical study, Statistics in Toxicology and Methodologies in Confirmatory Trials. The third section consists entirely of new chapters including DNA Copy Number Variation Analysis, Transcriptome Analysis , Design and Analysis of Linkage Study, Genetic Structure of Human Population, and Data Integration in Genome Wide Association Study (GWAS). They cover very broad topics in modern statistical genetics, which has become one of the most fertile research areas since the publication of the first edition. The first two chapters introduce new methods in bioinformatics and the last three chapters discuss important statistical issues in design, analysis and result interpretation in GWAS and linkage studies. The last section contains substantially revised chapters on Causal Inference, Bayesian Analysis, Tree-based method, Valid Prior-free Probabilistic Inference and its Application in Medical Science, Stochastic Process and Their Applications in Medical Sciences, and Time-series Analysis and its Application. Statistical methods in these areas have undergone rapid change with the revolutionized theoretical as well as computing tools. The revised chapter removes the obsolete content and reflects the newest status of the field. We have also removed/replaced three old book chapters: Evaluation of Diagnostic Tests Accuracy in Presence of Verification Bias Statistics in Genetics, Maximum Likelihood Estimation From Incomplete Data via EM-Type Algorithm.

Although tightly related, all the book chapters are self-contained and can be read independently. The book chapter intends to provide a convenient launch pad for readers interested in learning a specific topic, applying the related statistical methods in their scientific research and seeking the newest references for in-depth research.

We thank many readers, especially Dr. Paul Johnson, who helped us to catch numerous errors in the first edition. We have done our utmost best to correct them and avoid new ones. We also appreciate chapter authors for their support and contributions. We especially thank V K Sanjeed for his patience and constant help in preparing the second edition of the book.

CONTENTS

Section 1

Statistics in Medicine and Epidemiology

CHAPTER 1

HISTORY OF STATISTICAL THINKING IN MEDICINE

TAR TIMOTHY CHEN

Timothy Statistical Consulting, 2807 Marquis Circle East, Arlington TX 76016, USA

tar_timothy_chen@yahoo.com

1. Introduction

Biostatistics is a very hot discipline today with biostatisticians in great demand in the United States. Medical researchers appreciate statistical thinking and applications. In laboratory science, clinical research and epidemiological investigation, statisticians' collaborations are highly sought after. In many medical journals, statisticians are asked to serve as reviewers. In NIH (National Institutes of Health) grant applications, statisticians are required to be collaborators and statistical considerations have to be incorporated. In pharmaceutical development, drug companies recruit statisticians to guide study design, analyze data, and prepare reports for submission to FDA (Food and Drug Administration). All in all, statistical thinking permeates medical research and health policy. But it was not this way in the beginning. This article describes the history of application of statistical thinking in medicine.

2. Laplace and His Vision

Near the time of American independence and the French Revolution, French mathematician Pierre-Simon Laplace (1749–1827) worked on probability theory. He published many papers on different aspects of mathematical probability including theoretical issues and applications to demography and vital statistics. He was convinced that probability theory could be applied to the entire system of human knowledge, because the principal means of finding truth were based on probabilities. Viewing medical therapy as a domain for application of probability, he said that the preferred method of treatment would manifest itself increasingly in the measure as the number of observations was increased.[1,2]

Laplace's view that the summary of therapeutic successes and failures from a group of patients could guide future therapy was hotly debated within the medical community. Many famous physicians like Pierre-Jean-Georges Cabanis (1757–1808) claimed that the specificity of each patient demanded a kind of informed-professional judgment rather than guidance from quantitative analysis. According to their view, the proper professional behavior for physicians in diagnosing and treating disease was to match the special characteristics of each patient with the knowledge acquired through the course of medical practice. Physicians were able to judge individual cases in all of their uniqueness, rather than on the basis of quantitative knowledge. Cabanis rejected quantitative reasoning as an intellectual distraction and viewed medicine as an "art" rather than as a "science."[3]

On the other hand, other prominent physicians like Philippe Pinel (1745–1826) said that physicians could determine the effectiveness of various therapies by counting the number of times a treatment produced a favorable response. He considered a treatment effective if it had a high success rate. He even claimed that medical therapy could achieve the status of a true science if it applied the calculus of probabilities. His understanding of this calculation, however, was restricted to counting; he did not understand the detailed nature of the probability theory being developed by Laplace.[4]

3. Louis and Numerical Method

Later another prominent clinician, Pierre-Charles-Alexandre Louis (1787–1872), considered that enumeration was synonymous with scientific reasoning. He followed Laplace's proposal that analytical methods derived from probability theory help to reach a good judgment and to avoid confusing illusions. His method consisted of careful observation, systematic record keeping, rigorous analysis of multiple cases, cautious generalizations, verification through autopsies, and therapy based on the curative power of nature. He said that the introduction of statistics into diagnosis and therapy would ensure that all medical practitioners arrive at identical results.[5]

In his study of typhoid fever, which collected patient data between 1822 and 1827, Louis observed the age difference between the groups who died (50 patients with mean age 23) and who survived (88 patients with mean age 21). He also compared the length of residency in Paris and concluded that the group which survived lived in Paris longer. More importantly, Louis studied the efficacy of bloodletting as a therapy for typhoid fever. Among the 52 fatal cases, 39 patients (75%) had been bled. The mean survival time for the bled cases was 25.5 days contrasted to 28 days for those who were not bled. Of the 88 recovery cases, 62 patients (70%) were bled, with the mean duration of disease being 32 days as opposed to only 31 days for those not bled.[6]

Louis also studied the efficacy of bloodletting in treating pneumonitis and angina tonsillaris, and found it not useful. At that time, the method of venesection was defended by Francois Joseph Victor Broussais (1772–1838), the chief physician at the Parisian military hospital and medical school. Broussais claimed that diseases could be identified by observing the lesions of organs. Then patients could be treated by bleeding the diseased organ and by low fat, since most diseases were the result of inflammation. Louis, in contrast with Broussais, emphasized quantitative results from a population of sick individuals rather than using pathological anatomy to observe disease in a particular patient. He contended that the difference between numerical results and words, such as "more or less" and "rarely or frequently," was "the difference of truth and error; of a thing clear and truly scientific on the one hand, and of something vague and worthless on the other." He also proposed the basic concept of controlled clinical trial.[7]

Louis's work created more debates before the Parisian Academies of Sciences and Medicine in the late 1830s. The triggering issue was the question of the proper surgical procedure for removing bladder stones. A new bloodless method for removing bladder stones (lithotrity) was investigated by the surgeon and urologist Jean Civiale (1792–1867). He argued that given the fallacy of human memory, surgeons tend to remember their successful cases more than their unsuccessful ones; errors result from inexact records. He published the relative rates of death from the traditional surgical procedure and the lithotrity. The death rate of the old procedure was 21.6% (1,237/5,715); the death rate for lithotrity was 2.3% (6/257).[3]

In response to Civiale's statistical results, the Academy of Sciences established a commission in 1835 including the mathematician Simeon-Denis Poisson (1781–1840) and the physician Francois Double (1776–1842). Rejecting the attempt to turn the clinician into a scientist through the statistical method, Double believed that the physician's proper concern should remain the individual patient. He claimed it was inappropriate to elevate the human spirit to that mathematical certainty found only in astronomy;

the eminently proper method in the progress of medicine was logical not numerical analysis.[8]

During that time, Lambert Adolphe Jacques Quetelet (1796–1874) proposed a new concept of the "average man," defined as the average of all human attributes in a country. It would serve as a "type" of the nation similar to the idea of a center of gravity in physics. He formulated this idea by combining his training in astronomy and mathematics with a passion for social statistics. He analyzed the first census of Belgium (1829) and was instrumental in the formation of the Royal Statistical Society. He maintained that the concept of statistical norms could be useful to medical practice as it had been to medical research.[9] At the same time, Poisson applied probability theory to the voting patterns of judicial tribunals. He used the "law of large numbers" to devise a 99.5% confidence interval for binomial probability.[10]

In 1837, in a lecture delivered before the French Academy of Medicine, physician Risueno d'Amador (1802–1849) used the example of maritime insurance to illustrate why the probability was not applicable to medicine. If 100 vessels perish for every 1,000 that set sail, one still could not know which particular ships would be destroyed. It depended on other prognostic variables such as the age of the vessel, the experience of the captain, or the condition of the weather and the seas. Statistics could not predict the outcome of particular patients because of the uniqueness of each individual involved. For d'Amador, the results of observation in medicine were often more variable than in other sciences like astronomy.[11]

In the ensuing debates, Double commented that a Queteletian average man would reduce the physician to "a shoemaker who after having measured the feet of a thousand persisted in fitting everyone on the basis of the imaginary model." He also claimed that Poisson's attempts to mathematize human decision-making were useless because of the pressing and immediate concerns of medical practice.

Louis-Denis-Jules Gavarret (1809–1890), trained in both engineering and medicine, addressed the criticism of d'Amador in 1840. He maintained that the probability theory merely expressed the statistical results of inductive reasoning in a more formal and exact manner. He emphasized that statistical results were useful only if certain conditions prevailed — namely, the cases must be similar or comparable, and there must be large enough observations. He followed Poisson's example in requiring a precision of 99.5% or 212:1. He commented on the insufficient sample size in Louis' study of typhoid fever.[12]

In responding to the work of Gavarret, Elisha Bartlett (1804–1855), a professor of medicine at the University of Maryland and a student of Louis, said that the value of the numerical method was exhibited by Louis, and its true principles were developed and demonstrated by Gavarret.[13] However, the British statistician William Augustus Guy (1810–1885) in his Croonian lecture before the Royal College of Physicians in 1860, said that Gavarret's confidence interval could only be applied in rare occasions, and the results obtained from averaging a small number of cases could generally be assumed to be accurate.[14] In Germany, an ophthalmologist Julius Hirschberg (1843–1925), concerned about the number of observations required by Gavarret's assumption of 212:1 odds, modified the formula by using a lower standard of confidence of 11:1 or 91.6%.[15]

4. Statistical Analysis Versus Laboratory Investigation

In articles published in 1878 and 1881, German physician Friedrich Martius (1850–1923) commented that the dreams of Louis and Gavarret about a new era of scientific medicine had not been fulfilled due to the general "mathematical unfitness" of the medical profession as a whole. As one trained in laboratory methods, he said that the basis for science lay in laboratory experimentation rather than mere observation and the collection of numerical data.[3]

The legacy of Louis was in his claim that the clinical physician should aspire to become a scientist. But after Louis's retirement from the medical scene by the mid 1850s, some medical researchers began to argue that the compilation of numerical results might provide some useful insights about therapy; however, these results should not posses the authoritative status of "science." Friedrich Oesterlen (1812–1877) said that "scientific" results should be the discovery of knowledge which determined the causal connections, not just the discovery of the correlation.[16]

When Joseph Lister (1827–1912) published his pioneering work with antiseptic surgery in 1870, he noted that the average mortality rate was 45.7% (16/35) for all surgical procedures performed at the University of Edinburgh in the years 1864–1866 (before antiseptic methods were introduced). And it was 15% (6/40) for all surgical procedures performed in the three-year period 1867–1869 (after the introduction of antiseptic methods). Although he used this statistical result to show the efficacy of the new antiseptic method, he claimed that the science behind this was the germ theory of disease as proposed by Louis Pasteur (1822–1895).[17] Pasteur developed the germ theory and the concept of immunity. He carried out a clinical trial in 1881 to test his new vaccine against anthrax.

The founder of 19th century scientific positivism, Auguste Comte (1798–1857), believed that mere empiricism (as practiced by Louis) was not really useful for medicine.[18] Claude Bernard (1813–1878) proposed that the science of medicine resided in experimental physiology, rather than observational statistics. As a result of his laboratory-based orientation, he claimed that the experimental investigation of each individual patient could provide an "objective" scientific result. He agreed with Louis's vision of medicine as a science but saw the science of medicine as focused on the physiological measurements of individual patients.[19]

Other prominent clinicians at that time, like German Carl Wunderlich (1815–1877), tried to steer a middle ground between Louis and Bernard and synthesized both approaches. They collected a mass of quantifiable physiological data and tried to analyze it using numerical method. However, this approach was not accepted by the medical community in general, and many still opposed the process of quantification and remained focused on the individual patient.[20]

5. The Beginning of Modern Statistics

The founders of the Statistical Society in London in 1834 opted for the motto "Let others thrash it out," thus setting the general aim of statistics as the collection of data. Near the end of the 19th century, scientists began to collect large amounts of data in the biological world. Now they faced obstacles because their data had so much variation. Biological systems were so complex that a particular outcome had many causal factors. There was already a body of probability theory, but it was only mathematics. Prevailing scientific wisdom said that probability theory and actual data were separate entities and should not be mixed. Due to the work of the British biometrical school associated with Sir Francis Galton (1822–1911) and Karl Pearson (1857–1936), this attitude was changed, and statistics was transformed from an empirical social science into a mathematical applied science.

Galton, a half-cousin of Charles Darwin (1809–1882), studied medicine at Cambridge, explored Africa during the period 1850–1852, and received the gold medal from the Royal Geographical Society in 1853 in recognition of his achievement. After reading Charles Darwin's 1859 work *On the Origin of Species*, Galton turned to study heredity and developed a new vision for the role of science in society.[21] The late Victorian intellectual movement of scientific naturalism gave rise to the belief that scientifically trained persons must become leaders of British intellectual culture.

Galton accepted the evolutionary doctrine that the condition of the human species could be improved most effectively through a scientifically directed process of controlled breeding. His interest in eugenics led him to the method of correlation. He applied the Gaussian law of error to the intelligence of human beings and, unlike Quetelet, was more interested in the distribution and deviations from the mean than in the average value itself.

As a disciple of Galton, Karl Pearson, the founding father of modern statistics, created the statistical methodology and sold it to the world. Pearson changed statistics from a descriptive to an inferential discipline. He majored in mathematics at King's College, Cambridge. After Cambridge, he studied German literature, read law and was admitted to bar. He became professor of mathematics at King's College, London in 1881 and at University College, London in 1883. In June 1884 at age 27 he was appointed to Goldsmid Professor of Applied Mathematics at University College, London. Biologists at that time were interested in genetics, inheritance, and eugenics. In 1892 Pearson began to collaborate with zoologist WFR Weldon, Jodrell Chair of biology at University College, and developed a methodology for the exploration of life. Two years later Pearson offered his first advanced course in statistical theory, making University College the sole place for instruction of modern statistical methods before the 1920s.[22]

Following Galton, Pearson maintained that empirically determined "facts" obtained by the methods of science were the sole arbiters of truth. He argued for the almost universal application of statistical method, that mathematics could be applied to biological problems and that analysis of statistical data could answer many questions about the life of plants, animals, and men.[23] After a paper was rejected by the Royal Society, he founded the journal *Biometrika* in 1901 together with Galton and Weldon to provide an outlet for the works he and his biometrical school generated. Under Galton's generous financial support, Pearson transformed his relatively informal group of followers into an established research institute. Although he was interested in eugenics, he tried to do objective research using statistical methods and separated his institute from the social concerns of the Eugenics Education Society.

Pearson's emphasis on the relevance of statistics to the problems of biology had a very small audience. Mathematicians despised new endeavors to develop statistical methodology, and biologists thought mathematicians had no business meddling with such things. In 1903 Pearson wrote to Galton that there were only two subscribers of *Biometrika* in Cambridge, one a personal friend of Pearson and one of Weldon. Even though his major contributions were correlational methods and chi-square goodness-of-fit test, in 1906 the *Journal of the Royal Society* refused to publish a paper because they failed to see the biological significance of a correlation coefficient. In 1911 after Galton's death, Pearson became the first Galton Professor of Eugenics at University College, London.

Pearson also attempted to build an intellectual bridge to medicine by applying the statistical methods he developed. During his lifetime, the medical profession was divided in their opinion of the usefulness of statistical reasoning. Clinicians who continued to emphasize the "art" of medicine thought that statistics added little information beyond that supplied by experience. Those who argued for the existence of a "clinical science," basing diagnosis on physiological instruments or bacteriological observation, saw statistics as a way to make observation more objective, but did not consider statistics as "scientific" evidence.

6. The Beginning of Medical Statistics

Major Greenwood (1880–1949) was first to respond to Pearson's "crying need" for the medical profession to appreciate the importance of new statistical methods. At the age of 18, he entered medical school and read Pearson's *Grammar of Science.* He wrote to Pearson and applied statistical analyses to his research data while a student at London Hospital. During the academic year 1904–1905, after obtaining his license to practice medicine and publishing an article in *Biometrika*, he chose to study under Pearson. Despite Pearson's warning about the difficulty of earning a living as a biometrician, Greenwood decided to stake his professional career on the application of mathematical statistical methods to medical problems.

In debating with the bacteriologist Sir Almroth Wright (1861–1947) about the efficacy of vaccine therapy and a statistical measure called "opsonic index," Greenwood invoked the distinction between functional and mathematical error.[24] The former concerned errors in techniques of measurement, while the latter concerned inferential errors derived from the fact that data were a sample of population. When he pointed out that Wright had committed mathematical error, he got the attention of the medical community.[25] Consequently the Lister Institute for Preventive

Medicine in 1903 created the first department of statistics and named him its head. Greenwood characterized his department as dealing with problems of epidemiology and pathology, in contrast to Pearson's department at the University College, which dealt with heredity, eugenics and pure mathematical statistics. By training Greenwood, Pearson had helped to create the role of medical statistician, who as a researcher, understood both medical results and statistical methods.

Greenwood left the Lister Institute in 1920 for a position at the Ministry of Health and became affiliated with the newly created Medical Research Council (MRC). He saw his position at the medical establishment as instrumental in furthering the impact of statistical methods. Raymond Pearl (1879–1940) was Greenwood's American counterpart. He went to London to study under Pearson after finishing his PhD in biology at the University of Michigan. In 1918 Pearl began a long-standing relationship with The Johns Hopkins University as professor of biometry and vital statistics in the School of Hygiene and Public Health and as statistician at The Johns Hopkins Hospital.

By the early 1920's, Greenwood was not alone in arguing for application of modern statistics in medicine. One writer said in *the Journal of the American Medical Association* in 1920 that statistics was of great practical significance and should be required in the premedical curriculum.[26] Pearl in a 1921 article in the *Johns Hopkins hospital Bulletin* said that quantitative data generated by the modern hospital should be analyzed in cooperation with expert statistician. The arguments for using statistics in medicine were framed in terms of ensuring that medical research become "scientifically" grounded.[27]

7. Randomization in Experimentation

Besides Pearson, another founder of modern statistics was Sir Ronald A. Fisher (1890–1962). He also majored in mathematics at Cambridge and studied the theory of errors, statistical mechanics, and quantum theory.[28] By the age of 22, he published his first paper in statistics introducing the method of maximum likelihood, and three years later he wrote another paper deriving the exact sampling distribution of the Pearson correlation coefficient. He was also interested in applying mathematics to biological problems. Beginning in 1919, he spent many years at Rothamsted Experimental Station and collaborated with other researchers. He developed statistical methods for design and analysis of experiments, which were collected in his books *Statistical Methods for Research Workers*[29] and *The Design of Experiments*.[30] He proposed three main principles — the essentiality of replication and randomization, and the possibility of reducing errors by appropriate organization of the experiment.

Fisher's major contribution to science was using randomization to do experiments so that the variation in the data could be accounted for in the statistical analysis, and the bias of treatment assignment could be eliminated. Greenwood characterized Fisher's ideas as "epoch-making" in an article published in 1948, the year before Greenwood's death. For Fisher, statistical analysis and experimental design were only two aspects of the same whole, and they comprised all the logical requirements of the complete process of adding to natural knowledge by experimentation.[30] In other words, in order to draw inference, statisticians had to be involved in the design stage of experiments. Fisher, when addressing the Indian Statistical Congress in 1938, said, "To call in the statistician after the experiment is done may be no more than asking him to perform a post-mortem examination: he may be able to say what the experiment died of".

In addition to the new developments in statistical theory brought about by Fisher's work, changes within the organization of the MRC also facilitated the emergence of the modern clinical trial. Sir Austin Bradford Hill (1897–1991), one of Greenwood's proteges, was the prime motivator behind these Medical Research Council trials. He learned statistical methods from Pearson at University College and in 1933 became Reader in Epidemiology and Vital Statistics at the London School of Hygiene and Tropical Medicine, where Greenwood became the first professor of Epidemiology and Public Health in 1927. In 1937 the editors of *The Lancet*, recognizing the necessity of explaining statistical techniques to physicians, asked Hill to write a series of articles on the proper use of statistics in medicine. These articles were later published in book form as *Principles of Medical Statistics*.[31] Upon Greenwood's retirement in 1945, Hill took his place both as honorary director of MRC's Statistical Research Unit and as professor of medical statistics at the University of London.[32]

8. First Randomized Controlled Clinical Trial

The British Medical Research Council in 1946 began the first clinical trial with a properly randomized control group trial on the use of streptomycin in the treatment of pulmonary tuberculosis. This trial was remarkable for the degree of care exercised in its planning, execution and reporting. The trial involved patient accrual from several centers, and patients were randomized to two treatments — either streptomycin plus bed-rest, or bed-rest alone. Evaluation of patient X-ray films was made independently by two radiologists and a clinician. This blinded and replicated evaluation of a difficult disease end-point added considerably to the final agreed patient evaluation. Both patient survival and radiological improvement were significantly better on streptomycin.[33]

Hill's work set the trend for future clinical trials where both the insight of physicians and the statistical design of professional statisticians were combined. The convergence of these two separate disciplines constituted the *sine qua non* for the emergence of the probabilistically informed clinical trials. The Laplacian vision of the determination of medical therapy on the basis of the calculus of probability had finally found fulfillment.

Hill, a non-physician, acknowledged that the medical profession was responsible for curing the sick and preventing disease, but he emphasized that experimental medicine had the third responsibility of advancing human knowledge, and the statistically guided therapeutic trial was a useful way to discharge that responsibility. Unlike earlier advocates of statistical application in medicine, Hill's work became a rallying cry for supporters of therapeutic reform on both sides of Atlantic. Among many factors that contributed to this groundswell of support, one was the proliferation of new and potent industrially produced drugs in the postwar era. Supporters argued that randomized controlled clinical trials would permit doctors to select good treatments and prevent undue enthusiasm for newer treatments.

To those critics who believed in the uniqueness of the individual, whether patient or doctor, LJ. Witts, Nuffield Professor of Clinical Medicine of Oxford University, said in a conference in 1959, that neither patients nor doctors were as unique as they might have wanted to believe. Witts conceded that there was a conflict of loyalties between the research for truth and the treatment of the individual. However, he pointed out that similar conflict existed between the teaching of clinical students and the treatment of the patient.[34] At the same conference, Sir George Pickering, Regius Professor of Medicine at Oxford, praised the randomized controlled clinical trials and declared that, in contrast, clinical experience was unplanned and haphazard, and physicians were victims of the freaks of chance.[35]

Americans were not slow in following the British lead in applying statistics to controlled clinical trials. Americans carried out the largest and most expensive medical experiment in human history. The trial was done in 1954 to assess the effectiveness of the Salk vaccine as a protection against paralysis or death from poliomyelitis. Close to two million children participated, and the immediate direct cost was over 5 million dollars. The reason for such a large trial was that the annual incidence rate of polio was about 1 per 2000. In order to show that vaccine could improve upon this small incidence, a huge trial was needed. Originally, there was some resistance to the randomization, but finally about one quarter of the participants did get randomized. This randomized placebo controlled double-blind trial finally established the effectiveness of the Salk vaccine.[36]

9. Government Regulation and Statistics

Later in the early 1960s, the drug Thalidomide caused an outbreak of infantile deformity. The US FDA subsequently discovered that over two and a half million tablets had been distributed to 1,267 doctors who had prescribed the drugs to 19,822 patients, including 3,760 women of childbearing age. This evidence raised the question whether the "professional judgement" of the medical community could still be trusted. The outcry from the public led the US Congress to pass the Kefauver–Harris Bill, known as the Drug Amendments of 1962 and signed by President Kennedy on October 10, 1962. This law fundamentally altered the character of research both for the drug industry and for academic medicine. It transformed the FDA into the final arbiter of what constituted successful achievement in the realm of medical therapeutics. The FDA institutionalized clinical trials as the standard method for determining drug efficacy. By the late 1960s the double-blind methodology had become mandatory for FDA approval in the US, and the procedure had become standard in most of the other Western countries by the late 1970s.

The application of statistics in medicine has scientific authority and is seen as rising above individual opinions and possessing "objectivity" and "truth." The emergence of the randomized controlled clinical trials could be seen as a special case of a more general trend — the belief that "quantification is science." This also coincided with the change of definition about statistics as a discipline. In a book written by Stanford professors Chernoff and Moses in 1959, they said, "Years ago a statistician might have claimed that statistics deals with the processing of data. Today's statistician will be more likely to say that statistics is concerned with decision making in the face of uncertainty."[37]

Through the work of Hill, the father of the modern clinical trial, statistical methods slowly were adapted in medical research. The reason that clinical trials gained legitimacy was because that public at large realized that the decisions of the medical profession had to be regulated. Only when the issue of "medical decision making" was removed from the confines of professional medical expertise into the open arena of political debate could the statistical methods gain such wide acceptance. This ascendancy of the clinical trial method reflected the close connection between procedural objectivity and democratic political culture.

Above is the evolutionary history of statistical thinking in medicine. Medical research is much more than therapeutic research, but all medical research must lead to improvement of therapeutics or prevention. From this history one can see how the application of numerical methods in medicine has been debated throughout the past two hundred years. It shows that it took a long time for good concepts and procedures to prevail in science. The debates described could be applicable to the current problems about therapeutic research in alternative and complimentary medicine. Only through learning from past experience non-orthodox medicine can be modernized quickly.

10. Epilogue

Early landmarks in clinical investigation anticipated the current methodology.[38] For example, James Lind (1716–1794) in 1753 planned a comparative trial of the most promising treatment for scurvy. However, most pre-twentieth century medical experimenters had no appreciation of the scientific method. Trial usually had no concurrent control, and the claims were totally subjective and extravagant. The publication by Benjamin Rush (1745–1813) in 1794 about the success of treatment of yellow fever by bleeding was one example.

Statistics was very influential in the development of population genetics. Johann Gregor Mendel (1822–1884), a monk in the Augustinian order, studied botany and mathematics at the University of Vienna. He carried out experiments on peas to establish the three laws of genetics — uniformity, segregation and independence. After Darwin advanced the theory of evolution, there was a great debate between the evolutionists (biometricians) and those believing in the fixation of species (Mendelians). Pearson in his series of papers, *Contributions to the Mathematical Theory of Evolution, I to XVI*, gave mathematical form to the problems of genetics and evolution. However, he held the view of continuous change and never accepted Mendelism.[39]

After reading Pearson's papers while a student at Cambridge, RA Fisher made major contributions to the field of genetics. In particular he synthesized and reconciled the fixed inheritance theory of Mendel and the gradual evolution theory of Darwin.[40] He was considered as one of three founders of the population genetics, together with Sewall Wright and JBS Haldane, and he occupied an endowed chair of genetics at Cambridge University. Fisher's major contributions were the theoretical foundation of statistics including estimation and the testing of hypotheses, exact distributions of various statistics, and statistical models of natural phenomena.[41]

As mentioned in the debates between the numerical methods school and the physiological school, physiological measurement data were collected using precise instruments during the later half of the nineteenth century in conjunction with the creation of research universities. Statistical methods were developed to analyze the data coming from the laboratories. Later, the controversy between the biometrical school and the bacteriologists/immunologists in the laboratory led to further developments in correct statistical methods to analyze laboratory data.

Before the development of modern epidemiology, John Graunt (1620–1674) started to collect data on mortality, derived the life table based on survival, and thus created the discipline of demographic statistics. William Farr (1807–1883) further improved the method of the life table and created the best official vital statistics system in the world for Great Britain.[38]

In 1848, John Snow (1813–1858) carried out the first detailed investigation of the cholera epidemic of London. Development of the discipline of bacteriology was associated with the investigation of epidemics due to infectious agents. Mathematics and statistics were used in modeling and analysis of infectious epidemic data. Modern statistical methods were developed to investigate the epidemics of non-infectious diseases in the last half of the 20th century. Epidemiological research has become another field of statistical application. It has merged with statistical survey methods to carry out surveillance and disease monitoring, and is now called population science, in contrast to clinical and laboratory sciences.

In every field of medical research, statistical thinking and methods are used to provide insight to the data and to verify the hypotheses. The generation of new data and new hypotheses also propel developments of new statistical methodology. In the twentieth century, modern statistics as created by Pearson and Fisher has made a huge impact on the advancement of human knowledge, and its application to medicine richly demonstrates the importance of statistics.

Acknowledgment

The author would like to thank Dr. James Spivey for his input in this paper.

References

1. Laplace, P. S. (1951). *A Philosophical Essay on Probabilities*, 6th ed., trans. Frederick Wilson Truscott and Frederick Lincoln Emory. Dover, New York.
2. Todhunter, I. (1865). *A History of the Mathematical Theory of Probability*, Macmillan and Co, London.
3. Matthews, J. R. (1995). *Quantification and the Quest for Medical Certainty*, Princeton University Press, Princeton, New Jersey.
4. Pinel, P. (1809). *Traite medico-philosophique sur lalienation mentale*, 2nd ed., Paris.
5. Louis, P. C. A. (1836). *Pathological Researches on Phthisis*, trans. Charles Cowan. Hilliard, Gray, Boston.
6. Louis, P. C. A. (1836). *Anatomical, Pathological and Therapeutic Researches upon the Disease Known under the Name of Gastro-Enterite Putrid, Adynamic, Ataxic, or Typhoid Fever, etc., Compared with the Most Common Acute Diseases*, Vols. 1 and 2, trans. Henry I. Bowditch. Issac R. Butts, Boston.
7. Louis, P. C. A. (1836). *Researches on the Effects of Bloodletting in Some Inflammatory Diseases, and on the Influence on Tartarized Antimony and Vesication in Pneumonitis*, trans. C. G. Putnam. Hilliard, Gray, Boston.
8. Double, F. J. (1835). Statistique appliquee a la medecine. *Comptes rendus de lAcademie des Sciences* **1**: 281.
9. Quetelet, L. A. J. (1962). *A Treatise on Man and the Development of His Faculties*, trans. R. Knox. Research Works Series #247. Burt Franklin, New York.
10. Poisson, S. D. (1837). *Recherches sur la probabilite des jugements en matiere criminelle et en matiere civile*, Bachelier, Paris.
11. D'Amador, R. (1837). *Memoire sue le calcul des probabilites applique a la medecine*, Paris.
12. Gavarret, J. (1840). *Principes generaux de statistique medicale.* Libraries de la Faculte de Medecine de Paris.
13. Bartlett, E. (1844). *An Essay on the Philosophy of Medical Science.* Lea and Blanchard, Philadelphia.
14. Guy, W. A. (1860). The numerical method, and its application to the science and art of medicine. *British Medical Journal* **469**: 553.
15. Hirschberg, J. (1874). *Die mathematischen Grundlagen der Medicinischen Statistik, elementar Dargestellt*, Veit, Leipzig.
16. Oesterlen, F. (1852). *Medical Logic*, trans. G. Whitley. Sydenham Society, London.
17. Lister, J. (1870). Effects of the antiseptic system of treatment upon the salubrity of a surgical hospital, *The Lancet* **i**: 40.

18. Comte, A. (1864). *Cours de philosophie positive*, 2nd edn., Vol. 3, JB Bailliere, Paris.
19. Bernard, C. (1957). *An Introduction to the Study of Experimental Medicine*, trans. Henry Copley Greene. Dover, New York.
20. Wunderlich, C. A. (1871). *On the Temperature in Diseases: A Manual of Medical Thermometry*, trans. W. Bathurst Woodman. New Sydenham Society, London.
21. Stigler, S. M. (1986). *The History of Statistics: The Measurement of Uncertainty before 1900.* The Belknap Press of Harvard University Press, Cambridge.
22. Pearson, E. S. (1938). *Karl Pearson*, Cambridge University Press, London.
23. Pearson, K. (1911). *The Grammar of Science*, 3rd edn., Macmillan, New York.
24. Cope, Z. (1966). *Almroth Wright: Founder of Modern Vaccine-Therapy*, Thomas Nelson, London.
25. Greenwood, M. (1909). A statistical view of the opsonic index. *Proc. Royal Soc. Med.* **2**: 146.
26. Kilgore, E. S. (1920). Relation of quantitative methods to the advance of medical science. *J. Am. Med. Assoc.* **88**, July 10.
27. Pearl, R. (1921). Modern methods in handling hospital statistics. *The Johns Hopkins Hospital Bulletin* **32**: 185.
28. Box, J. E. (1979). *R. A. Fisher: The Life of a Scientist*, John Wiley and Sons, New York.
29. Fisher, R. A. (1958). *Statistical Methods for Research Workers*, 13th edn., Hafner, New York.
30. Fisher, R. A. (1960). *The Design of Experiments*, 7th edn., Hafner, New York.
31. Hill, A. B. (1991). Principles of Medical Statistics. 12th edn., Lancet Ltd., London.
32. Himsworth, Sir Harold. (1982). "Bradford Hill and Statistics in Medicine," *Statistics in Medicine* **1**: 301–302.
33. MRC. (1948). Streptomycin treatment of pulmonary tuberculosis: A Medical Research Council Investigation, *Br. Med. J.* **769**.
34. Witts, L. J. (1960). The ethics of controlled clinical trials. In *Controlled Clinical Trials*, Blackwell Scientific Publications, Oxford.
35. Pickering, Sir George. (1960). Conclusion: The Physician. In *Controlled Clinical Trials*, Blackwell Scientific Publications, Oxford.
36. Francis, T. Jr. *et al.* (1955). An evaluation of the 1954 poliomyelitis vaccines trials — Summary Report, *American Journal of Public Health* **45**(5): 1–63.
37. Chernoff, H. and Moses, L. E. (1957). *Elementary Decision Theory*, John Wiley and Sons, New York.
38. Gehan, E. A. and Lemak, N. A. (1994). *Statistics in Medical Research: Developments in Clinical Trials*, Plenum Publishing Co, New York.
39. Lancaster, H. O. (1994). *Quantitative Methods in Biological and Medical Sciences: A Historical Essay*, Springer-Verlag, New York.

40. Fisher, R. A. (1958). *The Genetical Theory of Natural Selection*, 2nd edn., Dover, New York.
41. Fisher, R. A. (1950). *Contributions to Mathematical Statistics*, ed. WA Shewhart, John Wiley and Sons, New York.

About the Author

Tar Timothy Chen, Ph.D., is currently in private consulting. He was Head of Biostatistics Section and Professor of Biostatistics at University of Maryland Greenebaum Cancer Center, 1998–2001; Mathematical Statistician, National Cancer Institute, 1989–1998. He received his Bachelor of Science in Mathematics from National Taiwan University in 1966, Master of Science in 1969, and Ph.D. in Statistics from University of Chicago in 1972. His research interests include categorical data analysis, epidemiological methods, and clinical trials methodology. He has authored and coauthored 102 research papers published in *Biometrics, JASA, Statistica Sinica, Statistics in Medicine, Controlled Clinical Trials, New England Journal of Medicine, Journal of Clinical Oncology, Surgery, Ophthalmology, Journal of National Cancer Institute* , and others. He is an elected fellow of American Statistical Association, and American Scientific Affiliation. He was the president of International Chinese Statistical Association (1999). His biosketch appeared in *Who's Who in America*, (1999, 2000, 2001), *American Men and Women of Science* (1989–1998), and *Marquis Who's Who in Cancer* (1985).

CHAPTER 2

DESCRIBING DATA, MODELING VARIATION, AND STATISTICAL PRACTICE

HONGYAN DU

Center for Clinical and Research Informatics
NorthShore University HealthSystem
1001 University Place Suite 100
Evanston, IL 60201, USA

MING T. TAN

Department of Biostatistics, Bioinformatics and Biomathematics
Georgetown University Medical Center
Georgetown Lombardi Comprehensive Cancer Center
4000 Reservoir Road NW Suite 180
Washington, DC 20057, USA
mttan@som.umaryland.edu

1. Introduction

In an era of rapid advances in molecular biology and genetics, medical research at all levels (from basic science, to translational research and to clinical and population research) produces a wealth of data at an amazing speed. These data themselves are useless unless converted into information and knowledge. What distinguishes Statistics as a scientific discipline is that it aims to make inference about the unknown population from analyzing the sample data. A key concept that is consistent in both statistical theory and practice is that of variability. It is inherent in our daily lives, our data and in statistical estimates derived from the data. Because every person is different, a wonderful drug or therapy may only work for some but not all patients. Our blood pressure varies all the time. It can be influenced by the time (i.e., morning or evening), the method (i.e., arm cuff or wrist cuff), the mood of the subject (i.e., anxiety, excitement), health status, taking medication or doing exercise, and some other unknown factors (*the random variation*). Random variation, also known as noise, cannot be explained.

In fact, controlling variability from different sources is the main subject of statistical experimental design. It is not possible to control all factors, and the random variation always exists. Statistical methods provide justifications to determine the sample size (number of subjects) that will be needed to separate noise from trends or patterns likely to be related to some specific factors. Statistical estimate of variability quantifies the uncertainty in biomedical findings. This knowledge can be further used to tailor the treatment strategy for individual patients. Such effort is the goal of personalized medicine based on genomics information.

Clearly, describing the data and understanding the variability is closely linked to the biomedical process, the data arisen and also the study design (the deliberate process of generating data for scientific investigation). Understanding the biological and medical process is essential for understanding and making sense of the data. Thus, methods and tools to describe and model the variability in a succinct way allow us to understand and appropriately convey the information in the data. The key is to understand the variability underlining the data. Common data analytical techniques are now well summarized in excellent first courses in statistics and biostatistics.[1,2] The focus of this chapter is to introduce some more advanced methods for best describing, understanding and accounting for variability. Thus the chapter will contain basic statistical techniques and cutting edge methodological developments such as mixed-effects dispersion models. In addition, we provide some general guidance useful in statistical practice from study design to statistical analysis addressing issues such as prediction and overfitting. Furthermore through reviewing the analysis of a large randomized trial with quality of life as the outcome where missing values presented additional challenges, we demonstrate the modeling process and emphasize the cares we need to take in statistical practice.

2. Methods for Describing Data

The first step toward understanding data and making any inference is to understand what type of data we are dealing with, since different types of data require different statistical methods for analysis. This is a fact sometimes easily overlooked by non-statisticians. We first review some common types of data in biomedical research with special emphasis on those not often discussed about in textbooks but appearing increasingly often in biomedical research. We also point out the methods that ought to be used to analyze them.

2.1. *Data type and measurement*

Although the data in biomedical research often are complex, they do fall into several common categories. Understanding them will guide us to choose the right methods for summarizing and analyzing the data. The type of data determines what methods shall be used for analyzing the data and making inference. In addition to reviewing the basic types of data[2] we describe other types of data increasingly common in modern biomedical research.

2.1.1. *Categorical data*

When a patient's characteristics or disease conditions are classified into different categories, those observations would give rise to categorical data (or sometimes called dichotomous or attribute data). The simplest examples are the two-category yes/no observations, such as, if a patient has responded to the cancer therapy, or whether the patient is a smoker or nonsmoker, or whether the patient has colon cancer or not. This type of data is sometimes under the name of binary data or 0–1 data. Data of three or more categories include blood types (A, B, AB, O), combined categories such as fcmalc and malc lcukcmia and non-leukemia patients. Since there is no inherent order among these categories (blood types, combined gender/disease classifications), this type of data is also called nominal data. They can be analyzed with methods for contingency tables or a generalized linear model. Another type of categorical data includes the classification of smokers (none, occasional, heavy), the stages of breast cancer (I, II, II, IV), the degree of improvement after therapy (none, moderate, great, full), and the degree of pain (minimal, moderate, severe, unbearable) as subjectively assessed. Since there is an inherent order among the categories, these data are called ordinal data. However, just like in nominal data, arithmetic does not make sense in ordinal data, e.g., it is hard to say unbearable pain is twice as bad as severe pain, although some of them may appear to be numeric, e.g., the stage of breast cancer (I, II, II, IV).

One case where such distinctions may become obscure is the score data where scores are assigned to certain outcomes, in this case, the scoring does indicate an equal increment from one point to one point higher.

2.1.2. *Continuous data*

Continuous data arise when some form of measurement is taken, e.g., body weight and temperature, blood pressures and most blood chemistry tests (bilirubin, hemoglobin, cholesterol etc.). Usually, these observations or their transformations (e.g., logarithmic or square root) are considered normally distributed. Statistical methods and models for analyzing continuous data are most comprehensively developed. However, the accuracy of these measurements and knowledge about the reliability of these measurements, is important to make valid inference.[3] Specifically, it should be noted that when these observations are used as independent variables in the analysis, an errors-in-variable (or measurement error) model may be necessary.[4] The influence and importance of measurement error are usually not well addressed in elementary textbooks. Recent methodological research has further extended the measurement error models in generalized linear models and survival models. Continuous data can further be specified as interval scaled such as a series of temperatures (i.e., 10, 20, 30), and ratio scaled such as age (i.e., 10, 20, 30). As implied by the names, it makes sense to interpret that an age of 30 is three times as old as an age of 10 ($30/10 = 3$), but it doesn't make sense to say a 30 degree of temperature is three times as hot as a 10 degree, since there is no absolute zero degree of temperature, one can only say a 30 degree is 20 ($30-10 = 20$) degrees hotter than a 10 degree.

2.1.3. *Ratios*

Ratio data arise when we take ratios of two variables. For example, ejection fraction, an important cardiac function index, is the ratio of the difference between end systolic and diastolic volumes to end systolic volume. Cardiac output and the percent change in renal function (e.g., the glomerular filtration rate (GFR)) from certain baseline are other examples. More recently, the microarray gene expression ratio has become a focus of much cutting-edge medical research. Microarray technology has allowed fast, large scale (up to thousands of genes) analysis of gene expression. In these experiments, the ratios of gene expression from the diseased tissue samples to that of reference samples are expressed as spots for each gene. The analysis of these gene expression ratios must take into account how the ratio is derived and an appropriate corresponding (in fact, Gamma) distribution should be used for analysis.[5,6]

2.1.4. *Continuous proportional data*

This is in fact a subtype of ratio data when the ratio is a percentage between 0 and 1, such as the percent decrease in renal functions at different follow-up times from the baseline, and percent changes from pre-treatment to post-treatment in terms of certain physiological variables or some molecular or genetic features. Statistical methods to directly model the means of the proportional responses have emerged[7,8] using the simplex distribution of Barndorff-Nielsen and Jorgensen,[9] which takes into account the fact that such responses are percentages restricted between 0 and 1 and may also have large dispersion.

2.1.5. *Repeated measures*

In medical studies, subjects are often followed over time either in natural history study of certain disease or therapeutic studies, or measurements are obtained within certain experimental units or clusters (e.g., eyes or limbs of an individual). These observations are called repeated measures data, or if they are obtained over different times from the same individual, they are also called longitudinal data. This kind of design is often necessary in order to assess how a patient's response variable of interest evolves over time. For example, we may be interested in how certain physiological (i.e., glomerular filtration rate) or genetic (i.e, telomere length) variables change over time, or whether certain events (e.g., ear infection) occur over time.

The key issue here is that the within-patient or within-cluster correlation needs to be accounted for in the experimental design and data analysis. For example, children who have ear infection in one of their ears may be more likely to have infection in the other ear. Thus, 10 patients with 2 repeated measures (2 ears for each patient) do not have the same power as 20 patients with one ear measured.

The response variable of interest with repeated measures could be continuous or categorical or ordinal, and different statistical models need to be used to analyze different types of repeated measures outcome. Generalized linear models (GLIM)[10] are used to analyze continuous and categorical outcomes, whereas the proportional odds model[11,12] is used to analyze ordinal outcomes.

2.1.6. *Censored and truncated data*

When we only know that an observation is beyond some threshold or point in time, the observation is defined as censored. In biomedical research, censored data are commonly known as survival data, with definition of time to the event, e.g., remission of cancer, or the death of a patient. Special techniques are needed in the analysis of time-to-event data, since survival data ingeneral are not symmetrically or normally distributed, it is more satisfactory to use an alternative distribution (i.e., log-normal, exponential,

Weibull) in the model. The feature in this type of study is, at the time of analysis, the survival endpoint (either death or remission of cancer) of some patients has not yet been observed, thus the survival status is censored and may never be known since some patients may be lost to follow up, or the study is designed to end at that time point.

2.2. *Variability*

Variability is one of the fundamentally important concepts that underlie all statistical theories and methods. As the world is full of uncertainty, it is necessary to use statistics to study uncertainty scientifically. Usually a biologically active agent only has 5% chance to make to the clinic due to the variability existing in experiment and mostly in human. Another related essential concept is the probability distribution that is used to describe and analyze the data. Often we assume that the observations are from a certain distribution with a known parametric form and some unknown parameters. The most prominent distribution is the normal distribution, which is fundamentally important in statistics because the central limit theorem suggests that most common statistics are asymptotically normally distributed. Methods that do not assume a parametric form are called nonparametric methods. The advantage of parametric methods lie in their simplicity and efficiency. Sometimes an intermediate (semi-parametric) approach is taken, assuming characteristics of main interest are of a parametric model. Parametric and semi-parametric methods are commonly used in medical research.

2.3. *Basic techniques*

The basic techniques for data description are computing means and standard deviations, which are associated with the parametric form of a normal distribution. The mean is a measure of the central location and the standard deviation is a measure of variability. Because of the importance of normal distribution based theory in statistical inference, these two measures have special importance. However, they do not necessarily give good inferential values, if the distribution of the variable under study is not normally distributed. Sometimes the variability is beyond what the assumed distribution can describe (the so-called *over-dispersion*).

The five-number summary statistics are commonly used to describe the data, minimum, maximum and 25% (1st quartile), 50% (the median) and 75% (3rd quartile) percentiles. Together with the mean and the standard deviation, the five-number summary statistics give a good summary about the distribution of the data. If the distribution is symmetric, the mean and the median should be equal. If the mean is greater than the median, the distribution is skewed to the right, otherwise the distribution is skewed to the left.

Example 1. is adopted from a phase I clinical trial of topotecan in solid tumors. Topotecan is a new molecular target based anti-cancer agent.[13,14] The goal of the study was to determine if variability in topotecan lactone systemic exposure, measured by the area under the plasma concentration-time curve (AUC), could be reduced by a dose adjustment strategy using pharmacokinetics (PK) guided dose escalation. The treatment was to give topotecan to 15 children with solid tumors 5 days a week for 2 consecutive weeks. Doses were adjusted in order to maintain a single day AUC in *the specified range*: 150 ± 30 ng/ml*hr (**Cohort #1 for the first 8 patients**) or 100 ± 20 ng/ml*hr (**Cohort #2 for 9 patients**),[15] where two patients who had been in Cohort 1 were moved to Cohort 2 (after day 10) due to excessive toxicities and the AUC target was lowered to 100 ± 20 ng/ml*hr in general for toxicity concerns. AUCs and clearances were measured on day 1, 3, 6, 8, 10 during the course of the treatment (see Box-plots in Figure 1).

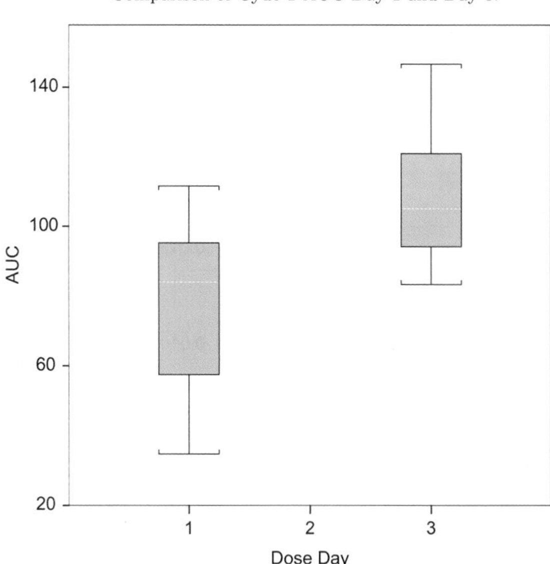

Fig. 1. Boxplot of AUC at different times.

2.4. *Graphic methods*

Graphic methods are commonly used in statistics and medical research to depict the distribution and variability of the data and to illustrate the methods, and indeed sometimes a picture is worth a thousand words.

For example, the five-number summary statistics are usually plotted as the box-and-whisker plot,[2] where the central line represents the median, the box represents the 25% and 75% percentiles (or the lower to the higher quartiles), and the whiskers are the minimum and the maximum. To see the variability and the overall distribution of AUC data for all the 15 patients, Figure 1 gives box-and-whisker plots for AUC at day 1 when the first dose was given and at day 3 when the second dose was given for these patients. As shown, the AUC is not symmetric on day 1 and is skewed to the right. At day 3, the AUC becomes more symmetric, which partly represents the effect due to dose targeting protocol based on PK data.

Histograms and smoothing techniques are also often used. The spline smoothing estimator, a nonparametric estimate of the density, provides a better description of the probability density of the distribution. With modern statistical software, it is easy to generate such estimates and overlay on the histogram. Figure 2 involves only the 8 patients in Cohort 1 in

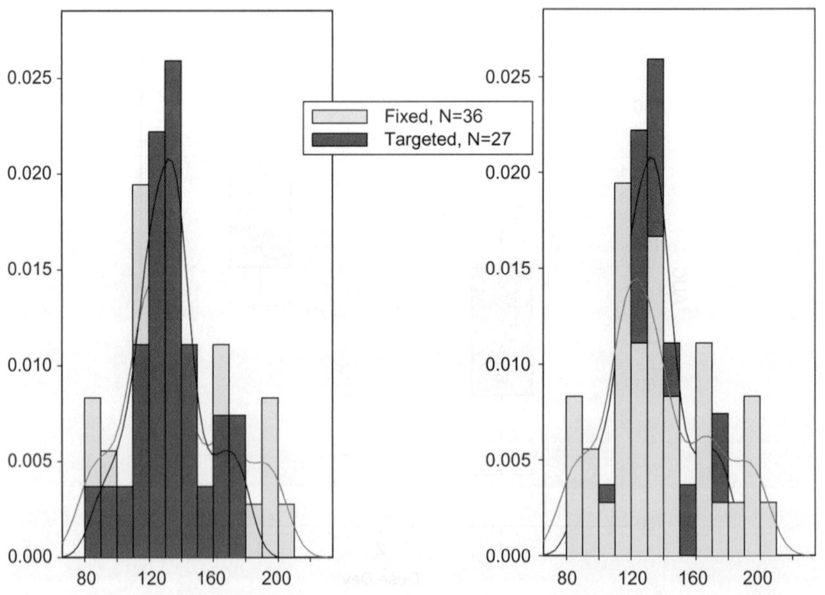

Fig. 2. Fixed and Targeted AUC 150.

Example 1 and displays the histograms and the fitted density curves for the AUCs. The "Fixed" refers to the 36 AUCs from the eight patients that were calculated alternatively using a fixed constant dose of 4 mg/m^2 divided by the patient's topotecan lactone clearance, and the "Targeted" refers to the 27 actual AUCs from the *same* eight patients that were dose-adjusted, however, the eight AUCs from the first dose and one AUC from the second dose were excluded.

3. Describing Data via Adjusting for Factors with a Model

Effective description of the data depends on the study design, and summarizing the data may not be straightforward because of the complicated design under which the data are produced, e.g., dependence of the observations (i.e, within-subject correlation) and missing values. In addition, a straightforward mean and standard deviation may be misleading. In Example 1, the fact that patients have multiple AUCs measured at multiple doses and some patients missed some AUCs, gives rise to an unbalanced repeated measures data structure. We used a mixed-effects model to estimate the PK parameters and compared those whose AUCs fell into the specified range and those whose AUCs did not. The summary statistics (such as the means and standard deviations) will need to account for within-patient correlation. Table 1 gives both the estimates that accounted for such correlation and those that did not. As shown in this table, the summary statistics using all the data based on the model are different from a straightforward

Table 1. Mean and standard deviation estimates according to dose adjustment requirements derived from a mixed effect model (p-values are for testing if the means are zero).

	Estimated mean (S.D.)		
PK Parameters	Adjusted	Unadjusted	p-value
Vc	31.67 (2.51)	30.90 (2.10)	0.76
Kel	1.28 (0.12)	1.21 (0.11)	0.30
Kcp	0.90 (0.13)	0.83 (0.13)	0.59
Kpc	0.68 (0.06)	0.65 (0.04)	0.54
Alpha	2.51 (0.27)	2.36 (0.25)	0.51
T1/2_alpha	0.34 (0.04)	0.37 (0.03)	0.44
Beta	0.34 (0.02)	0.33 (0.02)	0.44
T1/2_beta	2.28 (0.19)	2.34 (0.19)	0.58
CL	33.88 (1.62)	32.14 (1.30)	0.20
Vdss	66.13 (3.78)	64.55 (3.11)	0.55

calculation, thus the ones that accounted for the within-patient correlation should usually be considered for making inference if the model is reasonable.

More elaborate estimates based on models are often needed to avoid *bias*. There are several other examples where a mixed-effects spline model was used to estimate the mean glomerular filtration rate for diabetic patients at different stages of their lives and the associated standard errors.[16,17] We will discuss the model based approach for continuous proportional data and incomplete longitudinal data in Sections 4.4 and 5.

4. Over-Dispersion Issues

The term over-dispersion refers to the phenomenon that the observed variability (variance) is more than the nominal variability (variance) under a presumed model. Statistically speaking, over-dispersion shows that the mean-variance relationship of the assumed distribution is not correct. Although it is generally recognized that over-dispersion occurs in discrete data models under the binary and Poisson distribution assumptions, it also occurs in continuous proportional data.[7] The existence of over-dispersion was noticed a long time ago in statistics. Fisher noticed a lot of data in practice was over-dispersed.[8] Several natural questions arise such as what is the consequence of ignoring over-dispersion in the analysis and what are the appropriate techniques to detect and model the dispersion. In this section, we discuss the issues in several distributions including the more familiar binary and Poisson data and the developments on proportional data.

4.1. *Over-dispersed binomial data*

Binary outcome, e.g., success/failure of therapy, response to a cancer drug, etc., is one of the most common outcomes in medical research. Generically let the success probability be p and the binary (0–1) outcome Y_i of each of the n binary sequences (e.g., n cells, n mice, and perhaps n patients). Then the binomial outcome is $Y = \sum_{i=1}^{n} Y_i$. Over-dispersion arises when the empirical variance is greater than the binary variance $np(1-p)$, which is a function of the mean p. In this case, the distribution is completely determined by the mean parameter p. Then the variance of the binomial outcome is

$$\sum_{i=1}^{n} \text{var}(Y_i) + 2\sum_{i<j}^{n} \text{cov}(Y_i, Y_j) = np(1-p) + 2\sum_{i<j}^{n} \text{cov}(Y_i, Y_j).$$

Therefore, when the binary sequences are not independent of each other, namely, some $\text{cov}(Y_i, Y_j)$ is not zero, over-dispersion would occur. The consequence would depend on how much the over-dispersion is. Generally, over-dispersion can not be ignored.

Testing if over-dispersion presents can be done by using generalized linear models. With the development in generalized linear mixed effects model and Bayesian hierarchical model, over-dispersion can be accounted for directly in the modeling process.

4.2. *Over-dispersed Poisson data*

Similar to binomial data, Poisson distribution is determined by its mean parameter. Since Poisson model belongs to the generalized linear model, similar test statistics and modeling methods can be used in testing and modeling over-dispersion.

4.3. *Over-dispersed continuous proportional data*

The continuous data that have not been covered so much are the continuous proportional data and the directional data. The continuous proportional data arise when the response of interest is a percentage between 0 and 1, for instance, the percentage of decrease in renal functions at different follow-up times from the baseline, or the percentage of decrease in blood pressures from the baseline. The usual practice has been to just treat them as normal distributions. However, the variability in the response percentage is far beyond what the normal distribution can describe.[7] In fact, although the dispersion parameter is small, and the dispersion model is approximately normal,[9] real world data often have large dispersions.[19] In this case the normal model is usually not appropriate because although two variables are normally distributed, the ratio of the two is generally not.

Example 2. This was a prospective ophthalmology study on the use of intraocular gas in retinal repair surgeries.[16] The primary objective is to assess how quickly the gas is absorbed by patients over time and whether the absorption rate depends on the level of gas concentration. Three levels of gas concentration were administered in the study. The outcome variable was the percent of gas left in the eye. The gas was injected into the eye before surgery for a total of 31 patients. The patients were then followed three to eight (average of 5) times over a three-month period. The volume of the gas in the eye at the follow-up times was recorded as a percentage of the initial gas volume in that eye. An important issue was to estimate the kinetics of the disappearance of the gas (e.g., decay rate of the gas). Clearly the response variable here is confined between 0 and 1. Although, for instance, a logit transformation results in a transformed response in $(0, \infty)$, linear regression models with nonlinear transformed responses are often difficult to interpret. Particularly the serial correlation structure of the nonlinear transformed responses cannot be easily converted to that of the original responses. Our goal was to be able to model the dependence of gas decay on certain covariates directly. A common practice has been to assume that the response variable is normally distributed and ignore the fact that the responses are percentages confined between 0 and 1. However, as shown later, the variability in the response percentage is far beyond what the normal distribution can describe.

A moment estimator of the dispersion parameter σ^2 may be obtained by using the fact that the expected value of $d(Y;\mu) = \sigma^2$. Therefore,

$$\hat{\sigma}^2 = \frac{1}{\sum_{i=1}^{m} n_i - p} \sum_{i=1}^{n} \sum_{j=1}^{n_i} d(y_{ij}, \hat{\mu}_{ij}).$$

which is a consistent estimator of σ^2 as m tends to be infinity provided that $\hat{\mu}_{ij}$'s are consistent.

In **Example 2**, the estimate of dispersion parameter σ^2 is equal to 14.2. The p-value based on a χ^2 distribution with 2 degree of freedom is 0.0008, suggesting that the dispersion parameter is significantly greater than 0, that is, significantly greater than the dispersion of a normal distribution. Thus, the gas volume is not normally distributed at all. In fact, graphically, the simplex density function with this large dispersion parameter indicates the density has a dominant mass between 0.8 and 1, which is consistent with the feature of the data, that is, over 40% of observations are in this range. In addition, Song, Qiu and Tan examined how dispersion changes over time and other covariates and extended the marginal model to allow time-varying dispersion.[20] Therefore, indeed, the dispersion is needed to analyze this kind of data.

4.4. *Modeling dispersion in continuous proportional data*

In the example above, knowing the gas volume is not normally distributed and with over dispersion, the next question would be how to analyze such over-dispersed longitudinal data. A natural model would be a mixed effects model with outcomes observing a simplex distribution since an important objective is to make subject-specific inference. Qiu, Song and Tan proposed just such a simplex mixed-effects model (SMM)[21] and we will introduce it below briefly.

To specify the SMM, again let y_{ij} be the response for the ith subject at time j, let x_{ij} and z_{ij} be explanatory variables corresponding to the fixed and random effects, respectively, as in the usual mixed effects model with Gaussian outcome. Assume that, given a q-dimensional vector b; of random effects for subject i, the y_{ij} are conditionally independent with mean $\mu_{ij} = E(y_{ij}|b_i)$. With the outcome having a simplex distribution (see Appendix), we have $y_{ij}|b_i \sim S^-(\mu_{ij}, \sigma^2)$, where the conditional mean is related to the predictors (random and fixed effects) by

$$\eta_{ij} = g(\mu_{ij}) = x_{ij}^{\tau}\beta + z_{ij}^{\tau}b_i,$$

and g is the link function and β is a p-dimensional vector of fixed effects, and the random effects, $b_1, b_2, L, b_m \overset{i.i.d.}{\sim} N_q(0, D)$, with $D = D(\theta)$ depends on an unknown vector θ of variance components. The most commonly used link function for binary and continuous proportional data is the *logit* link given by $g(\mu) = \log\{\mu/(1-\mu)\}$. Denote $b = (b_1^{\tau}, b_2^{\tau}, \ldots, b_m)^{\tau}$ and $y = (y_1^{\tau}, y_2^{\tau}, \ldots, y_m)^{\tau}$, with $y = (y_{i1}, y_{i2}, \ldots, y_{im})^i$ for each subject i. The joint density function is

$$p(y, b) = \prod_{i=1}^{m}\left(\prod_{j=1}^{n_i} p(y_{ij}|b_i)p(b_i)\right),$$

where $p(y_{ij}|b_i)$ is the density of the simplex distribution and $p(b_i)$ is the density of the normal distribution. Then the log-likelihood function for parameters β, σ^2 and θ is proportional to

$$|D(\theta)|^{-m/2}\exp\left\{-\frac{1}{2\sigma^2}\sum_{i=1}^{m}\sum_{j=1}^{n_i} d(y_{ij};\mu_{ij}) - \frac{1}{2}\sum_{i=1}^{m} b_i^T D^{-1}(\theta)b_i\right\}.$$

Thus, integrating out the random effects gives the marginal log-likelihood of β and θ:

$$l(\beta, \theta) \infty - \frac{m}{2}\log|-D(\theta)| + \log\int_R e^{-h(b)}db,$$

where

$$h(b) = \sum_{i=1}^{m} h(b_i) \quad \text{with } h(b_i) = \frac{1}{2\sigma^2}\sum_{j=1}^{n_i} d(y_{ij};\mu_{ij}) + \frac{1}{2}b_i^{\tau}D^{-1}(\theta)b_i.$$

The marginal log-likelihood after integrating out the random effects from the augmented likelihood usually does not have explicit analytic expressions. To estimate the model, Qiu, Song and Tan proposed an extension[21] based on the approximate quasi-likelihood method (PQL/REML) proposed by Breslow and Clayton for generalized linear mixed effects model.[22] This approach is conceptually simple, numerically stable, and applicable to any number of random effects, q. It often results in fast computation algorithms, although the approximate inference can result in bias in parameter estimates. It is shown that when the fourth-order Laplace approximation is utilized, the estimation bias can be reduced to a satisfactory level.[21]

Example 2 (Continued). We analyzed the gas decay data using the SMM:

$$\text{logit}(\mu_{ij}) = \beta_0 + b_{0i} + \beta_1 \log(t_{ij}) + \beta_2 \log^2(t_{ij}) + \beta_3 x_{ij},$$

where the random intercept $b_{0i} \sim N(0, \theta_0)$. In addition, we considered another model including additionally random slopes $b_{1i} \sim N(0, \theta_1)$ as follows:

$$\text{logit}(\mu_{ij}) = \beta_0 + b_{0i} + \beta_1 \log(t_{ij}) + \beta_2 \log^2(t_{ij}) + (\beta_3 + b_{1j})x_{ij}.$$

where x_{ij} is the covariate of standardized gas concentration level with values 1, 0 or -1,[7] and t_{ij} is time covariate (days after surgery). We found that $\theta_0 = 0.26(0.19)$ and $\theta_1 = 0.09(0.25)$ using the adjusted PQL method. As the results showed the two variance parameters were insignificant — implying possibly an over-parameterization for the serial correlation — we used the simpler random intercept model as the model to make inference. Qiu, Song and Tan provide detailed analysis.[21] The PQLs analysis found the gas concentration level and the log-quadratic time covariate log2(*tij*) both significant ($p < 0.05$). However, if one uses the naïve approach of just taking *logit* transformation of the gas volume and proceed with a linear mixed effects model, gas concentration is not significant ($p = 0.14$).

5. Statistical Practice

In this section we discuss issues in statistical practice, especially, statistical applications in biomedical research, and discuss what an appropriate study design, rigorous analysis and proper inferences entail. The applications of statistics to biomedical studies usually follow three steps: we first determine the nature of the study design, specify research questions, and then determine the type of the data (measurement scale of the variables) and number of groups to be compared to form a statistical analysis plan.

5.1. *Study design*

A well designed study is essential, since no statistical process can effectively resurrect a poorly designed study. A study can be either experimental or observational. In an experimental study, investigators assign treatments or interventions to study subjects (i.e., patients, animals, or clinical sites) to determine whether the treatment or intervention has an effect. Randomization is typically used with the intent to generate comparable groups in all patients' characteristics such as age or gender except the treatment they receive. If the study shows group difference with respect to outcome of interest, the investigators will have confidence to conclude the treatment or intervention is efficacious. In addition, statistical significance may not translate to clinical meaningfulness (practical significance), e.g., 22 mg blood sugar improvement may not be meaningful among diabetic patients. It is hence important to specify a difference of practical significance in planning a study. For example, clinical trials are designed with adequate power (e.g., 80%) to detect such a predefined difference of practical significance, with a sample size no greater than necessary. On the other hand, in an observational study the assignment of the treatment or intervention under study is beyond the control of the investigators. Both experimental and observational studies have limitations which could be accounted for by the development of a rigid hierarchy of research design.[23] A study can also be designed as quasi-experimental, in which the investigators may have little or no control over the assignment of the treatments. In addition to determining whether the study is experimental or observational, we also need to clarify whether data are collected retrospectively or prospectively, and whether the data are obtained at one point in time (cross-sectional) or multiple point in time (longitudinal), since statistical approaches specifying correlation and covariance structures need to be utilized to analyze correlated observations generated from repeated measurements on the same subject.

5.2. *Research question*

The research question needs to be focused, clear and specific. In many cases, it should be easily translated into the two statistical hypotheses: null hypothesis and alternative hypothesis. The null hypothesis is a statement that is assumed true until sufficient contrary evidence is presented (e.g., treatment has no effect), whereas the alternative hypothesis is a statement that represents the investigators research interest (e.g., treatment has effect). Importantly, prior to performing any exploratory data analysis and statistical hypothesis testing, the significance (alpha) level needs to be specified, usually a $p < 0.05$ or <0.01 is regarded as statistically significant, and a $p < 0.10$ is regarded as marginally statistically significant. Typically, the investigators report confidence levels together with the statistical test of significance. The investigators' research interest or research question needs to be specific. For example, the investigators want to assess the relationship among variables, to evaluate the agreement between measures generated from different experimental methods, to detect difference between groups in terms of average measures at a certain point in time as well as change over time. It is important to clarify the research hypotheses before performing a statistical test, and by following a clearly designed protocol, the investigators will avoid pitfalls that can endanger the validity of research findings. Also, in some situations a lack of significance is as important as the significance investigators typically look for. To be effective, statisticians need to closely work with clinicians and medical researchers, to ensure everyone is on the same page about the analysis to be conducted. Therefore, in addition to rigorous statistical training, interdisciplinary training in biomedical sciences, collaborative research experiences, and communication skills are important.

The lack of clarity and understanding of the research question has resulted in much confusion about statistical inference recently with the explosion of both genetics and population data. It is important to keep in mind the research goal and to apply appropriate statistical modeling. One acute current issue is whether the research question is aiming to be explanatory or predictive, a question that has been overlooked in the ever rich tool box of statistical techniques. We discuss this issue in more detail in the following section.

5.3. *Is the research goal explanatory or predictive?*

Defined by the term itself, explanatory modeling is typically used to describe the relationship between a dependent variable and a set of explanatory variables where we are looking for correlation and association; a causal explanation can only be established if the causal factor occurs before the outcome response. On the other hand, predictive modeling is about applying a statistical model derived from the data in hand to predict future outcome (response) in new patients. Thus the explanatory power of a statistical model does not equal to its predictive power.

Traditionally, statistical modeling is to find the most parsimonious ones with least variables, with consideration of the model being numerically stable and easily generalizable. Clinical researchers working on epidemiology studies tend to include as many confounders as possible even they are not statistically significant, resulting in the model being more dependent in the given dataset. The advantage is that a model constructed in this way is usually a good fit, however it tends to result in 'overfitting' with enhanced parameter estimates but larger standard errors, since the more variables in the model, the larger the variation. Thus a model constructed in this way may have a high explanatory power but lacks predictive ability. Often in medical research, especially in diagnostic medicine about evaluating biomarkers for early cancer detection, constructing a prediction rule is emphasized beyond describing or explaining the relationships among the data.

Regression (both linear and nonlinear) analysis, commonly used in epidemiology studies, often reports R^2 (determinant coefficient) as the percentage of variance accounted for, which is a measure of the explanatory ability of the model. On the other hand, the same model may be used for different purpose. For example, logistic regression, a probability model for having certain disease, (i.e, colon cancer), is commonly used for disease classification in diagnostic medicine with a predictive goal. The area under receiver operating characteristic curve, AUC, also known as c-statistic or concordance probability from the Wilcoxon–Mann–Whitney test, is a good summary measure of predictive discrimination power. Resampling is usually needed to get an unbiased appraisal of the model's performance in future.

The distinction between explanatory modeling and predictive modeling can be subtle but important, Recently, Shmueli gave a thorough discussion in this regard,[24] declaiming both are necessary for generating and testing theories, but plays a different role, as the nature of uncertainty associated with explanation is different with that associated with prediction.[25] For example, epidemiological studies tend to assess associations while adjusting for all potential risk factors, while others involving a biomarker study may aim to predict outcome for a future patient. The statistical underpinning for the disparity between explanatory modeling and predictive modeling is the bias-variance trade-off. The estimated prediction error (EPE) is decomposed as noise, bias and estimation variance, namely,[26]

$$\text{EPE} = \text{Noise} + \text{Bias} + \text{Estimation Variance},$$

where noise is systematic error regardless of the correctness of the model and accuracy of its estimation, bias is how misspecifying the model is related to the given data set, and estimation variance is due to using a sample for model estimation, namely, sampling error with regards to the true model to measure similar data set. As a simple analogy to explain the concept, suppose a body temperature thermometer is not standardized, it will then constantly (systemically), and possibly accurately, measure someone's body temperature 1 degree higher — this systematic error is noise. Suppose there exists a thermometer (true model) to accurately measure the body temperature regardless of whether someone has a severe fever or a normal temperature, and there is a thermometer (model A) that performs well (less biased) on someone with lower temperature, and there is another thermometer (model B) that performs well (less biased) on someone with higher temperature. Although both models A and B are less biased, either one is regarded as a good predictive tool as the true model to measure someone in the future given his temperature is unknown in advance, and the difference between model A or B and the true model is the estimation variance. This equation shows the disparity between the *exploratory ability* derived from the given data set, which is represented by the *bias*, and the *predictive ability* to be assessed with future dataset, which is represented by the *estimation variance.* If the estimated prediction error (EPE) is a fixed value, and noise is under control, reducing the bias increases the estimation variance, and vice versa. Thus a model generated from exploratory purpose may not have good predictive power, and for prediction, avoiding overfitting is a key. Driven by the need to analyze large genomics data where the number of observations is typically much smaller than the number of predictors and overfitting can easily occur, numerous methods and several approaches have been developed. For example, the regularized regression or statistical learning have emerged to be a powerful tool for such analysis.[26] Recently, models that directly aim at maximizing a utility function of the receiver operating characteristics (ROC) curve such as the area under the ROC, the F-measure and linear combinations of sensitivity and specificity, have been developed in the setting of high dimensional.[27,28]

5.4. *Data distribution, normality assumption and robustness*

Once we have clarified the study design and the research questions, and have accurately translated them into statistical hypotheses, we start crunching the numbers. As previously described, the distribution of the data needs to be assessed to assure fulfillment of certain assumptions of the statistical test planned to run. An alternative test can be chosen if the assumptions on which the test is based are not met. For example, parametric statistical methods, such as student t test, ANOVA, and Pearson's correlation coefficient, require fulfillment of these three assumptions, normality, independence, and equality of variances; whereas nonparametric methods, such as Wilcoxon rank sum test, Kruskal–Wallis test, and Spearman correlation coefficient, are distribution free and do not require strict assumptions. In general, parametric methods are more sensitive with higher power but need bigger sample size, while non-parametric methods are less sensitive with lower power.

Should a parametric approach involving normal response be used, often the normality assumption in the model needs to be assessed. If normality had failed, appropriate data transformation, such as a logarithmic, a square root, and an inverse transformation need to be applied. A Box–Cox transformation, $T(Y) = (Y^{\lambda} - 1)/\lambda$, of the outcome variable (Y) with an optimal power coefficient λ may also be performed,[29] where the natural log-transformation is a special case for $\lambda = 0$.

Example 3. This is a randomized longitudinal clinical trial, with health related quality of life outcomes such as Trial Outcome Index (TOI) measured by the Functional Assessment of Cancer Therapy-Biologic Response Modifiers over 12 months for newly diagnosed patients with chronic myeloid leukemia.[30] Patients were randomly assigned to each of the two treatment groups at baseline. The TOI score ranged from 0 (worst) to 108 (best) and was measured up to nine times for each patient, including baseline and months 1, 2, 3, 4, 5, 6, 9, and 12 after randomization. The primary endpoint was to determine if there was a difference in mean TOI score between the two groups over time. The main covariates included treatment group (I vs. II), age (centered to mean) and gender. Among 1049 patients randomized at baseline, a total of 979 were identified as having baseline TOI score and be included in the analysis reported by Du *et al.*[31] The distribution of TOI was left skewed and a square root transformed in a double reverse fashion was made to correct for the left skewness, a situation in which a logarithmic transformation was not adequate whereas an inverse transformation tended to overcorrect. In addition, to make the assumption that the subjects observed only at baseline had a common distribution with those observed at follow up (month 6 or 9), the similarity of patient characteristics (age and gender) that were adjusted for in all the models with or without the outcome variable (TOI) was assessed at both month 6 and 9. Given the fact that more than 10% was missing data, the impact of missingness on estimation of health-related quality of life outcomes had to be assessed. A joint model for longitudinal TOI (mixed effects) with random effects assumed normal and time to dropout was developed for the analysis.

Although mixed effects model is widely used to analyze longitudinal and correlated data, where the random effects are commonly assumed to have a Gaussian distribution, examining the robustness to assumptions underlying such joint modeling is important. Several authors have examined this issue in linear mixed effects model.[32] Recently, McCulloch and Neuhaus examined such robustness in generalized linear mixed models used to analyze clustered or longitudinal data in a variety of inferences, including prediction, covariate effects, prediction of random effects and estimation of random effects variances based on examples, theoretical calculations and simulations.[33] They conclude that concerns over the misspecification of random effects distributions on inferences are often misplaced because (1) sensitivities are limited to aspects of the estimation that are not typically of interest, (2) the situations considered are too extreme, or (3) that published results do not actually support sensitivity to misspecification.

In the more complicated joint modeling of time to event and longitudinal outcomes for this quality of life data, Du *et al.* examined such robustness with respect to random effects.[31] We assessed how dense the longitudinal measurements were through the distribution of the number of longitudinal measurements utilizing theories and methods established for joint modeling of survival and longitudinal outcomes.[34, 35] This posterior of the random effects given the data TOIs and the fixed effects parameters approximates a normal density when the number of longitudinal measurements per subject is reasonably large. Since the random effect structure and longitudinal measurements (TOIs) are related to the survival parameters only through this posterior density, when the longitudinal measurements are dense the MLEs are robust against departures from the normal random effects assumption in the joint modeling of time to death/dropout and longitudinal data, whereas if the longitudinal measurements are sparse (e.g., with 3 observations per subject), the MLEs may be substantially biased.[34] We examined how dense the longitudinal measurements were through the distribution of the number of longitudinal measurements shown below (Table 2).

From Table 2, more than 90% of the patients had 4 or more observations. The median was more than 8 observations per subject. Stratified by group, about 56.5% of participants in group I and 39.2% of participants in group

Table 2. Distribution of the number of longitudinal measurements.

Number of longitudinal observations	Frequency	Percent	Cumulative Frequency	Cumulative Percent
1	27	2.76	27	2.76
2	14	1.43	41	4.19
3	23	2.35	64	6.54
4	25	2.55	89	9.09
5	50	5.11	139	14.2
6	70	7.15	209	21.35
7	113	11.54	322	32.89
8	188	19.2	510	52.09
9	469	47.91	979	100

II provided TOI score at all nine times. Therefore, the longitudinal TOI measurements are indeed rich and the MLE analysis is reasonably robust with respect to departures from random effects normality assumption.

For logistic regression with binary outcome, the continuous covariates need to fulfill the assumption of linearity in the *logit*.[36] Box–Tidwell transformation can be used to test the linearity in the *logit* by adding a variable in the model of the form x*log(x), and significance of the parameter estimate for this term indicates nonlinearity.

5.5. *Choosing the right statistical test*

In statistical practice choosing the right statistical test for the question to be addressed is obviously critical. In this section, we provide a summary and examples demonstrating how to choose the right statistical test according to the study design and research question; and pay special attention to methods that are scattered and sometimes overlooked in different textbooks.

5.5.1. *Evaluating relationship*

Correlation between two variables: When evaluating relationship between two variables that are measured for the same subject (e.g., imaging parameters and biomarkers), it is useful to display the data in a scatterplot and determine the correlation between the two variables, with the explanatory variable on the x axis and the response variable on the y axis. Scatterplot is a helpful tool to determine the overall pattern between the variables, once a linear relationship pattern is determined, the researchers further calculate the correlation coefficient to measure the strength and direction, and overlay a least-squares regression line that best represents the data.

Agreement between two measures: Bland and Altman have made the point that a high correlation does not imply a good agreement.[37] Bland–Altman approach for assessing agreement between two measures (i.e., by two methods, by two raters) on the same subject is by drawing a scatterplot of the difference between the two measures against the average of the two measures, and overlaying limits of agreement which is specified as average difference ± 1.96 standard deviation of the difference. For continuous measure, intraclass correlation coefficient (*ICC*) is computed to quantify the agreement, and for categorical measures a kappa statistic is computed.

Disease-Exposure relationship: in controlling for a confounder to assess exposure and disease relationship, Mantel–Hantzel test is usually used, and more sophisticated methods are also proposed.[38]

5.5.2. *Detecting group difference*

Cross-sectional measures: for two group comparison, a student t test is used given the assumptions (normality, independence, equality of variances) are fulfilled, otherwise a Wilcoxon rank-sum test is used; for three or more group comparison, analysis of variance (ANOVA) is used given the aforementioned assumptions are fulfilled, otherwise a Kruskall–Wallis test is used.

Longitudinal or repeated measures: in a longitudinal study each subject is measured multiple times thus the assumption of independence (observations are independent to each other, the value of one subject's measure is not affected by the value of another subject's measure) is violated, and methods accounting for within-subject correlation need to be utilized with appropriate variance-covariance structure specified. In addition, the group difference is expressed as not only the difference at each time point, but also the evolvement of the outcome variable over repeated measures (or over time if it's a longitudinal). For matched pair data, i.e., each subject is measured twice, a paired t test is used for continuous outcome given normality assumption is fulfilled, and a McNemar's test is used for binary outcome (i.e., yes vs. no). When repeated measurements are more than two, a repeated measures ANOVA, or a generalized mixed-effects model based on likelihood estimation for subject-specific inference, or a population average model based on generalized estimating equations (GEE) for inference at the population level can be used.[10] Specifically, for a study involving twins (both identical and non-identical), classic twin study methods with structural equation modeling can be used, such as an epidemiological study about the association of nongenetic factors with stress urinary incontinence,[39] in addition to GEE approach. In the classic twin model, differences in the phenotypic variance among identical and nonidentical twins are attributed to three basic factors: additive genetic influences, common environmental influences and individual-specific or unique environmental factors, assuming that identical twins share the same additive genetic variations, whereas nonidentical twins share just half of the additive genetic variations, and both sets of twins share the same common environmental variations.[40,41]

5.6. *Constructing a model*

5.6.1. *General steps*

A comprehensive and careful univaraite analysis needs to be performed as the first step in model building, to identify any interesting patterns, relationships, and associations. A main effect multivariable model is then constructed by initially including all candidate covariates whose p values are less than 0.25 in the univariate analysis, the candidate covariates are removed in a fashion of stepwise, backward, or forward, at a 0.05 cut-off. The magnitude of regression coefficient for each covariate in the multivariable model needs to be compared with that in the univariate analysis, to give an idea of whether an important covariate should not be excluded. Once the main effect multivariable model is determined, clinically meaningful interaction terms are tested and potential confounders are assessed. Note that a confounder can only be assessed but not statistically tested, and should be associated with both the outcome variable and the risk factor; usually a covariate is regarded as a confounder if adjusting for it, the magnitude of the effect of the primary risk factor changed 10% or more, i.e., the regression coefficient of smoking to low birth weight changed from 0.5 to 0.56 (>10% change) after adjusting for age, therefore age is considered as a confounder and should be included in the final multivariable model even age may not be statistically significant (i.e., $p > 0.05$) in some situations. Lastly, the adequacy and fit of the final model need to be evaluated before making statistical inferences.

Driven by the need to analyze high dimensional genomics data where the number of observations is typically much bigger than the number of variables/features, a large literature now exists on using statistical learning methods such as the LASSO for feature selection.[26] These methods are equally useful in more classic data analysis setting as well. Therefore, one can proceed with a lasso based variable selection procedure instead of the forward or backward selection procedures.

Furthermore, model building is often sequential. After examining the data and their distributions, more sophisticated modeling may be needed to analyze the data properly, and an easy to understand method (e.g., a graphical display) is important to convey the finding effectively to a broader audience. We illustrate this point and describe further modeling[31] for analysis of the data described in Example 3.

Example 3 (Continued). The first model for the analysis was the usual mixed effect model under MAR mechanism: $TOI_{ij} = X_{1i}^T(s)\beta_1 + W_{1i}(s_{ij}) + \varepsilon_{ij}$, where subject i was measured at time j $i = 1, \ldots, n$; and $j = 1, \ldots, k$, $X_{1i}^T(s)$ denotes the fixed effects, and $W_{1i}(s_{ij})$ denotes the subject-specific random effects, and $\varepsilon_{ij} \overset{iid}{\sim} N(0, \sigma_\varepsilon^2)$. In addition, a pattern-mixture model in which subjects were divided into groups depending on their missing patterns was constructed and the missing pattern was included into the longitudinal model as a between-subject variable. The model was the same as the first model while including dropout status as a covariate. Since the patterns without month 12 TOI were sparse, we treated all of these patterns as dropouts, the intermittent missing observations as MAR (missing at random), and defined completers as those with observations with last available TOI at month 12.[42] Since the time-to-dropout was potentially important, we constructed a shared parameter joint model, in which both the longitudinal TOI and the time-to-dropout process were modeled simultaneously. The time-to-dropout exponential regression model for hazard at time t (month) was specified as: $\lambda_i(t) = \exp(X_{2i}^T(t)\beta_2 + W_{2i}(t))$. Similarly $X_{2i}^T(s)$ denotes the fixed effects, and $W_{2i}(s_{ij})$ denotes the subject-specific random effects. The two models were linked by taking $W_{1i}(s) = U_{0i} + U_{1i}s$ and $W_{2i}(t) = \gamma_0 U_{0i} + \gamma_1 U_{1i}$, where γ_0 and γ_1 measure the association between the two models induced by the random intercepts and slopes respectively. Correlation between the intercept and slope was excluded for simplicity because its magnitude was negligible ($r < 0.013$). The censoring time was defined as the time between the baseline study date and the month 12 follow-up for completers. For dropouts, the time-to-dropout was defined as the time from the baseline study date to the midpoint between the date of the last HRQL collected and the scheduled date of the last visit. The covariates included age, gender and the 4th polynomial time with random intercept and slope with unstructured variance-covariance. An exponential distribution was assumed for the time-to-dropout component in the joint model. The joint model revealed significant ($p < 0.001$) between-group differences at each visit except for baseline. The parameter estimates[31] are similar to those as in the separate longitudinal and survival sub-models with a significant association parameter ($p = 0.039$) indicating negative association between slope of TOI and hazard of dropout and thus non-ignorable dropout. The study showed that joint modeling was a useful means to quantify the relationship between dropout and outcome when non-ignorable missing data existed in longitudinal data. In addition, it was a good practice to examine model sensitivity with respect to underlying model assumptions in complex longitudinal data with non-ignorable missing data.

Acknowledgments

The author thanks his collaborators Drs. Victor Santana and Clinton Stewart for making their data available for inclusion as an illustrative example, Dr. Peter Song for joint work on continuous proportional data and Kevin Liu and Catherine Billups for assistance with the data analysis. The author also acknowledges partial support by U.S. National Cancer Institute Cancer Center Support Grant P30 CA21765 and by American, Lebanese, Syrian Associated Charities (ALSAC).

Appendix

The density of a simplex distribution,[9] with mean (location parameter) $\mu \in (0,1)$ and dispersion parameter $\sigma^2 > 0$, is given by

$$p(y;\mu,\sigma^2) = [2\pi\sigma^2\{y(1-y)\}^3]^{-1/2}\exp\{-d(y;\mu)/(2\sigma^2)\}, y \in (0,1),$$

where

$$d(y;\mu) = \frac{(y-\mu)^2}{y(1-y)\mu^2(1-\mu)^2}.$$

The advantage of using this distribution is that the simplex distribution is a dispersion model,[9] where the response has density function of the form

$$a(y;\sigma^2)\exp\{-d(y;\mu)/(2\sigma^2)\}, y \in (0,1).$$

The density for this dispersion model seems analytically similar to that of a normal distribution[9] and it also includes a large class of distributions confined in (0, 1), ranging from highly skewed to very flat distributions (see, e.g., Figure 1.7 of Jorgensen).[9] The dispersion model is more general than the familiar generalized linear model based on exponential family of distributions.

References

1. Moore, D. S and McCabe, G. P. (1989). *Introduction to the Practice of Statistics*, W. H. Freeman, New York.
2. Altman, D. G. (1991). *Practical Statistics for Medical Research*, Chapman and Hall, London.
3. Gleser, L. J (1994). The importance of assessing measurement reliability in multivariate regression, *Journal of the American Statistical Association* **87**: 696–707.
4. Carroll, R., Ruppert, D. and Stefanski, L. A. (1995). *Measurement Error in Nonlinear Models*, Chapman and Hall, London.
5. Chen, Y, Dougherty, E. R., Bittner, M. L. (1997). Ratio-based decisions and the quantitative analysis of cDNA microarrays. *Nature Genetics Supplement* **21**: 33–37.
6. Newton, M. A., Kendziorski, C. M., Richmond, C. S., Blattner, F. R. and Tsui, K. W. (2001). On differential variability of expression ratios: Improving statistical inference about gene expression changes from microarray data. *Journal of Computational Biology*: **8**: 37–52.
7. Song, P. and Tan, M. (2000). Marginal model for continuous proportional data. *Biometrics* **56**: 496–502.
8. Tan, M. (2001). Using dispersion models in molecular pharmacology and genetics. Invited Presentation at *Joint Statistical Meetings*, Atlanta, GA, August 7.
9. Jorgenson, B. (1997). *Dispersion Models*. Chapman and Hall/CRC, London.
10. Diggle, P., Heagerty, P., Liang, K. Y. and Zeger, S. (1994). *Analysis of Longitudinal Data*. Oxford University Press, UK.
11. Qu, Y. and Tan, M. (1998). Analysis of clustered ordinal data with subclusters via a Bayesian hierarchical model. *Communications in Statistics A: Theory & Method* **27**: 1461–1475.
12. Tan, M., Qu, Y., Mascha, E. and Schubert, A. (1999). A Bayesian hierarchical model for multi-level repeated ordinal Data: Analysis of oral practice examinations in a large anesthesiology training program. *Statistics in Medicine* **18**: 1983–1992.
13. Houghton, P. J., Chesire, P. J., Myers, L. *et al.* (1992). Evaluation of 9-dimethylaminomethyl-10-hydroxycamptothecin against xenografts derived from adult and childhood solid tumors. *Cancer Chemother Pharmacol* **31**: 229–239.
14. Zamboni, W. C., Stewart, C. F., Thompson, J. *et al.* (1998). Relationship between topotecan systemic exposure and tumor response in human neuroblastoma xenografts. *Journal of National Cancer Institute* **90**: 505–511.
15. Santana, V. M., Zamboni, W. C., Kirstein, M. N., Tan, M., Liu, T., Gajjar, A., Houghton, P. J., Stewart, C. F. (2003). A pilot study of protracted topotecan dosing using a pharmacokinetically guided dosing approach in children with solid tumors. *Clinical Cancer Research* **9**: 633–640.
16. Meyers, S., Ambler, J. S., Tan, M., Werner, J. C. and Huang, S. S. (1992). Variation of perfluoropropane disappearance after vitrectomy. *Retina* **12**: 359–363.

17. Nelson, R. G., Bennett, P. H., Beck, G. J., Tan, M., Knowler, W. C., Mitch, W. E., Hirschman, G. H. and Myers, B. D. (1996). Development and Progression of Renal Disease in Pima Indians with Non-Insulin-Dependent Diabetes Mellitus. *New England Journal of Medicine* **335**: 1636–1642.
18. Fisher, R. A. (1950). The Significance of Deviations From Expectation in a Poisson Series. *Biometrics* **6**: 17–24.
19. Fisher, R. A. (1953). Note on the Efficient Fitting of the Negative Binomial. *Biometrics* **9**: 197–199.
20. Song, P., Qiu, Z. and Tan, M. (2004). Modeling heterogeneous dispersion in marginal simplex models for continuous longitudinal proportional data. *Biometrical Journal* **46**: 540–553.
21. Qiu, Z., Song, P. X. K., Tan, M. (2008) Simplex Mixed-Effects Models for Longitudinal Proportional Data. *Scandinavia Journal of Statistics* **35**: 577–596.
22. Breslow, N. E. and Clayton, D. G. (1993). Approximate Inference in Generalized Linear Mixed Models. *Journal of the American Statistical Association* **88**(421): 9–25.
23. Concato, J. (2004). Observational *Versus* Experimental Studies: What's the Evidence for a Hierarchy?.*NeuroRx: The Journal of the American Society for Experimental NeuroTherapeutics* **1**: 341–347.
24. Shmueli, G. (2010). To Explain or to Predict? *Statistical Science.* **25**: 289–310.
25. Helmer, O. and Rescher, N. (1959). On the epistemology of the inexact sciences. *Manag. Sci.* **5**: 25–52.
26. Hastie, T., Tibshirani, R. and Friedman, J. H. (2009). *The Elements of Statistical Learning: Data Mining, Inference, and Prediction*: pp. 23, 2nd ed. Springer, New York.
27. Liu, Z. and Tan, M. (2008). ROC based utility function maximization for feature selection and classification with application to high dimensional protease data. *Biometrics* **64**: 1155–1161.
28. Liu, Z., Chen, X., Gartenhaus, R. B., Howell, C. D., Tan, M. (2009). Survival Prediction and Gene Identification with Penalized Global AUC Maximization. *Journal of Computational Biology* **16**: 1661–1670.
29. Box, G. E. P. and Cox, D. R.(1964). An analysis of transformations. *Journal of the Royal Statistical Society. Series B*, **26**: 211–252.
30. Bacik, J., Mazumdar, M., Murphy, B. A., Fairclough, D. L., Eremenco, S., Mariani, T., Motzer, R. J., Cella, D. (2004). The functional assessment of cancer therapy-BRM (FACT-BRM): a new tool for the assessment of quality of life in patients treated with biologic response modifiers. *Qual Life Res* **13**: 137–54.
31. Du, H., Hahn, E. A. and Cella, D. (2011). The impact of missing data on estimation of health-related quality of life outcomes: an analysis of a randomized longitudinal clinical trial. *Health Services and Outcomes Research Methodology* **11**: 134–144.
32. Zhang, D. and Davidian, M. (2001). Linear mixed models with flexible distributions of random effects for longitudinal data. *Biometrics* **57**: 795–802.

33. McCulloch, C. E. and Neuhaus, J. M. (2011). Misspecifying the Shape of a Random Effects Distribution: Why Getting It Wrong May Not Matter. *Statistics Science* **26**; 388–402.
34. Hsieh, F., Tseng, Y. K., Wang, J. L.(2006). Joint modeling of survival and longitudinal data: likelihood approach revisited. *Biometrics* **62**: 1037–1043.
35. Huang, X., Stefanski, L. A., Davidian, M. (2009). Latent-model robustness in joint models for a primary endpoint and a longitudinal process. *Biometrics* **65**: 719–727.
36. Hosmer, D., Lemeshow, S. (2000). *Applied Logistic Regression.* 2nd ed. John Wiley & Sons, Inc. New York.
37. Bland, J. M. and Altman, D. G. (1986). Statistical methods for assessing agreement between two methods of clinical measurement. *The Lancet* **1**(8476): 307–310.
38. Kosinski, A. S., Flanders, W. D. (1999). Evaluating the exposure and disease relationship with adjustment for different types of exposure misclassification: a regression approach. *Stat Med.* **18**: 2795–2808.
39. Nguyen, A., Sarit, A., Sand, P., Du, H., Botros, S., Gamble, T., Kuo, R., Goldberg, R. (2011). Nongenetic factors associated with stress urinary incontinence. *American Journal of Obstetrics & Gynecology.* **117**: 251–255.
40. Neale, M. C., Boker, S. M., Xie, G., Maes, H. H. (2003). *Mx: Statistical Modeling.* 6th ed. VCU Box 900126, Richmond, VA 23298: Department of Psychiatry.
41. Neale, M. C. and Maes, H. M. (2004). *Methodology for genetics studies of twins and families.* Kluwer Academic, Dordrecht (The Netherlands).
42. Hedeker, D. and Gibbons, R. D. (1997). Application of random-effects pattern-mixture models for missing data in longitudinal studies. *Psychol. Methods* **2**: 64–78.

About the Authors

Hongyan Du, MB, MS, PStat®, is a statistician at the Center for Clinical and Research Informatics, NorthShore University HealthSystem, a teaching affiliate of University of Chicago Pritzker School of Medicine. She has extensive collaborative research experience in the design and analysis of laboratory, translational, clinical, and health outcomes studies. In the past 10 years, she has collaborated with investigators in cancer, diabetes, chronic kidney disease, HIV and other complex diseases. She has more than 70 publications in biomedical and statistical journals including *Cancer Research, Stroke, Clinical Trials, Statistics in Medicine* and *Health Services and Outcomes Research Methodology.* She has research interests in longitudinal models with nonignorable missing data, biomarker evaluation (ROC etc) and prognostic modeling. She also serves on the IRB of the NorthShore University HealthSystem. She qualified in medicine at West China University of Medical Sciences in 1993, and gained a Master of Science in Biostatistics at University of Illinois at Chicago in 2003. She is an Accredited Professional Statistician™ (PStat®), by the American Statistical Association.

Ming T. Tan, Ph.D., is Professor and Chairman at the Department of Biostatistics, Bioinformatics and Biomathematics at Georgetown University Medical Center and Georgetown Lombardi Comprehensive Cancer Center. Previously he was Professor of Epidemiology and Public Health (Biostatistics) and Director of the Division of Biostatistics and Bioinformatics, University of Maryland School of Medicine, and Director of Biostatistics at the University of Maryland Greenebaum Cancer Center. He was Associate Member/Professor of Biostatistics at the Department of Biostatistics, St. Jude Children's Research Hospital and biostatistics director for its Developmental Therapeutics for Solid Malignancies Program. He was Assistant (1990–1996) and Associate Staff/Professor (1996–1997) of Biostatistics at the Department of Biostatistics and Epidemiology at The Cleveland Clinic. He earned his PhD in Statistics from Purdue University in 1990. His current research interests include design and analysis of multi-drug combinations, the evaluation of biomarkers and diagnostic tests, adaptive clinical trial designs, random-effects and Bayesian models for longitudinal data. He has served as associate editor for *Biometrics* and *Statistics in Medicine*, US FDA (Food and Drug Administration) advisory committee and multiple US National Institutes of Health Panels. He is an elected Fellow of the American Statistical Association.

CHAPTER 3

COVARIATE-SPECIFIC AND COVARIATE-ADJUSTED PREDICTIVE VALUES OF PROGNOSTIC BIOMARKERS WITH SURVIVAL OUTCOME

YUNBEI MA

*Department of Finance and Economics, School of Statistics,
Southwest University of Finance and Economics,
Chengdu 611130, China*

XIAO-HUA ZHOU

*HSR&D Center of Excellence, Met Park West #1400,
Puget Sound Health Care
System; H-655E, HSB, Department of Biostatistics,
University of Washington, Seattle USA
azhou@Washington.edu*

KWUN CHUEN (GARY) CHAN

*Department of Biostatistics, 1959 NE Pacific St., H-655H,
School of Public Health, University of Washington,
Seattle, WA 98195, USA*

With rapid advances in genetic research, more and more genetic biomarkers are available for predicting the survival outcome of a patient after receiving a certain treatment. The predictive accuracy of these biomarkers may depend on a patient's characteristics. In this chapter, we first develop semi-parametric regression models for covariate specific predictive values of biomarkers, which have conditional interpretations. We then propose a marginalized covariate-adjusted predictive accuracy to represent a summary predictive measure of a biomarker in the whole population. We derive asymptotic results of the proposed estimators and demonstrate through simulation studies that the proposed methods perform well in finite sample sizes. We illustrate an application of the proposed method using the Multicenter AIDS Cohort Study (MACS) data.

1. Introduction

In medical research, especially in studies for cancer treatment, predicting future onset or progression of a disease is often a main focus, in order to avoid patients undergoing an unnecessary medical procedure. Biomarkers are often good indicators of future progression in a disease. Among many possible choices of continuous-scale biomarkers, we often need to evaluate and compare their predictive accuracies to make sure that the best predictive biomarker is selected. Common measures of predictive accuracy as opposed to discriminative accuracy, are positive and negative predicted values (PPV/NPV) when the outcome is binary. For a binary outcome, the PPV curve of a continuous-scale biomarker, which plots PPV among subjects with biomarker values greater than all thresholds defined by the percentile of the biomarker distribution, is a natural analogue of the ROC curve. The PPV (NPV) curve has a prospective interpretation as the probability of disease (non-disease) given a positive (negative) test result. The ROC curve, in contrast, has a retrospective interpretation. By plotting against percentiles instead of the actual threshold, the PPV curves for markers with different scales will all have the same domain $(0, 1)$, which allow standardized comparisons among biomarkers.

In many cases, we are interested in assessing the prognostic accuracy of a biomarker in predicting event times. For example, in the Multicenter AIDS Cohort Study (MACS), individuals with HIV-1 are followed until the termination of the study or death. The accuracy of the CD4 counts at baseline in predicting time-to-death is of interest. PPV curves have been extended to measure predictive accuracy for a survival outcome, which can be viewed as a time-dependent binary outcome.[1] The extension is called a time-dependent PPV curve. They have focused on an overall predictive measure of a biomarker in the whole population, and proposed a nonparametric and a semiparametric approach for estimating the time-dependent PPV curve for a survival outcome. This unadjusted time-dependent PPV curve assumes that no covariates, besides a biomarker, affect the distribution of the survival outcome, but in practice both biomarker and survival distributions could depend on other covariates as well. When covariates affect the distributions of a biomarker, survival outcome, or both, the unadjusted time-dependent PPV curve may be misleading. For example, in our motivational study (MACS), predictive accuracy of CD4 count may depend on age, race and antiviral drug use. On the other hand, individuals' CD4 counts may also be associated with their ages and races. First, when covariates affect biomarker observations but do not affect survival outcomes, the unadjusted time-dependent PPV curve, is biased relative to the covariate-specific time-dependent PPV curve. Second, when comparing predictive accuracy of biomarkers, using unadjusted time-dependent PPV curves may lead to an incorrect conclusion, as shown in Figure 4 of Section 4.3. In this case, marginal analysis of PPV curves needs to be covariate-adjusted.

In this chapter, we consider a semiparametric joint regression model for survival outcome and biomarker distributions and estimate covariate-specific time-dependent PPV curves. We model the survival outcome by a varying-coefficient Cox's model, and the biomarker outcome by a semiparametric location shift regression model. Although covariate-specific time-dependent PPV curves are useful in practice, a summary predictive measure in the whole population is also useful for comparing biomarkers and in small studies where covariate-specific time-dependent PPV curves can't be estimated with precision. To this end, this chapter further considers a covariate-adjusted marginalized summary of the predictive accuracy of the biomarker. We define the covariate-adjusted time-dependent PPV curve as a weighted average of covariate-specific time-dependent PPV curves. In our setting, the unadjusted and covariate-adjusted time-dependent PPV curves are different when covariates affect biomarker values and survival outcomes or when covariates affect biomarker values but do not survival outcomes. When a biomarker is independent of covariates, the covariate-adjusted time-dependent PPV curve reduces to the unadjusted time-dependent PPV curve defined in Zheng *et al.*[1]

This chapter is organized as follows. In Section 2, we propose a covariate-specific PPV curve, a measure of conditional predictive accuracy of the biomarker, and introduce the varying-coefficient Cox's model for a survival outcome and a semi-parametric location model for biomarker distribution. We then propose an estimation method for covariate-specific time-dependent PPV curves and derive asymptotic properties of the estimators. In Section 3, we define a covariate-adjusted time-dependent PPV curve, a measure of marginalized predictive accuracy of the biomarker, and propose an estimation method for covariate-adjusted time-dependent PPV curves, and derive asymptotic properties of the estimators. We then report simulation results and data analysis of a real-world example of the MACS in Sections 4 and 5, respectively. We give technical details of the asymptotic results in the Appendix.

2. Covariate-Specific Time-Dependent PPV Curves

Let T be an event time, where the event denotes death or disease progression. Let Y be a continuous biomarker, and let Z_1 and Z_2 denote vectors of covariates, which affect the biomarker distribution of Y and the survival distribution of event time T, respectively. Here we allow Z_1 and Z_2 to overlap.

Let $F_{z_1}(y) = P\{Y \leq y|Z_1 = z_1\}$ denote the conditional cumulative distribution function given $Z_1 = z_1$. Then we define covariate-specific time-dependent PPV curve as a plot of $\text{PPV}(v; t, z_1, z_2) = P\{T \leq t|F_{z_1}(y) \geq v, Z_2 = z_2\}$ versus v, at $Z_1 = z_1$ and $Z_2 = z_2$, where v in an open interval of $(0, 1)$.

Since the distribution of Y only depends on Z_1, with some simple algebra, we show that

$$\begin{aligned} & PPV(v; t, z_1, z_2) \\ & = 1 - \frac{P\{T > t, F_{z_1}(y) \geq v|Z_2 = z_2\}}{P\{F_{z_1}(y) \geq v|Z_2 = z_2\}} \\ & = 1 - (1 - v)^{-1} \int_{F_{z_1}^{-1}(v)} S(t|y, z_2) dF_{z_1}(y), \end{aligned} \tag{1}$$

where $S(t|y, z_2) = P\{T > t|Y = y, Z_2 = z_2\}$ is the conditional survival distribution given $Y = y$ and $Z_2 = z_2$.

2.1. *Estimation of the conditional survival distribution based on the varying-coefficient Cox's model*

Suppose that there is a random sample of size n from an underlying population. Let T_i and C_i denote the event time and censoring time for the ith individual, respectively, where $i = 1, \ldots, n$. Then, $X_i = \min(T_i, C_i)$ is the observed time for this individual. Let Δ_i be an indicator, which is 1 if X_i is an event time and 0 otherwise. In addition, we assume that for $i = 1, \ldots, n$, T_i and C_i are conditional independent given biomarker and covariates. Without loss of generality, we let the observation period be $[0, \tau]$, where τ is a constant denoting the time for end of the study.

Although Cox's model is a very powerful method in survival analysis, covariate effects on event time may not satisfy the proportional hazard assumption. True covariate effects on event time can be more complex than a log-linear effect. Non-parametric approaches are obvious alternative methods, but the rate of convergence of non-parametric estimators typically decreases as the number of covariates in the model grows — this is the so called curse of dimensionality problem. One attractive and powerful alternative approach is to use a varying-coefficient model. To this end, we consider a varying-coefficient hazard ratio model[2–4] which allows (non-linear) interaction between the exposure variable and a confounding covariate. Let us assume that the important exposure variable w is a continuous-scale element of z_2. Without loss of generality, we let w and z_2^* denote the first and the rest elements of z_2, respectively. We assume that the hazard function follows the following model:

$$\lambda(t|y, z_2) = \lambda(t|y, w, z_2^*) = \lambda_0(t)\exp\{\theta_0^T(w)z_2^* + \alpha_0 y + \rho_0^T y z_2\}, \qquad (2)$$

where $\lambda_0(t)$ is an unspecified baseline hazard function, and $\theta_0^T(w)$ is a functional coefficient vector of w. We illustrate the relevance of model (2) by examples of MACS data in Section 5, where the exposure covariate is the patient's age.

It follows from the model (2) and $S(t|y, z_2) = \exp\{-\int_0^t \lambda(u|y, z_2)du\}$ that

$$S(t|y, z_2) = \exp\left\{-\Lambda_0(t)\exp\left\{\theta_0^T(w)z_2^* + \alpha_0 y + \rho_0^T y z_2\right\}\right\},$$

where $\Lambda_0(t) = \int_0^t \lambda_0(u)du$.

Model (2) has several attractive properties, such as having less modeling assumptions than the parametric approach, having less possibilities of distorting the underlying relationship between the event time, and allowing interactions between covariates. Furthermore, the model (2) also allows interactions between the biomarker and covariates.

The observed data structure is $\{X_i, \Delta_i, Y_i, Z_{1i}, Z_{2i}\}$, where $i = 1, \ldots, n$. When all the observations are independent, $\theta_0(w)$, α_0 and ρ_0 can be estimated by using a profile partial likelihood method, with local polynomial (linear) fitting.[2] To estimate $S(t|y, z_2)$, we let $N_i(t) = I(T_i \leq t, \Delta_i = 1)$ and $R_i(t) = I(X_i \geq t)$. Let $\widehat{\theta}(w)$, $\widehat{\alpha}$ and $\widehat{\rho}$ be the profile partial likelihood estimates of $\theta_0(w)$, α_0 and ρ_0, respectively. Then we can estimate $\Lambda_0(t)$ by

$$\widehat{\Lambda}_0(t) = \sum_{i=1}^n \int_0^t \frac{dN_i(u)}{\sum_{j=1}^n R_j(u)\exp(\widehat{\theta}^T(W_j)Z_{2j} + \widehat{\alpha}Y_j + \widehat{\rho}^T Y_j Z_{2j})},$$

which yields the following estimator of $S(t|y, z_2)$:

$$\begin{aligned}\widehat{S}(t|y, z_2) &= \widehat{S}(t|y, w, z_2^*)\\ &= \exp\left\{-\widehat{\Lambda}_0(t)\exp\{\widehat{\alpha}y + \widehat{\theta}^T(w)z_2^* + \widehat{\rho}^T y z_2\}\right\}.\end{aligned}$$

Here, for $i = 1, \ldots, n$, W_i and Z^*_{2i} are the first element and the rests of Z_{2i}, respectively.

2.2. *Semiparametric estimations of the conditional distribution of the biomarker and the covariate-specified time-dependent PPV curve*

We assume a semi-parametric location model for the biomarker, given as follows:

$$P\{Y \leq y|Z_1\} = H(y - \gamma_0^T Z_1), \tag{3}$$

where $H(\cdot)$ is an unspecified distribution function.

The distribution function $H(y)$ can be estimated by $\widehat{H}(y, \widehat{\gamma}) = \frac{1}{n}\sum_{i=1}^n I(Y_i - \widehat{\gamma}^T Z_{1i} \leq y)$, where $\widehat{\gamma}$ is an estimator of γ, obtained by solving the following estimating equation:

$$\sum_{i=1}^n (Y_i - \gamma^T Z_{1i}) Z_{1i} = 0.$$

It follows that

$$\widehat{F}_{z_1}(y) = \frac{1}{n}\sum_{i=1}^n I(Y_i - \widehat{\gamma}^T Z_{1i} \leq y - \widehat{\gamma}^T z_1).$$

Therefore, plugging $\widehat{F}_{z_1}(y)$ and $\widehat{S}(t|y, z_2)$ into (1), we obtain the following semiparametric estimator for the covariate-specified time-dependent PPV curve:

$$\widehat{PPV}(v; t, z_1, z_2) = 1 - (1 - v)^{-1} \int_{\widehat{F}_{z_1}^{-1}(v)} \widehat{S}(t|y, z_2) d\widehat{F}_{z_1}(y). \tag{4}$$

2.3. *Asymptotic properties*

Let $\mathcal{Y}$, $\mathcal{Z}_1$ and $\mathcal{Z}_2$ be the supports of Y, Z_1 and Z_2, respectively. The following Lemma 1 and Lemma 2 are required to derive the asymptotic properties of $\widehat{PPV}(v; t, z_1, z_2)$.

Lemma 1. *Under the conditions A.i-A.vi given in Appendix A, given* $z_1 \in \mathcal{Z}_1$, $\sqrt{n}\{\widehat{F}_{z_1}(y) - F_{z_1}(y)\}$, *as a process of* y, *converges to a mean zero Gaussian process on* $\mathcal{Y}$ *with the covariance being given in Appendix B.*

Lemma 2. *Let h be a bandwidth chosen for estimating $\widehat{\beta}(\cdot)$, $\widehat{\alpha}$, and $\widehat{\rho}$. Under the conditions A.i–A.vi given in Appendix A and $(z_2, t) \in \mathcal{Z}_2 \times [0, \tau]$, if $nh^2 \to \infty$ and $nh^4 \to 0$ as $n \to \infty$, then $\widehat{\Lambda}_0(t)$ is root-n consistent, and $\sqrt{nh}\{\widehat{S}(t|y, z_2) - S(t|y, z_2)\}$, as a process of y, converges to a mean zero Gaussian process on $\mathcal{Y}$ with the covariance being given in Appendix B.*

Proofs of Lemma 1 and Lemma 2 are given in Appendix B.

Theorem 1. *Under the conditions A.i–A.vi given in Appendix A, for $(z_1, z_2, t) \in \mathcal{Z}_1 \times \mathcal{Z}_2 \times [0, \tau]$, if $nh^2 \to \infty$ and $nh^4 \to 0$ as $n \to \infty$, then*

$$\sqrt{nh}\{\widehat{PPV}(v; t, z_1, z_2) - PPV(v; t, z_1, z_2)\},$$

as a process of v, converges to a Gaussian process on $(0, 1)$ with covariance, $\nu_0 cov\{\kappa^*(v_1, t, z_1, z_2), \kappa^*(v_2, t, z_1, z_2)\}$, where $\nu_0 = \int K^2(t)dt$, and $K(\cdot)$ is a symmetric density function, which is used as the kernel function for profile partial likelihood estimators $\widehat{\theta}(\cdot)$, $\widehat{\alpha}$ and $\widehat{\rho}$.

Proof of Theorem 1 and expression of $\kappa^*(v, t, z_1, z_2)$ are shown in Appendix C.

Although an estimator of variance for $\widehat{\text{PPV}}(v; t, z_1, z_2)$ can be obtained by the functional delta method, smoothing techniques are needed because of the unknown density functions contained in the variance. In simulation studies, we compute the standard errors and confidence limits using the bootstrap approach.

3. Covariate-Adjusted Time-Dependent PPV Curve

Besides covariate-specific time-dependent PPV curves, we are also interested in a summary predictive measure of biomarkers in the whole population. A time-dependent PPV curve has been defined as a plot of $PPV(v; t) = P\{T < t|F(y) \geq v\}$ to measure the predictive accuracy in the whole population, where $F(y)$ is the cumulative distribution function of Y.[1] An overall predictive measure is useful for comparing biomarkers. However, the overall predictive measure proposed ignored covariates effects on the predictive accuracy.[1] Therefore, the method[1] either suffers from loss of efficiency or leads to serious bias.[1] For example, in Figure 5 reported in Section 4.3, two biomarkers, Y_1 and Y_2, have the same covariate-specific time-dependent PPV curves. However, the unadjusted (pooled) time-dependent PPV curves incorrectly indicate that Y_1 and Y_2 have different predictive accuracies.[1]

We define an overall predictive accuracy, adjusted for covariates. The concept is similar to the covariate-adjusted ROC curve in the context of ROC curves.[5] We define the covariate-adjusted time-dependent PPV curve as $APPV(v;t) = E\{PPV(v;t,Z_1,Z_2)\}$, where the expectation is taken with respect to $Z = Z_1 \cup Z_2$. Equivalently, the covariate-adjusted PPV curve can be interpreted as a weighted average of covariate-specific time-dependent PPV curves,

$$\begin{aligned} &APPV(v;t) \\ &\quad = \int P\{T \le t | F_{z_1}(y) \ge v, Z_2 = z_2\} dF_Z(z) \\ &\quad = \int PPV(v;t,z_1,z_2) dF_Z(z) \\ &\quad = 1 - (1-v)^{-1} \int \left\{ \int_{F_{z_1}^{-1}(v)} S(t|y,z_2) dF_{z_1}(y) \right\} dF_Z(z), \end{aligned} \tag{5}$$

where $F_Z(z)$ is the joint cumulative distribution of $Z = Z_1 \cup Z_2$.

From (5) we can see that, when $Z_1 = Z_2 = Z$ and when the common covariates Z affect biomarker observations but do not affect the predictive accuracy, the covariate-adjusted time-dependent PPV is equal to the common covariate-specific time-dependent PPV curves. On the other hand, when $Z_1 \neq Z_2$, the covariate-adjusted time-dependent PPV reports a weighted average of covariate-specific PPV.

The covariate-adjusted time-dependent PPV curve also has some attractive properties, such as invariance with respect to monotone increasing transformations of Y and/or Z.

Note that the unadjusted time-dependent PPV curve defined in Zheng *et al.*[1] is

$$\begin{aligned} &PPV(v;t) \\ &\quad = E\left[P\{T < t | F(y) \ge v, Z_1, Z_2\}\right] \\ &\quad = 1 - \int \frac{\int_{F^{-1}(v)} S(t|y,z_2) dF_{z_1}(y)}{F_{z_1}(F^{-1}(y))} dF_Z(z). \end{aligned} \tag{6}$$

Hence when the biomarker Y is independent of all covariates, i.e for any $z_1 \in \mathcal{Z}_1$, $F(\cdot) \equiv F_{z_1}(\cdot)$, the covariate-adjusted time-dependent PPV curve (5) reduces to the unadjusted time-dependent PPV curve (6). Another note of the covariate-adjusted time-dependent PPV curve is that $APPV(v) = P\{T \le t | F_{Z_1}(y) \ge v\}$. The covariate-adjusted time-dependent PPV curve is contrasted with the unadjusted time-dependent PPV curve,[1] where subjects with biomarker values at or above the vth entire population quantile are considered as test positive (i.e. $F(y) \geq v$).

3.1. *Estimation*

From (4) and (5), we can estimate the covariate-adjusted time-dependent PPV curve, $APPV(v;t)$, by the following estimator:

$$\begin{aligned}\widehat{APPV}(v;t) &\\ &= \int \widehat{PPV}(v;t,z_1,z_2)d\widehat{F}_Z(z) \\ &= 1-(1-v)^{-1}\int\left\{\int_{\widehat{F}_{z_1}^{-1}(v)} \widehat{S}(t|y,z_2)d\widehat{F}_{z_1}(y)\right\}d\widehat{F}_Z(z), \qquad (7)\end{aligned}$$

where $\widehat{F}_Z(z)$ is an estimator of the cumulative distribution $F_Z(z)$ of $Z = Z_1 \cup Z_2$. If we use the empirical distribution to estimate $F_Z(z)$, we obtain the following estimator for $APPV(v;t)$:

$$\widehat{APPV}(v;t) = \frac{1}{n}\sum_{i=1}^{n} \widehat{PPV}(v;t,Z_{i1},Z_{i2}). \qquad (8)$$

3.2. *Asymptotic properties*

Let $\mathcal{Z}$ be the supports of Z. We first derive the large sample properties of the empirical distribution $\widehat{F}_Z(z)$ of $Z = Z_1 \cup Z_2$, which are given in Lemma 3 below.

Lemma 3. *Assume that $F_Z(z)$ is continuous over $\mathcal{Z}$, then for any $z \in \mathcal{Z}$, $\sqrt{n}\{\widehat{F}_Z(z) - F_Z(z)\}$ converges to a normal distribution. Furthermore, if $F_Z(z)$ is absolutely continuous, then* $\sup_z |\sqrt{n}\{\widehat{F}_Z(z) - F_Z(z)\}| = O_p(1)$.

The first part of Lemma 3 follows from Equation (4.5),[6] and the second part of Lemma 3 can be obtained directly by Theorem 3.[7]

Thus, according to (7), the asymptotic distribution of $\sqrt{n}\{\widehat{\text{APPV}}(v;t) - \text{APPV}(v;t)\}$ can be directly obtained by using Theorem 1 and Lemma 3.

Theorem 2. *Suppose that the survival model (2) holds. Under the conditions A.i–A.vi given in Appendix A, if $F_Z(z)$ is absolutely continuous over $\mathcal{Z}$, if $H(u)$ is absolutely continuous over $(-\infty,\infty)$, and if $nh^2 \to \infty$ and $nh^4 \to 0$ as $n \to \infty$, then*

$$\sqrt{n}\{\widehat{APPV}(v;t) - APPV(v;t)\},$$

as a process of v, converges to a Gaussian process on $(0,1)$ *with covariance* $cov\{\zeta^*(v_1,t),\zeta^*(v_2,t)\}$.

The proof of Theorem 2 and the expression of $\zeta_i^*(v,t)$ are given in Appendix C.

Remark 1. We derive Theorem 2 under the assumption that $F_Z(z)$ is absolutely continuous over $\mathcal{Z}$. When Z is a vector of discrete covariates, or some components of Z are discrete, we may still use (8) to estimate the covariate-adjusted time-dependent PPV curves. We demonstrate in the simulation studies that the finite-sample performance of the proposed estimators for discrete covariates is still good.

Remark 2. The standard Cox's model is a special case of the varying-coefficient Cox's model (2). It is known that if the standard Cox's model holds, then by using partial likelihood method, we can get a $\sqrt{n}$-consistent estimator of $S(t|y,z_2)$ [Andersen and Gill, 1982],and consequently a $\sqrt{n}$-consistent estimator of $PPV(v;t,z_1,z_2)$. On the other hand, according to Theorem 2, assuming a varying-coefficient structure in the hazard ratio function do not decrease the converge rate of our proposed estimator of the covariate-adjusted time-dependent PPV curve APPV$(v;t)$.

4. Simulation Studies

In this section, we report the results of our simulation studies for evaluating the performance of covariate-specific time-dependent PPV curves and covariate-adjusted time-dependent PPV curve. We than compare the relative performance of our new time-dependent PPV curves with the existing one. We use 200 simulations in each simulation study.

4.1. *Simulation study for covariate-specific time-dependent PPV curves*

We first conduct a simulation study to evaluate the finite-sample performance of the covariate-specified time-dependent PPV estimator, when the varying-coefficient Cox's model for the survival time holds. In this simulation study, we generate failure time data following a varying-coefficient hazard function $\lambda(t|Y,W,Z_2) = \lambda_0(t)\exp\{\alpha_0 Y + \theta_{10}(W)Z_1 + \theta_{20}(W)Z_2\}$, where $\lambda_0(t) \equiv 0.1$, $\theta_{10}(W) = W$, $\theta_{20}(W) = W^2$, and W is generated from a uniform distribution over $[0,1]$. The covariate Z_1 is generated from an exponential distribution with mean $1/2$, the covariate Z_2 is generated from a normal distribution with mean 0 and variance 1, and the outcome Y is generated from a conditional normal distribution with mean Z_1 and variance 0.25. The censoring distribution is a uniform distribution over $[c/2, 3c/2]$, where c is a constant, which is set to control the censoring rate. Here we take $c = 12.5$, which corresponds to approximately 20% censoring. For the sample size $n = 200$, we plot a covariate-specific time-dependent PPV curve for $Z_1 = 1$, $Z_2 = 0.25$, and $W = 0.5$ at $t = 2$. For $v = 0.1, 0.3, 0.5, 0.7, 0.9$, by using the bootstrap method with 200 bootstrap samples, we compute their logit standard errors (SEs) and 95% confidence limits as follows:

$$SE^2 = \frac{1}{200}\sum_{j=1}^{200}\{logit(\widehat{PPV}_j)\}^2 - \left\{\frac{1}{200}\sum_{j=1}^{200} logit(\widehat{PPV}_j)\right\}^2,$$

and

$$logit^{-1}\{logit(\widehat{PPV}) \pm 1.96 * SE\}.$$

The optimal bandwidth $\widehat{h}_{opt}$ is selected by using the method in Ref. 8.

To check the accuracy of the bootstrap-based SEs, we compare them against the empirical standard deviations (SDs). The results are shown in Figure 1 and Table 1. The estimated PPV curve captures the form of the true curves well and shows negligible bias. The estimated SEs are pretty close to the SDs, and the coverage probabilities (CPs) of 95% confidence

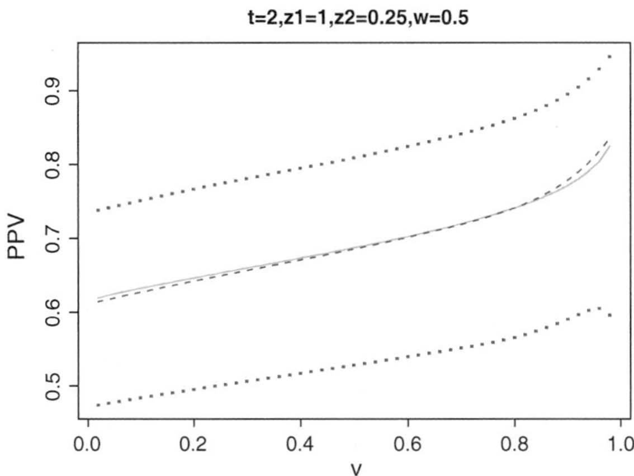

Fig. 1. The covariate-specific time-dependent PPV curves at $t = 2$. The solid and dashed lines are the true and estimated time-dependent PPV curves, respectively. The two dotted lines are 95% confidence limits for the estimated PPV curve.

Table 1. Simulation results for the covariate-specific time-dependent PPV(20% censoring rate).

	$z_1 = 1$, $z_2 = 0.25$, $w = 0.5$			
v	Bias	SD	SE	CP
0.1	−0.0053	0.2814	0.2980	0.955
0.3	−0.0042	0.3000	0.3175	0.960
0.5	−0.0036	0.3252	0.3399	0.960
0.7	−0.0039	0.3626	0.3733	0.975
0.9	0.0029	0.4627	0.4543	0.955

intervals are also close to the nominal level. All the results suggest that the proposed estimators for covariate-specified time-dependent PPV curves perform well.

4.2. *Simulation study for covariate-adjusted time-dependent PPV curves*

We conduct another simulation study to evaluate the finite-sample performance of the covariate-adjusted time-dependent PPV estimators. In this simulation study, we generate failure time data from the hazard function, $\lambda(t|Y, Z_1, Z_2) = \lambda_0(t)\exp\{\alpha_0 Y + \beta_0(W)Z_2 + \rho_0 Y Z_2\}$, where $\lambda_0(t) = 0.1$, $\alpha_0 = 1$, $\beta_0(W) = W^2$, and $\rho_0 = -1$, respectively. Here W is generated from a uniform distribution over $[0, 1]$. We first consider continuous covariates. We generate covariate Z_1 from a normal distribution with mean 0 and variance 1, covariate Z_2 from an exponential distribution with mean $1/5$, and the outcome Y from a conditional normal distribution with mean Z_1 and variance 1. The censoring time is also generated from a uniform distribution over $[c/2, 3c/2]$, where we take $c = 22$ corresponding to approximately 30% censoring. We plot the covariate-adjusted time-dependent PPV curves at $t = 1$, with their confidence limits, which are also derived by using a logit transformation as in Section 4.1. For the estimated APPV curves at $v = 0.1, 0.3, 0.5, 0.7, 0.9$, we also compute their SDs, SEs, and CPs of confidence intervals under 95% nominal level, by using the same method as the one in Section 4.1. For the sample size $n = 100$, the results are shown in Figure 2 and Table 2.

We next consider a case with discrete covariates, Z_1 and Z_2, where Z_1 is generated from a Poisson distribution with $\lambda = 1$, and Z_2 is generated from a binomial distribution with $p = 0.6$. Here we take $c = 12.5$, which corresponds to approximately 30% censoring. Results are represented in Figure 3 and Table 3.

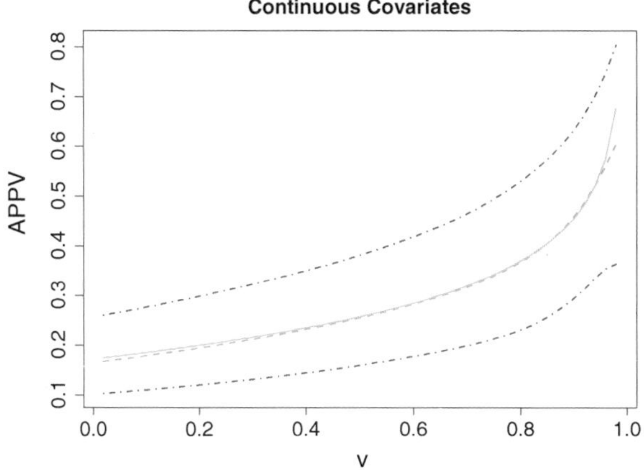

Fig. 2. The covariate-adjusted time-dependent PPV curves at $t = 1$ with continuous covariates. The solid and dashed lines are the true and estimated covariate-adjusted time-dependent PPV curves, respectively. The two dotted lines are 95% confidence limits for the estimated adjusted PPV curve.

Table 2. Simulation results for the APPV with continuous covariates (30% censoring rate).

v	Bias	SD	SE	CP
0.1	−0.007	0.299	0.287	0.955
0.3	−0.004	0.301	0.292	0.955
0.5	−0.002	0.304	0.300	0.955
0.7	−0.002	0.313	0.319	0.955
0.9	0.005	0.347	0.362	0.955

It can be seen from Tables 2–3 and Figures 2–3 that, no matter what covariates are, our proposed method can capture the form of the true APPV curves well. The estimated SEs are pretty close to the empirical SDs, and the coverage probabilities are also close to the nominal level. All the results suggest that the proposed estimators for covariate-specific time-dependent PPV curves perform well.

4.3. *Comparison with the covariate-unadjusted time-dependent PPV curves*

In this section, we report two sets of simulation studies that are used to compare our proposed covariate-adjusted time-dependent PPV (APPV) curves

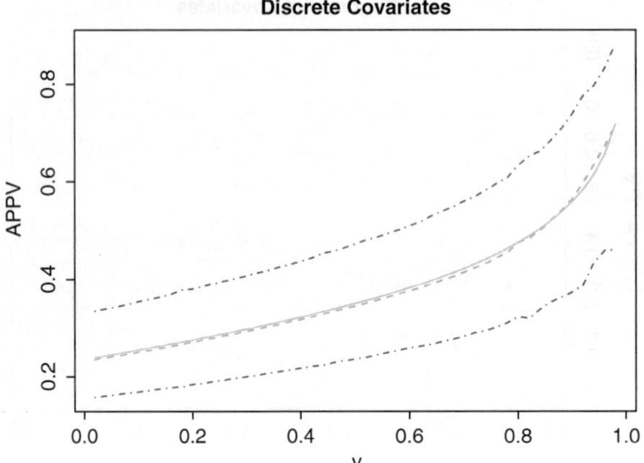

Fig. 3. The covariate-adjusted time-dependent PPV curves at $t = 1$ with discrete covariates. The solid and dashed lines are the true and estimated covariate-adjusted time-dependent PPV curves, respectively. The two dotted lines are 95% confidence limits for the estimated adjusted PPV curve.

Table 3. Simulation results for the APPV with discrete covariates (30% censoring rate).

v	Bias	SD	SE	CP
0.1	−0.014	0.231	0.253	0.960
0.3	−0.015	0.244	0.257	0.960
0.5	−0.017	0.263	0.272	0.960
0.7	−0.021	0.300	0.298	0.960
0.9	−0.012	0.453	0.398	0.960

with the unadjusted time-dependent PPV curves. We consider two scenarios, Scenario (I) with a need for covariate adjustment and Scenario (II) without a need for covariate adjustment.

In Scenario (I), we let Y_1 and Y_2 be two biomarkers, where the distribution of Y_1 is affected by a binary variable Z, whereas the distribution of Y_2 is not. Here $P(Z = 1) = 0.6$ and $P(Z = 0) = 0.4$. We generate Y_1 and Y_2 from a normal distribution with mean $2Z$ and variance 1 and the standard normal distribution, respectively. Hence Y_1 and Y_2 have same covariate-specific predictive accuracies, resulting in the same overall predictive accuracy. From Figure 5, it can be seen that failing to adjust for covariates leads to an incorrect conclusion on the relative performance of biomarkers.

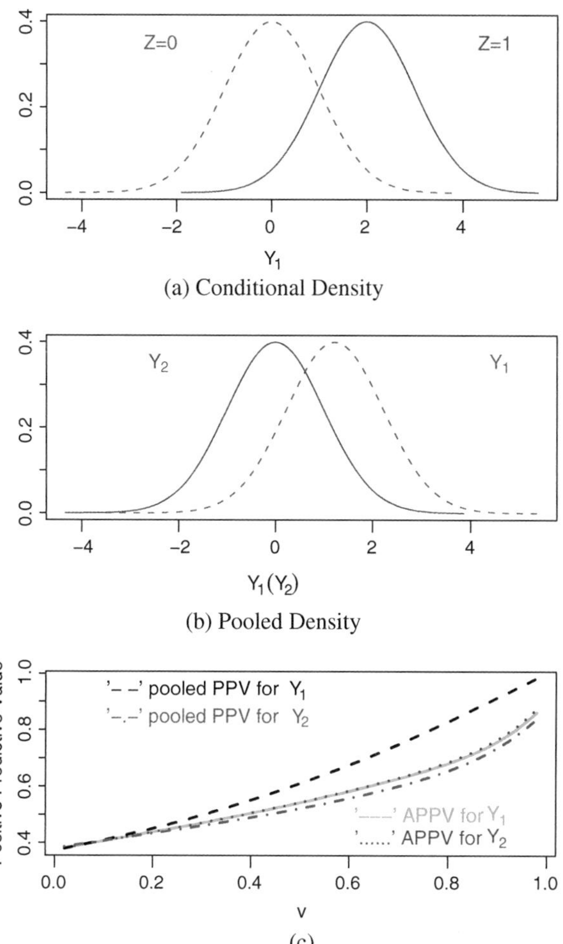

Fig. 4. (a) Density functions of Y_1 among $Z = 0$ and $Z = 1$, respectively; (b) density functions of Y_1 and Y_2 in the pooled data; (c) covariate-adjusted time-dependent PPV (APPV) curves for Y_1 and Y_2, unadjusted time-dependent PPV curves for Y_1 and Y_2.

In Scenario (II) with $APPV = PPV$, for continuous covariates, we compare our proposed method with the nonparametric method[1] to estimate the time-dependent PPV curves. We generate continuous covariates Z_1 and Z_2 from a normal distribution with mean 0 and variance 1 and an exponential distribution with mean $1/5$, respectively. The biomarker Y is generated from the standard normal distribution, and the survival and censoring times are generated in the same way as those in Section 4.2. Hence, in

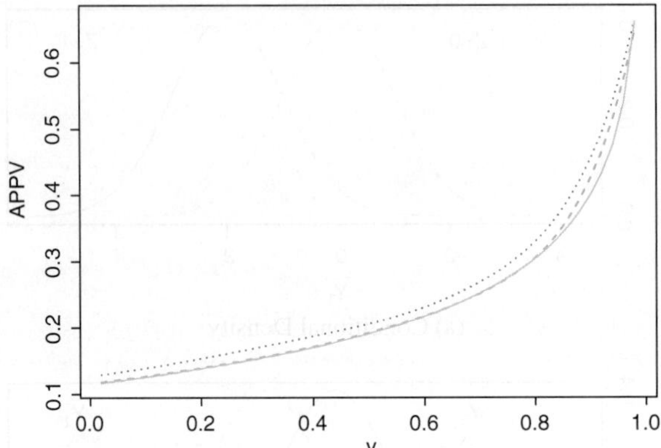

Fig. 5. The covariate-adjusted time-dependent PPV lines at $t = 1$ based on continuous covariates. The solid and dashed lines are the true and estimated covariate-adjusted time-dependent PPV curves, respectively. The dotted line is the unadjusted PPV curve in Ref. 1.

Table 4. Simulation results for the covariate-adjusted time-dependent PPV and nonparametric unadjusted time-dependent PPV curves for continuous covariates (27% censoring rate).

	APPV					Unadjusted PPV				
v	Bias	SD	SE	CP	IL	Bias	SD	SE	CP	IL
0.1	0.001	0.288	0.309	0.950	0.138	0.013	0.328	0.483	1	0.224
0.3	0.001	0.295	0.315	0.950	0.164	0.017	0.358	0.508	1	0.272
0.5	0.001	0.306	0.324	0.950	0.199	0.015	0.411	0.554	1	0.339
0.7	−0.001	0.328	0.348	0.950	0.255	0.017	0.441	0.634	1	0.452
0.9	0.025	0.402	0.410	0.930	0.375	0.054	0.576	0.956	0.980	0.724

this situation, the covariate-adjusted time-dependent PPV (APPV) curve reduces to the unadjusted time-dependent PPV curve. In this scenario, we estimate the overall time-dependent PPV curve by two method, our proposed method and the nonparametric method of.[1] Here the censoring rate is round 27%. For the sample size $n = 100$ and $v = 0.1, 0.3, 0.5, 0.7, 0.9$, we report the estimates for APPV with their SDs, SEs, and CPs of 95% confidence intervals in Figure 5 and Table 4.

From Figure 5 and Table 4, we see that the nonparametric unadjusted estimator shows poorer performance than the proposed method when some covariates, besides the biomarker, also affect the survival distribution.

Remark 3. Sections 4.2 and 4.3 reported the performance of the covariate-adjusted time-dependent PPV curves with univariate Z_1 and Z_2. On the other hand, we also conducted simulations for the APPV curves with high dimensional covariates, where Z_1 is a 3-dimensional covariate and Z_2 is a 7-dimensional covariate. The results showed that the estimated APPV curves still perform well. We omitted the results here for saving space.

5. Multicenter AIDS Cohort Study

The Multicenter AIDS Cohort Study (MACS) is an ongoing prospective study of the natural and treated histories of HIV-1 infection in homosexual and bisexual men. A total of 6,972 men have been enrolled. The public access data covers the first and the second enrollments from the beginning of the study through September 1996. Of the 5622 individuals enrolled, 2195 were HIV-positive at baseline. We are interested in the accuracy of the CD4 cell counts in predicting the time to death from any cause among HIV-infected individuals. Time-dependent PPV curves provide a graphical representation to achieve this goal. Since some factors may have an impact on the predictive accuracy of CD4 cell levels, we need to make adjustments on time-dependent PPV curves for those covariates.

Since HIV infection leads to a progressive reduction in the number of T cells possessing CD4 receptors, we let Y be the inverse of the CD4 cell counts (cells per cubic millimeter), so that a large value of Y is associated with a high risk of death. We let the important exposure covariate W be individual's age, and Z_2 be the treatment indicator, which is 1 if the individual took antiviral drugs before death or September 1996 and 0 otherwise. We let $Z_1 = (Z_{11}, Z_{12}, Z_{13}, Z_{14}, Z_{15})^T$ be the covariates which may impact on the CD4 cell levels. Here Z_{11} denotes age; Z_{12} is a race indicator, which is 1 for a White individual and 0 otherwise; Z_{13} is a race indicator, which is 1 for a Black individual and 0 otherwise; Z_{14} is a race indicator, which is 1 for a American Indian/Alaskan Native individual and 0 otherwise; and Z_{15} is a race indicator, which is 1 for a Asian/Pacific slander individual and 0 otherwise. We calculated the covariate-specific time-dependent PPV curves at survival time $T = 7$ years, and then compared the covariate-adjusted with unadjusted time-dependent PPV curves at survival times $T = 4$ and $T = 6$ years, respectively. Results are presented in Figures 6–7.

From Figure 6(A), we see that among HIV-infected individuals, White patients have the best responses to antiviral drugs. Figure 6(B) shows that

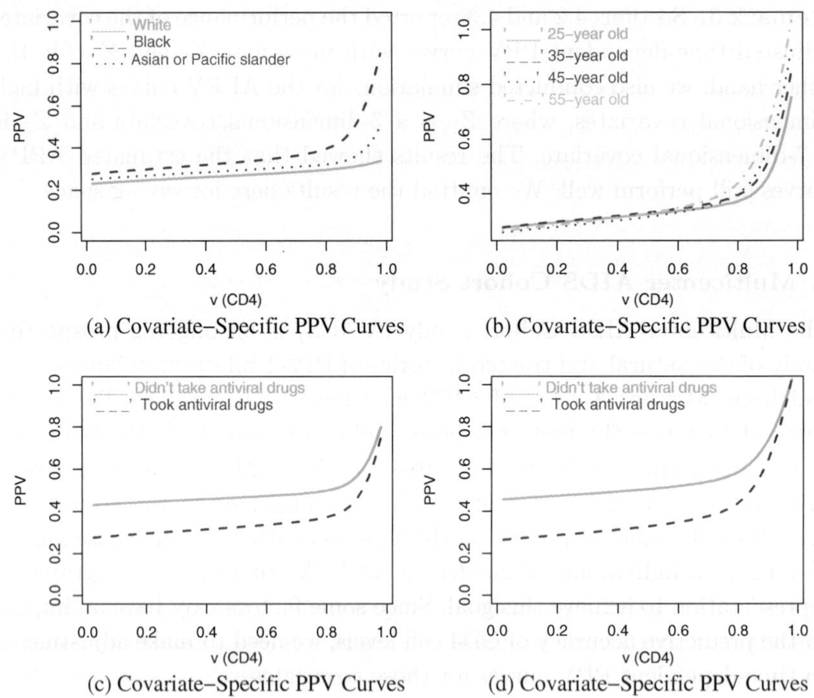

Fig. 6. Estimated covariate-specific time-dependent PPV curves at survival time $T = 7$ years. Figure (a) is for 35-year old individuals who had taken antiviral drugs; Figure (b) is for black who had taken antiviral drugs; Figure (c) is for 25-year old and black individuals; and Figure (d) is for 55-year old and black individuals.

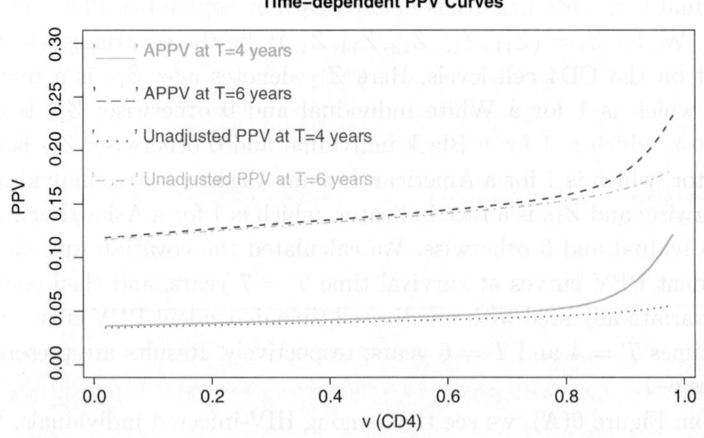

Fig. 7. Estimated covariate-adjusted and unadjusted time-dependent PPV curves at $T = 4, 6$ years.

the predictive accuracies of CD4 cell counts are similar for different ages. From Figure 6(C) and Figure 6(D), we see that antiviral drugs have dramatic effects on HIV-infected black individuals, especially when their CD4 cell counts are high. From Figure 7, we see that CD4 cell is able to predictive the time-to-death of HIV-infected individuals. Figure 7 also shows that there are dramatic differences between the covariate-adjusted and unadjusted time-dependent PPV curves, which provide the necessity of making adjustment for these covariates.

6. Discussion

In this chapter, we focus on predictive abilities of biomarkers rather than the risks of an event, which is the focus of standard survival models. We have developed new semi-parametric methodologies for assessing the accuracy of biomarkers for predicting the time to an event, taking into account covariate dependence on predictive accuracy. Our methods allow us to estimate covariate-specific and covariate-adjusted overall time-dependent PPV curves of a biomarker in assessing time to an event outcome. Compared with existing methods, we are making the following three contributions. First, we provide new semi-parametric methods to assess the effects of covariates on predictive ability of a biomarker in assessing time to an event. Second, we provide a better method than the existing one to assess and compare overall predictive abilities of biomarkers when either the distribution of a biomarker or the survival distribution depends on covariates. Third, by having functional coefficients in the survival model, we have less restrictions and allow the effects of some covariates on the survival model to be functions of another covariate. The validity of the proposed method depends on two semi-parametric regression models, one for the survival time and another for the distribution of the biomarker. Future research topics would be to develop statistical methods for assessing goodness-of-fit of the models, and the method of assessing predictive accuracy with multiple biomarkers.

Acknowledgment

This work was supported in part by the National Natural Science Foundation of China Grant (Grant No. 30728019) and U.S. Department of Veterans Affairs, Veterans Affairs Health Administration, Clinical R&D grant, entitled "Statistical Designs for Marker Validation Studies in Treatment Selection" (project grant number EPID-006-07F).

References

1. Zheng, Y., Cai, T., Pepe, M. and Levy, W. (2008). Time-dependent predictive values of prognostic biomarkers with failure time outcome. *Journal of American Statistical Association* **103**, 362–368.
2. Cai, J., Fan, J., Jiang, J. and Zhou, H. (2008). Partially linear hazard regression with varying-coefficients multivariate survival data. *Journal of the Royal Statistical Society, Series B* **70**, 141–158.
3. Cai, J., Fan, J., Zhou, H. and Zhou, Y. (2007). Hazard models with varying coefficients for multivariate failure time data. *The Annals of Statistics* **35**, 324–354.
4. Fan, J., Lin, H. and Zhou, Y. (2006). Local partial likelihood estimation for life time data. *The Annals of Statistics* **34**, 290–325.
5. Janes, H. and Pepe, M. (2009). Adjusted for covariate effects on classification accuracy using the covariate-adjusted receiver operating characteristic curve. *Biometrika* **96**, 371–382.
6. Neuhaus, G. (1971). On weak convergence of stochastic processes with multidimensional time parameter. *The Annals of Mathematical Statistics* **42**, 1285–1295.
7. Revesz, P. (1976). On strong approximation of the multidimensional empirical process. *The Annals of Probability* **4**, 729–743.
8. Fan, J. and Huang, T. (2005). Profile likelihood inferences on semiparametric varying-coefficient partially linear models. *Bernoulli* **11**, 1031–1057.
9. Andersen, P. K. and Gill, R. D. (1982). Cox's regression model for counting processes: A large sample study. *The Annals of Statistics* **10**, 1100–1120.

About the Authors

Dr. Yunbei Ma, Assistant Professor, joined the Southwestern University of Finance and Economics, China, in September 2012. She came to SWUFE from the Department of Operations Research and Financial Engineering at Princeton University, where she was Postdoctoral Research Associate of Statistics. Before then, she was Postdoctoral Senior Fellow at the Department of Biostatistics of the University of Washington. She received her PhD in Statistics from Chinese Academy of Science in 2009 and her MS in Statistics from Beijing University of Technology, China, in 2006. She is a young statistician with experience teaching statistical courses at both the master's and doctoral levels. At SWUFE, she teaches statistics courses for MS and PhD programs; she also teaches Econometrics for undergraduate students. Dr. Ma's research work focuses on High Dimensional Sparse Model, Nonparametric and Semi-parametric Modeling, Personalized Medicine and

Survival Analysis. She is the PI for an ongoing projects funded by National Natural Science Foundation of China.

Xiao-Hua (Andrew) Zhou, Ph.D., is currently Professor in the Department of Biostatistics at University of Washington and the Director of Biostatistics Unit in the U.S. Federal Government Department of Veterans Affairs (VA) Puget Sound Health Care System. Dr. Zhou received his B.Sc. in mathematics from Sichuan University in 1984, and his Ph.D in Biostatistics from Ohio State University in 1991. Dr. Zhou was a post-doctoral fellow in Biostatistics at Harvard University from 1991 to 1993. Dr. Zhou is well known for his research in the areas of diagnostic medicine and health service research, which include causal inference and analysis of missing data. Along with two co-authors, Dr. Zhou published the first textbook on statistical methods in diagnostic medicine in 2002. He has published 137 statistical papers in refereed journals and 55 medical papers in refereed medical journals. Dr. Zhou served as has been an associate editor for Biometrics and Statistica Sinica and is currently serving as Associate Editor for Statistics in Medicine. Jointly with Drs. Hirano, Imbens, and Rubin, Dr. Zhou received Mitchell Prize given annually by the International Society for Bayesian Analysis and Section on Bayesian Statistical Sciences of American Statistical Association (ASA) for the best Bayesian application paper. Dr. Zhou was elected to be a regular member in the International Statistical Institute (1998). He was elected to fellow of the ASA (2004). Dr. Zhou was elected to be Chair for the Section on Statistics in Epidemiology of ASA (2004). Dr. Zhou received a research career scientist award from U.S. federal government department of Veterans Affairs (2007). Dr. Zhou received an Advisory Committee Service Award from U.S. FDA (2008). Dr. Zhou was elected to be Chair for the Health Policy Statistics Section of ASA (2011). Currently, Dr. Zhou is serving as Chair of the mental health statistics section of ASA, the founding President of the VA Statisticians Association and a voting member of FDA Radiological Health Advisory Committee.

Dr. KC Gary Chan is currently the Associate Professor of the department of Biostatistics and department of Health Services at the University of Washington. He obtained his BSc degree from University of Hong Kong in 2004 and PhD degree in Biostatistics from Johns Hopkins University in 2008. Dr Chan's current research interests include Survival Analysis, Medical cost, Recurrent events, Clinical trials, Missing data, Causal Inference and Measurement error. Dr. Chan has received several awards for his outstanding research including the Distinguished Student Paper Award (International Biometric Society Eastern North American Region, 2008) and The Margaret Merrell Award (2008).

Appendix A: Regular Conditions

We first give some notations. Let $\mathcal{W}$ denote the support of W, for any $w \in \mathcal{W}$, let $\eta_0(w) = (\alpha_0, \theta_0^T(w), \rho_0^T)^T$, $\widehat{\eta}(w) = (\widehat{\alpha}, \widehat{\theta}^T(w), \widehat{\rho}^T)^T$. For $i = 1, \ldots, n$, let $b = (y, z_2^{*T}, yz_2^T)^T$ and $B_i = (Y_i, Z_{2i}^{*T}, Y_i Z_{2i}^T)^T$. For $k = 0, 1, 2$, define

$$\begin{aligned} & Q_k(\eta_0(w), s) \\ & = \frac{1}{n}\sum_{i=1}^n K_h(W_i - w) R_i(s) \exp\{\eta_0(W_i) B_i\}(B_i)^{\otimes k}, \\ & Q_k^*(s) \\ & = \frac{1}{n}\sum_{i=1}^n R_i(s) \exp\{\eta_0(W_i) B_i\}(B_i)^{\otimes k}, \end{aligned}$$

where $K_h(w) = K(w/h)/h$. Here $a^{\otimes k} = 1, a, aa^T$ for $k = 0, 1, 2$.

The following conditions are imposed to derive the proofs of Lemma 1, Lemma 2, Theorem 1, and Theorem 2.

(A.i) Failure time T and censoring time C are independent given Z_1 and Z_2.

(A.ii) $\int_0^\tau \lambda_0(u)du < \infty$.

(A.iii) The density of W is of compact support $\mathcal{W}$ and has a bound second-order derivative. The function $\theta(w)$ is absolutely continuous and has continuous second-order derivatives on $\mathcal{W}$.

(A.iv) For any $w \in \mathcal{W}$,

$$\begin{aligned} & E\{\sup_{\eta \in \mathcal{N}(\eta_0(w))} \exp\{\eta_0(w)B\}(B)^{\otimes 2}\} < \infty; \\ & \Pi(\eta_0) \\ & = \int_0^\tau \frac{EQ_2(\eta_0(w), s)EQ_0(\eta_0(w), s) - \{EQ_1(\eta_0(w), s)\}^{\otimes 2}}{EQ_0^2(\eta_0(y), s)} dEN(s) \end{aligned}$$

is positive definite; $EQ_0(\eta_0(w), s)$ and $EQ_0^*(s)$ are bounded away from zero.

(A.v) Given $(y, z_2) \in \mathcal{Y} \times \mathcal{Z}_2$, $S(t|y, z_2)$ is absolutely continuous for t over $[0, \tau]$.

(A.vi) The function $H(u)$ is bounded and has bounded first and second derivatives $H'(u)$ and $H''(u)$ for $u \in (-\infty, \infty)$.

Appendix B: Proof of Lemma 1 and Lemma 2

Proof of Lemma 1. Note that the semiparametric location model is equivalent to the following transformation model:

$$Y = \gamma_0^T Z_1 + \epsilon,$$

where ϵ has a distribution $H(\cdot)$. Under Conditions (A.iii) and (A.vi), the estimator $\widehat{\gamma}$ is consistent and asymptotically normal with

$$\begin{aligned} & n^{-\frac{1}{2}}(\widehat{\gamma} - \gamma_0) \\ & = n^{-\frac{1}{2}} \sum_{i=1}^{n} \Gamma^{-1}(Z_{1i}Y_i - Z_{1i}Z_{1i}^T\gamma_0) + o_p(1), \end{aligned} \tag{9}$$

where $\Gamma = E(Z_1 Z_1^T)$. Letting $B(\gamma) = E[H\{y + \gamma^T(Z_1 - z_1) - \gamma_0^T Z_1\}]$, since

$$\begin{aligned} & n^{\frac{1}{2}}\{\widehat{H}(y - \gamma^T z_1, \gamma) - B(\gamma)\} \\ & = n^{\frac{1}{2}}\Bigg[n^{-1}\sum_{i=1}^{n} I(Y_i \le y + \gamma^T Z_{1i} - \gamma^T Z_1) \\ & \quad - EH\{y + (\gamma^T - \gamma_0^T)Z_1 - \gamma^T z_1\}\Bigg], \end{aligned}$$

by the functional central limit theorem, we can show that $n^{\frac{1}{2}}\{\widehat{H}(y - \gamma^T z_1, \gamma) - B(\gamma)\}$ converges to a mean zero Gaussian process on $(y, \gamma) \in \mathcal{Y} \times \mathcal{N}(\gamma_0)$. It follows from the equicontinuity of the foregoing process and the consistency of $\widehat{\gamma}$ that

$$\begin{aligned} & \sup_{y \in \mathcal{Y}} |n^{\frac{1}{2}}\{\widehat{H}(y - \widehat{\gamma}^T z_1, \widehat{\gamma}) - B(\widehat{\gamma})\} \\ & \quad - n^{\frac{1}{2}}\{\widehat{\widehat{H}}(y - \gamma_0^T z_1, \gamma_0) - H(y - \gamma_0^T)\}| = o_p(1), \end{aligned}$$

which yields that

$$\begin{aligned} & n^{\frac{1}{2}}\{\widehat{H}(y - \gamma^T z_1, \gamma) - H(y - \gamma_0^T)\} \\ & \quad = n^{\frac{1}{2}}\{\widehat{H}(y - \gamma_0^T z_1, \gamma_0) - H(y - \gamma_0')\} \\ & \quad + n^{\frac{1}{2}}\{B(\widehat{\gamma}) - H(y - \gamma_0^T)\} + o_p(1) \end{aligned} \tag{10}$$

uniformly for $y \in \mathcal{Y}$. According to Taylor expansion, the second term on the right-hand side of (10) can be expressed as

$$\begin{aligned} & n^{\frac{1}{2}} E\left[H\{y + (\gamma - \gamma_0)^T Z_1 - \gamma^T z_1\} - H(y - \gamma_0^T z_1)\right] \\ & \quad = n^{\frac{1}{2}} H'(y - \gamma_0^T z_1)(\widehat{\gamma} - \gamma_0)^T (EZ_1 - z_1) + o_p(1) \end{aligned}$$

uniformly for $y \in \mathcal{Y}$. This together with (9) yields that

$$\begin{aligned} & n^{\frac{1}{2}}\{\widehat{H}(y-\widehat{\gamma}^T z_1, \widehat{\gamma}) - H(y-\gamma_0^T)\} \\ & \quad = n^{-\frac{1}{2}} \sum_{i=1}^{n} \xi_1(\gamma_0, y, z_1, Z_{1i}, Y_i) + o_p(1). \end{aligned}$$

Here

$$\begin{aligned} & \xi_1(\gamma_0, y, z_1, Z_{1i}, Y_i) \\ & \quad = \{I(Y_i - \gamma_0^T z_1 \le y - \gamma_0^T z_1) - H(y - \gamma_0^T z_1)\} \\ & \qquad + \{H'(y-\gamma_0^T z_1)(EZ_1 - z_1)^T \Gamma^{-1}(Z_{1i}Y_i - Z_{1i}X_i^T \gamma_0)\}, \end{aligned}$$

for $i = 1, 2, \ldots, n$.

Hence, $n^{\frac{1}{2}}\{\widehat{H}(y-\widehat{\gamma}^T z_1, \widehat{\gamma}) - H(y-\gamma_0^T)\}$ converge to a mean zero Gaussian process with covariance $Cov\{\xi_1(\gamma_0, y_1, z_1, Z_{1i}, Y_i),\ \xi_1(\gamma_0, y_2, x_1, Z_{1i}, Y_i)\}$.

Proof of Lemma 2. It is known that $\widehat{\Lambda}(t)$ is consistent. We first prove that $\widehat{\Lambda}(t)$ is $\sqrt{n}$-consistent. According to Cai *et al.* [2008], we can find a mean zero i.i.d. random vector $\{\xi_3(u, Z_{2i}, W_i, W_j)\}_{i=1}^n$, such that for each W_j, $j = 1, \ldots, n$,

$$\begin{aligned} & \widehat{\eta}(W_j) - \eta_0(W_j) \\ & \quad = \frac{1}{n}\sum_{i=1}^{n}\int_0^{\tau} K_h(W_i - W_j)\xi_3(u, Z_{2i}, Y_i, W_j)dM_i(u) \\ & \qquad + O_p(h^2). \end{aligned} \tag{11}$$

Hence, we have

$$\begin{aligned} & \sqrt{n}\{\widehat{\Lambda}(t) - \Lambda_0(t)\} \\ & \quad = \frac{1}{\sqrt{n}}\sum_{i=1}^{n}\int_0^{\tau}\frac{dM_i(s)}{Q_0^*(s)} - \frac{1}{\sqrt{n}}\int_0^{\tau}\frac{\Phi(s)}{Q_0^*(s)}d\Lambda_0(s) \\ & \qquad + O_p(\sqrt{n}h^2) \\ & \quad = \frac{1}{\sqrt{n}}\sum_{i=1}^{n}\int_0^{\tau}\frac{dM_i(s)}{EQ_0^*(s)} - \frac{1}{\sqrt{n}}\int_0^{\tau}\frac{\Phi(s)}{EQ_0^*(s)}d\Lambda_0(s) \\ & \qquad + O_p(\sqrt{n}h^2) + o_p(1), \end{aligned}$$

where $\Phi(s) = \sum_{j=1}^{n} R_j(s)\exp\{\eta_0^T(W_j)B_j\}B_j^T\{\widehat{\eta}(W_j) - \eta_0(W_j)\}$. Combining the second term on the right-hand side with (11) yields that

$$
\begin{aligned}
&-\frac{1}{\sqrt{n}}\int_0^\tau \frac{\Phi(s)}{EQ_0^*(s)}d\Lambda_0(s)\\
&\quad= -\frac{1}{\sqrt{n}}\int_0^\tau \frac{n^{-1}\sum_{j=1}^{n} R_j(s)\exp\{\eta_0^T(W_j)B_j\}B_j^T}{EQ_0^*(s)}\\
&\quad\left\{\sum_{l=1}^{n}\int_0^\tau K_h(W_l - W_j)\xi_3(u, Z_{2l}, Y_l, W_j)dM_l(u)\right\}d\Lambda_0(s)\\
&\qquad + O_p(\sqrt{n}h^2)\\
&\quad= -\frac{1}{\sqrt{n}}\sum_{l=1}^{n}\int_0^\tau\int_0^\tau \frac{n^{-1}\sum_{j\neq l}^{n} R_j(s)\exp\{\eta_0^T(W_j)B_j\}B_j^T}{EQ_0^*(s)}\\
&\qquad \{K_h(Y_l - W_j)\xi_3(u, Z_{2l}, Y_l, W_j)\}d\Lambda_0(s)dM_l(u)\\
&\qquad + O_p(\sqrt{n}h^2) + O_p\left(\frac{1}{\sqrt{n}}\right)\\
&\quad= O_p(\sqrt{n}h^2) + O_p(1).
\end{aligned}
$$

Thus, if $nh^2 \to \infty$ and $nh^4 \to 0$ as $n \to \infty$, we have for any $t \in (0, \tau]$, $\sqrt{n}\{\widehat{\Lambda}(t) - \Lambda_0(t)\} \xrightarrow{P} 0$. Furthermore, according to,[3] $\widehat{\Lambda}(t) \longrightarrow \Lambda_0(t)$ uniformly on $(0, \tau]$ in probability.

Next we prove the asymptotic normality of $\sqrt{nh}\{\widehat{S}(t|y, z_2) - S(t|y, z_2)\}$. Note that

$$
\begin{aligned}
&\sqrt{nh}\{\widehat{S}(t|y, z_2) - S(t|y, z_2)\}\\
&\quad= \sqrt{n}\exp\{-\Lambda(t|y, z_2)\}\{\Lambda(t|y, z_2) - \widehat{\Lambda}(t|y, z_2)\} + o_p(1)\\
&\quad= \sqrt{nh}S(t|y, z_2)\exp\{b^T\eta_0(w)\}b^T\\
&\qquad \Lambda_0(t)\{\widehat{\eta}(w) - \eta_0(w)\} + o_p(1)\\
&\quad= \sqrt{\frac{h}{n}}\sum_{i=1}^{n}\int_0^\tau K_h(W_i - w)S(t|w, z_2)\exp\{b^T\eta_0(w)\}b^T\\
&\qquad \Lambda_0(t)\xi_3(u, Z_{2i}, Y_i, w)dM_i(u) + o_p(1)\\
&\quad\equiv \sqrt{\frac{h}{n}}\sum_{i=1}^{n} K_h(W_i - w)\xi_4(\eta_0(w), y, z_2, Z_{2i}, Y_i, t) + o_p(1). \qquad (12)
\end{aligned}
$$

Here, $E[\xi_4(\eta_0(w), y, z_2, Z_{2i}, Y_i, t)] = 0$. Thus, $\sqrt{nh}\{\widehat{S}(t|y, z_2) - S(t|y, z_2)\}$ converges to a mean zero Gaussian process with covariance $\nu_0 Cov\{\xi_4(\eta_0(w), y_1, z_2, Z_{2i}, Y_i, t),\ \xi_4(\eta_0(w), y_2, z_2, Z_{2i}, Y_i, t)\}$.

Appendix C: Proof of Theorems 1–2

Proof of Theorem 1. Note that $\sup_y |\widehat{F}(y|z_1) - F(y|z_1)| + \sup_y |\widehat{F}^{-1}(y|z_1) - F^{-1}(y|z_1)| = o_p(n^{-\frac{1}{4}})$ and $\sup_y |\widehat{S}(t|y, z_2) - S(t|y, z_2)| = O_p(\frac{\log h}{\sqrt{nh}} + h^2)$, hence it follows from Lemma 2 that

$$
\begin{aligned}
&\sqrt{nh}\{\widehat{PPV}(v; t, z_1, z_2) - PPV(v; t, z_1, z_2)\} \\
&= \sqrt{nh}(1-v)^{-1}\left\{\int_{\widehat{F}_{z_1}^{-1}(v)} \widehat{S}(t|y, z_2) d\widehat{F}_{z_1}(y)\right. \\
&\quad \left. - \int_{F_{z_1}^{-1}(v)} S(t|y, z_2) dF_{z_1}(y)\right\} \\
&= \sqrt{nh}(1-v)^{-1}\left\{\int_{\widehat{F}_{z_1}^{-1}(v)} \widehat{S}(t|y, z_2) d\widehat{F}_{z_1}(y)\right. \\
&\quad \left. - \int_{F_{z_1}^{-1}(v)} \widehat{S}(t|y, z_2) dF_{z_1}(y)\right\} \\
&\quad + \frac{\sqrt{nh}}{(1-v)}\left\{\int_{F_{z_1}^{-1}(v)} \{\widehat{S}(t|y, z_2) - S(t|y, z_2)\} dF_{z_1}(y)\right\} \\
&= \sqrt{\frac{h}{n}}\sum_{i=1}^{n}(1-v)^{-1}\int_{F_{z_1}^{-1}(v)} \xi_4(\eta_0(w), y, z_2, Z_{2i}, Y_i, t) \\
&\quad K_h(W_i - w) dF_{z_1}(y) + o_p(1) \\
&\equiv \sqrt{\frac{h}{n}}\sum_{i=1}^{n} K_h(W_i - w)\kappa_i^*(v, t, z_1, z_2) + o_p(1),
\end{aligned} \tag{13}
$$

where $E[\kappa_i^*(v, t, z_1, z_2)] = 0$. Therefore Theorem 1 follows.

Proof of Theorem 2. Notice that after some algebra manipulations, we obtain the following equations:

$$
\begin{aligned}
&\sqrt{n}\{\widehat{APPV}(v;t) - APPV(v;t)\} \\
&\quad = \sqrt{n}\int\{\widehat{PPV}(v;t,z_1,z_2) - PPV(v;t,z_1,z_2)\}dF_Z(z) \\
&\quad + \sqrt{n}\int\{\widehat{PPV}(v;t,z_1,z_2) - PPV(v;t,z_1,z_2)\} \\
&\quad d\{\widehat{F}_Z(z) - F_Z(z)\} \\
&\quad + \sqrt{n}\int PPV(v;t,z_1,z_2)\}d\{\widehat{F}_Z(z) - F_Z(z)\}. \qquad (14)
\end{aligned}
$$

Note that, since $\theta(w)$ is absolutely continuous and has the continuous second-order derivative on $\mathcal{W}$, we can show that $\sup_z |\widehat{PPV}(v;t,z_1,z_2) - PPV(v;t,z_1,z_2)| = O_p(\frac{\log h}{\sqrt{nh}} + h^2)$. Then by Lemma 3 we can show that the second term on the right-hand side of (14) converges to zero in probability. It follows from Theorem 1 that

$$
\begin{aligned}
(14) &= \frac{1}{\sqrt{n}}\sum_{i=1}^{n}\int K_h(W_i - w)\kappa_i^*(v,t,z_1,z_2)dF_Z(z) \\
&\quad + \frac{1}{\sqrt{n}}\sum_{i=1}^{n}\{PPV(v;t,Z_{i1},Z_{i2}) - APPV(v;t)\} \\
&\quad + o_p(1) \\
&\equiv \frac{1}{\sqrt{n}}\sum_{i=1}^{n}\zeta_i^*(v;t) + o_p(1),
\end{aligned}
$$

where $E\{\zeta_i^*(v;t)\} = 0$. Hence Theorem 2 follows.

CHAPTER 4

STATISTICAL METHODS FOR PERSONALIZED MEDICINE

LU TIAN

Department of Health Research and Policy
Stanford University
Palo Alto, CA 94301, USA
lutian@stanford.edu

XIAOGUANG ZHAO

Department of Bone and Joint Surgery
The First Affiliated Hospital of Xi'an Medical University,
Xiŭan 710077, Shaanxi Province, P.R. China
xgzhao85@gmail.com

1. Introduction

There has been a lot of interest in advancing personalized medicine in medical research as well as clinical practice recently. The basic concept of personalized medicine is to tailor the treatment for a patient based on his or her genetic makeup, clinical conditions and other personal characteristics to improve treatment efficacy and safety.[1–3] The idea of personalized medicine is not entirely new in that most clinical decisions should be — and to some extent have been — made on an individual basis. However, rich omics information available only recently enables us to characterize individuals in fine detail and make the "personalized" clinical decision truly personalized.[4] For example, the completion of the human genome project and continuously decreasing cost of genetic tests have opened up a world with immense possibility for doctors to estimate the future risk or treatment response for a patient using his/her own genetic information. Personalized medicine has great potential for improving disease prevention, diagnosis and treatment. Genetic test guided Warfarin dosing selection is a good example.[5,6] The statistical challenges associated with personalized medicine related clinical research revolve around the task of providing effective tools for constructing and evaluating evidence-based personalized intervention strategy, i.e., based on observed data. Depending on the clinical question of interest, different statistical methods are needed. In general, there are two types of objectives: (a) developing a personalized risk stratification method which can be used to guide the selection of appropriate prevention and treatment strategy for individual patient; (b) estimating the personalized treatment effect which can be used to identify subgroups of patients who may benefit the most from a treatment. In the next two sections, we will discuss and review the most recent developments in statistical methodology for these two types of research.

2. Personalized Risk Prediction

In disease prevention, it is crucial to accurately identify high risk population and administrate special intervention accordingly. Therefore, it is important to accurately predict future risk of a given disease for example, it is known that aspirin can effectively reduce risk of cardiovascular disease. However, considering the cost and potential side effect including gastrointestinal ulcers and stomach bleeding, it may not be economical to prescribe the medicine to the entire population. On the other hand, it is generally accepted that if the 10-year risk of experiencing a cardiovascular event is higher than a threshold such as 10%, then the benefit of taking aspirin outweighs the potential cost. To implement such a prevention strategy, the clinician needs to estimate a patient's 10-year risk of having cardiovascular events with available information .[7] From the statistical perspective, it is a regression problem. Normally, the regression analysis is used for characterizing the association between a set of exposure variables and outcome of interest. The main focus of the regression analysis is on the efficient estimation of the model parameter summarizing the association under the assumption that the model is correctly specified.[8] Consequently, it is also important to examine the validity of the model assumption based on the observed data. In our case, however, the main objective is to make accurate outcome predictions based on the imposed regression model. Therefore, one doesn't need to assume that the regression model is correctly specified and the main criterion for evaluating and selecting different regression models should be their prediction performance for future observations.[9]

In the following, we will illustrate the general procedure for building and evaluating a prediction model with survival outcomes. Suppose that T and

X are survival time and covariate vector of interest, respectively. In most clinical studies, survival time may be right censored by an independent censoring time C and is not completely observable.[10] Instead of T, we only observe $\{U = \min(T, C), \Delta = I(T \leq C)\}$, where $I(\cdot)$ is the indicator function. Due to right censoring, the entire distribution of T oftentimes is not estimable without strong unverifiable parametric assumptions regardless of the sample size. Thus, one may not be able to predict the survival time T itself. In practice, one may restrict the attention to a transformation of T, Y, the new outcome of clinical interest whose distribution is estimable based on right-censored data. For example, Y could be $I(T \geq \tau)$, the binary survival status at time τ, or $\min(T, \tau)$, the restricted survival time up to time τ. For chosen Y, we may want to build a regression model for the conditional expectation $\mu(x) = E(Y|X = x)$, which can be used to predict the future outcome.

2.1. *Model building in personalized risk prediction*

Suppose that the observed data consists of n independent identically distributed observations $\{(U_i, \Delta_i, X_i), i = 1, \ldots, n\}$. Our objective is to build a regression model giving a prediction rule for future Y. When X is one-dimensional, the nonparametric smoothing method can be used to estimate $\mu(\cdot)$ without any specific assumption on its functional form. However, when the dimension of X is greater than one, nonparametric smoothing may not be feasible due to the curse of dimensionality and additional assumption for $\mu(\cdot)$ needed. For example, a simple working model is to assume that

$$\mu(x) = g\{\beta' W(x)\} \tag{1}$$

where $g(\cdot)$ is a given monotone link function, the vector $W(x)$ including the intercept is a known transformation of original covariate vector X and β is the unknown regression parameter of interest. Then β can be estimated by $\hat{\beta}$, the root of the inverse probability weighted estimating equation

$$\sum_{i=1}^{n} \frac{\Delta_i}{\hat{G}_C(U_i)} W_i\{Y_i - g(\beta' W_i)\} = 0,$$

where $\hat{G}_C(\cdot)$ is the Kaplan-Meier estimator for the censoring distribution and $W_i = W(X_i)$. Here the weight $\Delta_i/\hat{G}_C(U_i)$ is used to correct the bias caused by right censoring.[11] Once $\hat{\beta}$ is obtained, the outcome of a future patient with covariate x can be predicted as $\hat{Y}(x) = g\{\hat{\beta}' W(x)\}$. One appealing feature of this simple approach is that under mild regularity conditions, $\hat{\beta}$ converges to a constant vector β_0 as $n \to \infty$ even when model (1) is misspecified.[9] It implies that the derived prediction rule stabilizes as the sample size increases. Furthermore, the limiting rule does not depend on the censoring distribution.

Remarks

Other commonly used regression models can be employed as well. For example, one may fit the semiparametric proportional hazards[12] or accelerated failure time model[13,14] for the right censored outcomes. Based on the fitted model, the corresponding prediction rule for Y can be derived.[15,16] However those resulting prediction rules in general depend on the censoring distribution when the corresponding model assumptions are violated.[17,18]

2.2. *Model evaluation in personalized risk prediction*

Since more than one prediction rule can be derived based on different working models, it is important to select the optimal prediction rule/regression model in practice. For a typical regression analysis, one common approach for model evaluation is to construct a goodness of fit test statistics and derive the its distribution assuming that the model is correctly specified. The formal statistical test is then performed and a significant p-value is treated as an indication of the model mis-specification.[19,20] However, our purpose here is not to verify specific model assumptions, which are often chosen for mathematical convenience in estimating the model parameters. Since the ultimate goal is to predict future outcomes, the sensible approach for evaluating a model is to estimate the prediction error of the derived prediction rule in the targeted population. To this end, one needs to define a loss function reflecting the distance between the predicted and true outcomes. Ideally, the scale of the loss function is readily interpretable for clinical researchers. For example, one may use the expected absolute prediction error $E\{L(Y, \hat{Y})\} = E\{|Y - \hat{Y}(X)|\}$ to measure the prediction accuracy of the prediction rule $\hat{Y}(\cdot)$.[9] It degenerates into the simple misclassification error for binary responses. With the observed data, one simple estimator for this expected loss is

$$n^{-1} \sum_{i=1}^{n} \frac{\Delta_i}{\hat{G}_C(U_i)} |Y_i - \hat{Y}(X_i)|.$$

However, it is well known that this "apparent error" type estimator may be downward biased because the same data is used to derive and evaluate the prediction rule.[21,22] A more reliable estimator for the absolute prediction error is based on cross-validation method.[23,24] Specifically, we randomly split the data set into K disjoint subsets of approximately equal sizes, denoted by $\{\mathcal{I}_k, k = 1, \ldots, K\}$. For each k, we use all observations not in $\mathcal{I}_k$ to obtain a model-based prediction rule $\hat{Y}_{(-k)}(x)$ for subject with $X = x$, and then estimate the total absolute prediction error for observations in $\mathcal{I}_k$ by

$$\hat{D}_k = \sum_{i \in \mathcal{I}_k} \frac{\Delta_i}{\hat{G}_C(T_i)} \left| Y_i - \hat{Y}_{(-k)}(X_i) \right| .$$

Then the final estimate for the mean absolute prediction error is

$$\hat{D}^{(cv)} = \frac{1}{n} \sum_{k=1}^{K} \hat{D}_k .$$

This estimator can be used to evaluate the performance of a given prediction rule.

In the presence of multiple prediction rules, in general the rule with the smallest cross-validated estimator for the absolute prediction error should be chosen. However, in practice one may also prefer a simple prediction rule to a complicated one, if the difference in prediction accuracy between the two is not clinically important. Once the optimal prediction rule/working model is selected based on interpretability, complexity and estimated prediction error, the final prediction rule can then be derived using the entire data set and for making and then used fresh predictions.

2.3. *Additive value of biomarkers in personalized risk prediction*

It is oftentimes cortrovesal whether or not additional measurement of a novel biomarker (potentially expensive or invasive) can substantially improve the performance of an existing prediction rule based on old biomarkers.[25–27] Traditionally, this problem is tackled by fitting a multivariate regression model including both old and new biomarkers as covariates and testing the significance of the adjusted association between the new biomarker and clinical outcome of interest.[25] However, besides the validity of the assumed regression model, the significance level alone fails to quantify the incremental value of the new biomarker in a clinically meaningful way. Alternatively, one may estimate the mean absolute prediction error for both the existing prediction rule based on traditional biomarkers only and a new prediction rule based on both traditional and novel biomarkers derived from the method presented in Section 2.2. Denote the estimated prediction error of the old and new prediction rules by $\hat{D}_{old}$ and $\hat{D}_{new}$, respectively, one may quantify the additional value of the novel biomarker by an appropriate contrast of the estimated prediction errors, such as $\hat{D}_{old} - \hat{D}_{new}$.[9,28] The 95% confidence interval for the difference can be constructed as well. This approach provides a very transparent message on how much improvement in prediction performance the novel biomarker can bring in practice and thus helps the decision markers to determine on the "value" of the new biomarker.

Sometimes, it is only worthwhile to measure the new biomarker for a subgroup of a population for improving the prediction performance. To identify the appropriate subgroup, one may estimate the difference in prediction error between old and new prediction rules in different subgroups of patients.[29] For example, one may estimate

$$G(s) = E\{(|Y - \hat{Y}_{old}| - |Y - \hat{Y}_{new}|) \mid \hat{Y}_{old} \in [s - d, s + d]\}$$

by applying the cross-validation procedure to patients with $\hat{Y}_{old} \in [s - d, s + d]$, where $\hat{Y}_{old}$ and $\hat{Y}_{new}$ denote the predicted values from old and new prediction rules, respectively. One may then select the appropriate subgroup of patients who may benefit the most from measuring the new biomarker by examining the estimated function $G(s)$.

2.4. *Statistical inference for the scoring system used for personalized risk prediction*

The final prediction rule yields the predicted outcome for each individual and can be viewed as a scoring system. The main application of such a scoring system is to make personalized risk prediction and identify high or low risk patients based on "baseline" information. Naturally, the next step is to make statistical inference on the "true" association between the constructed score and future outcome.[30,35] Since the final prediction rule is selected from a group of candidates, one needs to use fresh data without any overlapping that used for selecting and constructing the scoring system to make the "honest" inference. Ideally, the fresh data is from an independent study with patient population mimicking the targeted population to which the risk stratification rule will be applied. Alternatively, one may split one big data set into training and holdout sets. The former is used for building the scoring system (including model selection via cross-validation procedure) and the latter is used for making statistical inference for the resulting scoring system. Since the score is one-dimensional, the nonparametric inference with minimum model assumption can be implemented. Specifically, assuming that the data in the holdout set consists of m, i.i.d observations $\{(\tilde{U}_i, \tilde{\Delta}_i, \tilde{X}_i, \tilde{V}_i), i = 1, \ldots, m\}$, where $\tilde{V}_i = \hat{Y}(\tilde{X}_i)$ and $\hat{Y}(\cdot)$ is the scoring system of interest. The objective of the inference at this stage can be for example to estimate the conditional expectation

$$\eta(\tilde{v}) = E(\tilde{Y}|\tilde{V} = \tilde{v}),$$

where $\tilde{Y}$ is the corresponding outcome of interest in the holdout set. Under the reasonable assumption that $\eta(\cdot)$ has a continuous second derivative over the support of $\tilde{V}$, one may employ the standard local linear smoothing method.[31 32] Specifically, $\eta(\tilde{v})$ can be estimated by $a(\tilde{v})$, where $\{a(\tilde{v}), b(\tilde{v})\}'$ is the solution to the estimating equation

$$\frac{1}{m}\sum_{i=1}^{m} \frac{\tilde{\Delta}_i}{\hat{G}_{\tilde{C}}(\tilde{U}_i|\tilde{v})} \begin{pmatrix} 1 \\ \tilde{V}_i - \tilde{v} \end{pmatrix} K_h(\tilde{V}_i - \tilde{v}) \left\{\tilde{Y}_i - a - b(\tilde{V}_i - \tilde{v})\right\} = 0,$$

where $K_h(x) = K(x/h)/h$, $K(\cdot)$ is a smooth kernel function with finite support, $h = o_p(1)$ is the smoothing bandwidth,

$$\hat{G}_{\tilde{C}}(t|\tilde{v}) = \exp\left\{-\sum_{i=1}^{m}\int_0^t \frac{d\tilde{N}_i^{\tilde{C}}(u)K_h(\tilde{V}_i - \tilde{v})}{\sum_{j=1}^{n}(\tilde{U}_j \geq \tilde{u})K_h(\tilde{V}_i - \tilde{v})}\right\}$$

is the local nonparametric estimator for the survival function of $\tilde{C}$[32, 33] and $\tilde{N}_i^C(u) = I(\tilde{U}_i \leq u)(1 - \tilde{\Delta}_i)$. Since we assume that the censoring time $\tilde{C}_i$ and $\tilde{V}_i$ are independent, the regular Kaplan-Meier estimator based on the entire sample and the local estimator $\hat{G}_{\tilde{C}}(t|\tilde{v})$ converge to the same limit. However, the latter may improve the efficiency of the resulting estimator $\hat{\eta}(\tilde{v}) = a(\tilde{v})$. If $(mh)^{-1} = o_p(1)$, then $\hat{\eta}(\tilde{v})$ converges to $\eta(\tilde{v})$ uniformly in probability for $\tilde{v} \in [v_1, v_2]$, where $[v_1, v_2]$ is within the support of $\tilde{V}$. Furthermore, if $mh^5 = o_p(1)$, then $(mh)^{1/2}\{\hat{\eta}(\tilde{v}) - \eta(\tilde{v})\}$ converges weakly to a mean zero Gaussian distribution with a variance of

$$\nu_2 E(\{\tilde{Y} - \eta(\tilde{v})\}^2|\tilde{V} = \tilde{v}) f_{\tilde{V}}(\tilde{v})^{-1}, \tag{2}$$

where $\nu_2 = \int_{-\infty}^{\infty} K^2(v)dv$ and $f_{\tilde{V}}(\cdot)$ is the density function of $\tilde{V}$. The variance of $\hat{\eta}(\tilde{v})$ can be estimated analytically based on (2). On the other hand, a more automatic and reliable variance estimation procedure is based on the resampling method.[30,34,35] Operationally, one may let $\eta^*(\tilde{v})$ be the solution of the perturbed estimating equation

$$\frac{1}{m}\sum_{i=1}^{m} B_i \frac{\tilde{\Delta}_i}{\hat{G}^*_{\tilde{C}}(\tilde{U}_i|\tilde{v})}\begin{pmatrix}1\\ \tilde{V}_i - \tilde{v}\end{pmatrix} K_h(\tilde{V}_i - \tilde{v})\left\{\tilde{Y}_i - a - b(\tilde{V}_i - \tilde{v})\right\} = 0,$$

where

$$\hat{G}^*_{\tilde{C}}(t|\tilde{v}) = \exp\left\{-\sum_{i=1}^{m} B_i \int_0^t \frac{d\tilde{N}_i^{\tilde{C}}(u) K_h(\tilde{V}_i - \tilde{v})}{\sum_{j=1}^{n}(\tilde{U}_j \geq \tilde{u}) K_h(\tilde{V}_i - \tilde{v})}\right\}$$

and $\{B_1, \ldots, B_m\}$ are m independent unit exponential random variables externally generated by the user. After generating $\{B_1, \ldots, B_m\}$ and obtaining $\eta^*(\tilde{v})$ repeatedly, the empirical variance of $\eta^*(\tilde{v})$ can then be used to approximate $\text{var}\{\hat{\eta}(\tilde{v})\}$. Let $\hat{\sigma}^2(\tilde{v})$ denote the variance estimator, the 95% confidence interval of $\eta(\tilde{v})$ can be constructed as $[\hat{\eta}(\tilde{v}) - 1.96\hat{\sigma}(\tilde{v}), \hat{\eta}(\tilde{v}) + 1.96\hat{\sigma}(\tilde{v})]$. The point estimator $\hat{\eta}(\tilde{v})$, coupled with its 95% confidence interval (or band), characterizes the underlying relationship of the score used for individual prediction and the real outcome. It may guide the risk stratification practice, for example, by setting appropriate threshold value of the score to identify high risk individuals for whom the aggressive intervention is needed.

To implement the aforementioned inference procedure, one needs to select the smoothing bandwidth, which is often achieved by implementing the cross-validation procedure. The resulting bandwidth normally is in the order of $O_p(m^{-1/5})$. To make the asymptotical bias ignorable, undersmoothing with bandwidth $h = o_p(m^{-1/5})$ is needed. One simple remedy is to multiply the bandwidth selected via cross-validation by a factor converging to zero as sample size increases, for example $m^{-1/10}$.

2.5. *Summary for statistical methods used in personalized risk prediction*

We have described the general statistical methods for developing scoring systems used for stratifying patients according to his/her individual risk and guiding the choice of clinical interventions. Unlike traditional statistical modeling, the main purpose of the data analysis here is to generate an accurate prediction rule for future outcome of clinical interest. To this end, various regression models can be used to derive specific prediction rules regardless of whether their assumptions are valid for the current data or not. The optimal prediction rule should then be selected by minimizing a clinical interpretable loss function measuring the prediction accuracy. The cross-validation procedure is recommended on the grounds of bias reduction. Furthermore, one may want to characterize the underlying relationship between the constructed score and future outcome. To this end, nonparametric regression methods with minimum model assumption can be implemented on a fresh holdout set.

3. Personalized Treatment Selection

For a given treatment, the effect on the patients may very heterogeneous, i.e., some patients may be benefit substantially more than others from the treatment. In a typical randomized clinical trial aiming to prove the efficacy of a treatment, the final conclusion is drawn for the average treatment effect in the entire study population. In other words, it is possible that while the average treatment effect is near zero, the treatment may still be beneficial to a subgroup of patients. The opposite may be true as well: the positive overall treatment effect does not rule out the possible presence of subgroup of patients for whom the treatment has null or even negative effect. In the causal inference framework, we may assume that every patient has a pair of potential responses $(Y^{(1)}, Y^{(-1)})$, where $Y^{(1)}$ and $Y^{(-1)}$ are outcomes if the patient receives the treatment and placebo (or other standard care intervention in the comparison), respectively.[36] In practice, we can only observe $Y = Y^{(1)}$ or $Y^{(-1)}$ depending on the actual treatment assignment. The traditional analysis for randomized clinical trial targets the estimation the expectation of a contrast between $Y^{(1)}$ and $Y^{(-1)}$ measuring the treatment effect such as $E(Y^{(1)} - Y^{(-1)})$. When the potential stratification of the patient population is given before the data analysis, the simple subgroup analysis adjusted for multiple testing can be used.[37,38] On the other hand, in the statistical analysis assisting the development of the unknown personalized treatment strategy, the parameter of interest is the "personalized" treatment effect $\mu(x) = E(Y^{(1)} - Y^{(-1)}|X = x)$, where X is a set of baseline covariates measured prior to intervention. For this type of analysis, there are two objectives. Firstly, one may want to estimate the sign of $\mu(x)$ such that one can identify the optimal treatment for individual patient. Secondly, one may want to estimate $\mu(x)$ itself, which completely quantifies the personalized treatment effect. In the following, we will illustrate the operational procedure for achieving these two aims with examples in sequence.

It is worthy to point out that although "personalized medicine" is the buzzword in media, a more appropriate word describing the approach should probably be "group specific medicine" or "precision medicine", since the "average" treatment effect for the subgroup of patients with the same covariate X is the best we can estimate from the observed data. In other words, we may know the optimal treatment for this subgroup of patients but that treatment may still not be the optimal choice for all individuals in the subgroup. When a richer set of biomarkers characterizing patients becomes available, one may further divide the existing subgroup into smaller subgroups and seek optimal treatment strategy for each of them. Nevertheless, we still will never know the "best" treatment for individual patients, since ultimately each patient is unique!

3.1. *Estimation of the personalized treatment effect*

When X is a vector with more than 2 dimensions, $\mu(x)$ in general cannot be consistently estimated without specific model assumptions. Therefore, to directly estimate $\mu(x)$, one often needs to assume a joint model for the conditional distributions $Y^{(1)}|X = x$ and $Y^0|X = x$. We will use survival data to illustrate this approach. Specifically, we assume that the observed data consists of $\{(U_i, \Delta_i, R_i, X_i), i = 1, \ldots, n\}$, where $R_i = \pm 1$ is the treatment indicator. Again Y, a given transformation of T, is the outcome of interest. For illustration purpose, we let $Y = \min(T, \tau)$, where τ is a given constant such that $P(U > \tau | R = r) > 0$ for $r \in \{-1, 1\}$.[39,40] Other choices of Y are also possible. With these notations, $Y = Y^{(R)}, R = \pm 1$. Furthermore, R and X are independent due to the randomization. Without loss of generality, we also assume that $\text{pr}(R = 1) = \text{pr}(R = -1) = 0.5$. Firstly, we may assume the commonly used proportional hazards regression model in both arms separately:

$$\lambda(t|R, X) = \lambda_R(t) \exp\{\beta_R' W(X)\},$$

where $W(x)$ is a given transformation of x and $\lambda_r(t)$ is the baseline hazard function in arm r. With the observed data, one may estimate β_r by maximizing the partial likelihood function with observations in the corresponding arm. Furthermore, one may estimate the cumulative hazard function $\Lambda_r(t) = \int_0^t \lambda_r(u)du$ by the Breslow estimator.[41] Denote the resulting estimators by $\hat{\beta}_r$ and $\hat{\Lambda}_r(\cdot)$ for the regression coefficient and cumulative baseline hazard function, respectively. The personalized treatment effect $\mu(x)$ can be estimated by

$$\hat{\mu}(x) = \int_0^\tau \exp\{-\hat{\Lambda}_1(t) e^{\hat{\beta}_1' W(x)}\} dt - \int_0^\tau \exp\{-\hat{\Lambda}_{-1}(t) e^{\hat{\beta}_{-1}' W(x)}\} dt.$$

When the proportional hazards model is correctly specified, the above estimator is consistent.

The proportional hazards regression model is by no means unique here and one may assume other convenient regression models for estimating $\mu(x)$. For example, one can assume that

$$E(Y|R, X = x) = \gamma_R' W(x)$$

and $\mu(x) = (\gamma_1 - \gamma_{-1})' W(x)$ under this model. The regression coefficient γ_r can be estimated by $\hat{\gamma}_r$, the solution of the estimating equation

$$\sum_{i=1}^{n} \frac{\Delta_i}{\hat{G}_r(U_i)} W(X_i)\{Y_i - \gamma_r' W(X_i)\} I(R_i = r) = 0,$$

for $r \in \{-1, 1\}$, where $\hat{G}_r(\cdot)$ is the Kaplan-Meier estimator for the survival function of the censoring time C in arm r. As a result, $\mu(X)$ can be simply estimated by

$$\hat{\mu}(x) = (\hat{\gamma}_1 - \hat{\gamma}_{-1})' W(x).$$

Sometimes, one may not need to completely model the conditional distribution $Y^{(r)}|X = x$. For example, one could directly assume that

$$\mu(x) = \beta' W(x),$$

where the parameter β can be estimated by minimizing the least square objective function

$$\sum_{i=1}^{n} \frac{\Delta_i}{\hat{G}_{R_i}(U_i)} \{Y_i - \beta' W(X_i) R_i/2\}^2$$

This amounts to fitting a standard linear regression model on Y with modified covariates $W(X)R$. Performing regression analysis with modified covariates is a general approach for generating a scoring system measuring the treatment effect.[42] For example, one may maximize the partial likelihood function from the proportional hazards model

$$\lambda(t|X, R) = \lambda_0(t) e^{\beta' W(X) R}$$

with the similarly modified covariate $W(X)R$. One can show that the resulting scoring system $\hat{\beta}' W(X)$ can serve as a surrogate to the treatment effect even when the above proportional hazards model is incorrectly specified.

All aforementioned statistical models in essence use different methods to characterize the interaction between the treatment and baseline covariates and therefore other models with specified interaction terms can be used as well.[43–45]

3.2. *Estimation of the direction of personalized treatment effect*

To determine the optimal treatment to individual with covariate $X = x$, one needs and only needs to know the sign of $\mu(x)$. Specifically, one may be satisfied in identifying the regions $R^+ = \{x \mid \mu(x) > 0\}$ and $R^- = \{x \mid \mu(x) < 0\}$. Assuming $\mu(x) > 0$ represents the positive treatment effect as in the survival analysis example with $Y = \min(T, \tau)$, the optimal treatment choice for patients with $x \in R^+$ and R^- would be $r = 1$ and $r = -1$, respectively. Therefore, estimating the sign of $\mu(x)$ is equivalent to finding the optimal treatment assignment for every patient. If every patient receives his/her optimal treatment, the total "utility" of the entire population is maximized. Thus one may identify the optimal treatment assignment by maximizing the overall utility $E\{Y|R = \hat{R}(X)\}$ with respect to an treatment assignment rule $\hat{R}(X) : R^q \rightarrow \{-1, 1\}$.[46] When there is no censoring, the empirical counterpart of the overall utility is simply

$$\frac{2}{n}\sum_{i=1}^{n} Y_i I\{R_i = \hat{R}(X_i)\}. \tag{3}$$

Maximizing (3) is equivalent to minimizing the weighted misclassification error

$$\sum_{i=1}^{n} Y_i I\{R_i \neq \hat{R}(X_i)\}.$$

In the presence of right censoring, Y_i is not always observable, one may instead minimize

$$\sum_{i=1}^{n} \frac{\Delta_i}{\hat{G}_{R_i}(U_i)} Y_i I\{R_i \neq \hat{R}(X_i)\}.$$

Many different data-mining techniques can be employed to solve this weighted classification problem. For example, after representing $\hat{R}(x)$ in the form of $\text{sign}\{\hat{\mu}(x)\}$, one may replace the indicator function by a convex hinging loss function as its surrogate.[47,48] The modified objective function becomes

$$\sum_{i=1}^{n} \frac{\Delta_i}{\hat{G}_{R_i}(U_i)} Y_i \left[1 - R_i\hat{\mu}(X_i)\right]_+ ,$$

where $[x]_+ = |x|I(x \geq 0)$. Operationally, one may approximate $\hat{\mu}(x)$ by $\gamma_0 + \sum_{k=1}^{K} \gamma_k W_k(x)$, a linear combinations of given basis functions

$\{W_1(x), W_2(x), \ldots, W_K(x)\}$. When K is not small, appropriate penalty for γ_k can be included as in the standard support vector machine. The resulting problem is a convex optimization problem and one may let the estimated treatment assignment rule be

$$\text{sign}\left\{\hat{\gamma}_0 + \sum_{k=1}^{K} \hat{\gamma}_k W_k(x)\right\},$$

where $\hat{\gamma}_k, k = 0, \ldots, K$ are minimizer of the objective function. In the end, one may assign patients with

$$X_i \in \hat{R}^+ = \left\{x \,\middle|\, \hat{\gamma}_0 + \sum_{k=1}^{K} \hat{\gamma}_k W_k(X_i) > 0\right\}$$

to treatment $r = 1$ and

$$X_i \in \hat{R}^- = \left\{x \,\middle|\, \hat{\gamma}_0 + \sum_{k=1}^{K} \hat{\gamma}_k W_k(X_i) < 0\right\}$$

to treatment $r = -1$. Furthermore, as a byproduct of this support vector machine approach, $\hat{\gamma}_0 + \sum_{k=1}^{K} \hat{\gamma}_k W_k(x)$ can be thought of as a surrogate for $\hat{\mu}(x)$.

Remarks

In Sections 3.1 and 3.2, we have presented several approaches for estimating either $\mu(x)$ or $\text{sign}\{\mu(x)\}$. When the working model deriving the estimators is correctly specified, the consistency of the resulting estimator is assured. However, in practice, all working models are at the best approximation to the complicated underlying relationship between the treatment and outcome and therefore all the estimators do not necessarily converge to the true parameter even as the sample size goes to infinity. Given this limitation, the obtained estimators can still be viewed as a scoring system used to rank patients according to their personalized treatment effect and select subgroups of patients who may or may not benefit from the treatment of interest. Therefore, it is important to determine the effectiveness of the scoring system in stratifying the patient population in terms of treatment effect with minimum model assumptions. We will discuss related methods in the next two sections.

3.3. *Model evaluation for personalized treatment effect prediction*

There are multiple ways to construct a scoring system estimating the personalized treatment effect. Therefore it is crucial to evaluate and compare their performance in the targeting population. There are two classes of criteria for measuring the quality of a scoring system. The first class is to measure the distance or concordance between the constructed score and $\mu(x)$, the true personalized treatment effect unknown to us. The second class relies on how effective the scoring system can select subgroups of patients with desirable treatment effect. As we will demonstrate next, these two classes of criterions are closely related.

Formally, assuming that $\hat{\mu}_1(\cdot), \hat{\mu}_2(\cdot), \ldots, \hat{\mu}_J(\cdot)$ are J scoring systems measuring treatment effect and we are interested in selecting the optimal one from the pool. Firstly, we need to define a reasonable optimality criterion. Since the score $\hat{\mu}_j(x)$ targeting on approximating $\mu(x)$,

$$\xi_j = E[\{\mu(X) - \hat{\mu}_j(X)\}^2],$$

the L_2 distance between them is a natural measure for the performance of scoring system j. However, $\xi_j, j = 1, \ldots, J$ are not estimable with the observed data, since the true treatment effect $\mu(\cdot)$ is unknown. Instead, we can directly estimate the pair-wise difference between ξ_m and ξ_l by

$$\hat{D}_{ml} = \frac{1}{n} \sum_{i=1}^{n} \frac{\Delta_i}{\hat{G}_C(U_i)} \left[\{2Y_i R_i - \hat{\mu}_m(X_i)\}^2 - \{2Y_i R_i - \hat{\mu}_l(X_i)\}^2 \right],$$

which can be used to compare the score systems m and l. The rational is that under certain regular conditions,

$$\hat{\xi}_j = n^{-1} \sum_{i=1}^{n} \frac{\Delta_i}{\hat{G}_C(U_i)} \{2Y_i R_i - \hat{\mu}_j(X_i)\}^2$$

is a consistent estimator for ξ_j up to a constant, which does not depend on the scoring system.[49] When the scoring systems are constructed based on the same data set used for estimating ξ_j, $\hat{D}_{ml}$ may be biased since $\hat{\xi}_j, j = 1, \ldots, J$ tend to downward biased for estimating ξ_j + const to different degrees. Therefore, the cross-validation needs to be used to correct the potential bias. Specifically, we randomly split the data set into K disjoint subsets of approximately equal sizes, denoted by $\{\mathcal{I}_k, k = 1, \ldots, K\}$. For each k, we use all observations not in $\mathcal{I}_k$ to re-construct the scoring systems

$\hat{\mu}_m^{(-k)}(\cdot)$ and $\hat{\mu}_l^{(-k)}(\cdot)$ and then estimate the difference between ξ_m and ξ_l using observations in $\mathcal{I}_k$ by

$$\hat{D}_{kml} = \frac{K}{n} \sum_{i \in \mathcal{I}_k} \frac{\Delta_i}{\hat{G}_C(U_i)} \left[\left\{ 2Y_i R_i - \hat{\mu}_m^{(-k)}(X_i) \right\}^2 - \left\{ 2Y_i R_i - \hat{\mu}_l^{(-k)}(X_i) \right\}^2 \right].$$

The cross-validated estimator for $\xi_m - \xi_l$ is

$$\hat{D}_{ml}^{(cv)} = \frac{1}{K} \sum_{k=1}^{K} \hat{D}_{kml}.$$

The resulting $\{\hat{D}_{ml}^{(cv)}, 1 \leq m < l \leq J\}$ can then be used to rank J scoring systems and identify the scoring system with the smallest square error in predicting the personalized treatment effect.

In general, a scoring system derived from a working model cannot consistently estimate the treatment effect. However, one may still expect that the scoring system can rank the patients according to the individualized treatment effect reasonably well. In practice, one may align the patients according to the estimated scores and identify subgroup of patients with top scores as patients who may benefit the most from the treatment. This motivates the following approach: for scoring system j, denote the subgroup of patients with top $100(1-\alpha)$ percent of the scores by I_α^j, where the proportion $\alpha \in (0,1)$; nonparametrically estimate the treatment effect within the subgroup I_α^j by

$$\hat{AD}_j(\alpha) = \frac{1}{n(1-\alpha)} \sum_{i \in I_\alpha^j} \frac{\Delta_i}{\hat{G}_C(U_i)} 2Y_i R_i.$$

More formally, we may let

$$\tilde{AD}_j(\mu) = \frac{\sum_{i=1}^n I(\hat{\mu}_j(X_j) \geq \mu) \frac{\Delta_i}{\hat{G}_C(U_i)} 2Y_i R_i}{\sum_{i=1}^n I(\hat{\mu}_j(X_i) \geq \mu)}$$

and

$$\hat{AD}_j(\alpha) = \tilde{AD}_j\{\hat{F}_j^{-1}(\alpha)\}$$

where $\hat{F}_j(\cdot)$ is the empirical cumulative distribution function of $\{\hat{\mu}_j(X_1), \ldots, \hat{\mu}_j(X_n)\}$. When $\alpha = 0$, $\hat{AD}_j(\alpha)$ is the estimated treatment effect in the entire study population. When $\alpha \approx 1$, $\hat{\mu}_j(\alpha)$ is the estimated treatment effect for the most promising patients according to the given scoring system. If the jth scoring system can rank patients well, it is expected that $\hat{\mu}_j(\alpha)$ is monotone increasing. This suggests that we may plot the estimated average difference (AD) curve (α versus $\hat{AD}_j(\alpha)$) and evaluate the performance of the scoring systems graphically. For example, if we want to compare scoring systems m and l, we may plot their treatment effect curves in the same graph and choose the AD curve with a more steep slope.

Note that $\hat{AD}_1(0) = \cdots = \hat{AD}_J(0)$, i.e., all AD curves share the same starting point. Thus, the area between the treatment effect curve $\hat{AD}_j(\alpha)$ and the horizontal line $\hat{AD}_j(0)$ can be used to quantify the average "height" of the treatment effect curve. Indeed, one can show that the area between these two curves approximates

$$\text{cov}\left(\psi[F_j\{\hat{\mu}_j(X)\}], \mu(X)\right) = const \times \text{cor}\left(\psi[F_j\{\hat{\mu}_j(X)\}], \mu(X)\right),$$

where $\psi(\cdot)$ is a monotone increasing function and $F_j(\cdot)$ is the cumulative distribution function of $\hat{\mu}_j(X)$. Since $F_j\{\hat{\mu}_j(X)\}$ always follows $U(0,1)$, the universal constant above is independent of the choice of the specific scoring system. Furthermore, the weighted area between two curves

$$\int_0^1 (1-\alpha)\left\{\hat{AD}_j(\alpha) - \hat{AD}_j(0)\right\} d\alpha \approx const \times \text{cor}\left(F_j\{\hat{\mu}_j(X)\}, \mu(X)\right),$$

the correlation coefficient between the ranks of the construct score and true individualized treatment effect up to multiplying an universal constant .[50] Therefore, the (weighted) area between two curves indeed provides a concordance measure between the ranking induced by the scoring system and the true individualized treatment effect. For example, to compare scoring systems $\hat{\mu}_m(\cdot)$ and $\hat{\mu}_l(\cdot)$, the ratio

$$\hat{R}_{ml} = \frac{\int_0^1 (1-\alpha)\left\{\hat{AD}_m(\alpha) - \hat{AD}_m(0)\right\} d\alpha}{\int_0^1 (1-\alpha)\left\{\hat{AD}_l(\alpha) - \hat{AD}_l(0)\right\} d\alpha} \approx \frac{\text{cor}\left(F_m\{\hat{\mu}_m(X)\}, \mu(X)\right)}{\text{cor}\left(F_l\{\hat{\mu}_l(X)\}, \mu(X)\right)}$$

can be used to quantify their relative performance. Again when the same data set is used for both scoring system construction and evaluation, the cross-validation method should be used in the evaluation step to avoid the "self-serving" bias. To be specific, one may randomly separate the data set into training and evaluation sets. We construct the scoring system $\hat{\mu}_j(\cdot)$ in the training set and construct $\tilde{AD}_j(\cdot)$ and $\hat{AD}_j(\cdot)$ in the evaluation set. We repeat this process B times. In the bth iteration, $b = 1, \ldots, B$, let $\tilde{AD}_j^b(\cdot)$ and $\hat{F}_j^b(\cdot)$ be the counterparts of $\tilde{AD}_j(\cdot)$ and $\hat{F}_j(\cdot)$ based on the evaluation set. The cross-validated AD curve for the jth scoring system can then be constructed as

$$\hat{AD}_j^{(cv)} = \tilde{AD}_j^{(cv)}\left\{(\hat{F}_j^{(cv)})^{-1}(\alpha)\right\},$$

where $\tilde{AD}_j^{(cv)}(\mu) = B^{-1}\sum_{b=1}^{B}\tilde{AD}_j^{b}(\mu)$ and $\hat{F}_j^{(cv)}(\mu) = B^{-1}\sum_{b=1}^{B}\hat{F}_j^{b}(\mu)$. Based on the estimated AD curves $\hat{AD}_j^{(cv)}(\alpha)$ via cross-validation, one may also estimate the ratio between the areas between two curves for any pair of scoring systems $\{\hat{R}_{lm}^{(cv)}, 1 \leq l < m \leq J\}$. We then can select the "best" scoring system accordingly.

3.4. *Statistical inference for the scoring system estimating the personalized treatment effect*

The chosen scoring system can be used to stratify future patients. The next step is to make statistical inference on the association between the constructed score and the true treatment effect. Since the construction of the final scoring system may involve complex model fitting and selection steps, one needs to use fresh data without overlapping the one used for estimating the scoring system to make valid statistical inference.[51] As in the previous section, ideally the fresh data used for statistical inference on the scoring system is from an independent study. Since the score is one-dimensional, the nonparametric inference with minimum model assumption can be implemented. Specifically, assuming the data in the holdout set consists of $\{(\tilde{U}_i, \tilde{\Delta}_i, \tilde{R}_i, \tilde{X}_i\tilde{S}_i), i = 1, \ldots, m\}$, where $\tilde{S}_i = \hat{\mu}(\tilde{X}_i)$ and $\hat{\mu}(\cdot)$ is the final scoring system of interest. The objective of the inference at this stage can be the conditional expectation

$$\zeta(\tilde{s}) = E(\tilde{Y}^{(1)} - \tilde{Y}^{(-1)}|\tilde{S} = \tilde{s}),$$

where $\tilde{Y}^{(1)}$ and $\tilde{Y}^{(-1)}$ are the corresponding potential outcomes under treatment and control, respectively. Under mild assumptions, one may employ the standard local linear smoothing method. Specifically, $\zeta(\tilde{s})$ can be estimated by $\hat{\zeta}(\tilde{s}) = a(\tilde{s})$, where $\{a(\tilde{s}), b(\tilde{s})\}'$ is the solution to the estimating equation

$$\frac{1}{m}\sum_{i=1}^{m}\frac{\tilde{\Delta}_i}{\hat{G}_{\tilde{C}}(\tilde{U}_i|\tilde{s})}\begin{pmatrix}1\\ \tilde{S}_i - \tilde{s}\end{pmatrix}K_h(\tilde{S}_i - \tilde{s})\left\{2\tilde{Y}_i\tilde{R}_i - a - b(\tilde{S}_i - \tilde{s})\right\} = 0,$$

where $\hat{G}_{\tilde{C}}(t|\tilde{s})$ is the local nonparametric estimator for the survival function of $\tilde{C}|\tilde{S} = \tilde{s}$. If $(mh)^{-1} = o_p(1)$ and $h = o_p(1)$, then $\hat{\zeta}(\tilde{v})$ converges to $\zeta(\tilde{v})$

uniformly in probability for $\tilde{s} \in [s_1, s_2]$, where $[s_1, s_2]$ is within the support of $\tilde{S}$. Furthermore, if $mh^5 = o_p(1)$, then $(mh)^{1/2}\{\hat{\zeta}(\tilde{s}) - \zeta(\tilde{s})\}$ converges weakly to a mean zero Gaussian with a variance of

$$\nu_2 E(\{2\tilde{Y}\tilde{R}_i - \eta(\tilde{s})\}^2 | \tilde{S} = \tilde{s}) f_S(\tilde{s})^{-1}$$

where $f_S(\cdot)$ is the density function of $\tilde{S}$. The variance of $\hat{\zeta}(\tilde{s})$ can be estimated via an automatic resampling method. Operationally, one may let $\zeta^*(\tilde{v})$ be the solution of the perturbed estimating equation

$$\frac{1}{m}\sum_{i=1}^{m} B_i \frac{\tilde{\Delta}_i}{\hat{G}^*_{\tilde{C}}(\tilde{U}_i|\tilde{s})} \begin{pmatrix} 1 \\ \tilde{S}_i - \tilde{s} \end{pmatrix} K_h(\tilde{S}_i - \tilde{s}) \left\{2\tilde{Y}_i\tilde{R}_i - a - b(\tilde{S}_i - \tilde{s})\right\} = 0,$$

where $\hat{G}^*_{\tilde{C}}(t|\tilde{s})$ is the perturbed "local" Kaplan-Meier estimator for the survival function of $\tilde{C}$ and $\{B_1, \ldots, B_m\}$ are m independent unit exponential random variables. The empirical variance of $\zeta^*(\tilde{s})$ can be used to approximate the variance of $\hat{\zeta}(\tilde{s})$. The 95% confidence interval of $\zeta(\tilde{s})$ can be constructed accordingly. The point estimator and its confidence interval/band provide useful information for quantifying the treatment effect for patients sharing similar scores. The smoothing bandwidth used in the aforementioned procedure can be selected via cross-validation procedure. Similar to the case in Section 2.4, under-smoothing with a smaller bandwidth needs to be introduced to avoid estimating the asymptotical bias in making statistical inferences on $\hat{\zeta}(\tilde{s})$.

3.5. *Summary for statistical methods used in personalized treatment effect prediction*

We have described the general statistical methods for developing scoring systems used for stratifying patients according to his/her individual treatment effect. Similar to the statistical methods assisting personalized risk stratification presented in section 2, the objective here is to predict the personalized treatment effect. The implicit assumption is that the treatment effect may vary depending on a set of baseline covariate. To this end, various regression models allowing interaction between treatment and covariate can be employed to derive the scoring system estimating the personalized treatment effect. Alternatively, one may directly estimate the optimal treatment allocation rule by maximizing the overall utility with respect to the treatment assignment rule. There are special challenges for evaluating the resulting scoring system due to the fact that the individualized treatment effect is neither observable nor estimable nonparametrically in practice. The consequence is that we cannot estimate the prediction error of the scoring system itself. Instead, we only can estimate the difference between the mean squared prediction errors of two scoring systems or the ratio between correlation coefficients (between the rank of the score and true personalized treatment effect) of two scoring systems. The inference on the underlying relationship between the constructed score and future outcome can be made nonparametrically using a fresh data set.

4. Discussion

In this chapter, we have reviewed statistical methodology for assisting the development of personalized risk stratification and treatment selection procedures, which can be used in future clinical practice. The main theme is that the objective of the statistical analysis is to construct, evaluate and select scoring systems, which can accurately predict either the clinical outcome of interest or the treatment effect for individual patients. In general, there are three stages in the analysis:

(1) Construct the scoring systems via fitting working models;
(2) Evaluate and select the optimal scoring system via cross-validation;
(3) Make statistical inference on the selected scoring system using fresh data.

At the first stage, the regression working model is merely a vehicle employed to derive the scoring system and does not need to be correctly specified. When the dimension of the covariate is big relative to the sample size, appropriate regularization method can be used to generate a stable and parsimonious solution.[52–54] At the second stage, it is crucial to use cross-validation method to avoid the self-serving bias associated with the "apparent error" type estimator. Lastly, once a final scoring system is obtained, the traditional statistical inference can be made conditional on the scoring system with a new data set. At first glance, it seems odd to ignore the variability in the construction of the scoring system. However, it is consistent with the observation that the scoring system such as Framingham risk score is fixed and thus not random once it is constructed and accepted by the medical community.[55] It is worth to note that the presented methods are mainly for the analysis of the data already collected. There are a lot of interesting developments for novel study design in the context of personalized medicine.[56–61] Statistical method related to developing optimal dynamic treatment regimes is another hot topic not covered here.[62–64]

References

1. Arnedos, M., Andre, F., Farace, F., *et al.* (2012). The challenge to bring personalized cancer medicine from clinical trials into routine clinical practice: the case of the institut gustave roussy. *Mol Oncol* **6**:204–210.
2. Ziegler, A., Koch, A., Krockenberger, K., and Grobhennig, A. (2012). Personalized medicine using dna biomarkers: a review. *Human Genetics* **131(10)**:1627–1638.
3. Jungic, S., Tubic, B., and Skrepnik, T. (2012). The roble of biomarkers in the development of novel cancer therapies. *Drug Metablo Durg Interct.* **27(2)**: 89–99.
4. Fernald, G., Capriotti, E., Daneshjou, R., *et al.* (2011). Bioinformatics challenges for personalized medicine. *Bioinformatics* **27(13)**:1741–1748.
5. Gage, B., Johnson, J., Deych, E., *et al.* (2008). Use of pharmacogenetic and clinical factors to predict the therapeutic dose of warfarin. *Clin Pharmacol Ther* **84**:326–331.
6. Lenzini, P., Wadelius, M., Kimmel, S., *et al.* (2010). Integration of genetic, clinical, and laboratory data to refine warfarin dosing. *Clin Pharmacol Ther* **87**:572–578.
7. Lloyd-Jones, D. (2010). Risk prediction in cardiovascular medicine. *Circulation* **121**:1768–1777.
8. Draper, N. and Smith, H. (1998). *Applied regression Analysis (3rd Edition).* John Wiley & Son.
9. Tian, L., Cai, T., Goetghebeur, E., and Wei, L. (2007). Model evaluation based on the sampling distribution of estimated absolute prediction error. *Biometrika* **94(2)**:297–311.
10. Fleming, T. and Harrington, D. (1991). *Counting processes and survival analysis.* John Wiley & Son.
11. Zhao, H. and Tsiatis, A. (1997). A consistent estimator for the distribution of quality adjusted survival time. *Biometrika* **84(2)**:339–348.
12. Cox, D. (1972). Regression models and life-tables. *Journal of the Royal Statistical Society (Series B)*, 34(2):187–220.
13. Buckley, J. and James, I. (1979). Linear regression with censored data. *Biometrika* **66(3)**:429–436.
14. Wei, L. (1992). The accelerated failure time model: A useful alternative to the cox regression model in survival analysis. *Statistics in Medicine* **11(14)**:1871–1879.
15. Lin, D., Fleming, T., and Wei, L. (1994). Confidence bands for survival curves under the proportional hazards model. *Biometrika* **81**:73–81.
16. Park, Y. and Wei, L. (2003). Estimating subject-specific survival functions under the accelerated failure time model. *Biometrika* **90**:717–723.
17. Lin, D. Y. and Wei, L. J. (1989). The robust inference for the cox proportional hazards model. *Journal of American Statistical Association* **84**:1074–1078.
18. Xu, R. and O'Quigley, J. (2000). Estimating average regression effect under non-proportional hazards. *Biostatistics* **1(4)**:423–439.

19. Fan, J. and Huang, L. (2001). Goodness-of-fit tests for parametric regression model. *Journal of the American Statistical Association* **96(454)**:640–652.
20. Lin, D., Wei, L., and Ying, Z. (2002). Model-checking techniques based on cumulative residuals. *Biometrics* **58(1)**:1–12.
21. Stone, M. (1974). Cross-validatory choice and assessment of statistical predictions. *Journal of Royal Statitical Society. (Series B)* **36**:111–147.
22. Geisser, S. (1975). The predictive sample reuse method with applications. *Journal of American Statistical Association* **70**:320–328.
23. Efron, B. and Tibshirani, R. (1997). Improvements on cross-validation: the .632+ bootstrap method. *Journal of the American Statistical Association* **92**:548–560.
24. Efron, B. (2004). The estimaton of prediction error: covariance penalties and cross-validation. *Journal of the American Statistical Association* **99**:619–632.
25. Ridker, P., Glynn, R., and Hennekens, C. (1998). C-reactive protein adds to the predictive value of total and hdl cholesterol in determining risk of first myocardial infarction. *Circulation* **97**:2007–2011.
26. Ridker, P. (2007). C-reactive protein and the prediction of cardiovascular events among those at intermediate risk: Moving an inflammatory hypothesis toward consensus. *Journal of the American College of Cardiology* **49(21)**:2129–2138.
27. Uno, H., Cai, T., Tian, L., and Wei, L. (2011). Graphical procedures for evaluating overall and subject-specfic incremental values from new predictors with censored event time data. *Biometrics* **67**:1389–1396.
28. Uno, H., Cai, T., Tian, L., and Wei, L. (2007). Evaluating prediction rules for t-year survivors with censored regression models. *Journal of the American Statistical Association* **102(478)**:527–537.
29. Tian, L., Cai, T., and Wei, L. (2009). Identifying subjects wo beneift from additional information for better prediction of the outcome variables. *Biometrics* **65(3)**:894–902.
30. Cai, T., Tian, L., Uno, H., Solomon, S., and Wei, L. (2010). Calibrating parametric subject-specific risk estimation. *Biometrika* **97(2)**:389–404.
31. Fan, J. and Gijbels, I. (1996). *Local Polynomial Modelling and its Applications*. Chapman and Hall, London.
32. Dabrowska, D. (1987). Non-parametric regression with censored survival time data. *Scandinavian Journal of Statistics* pages 181–197.
33. Dabrowska, D. (1989). Uniform consistency of the kernel conditional kaplan-meier estimate. *The Annals of Statistics* **17(3)**:1157–1167.
34. Gilbert, P., Wei, L., Kosorok, M., and Clemens, J. (2002). Simultaneous inferences on the contrast of two hazard functions with censored observations. *Biometrics* **58(4)**:773–780.
35. Li, Y., Tian, L., and Wei, L. (2011). Estimating subject-specific dependent competing risk profile with censored event time observations. *Biometrics* **67(2)**:427–435.
36. Rubin, D. (1974). Estimating casual effects of treatments in randomized and nonrandomized studies. *Journal of Educational Psychology* **66**:688–701.

37. Wang, S., ONeill, R., and Hung, H. (2007). Approaches to evaluation of treatment effect in randomized clinical trials with genomic subset. *Pharm Stat* **6**:227–244.
38. Alosh, M. and Hugue, M. (2009). A flexible strategy for testing subgroups and overall population. *Statistics in Medicine* **15**:3–23.
39. Andersen, P., Hansen, M., and Klein, J. (2004). Regression analysis of restricted mean survival time based on pseudo-observations. *Lifetime Data Analysis* **10(4)**:335–350.
40. Zhao, L., Tian, L., Uno, H., Solomon, S., Pfeffer, M., Schindler, J., and Wei, L. (2012a). Utilizing the integrated difference of two survival functions to quantify the treatment contrast for designing, monitoring, and analyzing a comparative clinical study. *Clinical Trials* **9(5)**:570–577.
41. Breslow, N. (1972). Discussion of the paper by d.r. cox. *Journal of Royal Statistical Socienty (Series B)* **34**:216–217.
42. Tian, L., Alizadeh, A., Gentles, A., and Tibshirani, R. (2012). A simple method for detecting interactions between a treatment and a large number of covariates. *Technical Report (Stanford University)* pages http://www–stat.stanford.edu/ tibs/ftp/interactionpaper.pdf.
43. Su, X., Zhou, T., Yan, X., Fan, J., and Yang, S. (2008). Interaction trees with censored survival data. *The International Journal of Biostatistics*, **4(1)**: Article 2.
44. Royston, P. and Sauerbrei, W. (2008). Interactions between treatment and continuous covariates: A step toward individualizing therapy. *Journal of Clinical Oncology* **26(9)**:1397–1399.
45. Tian, L. and Tibshirani, R. (2011). Adaptive index models for marker-based risk stratification. *Biostatistics* **12(1)**:68–86.
46. Zhao, Y., Zeng, D., Rush, A., and Kosorok, M. (2012b). Estimating individualized treatment rules using outcome weighted learning. *Journal of the American Statistical Asssociation* **107**:1106–1118.
47. Hastie, T. and Zhu, J. (2006). Discussion of "support vector machines with applications" by Javier Moguerza and Alberto Munoz. *Statistical Science* **21(3)**:352–357.
48. Zhao, X., Dai, W., Li, Y., and Tian, L. (2011b). Auc-based biomarker ensemble with an application on gene scores predicting low bone mineral density. *Bioinformatics* **27(21)**:3050–3055.
49. Sinovitch, J. (2008). Ph.d thesis. *Harvard University.*
50. Zhao, L., Tian, L., Cai, T., Claggett, B., and Wei, L. (2011a). Effectively selecting a target population for a future comparative study. *Harvard University Biostatistics Working Paper Series.* 134:http://biostats.bepress.com/ harvardbiostat/paper134.
51. Cai, T., Tian, L., Wong, P., and Wei, L. (2011). Analysis of randomized comparative clinical trial data for personalized treatment selections. *Biostatistics* **12(2)**:270–282.
52. Friedman, J. (1991). Multivariate adaptive regression splines (with discussion). *Annals of Statistics* **19(1)**:1–141.

53. Tibshirani, R. (1996). Regression shrinkage and selection via the lasso. *Journal of the Royal Statistical Society, Series B* **58**:267–288.
54. Zou, H. and Hastie, T. (2005). Regularization and variable selection via elastic net. *Journal of Royal Statistical Socienty. B* **67**:301–320.
55. Wilson, P., D'Agostino, R., Levy, D., *et al.* (1998). Prediction of coronary heart disease using risk factor categories. *Circulation* **97(18)**:1837–1847.
56. Sargent, D., Conley, B., Allegra, C., and Collette, L. (2005). Clinical trial designs for predictive marker validation in cancer treatment trials. *J Clin Oncol* **23**:2020–2027.
57. Simon, R. (2008). The use of genomics in clinical trial design. *Clin Cancer Res* **14**:5984–5993.
58. Zhao, Y., Kosorok, M., and Zeng, D. (2009). Reinforcement learning design for cancer clinical trials. *Statistics in Medicine* **28(26)**:3294–3315.
59. Arkenau, H., Barriuso, J., Olmos, D., *et al.* (2009). Prospective validation of a prognostic score to improve patient selection for oncology phase i trials. *J Clin Oncol* **27**:2692–2696.
60. Frech, B., Joo, J., Geller, N., *et al.* (2010). Statistical design of personalized medicine interventions: The clarification of optimal anticoagulaiton through genetics(coag) trial. *Trials* **11**:108–116.
61. Le Tourneau, C., Kamal, M., Tredan, O., Delord, J., *et al.* (2012). Designs and challenges for personalized medicine studies in oncology: focus on the shiva trial. *Target Oncol.* **7(4)**:253–265.
62. Murphy, S. (2003). Optimal dynamic treatment regimes. *Journal of the Royal Statistical Society (Series B)*, **65(2)**:331–366.
63. Moodie, E., Richardson, T., and Stephens, D. (2007). Demystifying optimal dynamic treatment regimes. *Biometrics* **63**:447–455.
64. Chakraborty, B., Murphy, S., and Strecher, V. (2010). Inference for non-regular parameters in optimal dynamic treatment regimes. *Stat Methods Med Res* **19(3)**:317–343.

About the Authors

Lu Tian, Bachelor degree in Mathematics from Nankai University (1995); Master degree in Applied Mathematics from Nankai University (1998); Doctor of Science degree in Biostatistics from Harvard University (2002). His graduate study was supported by Howard Hughes Fellowship. He was awarded the Robert B. Reed Award for Excellence in Biostatistics at Harvard University. He had been working at the Department of preventive medicine, northwestern university (2004–2008) as Assistant Professor. He is currently Associate Professor at the Department of Health Research and Policy, Stanford University. He has rich experience in conducting statistical methodological research, planning large epidemiological studies, running data management for randomized clinical trials and conducting applied data analysis. His current research interest is in developing statistical methods in semiparametric regression modeling, survival analysis and high throughput data analysis.

Xiaoguang Zhao, Bachelor degree in clinical medicine from Xi'an Medical University (1995). He is currently the director of the department of Bone and joint surgery, the first affiliated hospital of Xian medical university. He is specialized in complex spinal fracture and fracture, hip replacement surgery. He has published numerous papers in the core medical journals and participated in research project on spinal cord ischemia-reperfusion injury. He is also the member of Shanxi Branch of the Chinese Medical Association. His methodological research interest is mainly on personalized medicine and clinical outcome predictions.

CHAPTER 5

STATISTICS USED IN QUALITY CONTROL, QUALITY ASSURANCE, AND QUALITY IMPROVEMENT IN RADIOLOGICAL STUDIES

YING LU

Department of Health Research and Policy,
Stanford University School of Medicine,
Stanford, CA 94305-5405, USA
Ying.Lu@va.gov

SHOUJUN ZHAO

Department of Surgery, University of California,
San Francisco, CA 94143-0104, USA

1. Introduction

Quality control, quality assurance, and quality improvement in medical studies are active and large topics. From 1995–2000, there were more than 40,000 articles in MEDLINE database that had key words of at least one of these three terms. Quality has many connotations. The term "total quality management" (TQM) is given to an approach that related to the daily functioning of medical practices or medical research processes. All participated personnel and operational aspects are involved. Quality control is a very limited function that "controls" the product, primarily by testing, while quality assurance regulates the systems and methods for "assuring" the quality of the product.[1]

Every aspect of medical practice and research requires quality control and quality assurance. Although the statistical principles presented here can apply to other fields such as laboratory medicine, etc. this chapter is limited to quality control and quality assurance specifically in radiology. There are several reasons for this focus. First, this is the field in which the authors have the most experience. Second, radiology evaluation relies on radiological equipment, whether X-ray, ultrasound, CT, or MRI machines. As with all machinery, products of different manufacturers vary in quality. Over time, machine may draft and age can affect performance. Furthermore, precision errors are always to be expected in any radiological equipments or technique; even when the same patient is scanned under identical conditions the results will be different. Last but not least, many radiological assessments are based on the experience of reader and are relatively subjective. It is common to have different readers to give different interpretations of the same image. Therefore, many factors will affect the results of radiological assessments. The statistical principles discussed here can resolve the conflicts among results from different devices and improve interpretation of the results.

Radiology has been used to help decisions in disease diagnosis and management of patients. Its use as tools for population screening and for drug development is increasing. The newly developed response evaluation criteria in solid tumors (RECIST) uses changes in unidimensional CT measurement of tumor lesions to define the treatment response rates.[2] Osteoporosis is defined by bone mineral density (BMD) measured by dual X-ray absorptiometry (DXA) scans[3] and osteoporosis prevention drugs are assessed according to their effect on BMD.[4] In fact, medical imaging has been used as surrogate endpoint or biomarkers in many therapeutic and diagnostic clinical trials, and radiologists are increasingly involved in these clinical trials.

Good Clinical Practice (GCP) is an international quality standard for the design, conduct, recording, and reporting of clinical trials with human subjects. GCP guidelines not only provide a framework for protecting the rights of participating patients or volunteers, they also set standards to safeguard the integrity of data that are used to evaluate treatment efficacy and submitted to regulatory agencies.[5] In radiology, GCP includes training documents and standard operating procedures, imaging device quality control, image acquisition protocols, software validation, record keeping, and reporting, etc.[6] Obviously, this is not only a statistical process. Successful quality control and quality assurance require good leadership from department chairs or principal investigators and, importantly, a team of multi-disciplinary experts. The expert team should always include a statistician. Statisticians are important in planning quality control, including determining appropriate sampling to avoid bias in selecting test samples, calculating the sample sizes, analyzing results to identify deficiencies, planning the processing control charts for monitoring machine performance, reassessing the results of quality improvement, and in reporting data and study results.

There are many aspects of quality control and quality assurance that are not directly related to statistics.[7–9] This chapter presents some statistical tools used in radiological or osteoporosis research based on the experience of the authors. It is beyond the scope of this book to present a complete picture of quality control and quality assurance for all radiological studies.

This chapter is organized into 5 sections. In the next section, we introduce definitions of different measurement errors for continuous radiological results and different ways to evaluate these errors. In Sec. 3, we present applications of process control-charts to monitoring measurement errors over time. In Sec. 4, we review the statistics of measurement agreement. In Sec. 5, we discuss the calibration problem.

2. Measurement Errors

Radiological techniques are used to measure physical or mechanical properties that relate to disease status or progression. We use statistical techniques or procedures to transform our observations of a variable of interest into a particular category or number. This is the measurement process. For a categorical variable, we try to assign a subject into a particular, unambiguous category, as in the assessment of treatment response of solid tumors[2] or evaluation of spine fracture severity.[10] In other cases, we derive a numerical value that reflects the underlying physical quantity, such as tumor volume, bone mineral content or density, etc.

Measurement errors describe the limits of a quantitative or qualitative assessment of a disease using a particular technique or procedure. Measurement errors have many sources. This section focuses on 2 types of measurement errors — precision and accuracy — and their applications to the diagnosis of osteoporosis and monitoring changes in bone status. The implications of precision on monitoring changes are emphasized, including the concepts of standardized precision, longitudinal sensitivity, and their applications to patient measurements and quality assurance, i.e. the monitoring of machine performance.

2.1. *Measurement errors in radiological instruments*

Many sources of errors can affect the measurement and cause varying results, even when they are from the same region of interest in the same subject. Some of these variations can be controlled to minimize their impact.

Some of the error sources are — in part — uncontrollable. Controllable variations are called fixed factors. Our interests, however, are usually on the uncontrollable random variations.

Errors of measurement are the differences between observed values recorded under identical conditions and a fixed true value. In osteoporosis studies, we always assume there are true quantities for densitometry parameters for each measured subject, even though we don't always know their values. Measurement errors should be random in nature and can be attributed to two different sources: accuracy errors and precision errors.[11]

2.1.1. *Accuracy errors*

Accuracy errors here are used as equivalent to the term bias. They reflect the degree to which the measured results deviate from the true values. To evaluate accuracy errors, we need to know the true values of the measured parameters. It is not always possible, however, to measure the accuracy errors because sometimes the true values of the measured parameters cannot be verified. For example, quantitative ultrasound (QUS) bone measurements are affected by a number of quantitative and qualitative factors, and there is no single correlate for any QUS measurement. Therefore, we cannot define a single accuracy error for QUS.[12]

For clinical applications only the part of the accuracy error that varies from patient to patient in an unknown fashion is relevant. The other part, i.e. the one that is constant, can be averaged across subjects e.g. the average underestimation of bone density due to the average fat content of bone marrow in Quantitative Computed Tomography (QCT), can be ignored. There are two reasons: First, for diagnostic uses, the reference data will be affected by the same error so the difference between healthy and diseased subjects is constant. Second, the error is present at both baseline and follow-up measurements, and does not contribute to measured changes. Therefore, when discussing the impact of accuracy errors only that part of the error that changes from patient to patient in an unknown and uncontrollable fashion is of interest.[13] For this reason, small accuracy errors are of little clinical significance provided they remain constant.[14] In general they are more relevant to diagnosis and risk assessment than to monitoring.

2.1.2. *Precision errors*

They reflect the reproducibility of the technique. They measure the ability of a method to reproducibly measure a parameter for the purpose of reliably monitoring changes in bone status over time. Precision errors can be further separated into *short-term* and *long-term* precision errors. Short-term precision errors characterize the reproducibility of a technique and are useful for describing the limitations of measuring changes in skeletal status. If they are large they may affect the diagnostic sensitivity of a technique. Long-term precision errors are used to evaluate instrument stability. Because long-term precision errors include additional sources of random variation attributable to small drifts in instrumental calibration, variations in patient characteristics, and other technical changes related to time, they provide a better measure of a technique's ability to monitor parameter changes than the short-term precision errors do. For patient measurements, estimates of long-term precision usually also include true longitudinal variability of skeletal status. For both of these reasons long-term precision errors normally are larger than short-term errors. While precision errors are easy to define, there are many ways to describe them depending on the purpose at hand, and there is no universal consensus on which definition is most appropriate.

Mathematically, let θ be the theoretical true value in which we are interested, and let X be the observed value. The difference of $\xi = X - \theta$ is the measurement error. Furthermore, if X follows a normal distribution $N(\mu, \sigma^2)$, the accuracy error is $\mu - \theta$ and precision error is σ. Here, θ is considered a gold standard.

Figure 1 illustrates the differences between precision and accuracy errors. If an archer consistently hits the target board close to the bull's-eye, but with the arrows spread out around it, it is good accuracy but poor precision. If the archer consistently hits the board far off the bull's-eye, but with all of the arrows in approximately the same location, it is poor accuracy but good precision.

2.2. *Absolute precision errors*

Although there are many different ways to describe precision errors, they can be classified as absolute or relative. For the following descriptions of precision errors, we introduce some notations. Let $X_{i,j}$ be the quantitative results (such as BMD) of the jth measurement for the ith individual, $i = 1, \ldots, m$ and $j = 1, \ldots, n_i$. Because individual subjects have different underlying true values due to biological variation, it is necessary to measure individual subjects repeatedly to evaluate precision errors. We use n_i to denote the total number of measurements for the ith individual. The standard deviation (SD) of bone densitometry parameters from an individual

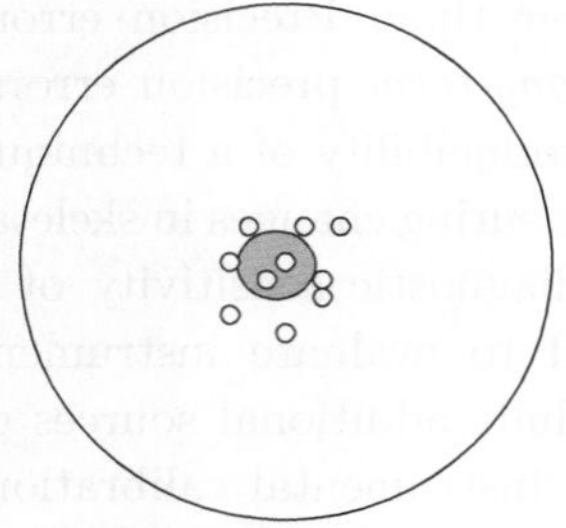
Good Accuracy and Precision
Good for Diagnosis and Monitoring

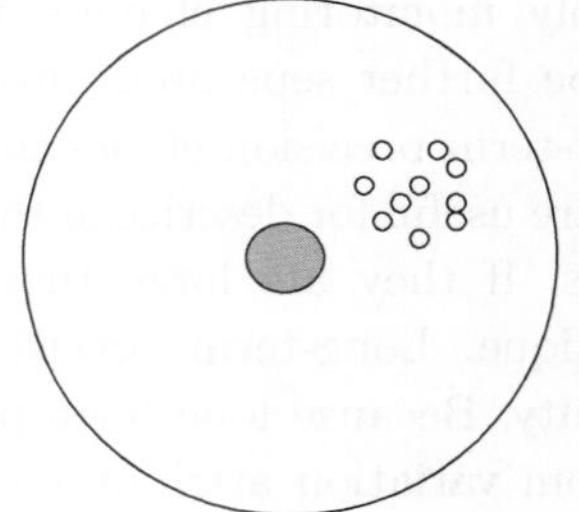
Poor Accuracy and Good Precision
Acceptable for Monitoring

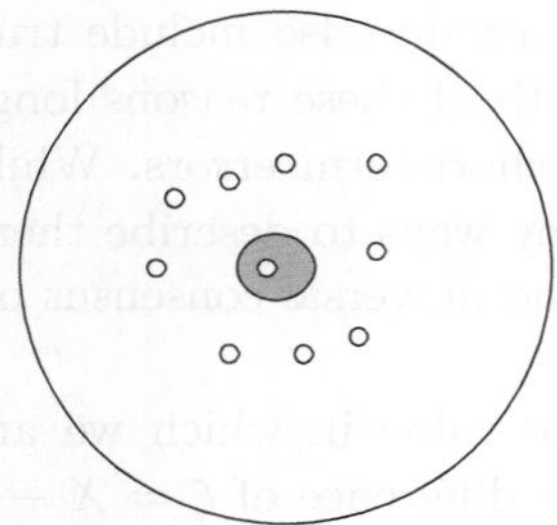
Good Accuracy and Poor Precision
Unacceptable for Monitoring

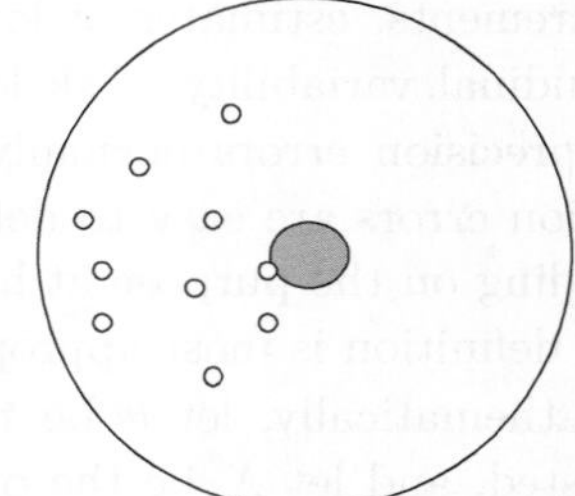
Poor Accuracy and Precision
Unacceptable for Diagnosis and Monitoring

Fig. 1. Precision and accuracy.

subject i as a measure of short-term reproducibility is defined as the average distance of individual $X_{i,j}$ to the mean value for that subject, $\bar{X}_i$. Mathematically, it is the sample standard deviation:

$$\mathrm{SD}_i = \sqrt{\sum_{j=1}^{n_i}(X_{i,j} - \bar{X}_i)^2/(n_i - 1)}. \tag{1}$$

Individual precision may vary. To estimate the reproducibility of a parameter in clinical use, we need to measure a representative set of individuals and combine their individual precision errors using the root-mean-square average of individual SD values (RMS SD) or in other words, within the mean squared errors in Analysis of Variance terms. Mathematically,

$$\text{RMS SD} = \sqrt{\frac{\sum_{i=1}^{m}\sum_{j=1}^{n_i}(X_{i,j} - \bar{X}_i)^2}{\sum_{i=1}^{m}(n_i - 1)}} = \sqrt{\frac{\sum_{i=1}^{m}(n_i - 1)\mathrm{SD}_j^2}{\sum_{i=1}^{m}(n_i - 1)}}, \tag{2}$$

where m is the number of subjects measured for precision evaluation. When each subject has the same number of measurements, the RMS SD = $\sqrt{\sum_{i=1}^{m} \mathrm{SD}_i^2/m}$.

With long-term precision, the underlying parameter can change for individual subjects over time. Therefore, instead of measuring the distance from the observed individual values to the mean of the individual subject, we use the distances from the observed individual values to the expected value of the parameter at the time of measurement. In many situations we assume that the change of the parameter over time is linear for mathematical convenience. Thus, we can fit a regression line for observed individual measurements over time, i.e. $\hat{X}_{i,j} = \hat{a}_i + \hat{b}_i t_{i,j}$ with $t_{i,j}$ as the time of the jth measurement for the ith subject. The variation around the regression line is the standard error of the estimate (SEE):

$$\mathrm{SEE}_i = \sqrt{\frac{\sum_{j=1}^{n_i}(X_{i,j} - \hat{X}_{i,j})^2}{n_i - 2}}. \tag{3}$$

In this case, SEE rather than SD should be taken as the estimate of the long-term precision error for an individual subject. For precision errors of a group of subjects, we use the root-mean-square SEE (RMS SEE) to evaluate the long-term precision error for clinical use.

$$\mathrm{RMS\ SEE}_i = \sqrt{\frac{\sum_{i=1}^{m}(n_i - 2)\mathrm{SEE}_i}{\sum_{i=1}^{m}(n_i - 2)}}. \tag{4}$$

The confidence intervals of RMS SD and RMS SEE can be derived using transformation of a Chi-squared distribution. The generic formula of $(1 - \alpha) \bullet 100\%$ confidence interval is

$$\left(\sqrt{\frac{df}{\chi^2_{1-\frac{\alpha}{2},df}}} \cdot \text{Absolute Precision}, \sqrt{\frac{df}{\chi^2_{\frac{\alpha}{2},df}}} \cdot \text{Absolute Precision}\right). \tag{5}$$

Thus, for short-term precision, $df = \sum_{i=1}^{m}(n_i - 1)$ and the absolute precision error is RMS SD. For long-term precision, $df = \sum_{i=1}^{m}(n_i - 2)$ and the absolute precision error is RMS SEE. The values of $\chi^2_{1-\frac{\alpha}{2},df}$ and $\chi^2_{\frac{\alpha}{2},df}$ can be obtained from most software and tables from statistics text books.

The absolute precision error depends on the unit of measurement. While it gives important information on measurement errors, it is inadequate for comparing precision errors across several techniques or measurements. For diagnosis or for monitoring longitudinal changes, we are usually more interested in the relative precision of a technique than in the absolute minimum measurement errors.

2.3. *Relative short-term precision errors*

2.3.1. *Short-term coefficient of variation*

The most commonly used measure of relative precision error is the coefficient of variation (CV), defined as the ratio of the standard deviation to the mean measurement. It is usually given on a percentage basis. CV is unit free and therefore can be used with different techniques and instruments.

CV has a long history as a measure of reproducibility. It was first proposed by Karl Pearson in 1895 to measure the variability of a distribution. The distribution of CV is complicated. The simplest case is one individual with repeated measurements. Assuming that $X_{i,j}$ obtained from the ith individual are independent identical samples from a normal distribution $N(\mu_i, \sigma_i^2)$, the density functions for CV_i is:[15]

$$f_{\mathrm{CV}_i}(x; n_i, \lambda_i) = \begin{cases} \dfrac{e^{-n_i\lambda_i^2/2}}{\sqrt{\pi}\,\Gamma(\frac{n_i-1}{2})} \displaystyle\sum_{k=0}^{\infty} \dfrac{(\sqrt{2n_i}\lambda_i)^k}{k!}\Gamma\left(\dfrac{n_i+k}{2}\right) \dfrac{x^{n_i-2}}{(1+x^2)^{\frac{n_i+k}{2}}}, & x \geq 0, \\ \dfrac{e^{-n_i\lambda_i^2/2}}{\sqrt{\pi}\,\Gamma(\frac{n_i-1}{2})} \displaystyle\sum_{k=0}^{\infty} \dfrac{(-\sqrt{2n_i}\lambda_i)^k}{k!}\Gamma\left(\dfrac{n_i+k}{2}\right) \dfrac{|x|^{n_i-2}}{(1+x^2)^{\frac{n_i+k}{2}}}, & x < 0, \end{cases} \tag{6}$$

with $\lambda_i = \sigma_i/\mu_i$. Asymptotically, the variance of CV_i is $\lambda_i\sqrt{\frac{1}{n}(\frac{1}{2}+\lambda_i^2)}$.[16]

This individual CV is only meaningful if the subject has multiple measurements. When all individuals in a study have only one measurement, a population CV can be defined similarly to the ratio of population standard deviation and population mean. Such a CV is no longer related solely to measurement errors but to a combination of measurement errors and population variations. Feltz and Miller[17] gave an asymptotic χ^2-test (DAD test) to compare the CV from k-populations. Fung and Tsang[18] compared the DAD test with the likelihood ratio test (LRT), and the squared ranks test (SRT) in a simulation study. They concluded that the DAD test is a very good test for CVs from k-populations of normal distributions, although it is not robust, for a symmetric distribution with heavy tails. The LRT does not control type I errors correctly, although it is very powerful. The SRT is slightly liberal, but rather robust. In radiological studies, the population CV is rarely of interest, and it will not be discussed in detail here.

An alternative CV for non-normal distributions is the non-parametric CV, defined as the ratio of inter-quartile range over the median of the population.[19] The confidence interval and hypothesis testing for the non-parametric CV can be derived using bootstrap or jackknife resampling techniques.[20, 21]

In radiology, we are more interested measurement errors in a random effects model. Here, we assume that

$$X_{i,j} = \theta_i + e_{i,j}, \tag{7}$$

where θ_i is the unobserved true (expected) value for the ith subject that follows a $N(\mu, \tau^2)$, and $e_{i,j}$ are independent measurement errors that follow $N(0, \sigma^2)$. As in Sec. 2.2, the RMS SD in (2) is the best estimate of σ. Thus, for short-term precision, CV is defined as

$$\text{CV} = 100 \times \frac{\text{RMS SD}}{\bar{X}}\%, \tag{8}$$

Where $\bar{X}$ is the mean of $X_{i,j}$. This is also called within-batch CV in laboratory medicine.[22] The distribution of this short-term precision is much more complicated because means of subjects θ_i's also follow a normal distribution. Quan and Shih[23] derived the asymptotic sample variances for short-term CVs. The derivation requires two assumptions: (1) the number of repeated measurements of a patient n_i will not be more than a positive number C; (2) the proportion of subjects with $n_i = l$ converges to a constant $0 \leq p_l \leq 1$, as $m \to \infty$. Under these two concditions, the asymptotic standard deviation of moment estimator of short term CV defined in formula (8) is

$$\sqrt{\frac{\sigma^2}{\mu^4} \frac{(\sum_{i=1}^m n_i)\sigma^2 + (\sum_{i=1}^m n_i^2)\tau^2}{(\sum_{i=1}^m n_i)^2} + \frac{\sigma^2}{2\mu^2 \sum_{i=1}^m (n_i - 1)}}, \tag{9}$$

for $m \to \infty$. The sample variation when $X_{i,j}$'s follow log-normal distribution can also be found in Quan and Shih.[23]

It is often useful to compare the CVs of different techniques, or of the same techniques at different research centers. When comparing the same technique at different centers, the measured subjects in different centers are independent so it is appropriate to use the DAD test similar to Feltz and Miller.[17] When comparing the CVs of different techniques, however, it is preferable to apply the techniques to the same set of subjects to control for confounding factors. This resulted correlated estimated CV and testing can be complicated. A two-step bootstrap algorithm can be used to compare two or more CVs:

Step 1. Draw m random samples with replacement from the study subjects.
Step 2. For each selected subject (possibly selected multiple times but treating each measurement as an independent sample) in Step 1, draw n_i random samples with replacement from his/her corresponding measurements.
Step 3. Calculate the difference of the two CV's based on data in Step 2.
Step 4. Repeat Steps 1 to 3 many times (1,000–2,000 times).
Step 5. Calculate the 95% bootstrap confidence intervals of the differences. If the 95% bootstrap confidence interval excludes 0, the null hypothesis that the two CVs are equal is rejected.

2.3.2. *Alternative forms of short-term coefficient of variation*

Intuitively, the larger the CV, the larger the precision errors and the poorer the technique's ability to monitor changes. However, this is not always true. To use CV, the value 0 of a measurement should have some physical meaning. For example, 0 bone mineral content and density have clear physical meanings. On the other hand, 0 value in speed of sound (SOS) in quantitative ultrasound has no physical meaning — the lower limit for speed of sound in water is around 1500 m/s. When the value 0 has no physical meaning, the origin of the parameters can be moved up or down so that CV has no physical meaning. Secondly, using CV to characterize the precision error of a technique implies that the precision error is proportional to the quantity of measurements. This is not true for many bone densitometry measurements. Normally, we see that the lower the bone density, the higher the relative precision errors (actually, even the absolute precision error increases with decreasing BMD). Thus, CV is not always a robust parameter for evaluating precision, at least for bone densitometry in osteoporosis research. Third, the mean value of the measured quantity, in many cases, is not the primary interest. We are more interested in discriminating between patients and normal controls, monitoring changes in bone status, or evaluating treatment responses, and CV is inadequate for these purposes. A major limitation of CV is that it does not take into account the impact of the technique's responsiveness to changes caused by disease or disease progression. When a technique has a very low precision error (i.e. a very "good" precision) but an even lower responsiveness (e.g. differences between healthy and diseased subjects or changes as a result of disease progression or treatment) it will not have a good longitudinal sensitivity to detect changes caused by disease over short time periods. Therefore, several approaches to adjust for differences in responsiveness have been proposed.

Miller *et al.*[24] proposed a standardized coefficient of variation (SCV) as the ratio of absolute precision over the range (5th to 95th percentiles) of parameters. The range can be obtained from manufacturer's normative data or from the observed study subjects when the sample size is large enough and sampling procedures are appropriate. Mathematically,

$$\begin{aligned} \text{SCV} &= \frac{\text{Absolute Precision}}{\text{Range}} \bullet 100\% \\ &= \frac{\text{Absolute Precision}}{95\%\ tile - 5\%\ tile} \bullet 100\%. \end{aligned} \tag{10}$$

Alternatively, Blake *et al.*[25] proposed using the population standard deviations as the measure for the range of the measure. Thus, the precision error is measured by the ratio of standard deviation of measurement errors over measured population standard deviation (including both measurement errors and population variations), which we call it SCV2. SCV2 relates to the attenuation parameter in the measurement error models[26] that measures the bias caused by measurement errors in linear and nonlinear regression analysis. Because the width of the 90th percentile range in SCV is about 3.3 times the population standard deviation, SCV is approximately a third of SCV2.

Machado *et al.*[27] proposed a similar standardized precision measurement by replacing the range in the above formula with the differences in mean values of parameters for diseased and normal subjects, which we call SCV3. It is important to note that all these standardized CVs are also unit free.

In osteoporosis research, the population range or standard deviations of BMD change across different age groups. To adjust for the age effects on precision errors, Langton[28] proposed a precision parameter, ZSD. A ZSD is the standard deviation of an individual's Z-scores, $z_{i,j}$'s, a transformation of the observed measurement $X_{i,j}$'s. This Z-score is different from Z-statistics in statistical literature. Here, Z-score is defined as $z_{i,j} = \frac{X_{i,j} - \mu(age_i)}{\sigma(age_i)}$ where $\mu(age_i)$ and $\sigma(age_i)$ are the BMD mean and standard deviation of the age group for the ith subject. Therefore, a Z-score is the number of population standard deviations by which a subject's value varies from the population age-matched mean. It is unit free. A RMS ZSD will be a measurement for a technique.

The standard deviation of $z_{i,j}$ is $\text{ZSD}_i = \frac{\text{SD}_i(X_{i,j})}{\sigma(age_i)} \times 100\%$. Thus, ZSD_i for the ith subject is actually an age matched SCV2. A RMS ZSD is a RMS average of individual SCV2'S.

The SCV proposed by Miller *et al.*[24] is an important step in recognizing the limitations of a traditional CV. SCV often provides different information than CV. For example, PA spine BMD measured by a DXA scanner such as the Hologic QDR-1000 has a higher short term CV (1%) than speed of sound (SOS) (0.3%) measured by quantitative ultrasound machines like the Hologic Sahara. However, defining the SCV as the ratio of RMS SD over the young adult population SD gives the opposite result: the SCV of PA spine BMD is 8% and SOS is 20%.[25] Rather than using the population standard deviation, ZSD uses the age specific population standard deviation. ZSD has advantages when the population variance varies for different age groups, and the purpose of the technique is to determine the differences of individual subjects from their corresponding age group means.

An important limitation of SCV and SCV2 is their dependence on the normative data. In most cases, normative data from different equipment manufacturers are not comparable. Different manufacturers have different normative data based on different selection criteria. The procedures for collecting data may not always follow appropriate statistical sampling procedures and thus may not represent the true population distribution of the parameters. Comparing two SCVs based on two different normative data sets can be like comparing apples to oranges. Many precision studies have small sample sizes and subjects are recruited from convenient samples. The study sample may not be compatible with normative populations. These logistic difficulties severely limit the scientific validity of SCVs.

Statistical properties and hypothesis testing procedures for all the SCVs are complicated and have not been fully studied. In all these cases, the bootstrap method can be applied to resolve the real application needs.

2.3.3. *Sample size for short-term precision studies*

When planning for a short-term precision study, there are always trade-offs between the number of study subjects and the number of measurements. In most cases, we plan to have the same number of measurements n for all the m study subjects. Sample size calculations can be based on the width of the confidence intervals or on the null hypothesis. In both cases, one should have some idea of the ratio between population standard deviation τ and population mean μ.

For a given n, the asymptotic $(1-\alpha) \bullet 100\%$ confidence width for estimated CV λ is

$$2z_{1-\alpha/2}\frac{\lambda}{\sqrt{m}}\sqrt{\frac{\lambda^2}{n}+\frac{\tau^2}{\mu^2}+\frac{1}{2(n-1)}}. \tag{11}$$

This is obtained by rearranging formula (9). A similar argument for the sample size to test the hypothesis $H_0 : \lambda = \lambda_0$ versus $H_1 : \lambda \neq \lambda_0$ is given as

$$m = \frac{\left(z_{1-\alpha/2}\lambda_0\sqrt{\frac{\lambda_0^2}{n}+\frac{\tau_0^2}{\mu_0^2}+\frac{1}{2(n-1)}}+z_{1-\beta}\lambda_1\sqrt{\frac{\lambda_1^2}{n}+\frac{\tau_1^2}{\mu_1^2}+\frac{1}{2(n-1)}}\right)^2}{(\lambda_1-\lambda_0)^2}. \tag{12}$$

Here, α and β are the types I and II errors; λ_1 is the alternative CV; and τ_i and μ_i are population standard deviation and means under the null $(i = 0)$ and alternative $(i = 1)$ hypotheses.

Equation (12) shows that the sample size m decreases as number of measurements n increases. In practice, recruiting subjects is more difficult and costly than repeating measurements. However, many factors can influence precision errors and selecting a small number of patients can either over- or under-state the true precision of the technique in clinical use. For example, measuring only healthy young women to evaluate DXA scanner precision will give smaller precision errors and will overstate the precision of the scanner. Measuring only elderly osteoporotic women will give larger precision errors and will understate the precision of the scanner. Some balance of confounding factors for precision errors must be achieved to represent the clinical population to which the machine or technique will be applied.[11] Within the given cost constraints, one should try to reach as many subjects as possible.

2.4. *Relative long-term precision errors and sensitivity of monitoring changes*

Short-term precision is useful for evaluating the utility of a diagnostic technique. The smaller the precision error, the easier to separate diseased and normal subjects. This is particularly true for standardized precision errors. They cannot, however, describe the ability of a technique to monitor changes.

2.4.1. *Longitudinal CV*

Like the limitation of short-term absolute precision errors, RMS SEE depends on the measurement unit and is not appropriate to compare across techniques. Correspondingly, we can define a longitudinal CV as

$$\mathrm{CV} = 100 \times \frac{\mathrm{RMS\ SE}}{\bar{X}}\%^E. \tag{13}$$

If we assume that the changes of measurements for individual subjects over time follows a linear model, that is

$$X_{i,j} = a_i + b_i t_{i,j} + e_{i,j}, \tag{14}$$

with $t_{i,j}$ the measurement time for the jth measurement of the ith subject, the longitudinal CV is

$$\mathrm{CV} = \frac{\sqrt{\sum_{i=1}^{m}\sum_{j=1}^{n_i}(X_{i,j} - \hat{a}_i - \hat{b}_i t_{i,j})^2 / \sum_{i=1}^{m}(n_i - 2)}}{\sum_{i=1}^{m}\bar{X}_i/m}. \tag{15}$$

Here, $\hat{a}_i$ and $\hat{b}_i$ are the estimated intercept and slop and $\bar{X}_i$ is the average for the ith subject. Derivation of asymptotic standard deviations of Eq. (15) has not yet been reported in the literature.

Although, it is inexplicitly, the longitudinal CV depends on the length of time that the measurement performed. If the length of time and frequency of measurements are different for the same technique and same subjects, the CV may be different. This is because that $\bar{X}_i \cong a + b\bar{t}_i$, which is not the case for the absolute precision. Therefore, to compare the same technique on different machines, the absolute longitudinal precision in RMS SEE is more appropriate. When comparing different techniques, the measurement times should be identical. The best plan is to measure the same subjects at the same time. Otherwise, their longitudinal CVs will not be comparable.

2.4.2. *The least significant change*

For clinical decision making it is important to know the minimum magnitude of measured change that is not caused by measurement errors. The least significant change (LSC) is defined as 2.8 times the longitudinal absolute precision,[29] i.e.

$$\mathrm{LSC} = 2.8 \times \mathrm{RMS\ SEE}. \tag{16}$$

More specifically, if we observe a change of a subject more than LSC, we will have 95% confidence that the change is beyond measurement errors.

The derivation of the LSC is based on the following argument. Let X_1 and X_2 be two successive measurements of a subject. If there is no change in the two measurements, the difference between them is the result of longitudinal measurement errors. If we assume the longitudinal measurement variation is σ, as estimated by RMS SEE in Eq. (4), $\Pr(|X_1 - X_2| > z_{1-\alpha/2}\sqrt{2}\sigma) = \alpha$. The least significant change is also called the "biologically significant change" in laboratory medicine.[22]

The longitudinal precision error must be used to evaluate the LSC rather than the short-term precision error, which is normally smaller than the longitudinal precision error.

The significance level of 5% has no clinical meaning. Therefore, there is no need to insist on 95% confidence when evaluating the LSC. To treat patients early, before the disease progresses, lower confidence levels can be chosen. Another parameter trend assessment margin (TAM) was proposed as $1.8 \times$ RMS SEE, which was calculated as corresponding to an 80% confidence level.[30] The LSC and TAM can also be approximately calculated in percentages based on longitudinal CV's.

2.4.3. *Follow-up time interval*

Radiological variables are often used as monitoring tools for individual patients. To assess the sensitivity of a technique for monitoring patients, Gluer[30] introduced the concept of "monitoring time interval" (MTI). The MTI for assessment of disease progression or treatment response is an estimate of the time period after which a patient will have a 50% chance of showing changes that exceed the LSC. Thus,

$$\text{MTI} = \text{LSC}/\text{Median Changes Per-Annual}. \tag{17}$$

The changes here can be caused by age, disease progression or treatment efficacy depending on the purpose of the study. The change also should be consistent with the units of the LSC. That is, if LSC is expressed as absolute precision, the change should be expressed as absolute changes. If the LSC is expressed as a percentage, a percentage change should be used. It is important to note that the unit of MTI is a year.

Similarly to TAM, Gluer[30] also suggested the "trend assessment interval" (TAI) an estimate of the follow-up time after which a subject will have 50% chance of changes exceeding TAM.

The determination of appropriate monitoring time intervals always represents a tradeoff between frequent visits with patient discomfort and additional costs, and fewer visits with the risk of substantial disease progress in the interval. MTI requires the usual 95% confidence level, which means the corresponding monitoring time interval would be almost double the TAM. This shows that MTI and TAI, as applications of longitudinal precision, when defined in this fashion, have a direct and very intuitive meaning closely related to recommended monitoring time intervals. However, one should note that there is no single MTI (TAI) for each technique. They will differ substantially depending on the expected response of the patients. For their purpose, this is not a disadvantage, since it directly reflects that the frequency of follow-up measurements will depend on the type of patient examined. In osteoporosis clinics, for example, fast bone losers should have MTIs shorter than average postmenopausal women.

2.5. *Examples of applications of precision errors*

In this subsection, we give some examples of calculating absolute and relative precision as described in the previous subsections.

2.5.1. *Example* 1

The short-term precision errors of two quantitative ultrasound scanners for osteoporosis from two different manufacturers were compared. Twenty healthy elderly volunteers participated in the study. Speed of sound (SOS) at the calcaneus was measured twice on the same day for each subject. The data is given in Table 1.

Therefore, we have $m = 20$ and $n_1 = \cdots = n_{20} = 2$. The results are summarized in the following Table 2.

SCV2 was defined in Sec. 2.3.2, immediately after Eq. (10). We did not calculate SCV3 and ZSD here because SCV3 requires information from individual disease status and ZSD requires manufacturer's normative data, and neither were available. It is worth-noting that classical CV for SOS is very low compared to BMD measured by DXA (CV range from 1% to 6%). However, this does not mean that SOS is more precise in clinical use. The clinically useful range of SOS does not begin with zero and, in fact, zero is not defined here. That is why SCV and SCV2 are more meaningful in this example. The reported SCV2 for BMD measured by DXA ranged from 8% to 11%,[25] far less than SOS on a quantitative ultrasound scanner.

2.5.2. *Example* 2

Five normal volunteers participated in a longitudinal quality evaluation study for two new quantitative ultrasound (QUS) devices from different manufacturers with in one year. Table 3 lists their SOS measurements.

Table 1. SOS (m/sec) at calcaneus of 20 volunteers.

Subject	Manufacturer 1		Manufacturer 2	
ID	Measure 1	Measure 2	Measure 1	Measure 2
1	1499	1505	1579	1586
2	1487	1488	1594	1590
3	1471	1465	1543	1556
4	1468	1467	1536	1545
5	1501	1504	1587	1588
6	1516	1517	1618	1605
7	1490	1491	1580	1587
8	1569	1565	1670	1683
9	1534	1543	1641	1641
10	1464	1468	1547	1558
11	1509	1510	1591	1593
12	1567	1541	1621	1647
13	1514	1509	1605	1625
14	1539	1540	1619	1614
15	1540	1537	1632	1648
16	1532	1535	1616	1617
17	1544	1531	1629	1636
18	1578	1574	1637	1644
19	1484	1482	1574	1576
20	1518	1522	1606	1610

Table 2. Short-term precisions and related parameters.

	Statistics (and equation number)				
Manufacturer	RMS SD (2)	CV (8)	SD for CV (9)	SCV (10)	SCV2
1	5.30	0.35%	0.06%	5.33%	16.28%
2	7.59	0.47%	0.07%	8.29%	21.62%

Table 4 displays the longitudinal precision. Although not all subjects demonstrated linear changes over time — Subject 3 in particular had some non-linear changes in Machine 1 — we applied only linear trends to all individuals. Also, as pointed out in Example 1, CV is not an appropriate measurement for SOS in QUS. CV is included in Table 4 only for demonstration.

Thus, although Machine 2 has higher precision errors, it is more sensitive to changes in age and may be a better choice for longitudinal follow-up. Of course, the sample size in this study is too small to reliably determine the monitoring time intervals.

Table 3. Longitudinal QC data for 5 normal volunteers.

		SOS (m/sec)				SOS (m/sec)	
Subject	Date	Machine 1	Machine 2	Subject	Date	Machine 1	Machine 2
1	09/21/97	1554	1636	3	05/07/98	1588	1698
1	10/04/97	1563	1642	3	06/01/98	1586	1717
1	11/05/97	1546	1634	3	07/24/98	1587	1708
1	11/18/97	1554	1635	3	09/23/98	1588	1708
1	12/29/97	1560	1656	4	09/22/97	1598	1709
1	01/09/98	1551	1626	4	10/04/97	1595	1694
1	02/04/98	1556	1648	4	10/29/97	1601	1698
1	02/24/98	1548	1642	4	11/17/97	1585	1677
1	03/22/98	1552	1658	4	12/12/97	1590	1696
1	04/11/98	1562	1665	4	12/28/97	1608	1720
1	05/07/98	1544	1637	4	01/25/98	1593	1691
1	07/11/98	1548	1653	4	02/20/98	1595	1692
1	08/13/98	1567	1672	4	03/11/98	1586	1688
1	08/26/98	1563	1658	4	03/23/98	1593	1718
1	09/21/98	1554	1646	4	04/24/98	1594	1722
2	09/22/97	1560	1654	4	06/13/98	1602	1727
2	10/05/97	1565	1660	4	06/26/98	1600	1733
2	11/06/97	1563	1643	4	07/27/98	1598	1708
2	11/19/97	1562	1652	4	08/09/98	1591	1719
2	12/22/97	1558	1663	4	09/21/98	1594	1714
2	01/04/98	1572	1680	5	09/22/97	1591	1664
2	02/05/98	1567	1674	5	11/14/97	1586	1678
2	02/19/98	1566	1667	5	12/17/97	1587	1677
2	03/23/98	1568	1677	5	12/29/97	1605	1703
2	04/12/98	1572	1663	5	02/01/98	1587	1682
2	05/08/98	1569	1661	5	02/15/98	1586	1681
2	07/12/98	1573	1650	5	03/20/98	1588	1688
2	09/21/98	1576	1695	5	04/02/98	1594	1693
3	09/22/97	1579	1654	5	05/05/98	1594	1682
3	11/17/97	1575	1666	5	05/19/98	1593	1684
3	12/15/97	1576	1667	5	06/27/98	1594	1695
3	01/13/98	1571	1669	5	07/11/98	1596	1677
3	01/29/98	1573	1670	5	08/13/98	1594	1675
3	03/03/98	1579	1676	5	08/26/98	1596	1701
3	03/27/98	1580	1690	5	09/21/98	1594	1689

Table 4. Longitudinal precision for 2 QUS machines.

		Machine 1			Machine 2		
Subject	d.f	SEE	Mean	CV	SEE	Mean	CV
1	13	7.11	1555	0.46%	10.87	1647	0.66%
2	11	3.25	1567	0.21%	12.74	1665	0.77%
3	9	4.07	1580	0.26%	8.17	1684	0.49%
4	14	6.14	1595	0.39%	13.67	1707	0.80%
5	13	4.91	1592	0.31%	10.00	1685	0.59%
Total	60	5.43	1578	0.34%	11.49	1678	0.69%
LSC (m/sec)			15.21			32.18	
MTI (yr)			2.5			1.3	

3. Statistical Process Control Charts

In Sec. 2, we introduced the concept of measurement errors and the statistics to evaluate them. Precision errors are usually evaluated whenever new techniques or new devices are developed. Precision errors are also evaluated immediately after a device is installed in clinical sites to assure that the equipment is performing according to the manufacturer's specifications at baseline. Precision errors also are always assessed before the beginning of clinical trials or longitudinal studies.[7,31] Although the manufacturer's service personnel can set up the device so that precision errors are within appropriate limits at baseline, it is very important to monitor the equipment to assure that imprecision remains within acceptable limits. Despite the remarkable accuracy and reproducibility of radiological equipment, measurements can still vary because of changes in equipment, software upgrades, machine recalibration, X-ray source decay, hardware aging and/or failure, or operator errors.

In an ideal setting, a well maintained equipment produce values that are randomly spread around a reference value. A change point is defined as the point in time at which the measured values start to deviate from the reference value. To evaluate measurement stability and identify change points, radiologists develop phantoms that simulate human measurements but, unlike humans, do not change over time.[7,32,33] Variations in phantom measurements should reflect variations in human measurements. Phantoms are measured regularly to detect one or more of the following events: (1) The mean values before and after the change point are statistically significantly different; (2) The standard deviations of measurements before and after the

Table 5. AP spine BMD of a hologic phantom in a QC study (13 March 1989 to 15 May 1989).

i	Date	BMD (X_i)	μ_0	$\sigma(=\mu\times 0.5\%)$
41	03/13/89	1.039	1.033	0.00517
42	03/15/89	1.039	1.033	0.00517
43	03/21/89	1.029	1.033	0.00517
44	03/22/89	1.036	1.033	0.00517
45	03/23/89	1.030	1.033	0.00517
46	03/27/89	1.033	1.033	0.00517
47	03/28/89	1.036	1.033	0.00517
48	03/29/89	1.038	1.033	0.00517
49	03/30/89	1.036	1.033	0.00517
50	04/03/89	1.033	1.033	0.00517
51	04/04/89	1.036	1.033	0.00517
52	04/05/89	1.034	1.033	0.00517
53	04/06/89	1.029	1.033	0.00517
54	04/07/89	1.033	1.033	0.00517
55	04/10/89	1.037	1.033	0.00517
56	04/14/89	1.042	1.033	0.00517
57	04/17/89	1.044	1.033	0.00517
58	04/18/89	1.041	1.033	0.00517
59	04/19/89	1.040	1.033	0.00517
60	04/20/89	1.036	1.033	0.00517
61	04/28/89	1.039	1.033	0.00517
62	05/01/89	1.035	1.033	0.00517
63	05/02/89	1.047	1.033	0.00517
64	05/03/89	1.028	1.033	0.00517
65	05/04/89	1.035	1.033	0.00517
66	05/05/89	1.038	1.033	0.00517
67	05/09/89	1.031	1.033	0.00517
68	05/10/89	1.041	1.033	0.00517
69	05/12/89	1.043	1.033	0.00517
70	05/15/89	1.034	1.033	0.00517

change point are statistically significantly different; (3) The measurements after the change point show a gradual but significant departure from the reference value.

In Table 5, we introduce our third example, which is roughly two months of quality control data from a DXA scanner. In this example, a Hologic spine phantom was scanned about three times a week. The purpose of the study was to monitor the stability of the DXA scanner. If the scanner is functioning acceptably, the coefficient of variation should be less than 0.5%

in the total AP spine BMD values. (Information on this data set can be found in Lu *et al.*[34]). In Table 5, i is an indicator of the observation number; date is the date the scan was performed; BMD is the ith measurement; μ_0 is the reference value based on historical QC data; and σ is the standard deviation based on 0.5% CV. We will use this data to illustrate statistical process control charts.

Statistical process control (SPC) is a powerful collection of problem solving tools for achieving process stability and improving capacity through reduction of variability.[35] There are several statistical methods for identifying change points. One is to visually check the retrospective data to determine the change points and then to verify these changes by a t-test for means and an F-test for variances. An alternative is to use statistical process control charts.[34,36] In this section, we introduce these methods and provide examples of their application in monitoring BMD measured by DXA scanners in osteoporosis studies.

3.1. *Visual inspection*

Potential change points in the data can be determined after careful visual inspection. This can be done by plotting longitudinal phantom data over time and using visual judgment to identify the potential change points created by drifts or sudden jumps. Statistical tests, such as the t-test, can be used to confirm the significance of the changes. It is important to note that there can be multiple potential change points observed for a given period of time. Careful control for type one errors for repeated tests is recommended for the t-tests.

Only experienced medical physicists or radiologists should perform periodic visual inspections. The role of primary evaluator should always be taken by the same individual to avoid subjective variations. The selection of the change points is based on the scatter plot in the most recent data. Once a change point has been identified, its cause should be investigated to determine if the change is machine related.

Visual inspection is not recommended because its efficiency depends on the experience of the reviewer and may not be reproducible.

3.2. *Shewhart control chart*

A Shewhart chart is a graphic display of a quality that has been measured over time. The chart contains a central horizontal line that represents the mean reference value. Three horizontal lines above and three below the central line indicate 1, 2, and 3 standard deviations from the reference value. By plotting the observed quality control measurements on the chart, we can determine if the machine is operating within acceptable limits.

The reference values can be derived from theoretical values for the phantom, or from the first 25 observations measured at baseline. The reference value changes whenever the Shewhart chart indicates an out of control signal and the machine is recalibrated. The new reference value will then be the mean of the first 25 observations after recalibration. The number of observations needed to calculate the reference value may vary; the number 25 was chosen based on practical experience to balance the stability of the reference value with the length of time needed to establish it.

The standard deviation varies among individual devices, and manufacturers should be selected accordingly. For example, in one osteoporosis study, we sometimes use the BMD of a Hologic phantom to monitor DXA scanner performance. We usually assume the coefficient of variation for Hologic machines to be 0.5% and Lunar to be 0.6%, based on reported data on long-term phantom precision.[37] Therefore, the standard deviation for the scanner was calculated as 0.005 and 0.006 times the reference value for Hologic and Lunar machines respectively.

The original Shewhart chart will signal that there is a problem if the observed measurement is more than 3 standard deviations from the reference value. Although intuitive and easy to apply, the chart is not very sensitive to small but significant changes.[35] Therefore, a set of sensitizing tests for assignable causes has been developed to improve the sensitivity of Shewhart charts. Eight of the tests are available in the statistical software package SAS.[38] The tests are listed in Table 6.

The sensitizing rules can be used in toto or in part depending on the underlying processes of interest. For example, for quality control of DXA machines, we used four tests — 1, 2, 5 and 6.[34] Once a change point has been identified by any one of the tests, the manufacturer's repair service should be called to examine the causes and to recalibrate the machine. We then use the next 25 observations to generate new reference values and apply the tests to the subsequent data according to the new reference value.

Figure 2 shows the application of a Shewhart chart for Example 3. In this chart, the dots are the observed BMD. The six lines are the control limits 1, 2 and 3 standard deviations away from the central reference line. There is a problem with Test 2 from April 10, 1989.

The sensitizing rules increase the sensitivity of the Shewhart chart, but also increase the number of clinically insignificant alarms, which is not

Table 6. Definition of tests for assignable causes for Shewhart charts.

Tests	Pattern Description
1	One point is more than 3 standard deviation from the central line.
2	Nine points in a row on one side of the central line.
3	Six points in a row steadily increasing or steadily decreasing.
4	Fourteen points in a row alternating up and down.
5	Two out of 3 points in a row more than 2 standard deviation from the central line.
6	Four out of 5 points in a row more than 1 standard deviation from the central line.
7	Fifteen points in a row all within 1 standard deviation from the central line on either or both sides of the line.
8	Eight points in a row all beyond 1 standard deviation from the central line on either or both sides of the line.

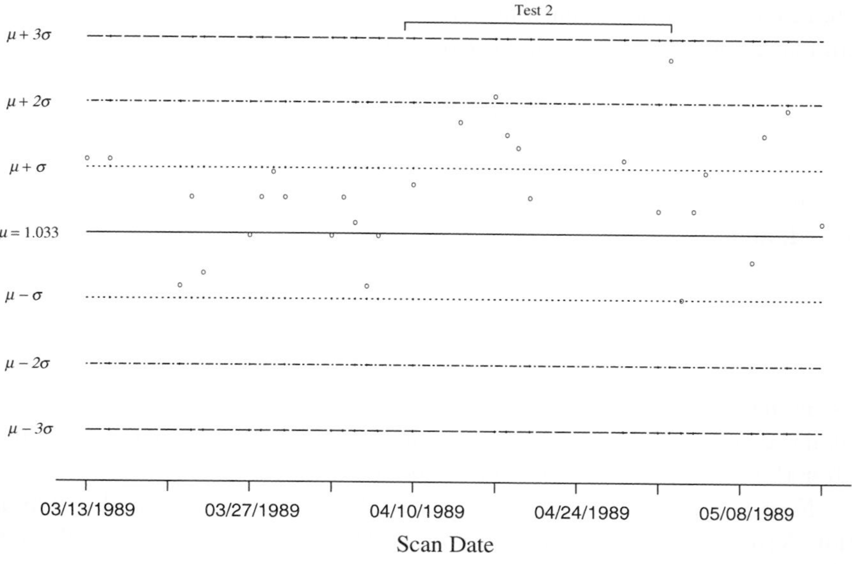

Fig. 2. Shewhart chart for QC data in Example 3.

desirable. To overcome this problem, a threshold based on the magnitude of the mean shift can also be implemented. For example, we can select ten consecutive scans from after the possible change point identified on the Shewhart chart, and then calculate their mean values. If the mean differs by more than one standard deviation (which equals 0.5% times the reference value, in our example) from the reference value, the change point is confirmed as a true change point. Otherwise, the signal from the Shewhart chart is ignored and the reference value is unchanged. This approach filters out small and clinically insignificant changes. However, the true difference must be more than one standard deviation for this approach to be effective, and this approach can delay the recognition of true change points.

3.3. *Moving average chart*

An alternative method is to determine the means and standard deviations of 25 consecutive measurements and then plot them over time. Control limits can be based on the assumption of a constant coefficient of variation during the process (0.5% times the reference mean) and a type one error rate comparable to the original Shewhart method (0.27%).[35] More specifically, we use X_i, for $i = 1, 2, \ldots, n$, the measured QC values of n longitudinal phantom scans from a machine. We define the moving average mean and standard deviation based on 25 scans as:

$$M_i = \sum_{j=i-24}^{i} X_j \Big/ 25, \quad i = 25, 26, \ldots, n \tag{18}$$

as the moving average of 25 scans to the date when the ith scan was collected, and

$$S_i = \sqrt{\sum_{j=i-24}^{i} (X_j - M_i)^2 \Big/ 24}, \quad i = 25, 26, \ldots, n \tag{19}$$

as the moving standard deviation of the 25 scans to the date when the ith scan was collected. Note that the first moving average can only be calculated after the first 25 scans have been collected.

Now if we assume that X_i's independently follow a normal distribution $N(\mu, \sigma^2)$, it can be shown that the M_i's follow a normal distribution $N(\mu, \sigma^2/25)$ and $24\ S_i^2/\sigma^2$'s follow a chi-square distribution with 24 degrees of freedom denoted by χ^2_{24}. However, note that both M_i's and $24\ S_i^2/\sigma^2$'s are not independent samples from the normal distribution and the chi-square distribution, respectively, for different i's.

Let μ_0 be the reference mean. If the machine is operating correctly, we should accept the null hypothesis, $H_0 : \mu = \mu_0$. If the machine is not operating correctly, we will accept the alternative hypothesis, $H_1 : \mu \neq$

μ_0. We select a type one error level of 0.0027 to be comparable to the original Shewhart method. We will reject the null hypothesis if $|M_i - \mu_0| > z_{1-\alpha/2}\frac{\sigma}{5} = 0.5991\sigma$. Thus, the control limits for the moving average are $\pm 59.91\%$ of the standard deviation from the reference mean.

We assumed that the CV for the machine is constant. Therefore, if it is functioning correctly, we can derive the standard deviation as equal to the reference mean times the CV. To check whether the precision of the machine is acceptable, we will test the null hypothesis, $H_0 : \sigma = \sigma_0$, versus the alternative that $H_1 : \sigma > \sigma_0$. With the same level of type one error rate as the mean difference, we will reject the null hypothesis if 24 $S_i^2/\sigma_0^2 > \chi^2_{24,1-\alpha}$, or equivalently, if $S_i > 1.41\sigma_0$. Thus, the control limit of the moving standard deviation is 1.41 times the standard deviation.

Note that there is only an upper limit for the moving standard deviation chart, as we are interested only in the increase in the standard deviation. In other words, we are looking for quality control but not quality improvement. Once the moving average moves out of the control limit, the value of the moving average at that point is used as the new reference value for scans performed after that date.

The number of scans used to calculate the moving average will affect performance of the method. Twenty-five scans were selected based on power analysis, so that the moving average chart has less than a 0.27% chance of a false alarm and a 98% chance of detecting an increase in the mean of one standard deviation. Also, the moving standard deviation chart has a 98% chance of picking up a 100% increase in the standard deviation.[34] Twenty-five scans is also a typical month's worth of quality control measurements.

3.4. *CUSUM chart*

CUSUM chart is short for Cumulative Sum Chart. In applications, we recommend a version of CUSUM known as Tabular CUSUM[35] because it can be presented with or without graphs. Mathematically, we define an upper one-sided tabular CUSUM $S_H(i)$ and a lower one-sided tabular CUSUM $S_L(i)$ for the ith QC measurement as the following:

$$S_H(i) = \max\left[0, \frac{X_i - \mu_0}{\sigma} - k + S_H(i-1)\right], \tag{20}$$

$$S_L(i) = \max\left[0, \frac{\mu_0 - X_i}{\sigma} - k + S_L(i-1)\right]. \tag{21}$$

Here, μ_0 is the reference mean, σ is the standard deviation, and k is a parameter to filter out insignificant variations and is usually set at 0.5. The initial values of $S_H(0)$ and $S_L(0)$ are 0. The chart sends an alarm message if $S_L(i)$ or $S_H(i)$ is greater than 5. In other words, when the standardized BMD value deviates more than k from zero, the cumulative upper bounded sum increases by the amount of deviations above k. On the other hand, if the deviation is less than k, the cumulative sum will be reduced accordingly. When the cumulative sum is less than zero, we ignore the past data and set the cumulative sum as zero. However, a cumulative sum greater than 5 is a strong indication of a deviation from the reference mean in the data.

CUSUM also estimates when the change occurred and the magnitude of the change. We use the estimated magnitude of change to establish the new reference values.

Table 7 demonstrates the application of CUSUM chart to Example 3.

In this table, $S_H(i)$ and $S_L(i)$ are defined in Eqs. (20) and (21), and we selected $k = 0.5$ to detect a mean change of one standard deviation.[35] Along with the sequences $S_H(i)$ and $S_L(i)$, sequences $N_H(i)$ and $N_L(i)$ denote the number of scans since the last positive observation of $S_H(i)$ and $S_L(i)$, respectively. For example, from records one to four, the $S_H(i)$'s were positive, so that $N_H(i)$ goes from 41 to 44. However, $S_H(45)$ was zero. Therefore, the corresponding $N_H(45) = 0$. A similar rule applies for $N_L(i)$.

As explained, the initial reference value was obtained from the mean of the first 25 observations. However, once $S_H(i)$ or $S_L(i)$ exceeded 5, we concluded that the scanner was malfunctioning. For example, on April 20, 1989, $S_H(60) > 5$, suggesting that the BMD values were too high. We estimate that this event could have started on April 10, 1989, by noting the last date when $N_H(i) = 1$. Therefore, the investigation of assignable causes should focus around that time. The magnitude of change from the reference value can be estimated as $\sigma[k + S_H(i)/N_H(i)]$, which equals the average difference.[35]

Once we know the machine is malfunctioning, we will establish new reference values. If the manufacturer was involved in correcting the machine, the new mean should be established by the first 25 observations after the correction. However, if there is no intervention by the manufacturer or, as in our case, when performing retrospective data analysis, the new reference value can be estimated by $\mu_0 + \sigma[k + S_H(i)/N_H(i)]$, if the new BMD values are greater than the reference value, or by $\mu_0 - \sigma[k + S_H(i)/N_H(i)]$ when the new BMD values are smaller than the reference value. This results in a new μ_0 after the 60th scan of 1.040 mg/cm^2.

Table 7. CUSUM table (from 13 March 1989 to 15 May 1989).

i	Date	X_i	μ_0	σ $(0.5\%_{\mu_0})$	$\frac{X_i-\mu_0}{\sigma}-0.5$	$S_H(i)$	$N_H(i)$	$\frac{\mu_0-X_i}{\sigma}-0.5$	$S_L(i)$	$N_L(i)$
41	03/13/89	1.039	1.033	0.00517	0.65	0.65	1	−1.65	0.00	0
42	03/15/89	1.039	1.033	0.00517	0.65	1.29	2	−1.65	0.00	0
43	03/21/89	1.029	1.033	0.00517	−1.29	0.00	3	0.29	0.29	1
44	03/22/89	1.036	1.033	0.00517	0.07	0.07	4	−1.07	0.00	0
45	03/23/89	1.030	1.033	0.00517	−1.10	0.00	0	0.10	0.10	1
46	03/27/89	1.033	1.033	0.00517	−0.52	0.00	0	−0.48	0.00	0
47	03/28/89	1.036	1.033	0.00517	0.07	0.07	1	−1.07	0.00	0
48	03/29/89	1.038	1.033	0.00517	0.45	0.52	2	−1.45	0.00	0
49	03/30/89	1.036	1.033	0.00517	0.07	0.58	3	−1.07	0.00	0
50	04/03/89	1.033	1.033	0.00517	−0.52	0.07	4	−0.48	0.00	0
51	04/04/89	1.036	1.033	0.00517	0.07	0.13	5	−1.07	0.00	0
52	04/05/89	1.034	1.033	0.00517	−0.32	0.00	0	−0.68	0.00	0
53	04/06/89	1.029	1.033	0.00517	−1.29	0.00	0	0.29	0.29	1
54	04/07/89	1.033	1.033	0.00517	−0.52	0.00	0	−0.48	0.00	0
55	04/10/89	1.037	1.033	0.00517	0.26	0.26	1	−1.26	0.00	0
56	04/14/89	1.042	1.033	0.00517	1.23	1.49	2	−2.23	0.00	0
57	04/17/89	1.044	1.033	0.00517	1.61	3.10	3	−2.61	0.00	0
58	04/18/89	1.041	1.033	0.00517	1.03	4.13	4	−2.03	0.00	0
59	04/19/89	1.040	1.033	0.00517	0.84	4.97	5	−1.84	0.00	0
60	04/20/89	1.036	1.033	0.00517	0.07	5.04	6	−1.08	0.00	0

(*Continued*)

Table 7. *(Continued)*

i	Date	X_i	μ_0	σ $(0.5\%_{\mu_0})$	$\frac{X_i-\mu_0}{\sigma} - 0.5$	$S_H(i)$	$N_H(i)$	$\frac{\mu_0-X_i}{\sigma} - 0.5$	$S_L(i)$	$N_L(i)$
61	04/28/89	1.039	1.040	0.00520	−0.69	0.00	0	−0.31	0.00	0
62	05/01/89	1.035	1.040	0.00520	−1.46	0.00	0	0.46	0.46	1
63	05/02/89	1.047	1.040	0.00520	0.85	0.85	1	−1.85	0.00	0
64	05/03/89	1.028	1.040	0.00520	−2.81	0.00	0	1.81	1.81	1
65	05/04/89	1.035	1.040	0.00520	−1.46	0.00	0	0.46	2.27	2
66	05/05/89	1.038	1.040	0.00520	−0.88	0.00	0	−0.12	2.15	3
67	05/09/89	1.031	1.040	0.00520	−2.23	0.00	0	1.23	3.38	4
68	05/10/89	1.041	1.040	0.00520	−0.31	0.00	0	−0.69	2.69	5
69	05/12/89	1.043	1.040	0.00520	0.08	0.08	1	−1.08	1.62	6
70	05/15/89	1.034	1.040	0.00520	−1.65	0.00	0	0.65	2.27	7

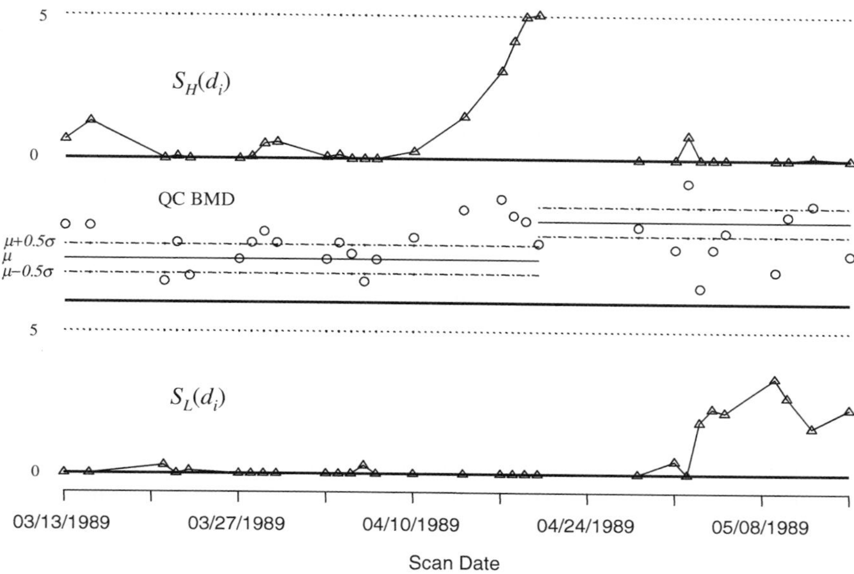

Fig. 3. CUSM chart for QC data in Example 3.

Graphical presentation of the CUSUM chart was shown in Fig. 3. In some senses, it is easier to review the Table 7 than the chart for identifying change points.

A separate CUSUM chart can be constructed for a one-sided change in variance. The one-sided variance chart was constructed according to Ryan.[39] In this approach, the observed difference of two successive scans $X_i - X_{i-1}$ was transformed to $Z_i = \{|[(X_i - X_{i-1})/\sqrt{2\sigma^2}|^{1/2} - 0.82218\}/0.34914$, which approximately follows a standard normal distribution $N(0,1)$. For the variance chart, we selected $k = 0.75$ to reduce the number of alarms due to single outliers. When an alarm for a change in variance is identified, we will investigate the causes of the alarm and may need to recalibrate the machine.

Table 8 is a variance chart for Example 3. The table has calculated values of Z_i. Since Z_i follows a standard normal distribution, the upper side CUSUM for variance is $S_H(i) = \max[0, Z_i - 0.75 + S_H(i-1)]$, which is given in the eighth column. As before, $N_H(i)$ indicates when a positive cumulative sum occurs and is useful for finding the assignable causes. The graphic presentation is similar to Fig. 3 and is not presented here.

Table 8. CUSUM table for change of variance for Example 3.

i	Date	X_i	$X_i - X_{i-1}$	$\sigma(0.5\%_{\mu_0})$	Z_i	$Z_i - 0.75$	$S_H(i)$	$N_H(i)$
55	04/10/89	1.037	0.004	0.00517	−0.24	−0.99	0.000	0
56	04/14/89	1.042	0.005	0.00517	0.01	−0.74	0.000	0
57	04/17/89	1.044	0.002	0.00517	−0.86	−1.61	0.000	0
58	04/18/89	1.041	−0.003	0.00517	−0.52	−1.27	0.000	0
59	04/19/89	1.040	−0.001	0.00517	−1.30	−2.05	0.000	0
60	04/20/89	1.036	−0.004	0.00517	−0.24	−0.99	0.000	0
61	04/28/89	1.039	0.003	0.00520	−0.52	−1.27	0.000	0
62	05/01/89	1.035	−0.004	0.00520	−0.24	−0.99	0.000	0
63	05/02/89	1.047	0.012	0.00520	1.30	0.55	0.554	1
64	05/03/89	1.028	−0.019	0.00520	2.25	1.50	2.053	2
65	05/04/89	1.035	0.007	0.00520	0.44	−0.31	1.742	3
66	05/05/89	1.038	0.003	0.00520	−0.53	−1.28	0.467	4
67	05/09/89	1.031	−0.007	0.00520	0.44	−0.31	0.156	5
68	05/10/89	1.041	0.010	0.00520	0.99	0.24	0.391	6
69	05/12/89	1.043	0.002	0.00520	−0.86	−1.61	0.000	0
70	05/15/89	1.034	−0.009	0.00520	0.81	0.06	0.060	1

The general procedure for deriving the algebraic boundaries of the CUSUM chart is given in Montgomery[35] and Rice[39] and theoretical comparisons of Shewhart and CUSUM can be found in both books.

The V-mask chart is another form of CUSUM chart and is essentially the same as the Tabular CUSUM.[35,40]

3.5. *Comparison of statistical process control charts in osteoporosis studies*

Lu *et al.*[34] compared several statistical process control procedures and their applications to monitoring DXA scanners based on daily scans of a Hologic spine phantom. The comparisons were based on their results on longitudinal quality control data from 5 clinical trial sites as well as simulation studies. They concluded that visual inspection is relatively subjective and depends on the operator's experience and alertness. The regular Shewhart chart with sensitizing rules has a high false alarm rate. The Shewhart chart with sensitizing rules and an additional filter of clinically insignificant mean changes has the lowest false alarm rate but relatively low sensitivity. This method does not require a lot of statistics and can be easily applied to clinical study sites. The CUSUM approach has the best combination of sensitivity, specificity, and identification of the time and magnitude of change. It is recommended for use in quality control centers in clinical trials, especially if patient data must be recalculated to adjust for change points.[41] Combining a moving average chart and a moving standard deviation chart comes closest to the performance of the CUSUM method as a quality control procedure for monitoring DXA scanner performance.

3.6. *Other charts*

In all the above procedures, we assumed that there is no autocorrelation between consecutive measurements. This is rarely true for longitudinal quality control for radiological equipment. The effects of such an assumption on the use of statistical process control charts and their decision structures are rather debatable. At one extreme, Wheeler[42] argues that the usual control limits are contaminated "only when the autocorrelation becomes excessive (say 0.80 or larger)." He concludes that "one need not be overly concerned about the effects of autocorrelation upon the control chart." Our personal experience with Shewhart or CUSUM charts and DXA quality control has been positive. This does not preclude autocorrelation from being a problem for other applications. Johnson and Bagshaw[43] concluded that the problem is potentially quite serious. Strike suggested "clever use" of CUSUMs in laboratory medicine, such as process control for assays.[22]

Statistical approaches for dealing with autocorrelation are to construct process charts based on residuals after removing the autocorrelation or the use of an exponentially weighted moving-average (EWMA) control chart.[35] EWMA is a flexible approach to statistical process control applications. When applied to uncorrelated data, it is a good alternative to the CUSUM chart. Applied to autocorrelated data, it can be adapted to form a control chart that eliminates the excessive false alarm problem associated with traditional control charts. Details of EWMA can be found in most books on quality control.[35,39]

While all the statistical process control charts presented here are for univariate continuous measurements, there are other types of charts for proportions and rates,[44,45] and other quality control and improvement techniques from multivariate approaches.[35,46]

4. Assessment of Agreement

In quality control for clinical trials, we must always assess the agreement of measurements. For example, during a longitudinal osteoporosis trial, a study site might upgrade its DXA machine. Because the change of

BMD from baseline is the key measurement, we must be certain that the BMD values measured by the old and new machines are equivalent or in agreement. Also in clinical trials that require a radiologist's assessment of outcomes, we must be certain that readings from different radiologists are the same, and that readings at the beginning and the end of the study are similar. All these require assessment of agreement.

After a DXA scanner upgrade, multiple phantoms scans should be performed, and if possible, a group of volunteers should be scanned on both the old and new devices. If human data is available, it can be used data to assess the agreement rather than phantom data. We hope the volunteers present a range of BMD wide enough to cover the spectrum of clinical uses. Before upgrading a machine that is being used in a clinical trial, the site must first inform the trial sponsors and quality assurance centers for their approval and must rely on manufacturers to assure proper installation and calibration. The site must maintain proper documentation for machine upgrades.

Assessment of inter-reader agreement among radiologists in a clinical trial and intra-reader longitudinal consistency during a trial, normally requires group training before the trial starts. A database of representative images is assembled into a database. Potential readers for the study read the images together and discuss the grading criteria. Only trained radiologists can be readers. The group training should be documented. After training, inter-reader agreement should be assessed. If the agreement does not satisfy the requirements of the sponsors or protocols, the readers will be re-trained and a new set of test cases used to test for agreement. The trial cannot start until reader agreement reaches the pre-specified requirements. During the trial, the radiologists are required to re-read the test sets periodically to assess the agreement of their current readings with their baseline readings. This is necessary to assure longitudinal consistency. All tests for reader agreement should be documented and archived for auditing purposes.

Evaluation of agreement is also important for other purposes, such as validation of diagnostic methods or radiological devices. In these cases, a gold standard will be selected and validation is performed to assure the new measurements agree with the gold standard.

4.1. *Association versus agreement*

The concepts of agreement and association are related but different. Agreement means interchangeability of two measurements. In other words, a patient's BMD should be the same whether measured on an old DXA scanner or a new one; and the spine fracture grade of a vertebra should be the same regardless by whom or when it is read. An association, on the other hand, suggests that two machines or two readers tend to agree in the same directions. In other words, for two patients with different BMD values, both DXA machines will find the same lower and higher BMD subjects but their BMD measurements can be different.

The best example of the difference between agreement and association is the correlation coefficient of two continuous variables.[47,48] A correlation coefficient can apply to any two continuous variables regardless of their scales, such as height and weight. Even if there is a high association between height and weight, they are not interchangeable because they measure completely different things. Even when X and Y are two continuous variables that measure the same physical properties in the same units, an association still cannot indicate agreement. In fact, $cor(X, Y) = cor(a + bX, Y)$. Thus, the correlation is invariant for a shift of mean or a change of scale. Further, the estimation of the correlation depends on the range of the true quantity in the sample: the wider the range, the higher the correlation coefficient. Also, the null hypothesis in testing for a correlation coefficient is the more independent of two variables, which is not relevant to the agreement. Therefore, the use of correlation to assess agreement is inappropriate. On the other hand, a high correlation of two continuous variables in the same scale suggests that it is possible to calibrate variables so that they agree with each other.

4.2. *Assessment of agreement of two continuous variables*

As discussed above, only when two variables measure the same physical property using the same units can they be assessed for agreement. Let Y_1 and Y_2 be such continuous variables that follow normal distributions $N(\mu_{Y_1}, \sigma^2_{Y_1})$ and $N(\mu_{Y_2}, \sigma^2_{Y_2})$. They are measured from the same subjects. The correlation coefficient between Y_1 and Y_2 is ρ. Let $D = Y_1 - Y_2$ and $A = (Y_1 + Y_2)/2$. We want to perform a regression analysis of $D = \alpha + \beta A + \varepsilon$. We are interested in $\alpha = \beta = 0$.[47]

It is easy to verify that

$$\beta = \mathrm{cov}(D, A)/\sigma^2_A = 0.5(\sigma^2_{Y_1} - \sigma^2_{Y_2})/(\sigma^2_{Y_1} - \sigma^2_{Y_2} + 2\rho\sigma_{Y_1}\sigma_{Y_2}), \tag{22}$$

and

$$\alpha = (\mu_{Y_1} - \mu_{Y_2}) - \frac{\mu_{Y_1} + \mu_{Y_2}}{2}\beta. \tag{23}$$

Therefore, $\alpha = \beta = 0$ implies that $\mu_{Y_1} = \mu_{Y_2}$ and $\sigma_{Y_1} = \sigma_{Y_2}$, i.e., the two measurements have the same distribution parameters.

Bland and Altman[47] further suggested plotting the difference D against average A and calculating the standard deviation of D (σ_D). With 95% confidence, the differences between paired data are between $\pm 2\sigma_D$. If this σ_D is less than or equal to the precision errors of Y_1 and Y_2, then these two measurements are exchangeable and therefore, equivalent. Also, if $\sigma_D/\bar{A} \times 100\%$ is less than the CVs for Y_1 and Y_2, they should be equivalent. Here we use a bar to denote sample means.

Noting that both D and A are random variables, Bartko[49] proposed a bivariate confidence ellipse for the Bland-Altman plot. The equation of the 95% ellipse is

$$\begin{aligned}(A - \bar{A})^2/\sigma_A^2 - 2r(A - \bar{A})(D - \bar{D})^2/\sigma_A\sigma_D + (D - \bar{D})^2/\sigma_D^2 \\ = q_{\chi^2}(0.95, 2)(1 - r^2).\end{aligned} \tag{24}$$

Here, $q_{\chi^2}(0.95, 2) = 5.991$ is the 95% quantile of the χ^2-distribution with 2 degrees of freedom and r is the sample correlation coefficient of D and A.

The hypothesis $\alpha = \beta = 0$ can be tested using the Bradley-Blackwood procedure.[50] The test statistic is

$$F = (n-2)\frac{\left(\sum_{i=1}^n D_i^2 - \sum_{i=1}^n (D_i - \hat{\alpha} - \hat{\beta}A_i)^2\right)}{\left(2\sum_{i=1}^n (D_i - \hat{\alpha} - \hat{\beta}A_i)^2\right)} \sim F(2, n-2), \tag{25}$$

which simultaneously tests for the zero intercept and slope.

Table 9 shows a dataset of AP Spine BMD (mg/cm^2) from 10 normal volunteers measured on three different DXA scanners. We are interested in the equivalence of Scanner 1 and the other two scanners.

As shown in Table 9, we can accept the null hypothesis that there is no difference in means and standard deviations between Scanners 1 and 2 by the Bradley-Blackwood test. There is, however, a significant difference between Scanners 1 and 3. Further examination of the data shows that Scanners 1 and 2 have different standard deviations. Using Bland and Altman's method, we can plot the comparison of Scanners 1 versus 2 and Scanners 1 versus 3 (Fig. 4). The dashed line shows that the 95% confidence interval is the most important measurement of these figures. Even though there is a significant non-zero intercept or slope in the Bland-Altman regression, we may still be able to treat the two measurements as interchangeable if the variation of differences is less than the *in vivo* short-term

Table 9. AP spine BMD of 10 patients by three DXA scanners.

	Observed BMD Data			Comparison Scanners 1 and 2		Comparison Scanners 1 and 3	
Subject	Scanner 1	Scanner 2	Scanner 3	D_1	A_1	D_2	A_2
1	1.342	1.328	1.352	0.014	1.335	−0.010	1.347
2	1.303	1.312	1.317	−0.009	1.308	−0.014	1.310
3	1.093	1.100	1.078	−0.007	1.096	0.015	1.085
4	1.092	1.116	1.087	−0.024	1.104	0.005	1.089
5	1.215	1.215	1.216	0.000	1.215	−0.001	1.216
6	1.155	1.157	1.137	−0.002	1.156	0.018	1.146
7	1.125	1.117	1.097	0.008	1.121	0.028	1.111
8	1.434	1.437	1.447	−0.003	1.436	−0.013	1.441
9	1.230	1.225	1.231	0.005	1.228	−0.001	1.231
10	1.326	1.324	1.313	0.002	1.325	0.013	1.320
σ_D				0.0104		0.0141	
Bradley-Blackwood Test			F	0.6733		5.3645	
			p-value	0.5367		0.0333	

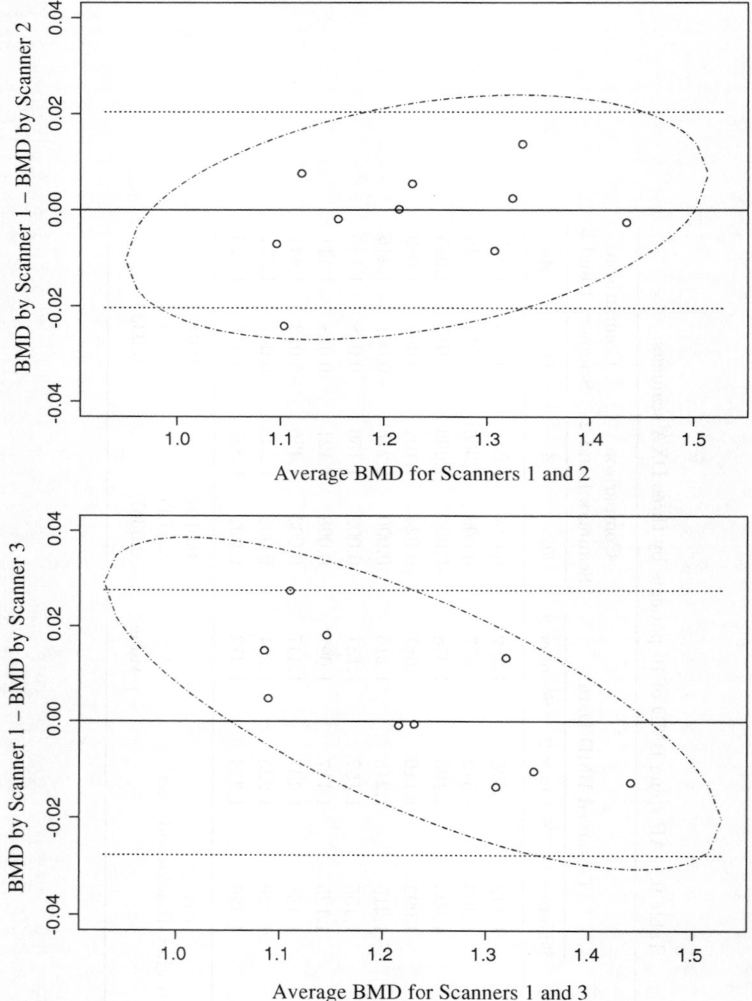

Fig. 4. Examples of Bland-Altman plots for equivalence of 3 scanners. The dashed lines are the 95% confidence intervals for the differences between two Scanners. The ellipses are the 95% bivariate confidence ellipses.

precision error. The 95% confidence ellipse of a Bland-Altman plot is useful for indicating the differences between sample variances.

A bivariate normal distribution has 5 parameters: two means, two standard deviations, and a correlation coefficient. The Bland-Altman regression compares four of the five parameters. We can have two normal random variables with the same mean and standard deviation but a negative correlation coefficient, such as Y and $-Y$, when mean Y is 0. Thus, the Bland-Altman regression alone is inadequate for evaluating agreement. We still need to examine the correlation coefficient between the two measurements, in addition to the Bland-Altman regression. Only a high correlation with a zero intercept and slope in the Bland-Altman regression can suggest that the two measurements are equivalent.

4.3. *Intraclass correlation coefficient*

An alternative measurement for agreement is the intraclass correlation coefficient (ICC),[51] which is simply the percentage of between readers/techniques variance in the total variance of the sum of between and within reader/technique variations. More specifically, we assume that $Y_{ij} = \mu + p_i + r_j + (pr)_{ij} + \varepsilon_{ij}$, with i representing the ith individual ($i = 1, \ldots, N$) and j representing the jth reader/devices ($j = 1, \ldots, K$). Here, Y_{ij} is the observation of the ith individual measured by jth reader/scanner/machine; μ is the overall effect common to all observations; p_i is the random patient effect; r_j is the random reader/device effect; $(pr)_{ij}$ is the interaction between patient and reader/device; and ε_{ij} is the measurement error. Here, we assume that p_i and r_j are independent and follow normal distributions $N(0, \sigma_P^2)$ and $N(0, \sigma_R^2)$, respectively, and ε_{ij} is independent of p_i and r_j and follows $N(0, \sigma_e^2)$. Without duplicate observations, the interaction term $(pr)_{ij}$ cannot be separated from measurement error and can be dropped. An intraclass correlation coefficient is defined as

$$\mathrm{ICC} = \frac{\sigma_P^2}{\sigma_P^2 + \sigma_R^2 + \sigma_e^2}. \tag{26}$$

Thus, a high ICC means less difference between two readers as well as less measurement error. Lee *et al.* suggested a cut-off value of 0.75 beyond which the readers or measurement devices are considered to be in agreement.[51]

The ICC can be estimated based on the output of an ANOVA table of the two-way mixed model as the following.

$$\rho_{\mathrm{ICC}} = \frac{N(\mathrm{MSB} - \mathrm{MSE})}{N\,\mathrm{MSB} + K\,\mathrm{MSR} + (KN - K - N)\mathrm{MSE}}. \tag{27}$$

Here, MSB, MSR, and MSE are the mean squared between subject, between reader/device, and error respectively.

Fleiss and Shrout[52] derived an approximate formula for the confidence interval of ρ_{ICC}. Let F_U and F_L be the upper and lower $100(1 - \alpha/2)\%$

percentiles, respectively from F distribution with degrees of freedom $(N-1)$ and v, where

$$v = \frac{(K-1)(N-1)\{K\rho_{\text{ICC}}\text{MSR}/\text{MSE} + N[1+(K-1)\rho_{\text{ICC}}] - K\rho_{\text{ICC}}\}^2}{(N-1)K^2\rho_{\text{ICC}}^2\text{MSR}^2/\text{MSE}^2 + \{N[1+(K-1)\rho_{\text{ICC}}] - K\rho_{\text{ICC}}\}^2}. \tag{28}$$

The approximate upper and lower bounds, ρ_U and ρ_L, respectively, for the $100(1-\alpha)\%$ confidence bounds of ρ_{ICC} are given as following.

$$\rho_U = \frac{N(\text{MSB} - F_L\text{MSE})}{F_L[K\,\text{MSR} + (NK - L - N)\text{MSE}] + N\,\text{MSB}} \tag{29}$$

and

$$\rho_L = \frac{N(\text{MSB} - F_U\text{MSE})}{F_U[K\,\text{MSR} + (NK - L - N)\text{MSE}] + N\,\text{MSB}}. \tag{30}$$

Table 10 shows ANOVA tables for comparison of scanners in Example 4, and the corresponding intraclass correlation coefficients.

It is clear from this example that ICC is less sensitive to agreement between two scanners. The ICC for Scanners 1 and 3 is much higher but the Bland-Altman regression shows significant disagreement. Bland and Altman[53] list other deficiencies of ICC for evaluation of agreement, including its dependence on sample variations. On the other hand, it is easier to use ICC to evaluate agreement among three or more readers or devices. Bartko[49] developed an altered version of ICC, which is simplified and has an exact formula for confidence intervals.

4.4. *Kappa statistics for agreement of categorical variables*

Like continuous measurements, agreement between two categorical variables is only meaningful when the two categorical variables have the same biological or physical meanings. Agreement of categorical variables is most commonly applied to qualitative evaluations of health or disease status by two readers or by the same reader at two different sessions, which are referred as inter-reader and intra-reader agreement respectively. In clinical studies using qualitative assessments by multiple readers, we hope that all readers will produce consistent readings, and that their assessments will remain consistent during the study period. Thus, periodic review of inter- and intra-reader agreement should be a part of quality control of clinical trials. If the readers do disagree with each other, re-training is necessary.

Table 10. ANOVA Tables and ICC for Data in Example 4.

Agreement for	Scanners 1 and 2		Scanners 1 and 3		All 3 Scanners	
Source	d.f	MS	d.f	MS	d.f	MS
Between-subject	9	MSB $= \sigma_2^2 + K\sigma_P^2 = 0.02660$	9	MSB $= 0.02992$	9	MSB $= 0.04278$
Between-scanner	1	MSR $= \sigma_2^2 + N\sigma_R^2 = 0.00001$	1	MSR $= 0.00008$	2	MSR $= 0.00008$
Residual	9	MSE $= \sigma_2^2 = 0.00005$	9	MSE $= 0.00010$	18	MSE $= 0.00010$
Total	19		19		29	
v		9.3622		9.9615		19.9237
ICC and 95% C.I.		0.9963 (0.9865, 0.9991)		0.9935 (0.9755, 0.9983)		0.9931 (0.9807, 0.9981)

Table 11. Joint distribution of outcomes of two binary variables.

		X_2		
		Health ($X_2 = 0$)	Diseased ($X_2 = 1$)	Total
X_1	Health ($X_1 = 0$)	P_{00}	P_{01}	P_{0+}
	Diseased ($X_1 = 1$)	P_{10}	P_{11}	P_{1+}
Total		P_{+0}	P_{+1}	1

The simplest way to display categorical variables of two readers is a 2×2 table, displayed in Table 11. Here, X_1 and X_2 are results from two readers, with 0 indicating healthy and 1 indicating diseased, and P_{ij} representing the probability of the event. There are many ways to measure the agreement of two readers. The probability of agreement, i.e., $P(X_1 = X_2) = P_{00} + P_{11}$ is the most direct measurement. Analysis of the probability of agreement is just like analysis of binary probability. Sample size calculations for reader agreement based on duplicated readings were presented by Freedman, Parmar, and Baker.[54]

The drawback of the probability of agreement is a positive chance of agreement even when the two readers are independent. As a result, Cohen proposed the use of Kappa statistics,[55] which offer a means of correcting measurement of agreement, defined as the following.

$$\kappa = \frac{P_{00} + P_{11} - P_{0+}P_{+0} - P_{1+}P_{+1}}{1 - P_{0+}P_{+0} - P_{1+}P_{+1}} = \frac{P_O - P_E}{1 - P_E}. \tag{31}$$

Here, $P_O = P_{00} + P_{11}$ is the observed probability of agreement and $P_E = P_{0+}P_{+0} + P_{1+}P_{+1}$ is the probability of agreement due to changes when X_1 and X_2 are independent. κ can reach 100% if there is perfect agreement and can be as low as $-P_E/(1 - P_E)$, when X_1 and X_2 are completely different.

If we use n_{ij} to denote the observed number of subjects in each category of Table 11, the maximum likelihood estimates for P_{ij}, P_{i+} and P_{+j} are $\hat{p}_{ij} = n_{ij}/n$, $\hat{p}_{+j} = n_{i+}/n$ and $\hat{p}_{+j} = n_{+j}/n$, respectively, with n as the total number of subjects. Through algebra operations, we can estimate κ by substituting the maximum likelihood estimates of the probabilities into Eq. (31).

$$\hat{\kappa} = \frac{2(n_{00}n_{11} - n_{01}n_{10})}{n_{0+}n_{+1} + n_{+0}n_{1+}}. \tag{32}$$

There are several methods for calculating the sample variations for MLE estimates in Eq. (32). Using the delta method, Fleiss *et al.*[56] derived a large sample variance of the estimator.

$$\mathrm{var}(\hat{\kappa}) = \frac{1}{n(1 - P_{0+}P_{+1} - P_{1+}P_{1+})^2}$$
$$\times \left\{ \sum_{i=0}^{1} P_{ii}[1 - 2(P_{i+} + P_{+i})(1 - \kappa)] \right.$$
$$+ (1 - \kappa)^2 \sum_{i=0}^{1} \sum_{j=0}^{1} P_{ij}(P_{+i} + P_{j+})^2$$
$$\left. - [\kappa - (P_{0+}P_{+0} + P_{1+}P_{+1})(1 - \kappa)]^2 \right\}. \tag{33}$$

Alternatively, Kraemer[57] and Fleiss and Davies[58] proposed the use of jackknife technique to calculate the variance of the estimated κ. Let $\hat{\kappa}_{ij}$ be the MLE of κ when one observation in the (i, j)th cell is excluded, and $J_{ij}(\hat{\kappa}) = n\hat{\kappa} - (n - 1)\hat{\kappa}_{ij}$. The jackknife estimator of κ is given by

$$\hat{\kappa}_J = \sum_{i=0}^{1} \sum_{j=0}^{1} n_{ij} J_{ij}(\hat{\kappa})/n, \tag{34}$$

which should be a less biased estimator than $\hat{\kappa}$. The jackknife variance can be estimated by

$$\mathrm{var}(\hat{\kappa}_J) = \sum_{i=0}^{1} \sum_{j=0}^{1} n_{ij}[J_{ij}(\hat{\kappa}) - \hat{\kappa}_J]^2/[n(n - 1)]. \tag{35}$$

Conditioned on marginal distributions of the 2×2 table in Table 11, Garner[59] proposed the following simpler formula:

$$\mathrm{var}(\hat{\kappa}) = \frac{4}{n^2(1 - \hat{p}_{0+}\hat{p}_{+0} - \hat{p}_{1+}\hat{p}_{+1})^2(\sum_{i=0}^{1}\sum_{j=0}^{1} 1/(n_{ij} + 1))}. \tag{36}$$

Although all these formulas are asymptotically equivalent, there are still differences when using them for small samples. A simulation study[60] compared the different estimates for $\hat{\kappa}$ and gave guidance in methods to estimate and construct confidence intervals for Cohen's $\hat{\kappa}$ for small samples as indicated in Table 12. In this table, the "(" and ")" indicate the open-ends of an interval and "[" and "]" the closed ends of an interval. Landis and Koch[61]

Table 12. Guidance in selecting a method for constructing confidence intervals for Cohen's $\hat{\kappa}$.[60]

Kappa ($\hat{\kappa}$)	Agreement[61]	Prevalence[62]	Sample Size	Equations
[0, 0.2)	Slight	(0.1, 0.9)	$n \geq 20$	(33)
[0.2, 0.4)	Fair	[0.1, 0.9]	$n \geq 20$	(33) or (35)
[0.4, 0.6)	Moderate	(0.2, 0.8)	$20 \leq n < 40$	(36)
		(0, 0.2] or [0.8, 1)	$n \geq 40$	(35)
[0.6, 1)	Substantial to almost perfect	(0.1, 0.9)	$n \geq 20$	(36)

provided guidelines for interpreting kappa values as the level of agreement among readers. Prevalence was defined as $(2n_{11} + n_{10} + n_{01})/(2n)$.[62] The last column indicates the preferred equations for estimating the sample variance.

The use of Kappa statistics in quality control and quality assurance is mainly for estimation rather than hypothesis testing. We want to ensure that the inter-reader agreement is above an acceptable pre-specified level before we start the study. We also want to be certain that the longitudinal intra-reader Kappa statistics are beyond that given level. However, the subject of Kappa applications is very broad and goes far beyond quality assurance. The extensive literature on Kappa statistics includes agreement for ordinal or multinomial data;[63–66] for case-control studies;[67] for multiple readers or correlated samples;[68–70] and for using logistic regression models to adjust for the effects of covariates on Kappa statistics.[71] These topics are far beyond the scope of this chapter; interested readers should investigate the literature.

4.5. *Log-linear models for agreement of categorical variables*

Log-linear models can express agreement in terms of components, such as chance agreement and beyond-chance agreement. They can also display patterns of agreement among several observers, or compare patterns of agreement when subjects are stratified by values of a covariate.[72] The later is particularly useful for quality improvement to identify factors that have an affect on reader agreement.

Let $\{m_{ij} = nP_{ij}\}$ denote expected frequencies for ratings (i, j) of n subjects by two observers A and B. Chance agreement, or statistical independence of the ratings, has log-linear model representation

$$\log m_{ij} = \mu + \lambda_i^A + \lambda_j^B. \tag{37}$$

An extension of this independent model is the quasi-independent model[73]

$$\log m_{ij} = \mu + \lambda_i^A + \lambda_j^B + \delta_i I_{(i=j)}, \tag{38}$$

where the indicator $I_{(i=j)}$ equals 1 when $i = j$ and 0 otherwise. Constrains on the model parameters are $\sum_i \lambda_i^A = \sum_j \lambda_j^B = 0$. Conditional on disagreement by the observers, the rating by A is statistically independent of rating by B. When $\delta_i > 0$, more agreements regarding outcome i occur than would be expected by chance. The model is easy to fit by most statistical software. When we assume a constant $\delta_i = \delta$, a Kappa-like index of chance-corrected agreement[74] is

$$\kappa_A = (P_{00} + P_{11})(1 - e^{-\delta}) = (P_{00} + P_{11})(1 - 1\sqrt{OR}). \tag{39}$$

Graham extended above model to allow binary covariates.[75] Let X be the binary covariate with value 0 and 1. Let $\{m_{ijk} = nP_{ij}(X = k)\}$ be the frequencies of observing (i, j) by readers A and B when covariate X equals k. The extended model is

$$\log m_{ijk} = \mu + \lambda_i^A + \lambda_j^B + \lambda_k^X + \lambda_{ik}^{AX} + \lambda_{jk}^{BX} + \delta^{AB} I_{(i=j)} + \delta_k^{ABX} I_{(i=j)}. \tag{40}$$

Here, terms with single superscripts and subscripts correspond to main effects. Terms with double superscripts and subscripts represent partial associations between the superscripted variables, controlling for the variable omitted from the superscript. As with other log-linear models, we impose the constraints of zero sums on the main effects and partial associations, respectively. In this model, δ^{AB} represents the overall agreement between two readers and δ_k^{ABX} represents the additional chance corrected agreement associated with covariate X when $X = k$. A model constraint is zero sum of δ_k^{ABX}. This model readily extends to multiple covariate situations, and estimates can be obtained using the SAS CATMOD procedure.

In model (40), δ_k^{ABX} is an interpretation of the estimates of the average of the two conditional agreement log odds ratios, $\log[(m_{iik}/m_{jik})/(m_{ii0}/m_{ji0})]$ and $\log[(m_{jjk}/m_{ijk})/(m_{jj0}/m_{ij0})]$, for any pair of distinct categories i and j. In his paper,[75] Graham applied this model to a study of the effects of age, sex, and proxy type on agreement between the primary and proxy respondents regarding the primary respondent's participation in vigorous leisure time activity.

Table 13. Probability in a 2 × 2 table with latent classification model.

Rater A	Rater B: Positive	Rater B: Negative	Total
Positive	$Kp + (1-K)\pi^2$	$(1-K)(1-\pi)\pi$	$Kp + (1-K)\pi$
Negative	$(1-K)(1-\pi)\pi$	$K(1-p) + (1-K)(1-\pi)^2$	$K(1-p) + (1-K)(1-\pi)$
Total	$Kp + (1-K)\pi$	$K(1-p) + (1-K)(1-\pi)$	1

4.6. *Latent class models*

In a latent class analysis of observer agreement, it is assumed that the ratings of observers appear related because they are, in fact, related to some latent classification of items that explains all associations in the observed agreement table. For example, we can assume that there are three types of subjects in the study population: those that all readers classify as positive or negative, and those inconclusive subjects that are rated as positives or negatives by chance by each reader.[76] Let K be the prevalence of those "agreements beyond chance" and p be the probability of conclusive items belonging to the positive category. Let π be the probability of positively rating for inconclusive subjects. With the assumption of independent rating by the two readers for inconclusive subjects, the following Table 13 gives the probability distribution of the 2 × 2 table.

Thus, if $p = \pi$, K is the Cohen's Kappa statistics. If $p/(1-p) = \pi^2/(1-\pi)^2$, K equals Aickin's Kappa in Eq. (39).

Latent classification models have many uses.[76] Baker, Freedman, and Parmar[77] proposed a model with duplicate observations that allows a separation of intra- and inter-reader agreement simultaneously for binary measures.

5. Clibration and Standardization

The most important mission of quality assurance is to prevent measurement errors from exceeding a pre-specified level. For this purpose, we evaluate the performance of instruments to ensure that their precision and accuracy are acceptable for clinical diagnosis or clinical monitoring. Once we have chosen the particular devices or methods to measure study parameters, we want to be sure that they are equivalent to each other. During the study, we use the quality process control charts to monitor whether the instruments are still providing the required precision and/or whether the readers are giving consistent readings. With each step, we may still find disagreements between instruments or readers. Once we have chosen one of them as the reference standard, the process of assigning values for other instruments or readers to correct their differences from the reference standard is called calibration.

In the example of multi-center studies, we normally choose the coordinating center as the reference standard. Thus, any site/machine that produces readings or measurements that are different from the reference standards will be calibrated. This is called cross-calibration in the literature on quality control of clinical trials.[41] Although mathematically any site can be chosen as the reference standard, in practice, selection of a reference standard should take into consideration the qualifications and quality control history of the selected site. Sometimes, multiple reference standards are needed. For example, in a clinical trial of osteoporosis that uses DXA scanners from different manufacturers, one option is to select reference standards for each manufacturer and then calibrate devices at the other study sites to the corresponding reference standards. The next step of calibration is to standardize among the reference standards.

Calibration can also occur for a single radiological machine. In the longitudinal quality control process mentioned in Sec. 3, a radiological machine was compared to a standard defined by a phantom. We normally look for the mean and variance changes in reference to the baseline value. One may also be interested in scale differences, i.e. changes in measurement unit. For DXA scanners, phantoms with different linear scaled densities can be used to serve as reference standard and calibration of a scanner may be needed if there are clinically significant deviations from that standard.

5.1. *Calibration of measurements to a standard*

To calibrate radiological equipment to the chosen standard, we need to measure the standard. One method is to measure phantoms with known theoretical measurement values.[32] Another method is to measure a set of phantoms or a group of sampled subjects to examine the differences between the reference standard device and all other study instruments, referred as cross-calibration in multi-center clinical trials.[7] In all cases, we observe pairs of data (X_i, Y_i) with X_i representing the reference standard and Y_i representing measurement of the instrument to be calibrated.

The practical question is how to assign a correct X (standard value) based on measurement Y. A naïve solution is to perform a (linear or non-linear) regression of X_i on Y_i and use that regression model to correct future readings of Y. This solution may be adequate, but it has statistical flaws.

When we choose the standard, we assume that the standard should be accurate, that is its measurement error can be ignored. Thus, the measurement error should be associated only with Y not X. A proper linear relationship should be $Y = \alpha + \beta X + \varepsilon$, with α and β as regression parameters and ε as the random measurement error for Y. These regression parameters α and β are also referred as constant bias and relative (scale) bias.

Maximum likelihood estimates of regression parameters, denoted as $\hat{\alpha}$ and $\hat{\beta}$, and their covariance matrix as well as model RMSE are easily available by many statistical software packages. Based on these estimates, for a given observation of y, we can calibrate it to the standard by $\hat{x} = (y - \hat{\alpha})/\hat{\beta}$.

The predicted value $\hat{x}$ is a biased estimate of true value x except when $x = \bar{X}$.

$$E(\hat{x}|y) = x + [S_e^2(x - \bar{X})]/S_{XX}\hat{\beta}^2). \tag{41}$$

Here, S_e is the RMSE of the regression line and $\bar{X}$ and S_{XX} are the sample mean and sample variance of X_i's used to derive calibrations. This is because $\hat{x}$ is estimated by ratio of correlated normal variables. In most cases, such bias can be ignored for large $\hat{beta}$. More specifically, when

$$g = (t_{n-2,0.05}^2 S_e^2)/(S_{XX}\hat{\beta}^2) < 0.05. \tag{42}$$

When $g > 0.2$, we are not able to calibrate Y to the standard X with acceptable accuracy.[22] Details of the 95% confidence interval of calibrated $\hat{x}$ as well as simultaneous tolerance interval for it can be found in the same reference.

When we allow measurement errors for standard X, we are dealing with the calibration problem as a regression with measurement errors, and the regression and calibration problems are equivalent mathematically. Rearrangement of the linear regression gives the following relationship between X and Y:

$$X = \gamma_0 + \gamma_1 Y + \delta. \tag{43}$$

The difference between this calibration model and regular regression model is that Y is a random variable with $Y = U + \varepsilon$. This regression is not always identifiable unless under certain conditions.[78] When we assume that the measurement error ε and underlying true U are independent and ε has mean zero and a known variance σ_ε^2 (such as estimated through repeated measurements), the calibration formula is

$$\hat{x} = \mu_X + \hat{\gamma}_1\sigma_Y^2/(\sigma_Y^2 - \sigma_\varepsilon^2)(y - \mu_Y) = \mu_X + \hat{\gamma}_1(\sigma_U^2 - \sigma_\varepsilon^2)/\sigma_U^2(y - \mu_Y). \quad (44)$$

Here, $\hat{\gamma}_1$ is the least squared estimate of slope based on observed Y with measurement errors.

5.2. *Comparative calibrations and latent structure models*

Barnett[79] first considered a model to assess "the relative calibration and relative accuracies of a set of p instruments, each designed to measure the same characteristic, on a common group of individuals." It is common for several manufacturers to produce similar machines that measure the same physical properties. For various reasons, these machines will not produce identical measurements for the same subjects. Converting measurements from different manufacturers is important for clinical studies to reduce machine introduced variations improving study efficiency and facilitating comparisons among different studies.

For the ith subject, let a vector $\overrightarrow{Y_i} = (Y_{1i}, Y_{2i}, \ldots, Y_{pi})^T$ to denote the measurements by p instruments for the subject. Here, superscript T represents "transpose." Statistically, we assume that $\overrightarrow{Y_i}$ measures the underlying unobservable quantity X_i from an unknown normal distribution $N(\mu, \sigma_0^2)$. The relationship between $\overrightarrow{Y_i}$ and X_i is that

$$\overrightarrow{Y_i} = \overrightarrow{a} + \overrightarrow{b}X_i + \overrightarrow{\varepsilon_i} \quad (45)$$

with unknown regression parameters $\overrightarrow{a}$ and $\overrightarrow{a}$, and $\overrightarrow{\varepsilon_i}$ as a p-dimensional random measurement errors following $N(\overrightarrow{0}, \Sigma)$.

The difference between this model and the regular calibration model is that X_i can be observed in a regular problem, while X_i is unknown in comparative calibration problems.[80]

The number of sufficient statistics based on observations of $\overrightarrow{Y_i}$ is p means and $p(p+1)/2$ covariance matrix. The number of unknown parameters are 2 for distribution of X, $2p$ for regression coefficients, and $p(p+1)/2$ for the covariance matrix for measurement errors. Thus, for $p < 3$, comparative calibration is unidentifiable. Even for $p \geq 3$, we still need additional assumptions to make the model identifiable.

Barnett[79] assumed $a_1 = 0$ and $b_1 = 1$, and the covariant matrix of measurement errors Σ as a diagonal matrix. He used moment estimates to obtain MLE for the modal parameters. Other authors have studied similar problems.[81–84] The following EM algorithm is a shorter form of a more extended model by Lu *et al.*[85]

Like Barnett, we assume that Σ is a diagonal matrix. When we do not observe X_i, the log-likelihood of our model is pretty complicated. The log-likelihood function of observations $\vec{Y}_i$ is

$$C - \frac{p}{2}\sum_{i=1}^{n} \log(|\vec{b}\,\vec{b}^T\sigma_0^2 + \Sigma|]$$

$$-\frac{1}{2}\sum_{i=1}^{n}(\vec{Y}_i - \vec{a} - \vec{b}\,\mu_0)^T(\vec{b}\,\vec{b}^T\sigma_0^2 + \Sigma)^{-1}(\vec{Y}_i - \vec{a} - \vec{b}\,\mu_0). \tag{46}$$

To make the model identifiable, we also impose linear constrains on regression parameters as $\vec{l}^T\vec{a} = c_1$ and $\vec{l}^T\vec{b} = c_2$. When $\vec{l} = (1, 0, \ldots, 0)^T$ and $c_1 = c_2 = 0$, the model is similar to Barnett.[79] When $\vec{l} = (1, 1, 1)^T$, $c_1 = 0$ and $c_2 = 2.912$, the model is similar to Lu *et al.*[84] While the log-likelihood function is complicated, the likelihood function for known X_i is rather simple:

$$C - \frac{p}{2}\log(|\Sigma|) - \frac{1}{2}\log\sigma_0^2 - \frac{1}{2}(\vec{Y}_i - \vec{a} - \vec{b}\,X_i)^T$$

$$\times\,\Sigma^{-1}(\vec{Y}_i - \vec{a} - \vec{b}\,X_i) - \frac{(X_i - \mu_0)^2}{2\sigma_0^2}. \tag{47}$$

Thus, we can treat X_i as missing data and use the EM algorithm to derive the MLE of model parameters. The EM algorithm has the following steps:

Step 0. Set the initial values of the model parameters $\vec{a}, \vec{b}, \Sigma$, μ_0 and σ_0^2.

Step 1. E-Step: Calculate the conditional expectation of the sufficient statistics for the complete likelihood function. They are

$$V = \mathrm{var}(X_i|\,\vec{Y}_i, \vec{a}, \vec{b}, \Sigma, \mu_0, \sigma_0^2) = (\vec{b}^T\Sigma^{-1}\vec{b} + 1/\sigma_0^2)^{-1}, \tag{48}$$

$$E(X_i|\,\vec{Y}_i, \vec{a}, \vec{b}, \Sigma, \mu_0, \sigma_0^2) = \mu_0 + V\,\vec{b}^T\,\Sigma^{-1}(\vec{Y}_i - \vec{a} - \vec{b}\,\mu_0). \tag{49}$$

Step 2. M-Step: Calculate the MLEs by replacing the conditional sufficient statistics into the following MLE formulas.

$$\hat{\vec{b}} = \frac{S_{Y,X} - (\lambda_1\bar{X} + \lambda^2)\Sigma^{-1}\vec{l}}{S_{XX}}, \tag{50}$$

$$\hat{\vec{a}} = \bar{\vec{Y}} - \hat{\vec{b}}\bar{X} - \lambda_1 \Sigma \vec{l}, \tag{51}$$

$$\hat{\Sigma} = \frac{1}{n}\sum_{i=1}^{n} \text{diag}[(\vec{Y}_i - \hat{\vec{a}} - \hat{\vec{b}}X_i)(\vec{Y}_i - \hat{\vec{a}} - \hat{\vec{b}}X_i)^T], \tag{52}$$

$$\hat{\mu}_0 = \bar{X}, \tag{53}$$

$$\hat{\sigma}_0^2 = \sum_{i=1}^{n}(X_i - \hat{\mu}_0)^2/n. \tag{54}$$

Here, $\bar{\vec{Y}}$ and $\bar{X}$ are the sample means for $\vec{Y}_i$ and X_i, respectively; $S_{Y,X} = \frac{1}{n}\sum_{i=1}^{n}(X_i - \bar{X})\ (\vec{Y}_i - \bar{\vec{Y}})$; and λ_1 and λ_2 are the Lagrange-coefficients for conditional maximization with $\lambda_1 = (\vec{l}\,\bar{\vec{Y}} - c_1 - c_2\bar{X})/\vec{l}^{\,T}\Sigma\vec{l}$ and $\lambda_2 = [\vec{l}^{\,T} S_{Y,X} + \vec{l}^{\,T}\bar{\vec{Y}}\bar{X} - (c_1 + c_2)\bar{X} - c_2 S_{X,X}]/\vec{l}^{\,T}\Sigma\vec{l}$.

Step 3. Check the convergence of the unconditional log-likelihood function and decide to stop or go back to Step 1.

Based on the MLE, we can calibrate the unobserved underlying X based on measures from any one instrument by inverse linear calibration. Moreover, this model allows us to calibrate measures from instruments k to l by the following formula:

$$\hat{Y}_{i,l} = a_l + b_l(Y_{i,k} - a_k)/b_k. \tag{55}$$

Here, subscript i indicates the ith subject and k, l indicate the instruments; a_k, a_l, b_k, and b_l are the kth and lth components in the vectors $\vec{a}$ and $\vec{b}$, respectively.

A much simpler model is for $p = 3$, where the closed forms of MLEs can be derived and asymptotic covariance of the MLEs can be obtained explicitly.[84] This model has been used for standardization of bone mineral densities measured by three different manufacturers.[84, 86, 87]

5.3. *Least square approach for comparative calibrations*

Alternatively, we define $\vec{Y}'_i = \vec{Y}_i - \bar{\vec{Y}}$ and $\vec{X}_i = G\vec{Y}'_i + k$. Here, k is a real number and G is a $p \times p$ diagonal matrix, $G = \text{diag}(g_j)$ with $g_j \geq 0$. If $\vec{X}_i$ is the standard references for instruments, there should be no differences between any pairs of its components. Let H be a $p \times p$ matrix

$$H = \begin{bmatrix} 1 & -1 & 0 & \cdots & 0 & 0 \\ 0 & 1 & -1 & \cdots & 0 & 0 \\ \cdots & \cdots & \cdots & \cdots & \cdots & \cdots \\ 0 & 0 & 0 & \cdots & 1 & -1 \\ -1 & 0 & 0 & \cdots & 0 & 1 \end{bmatrix}.$$

Hui *et al.*[88] proposed to find g_j's that minimize the differences between components in vector $\overrightarrow{X}_i$[88]:

$$\min \sum_{i=1}^{n} \overrightarrow{X}_i^T H^T H \overrightarrow{X}_i = \min \sum_{i=1}^{n} (\overrightarrow{Y}_1 - \overline{\overrightarrow{Y}})^T G^T H^T H G (\overrightarrow{Y}_i - \overline{\overrightarrow{Y}}) \tag{56}$$

under constrains $\sum_{j=1}^{p} g_j^2 = p$. Because of the quadratic constrains, the solution for minimization Eq. (56) is not in a closed form. Symbolic programming languages, such as Maple, can be used to calculate the numeric solutions.

Like the latent structure models in the previous subsection, this model needs two constraints in order to make the model identifiable. The constant parameter k can be determined by a linear constraint as demonstrated in Hui *et al.*[88]

After we derive the solutions for g_j's, we can use the following formula to calibrate values between instruments:

$$Y_{i,j} = \bar{Y}_{.,j} + g_k/g_j(Y_{i,k} - \bar{Y}_{.,k}). \tag{57}$$

For $p = 3$, the calibration conversion formulas between instruments are the same for the least square approach [Eq. (57)] and latent structure model [Eq. (55)] if and only if the measurement errors of instruments in latent structure model σ_j^2 are equal.[84]

6. Conclusions

Radiological instrument quality is important for both clinical diagnosis of disease and clinical monitoring of patient changes. Quality assurance and quality improvement need efforts of people who involve in the processes of manufacturing, maintaining, and operating the equipment as well as statisticians who involved in assessing the quality, monitoring the changes in quality and identifying areas for quality improvement. In this chapter, we have introduced some statistical concepts and methods that are commonly used in quality assurance of radiology studies. There are many other materials and considerations that could not be covered because of the limitation of the space. The methods discussed in this chapter have applications beyond radiological studies and are relevant to most clinical studies. Quality assurance and quality control is rather a practice than a theoretical discussion. Successful quality assurance can have visible and immediate effects. Statisticians should actively participate in quality assurance. While it is important for clinicians and biomedical researchers to realize the importance of statistics in their quality control and quality assurance practice, it is also important for biostatisticians to understand the subject issues and communicate effectively statistical principles to scientists from different backgrounds. The collaborations between statisticians and biomedical researchers in other fields will not only benefit clinical researches but also lead to new challenges for research and development of new statistical methods.

References

1. Huxsoll, J. F. (1994). Organization of quality assurance. In *Quality Assurance for Biopharmaceuticals*, ed. J. F. Huxsoll, John Wiley and Sons, Inc., New York: 2–13.
2. Therasse, P. A., Arbuck, S. G., Eisenhauer, E. A., Wanders, J., Kaplan, R. S., Rubinstein, L., Verweij, J., Van Glabbeke, M. van Oosterom, A. T., Christian, M. C. and Gwyther, S. G. (2000). New guidelines to evaluate the response to treatment in solid tumors. *Journal of the National Cancer Institute* **92**(3): 205–216.
3. WHO. (1994). Assessment of fracture risk and its application to screening for postmenopausal osteoporosis. *Report of a WHO Study Group*. World Health Organization, Geneva.
4. Siris, E. (2000). Alendronate in the treatment of osteoporosis: A review of the clinical trials. *Journal of Womens Health and Gender-Based Medicine* **9**(6): 599–606.
5. Switula, D. (2000). Principles of good clinical practice (GCP) in clinical research. *Sciences Ethics and Engineering* **6**(1): 71–77.
6. van Kuijk, C. (1998). Good clinical practice in clinical trials: What does it mean for a radiology department? *Radiology* **209**(3): 625–627.
7. Fuerst, T., Lu, Y., Hans, D. and Genant, H. K. (1998). Quality assurance in bone densitometry. In *Bone Densitometry and Osteoporosis*, eds. H.K. Genant, G. Guglielmi and M. Jergas, Springer-Verlag, New York: 461–476.
8. Fraass, B. D. K., Hunt, M., Kutcher, G., Starkschall, G., Stern, R. and Van Dyke, J. (1998). American Association of Physicists in Medicine Radiation

Therapy Committee Task Group 53: Quality assurance for clinical radiotherapy treatment planning. *Medical Physics* **25**(10): 1773–1829.

9. Laurila, JS-N. C. G., Suramo, I., Tolppanen, E. M., Tervonen, O., Korhola, O. and Brommels, M. (2001). The efficacy of a continuous quality improvement (CQI) method in a radiological department. Comparison with non-CQI control material. *Acta Radiologica* **42**(1): 96–100.
10. Genant, H., Wu, C., van Kuijk, C. and Nevitt, M. (1993). Vertebral fracture assessment using a semiquantitative technique. *Journal of Bone and Mineral Research* **8**(9): 1137–1148.
11. Gluer, C., Blake, G., Lu, Y., Blunt, B., Jergas, M. and Genant, H. (1995). Accurate assessment of precision errors: How to measure the reproducibility of bone densitometry techniques. *Osteoporosis International* **5**: 262–270.
12. Njeh, C. F., Nicholson, P. H. F. and Langton, C. M. (1999). The physics of ultrasound applied to bone. In *Quantitative Ultrasound: Assessment of Osteoporosis and Bone Status.* eds. C.F. Njeh, D. Hans, T. Fuerst, C.C. Gluer and H.K. Genant, Martin Dunitz Ltd., London: 420.
13. Gluer, C. and Genant, H. (1989). Impact of marrow fat on accuracy of quantitative CT. *Journal of Computer Assistant Tomographics* **13**(6): 1023–1035.
14. Jergas, M. and Uffmann, M. (1998). Basic considerations and definitions in bone densitometry. In *Bone Densitometry and Osteoporosis*, eds. H. Genant, G. Guglielmi and M. Jergas, Springer, New York: 269–290.
15. Liu, C.-Y. and Zheng, Z.-Y. (1989). Stabilization coefficient to random variable. *Biometrical Journal* **31**(4): 431–441.
16. Miller, G. E. (1991). Asymptotic test statistics for coefficients of variation. *Communication in Statistics — Theory and Methods* **20**(10): 3351–3363.
17. Feltz, C. J. and Miller, G. E. (1996). An asymptotic test for the equality of coefficient of variation from *k* populations. *Statistics in Medicine* **15**: 647–658.
18. Fung, W. K. and Tsang, T. S. (1998). A simulation study comparing tests for the equality of coefficients of variation. *Statistics in Medicine* **17**: 2003–2014.
19. Arenson, R., Lu, Y., Elliott, S., Jovais, C. and Avrin, D. (2001). Measuring the academic radiologist's clinical productivity. *Academic Radiology* **8**: 524–532.
20. Efron, B. and Tibshirani, R. J. (1993). *An Introduction to the Bootstrap*, Chapman and Hall, San Francisco.
21. Shao, J. and Tu, D. (1995). *The Jackknife and Bootstrap*, Springer-Verlag, New York.
22. Strike, P. W. (1991). *Statistical Methods in Laboratory Medicine*, Butterworth-Heinemann Ltd., Oxford.
23. Quan, H. and Shih, W. J. (1996). Assessing reproducibility by the within-subject coefficient of variation with random effects models. *Biometrics* **52**(4): 1195–1203.
24. Miller, C. G., Herd, R. J., Ramalingam. T., Fogelman, I. and Blake, G. M. (1993). Ultrasounic velocity measurements through the calcaneus: Which velocity should be measured? *Osteoporosis International* **3**(1): 31–35.

25. Blake, G. M. and Fogelman, I. (1997). Technical principles of dual X-ray absorptiometry. *Seminar in Nuclear Medicine* **27**(3): 210–228.
26. Carroll, R. J., Ruppert, D. and Stefanski, L. A. (1995). *Measurement Error in Nonlinear Models*, Chapman and Hall, London.
27. Machado, A., Hannon, R., Henry, Y. and Estell, R. (1997). Standardized coefficient of variation for dual X-ray absorptiometry (DXA), quantitative ultrasound (QUS) and markers of bone turnover (Abstract). *Journal of Bone and Mineral Research* **12**(Suppl. 1): S258.
28. Langton, C. M. (1997). ZSD: A universal parameter for precision in the ultrasonic assessment of osteoporosis. *Physiological Measurement* **18**: 67–72.
29. Cummings, S. R. and Black, D. (1986). Should perimenopausal women be screened for osteoporosis? *Annals of Internal Medicine* **104**: 817–823.
30. Glüer C. (1999). Monitoring skeletal changes by radiological techniques. *Journal of Bone and Mineral Research* **14**(11): 1952–1962.
31. Faulkner, K. M., MR. (1995). Quality control of DXA instruments in multicenter trials. *Osteoporosis International* **5**(4): 218–227.
32. Kalender, W., Felsenberg, D., Genant, H. K., Fischer, M., Dequeker, J. and Reeve, J. (1995). The European spine phantom — A tool for standardization and quality control in spine bone mineral measurements by DXA and QCT. *European Journal of Radiology* **20**: 83–92.
33. Anderson, J. W. and Clarke, G. D. (2000). Choice of phantom material and test protocols to determine radiation exposure rates for fluoroscopy. *Radiographics* **20**(4): 1033–1042.
34. Lu, Y., Mathur, A. K., Blunt, B. A. *et al.* (1996). Dual X-ray absorptieometry quality control: Comparison of visual examination and process-control charts. *Journal of Bone and Mineral Research* **11**(5): 626–637.
35. Montgomery, D. C. (1992). *Introduction to Statistical Quality Control*, 2nd edn., Wiley, New York.
36. Orwoll, E. S., Oviatt, S. K. and Biddle, J. A. (1993). Precision of dual-energy X-ray absorptiometry: Development of quality control rules and their application in longitudinal studies. *Journal of Bone and Mineral Research* **8**(6): 693–699.
37. Jergas, M. and Genant, H. K. (1993). Current methods and recent advances in the diagnosis of osteoporosis. *Arthritis and Rheumatism* **36**(12): 1649–1662.
38. SAS/QC (2000). *User's Guide* (for SAS V8), SAS Research Institute, Cary, North Carolina.
39. Ryan, T. P. (1989). *Statistical Methods for Quality Improvement*, Wiley, New York.
40. Pearson, D. C. and Gawte, S. A. (1997). Long-term quality control of DXA: A comparison of Shewhart rules and Cusum charts. *Osteoporosis International* **7**(4): 338–343.
41. Lu, Y., Mathur, A. K., Gluer, C. C. *et al.* (1995). Application of statistical quality control method in multicenter osteoporosis clinical trials. *International Conference on Statistical Methods and Statistical Computation for Quality and Productivity Improvement*, Seoul, Korea, 474–480.

42. Wheeler, D. J. (1991). Shewhart's Chart: Myths, Facts, and Competitors. *45th Annual Quality Congress Transactions*: *American Society for Quality Control*, 533–538.
43. Johnson, R. A. and Bagshaw, M. (1974). The effect of serial correlation on the performance of CUSUM tests. *Technometrics* **16**: 103–112.
44. Kaminsky, F. C., Maleyeff, J., Providence, S., Purinton, E. and Waryasz, M. (1997). Using SPC (statistical process control) to analyze quality indicators in a healthcare organization. *Journal of Healthcare Risk Management* **17**(4): 14–22.
45. Quesenberry, C. P. (2000). Statistical process control geometric Q-chart for nosocomial infection surveillance. *American Journal of Infection Control* **28**(4): 314–20.
46. Thompson, J. R. and Koronachi, J. (1993). *Statistical Process Control for Quality Improvement*, Chapman and Hall, New York.
47. Bland, J. M. and Altman, D. G. (1986). Statistical methods for assessing agreement between two methods of clinical measurement. *The Lancet* **i**: 307–310.
48. Bland, J. M. and Altman, D. G. (1995). Comparing two methods of clinical measurement: A personal history. *International Journal of Epidemiology* **24**(Suppl. 1): S7–S14.
49. Bartko. J. J. (1994). General methodology II measures of agreement: A single procedure. *Statistics in Medicine* **13**: 737–745.
50. Bradley, E. L. and Blackwood, L. G. (1989). Comparing paired data: A simultaneous test of means and variances. *The American Statistician* **43**: 234–235.
51. Lee, J., Koh, D. and Ong, C. N. (1989). Statistical evaluation of agreement between two methods for measuring a quantitative variable. *Computers in Biology and Medicine* **19**: 61–70.
52. Fleiss, J. L. and Shrout, P. E. (1978). Approximate interval estimation for a certain intraclass correlation coefficient. *Psychometrika* **43**: 259–262.
53. Bland, J. M. and Altman, D. G. A note on the use of the intraclass correlation coefficient in the evaluation of agreement between two methods of measurements. *Computers in Biology and Medicine* **20**(5): 337–340.
54. Freedman, L. S., Parmar, M. K. B. and Baker, S. G. (1993). The design of observer agreement studies with binary assessements. *Statistics in Medicine* **12**: 165–179.
55. Cohen, J. A. (1960). A coefficient of agreement for nominal scales. *Educational and Psychological Measurement* **20**: 37–46.
56. Fleiss, J. L, Cohen, J. and Everitt, B. S. (1969). Large-sample standard errors of kappa and wieghted kappa. *Psychological Bulletin* **72**: 323–327.
57. Kraemer, H. C. (1980). Extension of the kappa coefficient. *Biometrics* **36**: 207–216.
58. Fleiss, J. L. and Davies, M. (1982). Jackknifing functions of multinomial frequencies, with an application to a measure of concordance. *American Journal of Epidemiology* **115**: 841–845.

59. Garner, J. B. (1991). The standard error of Cohen's Kappa. *Statistics in Medicine* **10**: 767–775.
60. Blackman, NJ.-M. and Koval, J. J. (2000). Interval estimation for Cohen's kappa as a measure of agreement. *Statistics in Medicine* **19**: 723–741.
61. Landis, J. R. and Koch, G. G. (1977). The measurement of observer agreement for categorical data. *Biometrics* **33**: 159–174.
62. Block, D. A. and Kraemer, H. C. (1989). 2 × 2 kappa coefficients: Measures of agreement or association. *Biometrics* **45**: 269–287.
63. Cohen, J. (1968). Weighted kappa: Nomial scale agreement with provision for scaled disagreement or partial credit. *Psycological Bulletin* **70**(4): 213–219.
64. Fleiss, J. L. (1981). *Statistical Methods for Rates and Proportions*, 2nd edn., Wiley, New York.
65. Barlow, W., Lai, M.-Y. and Azen, S. P. (1991). A comparison of methods for calculating a stratified kappa. *Statistics in Medicine* **10**: 1465–1472.
66. Donner, A. and Eliasziw, M. (1997). A hierachical approach to inferences concerning interobserver agreement for multinomial data. *Statistics in Medicine* **16**: 1097–1106.
67. Kraemer, H. C. and Bloch, D. A. (1990). A note on case-control sampling to estimate kappa coefficients. *Biometrics* **46**(1): 49–59.
68. Posner, K. L., Sampson, P. D., Caplan, R. A., Ward, R. J. and Cheney, F. W. (1990). Measuring interrater reliability among multiple raters: An example of methods for nominal data. *Statistics in Medicine* **9**: 1103–1115.
69. Oden, N. L. (1991). Estimating kappa from binocular data. *Statistics in Medicine* **10**: 1303–1311.
70. Shoukri, M. M. and Martin, S. W. (1995). Maximum likelihood estimation of the kappa coefficient from models of matched binary responses. *Statistics in Medicine* **14**: 83–99.
71. Shoukri, M. M. and Mian, I. U. H. (1996). Maximum likelihood estimation of the kappa coefficient from bivariate logistic regression. *Statistics in Medicine* **15**: 1409–1419.
72. Agresti, A. (1992). Modelling patters of agreement and disagreement. *Statistical Methods in Medical Research* **1**: 201–218.
73. Tanner, M. A. and Young, M. A. (1985). Modelling agreement among raters. *Journal of American Statistical Association* **80**: 175–180.
74. Aickin, M. (1990). Maximum likelihood estimation of agreement in the constant predictive probability model, and its relation to Cohen's kappa. *Biometrics* **46**: 293–302.
75. Graham. P. (1995). Modelling covariate effects in observer agreement studies: The case of nomial scale agreement. *Statistics in Medicine* **14**: 299–310.
76. Guggenmoos-Holzmann, I. and Vonk, R. (1998). Kappa-like indices of observer agreement viewed from a latent class prespective. *Statistics in Medicine* **17**: 797–812.
77. Baker, S. G., Freedman, L. S. and Parmar, M. K. B. (1991). Using replicate observations in observer agreement studies with binary assessments. *Biometrics* **47**(4): 1327–1338.

78. Cheng, C.-L. and Van Ness, J. W. (1999). *Statistical Regression with Measurement Error*, Arnold, London.
79. Barnett, D. V. (1969). Simultaneous pairwise linear structural relationships. *Biometrics* **28**: 129–142.
80. Theobald, C. M. and Mallinso, J. R. (1978). Comparative calibration, linear structural relationships and congeneric measurements. *Biometrics* **34**: 39–45.
81. Fuller, W. A. (1987). *Measurement Error Models*, Wiley, New York.
82. Dunn, G. (1989). *Design and Analysis of Reliability Studies*, Oxford University Press, New York.
83. Kimura, D. K. (1992). Functional comparative calibration using EM algorithm. *Biometrics* **48**: 1263–1271.
84. Lu, Y., Ye, K., Mathur, A., Hui, S., Fuerst, T. P. and Genant, H. K. (1997). Comparative calibration without a gold standard. *Statistics in Medicine* **16**: 1889–1905.
85. Lu, Y., Ye, K., Mathur, A. K., Srivastav, S. K., Yang, S. and Genant, H. K. (1997). Application of random effects models in comparative calibration. *Proceedings of the Biometrics Section of American Statistical Association*, 170–176.
86. Hanson, J. (1997). Standardization of femur BMD [letter]. *Journal of Bone and Mineral Research* **12**(8): 1316–1317.
87. Lu, Y., Fuerst, T., Hui, S. and Genant, H. K. (2001). Standardization of bone mineral density at femoral neck, trochanter and Ward's triangle. *Osteoporosis International* **12**: 438–444.
88. Hui, S. L., Gao, S., Zhou, X.-H. *et al.* (1997). Universal standardization of bone density measurements: A method with optimal properties for calibration among several instruments. *Journal of Bone and Mineral Research* **12**(9): 1463–1470.

About the Author

Ying Lu, Ph.D., is a Professor of Biostatistics, Department of Health Research and Policy, Stanford University and Director of the Palo Alto VA Cooperative Studies Program Coordinating Center at Palo Alto Veterans Affairs Health Care System. He received his Bachelors of Science in Mathematics from Fudan University 1982, Master of Science in Applied Mathematics from Shanghai Jiao Tong University 1984, both in Shanghai, China, and his Ph.D. in Biostatistics from the University of California, Berkeley, 1990, California, USA. After graduation, he worked as an assistant professor at the University Miami School of Medicine 1990–1994, assistant, associate and full professor at the University of California, San Francisco, from 1994–2009, and professor in biostatistics at the Stanford University. Dr. Lu's research focuses on biostatistics methodology development and application to address clinical questions, in particular, in medical diagnosis, clinical trial design, and medical decision making. He is a fellow of the American Statistical Association (2011) and president elect of the International Chinese Statistical Association 2013. Further information is available from: http://med.stanford.edu/profiles/Ying_Lu/.

Shoujun Zhao, Ph.D., studied medicine from 1977 to 1982, and got his biostatistics master degree in Shanxi Medical College in 1986, then he received his PhD. degree of epidemiology from Shanghai Medical University in 1993, and worked there as an associate professor for three years. Dr Zhao participated in hepatitis A and B studies of Chinese National 8/5 and 9/5 Projects and received the prestigious China National Science and Technology Progress Award in 2000. Dr Zhao finished his post-doctoral training in the Department of Radiology at the University of California, San Francisco in 2000. Since then, he has been working as a biostatistics specialist in medical research areas, including clinical trial design, data quality control, large scale medical database management and analysis. His main interests are in the areas of infectious disease transmission model, multivariate statistical mode application and diagnostic statistical methods.

CHAPTER 6

APPLICATIONS OF STATISTICAL METHODS IN MEDICAL IMAGING

JESSE S. JIN

Department of Computer Science,
University of Sydney NSW 2006, Australia
Jesse.Jin@newcastle.edu.au

Medical images are two-dimensional stochastic signals. There are many common issues of stochastic signals such as noise removal, signal restoration, signal sampling, etc. There are also many special issues which are relevant to high dimensional signals only, such as segmentation, clustering, etc. This chapter discusses issues of medical imaging. In particular, we will discuss the application of statistical methods in this area.

1. Introduction

Medical imaging is a fast growing area with the richest source of information and variety of modalities such as Magnetic Resonance Imaging (MRI), X-ray Transmission Imaging (X-ray), Computerised Tomography (CT), ultrasound images (both 2D and 3D), Positron Emission Tomography (PET), Single-Photon Computed Tomography (SPECT), Magnetic Source Imaging (MSI), Electrical Source Imaging (ESI), X-ray Mammography (MG), Orthopantomograms (OPG), and many others.

MRI is one of the most powerful non-invasive techniques in diagnostic clinical medicine and biomedical research. The technique is an application of nuclear magnetic resonance (NMR), a well-known analytical method of chemistry, physics and molecular structural biology. MRI is primarily used as a technique for producing anatomical images, but MRI also gives information on the physical-chemical state of tissues, flow diffusion and motion information. Magnetic Resonance Spectroscopy (MRS) gives chemical/composition information. MRI has revolutionised imaging of the brain, spine and the musculoskeletal system. Superb soft tissue contrast and spatial resolution have made MRI the investigation of choice in many neurologic and orthopaedic diseases.

X-rays are generated by the interaction of accelerated electrons with a target material (usually tungsten). X-rays are deflected and absorbed to different degrees by the various tissues and bones in the patient's body. The amount of absorption depends on the tissue composition. For example, dense bone matter will absorb many more X-rays than soft tissues, such as muscle, fat and blood. The amount of deflection depends on the density of electrons in the tissues. Tissues with high electron densities cause more X-ray scattering than those of lower density. Thus, since less photons reach the X-ray film after encountering bone or metal rather than tissue, the X-ray will look brighter for bone or metal.

CT became generally available in the mid 1970s and is considered one of the major technological advances of medical science. X-ray CT gives anatomical information on the positions of air, soft tissues, and bone. Three-dimensional imaging is achieved by rotating an X-ray emitter around the patient, and measuring the intensity of transmitted rays from different angles.

Ultrasound, as currently practiced in medicine, is a real-time tomographic imaging modality. Not only does it produce real-time tomograms of the position of reflecting surfaces (internal organs and structures), but it can be used to produce real-time images of tissue and blood motion.

The history of PET can be traced to the early 1950s, when workers in Boston first realized the medical imaging possibilities of a particular class of radioactive isotopes. Whereas most radioactive isotopes decay by release of a gamma ray and electrons, some decay by the release of a positron. A positron can be thought of as a positive electron. Widespread interest and an acceleration in PET technology was stimulated by development of reconstruction algorithms associated with X-ray CT and improvements in nuclear detector technologies. By the mid-1980s, PET had become a tool for medical diagnosis, for dynamic studies of human metabolism and for studies of brain activation.

PET has a million fold sensitivity advantage over other techniques used to study regional metabolism and neuroreceptor activity in the brain and other body tissues. In contrast, magnetic resonance has exquisite resolution for anatomic studies and for flow or angiographic studies. In addition, magnetic resonance spectroscopy has the unique attribute of evaluating chemical composition of tissue but in the millimolar range rather than the nanomolar range. Since the nanomolar range is the concentration range of most receptor proteins in the body, positron emission tomography is ideal for this type of imaging. The major clinical applications of PET have been in cancer detection of the brain, breast, heart, lung and colorectal tumors. Another application is the evaluation of coronary artery disease by imaging the metabolism of heart muscle.

SPECT, like PET, acquires information on the concentration of radionuclides introduced to the patients body. SPECT dates from the early 1960s, when the idea of emission traverse section tomography was introduced by D. E. Kuhl and R. Q. Edwards prior to either PET, X-ray CT, or MRI.

Iron currents arising in the neurons of the heart and the brain produce magnetic fields outside the body. These fields can be measured by arrays of SQUID (Superconducting QUantum Interference Device), detectors that are placed on or near the head or chest. The recording of magnetic fields of the head is known as MagnetoEncephaloGraphy (MEG) while that of the heart is called MagnetoCardioGraphy (MCG). Magnetic Source Imaging (MSI) is the general term for the reconstruction of current sources in the heart or brain from the measurements of external magnetic fields.

Electrical source imaging (ESI) is an emerging technique for reconstructing electrical activity in the brain or heart from electric potentials measured on the scalp or torso. Standard ElectroEncephaloGraphic (EEG), ElectroCardioGraphic (ECG) and VectorCardioGraphic (VCG) techniques are limited in their ability to provide information on regional electrical activity or localize bioelectrical events within the brain and heart. Noninvasive ESI of the brain requires simultaneous electric potential recordings from 20 or more electrodes for the brain and 100 to 250 torso electrode sites to map the body surface potential from the heart.

X-ray mammography (MG) is an effective method to diagnose the breast cancer. A low dose X-ray screening mammograms are performed on a woman's breasts with no symptoms to detect breast cancer at an early stage. The practice can perform diagnostic mammography. Breast needle localisation prior to surgery can be performed to provide location information and fine tissue information.

Orthopantomograms (OPG) and lateral cephalograms are the latest techniques for dental or orthodontic assessment.

Medical images are 2D stochastic signals. There are many common issues of stochastic signals such as noise removal, signal restoration, signal sampling, etc. There are also many special issues which are relevant to high dimensional signals only, such as segmentation, clustering, etc. We will discuss issues of medical imaging. In particular, we will discuss the image sampling and compression in Sec. 2, filtering in Sec. 3, segmentation in Sec. 4 and registration in Sec. 5. Finally, there is a conclusion.

2. Sampling and Compression Using Statistical Features of Images

Computer-based advanced medical imaging techniques such as Positron Emission Tomography (PET) have been playing a crucial and expanding role in modern medical research and diagnosis. However, these powerful techniques have being accompanied by the growing size of image data sets as well. For example, a routine dynamic PET study using the CTI 951 scanner usually acquires 31 cross-sectional image planes of 128×128 pixels each, at 20 to 30 time points. It results a 4D data set containing up to 11 million data points with approximately 22 Mbytes storage space. As the resolution of current PET imaging improves, the large volume of related data will further increase. It has therefore, prompted significant recent interest in developing efficient image compression techniques which can contribute to the current expansion in medical digitalization, image database management and telemedicine.

Taking advantage of domain specific physiological kinetic knowledge related to dynamic PET images and physiological tracer kinetic modeling, this paper presents a novel knowledge-based near-lossless data compression algorithm for dynamic PET images. The proposed compression algorithm consists of three stages: (a) compression in the temporal domain using optimal image sampling schedule design; (b) compression in the spatial domain through cluster analysis; and (c) index image compression using standard still image compression techniques. In this section, clinical human brain PET studies using the $[^{18}F]$ *2-fluoro-deoxy-glucose* (FDG) tracer are presented to illustrate the proposed compression algorithm. The technique can be easily applied to other PET studies with different tracers. The conventional[22] and proposed techniques are implemented on clinical dynamic PET images. Empirical results are given to illustrate the compression performance and the image quality.

2.1. *Tracer kinetic modeling and functional imaging*

Tracer kinetic techniques with PET are widely applied to extract valuable information from dynamic processes in the body. This information is usually defined in terms of a mathematical model $u(\boldsymbol{t}|\boldsymbol{p})$, where $\boldsymbol{t} = 1, 2, \ldots, T$ and $\boldsymbol{p}$ are the model parameters. The parameters describe the delivery, transport and biochemical transformation of the tracer. The driving function for the model is the plasma blood input function, which is often obtained from blood sampling.[22] Measurements acquired by PET define the tissue time activity curve (TAC), or output function, denoted $z_i(\boldsymbol{t})$, where $\boldsymbol{t} = 1, 2, \ldots, T$ are discrete sampling times of the measurements, and $i = 1, 2, \ldots, I$ corresponds to the ith pixel in the imaging region. The purpose of dynamic PET image analysis is to obtain tracer TACs and parameter estimates for each pixel in the imaging region. These parameters can then be used to define physiological parameters, such as the local cerebral metabolic rate of glucose (LCMRGlc).

The conventional method uses the complete set of acquired PET projection data. Through the parameter estimation on a pixel-by-pixel basis using certain rapid estimation algorithms,[16, 22, 36] functional images can be generated. In this section, the Patlak method[35, 36] was used to generate the LCMRGlc functional images for the purpose of comparing the estimation accuracy of the original and compressed data.

2.2. *Sampling and compression in temporal and spatial domains*

The sampling and compression scheme using statistical features of tracer kinetics consists of three stages.[6]

2.2.1. *Stage* 1: *Compression in the temporal domain using optimal image sampling schedule*

In dynamic PET studies, the reliability of temporal frames is directly influenced by the sampling schedules and duration used to acquire the data. The longer the duration and greater the radio-activity counts, the more reliable the temporal frames. However, in order to obtain quantitative information from the dynamic processes, a certain number of temporal frames are required. Recently, it has been shown that the minimum number of temporal frames required is equal to the number of model parameters to be estimated.[26] Based on this, an algorithm that automatically determines optimal image sampling schedule (OISS) and maximizes the information content of the acquired PET data was developed.[26] The algorithm utilizes the accumulated/integral PET measurements.

In the design of OISS, a new objective function based on the *Fisher Information Matrix*,[10] was proposed to limit the loss of dynamic information. This objective function was used to discriminate between different experimental protocols and sampling schedules. OISS can be directly applied to acquisition of PET projection data. This reduces the number of temporal frames obtained and therefore, reduces data storage. Furthermore, as fewer temporal frames are reconstructed the computational burden posed by image reconstruction is reduced. Details of this algorithm can be found in Li *et al.*[26]

2.2.2. *Stage* 2: *Compression in the spatial domain through cluster analysis*

The prior knowledge has the form of tracer kinetic model to a time series of PET tracer uptake measurements. From the model, using cluster analysis, the image-wide TACs can be extracted and further classified into a certain numbers of TAC groups which corresponding to different tissue regions, according to the similarity of their kinetics.

Cluster analysis aims at grouping and classifying image-wide TACs, $z_i(t)$ (where $i = 1, 2, \ldots, I$), into C_j cluster groups (where $j = 1, 2, \ldots, J$ and $J \ll I$) by measuring the magnitude of natural association (similarity characteristics). It is expected that TACs with high degrees of natural association will belong to different groups.[8] It should be noted that each TAC must be assigned uniquely to a cluster group. In this paper, a hierarchical-agglomerative clustering algorithm based on the Euclidean distance measurement was used to classify the clinical dynamic PET image data.

Using the results of cluster analysis, an index table containing the mean TAC within each cluster and an indexed image can be formed. The indexed image represents a mapping from the cluster to its respective pixel TAC locations. This image together with the index table forms the basis of the compressed temporal/spatial data. With PET, the number of distinguishable clustering groups may generally not exceed 64. This means that an 8-bit indexed image is sufficient to represent the cluster mapping.

2.2.3. *Stage* 3: *Index image compression*

A lossless compression scheme is considered in this paper for further reduction of the indexed image. The PNG (Portable Network Graphics)[11] format was used to compress and store the indexed image obtained from cluster analysis. The coding technique presently defined and implemented for PNG is based on deflate/inflate compression with a 32-Kb sliding window. The PNG format was chosen over other lossless image compression file formats due to its portability, flexibility and being legally unencumbered. Details on the PNG format can be found in Crocker.[11]

Human dynamic FDG-PET brain studies were performed using an eight-ring, fifteen-slice PET scanner (GE/Scanditronix PC4096-15WB).

This scanner contains 4096 detectors and achieves axial and trans-axial resolutions of 6.5-mm full width at half maximum (FWHM) at the center of the field of view. Between 200 and 400 mBq (approximately 0.5 mg) of FDG was injected intravenously and arterial blood sampling commenced immediately thereafter. The blood samples (each 2–3 ml) were taken at 8×0.25 minute intervals for the first 2 minutes, then at 2.5, 3, 3.5, 7, 10, 15, 20, 30, 60, 90 and 120 minutes. These samples were immediately placed on ice and the plasma was subsequently separated for the determination of plasma FDG and "cold" glucose concentration. Figure 1(a) shows a set of temporal frames for the 15th plane from one patient study. Due to the lower tracer concentration in the first few frames, these images were scaled to be visible.

3. Noise Reduction Using Statistical Anisotropic Diffusion

Diffusion processes have been widely used in quantum physics, material science, fluid dynamics, nuclear science, medicine and chemical physics. Perona and Malik[38,39] introduced it to image processing and proposed a multi-scale smoothing and edge detection scheme. It has the good property of eliminating noise while preserving high frequency components, namely edges.[2]

Diffusion is an iterative process. The degree of diffusion depends on the threshold of diffusion, i.e. the contrast cut-off. A contrast above the threshold will be enhanced during the diffusion process and that below the threshold will be smoothed out. The selection of the threshold is vital to the filtering process. However, the threshold varies from image to image. The problem compounds with the contrast variation from region to region and with intensity distortion of the same region in an image. It is thus desirable to have an adaptive criterion for selecting a threshold.

The threshold in a diffusion process is closely correlated with the contrast of the edges in an image. Selecting the threshold is a process of analysing local contrast. In low contrast images, especially when noise is present and the signal-noise ratio (SNR) is low, the contrast between regions is not significant and will be very difficult to pick up. The difficulty lies in the noise presence, unknown distribution of a stochastic signal, and unknown combination of multiple interferences. In most of these cases, the histogram of the region shows a single peak. Many automatic threshold selection mechanisms require a bi-peak histogram such as Tsai and Chen[46] and Bhandari *et al.*[5] A bi-peak or multi-peak histogram may not exist in many cases. Luijendijk[29] proposed an automatic threshold selection

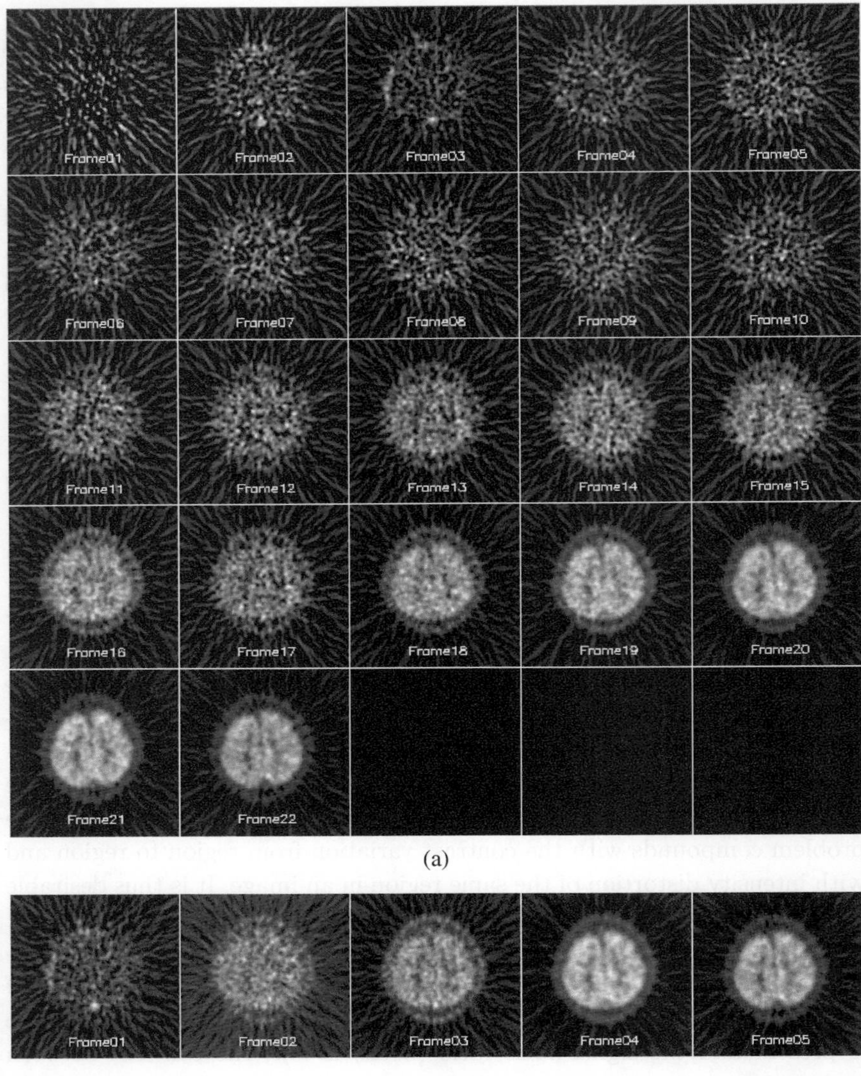

Fig. 1. Compression results. (a) A set of 22 temporal-frame images (scaled) for the 15th plane from one patient study. (b) Results of the proposed compression method in temporal domain: 5 temporal-frame images (scaled), obtained from 1(a).

using two histograms based on the count of 4-connected regions. Tseng and Huang[47] proposed to select the threshold using edge information, i.e. the intensity along edge intervals. Nagawa and Rosenfeld[33] fitted the histogram with two Gaussian functions, and Cho *et al.*[7] applied bias correction factors. Glaseby[18] combined them with an amendment using iteration. The assumption of Gaussian distribution is weak and correction does not make up this vital defect. Furthermore, iteration makes the computation very expensive.

Another difficulty is due to intensity distortion. The applicability of histogram analysis is based on the assumption that all image pixels which have a similar grey level correspond to one object or region of interest in the image. However, this assumption is not always true for most images. Rodriguez and Mitchell[41] used an adaptive thresholding method that extracts the background in two phases. The first step uses a global threshold to extract the structure of the regions and the second step refines the segmentation. Parker[34] used a local threshold to grow a region after finding a seed pixel in an object. Spann and Horne[44] grow regions from low resolution to high resolution in a quadtree structure. The adaptive scheme is a proper way to combat the distortion of intensity. However, the above mentioned methods have a try-and-error nature and do not have a solid theoretical foundation.

This section describes an adaptive diffusion scheme by applying the Central Limit Theorem. Regression is used to separate the distribution of the major object in a local window from other objects in a single-peak histogram. The separation will help to automatically determine the threshold. We have applied the algorithm to X-ray angiogram (XRA) images to extract brain arteries. The algorithm works well for single-peak distributions where there are no valleys in the histograms. It has also been used for filtering microscope images of kidneys where there are multiple visual objects and the contrast between objects is very low. The scheme shows that a fully automatic filtering process can be achieved. It works well with images which have texture patterns and are contaminated with noise while the distribution of noise is unknown. These kinds of images have posed a significant problem for traditional filtering schemes such as wavelet based de-noising.[13]

3.1. *Non-linear anisotropic diffusion*

Low-pass filters have been used to remove noise. Most filters are isotropic. Isotropic filtering tends to smear the corners and loses the accuracy of edges.

To examine the problem carefully, we notice that the gradient along an edge is not isotropic. It has the highest value perpendicular to the edge and is dilated along the edge. It is therefore proper to increase the smoothing function parallel to the edge and stop the smoothing perpendicular to the edge. Non-linear anisotropic diffusion provides such a function. It takes the form

$$\frac{\partial}{\partial t} I(x,y,t) = \operatorname{div}(g(\nabla I)\nabla I), \tag{1}$$

where $I(x, y, t)$ is the signal and $g(\nabla I)$ is a dilation function of gradients. There are two frequently used dilation functions:

$$g_1(x,y,t) = \frac{1}{1 + \frac{\nabla I(x,y,t)}{k}}, \tag{2}$$

$$g_2(x,y,t) = \exp\left\{-\left(\frac{\nabla I(x,y,t)}{k}\right)^2\right\}. \tag{3}$$

Calculation of diffusive filtering can be performed by a difference operation

$$\begin{aligned}
\frac{\partial}{\partial t} I(x,y,t) &= \operatorname{div}[g(x,y,t) * \nabla I(x,y,t)] \\
&= \frac{\partial}{\partial t}\left[g(x,y,t) * \frac{\partial}{\partial x} I(x,y,t)\right] + \frac{\partial}{\partial y}\left[g(x,y,t) * \frac{\partial}{\partial y} I(x,y,t)\right] \\
&= g(x+1,y,t)[I(x+1,y,t) - I(x,y,t)] \\
&\quad + g(x,y,t)[I(x-1,y,t) - I(x,y,t)] \\
&\quad + g(x,y+1,t)[I(x,y,+1,t) - I(x,y,t)] \\
&\quad + g(x,y,t)[I(x,y,-1,t) - I(x,y,t)] \\
&= \Phi'_e + \Phi'_w + \Phi'_s + \Phi'_n\,.
\end{aligned} \tag{4}$$

Diffusion encourages intra-region smoothing in preference to smoothing across boundaries. The basis of this method is to suppress smoothing at boundaries by selecting locally adaptive diffusion strengths. The parameter κ plays an important role in diffusion. If the κ value is set to too high the filter will act as a smoothing filter, diffusing across the edge boundary; while if κ is too low, small dilation will result in many iterations. At some κ values, an extra edge will be introduced between the region of high intensity and region of low intensity. Therefore, the vital question in our design is the selection of κ.

3.2. *Selection of the cut-off contrast*

Images requiring processing often have very low contrast with many intensity layers. Determining an appropriate threshold for such images is difficult. Figure 2 shows an XRA image of the brain artery (a) and its histogram (b) which is a single peak histogram. The selection of a threshold value from such a histogram is ambiguous and not viable by trial and error. We have developed a region-based method to dynamically select a threshold using regression.

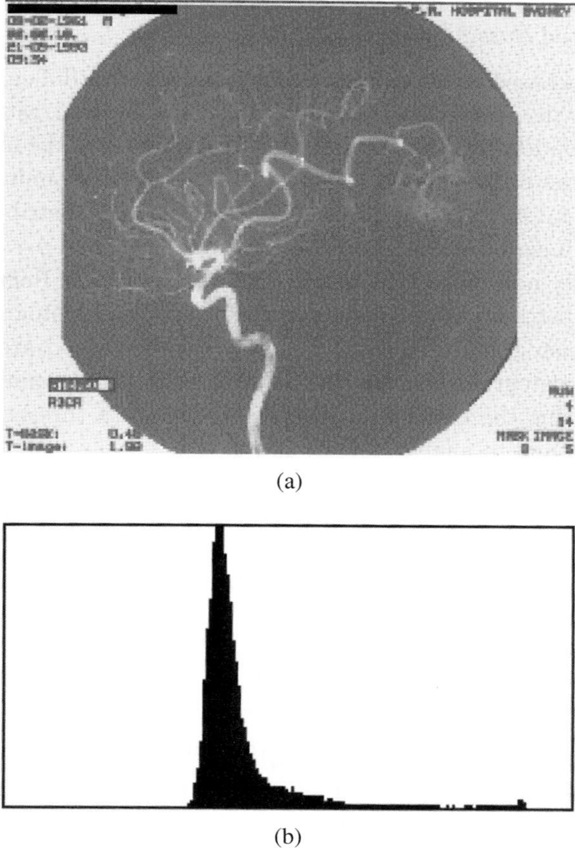

Fig. 2. Histogram analysis on background. (a) An XRA image; (b) Its histogram.

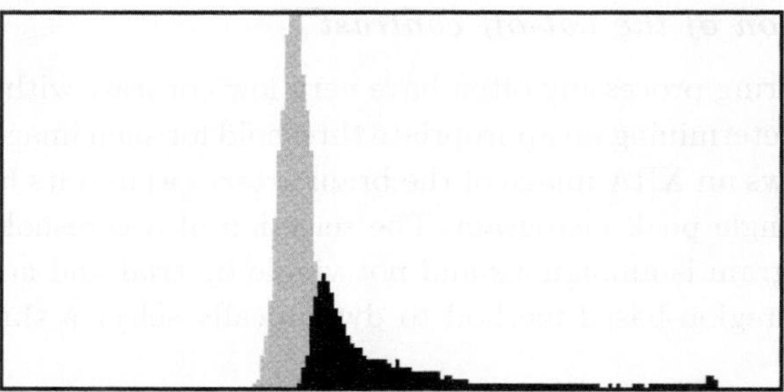

Fig. 3. Segmenting histogram using Gaussian regression.

3.2.1. *Selecting the threshold by regression and likelihood classification*

Our scheme is based on the Central Limit Theorem. It is difficult to segment brain arteries from the background because of the low contrast and an overwhelming proportion of the background. We do not know the histogram distribution of the background. However, from the Central Limit Theorem we know that if $x_1, x_2, \ldots, x_n$ are independent, identically distributed random variables with expectation μ and finite variance σ^2, then $y = \frac{1}{n}\sum_{i=1}^{n} x_i$ is asymptotically normal (μ, σ^2) when n is large enough.[42] Regression using a Gaussian distribution can separate the background histogram from the foreground histogram, as shown in Fig. 3, where shaded area shows the background histogram and the darker area is the foreground histogram. After separating the histogram, it is easy to select a threshold for image segmentation and to analyse foreground objects.

The sampling data for regression is obtained from partial histogram. We calculate the mean value of the histogram and take the half with less variance. Then we find the modal of that half histogram. The sampling data, $h_i, i \in S$, is on the same side with the modal against the mean value. The regression is obtained by

$$\begin{cases} \mu = \max\limits_{i \in s}(h_i) \\ \sigma = \sqrt{2 \sum\limits_{i \in_s} (h_i - \mu)^2} \,. \end{cases}$$

However, when the number of background pixels is not large enough, it is improper to use the Gaussian distribution in regression. Figure 4 shows another XRA image (a) and its histogram (b). Figure 4(c) is the histogram

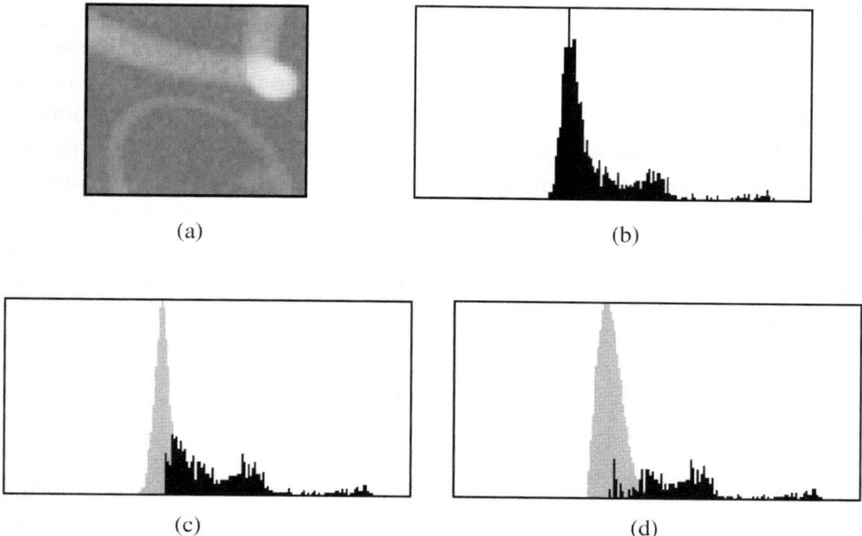

Fig. 4. Segmentation using regressions. (a) The original image; (b) Its histogram; (c) Gaussian regression does not show clear separation; (d) Rayleigh regression shows a clear separation.

after regression using Gaussian distribution over the background. It does not show a valley between two peaks as we expect, which means there is no clear separation. In this situation, we apply the Rayleigh distribution in regression. Probability theory states that when n is not large enough, $x = \bar{x}_n$ satisfies Rayleigh distribution:

$$f(x) = \begin{cases} \dfrac{x}{\mu^2} e^{\frac{x^2}{2\mu^2}} & x \geq 0 \\ 0 & x < 0 \,. \end{cases}$$

The Rayleigh regression is obtained by

$$\begin{cases} \mu = \sqrt{\dfrac{\pi}{2}} \max\limits_{i \in s}(h_i) \\ \sigma = \sqrt{\dfrac{4-\pi}{2} \mu^2} \,. \end{cases}$$

3.2.2. *Extracting a cut-off contrast*

The diffusion process is critically depended on the κ value in functions (2) and (3). The parameter κ can be associated with the contrast. The following discussion on extracting κ will be based on diffusion function (2) but it can be easily converted to function (3) by dividing κ by $\sqrt{2}$. Although we can obtain a proper estimation of the distribution of one visual object in the image, e.g. background in XRA images, we do not have information on other objects, e.g. vessels in XRA images. It is very difficult to estimate the average contrast between two objects. We use likelihood classification[45] to separate pixels from two objects after we separate the background histogram from the foreground histogram. These two histograms are used as the probability distributions of two clusters in likelihood classification. We calculate κ value from the following

$$\kappa = \left\{ l \,\middle|\, \max_{l\in\{0..255\}} \left(\sum_{P\in p}^{N_l} \nabla_p I(x,y)/N_l \right) \right\},$$

where N_l is the pixel number with gray level l, and P is a set of neighboring pixel pairs whose two pixels belong to different clusters. This calculation can be restricted to a local region. If two neighbor pixels belong to two clusters, we accumulate their difference into a difference histogram. The contrast can be extracted from the modal of differences within a local region.

4. Medical Imaging Segmentation

Segmentation is the process in which an image is divided into constituent objects or parts. It is often the first and most vital step in an image analysis task. Effective segmentation can usually dictate eventual success of the analysis. For this reason, many segmentation techniques have been developed by researchers worldwide.[19] Segmentation of intensity images usually involves four main approaches, namely thresholding, boundary detection, region-based and hybrid methods.

Thresholding techniques[43] are based on the postulate that all pixel whose value lie within a certain range belongs to one class. Such methods neglect all of the spatial information of the image and do not cope well with noise or blurring at boundaries.

Boundary-based methods are sometimes called edge-detection,[12] because they assume that pixel values change rapidly at the boundary between two regions. The basic method is to apply a gradient filter to the image. High values of this filter provide candidates for region boundaries, which must then be modified to produce closed curves representing the boundaries between regions.

Region-based segmentation algorithms postulate that neighbouring pixels within the same region have similar intensity values, of which the split-and-merge[21] technique based on homogeneity criterion is probably the most well know. It includes seeded region growing[32] and unseeded region growing.

Hybrid methods combine one or more of the above-mentioned criteria. This class includes the morphological watershed[32] segmentation, variable-order surface fitting[4] and active contour[24] methods.

This section presents two methods among which statistical features are used in segmentation.

4.1. *Probilistical segmentation using expectation-maximization*

Intensity-based classification of MR images has proven problematic, even when advanced techniques are used. Intra-scan and inter-scan intensity inhomogeneities are a common source of difficulty. While reported methods have had some success in correcting intra-scan inhomogeneities, such methods require supervision for the individual scan. This section describes a new method called adaptive segmentation that uses knowledge of tissue intensity properties and intensity inhomogeneities to correct and segment MR images. Use of the EM algorithm leads to a method that allows for more accurate segmentation of tissue types as well as better visualization of MRI data, that has proven to be effective in a study that includes more than 1000 brain scans. Implementation and results are described for segmenting the brain in the following types of images: axial (dual-echo spin-echo), coronal (3DFT gradient-echo T1-weighted) all using a conventional head coil; and a sagittal section acquired using a surface coil. The accuracy of adaptive segmentation was found to be comparable with manual segmentation, and closer to manual segmentation than supervised multi-variate classification while segmenting gray and white matter.

Advanced applications that use the morphologic contents of MRI frequently require segmentation of the imaged volume into tissue types. Such tissue segmentation is often achieved by applying statistical classification methods to the signal intensities[25, 49] in conjunction with morphological image processing operations.[9, 17]

Conventional intensity-based classification of MR images has proven problematic, however, even when advanced techniques such as non-parametric, multi-channel methods are used. Intra-scan intensity inhomogeneities due to

RF coils or acquisition sequences (e.g. susceptibility artifacts in gradient echo images) are a common source of difficulty. Although MRI images may appear visually uniform, such intra-scan inhomogeneities often disturb intensity-based segmentation methods. In the ideal case, differentiation between white and gray matter in the brain should be easy since these tissue types exhibit distinct signal intensities. In practice, spatial intensity inhomogeneities are often of sufficient magnitude to cause the distributions of signal intensities associated with these tissue classes to overlap significantly. In addition, the operating conditions and status of the MR equipment frequently affect the observed intensities, causing significant inter-scan intensity inhomogeneities that often necessitate manual training on a per-scan basis.

Intra- and inter-scan MRI intensity inhomogeneities is modeled with a spatially-varying factor called the *gain field* that multiplies the intensity data. The application of a logarithmic transformation to the intensities allows the artifact to be modeled as an additive *bias* field. If the gain field is known, then it is relatively easy to estimate tissue class by applying a conventional intensity-based segmenter to the corrected data. Similarly, if the tissue classes are known, then it is straightforward to estimate the gain field by comparing predicted intensities and observed intensities. It may be problematic, however, to determine either the gain or the tissue type without knowledge of the other. It will be shown that it is possible to estimate both using an iterative algorithm (that converges in five to ten iterations, typically).

A Bayesian approach is used to estimating the bias field that represents the gain artifact in log-transformed MR intensity data. First, a logarithmic transformation of the intensity data is computed as follows:

$$Y_i = g(X_i) = (\ln([X_i]_1), \ln([X_i]_2), \ldots, \ln([X_i]_m))^T \,, \tag{5}$$

where X_i is the observed MRI signal intensity at the ith voxel, and m is the dimension of the MRI signal.

Similar to other statistical approaches to intensity-based segmentation of MRI,[9,17] the distribution for observed values is modeled as a normal distribution (with the incorporation of an explicit bias field):

$$p(Y_i|\Gamma_i, \beta_i) = G_{\psi\Gamma_i}(Y_i) - \mu(\Gamma_i) - (\beta_i) \,, \tag{6}$$

where

$$G_{\psi\Gamma_i}(x) = (2\pi)^{-\frac{m}{2}} |\psi_{\Gamma_i}|^{-\frac{1}{2}} \exp\left(-\frac{1}{2}x^T \psi_{\Gamma_i}^{-1} x\right)$$

is the m-dimensional Gaussian distribution with variance ψ_{Γ_i} and where

Y_i is the observed log-transformed intensities at the ith voxel;
Γ_i is the tissue class at the ith voxel;
$\mu(x)$ is the mean intensity for tissue class x;
ψ_x is the covariance matrix for tissue class x;
β_i is bias field at the ith voxel.

Here, Y_i, $\mu(x)$, and β_i are represented by m-dimensional column vectors, while ψ_x is represented by an $m \times m$ matrix. Note that the bias field has a separate value for each component of the log-intensity signal at each voxel. In words, (6) states that the probability of observing a particular image intensity, given knowledge of the tissue class and the bias field is given by a Gaussian distribution centered at the biased mean intensity for the class.

A stationary prior (before the image data is seen) probability distribution on tissue class is used, it is denoted as $p(\Gamma_i)$.

If this probability is uniform over tissue classes, our method devolves to a maximum-likelihood approach to the tissue classification component. A spatially-varying prior probability density on brain tissue class has been studies.[23] Such a model might profitably be used within this framework.

The entire bias field is denoted by $\beta = (\beta_0, \beta_1, \ldots, \beta_{n-1})^T$, where n is the number of voxels of data. The bias field is modeled by a n-dimensional zero mean Gaussian prior probability density. This model allows us to capture the smoothness that is apparent in these inhomogeneities:

$$p(\beta) = G_{\psi_\beta}(\beta)\,, \tag{7}$$

where

$$G_{\psi_\beta}(\beta) = (2\pi)^{-\frac{n}{2}} |\psi_{\beta_i}|^{-\frac{1}{2}} \exp\left(-\frac{1}{2} x^T \psi_{\beta_i}^{-1} x\right)$$

is the n-dimensional Gaussian distribution. The $n \times n$ covariance matrix for the entire bias field is denoted ψ_β. Although ψ_β will be too large to manipulate directly in practice, tractable estimators can result when ψ_β is chosen so that it is banded.

It is assumed that the bias field and the tissue classes are statistically independent, this follows if the intensity inhomogeneities originate in the equipment. Using the definition of conditional probability the joint probability on intensity and tissue class can be obtained as follows:

$$p(Y_i, \Gamma_i | \beta_i) = p(Y_i | \Gamma_i, \beta_i) p(\Gamma_i)\,, \tag{8}$$

and we may obtain the conditional probability of intensity alone by computing a marginal over tissue class:

$$p(Y_i|\beta_i) = \sum_{\Gamma_i} p(Y_i, \Gamma_i|\beta_i) = \sum_{\Gamma_i} p(Y_i|\Gamma_i, \beta_i)p(\Gamma_i)\,. \tag{9}$$

This expression may be written more compactly as

$$\left[\sum_j W_{ij}[\psi_j^{-1}(Y_i - \mu_j - \beta_i)]_k + \frac{\frac{\partial}{\partial[\beta_i]_k}p(\beta)}{p(\beta)}\right]_{\beta=\hat{\beta}} = 0 \quad \forall i, \kappa \tag{10}$$

with the following definition of W_{ij}, (which are called the weights),

$$W_{ij} \equiv \frac{\lfloor p(\Gamma_i)G_{\psi_{\Gamma_i}}(Y_i - \mu(\Gamma_i) - \beta_i\rfloor_{\Gamma_i=\text{tissuee-class-}j}}{\sum_{\Gamma_i} p(\Gamma_i)G_{\psi_{\Gamma_i}}(Y_i - \mu(\Gamma_i) - \beta_i)}\,. \tag{11}$$

where subscripts i and j refer to voxel index and tissue class respectively, and defining

$$\mu_j \equiv \mu(\text{tissue-class-}j)$$

as the mean intensity of tissue class j. The mean residual is defined as

$$\bar{R}_i \equiv \sum_j W_{ij}\psi_j^{-1}(Y_i - \mu_j)\,, \tag{12}$$

and the mean inverse covariance is

$$\overline{\psi^{-1}}_{ik} \equiv \begin{cases} \sum_j W_{ij}\psi_j^{-1} & \text{if } j = \kappa \\ 0 & \text{otherwise}\,. \end{cases} \tag{13}$$

The result of the statistical modeling in this section has been to formulate the problem of estimating the bias field as a non-linear optimization problem embodied in

$$\bar{R} - \overline{\psi^{-1}}\hat{\beta} - \psi_\beta^{-1}\hat{\beta} = 0$$

or

$$\hat{\beta} \equiv (\overline{\psi^{-1}} + \psi_\beta^{-1})^{-1}\bar{R}\,. \tag{14}$$

This optimization depends on the mean residual of observed intensities and the mean intensity of each tissue class, and on the mean covariance of the tissue class intensities and the covariance of the bias field.

The expectation-maximization (EM) algorithm is used to obtain bias field estimates from the non-linear estimator of (10). The EM algorithm iteratively alternates evaluations of the expressions appearing in models (11) and (14),

$$W_{ij} \leftarrow \frac{\lfloor p(\Gamma_i) G_{\psi_{\Gamma_i}}(Y_i - \mu(\Gamma_i) - \beta_i) \rfloor_{\Gamma_i = \text{tissue-class-}j}}{\sum_{\Gamma_i} P(\Gamma_i) G_{\psi_{\Gamma_i}}(Y_i - \mu(\Gamma_i) - \beta_i)}, \tag{15}$$

$$\hat{\beta} \leftarrow (\overline{\psi^{-1}} + \psi_{\beta}^{-1})^{-1} \bar{R}. \tag{16}$$

In other words, model (15) is used to estimate the weights given an estimated bias field, then model (16) is used to estimate the bias, given estimates of the weights.

The adaptive segmentation can be applied to spin-echo and gradient-echo images. Examples are shown for the coronal (3DFT gradient-echo T1-weighted) images. All of the MR images shown in this section were obtained using a General Electric Signa 1.5 Tesla clinical MR imager [General Electric Medical Systems, Milwaukee, WI]. An anisotropic diffusion filter described in Sec. 3 was used as a pre-processing step to reduce noise.

Figure 5(a) shows the input image, a slice from a coronal 3DFT gradient-echo T1-weighted acquisition. The brain tissue ROI was generated manually. Figure 5(b) shows the final bias field estimate. The largest value of the input data was 85, while the difference between the largest and smallest values of the bias correction was about 10. Figure 5(c) shows the segmentation resulting from adaptive segmentation.

Note the significant improvement in the right temporal area. In the initial segmentation the white matter is completely absent in the binarization.

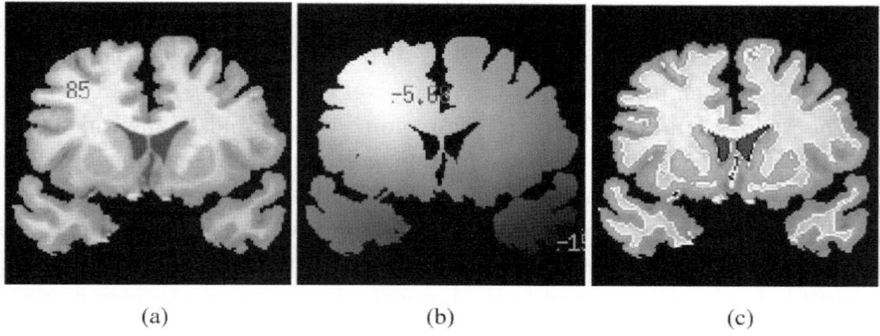

(a) (b) (c)

Fig. 5. Segmentation using expectation-maximization. (a) Original MRI brain slide; (b) Bias fied estimation; (c) Segmentation result.

4.2. *Unseeded region growing*

Unseeded region growing is similar to seeded region growing except that no explicit seed selection is necessary: the seeds can be generated by the segmentation procedure automatically. Therefore, this method can achieve fully automatic segmentation with the added benefit of robustness from being a region-based segmentation.

Formally, the segmentation process initializes with region A_1 containing a single image pixel, and the running state of the segmentation process consist of a set of identified regions, $A_1, A_2, \ldots, A_n$. Let T be the set of all unallocated pixels which borders at least one of these regions

$$T = \left\{ x \notin \bigcup_{i=1}^{n} A_i \wedge \exists k : N(x \cap A_k) \neq \emptyset \right\},$$

where $N(x)$ are immediate neighboring pixels of point x. Further, we define a difference measure

$$\delta(x, A_i) = |g(x)\text{-mean}_{y \in A_i}[g(y)]| ,$$

where $g(x)$ denotes the image value at point x, and i is an index of the region such that $N(x)$ intersect A_i.

The growing process involves selecting a point $z \in T$ and region A_j where $j \in [1, n]$ such that

$$\delta(x, A_i) = \min_{x \in T, \kappa \in [1,n]} \{\delta(x, A_i)\} .$$

If $\delta(z, A_j)$ is less than the predefined threshold t, then the pixel is added to A_j. Otherwise, we must choose the most substantially similar region $\boldsymbol{A}$ such that

$$\boldsymbol{A} = \arg\min_{A_k}\{\delta(x, A_k)\} .$$

If $\delta(z, \boldsymbol{A}) < t$, we can assign the pixel to $\boldsymbol{A}$. If neither of these two conditions above apply, then it is apparent that the pixel is significantly different from all the regions found so far, so a new region, A_{n+1} would be identified and initialized with pint z. In all three cases, the statistic of the assigned region must be updated once the pixel has been added to the region.

The URG segmentation procedure is inherently iterative, and the above process is repeated until all pixels have been allocated to a region. To ensure correct behavior with respect to the homogeneity criterion, the region growing operation requires the determination of the "best" pixel each time a region statistic is changed. The details of implementation can be found in Lin *et al.*[28] The segmentation results can be seen in Fig .6.

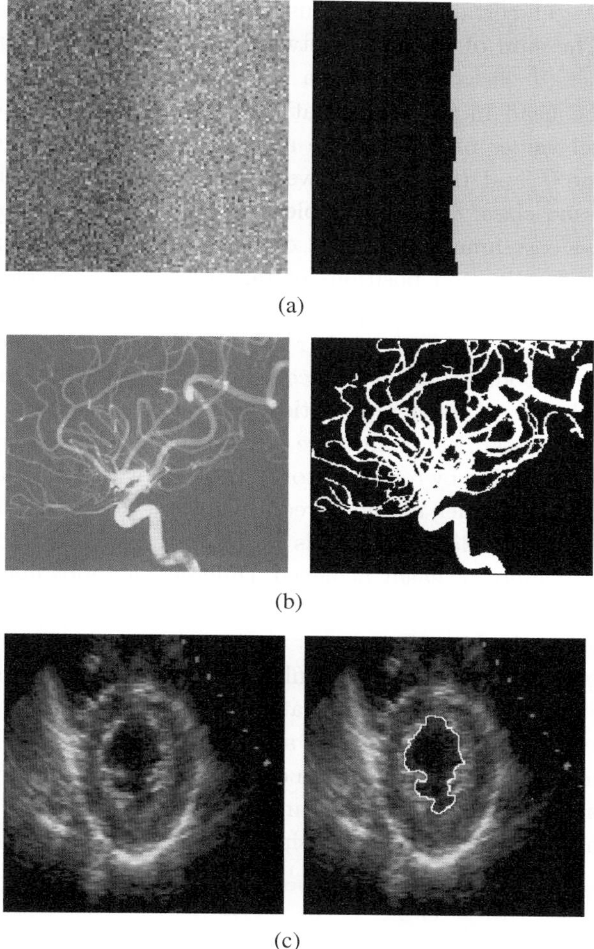

Fig. 6. Segmenation using unseeded region growing. (a) Noisy image ($\sigma = 10.0$); (b) X-ray angiogram; (c) Ultrasound heart image.

5. Improving Confidence Intervals of Image Registration Using 3-D Monte Carlo Simulations

Clinical diagnosis and treatment usually require registration of images with multiple modalities. Most of the medical image registration methods[30, 31, 48] minimize or maximize values of certain cost functions to achieve the global optimized match. These functions are usually the sum of squares of the distances between certain homogenous features in the two image sets to be registered. The sum of distances between homogenous point pairs of the two image sets,[15] distances between skin surfaces of CT, MR and PET images of the head in the "head-hat" method,[37] the absolute difference between pixel values of PET image and pixel values of image simulated by MR image,[28] and the ratio between pixel values and their means in the same tissue class[3, 51] are examples of these cost functions. However, most of these cost functions do not directly reflect the distance between the actual and estimated positions of targets, i.e. the target registration error (TRE). Most medical applications demand accuracy and precision assessment methods to justify their results. Internal consistency measures were used by Woods *et al.*[51] to place limits on registration accuracy for MRI data. Almost all other registration accuracy assessment methods fall into two broad categories: qualitative evaluations by visual inspection and quantitative evaluation by reference to results from a gold standard registration method. The former methods require special expertise and extensive experience, while the latter methods require an extremely accurate gold standard that cannot be easily achieved. Different methods may not always be comparable to each other under identical criteria.

Using the terminology of nonlinear regression analysis,[14] we can refer the problem of image registration as a nonlinear least sum of squares estimation of the transformation parameters that result in the optimal fitting of one set of image (function) to the other set of image (data). For least square estimation methods, the cost function could be assumed to be linear around the neighborhood of the current parameter values. So that we can calculate the confidence intervals or regions using the following equation:[14]

$$(\theta - \theta_0)\sum(f') \leq (\sigma^2(n-1))F(p, n-p, 1-\alpha)\,, \tag{17}$$

where F is a chosen F-test value of the corresponding confidence level, σ^2 is the residual sum of squares (registration cost function) value at the location of the estimated parameters, and $\sum(f')$ represents the sum of the derivatives of the reference model image to the transformation parameters. θ and θ_0 are the parameters corresponding to the confidence level and the optimal parameters found by the registration procedure, respectively.

Since all the data points involved in the calculation of (17) should be statistical independent to each other, and the data points in the images are correlated, the number of points in the image could not be used directly as n and the effective number of independent data points needs to be estimated.

To determine the effective number of independent data points involved in the estimation of confidence intervals, we first used one Monte Carlo simulation study based on normal conditions. The same number n selected according to this simulation results was found to be consistent for both the 95% and 90% confidence levels. We have further investigated the validity of the selected number n in various simulated conditions in other parts of the study.

Monte Carlo studies to simulate 2D PET images and subsequent registrations of the simulated images were conducted. The resulted distributions of the estimated transformation parameters were used to assess the consistency of 90%, 95% and 99% confidence intervals with the distributions in the parameter space. 2D grey matter and white matter sinograms of the segmented 2D Hoffman brain phantom[20] were combined with the grey-to-white ratios of 2:1, 3:1 and 4:1 before reconstruction to see whether the discrepancies of the ratios in two images can affect the confidence intervals. Then, filtered back-projection reconstruction programs with various filters (i.e. Hanning, Ramp, Butter-worth, Ham, Parzen and Shepp-Logan filters) were employed to reconstruct images of size 128×128. Various amounts of spatial displacements (i.e. rotations of 0.3, 0.8, 1.2 and 3.3 degrees, and translations of 0.16, 0.8, 1.6 and 2.4 mm) were introduced. Various levels of Poisson noise (i.e. total counts of 5×10^5, 1×10^6 and 2×10^6) were simulated. A Gaussian smoothing filter with a FWHM of 5 mm is applied to both sets of images before registration. The Powell's algorithm[40] was selected as the optimization procedure.

In the cases of extreme noise conditions and large contrast discrepancies, the residual sum of squares (RSS) consists of two parts: the systematic error and the error due to statistical noise:

$$RSS = RSS_{\text{system}} + RSS_{\text{noise}} \,. \tag{18}$$

The systematic error is contributed by the innate difference between the two images, inappropriate registration method, precision error of the program, etc. Such errors are independent of the initial displacements and noise. The second part of the residual sum of squares is due to statistical noise. If the systematic error is relatively large compared to the noise term, i.e. for cases with very low noise levels and high grey-to-white ratio discrepancies, the estimated residual sum of squares needs to be adjusted for systematic error.

Since the systematic component in RSS is much less sensitive to spatial smoothing than the other component in Eq. (18), it can be estimated by applying smoothing filters to both sets of images with relatively large

FWHMs when the parameters are found. By removing the systematic component, the result RSS provides an estimation of the noise component in Eq. (18).

The calculated confidence intervals based on statistical regression are consistent with the simulation results for sample distributions of the transformation parameters of image co-registration. Varying the amount of displacement, reconstruction processes, noise levels, or tracer distributions have little impacts on the validity of the calculated confidence intervals. After adjusted for systematic errors in the estimated residual sum of squares, confidence intervals can be calculated accurately even for very noisy conditions and with large distribution discrepancies between the two sets of images. Since multi-modality registration can be viewed as mono-modality registration of one image set with another simulated from the other image modality, this method is also expected to be applicable to multi-modality registration. Hence, visual inspection and validations by experts are not necessary for assessing the precision of the registration results. The results indicate the use of statistical confidence intervals has a potential to provide an automatic and objective assessment of individual image registration.

6. Conclusion

We have attempted a brief summary of the applications of statistical methods in image processing in general and medical imaging in particular. The issues cover image sampling, compression, filtering, segmentation and registration. Methods have been discussed in theory and illustrated in empirical results. Statistical methods are powerful tools in many signal processing applications. We hope this summary will provide an insight for the further use of statistical methods in image processing.

References

1. Adam, R. and Bischof, L. (1994). Seeded region growing, *IEEE Transactions on Pattern Analysis and Machine Intelligence* **16**(6): 641–647.
2. Alvarze, L. and Mazorra, L. (1994). Signal and image restoration using shock filters and anisotropic diffusion. *SIAM Journal on Numerical Analysis* **31**(2): 590–594.
3. Ardekani, B. A., Braun, M. *et al.* (1995). A fully automatic multimodality image registration algorithm, *Journal Computer Assistant Tomography* **19**(4): 615–623.

4. Besl, P. J., and Jain, R. C. (1988). Segmentation through variable-order surface fitting, *IEEE Transaction on Pattern Analysis and Machine Intelligence* **10**(2): 167–192.
5. Bhandari, D., Pal, N. R. and Majumder, D. D. (1992). Fuzzy divergence, probability measure of fuzzy events and image thresholding. *Pattern Recognition Letter* **13**: 857–867.
6. Cai, W., Feng, D. and Fulton, R. (1998). Clinical investigation of a knowledge-based data compression algorithm for dynamic neurologic FDG-PET images, *Proceedings of the 20th Annual International Conference of the IEEE Engineering in Medicine and Biology Society (EMBS'98)*, Vol. 20, part 3, 1270–1273, Hong Kong, October 29–November 1.
7. Cho, S., Haralick, M. R. and Yi, S. (1989). Improvement of Kittle and Illingworth's minimum error thresholding. *Pattern Recognition* **22**: 609–617.
8. Ciaccio, E. J., Dunn, S. M. and Akay, M. (1994). Biosignal pattern recognition and interpretation systems: Methods of classification, *IEEE Engineering in Medicine and Biology* **13**: 129–135.
9. Cline, H. E., Lorensen, W. E., Kikinis, R. and Jolesz, F. (1990). Three-dimensional segmentation of MR images of the head using probability and connectivity. *JCAT* **14**(6): 1037–1045.
10. Cobelli, C., Ruggeri, A., DiStefano, III, J. J. and Landaw, E. M. (1985). Optimal design of multioutput sampling schedules — software and applications to endocrine–metabolic and pharmacokinetic models, *IEEE Transactions on Biomedical Engineering* **32**(4): 249–256.
11. Crocker, L. D. (1995). PGN: The portable network graphic format. *Dr. Dobb's Journal*, 36-49, July.
12. Davis, S. L. (1975). A survey of edge detection techniques. *Computer Graphics Image Processing* **4**: 248–270.
13. Donoho, D. L. (1995). De-noising by soft-thresholding. *IEEE Transaction Information Theory* **IT-41**: 613–627.
14. Draper, N. R. (1981). *Applied regression Analysis*, 2nd edn., Wiley, New York.
15. Evans, A. C., Marrett, S., Collins, L. and Peters, T. M. (1989). Anatomical-functional correlative analysis of the human brain using three dimensional imaging systems. In *Medical Imaging*: *Image Processing*, eds. R.H. Schneider, S.J. Dwyer III AND R.G. Jost, SPIE Press, Bellingham, WA., **1092**: 264–274.
16. Feng, D., Ho, D., Chen, K., Wu, L., Wang, J., Liu, R. and Yeh, S. (1995). An evaluation of the algorithms for constructing local cerebral metabolic rates of glucose tomographical maps using positron emission tomography dynamic date. *IEEE Transaction on Medical Imaging* **14**(4): 697–710.
17. Gerig, G., Kuoni, W., Kikinis, R. and Kubler, O. (1993). Medical imaging and computer vision: An integrated approach for diagnosis and planning. *Proceedings of the 11th DAGM Symposium*, 425–443.
18. Glaseby, C. A. (1985). An analysis of histogram based thresholding algorithms. *CVGIP*: *Graphical Models and Image Processing* **55**: 532–533.
19. Haralick, R. M. and Shapiro, L. G. (1985). Image segmentation techniques. *Computer Graphics Image Processing* **29**: 100–132.

20. Hoffman, E. J., Cutler, P. D., Guerrero, T. M., Digdy, W. M. and Mazziotta, J. C. (1991). Assessment of accuracy of PET utilizing a 3-D phantom to simulate the activity distribution of [18F] fluorodeoxyglucose uptake in the human brain. *Journal of Cerebral Blood Flow and Metabolism* **11**: 17–25.
21. Horowitz, S. L. and Pavlidis, T. (1974). Picture segmentation by a directed split-and-merge procedure. *Proceedings 2nd International Joint Conference On Pattern Recognition*, 424–433.
22. Huang, S. C., Phelps, M. E., Hoffman, E. J., Sideris, K., Selin, C. and Kuhl, D. E. (1980). Non-invasive determination of local cerebral metabolic rate of glucose in man. *American Journal of Physiology* **238**: E69–E82.
23. Kamber, M., Collins, D., Shinghal, R., Francis, G. and Evans, A. (1992). Model-based 3D segmentation of multiple sclerosis lesions in dual-echo MRI data. *SPIE Vol. 1808, Visualization in Biomedical Computing.*
24. Kass, M., Witkin, A. and Terzonpoulos, D. (1987). Snakes: Active contour models. *Proceedings International Conference On Computer Vision*, London.
25. Kohn, M., Tanna, N., Herman, G. *et al.* (1991). Analysis of brain and cerebrospinal fluid volumes with MR imaging. *Radiology* **178**: 115–122.
26. Li, X., Feng, D. and Chen, K. (1996). Optimal image sampling schedule: A new effective way to reduce dynamic image storage space and functional image processing time. *IEEE Transactions* **15**: 710–718.
27. Lin, J. Z., Jin, J. S. and Hugo, T. (2001). Unseeded region growing. *Proceedings Workshop on Visual Information Processing*, 2000, Sydney.
28. Lin, K. P., Huang, S. C. *et al.* (1994). A general technique for interstudy registration of multifunction and multimodality images. *IEEE Tran Nuclear Science* **41**(6): 2850–2855.
29. Luijendijk, H. (1991). Automatic threshold selection using histograms based on the count of 4-connected regions. *Pattern Recognition Letter* **12**: 219–228.
30. Maintz, J. B. A. and Viergever, M. A. (1998). A survey of medical image registration. *Medical Image Analysis* **2**(1): 1–36.
31. Maurer, C. R. and Fitzpatrick, J. M. (1993). A review of medical image registration, In *Interactive Imageguided Neurosurgery, American Association of Neurological Surgeons*, ed. R.J. Maciunas, Parkridge, IL, 17–44.
32. Meyer, F. and Beucher, S. (1979). Morphological segmentation. *Journal of Visual Communication And Image Representation* **1**: 21–46.
33. Nagawa, Y. and Rosenfeld, A. (1979). Some experiments on variable thresholding. *Pattern Recognition* **11**: 191–204.
34. Parker, J. R. (1991). Gray level thresholding in badly illuminated images. *IEEE Transaction PAMI* **13**: 813–819.
35. Patlak, C. S. and Blasberg, R. G. (1985). Graphical evaluation of blood to brain transfer constaints from multiple-time uptake data generalizations. *Journal of Cerebral Blood Flow and Metabolism* **5**: 584–590.
36. Patlak, C. S., Blasberg, R. G. and Fenstermacher, J. (1983). Graphical evaluation of blood to brain transfer constants from multiple-time uptake data. *Journal of Cerebral Blood Flow and Metabolism* **3**: 1–7.

37. Pelizzari, C. A., Chen, G. T. Y. *et al.* (1989). Accurate three-dimensional registration of CT, PET and/or MR images of the brain. *Journal Computer Assistant Tomography* **13**: 20–26.
38. Perona, P. and Malik, J. (1987). Scale-space and edge detection using anisotropic diffusion. *Proceedings IEEE Workshop Computer Vision*, Miami, FL, 16–22.
39. Perona, P. and Malik, J. (1990). Scale-space and edge detection using anisotropic diffusion. *IEEE Transaction PAMI* **12**: 629–639.
40. Powell, M. J. D. (1964). An efficient method for finding the minimum of a function of several variables without calculating derivatives. *Computer Juornal* **7**: 155–163.
41. Rodriguez, A. A. and Mitchell, O. R. (1991). Image segmentation by successive background extraction. *Pattern Recognition* **24**: 409–420.
42. Ross, S. M. (1987). *Introduction to Probability and Statistics for Engineers and Scientists*, John Wiley and Sons, NY.
43. Sahoo, P. K., Soltani, S. and Wong, A. K. C. (1988). A survey of threhsolding techniques. *Computer Graphics Image Processing* **41**: 230–260.
44. Spann, M. and Horne, C. (1989). Image segmentation using a dynamic thresholding pyramid. *Pattern Recognition* **22**: 719–732.
45. Tou, J. T. and Gonzalez, R. C. (1972). *Pattern Recognition Principle*, Addison-Wesley.
46. Tsai, D. M. and Chen, Y. (1992). A fast histogram-clustering approach for multi-level thresholding. *Pattern Recognition Letter* **13**: 245–252.
47. Tseng, D. C. and Huang, M. Y. (1993). Automatic thresholding based on human visual perception. *Image and Vision Computing* **11**: 539–548.
48. Van den Elsen, P. A., Pol, E. J. D. and Viergever, M. A. (1993). Medical image matching — A review with classification. *IEEE Engineering in Medicine and Biology* **12**: 26–39
49. Vannier, M., Butterfield, R., Jordan, D., Murphy, W. *et al.* (1985). Multispectral analysis of magnetic resonance images. *Radiology* **154**: 221–224.
50. Wells III., W. M., Grimson, W. E. L., Kikinis, R. and Jolesz, F. A. (1996). Adaptive segmentation of MRI data. *IEEE Transactions on Medical Imaging* **15**(4): 429–443
51. Woods, R. P., Grafton, S. T., Holmes, C. J., Cherry, S. R. and Mazziotta, J. C. (1998). Automated image registration: I. General methods and intrasubject, intramodality validation. *Journal Computer Assistant Tomography* **22**(1): 139–152.

About the Author

Dr. Jesse Jin graduated with a Bachelor in Engineering degree from Shanghai Jiao Tong University and a Ph.D. from University of Otago,

New Zealand. He was Associate Professor in the Department of Computer Science, University of Sydney and Professor in the School of Design, Communication and IT, University of Newcastle. Dr. Jin was also an Adjunct Associate Professor and the Director of the Visual Information Processing Laboratory at the School of Computer Science and Engineering, University of New South Wales. Dr. Jin is an international renowned expert on multimedia technology and visual information retrieval and processing. He has published numerous articles and books. He established a spin-off company and the company won the 1999 ATP Vice-Chancellor New Business Creation Award. He is a consultant for many companies such as Motorola, Computer Associates, ScanWorld, Proteome Systems, HyperSoft, etc. He was a visiting professor at MIT, UCLA, HKPU and Tsinghua University. He is also a Vice President of Ausinan Science & Technology Society.

CHAPTER 7

COST-EFFECTIVENESS ANALYSIS AND EVIDENCE-BASED MEDICINE

JIANLI LI

Department of Corporate Performance,
St Michael's Hospital, 30 Bond Street,
Toronto, Ontario, M5B 1W8, Canada
Tel: 416-864-5894; lij@smh.ca

1. Introduction

Over the past few decades, as pressures to control health care spending have accelerated, the term "cost-effectiveness" has increasingly entered common parlance. It is widely used by groups as disparate as the government, the congress, the business community, managed-care organizations, the pharmaceutical industry and the press.

The central purpose of cost-effectiveness analysis (CEA) is to compare the relative value of different interventions in creating better health and/or longer life. The results of such evaluations are typically summarized in a cost-effectiveness ratio, where the denominator reflects the gain in health from a candidate intervention (measured, for example, in term of years of life gained, premature birth averted, sight years gained, symptom-free days gained) and the numerator reflects the cost of obtaining the health gain. A cost-effectiveness analysis provides information that can help decision makers sort through alternatives and decide which one best serves their programmatic and financial needs. The decision maker may be federal, state or local. They may be in the private sector or the public sector. They may control dollars or they may run programs. CEA provides a framework within which decision makers may pose a range of questions.

Cost-effectiveness analyses furnish information that can be useful in a variety of settings. For example, a managed-care organization might wish to know the cost per low-birthweight birth averted as a consequence of a prenatal outreach program. Or it might wish to take the question further and ask the cost of this program per year of life saved for its enrolled population. Or, recognizing that programs that avert premature births may not primarily save lives but rather avert disability over the lifetime of an individual, it might want to know the cost of this intervention for each quality-adjusted life year (QALY) gained. This latter question is addressed by a particular type of CEA, sometimes termed "cost utility analysis," where adjustments for the value assigned to health-related quality of life are built into the calculation.

As another example, a pharmaceutical manufacturer might wish to use CEA in pricing and marketing a new cholesterol-lowering drug. It might ask the question — How much does our medication cost per year of life gained compare to a similar product manufactured by a different company? Or, if the clinical trials show clinically insignificant changes in cholesterol level between the two products but significantly decreased side effects associated with the new drug, a drug purchaser or payer might wish then to calculate the cost per quality-adjusted life year (QALY) gained in using the new drug. An industry investigator might decide to extend the considerations of the analysis and explore the cost per year of life or QALY gained when comparing pharmaceutical treatment with surgical treatment for coronary disease.

Or, an analysis of a state health department might wish to explore different strategies for control of blood lead levels in the population. It might choose to assess the cost-effectiveness of screening all children, compared to screening only those thought to be at particular risk for elevated lead levels by reason of housing or environment surrounding.

1.1. *Worked examples*

1.1.1. *Bypass angioplasty revascularization investigation*

Percutaneous transluminal coronary angioplastry was introduced in 1977 as a less invasive alternative to coronary-artery bypass surgery. Several randomized clinical trials of angioplasty and bypass surgery have compared the clinical outcomes of these procedures. The Bypass Angioplasty Revascularization Investigation (BARI) was a large trial of angioplasty and bypass surgery in US, which collected five years of follow-up data.

Mark A. Hlatky *et al.*[8] conducted a study on a total 934 of the 1829 patients enrolled in the randomized BARI. Detailed data on quality of life were collected annually, and economic data were collected quarterly.

They compared quality of life, employment, and medical care costs during five year of follow-up among patients treated with angioplasty or bypass surgery. They found that on average, functional status, which was assessed by scores on the Duke Activity Status Index, was improved more with bypass surgery than with angioplasty in the first three years ($p < 0.05$), whereas in other respects the quality of life was equivalent with either method of revascularization. Patient in the angioplasty group returned to work five weeks sooner than did patients in the surgery group ($p < 0.001$). The cost of angioplasty was initially $11,234 lower than that of bypass surgery (a 35% saving, $p < 0.001$), but higher subsequent costs for hospitalization and medication reduced the saving to $2,644 at five years (a 5% savings, $p = 0.047$). The five-year cost of angioplasty was significantly lower than that of surgery among patients with two-vessel disease ($52,930 versus $58,498, $p < 0.05$), but not among patients with three-vessel disease. After five years of follow-up, surgery had an overall cost-effectiveness ratio of $26,177 per year of life added, but unacceptable ratios of $100,000 or more per year of life added could not be excluded ($p = 0.13$). Surgery appeared particularly cost effective in treating patients with diabetes because of their significantly improved survival.

1.1.2. *Treatment of high blood cholesterol*

In 1985, in response to the first evidence from a randomized controlled trial that reducing cholesterol reduces the risk of death from heart disease,[10] the US National Institutes of Health created the National Cholesterol Education Program (NCEP). Three years later the NCEP published guidelines for the management of high blood cholesterol which recommended that all adults have their cholesterol checked at least every 5 years and that those with high levels (240 mg/dl) or higher), or borderline-high levels (200–239 mg/dl) plus other risk factors, be tested further. It was suggested that those whose low-density lipoproteins (LDL) levels were also high should be treated by changes in diet or with cholesterol-lowering drugs.[11] It has been estimated that more than one-third of the adult population requires dietary change and/or drugs when judged by these criteria.[15]

Cost-effectiveness analyses done in the wake of the 1988 guideline focused on the management of high blood cholesterol once detected. Both lovastatin, a frequently prescribed drug, and dietary counseling were shown to vary widely in cost-effectiveness depending on age and other risk factors for heart disease.

One study examined the use of lovastatin for people initially free of heart disease and for those who had already suffered a heart attack.[7] The authors found that, for healthy people, saving a year of life is much more costly among those with cholesterol as their only risk factor than it is for those with several risk factors, even when cholesterol is very high; the cost ranged up to $330,000 for men aged 35–44 with no other risk factor and up to $1.5 million for women in the same category. The cost was considerably lower for people with other risk factors, reflecting the widely accepted assumption that risk factors interact to make the adverse effects of any one greater when others are present. Lovastatin treatment was still more costly per life year gained for people with levels in the range 250–299 mg/dl.

In contrast, the study found that it is potentially very cost-effective to treat people with elevated cholesterol who have had heart attacks. Costs per life year gained are relatively low and for some, such as men aged 35–44, drug treatment might save money as well as extended life. Another study found similar results for a program of intensive diet therapy modeled after the one in the Multiple Risk Factor Intervention Trial (MRFIT).[18] For example, diet therapy costs more than $500,000 per year of life for 20-year-old men with initial cholesterol of 240 mg/dl and no other risk factors. For men with several risk factors, the cost per life year gained in much lower.

These results suggest that management of high cholesterol in people without heart disease is often very costly per life year saved. Since they show that treatment of people whose blood cholesterol levels are not far above 240 mg/dl can be extremely costly, they suggest that the same would be true for people with levels in the borderline-high range, although the studies did not analyze this group. Taken together, cost-effectiveness results suggest that resources might better be concentrated on those with very high cholesterol levels and/or other risk factors for heart disease (and on those in whom heart disease is already present). Revised guidelines, published by NCEP in 1993,[12] were somewhat more modest in their aims, in response to studies like these as well to ongoing debate over whether reducing cholesterol lengthens life in those without heart disease.

If NCEP's 1988 guidelines were followed to the letter, it would cost, depending on the effectiveness of diet in reducing blood cholesterol levels, $20 billion to $27 billion to provide lovastatin at dose of 20 mg per day, and $47 billion to $67 billion to provide a higher, more effective, dose of 80 mg per day.[6] The savings from a more selective strategy would be substantial, freeing up resources to be applied elsewhere. The CEA results suggest that more selective treatment strategies could be designed that would lose little in health benefits.

2. Foundations of Cost-Effectiveness Analysis

2.1. *What is cost-effectiveness analysis?*

Cost-effectiveness analysis is a method designed to assess the comparative impacts of expenditures on different health interventions. As Weinstein and Stason[19] state, it is based on the premise that "for any given level of resources available, society . . . wishes to maximize the total aggregate health benefits conferred." For example, we might wish to know whether spending a certain amount of money on a public campaign to stop smoking will have greater or lesser effect on health than spending the same amount on colorectal screening. Cost-effectiveness analysis can be in decision making at different levels, such as societal level and organizational level.

2.2. *The cost-effectiveness ratio*

The central measure used in CEA is the cost-effectiveness ratio. Implicit in the cost-effectiveness ratio is a comparison between alternatives. One alternative is the intervention under study, while the other is a suitably chosen alternative — "usual care," another intervention, or no intervention. The cost-effectiveness ratio for comparing the two alternatives at the population level can be the ratio of expected costs to expected effect (CER), $E(c)/E(e)$, and ratio of incremental expected costs to incremental expected effects (ICER), $(E(c_i) - E(c_j))/(E(e_i) - E(e_j))$ or $\Delta E(c)/\Delta E(e)$).

The ratio $\Delta E(c)/\Delta E(e)$ is essentially the incremental price of obtaining a unit health effect (such as dollars per year, or per quality-adjusted year, of life expectancy) from given health intervention when compared with an alternative.

The following situations can arise:

$\Delta E(c) < 0$, $\Delta E(e) > 0$; dominance; to accept the given intervention;
$\Delta E(c) > 0$, $\Delta E(e) < 0$; dominance; to reject the given intervention;
$\Delta E(c) > 0$, $\Delta E(e) > 0$; trade-off; consider magnitude of ratio of difference in costs to difference in effectiveness;
$\Delta E(c) < 0$, $\Delta E(e) < 0$; trade-off; consider magnitude of ratio of difference in costs to difference in effectiveness.

The expected ratio of cost to effect, $E(c/e)$, can be investigated at patient level.

2.3. *The effectiveness*

The effectiveness is the extent to which medical interventions achieve health improvements in real practice settings.

2.3.1. *Individual and social well-being*

By describing CEA as a tool for improving general welfare, it can be placed squarely within the context of welfare economics. The effectiveness measures could be quantified in term of utility, such as quality-adjusted life years (QALY); and in terms of health status measures, such as the number of symptom-free days.

2.3.2. *A metric of health effect: Quality-adjusted life years*

It may appear that CEA cannot even be used to compare interventions whose effects on health are qualitatively different, such as prevention of coronary artery disease and treatment of arthritis. However, such a comparison is possible if the measure of effectiveness is general enough to capture all of the important health dimensions of the effects of the interventions. Using the quality-adjusted life year (QALY) as the unit of effectiveness approaches this ideal within the framework of CEA, thus expanding considerably the range of application of CEA. The QALY is a measure of health outcome which assigns to each period of time a weight, ranging from 0 to 1, corresponding to the quality of life during that period, where a weight of 1 corresponds to perfect health and a weight of 0 corresponds to a health state judged equivalent to death. The number of quality-adjusted life years, then, represents the number of healthy years of life that valued equivalently to the actual health outcome.

2.3.3. *How to obtain evidence on effectiveness?*

The foundation for economic evaluation is valid data on the effectiveness of the intervention being evaluated relative to some alternative.

The true cost and effectiveness of an intervention usually are not known but estimated. The source of estimates may be direct measurement (sampling) or indirect (non-sampling) methods such as expert opinion and published literature. There could be two types of data; sampled data where the sampling variance may or may not be known, and non-sampled data such as discount rate which do not have sampling variation, although the true value of the parameter may be uncertain. These data can be used in various combinations in two models of analysis: stochastic analysis where inferences are drawn using standard statistical methods based on sampling variation, and deterministic analysis where inferences are drawn from point estimates of variables but interpretation is conditional upon the range of uncertainty from sensitivity analysis. The appropriateness of methods for analyzing uncertainty in costs or effects will depend upon the mix of sampled and non-sampled data. Cost-effectiveness analysis can be wholly deterministic, partially stochastic or wholly stochastic.

2.3.4. *Deterministic cost-effectiveness analysis*

This is used where cost and effect variables are analyzed as point estimates. Sampling variation may not be available because of the source of the data (e.g. secondary data) or the variable may not have been sampled (e.g. choice of discount rate, expert opinion). Deterministic CEA models arise frequently in the early assessment of a new medical technology, where only limited data are available but some analysis is required for policy setting. For example, in their analysis of the implantable defibrillator, Kupperman *et al.*[9] constructed a cost-effectiveness model where effect data were taken from reports of patient series in the literature as point estimates of survival probabilities and cost data were derived from a Medicare claims database and expert opinion. Given these data, it was not possible to present cost and effect differences with 95% confidence intervals, therefore a deterministic point estimate of cost-effectiveness was subject to detailed sensitivity analysis to explore the impact of uncertainty. Therefore a point estimate based on expert opinion of resource use was used as a proxy for variables that could be sampled in the future as part of a prospective study.

2.3.5. *Partially stochastic cost-effectiveness analysis*

This is used where effectiveness has been estimated from clinical trial(s) and can be expressed as a mean effect size with an associated variance, but analysis of costs is deterministic because data are non sampled. This combination is common in decision analytic models of economic appraisal. Some studies with such data report confidence intervals for cost-effectiveness where only variation in effects has been analyzed. For example a study in ulcer maintenance theory presented 95% confidence intervals around expected one-year therapy costs including relapse management. But no primary data had been collected to determine variation between patients in costs of managing relapse. The source of variation for the confidence interval was only the surrounding the estimated incidence of relapse on treatment and control.

2.3.6. *Wholly stochastic cost-effectiveness analysis*

This is used where both costs and effects are determined from data sampled from the same patients in a study. Although our discussion focused on the randomized controlled trials (RCT) these data might also be measured by non-experiment-design. If cost and effect data are sampled and variances are available then formal statistical tests can be performed on observed differences in costs (treatment-control) or effects.

Randomized controlled trials (RCT) are one valuable source of evidence on effectiveness, used either as single studies or combined in a meta-analysis. There are two general ways in which RCT data can be incorporated into economic evaluation: (i) combining RCT effectiveness data retrospectively with cost data from secondary non-trial sources into a decision analysis model; or (ii) collecting effectiveness and cost data on the same patients prospectively as part of an RCT.

The growing interest in trial-based prospective cost-effective studies has raised some interesting statistical questions of study design and analysis. Given the traditional use of non-sampled secondary data (e.g. published literature, insurance claims databases, expert opinion) in cost-effectiveness models the convention for analyzing uncertainty in results has been to use sensitivity analysis, where the robustness of results is explored over a range of what if alternative values for uncertain variables. This analytical approach is in marked contrast to the conventional analysis of RCT effectiveness data where standard principles of statistical inference are used to construct tests of hypotheses and estimate intervention effect sizes, and where uncertainty is quantified by a confidence interval which has precise meaning in terms of probability.

2.4. *Sensitivity analysis and beyond*

Before considering the adaptation of stochastic methods for economic evaluation, it is necessary to review the limitation of sensitivity analysis. This method is widely recommended for assessing problems of data uncertainty in economic appraisals of health care programs and allied evaluative techniques such as clinical decision analysis. The purpose is to examine the robustness of an estimated result over a range of alternative values for uncertain parameters. Weinstein and Stason (1977)[19] describe the method in the following way: "The most uncertain features and assumptions... are varied one at a time over a wide range of possible values. If the basic conclusions do not change when a particular feature or assumption is varied, confidence in the conclusions is increased."

Whereas the traditional CEA model utilize sensitivity analysis, the mean-variance data on costs and effects from a prospective trial presents the opportunity to analyze cost-effectiveness using conventional inferential statistical methods.[13] The statistical approach in CEA have been discussed by many literatures.

3. Statistical Approach

3.1. *Costs and effects as point estimates*

The deterministic analysis of effectiveness is a comparison of point estimates. If we consider a treatment that is both more costly and more effective than control, then a useful way to represent incremental cost-effectiveness is illustrated in Fig. 1. In this diagram, the x axis represents the difference in effects between the experimental and control therapy (Δe) and the y axis the difference in cost between experimental and control (Δc). The slope of the line extending from origin (the control) through our study point estimate, Δe, Δc, represents the incremental cost-effectiveness of the treatment relative to control. Clearly, the steeper the slope of the line $\Delta c/\Delta e$ the greater is the additional cost at which additional units of effectiveness are gained by treatment relative to control, and the less attractive the treatment becomes. In the absence of any data on sampling variation for

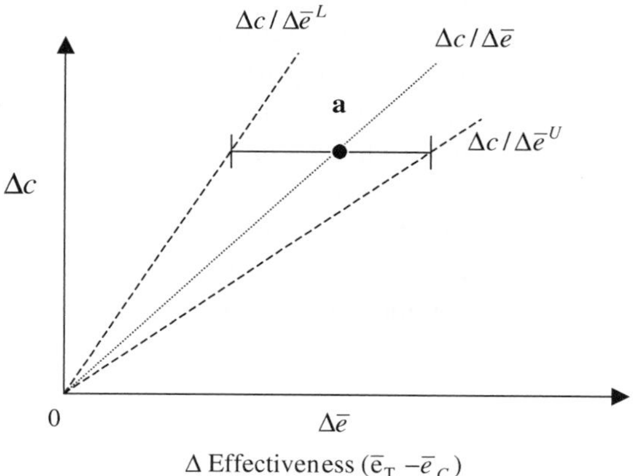

Fig. 1. Cost-effectiveness quasi-confidence interval: Deterministic analysis of cost differences and stochastic analysis of effectiveness differences.

costs or effects (point a) some form of sensitivity analysis would be useful to determine plausible ranges that may contain the true cost-effectiveness ratio.

3.2. *Sampled effectiveness and non-sampled costs*

In the analysis of sampled effect data (with sample variation) the null hypothesis is usually that there is no difference in outcomes between experimental and control therapy. This is tested against either a one-tailed alternative (usually that the experimental treatment more effective) or a two-tailed alternative (that the experimental treatment is more or less effective than control). For a continuos clinical variable such as blood pressure we assume, by convention, that the ratio of the difference in sample means $(\bar{e}_T - \bar{e}_C)$, where the subscript T stands for the treatment group and subscript C stands for the control group, to the pooled standard error of the difference follows some known probability distribution such as Z or t. Critical values of the test statistics are determined by the analyst's judgement about the acceptable risk of making a Type 1 (false-positive) error about a difference existing, this level conventionally being set to 5%.

A problem with hypothesis testing as a form of stochastic analysis is that an overemphasis tends to be placed on the statistical significance. The advantages of the confidence interval is two-fold. First it permits hypothesis testing as described above because if a 95% confidence interval for a difference includes zero, then the treatment groups are not significantly different at 5% level. Second, in addition to statistical significance, the confidence intervals yields information on the magnitude of the observed difference (quantitative significance or clinical importance). The relationship between these two parameters is important because a difference can be highly statistically significant but of no clinical importance, for example, a small difference (say, 0.25 mm/Hg) with $p < 0.0001$. Furthermore, the concept of a minimum clinically important difference δ to be detected is central to the design of a clinical experiment and determination of sample size.

A familiar two-tailed confidence interval for the treatment-effect size would be

$$(\bar{e}_T - \bar{e}_C) \pm t_{(n_T+n_C-2,1-\alpha/2)}\sqrt{\frac{S_{eT}^2}{n_T} + \frac{S_{eC}^2}{n_C}} \tag{1}$$

where S_{eT}^2 and S_{eC}^2 are the sample estimates of variances.

A confidence interval around (the mean effect size) has been drawn in Fig. 1. Given the confidence interval around $\Delta\bar{e}$, one approach to translating this into variation around the cost-effectiveness ratio is by creating an interval bounded by the ratio of cost difference to the lower bound of the effect interval ($\Delta_c/\Delta\bar{e}^L$) and the ratio of the cost difference to the effect upper bound of the effect interval ($\Delta_c/\Delta\bar{e}^U$). These upper and lower bounds for the cost-effectiveness ratio might be termed a quasi-confidence interval, because they are only based upon knowledge of sampling variation associated with the measurement of the denominator (effects). This reasoning can be applied analogously to a situation where we had stochastic costs but deterministic effects.

3.3. *Sampled effectiveness and sampled costs*

As we did in previous sections, we assumed that effects were measured from a trial and could be expressed as a confidence interval. However, we also assumed that resource use was measured to enable patient-specific costs to be estimated from j resources ($j = 1, \ldots, J$) in quantity Q_j at unit price P_j, then the costs for individual i can be expressed $c_i = \sum_{j=1}^{J} P_j Q_j$.

Summing over i patients ($i = 1, \ldots, n_T$) in the treatment group, mean cost per patient can be expressed as $\bar{c}_i = \frac{1}{n_T}\sum_{i=1}^{n_T} c_i$ with estimated variance

$$s_{EcT}^2 = \frac{1}{n_T(n_T-1)}\sum_{i=1}^{n_T}(c_i - \bar{c}_T)^2 . \tag{2}$$

Therefore the difference between the mean cost associated with treatment and control can be expresses as a confidence interval:

$$(\bar{c}_T - \bar{c}_C) \pm t_{(n_T+n_C-2,1-\alpha/2)}\sqrt{\frac{S_{cT}^2}{n_T} + \frac{S_{cC}^2}{n_C}} . \tag{3}$$

In this situation the incremental cost-effectiveness ratio is a ratio of two random variables, both of which can be expressed as a confidence interval (around a difference in means). If we initially assume zero covariance between costs and effects then one can conceptualize this ratio in the form of a two-dimensional confidence plane.

3.4. *Joint distribution of cost and effects*

It is assumed that in an RCT (or observational study in which valid inference can made) there are J interventions where n_j patients receive intervention j, $j = 1, 2, \ldots, J$. Costs and effects are viewed as vector random variables $\mathbf{c}_j$ and $\mathbf{e}_j - c_{ij}$ representing the costs incurred and e_{ij} the effects achieved by patient i on intervention j, $i = 1, 2, \ldots, n_j$, during a specified period. The joint probability distribution function of costs and effects on a patient level is modeled by the function $F_j(\mathbf{c}, \mathbf{e}; \mathbf{z})$. A vector of patient covariate, $\mathbf{z}$, such as diagnosis, gender and age, is introduced to cover the situation in which the cost-effect relationship of a intervention is expected to vary for different subgroups. It is assumed that $(c_{ij}(\mathbf{z}), e_{ij}(\mathbf{z}))$ are independently and identically distributed over the patients with covariates $\mathbf{z}$ receiving intervention j. The marginal distributions of F, which are the univariate distribution of cost and distribution of effect, are each associated with parameters such as expected cost $E(\mathbf{c})$, and expected effect, $E(\mathbf{e})$.

The expected cost and effect, $(E(\mathbf{c}), E(\mathbf{e}))$ could be estimated by the sample means of $\mathbf{c}$ and $\mathbf{e}$, that is, $(\bar{c}, \bar{e})$ and the covariance matrix of $(\bar{c}, \bar{e})$ could be presented as:

$$\begin{bmatrix} \dfrac{\widehat{\sigma}_c^2}{n} & \dfrac{\hat{\rho}\,\widehat{\sigma}_c\widehat{\sigma}_e}{n} \\ \dfrac{\widehat{\rho}\,\widehat{\sigma}_c\widehat{\sigma}_e}{n} & \dfrac{\widehat{\sigma}_e^2}{n} \end{bmatrix}, \tag{4}$$

where $\widehat{\sigma}_c$ and $\widehat{\sigma}_e$ are the estimated variances for cost and effect respectively and $\hat{\rho}$ is the estimated correlation coefficient between cost and effect.

The difference in expected cost and effect between two treatments/ interventions, $(\Delta E(\mathbf{c}), \Delta E(\mathbf{e}))$ could be estimated by the sample means of $\mathbf{c}$ and $\mathbf{e}$, that is, $(\bar{c}, \bar{e})$ and the covariance matrix of $(\Delta\bar{c}, \Delta\bar{e})$ could be expressed as:

$$\begin{bmatrix} \dfrac{\widehat{\sigma}_{ci}^2}{n_i} + \dfrac{\widehat{\sigma}_{cj}^2}{n_j} & \dfrac{\widehat{\rho}\,\widehat{\sigma}_{ci}\widehat{\sigma}_{ei}}{n_i} + \dfrac{\rho_j\widehat{\sigma}_{cj}\widehat{\sigma}_{ej}}{n_j} \\ \dfrac{\widehat{\rho}_i\widehat{\sigma}_{ci}\widehat{\sigma}_{ei}}{n_i} + \dfrac{\rho_j\widehat{\sigma}_{cj}\widehat{\sigma}_e}{n_j} & \dfrac{\widehat{\sigma}_{ei}^2}{n_i} + \dfrac{\widehat{\sigma}_{ej}^2}{n_j} \end{bmatrix}. \tag{5}$$

4. Statistical Inferences on Cost-Effectiveness Measures

4.1. *Parametric approaches to estimating the C-E ratio confidence interval*

4.1.1. *The confidence box approach*

A number of commentators advocated the cost-effectiveness plane (CE plane) for presenting the results of economic evaluation and for aiding policy decision. O'Brien and colleagues[13] showed how the CE plane could be used to present the confidence limits for the estimate of incremental cost-effectiveness under the assumption of zero covariance between costs and effects. The difference in effect between two interventions is shown on the horizontal axis with mean effect difference $\Delta\bar{e}$ and upper and lower confidence limits for the effect difference $(\Delta\bar{e}^U, \Delta\bar{e}^L)$. Similarly, the difference in cost between two interventions is shown on the vertical axis with mean cost difference $\Delta\bar{c}$ and upper and lower confidence limits for the effect difference $(\Delta\bar{c}^U, \Delta\bar{c}^L)$. These "I" bars intersect at point $(\Delta\bar{e}, \Delta\bar{c})$, hence the ray that connects this point of intersection to the origin has a slope equal to the value of the ICER. Under the assumption described above, the center of the two confidence intervals intuitively can be thought of as the maximum likelihood of the two-dimensional probability density function. O'Brien and colleagues[13] argue that combining the limits of the confidence intervals for costs and effects separately gives natural best and worst case limits on the ratio; that is, the upper limit of the cost difference over the lower limit of the effect difference $(\Delta\bar{c}^U/\Delta\bar{c}^L)$ gives the highest values of the ratio (worst case) and the lower limit of costs divided by the upper limit of effects $(\Delta\bar{e}^L/\Delta\bar{e}^U)$ gives the lowest (best) value of the ratio. Thus, in Fig. 1, the slope of the line from the origin through point *a* is a worst-case scenario for the incremental cost-effectiveness ratio based upon the upper 95% CI of the cost estimate and the lower 95% CI of the effect estimate. By similar reasoning, the line through point *c* is the best-case scenario. In contrast to Fig. 1, the slice of "pie" bounded from the origin by the best and worst cases scenarios has increased in size reflecting increased uncertainty about where the true cost-effectiveness ratio lies in this region.

There are two problems with this line of reasoning. The first is that the depiction of the two-dimensional confidence plane as being box-shaped is misleading. If costs and effects varied independently then the conditional probability of being at the lower 95% CI of both simultaneously would be less than 0.05. In principle we might expect such a bivariate probability density function to be elliptical in shape with lines of equi-probability central point-estimate (the maximum likelihood) much like an ordnance survey map of a mountain with height contours. Figure 3 illustrates how this general concept applies to the current problem. The second problem is the implicit assumption that costs and effects vary independently (i.e. have zero covariance). In principle we would expect covariance between costs and effects, and therefore we cannot assume that the numerator and

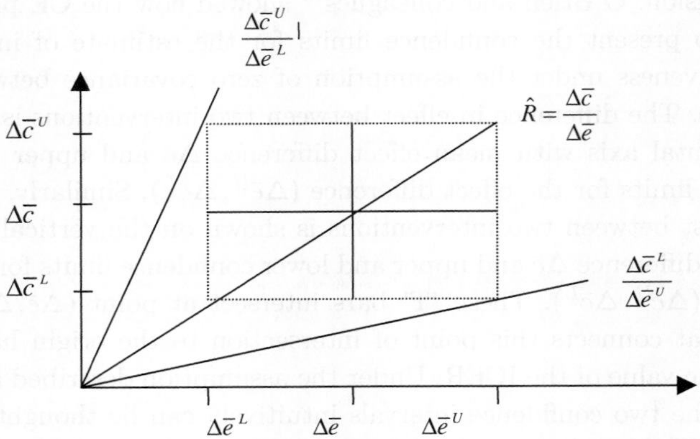

Fig. 2. Confidence limits on the cost-effectiveness plane and the "confidence box" approach to estimating confidence limits for the ICER.

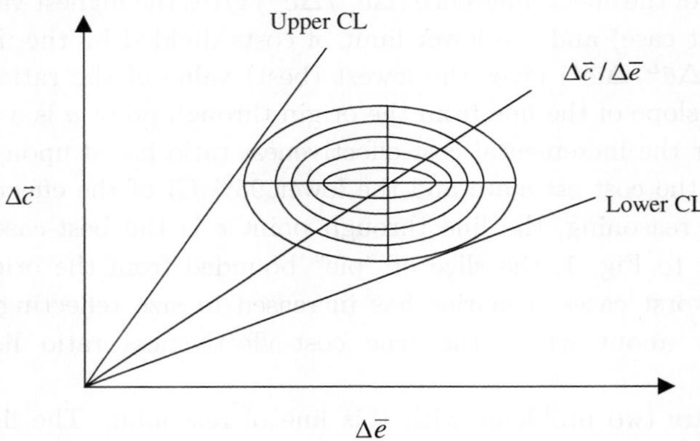

Fig. 3. Hypothetical probability density function around maximum likelihood point-estimate for cost-effectiveness.

denominator in the ratio are independent. This means that the bounds for the cost-effectiveness ratio depicted in Fig. 2 are still only a quasi-confidence interval because we have not taken account of all sampling variation. The challenge is whether a method exists for estimating the sampling distribution for the ratio of two random variables which may have nonzero covariance.

4.1.2. *The Taylor series approximation*

The Taylor approximation shows that where y is a function of two random variables x_1 and x_2, the variance of y can be expressed in term of the partial derivatives of y with respect to x_1 and x_2, weighted by the variances and covariance of x_1 and x_2. The Taylor series formula is

$$\begin{aligned}\operatorname{var}(y) \approx &\left(\frac{\partial y}{\partial x_1}\right)^2 \operatorname{var}(x_1) + \left(\frac{\partial y}{\partial x_2}\right)^2 \operatorname{var}(x_2)\\ &+ 2\left(\frac{\partial y}{\partial x_1}\right)\left(\frac{\partial y}{\partial x_2}\right) \operatorname{cov}(x_1, x_2)\,. \end{aligned} \tag{6}$$

For the ICER $\Delta E(c)/\Delta E(e)$, using the sample estimates of the means and variance, the variance of the ratio estimator can be given as follows:

$$\operatorname{var}(\hat{R}) \approx \frac{1}{\Delta\bar{e}^2}\operatorname{var}(\Delta\bar{c}) + \frac{\Delta\bar{c}^2}{\Delta\bar{e}^4}\operatorname{var}(\Delta\bar{e}) - 2\frac{\Delta\bar{c}}{\Delta\bar{e}^3}\operatorname{cov}(\Delta\bar{c}, \Delta\bar{e})\,. \tag{7}$$

Since the variance of difference in mean is equal to the sum of two sampling variances for those means, then we can simplify

$$\operatorname{var}(\Delta\bar{c}) = \frac{\hat{\sigma}_{c1}^2}{n_1} + \frac{\hat{\sigma}_{c2}^2}{n_2}, \quad \operatorname{var}(\Delta\bar{e}) = \frac{\hat{\sigma}_{e2}^2}{n_1} + \frac{\hat{\sigma}_{e2}^2}{n_2}, \tag{8}$$

and the covariance term can also be simplified

$$\operatorname{cov}(\Delta\bar{c}, \Delta\bar{e}) = \frac{\widehat{\operatorname{cov}}(c_1, e_1)}{n_1} + \frac{\widehat{\operatorname{cov}}(c_2, e_2)}{n_2} = \frac{\hat{\rho}_1\hat{\sigma}_{c1}\hat{\sigma}_{e1}}{n_1} + \frac{\hat{\rho}_2\hat{\sigma}_{c2}\hat{\sigma}_{e2}}{n_2}\,. \tag{9}$$

Combining these elements gives our expression for the variance of ratio

$$\begin{aligned}\operatorname{var}(\hat{R}) \approx &\left[\frac{\frac{\hat{\sigma}_{c1}^2}{n_1} + \frac{\hat{\sigma}_{c2}^2}{n_2}}{\Delta\bar{e}^2}\right] + \Delta\bar{c}^2\left[\frac{\frac{\hat{\sigma}_{e1}^2}{n_1} + \frac{\hat{\sigma}_{e2}^2}{n_2}}{\Delta\bar{e}^4}\right]\\ &- 2\Delta\bar{c}\left[\frac{\frac{\hat{\rho}_1\,\hat{\sigma}_{c1}\,\hat{\sigma}_{e1}}{n_1} + \frac{\hat{\rho}_2\,\hat{\sigma}_{c2}\,\hat{\sigma}_{e2}}{n_2}}{\Delta\bar{e}^3}\right]. \end{aligned} \tag{10}$$

Factoring $\hat{R}^2 = \Delta\bar{c}^2/\Delta\bar{e}^2$ from the right-hand side simplifies (7) to

$$\operatorname{var}(\hat{R}) \approx \hat{R}^2[(cv(\Delta\bar{c}))^2 + (cv(\Delta\bar{e}))^2 - 2\,\widehat{\rho}\,cv(\Delta\bar{c})cv(\Delta\bar{e})]\,, \tag{11}$$

where $cv(x)$ is the coefficient of variation for the random variable x and defined as $cv(x) = \sqrt{\operatorname{var}(x)}/\bar{x}$, and ρ_{xy} is the correlation coefficient between two random variables x and y and defined as $\rho_{xy} = \mathrm{cov}(x, y)/\sqrt{\mathrm{var}(x)\mathrm{var}(y)}$. The properties of this variance are intuitively appealing: the cost-effectiveness variance will increase with a greater difference in costs or effects, with a greater population mean cost between groups and with greater negative correlation between costs and effects. Conversely the ratio variance will decrease with greater sample size, with a greater difference in population mean effects between groups and a greater positive correlation between costs and effects.

The accuracy of the approximation in the equation above depends upon the random variables, $\Delta\bar{c}$ and $\Delta\bar{e}$, having small coefficients of variation. The coefficient of variation for each random variable is $(Z_{\alpha/2} + Z_\beta)^{-1}$, where the two-sided level test α of significance has $1 - \beta$ power against the true difference. For even a 50% power against the true difference the coefficient of variation would be $(1.96)^{-1} = 0.51$; small enough to ensure reasonable accuracy. The accuracy of the approximation begins to fail as the difference between treatments, with respect to cost or effect, approaches zero so that the power falls well below 50%.

Similarly, for the ratio $E(c)/E(e)$, we have

$$\mathrm{var}(\hat{R}) \approx \frac{1}{\bar{e}^2}\mathrm{var}(\bar{c}) + \frac{\bar{c}^2}{\bar{e}^4}\mathrm{var}(\bar{e}) - 2\frac{\bar{c}}{\bar{e}^3}\mathrm{cov}(\bar{c}, \bar{e}), \tag{12}$$

$$\mathrm{var}(\hat{R}) \approx \left[\frac{\widehat{\sigma}_c^2}{n}\Big/\bar{e}^2\right] + \bar{c}^2\left[\frac{\widehat{\sigma}_e^2}{n}\Big/\bar{e}^4\right] - 2\bar{c}\left[\frac{\widehat{\rho}\,\widehat{\sigma}_c\widehat{\sigma}_e}{n}\Big/\bar{e}^3\right], \tag{13}$$

$$\mathrm{var}(\hat{R}) \approx \hat{R}^2[(cv(c))^2 + (cv(e))^2 - 2\,\widehat{\rho}\,cv(c)cv(e)]\,. \tag{14}$$

Employing standard parametric assumptions gives the confidence interval as

$$\left(\hat{R} - z_{\alpha/2}\sqrt{\mathrm{var}(\hat{R})},\ \hat{R} + z_{\alpha/2}\sqrt{\mathrm{var}(\hat{R})}\right). \tag{15}$$

Knowledge of the variance of R would also enable some tests of hypotheses. For example, suppose we specified some *a priori* upper threshold for the cost-effectiveness ratio, $R_{\max}$, which was the maximum cost per unit effect that we would be willing to pay for this new treatment. Hence $R_{\max}$ would be the maximum acceptable slope of the cost-effectiveness line through the origin in Fig. 2. We might set up a one-tailed test of the hypothesis that the true ratio, R, was less than this maximum. Thus, we have a null hypothesis, $H_0 : R = R_{\max}$ which is to be tested against an alternative $H_A : R < R_{\max}$

and using our variance we might construct a test statistic of the general form:

$$Z = \widehat{R} - R_{\max}\sqrt{\operatorname{var}(\widehat{R})}\,.$$

In illustrating the possible use of $\operatorname{var}(\widehat{R})$ in estimation and hypothesis testing we have assumed that the distribution for $\widehat{R}$ will be statistically well-behaved such that some parametric distribution (e.g. normal) might be used in the large sample case. Although this is ultimately an empirical issue it seems a questionable assumption. For example, the distribution of a ratio of two differences may not be unimodal. While a non-parametric analogue of the approach might be developed using rank-order statistics a more practical alternative might be to generate an empirical distribution for $\widehat{R}$ by non-parametric bootstrapping.

4.1.3. *Fieller's method*

An alternative method of calculating confidence intervals around ratios has been described by Fieller.[5]

The advantage of Filler's method over the Taylor series expansion is that it takes into account the skew of the ratio estimator. The method assumes that the numerator and denominator of the ratio follow a joint normal distribution such that (in the case of the ICER) $\Delta\bar{c} - R\Delta\bar{e}$ is normally distributed. Hence, dividing through by the standard deviation equation follows the standard normal distribution:

$$\frac{\Delta\bar{c} - R\Delta\bar{e}}{\sqrt{\{\operatorname{var}(\Delta\bar{c}) + R^2\operatorname{var}(\Delta\bar{e}) - 2R\operatorname{cov}(\Delta\bar{c},\Delta\bar{e})\}}} \sim N(0,1)\,. \qquad (16)$$

Setting this expression equal to $z_{\alpha/2}$ and rearranging gives the following quadratic equation in R:

$$\begin{aligned}&\widehat{R}[1 - z^2_{\alpha/2}(cv(\Delta\bar{e}))^2] - 2R\,\hat{R}[1 - z^2_{\alpha/2}\,\rho cv(\Delta\bar{e})cv(\Delta\bar{c})]\\&\quad + \hat{R}^2[1 - z^2_{\alpha/2}\,cv(\Delta\bar{c})] = 0,\end{aligned} \qquad (17)$$

$$\begin{aligned}&\hat{R}\left[\frac{1 - z^2_{\alpha/2}\,\rho cv(\Delta\bar{c})cv(\Delta\bar{e})}{1 - z^2_{\alpha/2}[cv(\Delta\bar{e})]^2}\right]\\&\quad \pm z^2_{\alpha/2}\hat{R}\left[\frac{\sqrt{\begin{array}{l}[cv(\Delta\bar{c})]^2 + [cv(\Delta\bar{e})^2] - 2\rho cv(\Delta\bar{c})cv(\Delta\bar{e})\\ \quad - z^2_{\alpha/2}\{[cv(\Delta\bar{c})]^2[cv(\Delta\bar{e})^2] - \rho^2[cv(\Delta\bar{c})]^2[cv(\Delta\bar{e})]^2\}\end{array}}}{1 - z^2_{\alpha/2}[cv(\Delta\bar{e})]^2}\right].\end{aligned} \qquad (18)$$

Similarly, for the ratio $E(c)/E(e)$, we have

$$\frac{\bar{c} - R\bar{e}}{\sqrt{\{\text{var}(\bar{c}) + R^2\,\text{var}(\bar{e}) - 2R\,\text{cov}(\bar{c},\bar{e})\}}} \sim N(0,1)\,, \tag{19}$$

$$\hat{R}[1 - z^2_{\alpha/2}(cv(\bar{e}))^2] - 2R\,\hat{R}[1 - z^2_{\alpha/2}\,\rho cv(\bar{e})cv(\bar{c})] + \hat{R}^2[1 - z^2_{\alpha/2}cv(\bar{c})]\,, \tag{20}$$

$$\hat{R}\left[\frac{1 - z^2_{\alpha/2}\rho cv(\bar{c})cv(\bar{e})}{1 - z^2_{\alpha/2}[cv(\bar{e})]^2}\right]$$

$$\pm\, z^2_{\alpha/2}\,\hat{R}\left[\frac{\begin{array}{c}\sqrt{[cv(\bar{c})]^2 + [cv(\bar{e})^2] - 2\rho cv(\bar{c})cv(\bar{e})} \\ - z^2_{\alpha/2}\{[cv(\bar{c})]^2[cv(\bar{e})^2] - \rho^2[cv(\bar{c})]^2[cv(\bar{e})]^2\}\end{array}}{1 - z^2_{\alpha/2}[cv(\bar{e})]^2}\right]. \tag{21}$$

Siegel *et al.*[16] proposed that $\tau = \bar{c} - R\bar{e}$ is normally distributed with mean $E\tau = 0$ and $\text{var}(\tau) = (\text{var}(c) - 2R\,\text{cov}(c,e) + R^2\,\text{var}(e))/n$. Let $F_{1,n-1}$ denote the 95th percentile of an F distribution with 1 and $(n-1)$ degrees of freedom. The probability that

$$\tau^2/(\widehat{\text{var}}\,(c) - 2R\,\widehat{\text{cov}}(c,e) + R^2\,\widehat{\text{var}}\,(e)) < F_{1,n-1}(n-1)^{-1}$$

is 0.05 since the random variable of the left side of the inequality is distributed as an F distribution with 1 and $(n-1)$ degree of freedom. Multiplying both sides by the denominator and subtracting the right hand side from both sides of the inequality yields

$$\begin{aligned}(\bar{c}^2 - F_{1,n-1}(n-1)^{-1}\ \widehat{\text{var}}\,(c)) - 2R(\bar{c}\bar{e} - F_{1,n-1}(n-1)^{-1}\ \widehat{\text{cov}}(c,e)) \\ + R^2(\bar{e}^2 - F_{1,n-1}(n-1)^{-1}\ \widehat{\text{var}}\,(e)) \le 0\,.\end{aligned} \tag{22}$$

The set of values of R satisfying this inequality is a 95% confidence interval for the ratio $E(c)/E(e)$.

4.1.4. *Confidence interval for the expected cost to effect ratio* $E(c/e)$

Under an assumption of asymptotic normality, the expected value of the ratio $E(c/e)$ does not exist because ratios of normal random variables follow the Cauchy distribution. Therefore, in this case neither an estimator nor a confidence interval makes sense. The approximate distribution function of the random variable c/e, $F(y) = P(c/e < y\sigma_e/\sigma_c)$ is given by

$$\Phi((wE(e)/\sigma_e - E(e)/\sigma_c)(w^2 - 2\rho w + 1)^{-1/2}) \tag{23}$$

where $\Phi(\cdot)$ is the cumulative normal distribution with mean 0 and variance 1. Here, $w = y\sigma_e/\sigma_c$ where σ_e and σ_c are the population standard deviations of e and c respectively and ρ is the correlation between them. The median of this distribution is $E(c)/E(e)$. Thus, the ratio of expected costs to expected effects is the median of the distribution of the distribution of the patient level ratio of costs to effects. A 95% confidence interval for the median of this distribution may be obtained by applying the method based on Fieller's theorem.

For some data, rather than assuming that the distribution of F is multivariate normal, it may be more appropriate to assume that the distribution has a form for which $E(c/e)$ does exist. For example, under an assumption of asymptotic normality of the ratio, the sample mean of $\overline{c/e}$ and sample variance of the ratio $\widehat{\sigma}^2_{c/e}$ can be used to form a 95% confidence interval for the mean cost-weight ratio as follows:

$$\overline{c/e} + t_{n-1}\widehat{\sigma}_{c/e}\sqrt{n}\,, \tag{24}$$

where n is the number of patients.

4.2. *Bootstrap approaches to estimating the C-E ratio*

The bootstrap approach for the simple one sample case is straightforward. Suppose a particular population has a real but unobserved probability distribution F from which a random sample x of n observations is taken, and the statistic of interest $s(x)$ is calculated the concern of inferential statistics is to make statements about the population parameter θ based on the sample drawn from that population. In the "bootstrap world," the observed random sample x is treated as the empirical estimate of F by weighting observation in x by the probability $1/n$. Successive random samples of size n are then draw from x with replacement to give the bootstrap samples (re-sample from the original sample). The statistic of interest is calculated for each of these samples and these bootstrap replicates of the original statistic make up the empirical estimate of the sampling distribution for that statistic. This estimated sampling distribution can be used in a variety of ways to construct confidence intervals.

In principle, the bootstrap estimate of the ICER sampling distribution can be obtained in very similar way to that of the simple one sample case.

How ever, since the ICER is estimated on the basis of four estimators from two samples care must be taken to bootstrap each sample appropriately. For data structures which are more complicated than a one sample structure. Efron and Tibshirani[4] advocate that the bootstrap mechanism for the observed data mirror the mechanism by which those original data were obtained. In the case of the ICER, where data on resource use and outcome exists for two groups of patients of size n_i and n_j receiving treatments/interventions T_i and T_j, respectively this will involve a three-stage process:

(1) Sample with replacement n_i cost/effect pair from the sample of patients who received treatment T_i and calculate the bootstrap estimates $\bar{c}_i^*$ and $\bar{e}_i^*$ for the bootstrap sample.
(2) Sample with replacement n_j cost/effect pair from the sample of patients who received treatment T_j and calculate the bootstrap estimates $\bar{c}_j^*$ and $\bar{e}_j^*$ for the bootstrap sample.
(3) Calculate the bootstrap replicate of the ICER given by the equation

$$R^* = \frac{\bar{c}_i^* - \bar{c}_j^*}{\bar{e}_i^* - \bar{e}_j^*} = \frac{\Delta\bar{c}^*}{\Delta\bar{e}^*}\,. \tag{25}$$

Repeating this three-stage process many times gives a vector of bootstrap estimates, which is an empirical estimate of the sampling distribution of the ICER statistic.

Once the sampling distribution of the ICER has been estimated in this way, several approaches exit to estimate confidence limits using the bootstrap estimate of the sampling.

4.2.1. *Normal approximation*

One method for confidence interval estimation is to take the bootstrap estimate of standard error, given by

$$\hat{\delta}^* = \sqrt{\left\{\frac{1}{B-1}\sum_{b=1}^{B}(\bar{R}^* - \bar{R}^{*b})^2\right\}}\,, \tag{26}$$

(where B is the total number of bootstrap replications) and assume that the sampling distribution is normal. The resulting $100(1-\alpha)$ per cent confidence interval is

$$(\hat{R} - z_{\alpha/2}\hat{\delta}^*\,,\ \hat{R} + z_{\alpha/2}\hat{\delta}^*)\,. \tag{27}$$

4.2.2. *Percentile*

The percentile method avoids the problem by making direct use of the empirical sampling distribution. The $100(\alpha/2)$ and $100(1-\alpha/2)$ percentile values of the bootstrap sampling distribution estimate are used as the upper and lower confidence limits for the ICER. The attraction of this method is its simplicity and its avoidance of the assumption of normality for the ICER. However, skewed estimation can cause problems for the percentile method. In particular, in this context, the percentile method assumes that the bootstrap replicates of the ICER are unbiased, whereas it is known that ratio estimators are biased and that bootstrap replicates will magnify the bias of the sample estimate.[17]

4.2.3. *Bias-corrected and accelerated*

Efron[3] suggests a modification of the percentile method, which seeks to adjust for the bias and skew of the sampling distribution. This is the bias-corrected and accelerated (BCa) percentile method, which involves algebraic adjustments to the percentiles selected to serve as the confidence interval end points. The adjusted percentiles are given by

$$\begin{aligned}\alpha_1 &= \Phi\left(\hat{z} + \frac{\hat{z} + z_{\alpha/2}}{1 - \hat{a}(\hat{z} + z_{\alpha/2})}\right),\\ \alpha_2 &= \Phi\left(\hat{z} + \frac{\hat{z} + z_{(1-\alpha/2)}}{1 - \hat{a}(\hat{z} + z_{(1-\alpha/2)})}\right),\end{aligned} \tag{28}$$

where $\Phi(\cdot)$ is the standard normal cumulative distribution function and z_α is the 100α percentile point of standard normal distribution. Two adjustments to the percentiles are incorporated into Eq. (28): $\hat{z}$ adjusts the sampling distribution for the bias of the estimator, while $\hat{a}$ adjusts for the skew of the sampling distribution. Setting $\hat{a} = 0$ yields the adjustment for bias on the percentile chosen to serve as end points, and is equivalent to the bias-corrected method advocated by Chaudhary and Stearns[1]:

$$\begin{aligned}\alpha_1 &= \Phi(2\hat{z} + z_{\alpha/2}),\\ \alpha_2 &= \Phi(2\hat{z} + z_{(1-\alpha/2)}).\end{aligned} \tag{29}$$

The bias correction, $\hat{z}$, is given by $\hat{z} = \Phi^{-1}(Q)$ where Q is the proportion of bootstrap replicates which are less than the sample estimate, $\hat{R}$. Therefore, if the bootstrap sampling distribution has median $\hat{R}$, $Q = 0.5$ which gives $\hat{z} = 0$ and (in the absence of a skew adjustment) the percentiles from

Eq. (29) correspond to those from the straightforward percentile method. However, where the sampling distribution is not centered on $\hat{R}$ a correction is made for this bias. Notice that the nonlinear relationship between the z-score and its probability results in the percentile end points being shifted at unequal rates. It is also worth nothing that the bias correction adjustment of BCa method, while not employing distributional assumptions concerning the distribution of the ICER itself, does make use of parametric assumptions concerning the distribution of the observed bias. This reliance on parametric assumptions has been cited as a potential weakness of the BCa method (29).

The acceleration constant adjusts for the skew of the sampling distribution. Efron and Tibshirani[4] suggest using a jack-knife estimate for $\hat{\alpha}$:

$$\hat{\alpha}^{**} = \frac{\sum_{i=1}^{n}(\bar{R}^{**} - \hat{R}_i^{**})^3}{6[\sum_{i=1}^{n}(\bar{R}^{**} - \hat{R}_i^{**})^2]^{3/2}}, \tag{30}$$

where $\hat{R}_i^{**}$ is the jack-knife replicate of the ICER with the ith observation removed, $\bar{R}^{*}* = \sum \hat{R}_i^{**}/n$ for $i = 1$ to n and $n = n_t + n_c$. In terms of the adjustments to the percentiles given in Eq. (28). In the absence of a bias correction adjustment, the skew adjustment is given by

$$\begin{aligned} \alpha_1 &= \Phi\left(\frac{z_{\alpha/2}}{1 - \hat{a}z_{\alpha/2}}\right), \\ \alpha_2 &= \Phi\left(\frac{z_{(1-\alpha/2)}}{1 - \hat{a}z_{(1-\alpha/2)}}\right). \end{aligned} \tag{31}$$

Equation (30) shows that if the sampling distribution is symmetric, $\hat{a} = 0$ and Eq. (31) shows that no adjustment to the percentile interval end points is made.

4.2.4. *Parametric bootstrap*

Efron and Tibshirani[4] outline a simulation-based method of confidence interval estimation that they refer to as a parametric bootstrap approach. Notice that from the definition of ICER, the difference in cost on the numerator and the difference in effects on the denominator of the ICER are both simply the difference between two normally distributed. The parametric bootstrap approach involves using this property of the distribution of the numerator and denominator in combination with the observe means, variance and covariance to estimate the parameters of the sampling distribution of the cost and effect differences. Sampling from each of these two distributions, while allowing for the estimated covariance between them, gives an estimate of the ICER. Repeating this process many times generates an empirical estimate of the sampling distribution of the ICER. The $100(\alpha/2)$ and $100(1-\alpha/2)$ percentiles of this estimated distribution are used as estimstes for the upper and lower limits of the confidence interval, as with the percentile method.

5. Testing Difference Among the Populations

5.1. *Under assumption of normality of distribution*

5.1.1. *Testing on ICER*

Let R_0 be a specified value of the incremental cost-effectiveness ratio (ICER) R. It may be viewed as the maximum amount society is willing to pay to gain one unit of effectiveness by adopting the test intervention over the reference. We consider three tests of hypotheses on R:

(a) $H_0: R = R_0$ versus $H_A: R \neq R_0$;
(b) $H_0: R \geq R_0$ versus $H_A: R < R_0$;
(c) $H_0: \Delta E(e) \geq 0$ or $R \geq R_0$ versus $H_A: \Delta E(e) > 0$ and $R < R_0$.

In (b), rejection of the null hypothesis might be interpreted to mean that the test intervention is cost-effective, in the sense that the data supports a CER below the stipulated maximum R_0. Its two-tailed version, (a) tests whether the data are consistent with a specified value R_0 of the ICER. In (c), we test the joint hypothesis on effectiveness and cost effectiveness. If the null hypothesis is tenable, the test intervention is either not effective or not cost-effective. If the alternative is true, then the test intervention is both effective and cost-effective, relative to the referent intervention. The covariance matrix of $(\Delta\bar{c}, \Delta\bar{e})'$, Σ could be represented as follows

$$\Sigma = \begin{bmatrix} \widehat{\sigma}_c^2 \widehat{\rho}\,\widehat{\sigma}_c \widehat{\sigma}_e \\ \widehat{\rho}\,\widehat{\sigma}_c \widehat{\sigma}\,\widehat{\sigma}_e^2 \end{bmatrix} = \begin{bmatrix} \dfrac{\widehat{\sigma}_{c0}^2}{n_i} + \dfrac{\widehat{\sigma}_{c1}^2}{n_j} & \dfrac{\widehat{\rho}_i \widehat{\sigma}_{ci} \widehat{\sigma}_{ei}}{n_i} + \dfrac{\widehat{\rho}_j \widehat{\sigma}_{cj} \widehat{\sigma}_{ej}}{n_j} \\ \dfrac{\widehat{\rho}_i \widehat{\sigma}_{ci} \widehat{\sigma}_{ei}}{n_i} + \dfrac{\widehat{\rho}_j \widehat{\sigma}_{cj} \widehat{\sigma}_{ei}}{n_j} & \dfrac{\widehat{\sigma}_{ei}^2}{n_i} + \dfrac{\widehat{\sigma}_{e1}^2}{n_j} \end{bmatrix}. \tag{32}$$

Test of $H_0: R = R_0$ versus $H_A: R \neq R_0$.

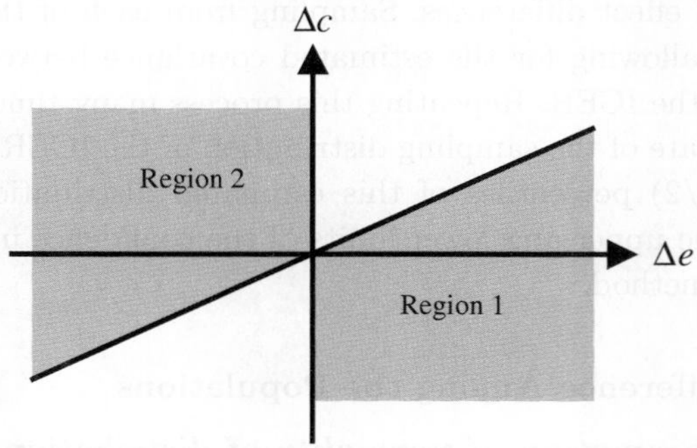

Fig. 4. Regions for one-sided test of effectiveness and cost-effectiveness. Region 1: test intervention both effective and cost-effective. Region 2: referent intervention effective and cost-effective.

We formulate our test in terms of the estimated net cost $\Delta\bar{c} - R_0\Delta\bar{e}$. Under H_0, the statistic

$$T = (\Delta\bar{c} - R_0\Delta\bar{e})/\{\mathrm{var}(\Delta\bar{c} - R_0\Delta\bar{e})\}^{1/2}$$

or

$$T = (\Delta\bar{c} - R_0\Delta\bar{e})/\{\mathrm{var}(\Delta\bar{c}) + R_0^2\ \mathrm{var}(\Delta\bar{e}) - 2R_0^2\ \mathrm{cov}(\Delta\bar{c}, \Delta\bar{e})\}^{1/2}$$

has an approximate standard normal distribution. The test rejects H_0 if $|T| > z_{(1-\alpha/2)}$ where $z_{(1-\alpha/2)}$ is the $100(1-\alpha/2)$ percentile of the standard normal distribution.

Test of $H_0 : R \geq R_0$ versus $H_A : R < R_0$
We would reject $H_0 : R \geq R_0$ if $\Delta\bar{c} - R_0\Delta\bar{e} < -z_{(1-\alpha/2)}\{\mathrm{var}(\Delta\bar{c}) + R_0^2\ \mathrm{var}(\Delta\bar{e}) - 2R_0^2\ \mathrm{cov}(\Delta\bar{c}, \Delta\bar{e})\}_{1/2}$
Test of $H_0 : \Delta E(e) \leq 0$ or $R \geq R_0$ versus $H_A : \Delta E(e) > 0$ and $R < R_0$.

In Fig. 4, the lower shaded region (region 1) in the C_E plane is where H_A holds. The complementary shaded region (region 2) in the second and third quadrants is where the referent intervention is both effective and cost-effective. Our one-sided test imposes asymmetry between the test and the referent interventions, and region 1 is the appropriate rejection region for our test.

Based on our previous discussion, an appropriate test would reject H_0 if $\Delta\bar{e} > c_1$ and $(\Delta\bar{c} - R_0\Delta\bar{e}) < c_2$ where the constants $c_1 > 0$ and $c_2 < 0$ need to be specified. The size of the test is

$$\alpha = \sup P[\Delta\bar{e} > c_1,\ (\Delta\bar{c} - R_0\Delta\bar{e}) < c_2],$$

where the supremum is taken over all $(\Delta\bar{e}, \Delta\bar{c})$ consistent with H_0. By normalization, we may express this in terms of the bivariate normal (Z_1, Z_2), with zero means, unit variances and correlation $-\rho^*$. Then

$$\alpha = \sup P\Bigg[Z_1 < \frac{-(c_1 - \Delta\bar{e})}{\sqrt{\text{var}(\Delta\bar{e})}},$$

$$z_2 < \frac{c_2 - (\Delta\bar{c} - R_0\Delta\bar{e})}{\{\text{var}(\Delta\bar{c}) + R_0^2\,\text{var}(\Delta\bar{e}) - 2R_0^2\,\text{cov}(\Delta\bar{c}, \Delta\bar{e})\}^{1/2}}\Bigg]$$

$$= \max\Bigg\{P\left[Z_1 < \frac{-c_1}{\sqrt{\{\text{var}(\Delta\bar{e})}}\right],$$

$$P\left[Z_2 < \frac{c_2}{\{\text{var}(\Delta\bar{c}) + R_0^2\,\text{var}(\Delta\bar{e}) - 2R_0^2\,\text{cov}(\Delta\bar{c}, \Delta\bar{e})\}^{1/2}}\right]\Bigg\}. \quad (33)$$

One solution to (33) is

$$c_1 = \sigma_1 z_{1-\alpha}\,,$$

$$c_2 = -\{\text{var}(\Delta\bar{c}) + R_0^2\,\text{var}(\Delta\bar{e}) - 2R_0^2\,\text{cov}(\Delta\bar{c}, \Delta\bar{e})\}^{1/2} z_{1-\alpha}\,. \quad (34)$$

5.1.2. *Testing on CER (cost-effectiveness ratio)*

If the cost-weight bivariate distributions are normal with mean vectors $(E(c_i), E(e_i))$ and common covariance matrix, the multivariate analysis of variance, MANOVA, can be used to test the hypothesis that the vectors of cost-efficiency measures are identical. If the MANOVA finds the means of the distributions of the populations to be equal and the $c - e$ measure is a function of the means, e.g. $E(c_i)/E(e_i)$, then it may be concluded that the $c - e$ measures do not differ.

A likelihood ratio test could be employed to test the hypothesis H_0 : $E(c_i)/E(e_i) = R_0$ for all i, that is, $E(c_i) - R_0E(e_i) = 0$.

An asymptotic α-level two sided test of H_0 may be obtained by first using likelihood theory for normal variables for testing the linear hypothesis that all ratios are equal to a specific value, say, R_0. The desired likelihood ratio test is found by maximizing the previous likelihood over all possible values of R_0.

Let n_i denote the number of bivariate observations of cost and effect for treatment i and let $n = \Sigma n_i$. The available data consists of the bivariate observations (c_{ij}, e_{ij}), $i = 1, 2, \ldots, I$, $j = 1, 2, \ldots, n_i$. Let $s_{11} = \Sigma_i\Sigma_j(c_{ij} - \bar{c}_i)^2/n$, $s_{22} = \Sigma_i\Sigma_j(e_{ij} - \bar{e}_i)^2/n$, and $s_{12} = \Sigma_i\Sigma_j(c_{ij} - \bar{c}_i)(e_{ij} - \bar{e}_i)/n$. Here, s_{ij} are the elements of the pooled covariance matrix, S. The hypothesis $E(c_i)/E(e_i) = R_0$ is equivalent to the hypothesis $E(c_i) - R_0E(e_i) = 0$ for all i. For a specific R_0 the classical test of the latter linear hypothesis is based on the Wilks' statistic, $W(R_0)$. The likelihood ratio statistic for the same linear hypothesis is given by $\Lambda(R_0) = W(R_0)^{n/2}$. Maximizing $\Lambda(R_0)$ over all possible values of R_0 yields the desired likelihood ratio test. The test rejects H_0 at the R_0 level if

$$-n\,\ln\chi_{\max} < \chi^2_{1-\alpha}(I-1)\,. \tag{35}$$

Here $\chi^2_{1-\alpha}(I-1)$ is the upper $1-\alpha$ percentage points of the chi-square distribution with $I-1$ degrees of freedom and $\chi_{\max}$ is the large of the two solutions of the following quadratic equation: $ax^2 + bx + c = 0$ where

$$\begin{aligned}
a &= \Sigma_i\Sigma_j c_{ij}^2 * \Sigma_i\Sigma_j e_{ij}^2 - (\Sigma_i\Sigma_j c_{ij}e_{ij})^2\,,\\
b &= [\Sigma_i\Sigma_j c_{ij}^2 * \Sigma_i(\Sigma_j e_{ij}^2 - n_i\bar{e}_i^2) + \Sigma_i\Sigma_j e_{ij}^2 * \Sigma_i(\Sigma_j c_{ij}^2 - n_i\bar{c}_i^2)\\
&\quad - 2(\Sigma_i\Sigma_j c_{ij}e_{ij}) * (\Sigma_i(\Sigma_j c_{ij}e_{ij} - n_i\bar{c}_i\bar{e}_i))]\,,\\
c &= \Sigma_i(\Sigma_j c_{ij}^2 - n_i\bar{c}_i^2) * \Sigma_i(\Sigma_j e_{ij}^2 - n_i\bar{e}_i^2) - (\Sigma_i(\Sigma_j c_{ij}e_{ij} - n_i\bar{c}_i\bar{e}_i))^2\,.
\end{aligned}$$

5.2. *Without assumption of normality of distribution*

The distribution of c/e is often skewed. The lifetime models can be widely applied to investigate the distributions of c/e and the difference in c/e between populations. A cost-effectiveness distribution function, or $c-e$ distribution function, could be defined as:

$$S(c_e) = \Pr(c/e > c_e)\,. \tag{36}$$

The parametric, semi-parametric and non-parametric methods are able to deal with the data, whose distributions do not meet the assumption of normality and with censored data.

The Weibull, gamma and log-normal distributions could be applied to estimate the $c-e$ distribution function and the difference in c/e between different populations.

The non-parametric approach, such as Kaplan–Meier method could be applied to estimate the $c-e$ function. The non-parametric tests such as Wilcoxon and logrank test can be used to test the equality of the different groups.

6. Power and Sample Size Assessment for Tests of Hypotheses on Cost-Effetiveness Ratios

6.1. *Test of $H_0 : R = R_0$ versus $H_A : R \neq R_0$*

The power $(= 1 - \beta)$ of this test at the alternative $H_A : R = R_A (\neq R_0)$ is given by

$$P[|\Delta\bar{c} - \bar{R}_0\Delta\bar{e}| < z_{1-\alpha/2}\{\mathrm{var}(\Delta\bar{c}) + R_0^2\,\mathrm{var}(\Delta\bar{e}) \\ - 2R_0^2\,\mathrm{cov}(\Delta\bar{c},\Delta\bar{e})\}^{1/2}|H_A] = \beta\,. \tag{37}$$

Under H_A, $E(\Delta\bar{c} - \bar{R}_0\Delta\bar{e}) = \delta(R_A - R_0)$, with $\delta(\neq 0)$ denoting the true incremental effectiveness. Assuming the covariance matrix of $(\Delta\bar{c}, \Delta\bar{e})'$, Σ, is known, Eq. (37) yields

$$P[-z_{1-\alpha/2} - \delta(R_A - R_0)\{\mathrm{var}(\Delta\bar{c}) + R_0^2\,\mathrm{var}(\Delta\bar{e}) \\ - 2R_0^2\,\mathrm{cov}(\Delta\bar{c},\Delta\bar{e}\}^{-1/2} < Z < z_{1-\alpha/2} \\ - \delta(R_A - R_0)\{\mathrm{var}(\Delta\bar{c}) + R_0^2\,\mathrm{var}(\Delta\bar{e}) \\ - 2R_0^2\,\mathrm{cov}(\Delta\bar{c},\Delta\bar{e}\}^{-1/2}] = \beta\,, \tag{38}$$

where Z is standard normal and $n_A = kn_0$. Depending on the sign of $\delta(R_A - R_0)$, the absolute magnitude of one of the limits on Z is usually large. In either case, we will get, approximately

$$|\delta(R_A - R_0)| \\ = (z_{1-\alpha/2} + z_{1-\beta})\{\mathrm{var}(\Delta\bar{c}) + R_0^2\,\mathrm{var}(\Delta\bar{e}) - 2R_0^2\,\mathrm{cov}(\Delta\bar{c},\Delta\bar{e})\}^{1/2}\,. \tag{39}$$

Routing algebraic steps gives

$$\mathrm{var}(\Delta\bar{c}) + R_0^2\,\mathrm{var}(\Delta\bar{e}) - 2R_0^2\,\mathrm{cov}(\Delta\bar{c},\Delta\bar{e}) = \widehat{\sigma}_c^2(1 - \widehat{\rho}^2)(1 + v_0)\,,$$

where $v_0 = \{R_0(\widehat{\sigma}_e/\widehat{\sigma}_c) - \widehat{\rho}\}^2/(1 - \widehat{\rho}^2)$. Supposing $n_1 = kn_0$, where n_0 and n_1 are the number of patients in the test intervention and referent intervention respectively, we have

$$n_0 = \frac{(\widehat{\sigma}_{c_0}^2 + k^{-1}\widehat{\sigma}_{c_1}^2)(z_{1-\alpha/2} + z_{1-\beta})^2(1 - \widehat{\rho}^2)(1 + v_0)}{\delta^2(R_A - R_0)^2} \tag{40}$$

Under the same design set-up, the sample size n_{0b} in the referent intervention needed to guarantee power of $1 - \beta$ to detect a difference δ in the test of $H_{01} : \Delta\bar{e} = 0$ is given by

$$n_{0b} = \delta^{-2}(\widehat{\sigma}_{e0}^2 + k^{-1}\widehat{\sigma}_{e1}^2)(z_{1-\alpha/2} + z_{1-\beta})^2\,.$$

Therefore,

$$n_0/n_{0b} = \frac{(\widehat{\sigma}_{c0}^2 + k^{-1}\widehat{\sigma}_{c1}^2)(1-\widehat{\rho}^2)(1+v_0)}{(\widehat{\sigma}_{e0}^2 + k^{-1}\widehat{\sigma}_{e1}^2)(R_A - R_0)^2}. \tag{41}$$

The parameter v_0 is a function of ρ^* between $\Delta\bar{e}$ and $(\Delta\bar{c} - R_0\Delta\bar{e})$. In fact,

$$\rho^* = -\{R_0(\widehat{\sigma}_e/\widehat{\sigma}_c) - \widehat{\rho}\}/\sqrt{(1-v^2)}(1+-v_0)\,.$$

Therefore, $|\rho^*| = \{v_0/(1+v_0)\}^2$. It will be very large if ρ^* is close to one and, consequently, the sample sizes in (40) and (41) will also be large. The correlation between the incremental cost and the incremental effectiveness is related through (32) to $\widehat{\rho}$ the individual correlations $\widehat{\rho}_0, \widehat{\rho}_1$ between cost and benefit in the two interventions. As is usually the case, $R_0 \geq 0$ and both (40) and (41) are monotonically decreasing in $\widehat{\rho}$ leading to a smaller sample size n_0 and relative size n_0/n_{0b} with increasing value of $\widehat{\rho}$. Finally, these sample size formulae are dependent on both the hypothesized CER R_0 and the difference $R_A - R_0$.

6.2. *Test of $H_0 : R \geq R_0$ versus $H_A : R < R_0$*

Analogous sample size calculations yield the following formula, which replaces (40):

$$n_0 = \frac{(\sigma_{c0}^2 + k^{-1}\sigma_{c1}^2)(z_{1-\alpha} + z_{1-\beta})^2(1-\rho^2)(1+v_0)}{\delta^2(R_A - R_0)^2}. \tag{42}$$

For the one-sided test $H_{01} : \Delta E(e) = 0$, with regard to their effectiveness and, therefore, should be compared on their costs. The ratio n_0/n_{0b} compares the sample size requirement of the test $H_0 : R = R_0$ with that for $H_{01} : \Delta\bar{e} = 0$, with the latter powered to detect the difference δ.

6.3. *Test of $H_0 : \Delta E(e) \leq 0$ or $R \geq R_0$ versus $H_A : \Delta E(e) > 0$ and $R < R_0$*

With the solution (34), the power $(1-\beta)$ of the test can be computed from the bivariate normal distribution of (Z_1, Z_2) and is given by

$$1 - \beta = P\Bigg[Z_1 < -z_{1-\alpha} + \frac{\delta}{\sigma_1},\ Z_2 < -z_{1-\alpha} + \frac{\delta|R - R_0|}{\{\mathrm{var}(\Delta\bar{c}) + R_0^2\,\mathrm{var}(\Delta\bar{e}) - 2R_0^2\,\mathrm{cov}(\Delta\bar{c}, \Delta\bar{e})\}^{-1/2}}\Bigg], \tag{43}$$

where $\delta > 0$ is the incremental effectiveness and $R(< R_0)$ is the true cost-effectiveness ratio. This parallels the power considerations leading to (39) for the test of cost-effectiveness only. The choice of c_1 and c_2 in (33) is optimal in order to gain maximal power for a given sample size and alternative. An implicit expression for the sample size n_0 corresponding to ( ) can be derived by making the substitutions $\sigma_e^2 = (\sigma_{e0}^2 + k^{-1}\sigma_{c1}^2)/n_0$, $\sigma_e^2 = (\sigma_{c0}^2 + k^{-1}\sigma_{c1}^2)/n_0$ and $\mathrm{var}(\Delta\bar{c}) + R_0^2\,\mathrm{var}(\Delta\bar{e}) - 2R_0^2\,\mathrm{cov}(\Delta\bar{c}, \Delta\bar{e}) = \sigma_c^2(1-\rho)(1+v_0)$. Note that the previous expression for n_0 in (42) is a lower bond for the sample size requirements for testing $H_0 : \Delta E(e) \le 0$ or $R \ge R_0$.

6.4. *Numerical computations*

In some special cases, simplification of (40)–(43) are possible. Suppose the costs (c_0, c_1) and benefit measures (e_0, e_1) in the two interventions have the same variance $\widehat{\sigma}_{c0}^2 = \widehat{\sigma}_{c1}^2 (= \widehat{\sigma}_c^2)$, $\widehat{\sigma}_{e0}^2 = \widehat{\sigma}_{e1}^2 (= \widehat{\sigma}_e^2)$, respectively. Then, assuming equal allocation to the two interventions ($k = 1$), we have $\widehat{\rho} = (\widehat{\rho}_0 + \widehat{\rho}_1)/2$ and the sample size n_0, n_{0b} in (40) and (41) reduce to

$$\begin{aligned} n_0 &= \frac{2\widehat{\sigma}_e^2(z_{1-\alpha/2} + z_{1-\beta})^2(R_0^2 + (\widehat{\sigma}_c/\widehat{\sigma}_e)^2 - 2\widehat{\rho}\,R_0(\widehat{\sigma}_c/\widehat{\sigma}_e))}{\delta^2(R_A - R_0)^2}, \\ n_{0b} &= \delta^{-2} 2\widehat{\sigma}_e^2(z_{1-\alpha/2} + z_{1-\beta})^2 . \end{aligned} \tag{44}$$

From (42), for one-sided testing, $z_{1-\alpha/2}$ must be replaced by $z_{1-\alpha}$. The effect size $\delta/\sigma_\varepsilon$ is the difference in effectiveness in units of standard deviation (SD). For the joint hypothesis test of $H_0 : \Delta E(e) \le 0$ or $R \ge R_0$, the power and sample size expression (43) becomes

$$\begin{aligned} 1 - \beta = P\Bigg[& Z_1 < -z_{1-\alpha} + \sqrt{\frac{n_0}{2}}\frac{\delta}{\widehat{\sigma}_e},\ Z_2 < -z_{1-\alpha} \\ & + \sqrt{\frac{n_0}{2}}\frac{\delta}{\widehat{\sigma}_e}\frac{|R - R_0|}{\{R_0^2 + (\widehat{\sigma}_c/\widehat{\sigma}_e)^2 - 2\widehat{\rho}\,R_0(\widehat{\sigma}_c/\widehat{\sigma}_e)\}^{-1/2}}\Bigg]. \end{aligned} \tag{45}$$

The sample size requirement for this joint test to ensure power $(1 - \beta)$ would be greater than the sample size needed for the one-sided test for effectiveness alone. For fixed n_0, the factor

$$\zeta = \frac{R_0^2 + (\widehat{\sigma}_c/\widehat{\sigma}_e)^2 - 2\rho R_0(\widehat{\sigma}_c/\widehat{\sigma}_e)\}^{-1/2}}{|R - R_0|}$$

would drive the power, with power decreasing with increasing ζ. This factor is the square-root of the sample size ratio n_0/n_{0b} in (41). Note that if

$|\widehat{\sigma}_c/\widehat{\sigma}_e - R_0| > |R_0 - R|$, irrespective of the value $\widehat{\rho}$ we always have $\zeta > 1$. Therefore, (45) should be used to calculate power of the joint test given a sample size that might be available for testing effectiveness. On the other hand, (44) is suitable for assessing the sample size needed to establish cost-effective. It should be noted that the right-hand side of (45) is dependent on $\widehat{\rho}$ through the correlation first decrease Z_1 and Z_2. In practice, we are likely to have $R_0 > \widehat{\sigma}_c/\widehat{\sigma}_e$, in which case this correlation $\widehat{\rho}$ first decreases with and then increase after the value $\widehat{\rho} = (R_0\sigma_e/\sigma_c)^{-1}$, therefore, in this circumstance, a strong positive correlation between cost and effectiveness would suggest a smaller sample size requirement for (45) to hold given β.

7. Examples

7.1. *Example* 1

We use summary data from Sacristan *et al.*[14] on a trial comparing two pharmacological agents in this example. Data on 150 patients using the test drug yield a mean cost of $200,000 (SD = $78,400). Health benefit measured in QALYs is 8 (SD = 2.1) corresponding values on 150 patients using the standard drug are $80,000 (SD = $27,343) for mean cost, and 5 QALYs (SD = 2.0) for mean health benefit. These values yield the following estimates: $\Delta\bar{e} = 3$, $\Delta\bar{c} = \$120,000$ and from (32) $\widehat{\sigma}_e = 0.237$ and $\widehat{\sigma}_c = 6779$. In the absence of a reported value for the correlation between cost and effectiveness, we consider values $\widehat{\rho}_0 = \widehat{\rho}_1 = 0.7$. From (32), we see that with zero correlations, the incremental cost and incremental effectiveness are uncorrelated ($\rho = 0$). For $\widehat{\rho}_0 = \widehat{\rho}_1 = 0.7$, we get $\widehat{\rho} = 0.638$ approximately.

7.1.1. *Hypothesis testing for the CER*

Suppose the hypothesized CER was $R_0 = \$50,000/\text{QALY}$. From the test of $H_0 : R = R_0$ versus $H_A : R \neq R_0$ section, the two-sided test of $H_0 : R = R_0$ based on the statistic $T = (\Delta\bar{c} - R_0\Delta\bar{e})/\{\text{var}(\Delta\bar{c} - R_0\Delta\bar{e})\}^{1/2}$ has a p-value of 0.03 if $\widehat{\rho}_0 = 0$ and approximately 0.001 if $\widehat{\rho}_0 = 0.7$. It can be shown that the p-values decrease with increasing values of $\widehat{\rho}_0$.

7.1.2. *Determining statistical power*

What power does this test have to detect an alternative CER, $R_0 = \$40,000/\text{QALY}$? We compute the power from (39) assuming an incremental effectiveness of 3 QALYs. If $\widehat{\rho}_0 = 0$ the power is about 59% and increases to 94% if $\widehat{\rho}_0 = 0.7$. A lower power may be acceptable in studies of cost-effectiveness.

7.1.3. *Testing the joint hypothesis on effectiveness and cost-effectiveness*

The power function of this one-sided test is given in (43). To test for significance of the difference in effectiveness (i.e. $H_{01} : \Delta E(e) = 0$), we would reject if $|\Delta\bar{e}/\widehat{\sigma}_e| > z_{1-\alpha/2}$. In this example, the difference δ being highly significant makes the right-hand side of (43) essentially

$$P\left[Z_2 < -z_{1-\alpha} + \frac{\delta|R - R_0|}{\{\mathrm{var}(\Delta\bar{c}) + R_0^2\,\mathrm{var}(\Delta\bar{e}) - 2R_0^2\,\mathrm{cov}(\Delta\bar{c}, \Delta\bar{e})\}^{-1/2}}\right].$$

The power at $\delta = 3$ and $R = \$40,000$ is about 0.71 for these data.

7.2. *Example* 2

Consider the simplifications leading to (44) and (45). To ensure a power of 80% to detect an effect size $\delta/\widehat{\sigma}_e = 0.5$ with a two-sided test of $H_{01} : \Delta E(e) = 0$ with $\alpha = 0.05$, we get $n_{0b} = 63$. Suppose the hypothesized ICER is $R_0 = \$80,000$/QALY and the relative SD $\widehat{\sigma}_c/\widehat{\sigma}_e = 5,000$ (\$/QALY). Correlation between the cost and effectiveness measures is likely to be positive. Let $\widehat{\rho} = 0.7$ and assume a known effect size $\delta/\widehat{\sigma}_e = 0.5$. The sample size n_0 needed to detect an ICER of \$50,000/QALY or less with 80% power requires $n_0 \geq 6.51 n_{0b}$. For two-sided testing, this yields $n_0 \geq 410$. The sensitivity of $\rho(> 0)$ to this relative sample size is small. A zero correlation increase this ratio to 7.1.

Now consider testing the joint hypothesis $H_0 : \Delta E(e) \leq 0$ or $R \geq R_0$ under the same constraints. Suppose we want 80% power to detect an effect size 0.5 and an ICER of \$50,000/QALY. Using (45), we will get $n_0 = 323$ when $\widehat{\rho} = 0.7$. Note that the joint hypothesis is formulated as one-sided. In comparison, a one-sided test for effectiveness would need approximately 50 subjects per arm to detect an effect size of 0.5 with 80% power. As noted after (45), the power is driven by the probability involving Z_2 because $\zeta > 1$ in this case.

7.3. *Example* 3

Sample size requirements for testing $H_0 : \Delta E(e) \leq 0$ or $R \geq R$ are given in Table 1 for some values of R_0 and effective sizes $\delta/\widehat{\sigma}_e$. The test is designed

Table 1. Sample size requirements for testing effectiveness and cost-effectiveness.

	Maximum ICER R_0 ($1000/QALY)					Effectiveness
Effective size	40	45	50	55	60	alone
0.3	1848	1060	748	586	490	175
0.4	1040	596	421	330	276	99
0.5	666	382	269	211	177	63
0.6	462	265	187	147	123	44

with $\alpha = 0.05$ and 80% power at $R = \$30,000$/QALY. We use (45) with $\widehat{\rho} = 0.7$ and $\widehat{\sigma}_c/\widehat{\sigma}_e = 5,000$ ($/QALY).

The last column of Table 1 gives the sample size requirement to ensure 80% power in the two-sided test of effectiveness alone. For example, to detect an effect size of 0.4 and a ICER of $30,000/QALY, when the maximum acceptable level is $50,000/QALY, we require a sample size of 421 for the test and referent groups. In comparison, for testing $H_{01} : \Delta E(e) = 0$, only 99 subjects are required to detect an effect size of 0.4.

Because of the relatively large sample size needed to test the joint hypothesis of cost-effectiveness and effectiveness, in practice power could be calculated from (10) using the sample size that is needed to demonstrate a difference in effectiveness between two treatments. For example, with 175 subjects per arm, we have 80% power to detect an effect size of 0.3. with this sample size, $\widehat{\rho} = 0.7$ and $R_0 = \$50,000$/QALY we will have 64% power to detect a ICER of $30,000/QALY at an effect size of 0.5 at an effect size of 0.3, the power is only 33%.

8. Modeling for Cost-Effectiveness Analysis

Cost-effectiveness analysis require estimation of the health effects and resource costs associated with an intervention and with the alternatives to which it will be compared. Modeling is frequently necessary since few studies provide information over sufficiently long periods or for all relevant costs, effects and population groups.

Cost-effectiveness analysis helps inform different types of decisions about health interventions. To begin, it can inform the decision to use an intervention at all by showing whether it is cost-effective enough compared to alternatives. More often decisions concern hoe to use the intervention. Should screening for hypertension be done every year, every two years, or every five years? If hypertension is diagnosed, and non-drug therapies are unsuccessful, which drugs should be used? Should folic acid supplementation be accomplished through diet, vitamin supplements, or fortification of cereal grains? If fortification, how many mg of folic acid per 100 grams of cereal grain product? Should every patient who presents at the emergency.

A model creates the framework for cost-effectiveness analysis. To serve its purpose, and enable decision makers to explore the implications of variation in the intervention, the condition, and the population, it must allow not only for substantial variation in those factors.

8.1. *Validating effectiveness estimates*

Accuracy is essential for a model. Eddy[2] described four levels of validation. First, the structure of the model should make sense to experts. Second, the model should reproduce the outcomes observed in the studies used to estimate its parameters. Third, the models' predictions could be compared with results from studies not used in its construction. Fourth, the model could be used to predict outcomes for a new program and the predictions compared with the outcomes when the program is implemented. The first and second steps are essential. For the third step, randomized clinical trials (RCTs) offer a challenging, but potentially persuasive, test of a models accuracy. While trials are usually the benchmark, the model may be accurate on specific points.

It is reasonable to expect a good model to match the results of trials available at the time of its construction, but not to predict the results of future trials. Models can and should accurately reflect the state of knowledge at the time they are created.

When is a model going too far beyond the data? The medical and public health practice are the best guides. Models can appropriately be used to analyze any circumstances in which the intervention is already being applied, or in which it is being seriously considered for application. If it is appropriate to use the intervention in the real world, on real people, it is an appropriate to analyze the implications of that use of a model.

8.2. *Modeling costs*

Eddys suggestions described above should be considered for the cost estimate as well.[2] Modelers need to pay attention to ensuring that the pathway of events described by a model represents costs as well as it does effects.

In part, the failure to validate cost estimates reflects the failure to take cost data as seriously as effectiveness data. A basic requirement for accurate predictions, often overlooked, is that both costs and effects should apply to the same population and the same circumstances. Further, data on resource use and cost need to be associated with the same care and subjected to the same sorts of consistency checks as effectiveness data — comparing one source with another, relating differences in costs to characteristics thought to be associated with those differences and so on.

In addition, the range of variation that could usefully be modeled is as wide for costs as for effects. An itervention's effectiveness differs across the country because populations differ in incidence of the condition, risk factors and co-morbidities. Costs differ across the country because of differences in wages and other costs, in practice patterns and in suitable production technologies. While one purpose of sensitivity analyses is to determine which parameters have a major influences on cost-effectiveness, it would also be useful to explore sets of assumptions that describe, as accurately as the data allow, circumstances in another part of the country or another delivery system.

The US panel on cost-effectiveness in Health and Medicine has urged the use of micro-costing for costing events important to an analysis. Micro-costing could yield a better understanding of the factors that underlie resource use and costs for various conditions, analogous to the understanding of effectiveness built up from epidemiological and clinical research. That understanding might reveal alternatives for making interventions more cost-effective by changing the way they are delivered, not just by targeting them to population subgroups.

Models should be flexible enough to permit exploration of a range of production possibilities and cost levels for an intervention. Analysts could then examine plausible differences in costs and production technologies. It would be useful to evaluate combinations of values that occur in the real world: conditions in Michigan versus those in San Francisco, conditions in an inner city, a suburb, or a rural area.

8.3. *Modeling form*

Models are built from estimates of risk — the probability that a condition will progress to the next stage, that a test is accurate, that a treatment will be effective. In medical research, the familiar and convenient mathematical forms for fitting risk relationships are the logistic and, more recently hazard models. Both forms incorporate an assumption that the risk relationship is multiplicative, and thus that the size of the risk reduction caused by changing one risk factor differs for different levels of the other risk factors. This assumption implies, for example, that the reduction in risk caused by lowering systolic blood pressure from 160 mmHg to 140 mmHg will be larger in people who also smoke, even though they continue to smoke, than in people whose only risk factor is high blood pressure. Similarly, the reduction in risk from smoking cessation will be greater in people who are hypertensive, even if their blood pressure is unchanged, than in non-smokers.

In turn, this implies that it will be more cost-effective to apply an intervention to people with several risk factors, not because the programme achieves economies by treating several risk factors, but because intervention against a single risk factor is more effective in these people. The point is clear in an analysis by Taylor *et al.*[18] of a dietary programme to lower serum cholesterol modeled after the one employed in MRFIT. Effectiveness was estimated using logistic coefficients reported from the Framingham study. Results were presented separately for low-risk men, whose only risk factors for heart disease were their gender and cholesterol level, and for high-risk men, who also smoked and had high blood pressure and low HDL levels. Although the cost of the intervention was the same, cost per life-year was approximately ten times higher for low-risk men because of the multiplicative assumption incorporated in the logistic form.

Logistic and hazard models play an important role in some of the situations for which models are particularly useful — examining differences in effectiveness and cost-effectiveness among subgroups. When analysts model the implications of targeting an intervention to subgroups, or extrapolate to explore its application to less-studied groups, they need to be aware of the implications of the conventional forms. Modelers cannot supply the data to resolve this issue, but they can draw attention to it by showing how estimates change when additive and multiplicative forms are used. The ultimate goal is to ensure that estimated differences among subgroups are not an artifact of a convenient statistical model.

References

1. Chaudhary, M. A. and Stearns, S. C. (1996). Estimating confidence intervals for cost-effectiveness ratios: An example from a randomized trial. *Statistics in Medicine* **15**: 1447–1458.

2. Eddy, D. M. (1985). Technology assessment: The role of mathematical modeling in committee for evaluating medical technologies. In *Clinical Use, Institute of Medicine, Assessing Medical Technologies*, National academy Press, Washington, D.C. 144–154.
3. Efron, B. (1987). Better bootstrap confidence interval. *Journal of the American Statistical Association* **82**: 171–200.
4. Efron, B. and Tibshirani, R. (1993). *An Introduction to the Bootstrap*, Chapman and Hall, New York.
5. Fieller, E. C. (1954). Some problems in interval estimation. *Journal of the Royal Statistical Society, Series* **B16**: 175–183.
6. Garber, A. M. and Leichter, H. M. (1991). Practice guidelines and cholesterol policy. *Health Affairs* **10**(2): 52–66.
7. Goldman, L., Weinstein, M. C., Goldman, P. A. and Williams, I. W. (1991). Cost-effectiveness of HMG — CoA reductase inhibition for primary and secondary prevention of coronary heart disease. *Journal of American Medical Association* **265**: 1145–1151.
8. Hlatky, M. A., Rogers, W. J., Johnstone, I. *et al.* (1997). Medical care costs and quality of life after randomization to coronary angioplasty or coronary bypass surgery. *New England Journal Medicine* **336**: 92–99.
9. Kupperman, M., Luce, B., McGovern, B. *et al.* (1990). An analysis of the cost-effectiveness of the implantable defibrillator. *Circulation* **81**: 91.
10. Lipid Research Clinic Program (1984). Lipid research clinics coronary primary trial results, II: The relationship of reduction in incidence of coronary heart disease to cholesterol lowering. *Journal of American Medical Association* **251**: 365–374.
11. National Cholesterol Education Program (NCEP) (1988). High blood cholesterol in adults: Report of the expert panel on detection, evaluation, and treatment. National Institutes of Health. Department of Health and Human Services, Bethesda, MD.
12. National Cholesterol Education Program (NCEP) (1994). The second report of the expert panel on detection, evaluation, and treatment of high blood cholesterol in adults. *Circulation* **89**: 1329–1445.
13. OBrien, B. J., Drummond, M. F., Lebelle, R. J. and Willan, A. (1994). In search of power and significance: Issues in the design and analysis of stochastic cost-effectiveness studies in health care. *Medical Care* **32**: 150–163.
14. Sacristan, J. A., Day, S. J., Navarro, O., Ramos, J. and Hernandez, J. M. (1995). Use of confidence intervals and sample size calculations in health economic studies. *Annals of Pharmacotherapy* **29**: 719–725.
15. Sempos, C., Fulwood, R., Haines, C., Carroll, M. *et al.* (1989). Prevalence of high blood cholesterol levels among adults in the United States. *Journal of American Medical Association* **262**: 45–52.
16. Siegel, C., Laska, E. and Meisner, M. (1996). Statistical methods for cost-effectiveness analyses. *Controlled Clinical Trials* **17**: 387–406.
17. Stinnett, A. (1996). Adjusting for bias in C/E ratio estimates. *Health Economics* **5**: 469–472.

18. Taylor, W. C., Pass, T. M., Shepard, D. S. and Komaroff, A. F. (1990). Cost effectiveness of cholesterol reduction for the primary prevention of coronary heart disease in men. In *Preventing Disease: Beyond the Rhetoric*, eds. R. B. Goldbloom and R. S. Lawrence, Springer-Verlag, NY, 437–441.
19. Weinstein, M. C. and Stason, W. B. (1977). Foundations of cost-effectiveness analysis for health and medical practices. *New England Journal of Medicine* **296**: 716–721.

About the Author

Jianli Li is working at St. Michael's Hospital, University of Toronto, Canada, as biostatistician. He worked in Ontario Joint Policy and Planning Committee, Ontario Ministry of health and Ontario Hospital Association, as statistical consultant working on the hospital funding models and performance assessment. He has been working in healthcare management for decades and making efforts to apply the new developments in statistics, medical information science, computer science and applied mathematics into the healthcare management. He published and presented papers and chapters, such as "An Application of Life Time Model in Estimation of Expected Length of Stay of Patient in Hospital", "Impact of the Complexity Methodology on an Ontario Teaching Hospital", "A System for Evaluating Inpatient Case Cost Efficiency in Hospital", "Data Mining in Health Care Organizations: A Source for Continuous Health Care Information" and "Hospital Performance and Funding". He was a visiting professor at the department of Preventive Medicine and Biostatistics, University of Toronto. He was associate professor and vice chairman at the department of Healthcare Management, Shanghai Second Medical University.

CHAPTER 8

QUALITY OF LIFE: ISSUES CONCERNING ASSESSMENT AND ANALYSIS

JIQIAN FANG[*,†] and YUANTAO HAO[‡]

Department of Medical Statistics and Community Medicine,
School of Public Health,
Sun Yat-Sen University, 74 Zhongshan Road II,
Guangzhou 510080, People's Republic of China
[†]*fangjq@gzsums.edu.cn*
[‡]*haoyt@mail.sysu.edu.cn*

1. The Concept of QOL and its Components

What is quality of life? There is no universally agreed definition. Quality of life (QOL) not only means different things to different people, but it also varies according to a person's current situation. When a person falls sick he thinks QOL is good health, when he is poor, QOL is wealth. To a town planner, for example, QOL might represent access to green space and other facilities. In the context of clinical trials we are rarely interested in QOL in such a broad sense, but are concerned only with evaluating those aspects that are affected by disease or treatment of disease. This may sometimes be extended to include indirect consequences of disease such as unemployment or financial difficulties. To distinguish between QOL in its more general sense and the requirements of clinical medicine and clinical trials, the term "health-related quality of life" (HRQOL) is frequently used in order to remove ambiguity.

There are a number of reasons for developing a quality of life assessment tool. The main reason is undoubtedly that in recent years there has been a broadening of focus of the measurement of health beyond traditional health indicators such as mortality and morbidity.[1] Indeed, the measurement of health may now includes assessment of the impact of disease and impairment on daily activities and behaviour,[2] perceived health measures[3] and disability/functional status measures.[4] These measures, whilst beginning to provide an indication of the impact of disease, do not access quality of life per se, which has been aptly described as "the missing measurement in health".[5] The increasingly mechanistic model of medicine, concerned only with the eradication of disease and symptoms, reinforces the need for the introduction of a humanistic element into health care. Health care is essentially a humanistic transaction in which the patient's well-being is the primary aim. By calling for QOL assessment in health care, attention is focused on this aspect of health, and resulting interventions will pay increased attention to the problem.

There still has not been a single, clear, universally accepted definition of HR-QOL. What domains should be included in QOL? There are five major domains of QOL which are generally referred to by most authors. These domains are physical status and functional abilities, psychological status and well being, social interactions, economic and/or vocational status and factors, and religious and/or spiritual status.

The World Health Organization (WHO) has developed an international quality of life assessment instrument (WHOQOL) which allows an enquiry into an individual's perception of own position in life in the context of the culture and value systems in which they live, and in relation to their goals, expectations, standards and concerns. The WHOQOL measures quality of life related to health and health care. It has been developed in the framework of a collaborative project involving numerous centres in different cultural settings.[6] QOL is defined by WHO as "individuals' perceptions of their position in life in the context of the culture and value systems in which they live and in relation to their goals, expectations, standards and concerns". It is a broad ranging concept incorporating in a complex way the persons' physical health, psychological state, level of independence, social relationships, personal beliefs and their relationships to salient features of the environment.

This definition reflects the view that quality of life refers to a subjective evaluation, which is embedded in a cultural, social and environmental context. As such, quality of life cannot be equated simply with the terms "health status", "life style", "life satisfaction", "mental state" or "well-being". Because the WHOQOL focuses upon respondents' "perceived" quality of life, it is not expected to provide a means of measuring in any detailed fashion symptoms, diseases or conditions, nor disability as objectively judged, but rather the perceived effects of disease and health interventions on the individual's quality of life. The WHOQOL is, therefore, an assessment of a multi-dimensional concept incorporating the individual's perception of health status, psycho-social status and other aspects of life.

It is anticipated that the WHOQOL assessment will be used in broad-ranging ways. It will be of considerable use in clinical trials, in establishing baseline scores in a range of areas, and looking at changes in quality of life over the course of interventions. It is expected that the WHOQOL assessment will also be of value where disease prognosis is likely to involve only partial recovery or remission, and where treatment may be more palliative than curative.

For epidemiological research, the WHOQOL assessments will allow detailed quality of life data to be gathered on a particular population, facilitating the understanding of diseases, and the development of treatment methods. The international epidemiological studies that would be enabled by instruments such as the WHOQOL-100 and the WHOQOL-BREF will make it possible to carry out multi-center quality of life research, and to compare results obtained in different centers. Such research has important benefits, permitting questions to be addressed which would not be possible in single site studies. For example, a comparative study in two or more countries on the relationship between health care delivery and quality of life requires an assessment yielding cross-culturally comparable scores. Sometimes accumulation of cases in quality of life studies, particularly when studying less frequent disorders, is helped by gathering data in several settings. Multi-center collaborative studies can also provide simultaneous multiple replications of a finding, adding considerably to the confidence with which findings can be accepted.

In clinical practice the WHOQOL assessments will assist clinicians in making judgements about the areas in which a patient is most affected by disease, and in making treatment decisions. In some developing countries, where resources for health care may be limited, treatments aimed at improving quality of life through palliation, for example, can be both effective and inexpensive. Together with other measures, the WHOQOL-BREF will enable health professionals to assess changes in quality of life over the course of treatment.

It is anticipated that in the future the WHOQOL will prove useful in health policy research and will make up an important aspect of the routine auditing of health and social services. Because the instrument was developed cross-culturally, health care providers, administrators and legislators who require a valid QOL instrument for use can be confident that data yielded by work involving the WHOQOL assessment will be genuinely sensitive to their setting.

A large number of instruments have been developed for QOL assessment and we can divide them into two categories: generic instruments and disease-specific instruments.[7] Generic instruments are intended for general use, irrespective of the illness or condition of the patient. These generic questionnaires may often be applicable to healthy people too. Some of the earliest ones were developed initially with population surveys in mind, although they were later applied in clinical trial settings.

There are many instruments that measure physical impairment, disability or handicap. Although commonly described as QOL scales, these instruments are better called measures of health status because they focus on physical symptoms. They emphasize the measurement of general health, and make the implicit assumption that poorer health indicates poorer QOL. One weakness about this form of assessment is that different patients may react differently to similar levels of impairment. Many of the earlier questionnaires such as the Sickness Impact Profile (SIP)[2] and the Nottingham Health Profile (NHP)[8] to some degree adopt this approach. Few of the earlier instruments had scales that examined the subjective non-physical aspects of QOL, such as emotional, social and existential issues. Newer instruments such as the Medical Outcomes Study 36-Item Short Form (SF-36),[9] however, emphasize these subjective aspects strongly, and also commonly include one or more questions that explicitly enquire about overall QOL. More recently, some brief instruments that place even less emphasis upon physical functioning have been developed. Two such instruments are the EuroQol,[10] which is intended to be suitable for use with cost-utility analysis, and the SEIQol,[11] which allows patients to choose those aspects of QOL that they consider most important to themselves.

Generic instruments, intended to cover a wide range of conditions, have the advantage that scores from patients with various diseases may be compared against each other and against the general population. On the other hand, these instruments fail to focus on the issues of particular concern to patient with disease, and may often lack the sensitivity required to detect differences that arise as a consequence of treatment policies that are compared in clinical trials. This has led to the development of disease-specific questionnaires, for example, the EORTC QLQ-C30 (European Organization for Research and Treatment of Cancer QLQ-C30).[12]

2. Methods of Developing QOL Measurements

The development of a new QOL instrument requires a considerable amount of detailed work, demanding patience, time and resources. Some evidence of this can be seen from the series of publications that are associated with such QOL instruments as the SF-36, the FACT and the EORTC QLQ-C30. These and similar instruments have initial publications detailing aspects of their general design issues, followed by reports of numerous validation and field-testing studies.

Many aspects of psychometric validation depend upon collecting and analysing data from samples of patients or others. However, the statistical and psychometric techniques can only confirm that the scale is valid in so far as it performs in the manner that is expected. These quantitative techniques rely on the assumption that the scale has been carefully and sensibly designed in the first place. To that end, the scale development process should follow a specific sequence of stages, and details of the methods and the results of each stage should be documented thoroughly. Reference to this documentation will, in due course, provide much of the justification for content validity. It will also provide the foundation for the hypothetical models concerning the relationships between the items on the questionnaire and the postulated domains of QOL, which are then explored as construct validity.

Next, we will discuss the steps in instrument development in detail.

2.1. *Specifying measurement goals*

Before embarking on the development of any new instrument, the investigator should define exactly what the instrument is to measure. This initial definition will help the investigator design appropriate development and testing protocols and will enable other users of the instrument to identify its applicability to their own patients and studies. This process will include specification of the objectives in measuring QOL, a working definition of what is meant by "quality of life", identification of the intended groups of respondents, and proposals as to the aspects or main dimensions of QOL that are to be assessed. The investigator should consider at least the following criteria.

2.1.1. *Patient population*

As in a clinical trial, there should be clear inclusion and exclusion criteria that identify the precise clinical diagnosis and basic patient characteristics.

A detailed definition might include age, literacy level, language ability, and presence of other illness that might have impact on QOL. An investigator may be thinking of a particular study in which the instrument is to be used, but constructing an instrument for too specific a population or function may limit its subsequent use. One can usually choose a patient population that is narrow enough to allow focus on important impairments in that disease or function but board enough to be valid for use in other studies.

2.1.2. *Primary purpose*

The investigator needs to decide whether the primary purpose of the instrument is going to be evaluative, discriminative, or predictive. Although some instruments may be capable of all three functions, it is difficult to achieve maximum efficiency in all three.

2.1.3. *Patient function*

In most disease-specific instruments, investigators want to include all areas of dysfunction associated with that disease (physical, emotional, social, occupational). However, there are some instruments that are designed to focus on a particular function (e.g. emotional function, pain, sexual function) within a broader patient population. The investigator should decide whether all or only specific functions are to be included.

2.1.4. *Other considerations*

The investigator should also decide on the format of the instrument. Will it be interviewer and/or self-administered? Does it need to be suitable for telephone/postal interviews? Approximately how many items will the instrument contain?

Once a working definition of quality of life and study protocol are developed, a further phase of work involved operationalizing the broad domains and individual facets of quality of life. Consultants and principal investigators should draft a provisional list of domains and constituent facets of quality of life. Each facet definition should consist of a conceptual definition, a description of various dimensions along which a rating can be made for that facet, and a listing of some example situations or conditions that might significantly affect that facet at various levels of intensity. Once facets of QOL are drafted, a series of focus groups should be held with patients, well persons and health professionals to consider the facet definitions drafted by health professionals and QOL researchers. On the basis of the focus group data, a revised set of facet or domain definitions are compiled to guide subsequent item generation.

2.2. *Item generation*

The first task in instrument development is to generate a pool of all potential relevant items. For this pool, the investigator will later select items for inclusion in the final questionnaire. The most frequently used methods of item generation include unstructured interviews with patients who have insight into their condition, patient focus group discussions, a review of the disease-specific literature, discussions with health care professionals who work closely with the patients, and a review of generic QOL instruments.

A question-writing panel should be assembled. The question-writing panel should consist of the principle investigator, the main focus group moderator, at least one person with good interviewing skills and experience, and a lay person, preferably someone who participates in one of the lay focus groups, to ensure that questions are framed in a way that is easy to understand.

2.3. *Item reduction: Reducing items on the basis of their frequency and importance*

Having generated a large item pool, the investigator must select the items that will be most suitable for the final instrument. QOL instruments usually measure health status from the patients' perspective and so it is appropriate that patients themselves identify the items that are most important to them. Investigators should ensure that the patients selected represent the full spectrum of those identified in the patient population. It is important to ensure that all of the subgroups are adequately represented.

One approach to item reduction is to ask patients to identify those items that they have experienced as a result of their illness. For each positively identified item, they rate the importance using a 5-point Likert type scale ("extremely important" to "not important"). Results are expressed as *frequency* (the proportion of patients experiencing a particular item), *importance* (the mean importance score attached to each item), and the *impact*, which is the product of frequency and importance.

Very occasionally, there are items that have absolutely no potential of changing over time either as a result of an intervention or though the natural course of the disease. If one is developing an evaluative instrument, one may consider excluding such unresponsive items because they will only add to the measurement noise and the time taken to complete the questionnaire. However, if such an item is considered very important by patients and therefore potentially a future target for therapy, exclusion because of apparent unresponsiveness to current therapies may be unwise.

A comprehensive set of items will inevitably include some redundancies. How does one decide whether to include them? One approach is to test whether the items are highly correlated. If Spearman rank order correlations are high one could consider omitting one of the items. This strategy is particularly appropriate for a discriminative instrument, for highly correlated items will, when taken together, give little information in terms of distinguishing between those with mild and severe quality of life impairment. It is somewhat riskier for evaluative instruments; just because items correlate with one another at the item reduction phase does not guarantee that they will change in parallel when measured serially over time.

Investigators can select the sample size for the item reduction process by deciding how precise they want their estimates of the impact of an item on the population. The widest confidence interval around a proportion (the frequency with which patients identify items) occurs when the proportion is 50%; any other value will yield a narrower confidence interval. If one recruits 25 subjects, and an item is identified by 50% of the population, the true prevalence of that item is somewhere between approximately 30% and 70%. If one recruit 50 subjects, the 95% CI around a proportion of 0.5 will be approximately from 0.36 to 0.64. For 100 subjects, the confidence interval will be from 0.4 to 0.6. It is recommended that researchers recruit at least 100 subjects for this part of the questionnaire development process.

There are some statistical methods we can use to determine which items should be included in the instrument. Factor analysis, cluster analysis, multiple regression, and discriminant analysis are methods often used.

2.4. *Questionnaire formatting*

2.4.1. *Selection of response options*

Response options refer to the categories or scales that are available for responding to the questionnaire items. For example, one can ask whether the subject has difficulty climbing stairs; two response options, yes and no, are available. If the questionnaire asks about the degree of difficulty, a wide variety of response options are available.

An evaluative instrument must be responsive to important changes even if they are small. To ensure and enhance this measurement property, investigators usually choose scales with a number of options, such as a 7-point scale where responses may range from 1 = no impairment to 7 = total impairment, or a continuous scale such as a 10-cm Visual Analogue Scale (VAS). The 7-point Likert scale is often preferred, because although both yield similar data, the Likert scale has practical advantages over the VAS, being both easier to administer and easier to interpret.

Likert scale and VAS can be used as discriminative and predictive instruments, and are likely to yield optimal measurement properties. However, Likert scale and VAS are more complex than a simple yes/no response and they are very difficult to use for telephone interviews. In health surveys, investigators requiring only satisfactory discriminative or predictive measurement properties of their instrument may choose a simple response option format.

2.4.2. *Time specification*

A second feature of presentation is time specification: patients should be asked how they feeling over a well-defined period of time. Two weeks is the time frame used by most instruments on the basis of the intuitive impression that patients can accurately recall. Time specification can be modified according to the study, and other investigators may have different impressions of the limits of their population's memory.

When a new questionnaire is developed, it is necessary to test its psychometric properties including validity, reliability, responsiveness and sensitivity. Validation of instruments is the process of determining whether there are grounds for believing that the instrument measures what it intends to measure, and that it is useful for its intended purpose. Reliability concerns the random variability associated with measurements. Ideally, patients whose QOL status has not changed should make very similar, or repeatable, responses each time they are assessed. If there is considerable random variability over time, the measurements are unreliable. Sensitivity is the ability of measurement to detect differences between patients or groups of patients. Sensitivity is important in clinical trials since a measurement is of little use if it cannot detect the differences in QOL that may exist between the randomised groups. We will discuss these properties in detail in Sec. 6.

3. Linguistic Validation of QOL Instrument

3.1. *Introduction*

Most health status measures and psychological tests are used only in the setting in which they were originally developed. Some are translated into other languages and used without making any adaptations, and yet this is necessary to ensure their usefulness in another culture or language. A very small number of instruments are produced in equivalent version in different languages, before assessing the instruments' validity and reliability that are prerequisites for the use of instrument in a new culture.

WHO has accrued considerable experience in translating health measurements. This has facilitated the development of a translation methodology which has significant advantages over the forward-translation and the translation-back-translation methodologies. We call this procedure "linguistic validation". The steps outlined below describe a sequence which has been used successfully in a number of studies. It is clear that variations of the method may well be necessary, and indeed desirable, in certain situations.

The aim of linguistic validation of a QOL questionnaire is to maintain, as far as possible, conceptual, semantic and technical equivalence between the target language and source language versions of the instrument. Conceptual equivalence refers to the same concepts underlying the questions in an instrument in both source and target languages. Semantic equivalence refers to the same denotative and connotative elements of words. Denotation refers to that which is implied by the word, and connotation refers to the emotional meaning of the word. That is to say, what the words indicate or are a sign for (denotation) or what is implied by the words in addition to their emotional meaning (connotation). Technical equivalence refers to two separate but overlapping issues: first, the equivalence of technical features of language and their relationship to the socio-cultural context; and secondly, the feasibility of the nature and mode of questioning of the instrument in both source and target culture.

The linguistic validation of a QOL questionnaire is a complex process which requires the recruitment of professional teams who are familiar with this type of work. The linguistic validation of a questionnaire is not a literal translation of the original questionnaire, but the production of a translation which is conceptually equivalent to the original, and culturally acceptable in the country in which the translation will be used.

In order to work towards an acceptable translation of an instrument in a given language the following points should be adhered to:

— The translation methodology should be adhered to and the different phases of the process should be summarised in a report
— The translated version of a questionnaire — obtained if possible in collaboration with its developer — should be recognised as the official version in the country concerned. This will avoid the proliferation of "pirate" versions and will help to facilitate the access to translations
— Ideally, a linguistic validation of a QOL questionnaire should be complemented by a psychometric validation of the questionnaire.

3.2. *Methodology*

The original language in which the questionnaire was developed is called **source language.** The language into which the questionnaire is translated is called **target language.**

After the recruitment of a QOL specialist in each country concerned, and having explained the concepts of a linguistic validation in detail, a QOL instrument is then ideally translated according to Table 1.

Table 1. Methodology for linguistic validation of a QOL questionnaire.

Steps	Source Questionnaire
1. "Forward" translation by two independent translators	forward version A1 and forward version A2
2. Reconciliation meeting between the 2 "forward" translators and the local project manager	forward version B
3. "Backward translation" by 1 independent translator	backward translation
4. Comparison of the source questionnaire with the "backward" translation by the local team	forward version C
5. Cognitive debriefing	forward version D
6. International harmonisation (if the original is translated into more than 1 language)	final version
7. Report	

Thus, in summary, the linguistic validation of a QOL questionnaire comprises 7 steps shown in the first column of Table 1.

The questionnaire should always be considered as a whole (i.e. the response choice could influence the translation of the items and vice verse).

It cannot be assumed that a questionnaire, however, extensively tested in the originating country, will be valid and reliable once it has been translated. No instrument for the assessment of psychological states of subjective perceptions is culture-free. In each instance the validity and other metric characteristics of the instrument must be assessed in the country of application. Important components of psychometric testing in cross-cultural quality of life studies include reliability, validity, responsiveness, and effect size interpretation.

4. Design Issues Relating to QOL Study

4.1. *Study objectives*

Clear study goals are prerequisites to developing appropriate design and analysis strategies that answer clinically relevant questions. Overly general objectives, such as "describe the QOL of..." do not adequately address aspects of study such as the comparison of the two treatment arms, whether the comparisons are limited to the period of therapy or extend across time within a treatment group. Without a focused objective, unnecessary assessments are often included in protocol designs. This increases problems of multiple comparisons and missing data, and increases the possibility that critical assessments will be omitted.

4.2. *QOL instruments*

QOL assessments should ideally be brief, using an uncomplicated and least complicated instrument or combination of instruments that adequately address primary research questions. Adding scales/instruments in order to obtain less relevant data will increase both the multiple comparisons problem and the likelihood that data will be incomplete. This will in turn potentially compromise the ability of the trial to achieve the primary objectives of the study.

4.3. *Timing of assessments*

The timing of QOL assessments must also be specified to achieve the goals of the study. Baseline measures that precede therapy allow for assessment of treatment-related changes within an individual. Depending on the goals of the study, it is also important to have a sufficiently long period of follow-up after therapy to allow for assessment of the long-term treatment effect and potential late sequelae. In the phase 3 treatment comparison setting, it is critical that QOL should be assessed regardless of treatment and disease status. Patients who have changes in status or who have discontinued treatment should still take part in QOL assessment, as the biggest differences in QOL may be in these patients. Without these measurements it will be difficult to derive summary measures and impossible to make unbiased comparisons of the effects of different therapeutic regimens on QOL. Procedures for obtaining assessments for patients who have changed status or discontinued therapy should be explicitly stated in protocols.

The timing of assessments should be chosen to minimize missing data. It is generally recommended that the frequency of assessments be minimized for ease of patient and staff burden. However, in some cases more frequent administration linked to the clinical routine (e.g. at the beginning of every treatment cycle) may result in more complete data because the pattern of assessment is established as part of the clinical routine.

4.4. *Sample size and power*

The sample size and power to detect meaningful differences for primary QOL hypotheses is critical to any study in which QOL is an important end point. In addition to the usual estimates of variation and correlations, the sensitivity of the QOL instrument to detect clinically significant changes is the most useful information that can be provided during the validation of a QOL instrument. Specific estimates of the changes in subscales and global scales related to clinical status give the statistician and the clinician a clear and familiar reference point for defining differences that clinically relevant. This is critical for insuring an adequate sample size for the study. It should be noted that because end points may involve repeated measurements at different times and/or combinations of subscales, both test-retest correlations and among-subscale correlations are useful and should be reported for validated instruments.

If the sample size requirements for the QOL component are substantially less than for the entire study, an unbiased strategy for selection of a subset of patients in which QOL will be assessed should be identified. For example, the first 500 patients enrolled in the study might be included in the QOL substudy. This may have an additional advantage in studies with a long duration of QOL follow-up. This strategy is being used in the design of an Eastern Cooperative Oncology Group (ECOG) study, in which patient entry is expected to take 5 years, an additional follow-up of 2.5 years is planned for the survival end point, and the desired duration of QOL assessment is 5 years. By limiting the patients in which QOL is assessed to those enrolled in the first 2.5 years, the QOL study is expected to be complete at the same time as the final analysis of the primary survival end points.

5. Characteristics of QOL Data and Statistical Issues

5.1. *Primary statistical issues*[14]

5.1.1. *Multiple comparisons*

Analysis of QOL data differs from the analysis of other clinical end points data. There are often a large number of measures resulting from both multiple dimensions of QOL (multiple instruments and/or subscales) and repeated assessments over time. Univariate tests for each subscale and time point can seriously inflate the type I error rate (false positive) for the overall trial such that the investigator is unable to distinguish between the true and false positive differences. Furthermore, it is often impossible to determine the number of tests performed at the end of analysis and adjust post hoc. Methods that allow summarization of multiple outcome both simplify the interpretation of the results and often improve the statistical power to detect clinically relevant differences, especially when small but consistent differences in QOL occur over time or across multiple domains. On the other hand, significant differences at a particular time or within a particular domain may be blurred by aggregation.

5.1.2. *Missing data*

Missing data refers to missing items in scales and missed and/or mistimed assessments. If the assessment was not completed for reasons that there are unrelated to the patient's QOL, the data are classified as "missing at random". Examples might be staff forgetting to administer the assessment, a missed appointment due to inclement weather, or the patient having moved out of the area. Data that are missing because the patient had not been on-study long enough to reach the assessment time point (i.e. the data are censored or incomplete) are also considered missing at random. Assessments may be mistimed if they are actually given but the exact timing does not correspond to the planned schedule of assessments for reasons unrelated to the patients' QOL. While these types of missing/mistimed data make analyses more complex and may reduce the power to detect differences, the estimates of QOL are unbiased even if they are based only on the observed QOL assessments.

Non-randomly missing or informatively censored data present researchers with a much more difficult problem. One example of this type of missing data is that due to death, disease progression, or toxicity where the QOL would generally be poorer in the patients who were not observed than in those who were observed. In the chronic disease setting, this relationship between QOL and missing data might manifest itself as study dropout due to lack of relief, presence of side effects, or, conversely, improvement in the condition. The difficulty occurs because analyses that inappropriately assume the data are randomly missing will result in biased estimates of QOL reflecting only the more limited population of patients who were assessed rather than the entire sample of population under study. One possibility is to limit the analysis, and thereby the inference, to patients with complete data. In most cases, however, this strategy is not acceptable to achieve the goal of comparing QOL assessment for all patients. Unless careful prospective documentation of the reasons for missing assessments is available in a clinical trial, it is generally impossible to know definitively whether the reason for the missing assessment is related to the patient's condition and/or to their QOL.

In scales based on multiple items, missing information results in a serious missing data problem. If only 0.1% of items are randomly missing for a 50-item instrument, 18% of the subjects will have one or more items missing over four assessments. If the rate is 0.5%, then only 37% of subjects will have complete data. Deletion of the entire case when there are missing items results in loss of power and potential bias if subjects with poorer QOL are more or less likely to skip an item. Individuals with a high level of non-response ($> 50\%$) should be dealt with on a case-by-case basis. Imputing missing items for an individual who has answered most questions would, in general, be preferable to deletion of the entire case or observation, although the method used for such imputing must be carefully considered. A simple method based solely on the patient's own data would use the mean of all non-missing items for the entire scale or the specific subscale. Methods based on other patients would include the mean of that item in individuals who had responded. Another method utilizing data from other participants is based on the high correlation of items within a scale or subscale and utilizes information about the individual's tendency for particular items to be scored higher or lower relative to other items. The procedure here is to regress the missing item on the non-missing items using data from individuals with complete data, and to then predict the value of the missing items using the information gained from the items that the individual has completed.

5.1.3. *Integration of QOL and survival data*

In clinical trials with significant disease-related mortality there is need to integrate survival with QOL. This was identified by the participants in the 1990 NCI QOL workshop who "acknowledged that the use of QOL data in clinical decision-making will not routinely occur until a larger body of QOL data is available and models for integrating medical and QOL information are available". In studies where both QOL (or toxicity) and clinical end points indicate the superiority of one treatment over another, the choice of the best treatment is clear. Similarly, if either QOL or the efficacy outcome demonstrates a benefit and there is no significant difference in the other, the choice of treatment is straightforward. The dilemma occurs when there is a conflict between the QOL and efficacy outcomes. This is often the case when there is significant toxicity associated with the more effective treatment.

5.2. *Statistical methods used to analyse QOL data*

5.2.1. *Univariate methods*

One approach to the reporting of QOL data has been descriptive univariate statistics such as means and proportions at each specific point in time. These descriptive statistics may be accompanied by simple parametric or nonparametric tests such as t-tests or Wilcoxon tests. While these methods are easy to implement and often used, they do not address any of the three previously identified issues. One recommended solution to the multiple comparisons problem is to limit the number of *a priori* end points in the design of the trial to three or less. The analyses of the remaining scales and/or time points can be presented descriptively or graphically. While theoretically improving the overall type I error rate for the study, in practice investigators are reluctant to ignore the remaining data and may receive requests from reviewers to provide results from secondary analyses with the corresponding significance level.

An alternative method of addressing the multiple comparisons problem is to apply a Bonferroni correction, which adjusts the test statistics on k end points so that the overall type I error is preserved for the smallest p value. The procedure is to accept as statistically significant only those tests with p value that are less than α/k where α is the overall type I error usually set equal to 0.05.

5.2.2. *Multivariate methods*

Multivariate analysis techniques include approaches such as repeated measures analysis of variance (ANOVA) or multivariate ANOVA (MANOVA). These techniques require complete data, which limits their use in settings where there is a low risk of mortality and very high compliance with QOL assessment. If the data are not complete, the inferences are restricted to a very select and generally non-representative group of patients. Multivariate statistics such as Hotelling's T are frequently used to control for type I error. These statistics, however, answer global questions such as "are any of the dimensions of QOL different?" or "are there differences in QOL at any point in time?" without considering whether the differences are in consistent directions. In general, the multivariate test statistics are not sensitive to differences in the same direction across the multiple end points.

The requirement for complete data can be relaxed by using repeated measures or mixed effects model with structured covariance. These methods assume that the data are missing for reasons unrelated to the patients QOL, such as staff forgetting to administer the assessment for example. If the missing assessment can reasonably be assumed to be missing at random, a likelihood-based analysis approach, such as mixed-effects models or EM (Estimation-Maximization) algorithm for repeated measures models, incorporates all patients with at least one assessment in the analysis. This approach has the additional advantages of estimation of within- and between-subject variation, inclusion of time varying variables, and of being able to test for significant changes over time.

Other methods often used to determine the risk factors related to QOL include multiple regression, stepwise discriminant analysis, canonical correlation, and Logistic regression.

5.2.3. *Other methods*

5.2.3.1. Quality-Adjusted Life Years (QALY)

An intuitive method of incorporating QOL and time would be to adjust life years by down-weighting time spent in periods of poor QOL. However, what would seem to be a simple idea has many methodological challenges.

The first of these challenges is the determination of weights. Torrance[14] describes several techniques for eliciting weights for states of health including direct ratings, time trade-offs, and standard gambles. In addition to the difficulties of administering some of these techniques in clinical trials, weights elicited by the different techniques or from different respondents may not result in equivalent measures. The choice of anchor points and content validity may mean that weights that are appropriate in one setting may be inappropriate in another. The other methodological difficulty occurs in trials with censored data. Although it might seem appropriate to undertake a standard survival analysis of individual quality-adjusted survival times, the usual product limit estimator of the survival function is biased because censoring is related by the future outcome. For example, if two groups have the same censoring time due to death, the group with the poorer QOL will be censored earlier on the QALY scale. This latter problem can be addressed by estimating the average time spent in each health state and then computing a weighted average of the time as is done in the Q-TwiST approach.

5.2.3.2. Q-TwiST

The objective of the Q-TwiST method is to evaluate therapies based on both quantity and quality of life. Q-TwiST stands for Quality-adjusted Time Without Symptoms of disease and Toxicity of treatment. It is based on the concept of quality-adjusted life years (QALYs) and represents a utility-based approach to QOL assessment in clinical trials. The starting point is to define QOL-oriented clinical health states, one of which represents relatively good health with minimal symptoms of disease or treatment associated toxicity (TWiST). Patients will progress through or skip these clinical health states, but will not back-track. The next step is to partition the area under the overall Kaplan–Meier survival curve and calculate the average time a patient spends in each clinical health state. The final step is to compare the treatment regimens using weighted sums of the mean duration of each health state, where the weights are utility based. If these utility weights are unknown, as is generally the case treatment comparisons can be made using sensitivity analyses, also called threshold utility analyses.

5.2.3.3. Markov and Semi-Markov Models

Markov and Semi-Markov models have been used to compare treatments based on estimates of the time spent in different health states and the probabilities of transitions between these states. The relevant health states must be identified and then each is weighted to reflect the relative value of a health state compared to perfect health. The treatments are then compared in terms of the total quality-adjusted time, the weighted sum of the health state durations. In general, to calculate the transition probabilities an underlying model must be assumed. The most commonly used model is the Markov chain, which assumes that the transitions from one QOL state to another are independent and continuous and only depend on the previous state. This requires that the assessments are made at time points independent of the patients' treatment schedule or health state. Discrete-time transient semi-Markov processes are used to model the health state transition probabilities corresponding to prolonged life, while a simple recurrent Markov process is used to derive the QOL state transition probabilities. In a semi-Markov process, the state changes from an embedded Markov chain and the times spent in different health states are mutually independent, and depend only on the adjoining states.

5.3. *Conclusions*

We have identified three characteristics of QOL studies that present challenges for analysis and interpretation. The first is the occurrence of random and non-random missing data. The analysis of random missing data is generally well documented with sufficient advice and guidelines for both practical and theoretical issues. In contrast, development of methods for analysis of non-random missing data is in its infancy, and we now require an enhanced knowledge and understanding to determine which methods are most practical and appropriate.

The second issue addressed is the multivariate nature of QOL studies. Not only is QOL a multi-dimensional concept measured by multiple scales, but most studies are longitudinal. Separate analyses of each domain at multiple time points may make it difficult to communicate the results in a manner that is meaningful for clinicians and patients. Summary measures may reduce the multi-dimensionality of the problem but may not make the interpretation much easier. The issue of weights that vary by technique and study also adds to the complexity of interpretation. In general, it would be advisable to perform the analyses using various assumptions to verify that the results are not sensitive to small changes in the assumptions.

The third issue addressed is the integration of survival data with QOL measures. This can be addressed from either the perspective of QOL or from the perspective of time. From a research perspective both approaches can be informative; however, currently time is the dimension that both clinicians and statisticians are most familiar with. Finally, interpretation of clinical trials may not always be helpful in guiding individual patient decisions. In theory, individual patients could utilize the threshold utility analysis of Q-TWiST, but this may require extensive patient education.

There are a number of statistical methodologies that can be employed in the analysis of QOL data, each of which is based on specific assumptions, yields a different summary measure, and thus emphasizes different aspects of QOL. When there is more than one analysis strategy that best anticipates the above issues should be considered. Analyses should be clearly and concisely reportable so that the relevant differences can be readily understood by those who will use the results.

6. The Validation Process: Psychometric Testing

The question of most concern relating to psychometrics is whether a measures both reliable and valid. Measurement is the process by which a concept is linked to one or more latent variables, and these are linked to observed variables. The concept can vary from one that is highly abstract, such as QOL, or intelligence, to one that is more concrete, such as age, sex, or race. One or more latent variables may be needed to represent the concept. The observed variables can be responses to questionnaire items, census figures, or any other observable characteristics.

The first step of the measurement process is to give the concept a theoretical definition. A theoretical definition explains in as simple and precise terms as possible the meaning of a concept. The second step is to identify the dimensions and latent variables that will represent it. The next step, of forming measures, depends on the theoretical definition. This is sometimes referred to as the operational definition. The operational definition describes the procedures to follow to form measures of the latent variables that represent a concept. In some situations the latent variables are operationalized as the responses to questionnaire items. The fourth step is construct the measurement model. A measurement model specifies a structural model connecting latent variables to one or more measures or observed variables. A simple measurement model for the latent variables influence on the two measures is

$$\begin{aligned} x_1 &= \lambda_{11}\xi + \delta_1 \,, \\ x_2 &= \lambda_{21}\xi + \delta_2 \,. \end{aligned} \tag{1}$$

where ξ represents the latent variable, x_1 and x_2 are its indicator. δ_1 and δ_2 are errors of measurement with expected values of zero and uncorrelated with ξ and with each other. All variables are in deviation form so that intercepts terms do not enter the equations.

In sum, the four steps in measurement are to give meaning, identify dimensions and latent variables, to form measures, and to specify a model. The theoretical definition assigns meaning to a term and the concept associated with it. On the basis of this definition, we can know a concept's dimensions. Each dimension is represented by one latent variable. Guided by theoretical definitions, we form measures, and hopefully two or more measures will be formed per latent variable. Finally, we formulate the structural relation between indicators and latent variables in the measurement model. Two important properties of measures are their validity and reliability.

6.1. *Validity*

Validity[15] is concerned with whether a variable measures what it is supposed to measure. For instance, does an IQ test measure intelligence? Does the WHOQOL-100 measure people's quality of life? These are questions of validity. They can never be answered with absolute certainty. Although we can never prove validity, we can develop strong support for it. Traditionally, psychologists have distinguished four types of validity: content validity, criterion validity, construct validity, and convergent and discriminant validity. Each attempts to show whether a measure corresponds to a concept, though their means of doing so differ. Content validity is largely a "conceptual test", whereas the other three types are empirically rooted. If a measure truly corresponds to a concept, we would expect that all four types of validity would be satisfied. Unfortunately, it is possible that a valid measure will fail one or more of these tests or that an invalid measure will pass some of them.

6.1.1. *Content validity*

Content validity is a qualitative type of validity where the domain of a concept is made clear and the analyst judges whether the measures fully represent the domain. To the extent that they do, content validity is met. A key question is, how do we know a concept's domain? For the answer we must return to the first step in the measurement process. That is, to know the domain of a concept, we need a theoretical definition that explains the meaning of a concept. Ideally, the theoretical definition should reflect the meanings associated with a term in prior research so that a general rather an idiosyncratic domain results. In addition the theoretical definition should make clear the dimensions of a concept.

Does it matter if our measures lack content validity? In general, the answer is yes. Just as a nonrepresentative sample of people can lead to mistaken inferences to the population, a nonrepersentative sample of measures can distort our understanding of a concept.

The major limitation of content validity stems from its dependence on the theoretical definition. For most concepts in the social sciences, no consensus exists on theoretical definitions. The domain of content is ambiguous. In this situation the burden falls on researchers not only to provide a theoretical definition accepted by their peers but also to select indicators that fully cover its domain and dimensions. In sum, content validity is a qualitative means of ensuring that indicators tap the meaning of a concept as defined by the analyst.

6.1.2. *Criterion validity*

Criterion validity is the degree of correspondence between a measure and a criterion variable, usually measured by their correlation. To assess criterion validity, we need an objective reliable standard measure with which to compare our measure. Suppose that in a survey we ask each employee in a corporation to report his or her salary. If we had access to the actual salary records, we could assess the validity of the survey measure by correlating the two. In this case employee records represent an ideal, or nearly ideal, standard of comparison.

The absolute value of the correlation between a measure and a criterion sometimes is referred to as the validity coefficient. Does this correlation of a measure and a criterion reveal the validity of a measure? If we represent the measure as x_1 and the criterion as c_1, the validity coefficient may be represent as $\rho_{x_1c_1}$. A simple model of the relation between x_1 and c_1, and the latent variable ξ_1 that they measure appears in the following equations:

$$\begin{aligned} x_1 &= \lambda_{11}\xi_1 + \delta_1\,, \\ c_1 &= \lambda_{21}\xi_1 + \delta_2\,, \end{aligned} \tag{2}$$

where δ_1 and δ_2 are uncorrelated with each other and with ξ_1, $E(\delta_1) = E(\delta_2) = 0$.

$$\rho_{x_1c_1} = \frac{\lambda_{11}\lambda_{21}\phi_{11}}{[\mathrm{var}(x_1)\ \mathrm{var}(c_1)]^{1/2}}\,. \tag{3}$$

As Eq. (3) reveals, the magnitude of $\rho_{x_1c_1}$ depends on factors other than the "closeness" of x_1 and ξ_1. This is made clearer if we standardize x_1, c_1, and ξ_1 to variances of one. In this case :

$$\begin{aligned}\rho_{x_1c_1} &= \lambda_{11}\lambda_{21},\\ \mathrm{Corr}(x_1,\xi_1) &= \lambda_{11},\\ \mathrm{Corr}(c_1,\xi_1) &= \lambda_{21}.\end{aligned} \tag{4}$$

The validity coefficient, $\rho_{x_1c_1}$, is affected not only by $\rho_{x_1\xi_1}(=\lambda_{11})$ but also by $\rho_{c_1\xi_1}(=\lambda_{21})$. Even if the correlation of x_1 with ξ_1 stays at 0.5 the validity coefficient would be 0.45, 0.35, or 0.25 if the correlation of c_1 and ξ_1, is 0.9, 0.7, or 0.5. Thus, even with one change in x_1's association with ξ_1, we obtain different values of validity, depending on the criterion's relation to ξ_1.

In sum, criterion validity as measured by $\rho_{x_1c_1}$, the validity coefficient, has several undesirable characteristics as a means to assess validity. It is not only influenced by the degree of random measurement error variance in x_1 but also by the error in the criterion. Furthermore different criteria lead to different "validity coefficient" for the same measure, leaving uncertainty as to which is an accurate reading of a measure's validity. Finally, for many measures no criterion is available.

6.1.3. *Construct validity*

Construct validity is a third type of validity. Many concepts within the social science are difficult to defined and formulated, and so content validity is difficult to apply. As mentioned earlier, appropriate criteria for some measures often do not exist. This prevents the computation of criterion validity coefficients. In these common situations construct validity is used instead.

Construct validity assesses whether a measure relates to other observed variables in a way that is consistent with theoretically derived predictions. Hypotheses may suggest positive, negative, or no significant associations between constructs. If we examine the relation between a measure of one construct to other observed variables indicating other constructs, we expect their empirical association to parallel the theoretically specified associations. To the extent that they do, construct validity exists.

The major steps in the process begin with postulating theoretical relations between constructs. Then the associations between measures of the constructs or concepts are estimated. Based on these associations, the measures, the constructs, and the postulated associations are re-examined.

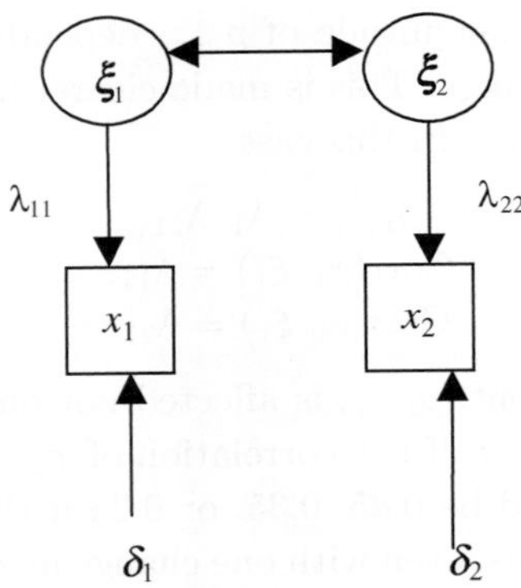

Fig. 1. Two constructs with one measure each.

Some of the difficulties with construct validity can be illustrated with a structural equation approach. As a simple example, consider Fig. 1. Assuming two constructs, ξ_1 and ξ_2. Each has one measure represented as x_1 and x_2. As usual δ_1 and δ_2 are random errors of measurement with expected values of 0, uncorrelated with each other and with ξ_1 and ξ_2. Suppose that the construct validity of x_1 is of interest. We hypothesize that the two constructs (ξ_1 and ξ_2) are positively correlated ($\phi_{12} > 0$). To test construct validity, we would compute the correlation between x_1 and x_2.

$$\rho_{x_1x_2} = (\rho_{x_1x_1}\rho_{x_2x_2})^{1/2}\rho_{\xi_1\xi_2}\,, \tag{5}$$

where $\rho_{x_ix_i}$ is the reliability of x_i. It is the squared correlation between x_i and ξ_i. The correlation of the two observed variables depends not only on the correlation of x_1 and ξ_1 but also on the correlation between the constructs ξ_1 and ξ_2 and the correlation of x_1 and x_2. Because of this, the interpretation of construct vability based on $\rho_{x_1x_2}$ is seriously complicated. For instance, if the correlation between ξ_1 and ξ_2 is relatively large and that x_1 has very high reliability but x_2 has low reliability. This would reduce $\rho_{x_1x_2}$, raising doubts about the construct validity of x_1.

In practical work, people usually use exploratory factor analysis or confirmatory factor analysis to test for construct validity. Confirmatory factor analysis is preferable than exploratory factor analysis, because its principle is similar to the definition of construct validity.

6.1.4. *Convergent and discriminant validity*

Convergent validity is another important aspect of construct validity, which is intended to show that for example, a postulated dimension of QOL correlates appreciably with all other dimensions that theory suggests should be related to it. That is, we may believe that some dimensions of QOL are related, and we therefore expect the observed measurements to be correlated. For example, one might anticipate that patients with severe pain are likely to be depressed, and that there should be a correlation between pain scores and depression ratings within group.

Many of the dimensions of QOL are interrelated. Very ill patients tend to suffer from a variety of symptoms, and have high scores on a wide range of psychological dimensions. As many dimensions of QOL are correlated with each other, assessment of convergent validity consists of predicting the strongest and weakest correlations, and confirming that subsequent observed values conform to the predictions. Analysis involves calculating all pairwise correlation coefficients between scores for different QOL scales.

Discriminant validity, or divergent validity, recognises that some dimensions of QOL are anticipated to be relatively unrelated, and that their correlations should be low. Convergent and discriminant validity represent the two extremes in a continuum of associations between dimensions of QOL. One problem when assessing discriminant validity (and to a lesser extent, convergent validity) is that two dimensions may correlate spuriously because of some third, possibly unrecognised, construct that links the two together. For example, if two dimensions are both affected by age, an apparent correlation can be introduced solely though the differing ages of the respondents. Another extraneous source of correlation could be that of social desirability, where patients may report a higher QOL on many dimensions simply to please staff or relative. When specific independent variables are suspected of introducing spurious correlations, the statistical technique of "partial correlation" should be used. This is a method of estimating the correlation between two variables, or dimensions of QOL, whilst holding other "nuisance" variables constant. In practice, there are usually many extraneous variables that contribute a little to the spurious correlations obtained.

Convergent validity and discriminant validity are commonly assessed across instruments. For convergent validity to exist, those scales from each instrument that are intended to measure similar constructs should have higher correlations with each other than with scales that measure unrelated constructs.

The multitrait-multimethod (MTMM) correlation matrix is a method for examining convergent and discriminant validity. The general principle of this technique is that two or more methods, such as different instruments,

Table 2. Template for the multitrait-multimethod (MTMM) correlation matrix.

	Instrument	Emotional function 1	Emotional function 2	Social function 1	Social function 2	Role function 1	Role function 2
Emotional	1	R					
function	2	C	R				
Social	1	D		R			
function	2		D	C	R		
Role	1	D		D		R	
function	2		D		D	C	R

are each used to assess the same traits, for example QOL aspects, items or subscales as estimated by the different methods. Various layouts are used for MTMM matrices, the most common being shown in Table 2.

In Table 2, the two instruments are methods, while the functioning scales are traits. Cells marked C show the correlations of the scores when different instruments are used to assess the same trait. Convergent validity is determined by the C cells. If the correlations in these cells are high, say above 0.7, this suggests that both instruments may be measuring the same thing. If the two instruments were developed independently of each other, this would support the inference that the traits are defined in a consistent and presumably meaningful manner.

Similarly, the D cells show the scale-to-scale correlations for each instrument, and these assess discriminant validity. Lower correlation are usually expected in these cells, because otherwise scales purporting to measure different aspects of QOL are in fact more strongly related than supposedly similar scales from different instruments. The main diagonal cells, marked R, can be used to show reliability coefficients, as described later. These can be either Cronbach's α for internal reliability or, if repeated QOL assessments are conducted on patients whose condition is stable, test-retest correlations. Since repeated values of the same trait measured twice by the same method will usually be more similar than values of the same trait measured by different instruments, the R cells containing test-retest repeatability scores should usually contain the most significant correlations.

One common variation on the theme of MTMM matrices is to carry out the patient assessments on two different occasions. The upper-right triangle of Table 2 can be used to display the correlations at time 1, and the correlations at time 2 can be shown the lower-left triangle that we have been describing above. The diagonal cells dividing the two triangles, marked R, should then show the test-retest repeatability correlations.

6.1.5. *Alternatives to classical validity measures*

Thus far we have reviewed four common types of validity: content, criterion, construct, and convergent and discriminant validity. Content validity is largely a theoretical approach to validation. Criterion validity is largely an empirical means of validating. Construct validity and convergent-discriminant validity are both theoretical and empirical. They are theoretical in the sense that theory suggests which constructs should correlate and which should not. The empirical aspect concerns the correlations of observed measures. The empirical aspect concerns the correlations between measures, although there are a number of limitations associated with this. One problem is that they rely on correlations rather than structural coefficients to test validity. Criterion validity examines the correlation between the criterion and the observed measure. Construct validity and convergent-discriminant validity are based on the correlation between measures of the same and different constructs. These correlations may have little to do with the validity of a measure. A second problem with these empirical tests is that they use only observed measures, rather than incorporating the latent variables into the analysis. The implicit assumption is that the correlation between two observed variables mirrors an association involving latent variables, so it is implicitly assumed that the correlation of the criterion and the measure adequately approximates the correlation between the latent variable and the measure. In construct and convergent-discriminant validities the correlation of observed measures is a proxy for the correlation of the latent constructs. But in fact, it can be a poor proxy under a number of conditions.

To overcome these limitations, Bollen[15] proposed an alternative definition that based on a structural equation approach. In his definition, the validity of a measure x_i of ξ_j is the magnitude of the direct structural relation between ξ_j and x_i. Therefore, for a measure to be valid, the latent and observed variable must have a direct link. Using this approach, a natural question is how to measure validity based on it? There is probably no one ideal measure of validity, but several correspond to this theoretical definition.

6.1.5.1. Unstandardized validity coefficient (λ)

One important gauge of validity, the direct structural relation between an and x_i and ξ_j, is λ_{ij} the unstandardized coefficient linking them. For instance,

$$x_1 = \lambda_{11}\xi_1 + \delta_1 , \tag{6}$$

where λ_{11} is the unstandardized coefficient, it provides the expected change in x_1 for a one-unit change in ξ_1. The λ_{ij} coefficients are in the Λ_x and Λ_y matrices.

As in multiple regression x_i may have a number of explanatory variables. Consider the following measurement model:

$$x_1 = \lambda_{11}\xi_1 + \lambda_{12}\xi_2 + \lambda_{13}\xi_3 + \delta_1 . \tag{7}$$

The validity of x_1 with respect to ξ_1 is indicated by λ_{11}. The λ_{11} coefficient is interpreted as the expected change in x_1 for one-unit change in ξ_1, holding constant ξ_2 and ξ_3. In addition the validity of x_1 with respect to ξ_2 and ξ_3 can be gauged by λ_{12} and λ_{13} respectively. Thus the unstandardized validity coefficient λ_{ij} is appropriate for measures that depend on one or more latent variables.

The unstandardized validity coefficient λ_{ij} is also useful for comparing samples from different populations. For example, the same observed variable may be measured in samples of males and females, samples from two different countries, or samples of some other groups. A comparison of validity could be made by comparing the corresponding $\hat{\lambda}_{ij}$ coefficients in the separate samples. They represent a better measure of the structural relation of the variables, and are less influenced by differences in population variances.

One disadvantage in comparing the unstandardized validity coefficients of measures that depend on the same latent variable is that the observed variables may be measured on very different scales. Direct comparison of the magnitude of λ's to determine the relative validity of measures generally is not appropriate.

6.1.5.2. The standardized validity coefficient, λ^s

The standardized validity coefficient λ^s is defined as

$$\lambda_{ij}^s = \lambda_{ij}\left[\frac{\phi_{jj}}{\mathrm{var}(x_i)}\right]^{1/2}, \tag{8}$$

where ϕ_{jj} is the variance of latent variable ξ_j.

Unlike λ_{ij}, λ_{ij}^s is one means to compare the relative influence of ξ_j on several x_i variables. For example, if x_1 and x_2 depend on ξ_j and λ_{1j}^s is 0.8 and λ_{2j}^s is 0.1, this would indicate that x_1 is more responsive to ξ_j than is x_2 in standard deviation units. In addition, if x_i depends on two or more latent variables the relative influence of the latent variables can be compared. The standardized λ_{ij}^s is less useful than λ_{ij} in comparing different populations because it is greatly influenced by the varying standard deviations of the variables in different populations.

6.1.5.3. Unique validity variance, $U_{x_i\xi_j}$

The unique validity variance measures that part of explained variance in x_i that is uniquely attributable to ξ_j. The formular for $U_{x_i\xi_j}$ is

$$U_{x_i\xi_j} = R^2_{x_i} - R^2_{x_i(\xi_j)}\,, \tag{9}$$

where $R^2_{x_i}$ is the squared multiple correlation coefficient or proportion of variance in x_i explained by all variables in a model that have a direct effect on x_i (excluding error terms) and $R^2_{x_i(\xi_j)}$ is the proportion of explained variance in x_i by all variables with a direct effect on x_i excluding ξ_j.

$U_{x_i\xi_j}$ always varies between zero and one. If only ξ_j has a direct effect on x_i, $U_{x_i\xi_j}$ equals the squared correlation between ξ_j and ξ_i. $U_{x_i\xi_j}$ is more general than $\rho^2_{x_i\xi_j}$ since it allows the observed variable to depend on more than one latent variable and it is zero if ξ_j has no direct effect on x_i. If multiple correlated latent variables underlie x_i, $U_{x_i\xi_j}$ will generally not equal $\rho^2_{x_i\xi_j}$ unless the latent variables are uncorrelated.

6.2. *Reliability*

Reliability is the consistency of measurement. It is not the same as validity since we can have consistent but invalid measures. To illustrate reliability, suppose that I wish to measure your level of education. I narrowly define education as completed years of formal schooling. I operationalize it by asking:" How many completed years of formal schooling have you had?" Next, I record your answer. If I had the ability to erase your memory of the question and the response you gave, I could repeat the same question and again, record your answer. Repeating this process an infinite number of times, I could determine the consistency of your response to the same question. The reliability of this education measure is the consistency in your response over the infinite trials. The greater the fluctuation across your answers, the lower the reliability of the measure.

It is possible to have a very reliable measure that is not valid. For example, repeatedly weighing yourself on a bathroom scale may provide a reliable measure of your weight but the scale is not valid if it always gives a weight that is 5 kg too light. A more extreme example would be obtaining a measure of intelligence by asking individuals their shoes size.

This may provide a very reliable measure, but it lacks validity as an intelligence measure. Thus the distinction between reliability and validity is a very important one.

Much of the social science literature on reliability originates in classical measurement theory from psychology. A fundamental equation of the theory is

$$x_i = \tau_i + e_i \,, \tag{10}$$

where x_i is the ith observed variable (or "test" score), e_i is the error term and τ_i is the true score that underlies x_i. It is assumed that $\text{cov}(\tau_i, e_i)$ is zero and that $E(e_i) = 0$. According to classical test theory, the errors of measurement for different items are uncorrelated. The correlation between two measures results from the association of their true scores. Thus the true scores are the systematic components that lead to the association of observed variables.

Parallel, τ-equivalent, and congeneric measures are the three major types of observed variables in test theory. They can be defined using two measures x_i and x_j as shown in the example below:

$$\begin{aligned} x_i &= \alpha_i \tau_i + e_i \,, \\ x_j &= \alpha_j \tau_j + e_j \,. \end{aligned} \tag{11}$$

The e_i and e_j are uncorrelated. Assume that the true scores are the same. If $\alpha_i = \alpha_j = 1$, $\text{var}(e_i) = \text{var}(e_j)$, then x_i and x_j are parallel measures. If $\alpha_i = \alpha_j = 1$, $\text{var}(e_i) \neq \text{var}(e_j)$, the measures are τ-equivalent. Finally, if $\alpha_i \neq \alpha_j$, $\text{var}(e_i) \neq \text{var}(e_j)$, then the measures are congeneric. Congeneric measures are the most general of the three types.

The reliability of a measure $\rho_{x_i x_i}$ is defined as

$$\rho_{x_i x_i} = \frac{\alpha_i^2 \, \text{var}(\tau_i)}{\text{var}(x_i)} \,. \tag{12}$$

For τ-equivalent or parallel measures, this simplifies to

$$\rho_{x_i x_i} = \frac{\text{var}(\tau_i)}{\text{var}(x_i)} \,. \tag{13}$$

Reliability is the ratio of true score's variance to the observed variable's variance. It is equals to the squared correlation of the observed variable and the true score:

$$\rho^2_{x_i \tau_i} = \frac{[\text{cov}(x_i, \tau_i)]^2}{\text{var}(x_i) \, \text{var}(\tau_i)}$$

$$= \frac{\alpha_i^2 [\text{var}(\tau_i)]^2}{\text{var}(x_i)\ \text{var}(\tau_i)}$$

$$= \frac{\alpha_i^2\ \text{var}(\tau_i)}{\text{var}(x_i)}$$

$$= \rho_{x_i x_i}\,. \tag{14}$$

Thus, $\rho_{x_i x_i}$ can be interpreted as the variance of x_i that is explained by τ_i with the remaining variance due to error.

A number of methods have been proposed for estimating the reliability of measures. Here will review the four most common: test-retest, alternative forms, split-halves, and Cronbach's α.

6.2.1. *Test-retest method*

The test-retest method is based on administering the same measure for the same observations at two points in time. The equations for the two measures are

$$\begin{aligned} x_t &= \alpha_t \tau_t + e_t\,, \\ x_{t+1} &= \alpha_{t+1}\tau_{t+1} + e_{t+1}\,, \end{aligned} \tag{15}$$

where t and $t+1$ are subscripts representing the first and second time periods for the x, α, τ and e. Here it is assumed that $E(e_t) = E(e_{t+1}) = 0$, that the true scores (τ_t, τ_{t+1}) are uncorrelated with errors (e_t, e_{t+1}), and that the errors are uncorrelated. In addition this method assumes that x_t, x_{t+1} are parallel measures and that the true scores are equal.
The reliability estimate is the correlation of x_t and x_{t+1}. Using the definition of the correlation between two variables and covariance algebra leads to

$$\rho_{x_t x_{t+1}} = \frac{\text{cov}(x_t, x_{t+1})}{[\text{var}(x_t)\ \text{var}(x_{t+1})]^{1/2}} = \frac{\text{var}(\tau_t)}{\text{var}(x_t)} = \rho_{x_t x_t}\,. \tag{16}$$

In fact, the correlation of any two parallel measures equals their reliability since all parallel measures have identical reliability.

Despite the intuitive appeal of the test-retest reliability technique, it has several limitations. First, it assumes perfect stability of the true score. In many cases the true score may change over time so that this assumption is not reasonable. If lack of equivalence of true scores is the only violated assumption, then $\rho_{x_t x_{t+1}}$ is less than the reliability. Secondly, memory effects are sometimes present. People's memories of response during the first interview can influence their response in a second interview. They may have the tendency to give the same responses.

In short, the test-retest method of estimating reliability has the advantage of simplicity, but it is dependent on assumptions that are unrealistic in practice.

6.2.2. *Alternative forms*

Another method for estimating reliability is that of alternative forms. This is similar to the test-retest method, except that different measures instead of the same measure are collected at t and $t+1$. The equations for the two measures are

$$\begin{aligned} x_1 &= \tau_t + e_t, \\ x_2 &= \tau_{t+1} + e_{t+1}. \end{aligned} \tag{17}$$

The x_1 variable is a measure of τ at time t, x_2 is a different measure at $t+1$, and x_1 and x_2 are parallel measures. Like the test-retest method it is assumed that τ_t equal τ_{t+1}, that the expected value of e_t and e_{t+1} are zero, and that the errors are uncorrelated with each other and with τ_t and τ_{t+1}. With these assumptions the correlation between x_1 and $x_2(\rho_{x_1,x_2})$ equals the reliability of both measures.

The alternative form does have two advantages. One is that compared to the test-retest, the alternative form measures are less susceptible to memory effects since time t and $t+1$ have different scales. Second, the errors of measurement for one indicator are less likely to correlate with a new measure at the second time period. Compared to test-retest, correlated errors of measurement are less likely to happen. Although the alternative forms estimate of reliability overcomes some of the limitations of the test-retest approach, several unrealistic assumptions remain there. For example, it is assumed that τ_t is still equal to τ_{t+1}. The assumption that the error variances are equal is less likely since x_1 and x_2 are different measures, that are administered at different time points.

6.2.3. *Split-halves*

A third means to estimate reliability is with split-halves. The split-halves method assumes that a number of items are available to measure τ. Half of these items are combined to form a new measure, say, x_1, and the other half to form x_2. Note that in contrast to the test-retest and alternative form, x_1 and x_2 are measures of τ in the same time period. It is still assumed that $E(e_1) = E(e_2) = 0$, $\text{cov}(e_1, e_2) = 0$, $\text{cov}(\tau_1, e_1) = \text{cov}(\tau_1, e_2) = 0$, and that x_1 and x_2 are parallel measures. The equations for x_1 and x_2 are

$$\begin{aligned} x_1 &= \tau_1 + e_1\,, \\ x_2 &= \tau_1 + e_2\,. \end{aligned} \tag{18}$$

The correlation of x_1 and x_2 equals to

$$\rho_{x_1 x_2} = \frac{\mathrm{cov}(x_1, x_2)}{[\mathrm{var}(x_1)\ \mathrm{var}(x_2)]^{1/2}} = \frac{\mathrm{var}(\tau_1)}{\mathrm{var}(x_1)} = \rho_{x_1 x_1} = \rho_{x_2 x_2}\,. \tag{19}$$

In many cases the unweighted sum of two halves forms a composite to measure τ_1 so that the reliability of $x_1 + x_2$ may be determined. As demonstrated earlier, in general the squared correlation of τ_1 with observed score represents the reliability of a measure. Employing this notion, the squared correlation of τ_1 with $x_1 + x_2$ is

$$\begin{aligned}
\rho^2_{\tau_1(x_1+x_2)} &= \frac{[\mathrm{cov}(\tau_1, x_1 + x_2)]^2}{\mathrm{var}(\tau_1)\ \mathrm{var}(x_1 + x_2)} \\
&= \frac{4[\mathrm{var}(\tau_1)]^2}{\mathrm{var}(\tau_1)[(\mathrm{var}(x_1) + \mathrm{var}(x_2) + 2\mathrm{cov}(x_1, x_2)]} \\
&= \frac{2\mathrm{var}(\tau_1)/\mathrm{var}(x_1)}{\mathrm{var}(\tau_1)/\mathrm{var}(x_1) + \mathrm{var}(x_1)/\mathrm{var}(x_1)} \\
&= \frac{2\rho_{x_1 x_1}}{1 + \rho_{x_1 x_1}}\,.
\end{aligned} \tag{20}$$

This formula is well known as the Spearman-Brown Prophey formula for gauging the reliability of a full test based on split-halves.

The split-halves test has several aspects more desirable than the test-retest and alternative forms methods. For one, the split-halves method does not assume perfect stability of τ since τ is only gauged in one time period. Secondly, the memory effects that can occur if the same item is asked at two points in time do not operate with this approach. Third, the correlated errors of measurement that are likely in test-retest approaches are less likely for split-halves. A practical advantage is that split-halves are often cheaper and more easily obtained than overtime data.

One disadvantage is that the split-halves must be parallel measures. Often we cannot know whether the variance of the measurement errors are equal, or whether α_1 and α_2 are equal to one. Another drawback is the way that the halves are allocated is somewhat arbitrary. There are many possible ways of dividing a set of items in half, and each split could lead to a different reliability estimate.

6.2.4. *Cronbach's α coefficient*

Cronbach's α coefficient overcomes some of the disadvantages of the split-halves method. The Coefficient α is the most popular reliability coefficient in social science research. It measures the reliability of a simple sum of τ-equivalent or parallel measures. For α, the observed variables $x_1, x_2, \ldots, x_q$ are summed. The x_i's should be scored so that they are all positively or all negatively related to τ_1. I will call this index H so that $\sum_{i=1}^{q} x_i = H$. The squared correlation of τ_1 and H or the reliability of H is

$$\begin{aligned}
\rho_{\tau_1 H}^2 &= \frac{[\text{cov}(\tau_1, H)]^2}{\text{var}(\tau_1)\ \text{var}(H)} \\
&= \frac{[\text{cov}(\tau_1, x_1 + x_2 + \cdots + x_q)]^2}{\text{var}(\tau_1)\ \text{var}(H)} \\
&= \frac{[\text{cov}(\tau_1, q\tau_1 + \sum_{i=1}^{q} e_i)]^2}{\text{var}(\tau_1)\ \text{var}(H)} \\
&= \frac{[q\ \text{var}(\tau_1)]^2}{\text{var}(\tau_1)\ \text{var}(H)} \\
&= \frac{q^2\ \text{var}(\tau_1)}{\text{var}(H)} \\
&= \rho HH\,. \qquad (21)
\end{aligned}$$

This equation provides a general formula for the reliability of the unweighted sum of q τ-equivalent or parallel measures. As the next equation shows, this can be manipulated so that it appears as the typical formula for Cronbach's α:

$$\begin{aligned}
\rho HH &= \frac{q^2\ \text{var}(\tau_1)}{\text{var}(H)} \\
&= \frac{q(q-1)q\ \text{var}(\tau_1)}{(q-1)\ \text{var}(H)} \\
&= \left(\frac{q}{q-1}\right)\left(\frac{q^2\ \text{var}(\tau_1) - q\ \text{var}(\tau_1)}{\text{var}(H)}\right) \\
&= \left(\frac{q}{q-1}\right)\left(\frac{q^2\ \text{var}(\tau_1) + \sum_{i=1}^{q} \text{var}(e_i) - q\ \text{var}(\tau_1) - \sum_{i=1}^{q} \text{var}(e_i)}{\text{var}(H)}\right) \\
&= \left(\frac{q}{q-1}\right)\left(\frac{\text{var}(H) - [q\ \text{var}(\tau_1) + \sum_{i=1}^{q} \text{var}(e_i)]}{\text{var}(H)}\right) \\
&= \left(\frac{q}{q-1}\right)\left(1 - \frac{\sum_{i-1}^{q} \text{var}(x_i)}{\text{var}(H)}\right). \qquad (22)
\end{aligned}$$

With these features the advantages of α over the other reliability measures should be evident. There are no assumptions needed for the stability of τ_1. The measures need not be parallel. The possibility of memory effects are remote since measures for only one time period are applied. There is no problem in selecting splits of items for testing since all measures can be treated individually. In addition, computation of α is relatively easy. However, two drawbacks to α are that it underestimates reliability for congeneric measures, and it is not suited to work with single indicators.

Measurement is a broad topic in social science research. This section emphasized the issues of measurement most relevant to a structural equations approach to measurement models. Most basic is the need to begin with a clear definition of the concepts to be measured. Without such a definition, we have little hope of identifying dimensions and latent variables. Validity and reliability are two basic characteristics of measures. Validity refers to the direct correspondence between a measure and a concept. Reliability refers to the consistency of a measure, regardless of whether it is valid. Many researchers have proposed empirical techniques to estimate validity and reliability. These often are based on correlation coefficients and restrictive assumptions about the properties of measures. Several alternative means have been shown here, that are more general than the traditional procedures, and they also fit well into a structural equations approach to measurement.

References

1. World Health Organization (1991). *World Health Statistics Annual.* WHO, Geneva.
2. Bergner, M., Bobbitt, R. A. and Carter, W. B. *et al* (1981). The sickness impact profile: Development and final revision of a health status measure. *Medical Care* **19**: 787–805.
3. Hunt, S. M., McKenna, S. P. and McEwan, J. (1989). *The Nottingham Health Profile. Users Manual*, Revised edition.
4. Ware, J. E., Snow, K. K., Kosinski, M. and Gandek, B. (1993). *SF-36 Health Survey: Manual and Interpretation Guide.* New England Medical Center, MA, USA.
5. Fallowfield, L. (1990). *The Quality of Life: The Missing Measurement in Health Care*, Souvenir Press.
6. The WHOQOL Group (1998). The World Health Organization Quality of Life Assessment (WHOQOL): Development and general psychometric properties. *Social Science and Medicine* **12**: 1569–1585.
7. Fayers, P. M. and Machin, D. (2000). *Quality of Life: Assessment, Analysis and Interpretation.* New York: John Wiley and Sons.
8. Hunt, S. M., McKenna, S. P. and McEwen, J. *et al.* (1981). The Nottingham Health Profile: Subjective health status and medical consultations. *Sosial Science and Medicine* **15A**: 221–229.

9. Ware, J. E. Jr, Snow, K. K. and Kosinski, M. *et al.* (1993). *SF-36 Health Survey Manual and Interpretation Guide*, New England Medical Centre, Boston, MA.
10. Brooks, R. and with the EuroQol group (1996). EuroQol: The current state of play. *Health Policy* **37**: 53–72.
11. Hickey, A. M., Bury, G. and O'Boyle, C. A. *et al.* (1996). A new short-form individual quality of life measure (SEIQol-DW): Application in a cohort of individuals with HIV/AIDS. *British Medical Journal* **313**: 29–33.
12. Bjordal, K., Hammerlid, E. and Ahlner-Elmqvist, M. *et al.* (1999). Quality of life in head and neck cancer patients: Validation of the European Organization for Research and Treatment of Cancer Quality of Life Questionnaire-H&N35. *Journal of Clinical Oncology* **17**: 1008–1019.
13. Spilker, B. (ed.) (1996) *Quality of Life and Pharmacoeconomics in Clinical Trials*. Lippincott Williams and Wilkins, Philadelphia.
14. Torrance G. W. (1986). Measurement of health state utilities for economic appraisal: A review. *Journal Health Econometrica* **5**: 1–30.
15. Bollen, K. A. (1989). *Structural Equations with Latent Variables*, John Wiley and Sons, NY.

About the Author

Jiqian Fang is Professor of Medical Statistics at Sun Yat-Sen University, Guangzhou, People's Republic of China. Due to his great contributions to statistical training in China, he was anointed with the "National Prominent Teaching Master" award in 2009, and "Outstanding Contributor to Preventive Medicine" award in 2010 by the Chinese Central Government. He obtained his Bachelor degree in Mathematics from Fu-Dan University, Shanghai, 1961, and Doctoral degree in Biostatistics from University of California, Berkeley, 1985. He was employed as the Chair Professor in Beijing Medical University 1985–1990 and then in Sun Yat-Sen University where he works presently. His research interests include multivariate analysis and stochastic modeling of life phenomenon. He was the Principal Investigator in the World Health Organization Quality of Life (WHOQOL) study in China. Since 2006, he has been interested in developing PRO instruments for different clinical fields, including Traditional Chinese Medicine. He is the chief editor for several published works including a textbook, *Medical Statistics and Computer Experiments* (1st and 2nd editions), a monograph, *Advanced Medical Statistics* in English, a series of Chinese textbooks on medical statistics, including *Health Statistics* (5th, 6th and 7th editions) for undergraduate students, and *Statistical Methods in Bio-medical Research* for post graduate students. He has trained many outstanding researchers and professors in medical statistics in Hong Kong and mainland China.

Hao Yuantao 郝元涛, is currently Dean, School of Public Health, Sun Yat-Sen University, Guangzhou, People's Republic of China. He received his undergraduate and graduate training in public health and preventive medicine at the West China University of Medical Sciences and his PhD in Biostatistics from Sun Yat-Sen University. Professor Hao's primary research interests are in the development of methods for assessing health-related quality of life, statistical methods for spatial-temporal analysis of infectious disease surveillance data, and reforms of public health education.

CHAPTER 9

META-ANALYSIS

XUYU ZHOU

Medical Information Institute, Sun Yat-Sen University, 74 Zhongshan Road II, Guangzhou 510080, PR China

JIQIAN FANG,* CHUANHUA YU and ZONGLI XU

Department of Medical Statistics, School of Public Health, Sun Yat-Sen University, 74 Zhongshan Road II, Guangzhou 510080, PR China

*Tel: 86-20-87330671; *fangjq@gzsums.edu.cn*

LU TIAN[†] and YING LU[‡]

Department of Health Research and Policy, Stanford University
Palo Alto, CA 94301, USA
[†]lutian@stanford.edu
[‡]Ying.Lu@va.gov

The best possible synthesis of available information is essential for medical researchers, health policy-makers, clinicians and other decision makers. With the explosion of information in the literature, literally hundreds of studies may exist on the same topics, and the designs, participants, outcomes, sample sizes, and interventions among these studies may differ. How can information derived from those studies be combined to arrive at a general conclusion? During the past 20 years, meta-analysis, a statistical procedure for systematically combining and analyzing the results of previous research, has been applied with increasing frequency to health-related contexts, especially in the field of clinical trials.

1. Introduction

1.1. *Definition*

The term "meta-analysis" was coined by psychologist Glass in 1976.[1] The prefix "meta" has several related meanings, including the ideas of occurring after something else, of transcending, or of being more comprehensive than the precursor. Glass' first definition of meta-analysis is the statistical analysis of a large collection of analyses results from individual studies for the purpose of integrating the findings. A useful definition was given by Huque: "...the term 'meta-analysis"' refers to a statistical analysis which combines or integrates the results of several independent clinical trials, considered by the analyst to be 'combinable'.[2]" Similar synonyms of meta-analysis include "overview", "quantitative review", "quantitative synthesis", and "pooling". But these alternative terms may be less specific or less poignant, and were not accepted broadly.

More recently, Evidence-Based Medicine (EBM) has been greatly developed. EBM, systematic review, and meta-analysis get widely used terms in medical journals. Systematic review denotes any type of review that has been prepared using strategies to avoid bias and that which includes a material and methods section. Systematic review may or may not include formal meta-analysis. The Cochrane Collaboration aims to prepare, maintain, and disseminate comprehensive and systematic reviews of the effects of health care. Systematic reviews provided by Cochrane Collaboration are regarded as the best evidence for practicing EBM.[3] Nowadays, meta-analysis is not limited to a statistical approach, and defined as a systematic approach to identifying, appraising, synthesizing, and (if appropriate) combining the results of relevant studies to arrive at conclusions about the body of research.[4]

1.2. *Historical notes*

The origins of pooling the results may be traced to statistician Karl Pearson in 1904, who was the first researcher to report the use of formal techniques to combine data from different samples. The first article which quantitatively synthesized the previous research in medicine, *The Powerful Placebo*, and written by Beecher, was published in 1955.[5] As a formal statistical technique to combine data from studies for the same topic, meta-analysis began to be applied to social sciences in the mid-1970s, particularly in educational and psychological research.

Widespread use of meta-analysis in medicine quickly followed its popularization in the social sciences, and mainly focused the research on the randomized clinical trials. In the late 1980s, there has been a rapid growth in interest and use of the method. At that time, descriptions of the method of meta-analysis and guidelines for its application appeared almost simultaneously in many general influential medical journals, such as the *New England Journal of Medicine*, *Lancet*, and *Annals of Internal Medicine*. Meta-analysis has been adopted by MEDLINE as a Medical Subject Heading (MeSH) term in 1989 and as a sort of Publication Type (PT) in 1993. Meta-analysis of observational studies has also been advocated.

Meta-analysis is now commonplace in a wide range of medical research contexts. Concurrent with the increased number of articles using meta-analysis in the last decade, there have been numerous articles relating to statistical issues or concerns. Many methods have been proposed and used, from crude "vote counting" of studies showing significant or non-significant results, through method for combination of effect size estimates based on fixed or random-effects models, to general linear mixed models and Bayesian methods. Meta-analysis has established itself as an influential branch of biostatistics.

With the sharp increasing use of meta-analysis, several unresolved issues concerning meta-analysis still remain. Incomplete or un-standardized reporting of results, and combing "apples and oranges and the occasional lemon" — failure to make allowance for varying nature and quality of the studies reviewed.[6] Therefore, both the uncritical synthesis of data from observational studies and the unconsidered synthesis of disparate results from randomized controlled trials can threaten to damage the validity and reliability of conclusions of meta-analysis. Other stubborn problems involved in meta-analysis may be biases, especially publication bias, and heterogeneity across studies.

1.3. *Objectives of meta-analysis*

Traditionally, research synthesis was done in a fairly simple way. The classic narrative reviews have several disadvantages that meta-analysis appear to overcome. The traditional review is a subjective method of summarizing research data and therefore prone to bias and error. Without guidance by formal rules, a narrative review expresses the personal opinions of their authors and depends heavily on the perspicacity and personal experience of the reviewer. Selective inclusion of studies that support the reviewer's view is common. On the other hand, a narrative review tends to present a series of effect measures in the narrative in most situations, and reviewers potential to ignore the factors that greatly influence the results of primary study, such as research design, sample size, and effect size. Meta-analysis provides a logical framework to research a review: Similar measures from

Table 1. Results of randomized trials of effect on mortality of intravenous streptokinase following acute myocardial infarction published before 1982.

Included Study	N Deaths/Total		Mortality (%)		Estimated relative Risk and its 95% CI
	Treated	Control	Treated	Control	
Avery (1969)	20/83	15/84	24.1	17.9	1.35(0.74–2.45)
European Working Party (1971)	69/373	94/357	18.5	26.3	0.70(0.53–0.92)
Heikinheimo (1971)	22/219	17/207	10.0	8.2	1.22(0.67–2.24)
Dioguardia (1973)	19/164	18/157	11.6	11.5	1.01(0.55–1.85)
Breddin (1973)	13/102	29/104	12.7	27.9	0.46(0.26–0.81)
Bett (1973)	21/264	23/253	8.0	9.1	0.88(0.50–1.54)
Aber (1979)	43/302	44/293	14.2	15.0	0.95(0.64–1.40)
UCSG for Streptokinase in AMI(1979)*	18/156	30/159	11.5	18.9	0.61(0.36–1.04)
			Summary relative risk		0.80(0.68–0.95)

*European Cooperative Study Group for Streptokinase in acute myocardial infarction.

comparable studies are listed systematically and the available effect measures are combined where possible.

For example, in 1982, use of thrombolytic agents after acute myocardial infarction was controversial. Table 1 presents the data of eight randomized clinical trials at that time, which examined the effects of a loading dose of at least 250,000 international units of intravenous streptokinase on mortality given a short time after an acute myocardial infarction had occurred. As shown in Table 1, two trials showed a higher risk of mortality in treated patients, with both 95% confidence intervals covering one, which means no statistical significance; five showed a lower risk, with four of those 95% confidence intervals covering one; and one showed same mortality rate in the treated and the control patients. The trials were all fairly small, and the difference in mortality between treated and controlled patients was statistically significant in only one trial. These studies were interpreted as inconclusive about the benefit of early treatment with intravenous streptokinase.

In a meta-analysis based on these trials, Stampfer estimated the relative risk of mortality in patients treated with intravenous streptokinase to be 0.80 with 95% confidence limits of 0.68 and 0.95, and draw the conclusion that streptokinase reduces the mortality following acute myocardial infarction.[7] The findings were published in the famous medical journal, *New England Journal of Medicine*, and were not accepted by clinician due to poor understanding of meta-analysis in early 1980s. Until 1986, a large clinical trial of intravenous streptokinase after acute myocardial infarction involving thousands of patients (GISSI 1985) confirmed the conclusion based on the meta-analysis, and streptokinase got to be widely used in clinical practice.

The objectives of meta-analysis are:

1.3.1. *To increase statistical power*

Meta-analysis effectively provides a gain in statistical power for average estimates. In clinical trials, meta-analysis offers an opportunity to observe more events of interest in the groups followed, when incidence or mortality is rare, and combined estimates are likely to be more precise. In some cases, a single study often cannot detect or exclude a modest, albeit clinical relevant, difference in the effects of two treatments with great confidence. For example, suppose a drug could reduce the risk of death from myocardial infarction by 10%, to detect such an effect with 90% confidence (that is, with a type II error of no more than 10%) over 10,000 patients in each treatment group would be needed. However, such large samples were difficult to recruit in a single study. Clearly, if data from more than one study are available and can be combined, the "sample size" and, thus, power increase, and relatively small effects can be detected or excluded with confidence.

1.3.2. *To improve estimate of effect size*

Meta-analysis has historically been useful in summarizing prior research based on randomized trials when individual studies are too small to yield a valid conclusion. Results from studies may disagree as to the magnitude of effects or, of more concern, as to the direction of effects. By integrating the actual evidence, meta-analysis allows a more objective appraisal, which can help to resolve uncertainties when the original researches, classic reviews, and editorial comments disagree. As an effective tool for quantitative synthesis, meta-analysis may resolve issues relating to inconsistent or conflicting results from studies, provide the pooled estimate of effect size with a more precise confidence interval, and draw an explicit conclusion.

1.3.3. *To assess the disagreement and generalizability of study results*

Studies for the same topic may use different eligibility criteria for participants, different definitions of disease, different methods of measuring or defining exposure, or different variations of treatment. It means there is heterogeneity between studies. When heterogeneity is large enough to be detected by a statistical test, it is important to explore its source. Meta-analysis also systematically assesses the biases and confounding in primary studies.

On the other hand, meta-analysis can contribute to considerations about the generalizability of study results. The findings of a particular study may be valid only for a specific population of patients with the same characteristics as those investigated in the trial. If many trials are available for different groups of patients, and show similar results, it can be concluded that the effect of the intervention under study has some generality. Furthermore, meta-analysis is also superior to individual trials when answering questions about whether an overall study result varies among subgroups — for example, among men and women, older and younger patients, or subjects with different degrees of severity of disease. These questions can be addressed in the analysis and often lead to insights beyond what is provided by the calculation of a single combined effect estimate.

1.3.4. *To answer new questions that were not previously posed in the individual studies*

Meta-analysis includes the epidemiological exploration and evaluation of results, new ideas (hypotheses) that were not posed in the individual studies can thus be developed and tested for further research and further original studies.

1.4. *The main steps involved in a meta-analysis*

Meta-analysis should be viewed as an observational study of the evidence. The steps involved are similar to any other research undertaking: Formulation of the problem to be addressed, collection and analysis of the data, and reporting of the results.

1.4.1. *Formulating the problem*

It is as important to carefully plan a study that involve in a meta-analysis as to carefully plan a clinical trial, a cross-sectional survey, and a case-control or a cohort study. Documentation of all aspects of study design and conduct of the study is a crucial and often overlooked step in carrying out the meta-analysis.

As with any research, a meta-analysis begins with a well-formulated question and design. Meta-analysis can, in general, be motivated by a number of factors. It can be conducted in an effort to resolve conflicting evidence, to answer the questions where the answer is uncertain or to explain variations in practice.

A well-formulated question is essential for determining the structure of a meta-analysis. Specifically, it will guide much of the meta-analysis process including strategies for locating and selecting studies or data, for critically appraising their relevance and validity, and for analyzing variation among their results.

There are several key components to a well-formulated question. A clearly defined question should specify the types of people (participants), types of interventions or exposures, types of outcomes that are of interest, and types of study design. In general the more precise one is in defining components, the more focused the meta-analysis.

The first step in planning the study is to define the problem. The problem definition is a general statement of the main questions that the study addresses. For examples, does the thrombolytic therapy lower the risk of death for patients with acute myocardial infarction? A meta-analysis for randomized clinical trials. Does the passive smoking increase the risk of lung cancer for women? A meta-analysis for case-control studies. These two topics are well-formulated questions that contain the main elements for a meta-analysis.

Once the problem is defined, developing a detail study protocol is essential. A protocol is the blueprint for conduct of the meta-analysis. The protocol should clearly state the objectives, the background, the hypotheses to be tested, the subgroups of interest, the proposed methods and criteria for identifying and selecting relevant studies, and extracting and analyzing information. The statement of objectives should be concise and specific.

1.4.2. *Searching for the relevant information*

A comprehensive, unbiased information search is one of the critical differences between a meta-analysis and a traditional review.

Systematic procedures for literature searching should be described in protocol in detail. Ideally, all of the relevant information, including the published literature, unpublished literature, uncompleted research reports, and work in progress, would be searched and identified in meta-analysis. In practice, the meta-analyst begins with searches of regular medical databases of published literature. Developing a search strategy is very important, which means to present the exact search terms and the search algorithm for each computer databases. Sometimes restrictions are necessary, such as language, study objects, publication year, or publication types, and it is easy to carry out in computer database search.

Skipping over important documents available in databases in searching process may affect the validity and reliability for the results of meta-analysis. The ability of a search algorithm to identify all of the pertinent literature can be improved by consultation with a professional librarian or an expert searcher. Two useful concepts in information retrieval can be used to describe the success of the search process: Sensitivity and precision. Sensitivity of a search is its ability to identify all of the relevant material. Precision (which is the positive predictive value of the search) is the amount of relevant material among the materials retrieved by the search. The overall strategy for searching is to maximize sensitivity and precision. But with the increase of the recall, the precision may be reduced. For meta-analysis, a higher percent sensitivity may be more important than precision.

MEDLINE is the most powerful bibliographic database that is the primary source of information on publication in the biomedical literature. It contains information on publications in over 3,500 and covers the period from 1966 to the present. MEDLINE provides more than 10 search entries and is very friendly to users. The use of MeSH (Medical Subject Headings) terms allows searches of MEDLINE to be focused and specific, which gives higher sensitivity and precision. Free access to MEDLINE through the Internet (`www.ncbi.nlm.nih.gov/PubMed`) greatly enhances the ability to conduct searches. Other broadly used biomedical databases include EMBASE, SCI (Web of Science), Cochrane Library, and specific databases, such as CANCERLINE, TOXLINE, etc.

The citations or abstracts in databases are browsed in search process, and those obviously unrelated to the topic are eliminated. The full-text of the remaining articles is then collected. These articles are read quickly, and those clearly irrelevant ones are excluded. The remaining publications are then systematically reviewed to determine whether they are eligible for the meta-analysis based on predetermined criteria for eligibility. The reference lists of the articles that contain useful information are searched for more references, then the new publications retrieved, and the process is repeated, until all potentially articles on the topic are identified.

Medical information is also presented in professional website, especially in the medical journal's website, and some of them also provide free full-text. Handsearching is often used. Scanning new information in key journals in the area of interest is an important supplement.

Furthermore, "fugitive" literatures, such as proceedings of conferences, dissertations and master's theses, books chapters, and government reports, are not included in MEDLINE and most other databases. To ignore these material have the potential to cause bias in the meta-analysis. One of the effective ways to obtain the information about publications in the fugitive literature is to consult experts.

Unpublished studies are the ultimate example of fugitive literature. The existence of large numbers of unpublished studies may cause publication bias, which will be discussed in detail in the final section in this chapter.

1.4.3. *Selecting the studies eligible for inclusion*

Studies are chosen for meta-analysis on the basis of inclusion and exclusion criteria. Inclusion criteria are ideally delineated at the stage of the development of the meta-analysis protocol, and should depend on the specific objectives of the analysis. The process of determining whether studies are eligible for inclusion in the meta-analysis should be systematic and rigorous. Each article must be assessed to see whether the inclusion criteria for the meta-analysis are met. To ensure reproducibility and minimize bias in selecting studies, the following six aspects should be addressed in almost all meta-analyses.

1.4.3.1. Study Population

What types of people should be included in meta-analysis? This involves deciding whether one is interested in a specific population group determined on the basis of factors such as age, sex, educational status, or presence of a particular condition such as the severity of disease and types of disease.

For example, in a meta-analysis of the effects of estrogen replacement therapy on the risk of breast cancer, the inclusion criteria for study population is limited to the women who experienced the natural menopause or who underwent premenopausal hysterectomy, with or without bilateral oophorectomy. The studies that included subjects with a previous history of breast cancer are excluded.

1.4.3.2. Study Design

In clinical trials, the effect of non-randomized controlled study is often overestimated compared with that of randomized study. The treat effect of single blind design may be different from that of double blind design, even though other aspects of the studies are the same. When both randomized and nonrandomized studies are available for a topic, estimates of effect size should be made separately for the randomized and the nonrandomized studies.

In observational studies, the results of case-control study and cohort study may be discrepant for identical problem due to the effects of confounding factors, the influence of biases, or both. The results of meta-analysis need to be reported respectively, according to the study design.

1.4.3.3. Intervention or Exposures

One of the key components about eligibility for a meta-analysis is to specify the intervention or exposure that is of interest, and what types of control groups that are acceptable also need to be defined. In other words, how similar intervention (exposure) should be to use them in the same analysis, such as studies with different doses of the same drug in clinical trials, and studies with the different intensity of exposures in observational data.

For example, a meta-analysis of low-dose aspirin for the prevention of pregnancy-induced hypertensive disease included the studies in which the intervention is aspirin in doses of less than 325 mg/day.

1.4.3.4. Outcomes

Researchers on primary studies often report more than one outcome, and may report the same outcome using different measures. When defining eligibility criteria for the meta-analysis, eligibility based on the similarity of the outcome will enhance the homogeneity of the studies. Generally, the end-points that are comparable, quantitative and reflecting the final outcomes are appropriate to be chosen for meta-analysis. For example, the chief endpoints, which included in the meta-analysis of randomized trials of angiotensin-converting enzyme (ACE) inhibitors on mortality and morbidity in patients with congestive heart failure (CHF), are total and cause-specific mortality (i.e. progressive heart failure, myocardial infarction, and sudden or presumed arrhythmic death) and hospitalization for CHF.

1.4.3.5. Inclusive dates of publication and English-language publication

Meta-analysis should be as up-to-date as possible, the cutoff date for identification of eligible studies should be specified in the report of the meta-analysis. The inclusive date of publication should be chosen based on consideration of the likelihood of finding important and useful information during the period that is chosen, but not simply on convenience, such as availability of MEDLINE.

A meta-analysis solely based on English-language publications has been shown to have the potential to cause bias. It is not valid to conduct a meta-analysis to rely only on the publications and reports that are easily found and understood.

1.4.3.6. Restriction on sample size or length of follow-up

Most of classical the statistical methods for meta-analysis are based on asymptotic. Normal under moderately large samples. The precision of small studies may tend to be overestimated. To avoid the problem of weighting small studies inappropriately in the meta-analysis, it is reasonable to make sample size an eligibility criteria for the meta-analysis. Small studies are excluded.

Sometimes, the length of follow-up may influence the likelihood of observing a true association in clinical trials. For observational studies, there are many situations where exposure would not affect the risk of disease until after a latent period. To avoid these problems, the length of follow-up could be a criterion for eligibility for the meta-analysis.

An alternative to making study size or length of follow-up an eligibility criterion is to estimate effect with and without small studies or with and without studies with short follow-up or low-dose exposure.

For example, in a meta-analysis of the efficacy of screening mammography, one of the inclusion criteria is, the length of follow-up is least 5 years and with minimum of 10 breast cancer mortality cases in each eligible study.

Generally, highly restrictive eligibility criteria tend to give meta-analysis greater validity. But the criteria may be so restrictive and require so much homogeneity as to limit the eligible studies to only one or two studies, which is conflicted with one of the goals of meta-analysis as a method to increase statistical power. However, less restrictive criteria may lead to the accusation that the meta-analysis "mixes apples and oranges".

1.4.4. *Abstracting the data*

The process of abstraction of information for meta-analysis from eligible studies should be reliable, valid, and free of bias. In order to enhance the reliability of data collection, a standardized form should be developed to record the information. The key components of a data collect form generally include study characteristic with methods, participants, interventions, outcome measures and results.

To avoid the selection bias, the abstraction of information should be done by two abstractors separately, and experts should be consulted for disagreement. Furthermore, the abstractors should be blinded to the information of the authors, the journals, and the funding sources. It is believed that these factors possibly influence the judgment of the abstractor.

1.4.5. *Assessing study quality*

It is important to systematically complete critical appraisal of all included studies, which primarily focus on the validity of studies. If the quality of original study is poor, the results of meta-analysis will be less reliable and valid.

The validity of a study is the extent to which its design and conduct are likely to prevent systematic errors, or bias. Generally, there are four sources of systematic errors in clinical trials: Selection bias, performance bias, attrition bias and detection bias. The randomization process, the measurement of patient compliance, the blinding of patients and observers, the statistical analyses, and the handling of withdrawals in each primary study should be examined. For non-experimental studies, control for confounding, measurement of exposure and completeness of follow-up are all the main factors that need to be greatly considered in the process of study quality assessment.

Because quality assessment is a subjective process, it may potential cause error and bias. There is not a "gold standard" for study quality appraise yet. So, the reliability of the quality rating scales in published meta-analysis is often not formally evaluated.

1.4.6. *Statistical analysis*

The process of quantitative combining the data is the key step for meta-analysis, which is distinguish from the traditional narrative review. The main procedures involved in the statistical analysis are: Defining the outcome; homogeneity test for the effect size; model choice (fixed-effects model or random-effects model); pooled estimate of effect size (point estimate and confidence interval estimate); hypothesis test for overall effect size and graphic display of the results.

1.4.7. *Sensitivity analysis*

The goal of sensitivity analysis in meta-analysis is to assess the robustness of conclusion when different assumptions are made in conducting the analysis. Sensitivity analysis is usually conducted to examine the change of the pooled estimate of effect size, when both fixed- and random-effects model are used. Sensitivity analysis is also often done including and excluding certain studies, which are controversial, have large effects and thus dominate the analysis, or cannot be determined to meet the eligibility criteria but whose exclusion may be problematic. When there is more than one estimate of effect size available from a study, sensitivity analysis can be performed using one estimate and then the other.

For example, Egger did a sensitivity analysis in the meta-analysis of β-blockade in secondary prevention after myocardial infarction.[8] Firstly, the overall effect was calculated by different statistical model, the results showed that the overall effect estimates are virtually identical and that confidence intervals are only slightly wider with random-effects model. Secondly, methodological quality was assessed in terms of how patients were allocated to treatment or control groups, how outcome was assessed, and how the data were analyzed. The results showed that the three low quality studies presented more benefit than high quality trials. Exclusion of these three studies, however, leaves the overall effect and the confidence intervals practically unchanged. Third, when stratifying the analysis by study size, the results showed the trials with smallest sample sizes have the largest effect. However, exclusion of such studies has little effect on the overall estimate. Thus, sensitivity analysis showed that the results from this meta-analysis were robust.

1.4.8. *Discussion of results*

As with any medical article, the last step in meta-analysis is discussion.

- Investigating and explaining the source of heterogeneity are critically important component of meta-analysis, when there is "statistically significant" heterogeneity across studies. Heterogeneity is easier to be observed in observational studies due to the diversity in their designs, the methods for collecting data, definitions of endpoints, and the degree of control for bias and confounding. Indeed, there are no statistical methods that can deal with the bias and confounding in the original studies. Meta-regression model and mixed model may adjust somewhat of heterogeneity by controlling the confounding, but it still cannot explain the source of heterogeneity. Sensitivity analysis and subgroup are useful for exploring the heterogeneity. It may not be appropriate with great difference.

- Subgroup analysis is necessary when treatment effect vary according to patient-level covariance or trial-level characteristics. For example, the effect of a given treatment is unlikely to be identical across different group of participant — for example, young people versus elderly people, those with mild disease versus with severe disease. A relationship between the underlying risk of patient and treatment effect may crucially affects decisions about which patients should be treated from a cost-effectiveness perspective: Patient at high risk with a small proportionate treatment benefit may be preferentially treated compared to low risk patients with a larger proportionate treatment benefit. Sometimes the treatment effect may be in the opposite direction for patients at low and high risk. Meta-analysis thus offers a sounder basis for subgroup analysis. But meta-analytic subgroup analyses are prone to bias and need to be interpreted with caution. Ideally, if individual patient data in each eligible study can be obtained, a standardized subgroup analysis can be performed.
- Meta-analysis is essentially viewed as an observational study. Bias can occur at multiple steps in the process of meta-analysis. Bias may seriously influence the validity and reliability of meta-analysis, and more attention needs to be paid to detect and assess of the bias.
- When reporting the conclusion, we should summarized the key finding, interpret the results in light of the total of available evidence, and suggest a future research agenda. But for meta-analysis of observational studies, generalization of the conclusions must be explained in caution, because bias and confounding may distort the findings as we have shown above.

For example, the hypothesis from ecological analyses that higher intake of saturated fat could increase the risk of breast cancer generated much observational research often with contradictory results. A comprehensive meta-analysis showed an association from case-control but not from cohort studies (odds ratio was 1.36 from case-control studies versus relative rate 0.95 from cohort study), and this discrepancy was also shown in two separate large collaborative meta-analyses of case-control and cohort studies. The most likely explanation for this situation is that biases in the recall of dietary items and in the selection of study participants have produced a spurious association in the case-control comparisons.[9]

2. Statistical Methods in Meta-Analysis

2.1. *Definition of the study outcome*

The primary studies included in the meta-analysis may report several different end points. Often the meta-analyst has little control over the choice of the study outcome, and it is very important to select pooled statistic that is comparable across all studies. In some situations this task will be impossible. Here, three classes of outcome measures are discussed: Measures based on discrete outcome data, that may generally be thought of as odds ratios, relative risks, or risk differences; those based on continuous data, such as mean difference, and standardized mean difference; and a miscellaneous set of outcome measures that may be based on test statistics.[10]

2.1.1. *Odds ratios, relative risks and risk differences*

Suppose there are K studies for binary discrete measurements included in the meta-analysis, whose data are in the form of 2×2 tables (see Table 2). Let i index study, in a typical one, clinical trials, let 1 denote treatment group, and 2 control group. We denote a_i, b_i, c_i, and d_i as the number of observations in each of the cells defined by the treatment and outcome table, with n_{1i} subjects in the treatment group and n_{2i} in the control group. p_{1i} and p_{2i}, are the proportions of having the characteristic under study, such as death, relapse or some other kind of failure. In an epidemiological case-control study, the two groups would be the cases and controls and the characteristic under study would be exposed to the hypothesized risk factor.

Table 2. Arrangement of data for 2×2 table.

	Treated (Exposed)	Not Treated (Not Exposed)	Total
Death (Case)	a_i	b_i	n_{1i}
Survival (Control)	c_i	d_i	n_{2i}
Total	m_{1i}	m_{2i}	T_i

Table 3. Parameter estimation for three binary measurements.

	Parameter	Estimator	Standard Error
Risk Difference	$D = P_1 - P_1$	$d_i = \hat{p}_{1i} - \hat{p}_{2i}$	$s_{di} = \left(\frac{p_{1i}(1-p_{1i})}{n_{1i}} + \frac{p_{2i}(1-p_{2i})}{n_{2i}}\right)^{\frac{1}{2}}$
Relative Risk	$R = P_1/P_2$	$r = \hat{p}_{1i}/\hat{p}_{2i}$	$S_{\text{Log}}(ri) = \left(\frac{(1-p_{1i})}{n_{1i}p_{1i}} + \frac{(1-p_{2i})}{n_{2i}p_{2i}}\right)^{\frac{1}{2}}$
Odds Ratio	$\Omega = \frac{P_1/(1-P_1)}{P_2/(1-P_2)}$	$\omega_I = \frac{\hat{p}_{1i}/(1-\hat{p}_{1i})}{\hat{p}_{2i}/(1-\hat{p}_{2i})}$	$s_{\text{Log}}(\omega i) = \left(\frac{1}{a} + \frac{1}{b} + \frac{1}{c} + \frac{1}{d}\right)^{\frac{1}{2}}$

Table 3 gives the formula of parameter inferences in three potential study summary statistics: The ratio of the odds for the treated group to the odds for the control group (odds ratio, OR), the ratio of two probabilities (relative risk, RR), and the difference between two probabilities (risk difference, RD). OR and RR are typically analyzed on logarithmic scale with normal distribution approximation, and the confidence intervals for OR and RR are also computed on the logarithmic scale, then transformed back to the original scale. In practice, OR is widely used as an outcome measure for its convenient mathematical properties, which allow for easily combining data and testing the significance of the overall effect. The OR will be close to the RR, if the end point occurs relatively infrequently, such as less than 20%. RD or absolute risk reduction is easy to interpret and defined for boundary values (proportions of 0 or 1), and is approximately normally distributed for the modest sample sizes. RD reflects both the underlying risk without treatment and the risk reduction associated with treatment. Taking the reciprocal of the RD gives the "number needed to treat" (the number of patients needed to be treated to prevent one event), which is very useful in making a decision in clinical practice.

2.1.2. *Means differences and standardized means differences*

When the primary studies report means as outcome measure on a continuous scale, there are two situations to be considered. First, all of the eligible studies use the same measure of effect, and mean difference may be used as summary measure to estimate pooled effect in the meta-analysis. Suppose the n_{1i} and n_{2i} are the sample sizes, x_{1i} and x_{2i} are the means, for treatment and control group, respectively. $Y_i = \bar{X}_{1i} - \bar{X}_{2i}$, with standard error, s_i, calculated as with

$$s_i^2 = s_{pi}^2\left(\frac{1}{n_{1i}} + \frac{1}{n_{2i}}\right) \quad \text{with} \quad s_{pi}^2 = \frac{(n_{1i}-1)s_{1i}^2 + (n_{2i}-1)s_{2i}^2}{n_{1i}+n_{2i}-2},$$

where s_{1i}^2 and s_{2i}^2 are the treatment and control group variance, respectively, of the ith study.

Second, all of the eligible studies address the same question, but the measure of effect is made using different instruments and thus different scales. When there is no direct measure common to all the studies, it may be feasible to transform the study-specific summary to a standardized (scale-free) statistic denoted as effect size. One common estimator of effect size is the standardized mean difference, which is calculated as the difference of means divided by the variability of the measures. If

$$Y_{ij}^1 \sim N(\mu^1, \sigma^2), \quad j = 1, 2, \ldots, n_{1i},$$
$$Y_{ij}^2 \sim N(\mu^2, \sigma^2), \quad j = 1, 2, \ldots, n_{2i},$$

then the standardized means difference is defined as

$$\delta = \frac{\mu^1 - \mu^2}{\sigma},$$

which denotes the gain (or loss) as the fraction of the measurements. The estimator of δ, Hedge's g, is defined as

$$h_i = \frac{\bar{Y}_i^1 - \bar{Y}_i^2}{s_p}.$$

Such standardization leads to a unitless effect measure. The results from the original studies, where "success" is measured in different ways, can be standardized to unitless measures and then pooled. The estimated variance of h_i is

$$Var(h_i) = \left(\frac{1}{n_{1i}} + \frac{1}{n_{2i}}\right) + \frac{h_i^2}{2(n_{1i} + n_{2i})}.$$

2.1.3. *Other measures*

When the summary data from the primary studies consist of test statistics, then it is sometimes possible to recover the estimated effect size if the appropriate pieces of information are also reported. For example, if the z-statistics is reported, the estimated standardized mean difference may be calculated as

$$\hat{\delta} = z\sqrt{\left(\frac{1}{n_{1i}} + \frac{1}{n_{2i}}\right)}.$$

2.2. *Model choice*

In meta-analysis, pooled effects and confidence intervals are usually obtained by using appropriate parametric statistical models. Just like ANOVA, analysis the sources of variation may be critical for the model used in meta-analysis.[11, 12]

There are at least two sources of variation to consider before combining summary statistics across studies. One is the inner- or within-study variation, which is derived from sampling error. Sampling error may vary with studies. In general, the sampling error may be relatively small for studies with large sample sizes, which means high degrees of precision and large weight would be given. The other is the inter- or between-study variation. The fixed-effects (FE) model assumes each study is measuring the same underlying parameter and there is no inter-study variation, in other words, the population from which the given studies were drawn comprises studies exactly like those in the sample, the only source of variation in the observations is due to within-study sampling. By contrast, the random effects (RE) model assumes each study is associated with a different but related parameter, which means the population believed to produce the sampled set of studies is a population of studies not exactly alike. For the RE model, each study's observed effect results from sampling variation about a random effect measure, which itself is "drawn" from a distribution of effect measures.

2.2.1. *Fixed-effects model*

A fixed-effects model assumes that each observed study effect, $Y_i (i = 1, 2, \ldots, K)$, is a realization of a population of independent studies with common parameters. Let θ be the parameter of interest, which quantifies the average treatment effect. Assume that Y_i is such that $E(Y_i) = \theta$ and let $s_i^2 = Var(Y_i)$ be the estimate of variance of the effect in the ith study. For moderately large study sizes, each Y_i should be asymptotically normal distributed (by the central limit theorem) and approximately unbiased. Thus,

$$Y_i \overset{\text{indep}}{\sim} N(\theta, s_i^2) \tag{1}$$

and s_i^2 is assumed known.

2.2.2. *Random-effects model*

The random-effects model framework postulates that each observed study effect, Y_i, is a draw from a normal distribution with a study-specific mean,

θ_i, and variance, s_i^2. θ_i is interpreted as the "true effect" in study i. Furthermore, θ_i is assumed to be a draw from some hyper-distributions of effects with mean θ and variance τ^2. θ is the true underlying effect of interest, represent the average treatment effect, and τ^2 is the inter-study variance, or heterogeneity parameter. Thus,

$$Y_i|\theta_i,\ s_i^2 \overset{\text{indep}}{\sim} N(\theta_i, s_i^2)\,, \tag{2}$$

$$\theta_i|\theta,\ \tau^2 \overset{\text{indep}}{\sim} N(\theta, \tau^2)\,. \tag{3}$$

Random-effects model "borrow strength" across studies when estimating study-specific effects, θ_i, as well as the population effect θ. RE model of (2) and (3) is refer to "hierarchic" model. This structure will be particularly useful in the development of the Bayesian paradigm.

2.3. *Statistical inference*

A test of homogeneity should be done before any further analysis. If no significant inter-study variation is found, a fixed-effects approach is adopted. Otherwise, the meta-analyst either adopts a random-effects approach or identifies study characteristics that stratify the studies into subsets with homogeneous effects. The test of heterogeneity is described next and followed by a description of inference for fixed-effects and random-effects models. Maximum likelihood, and restricted maximum likelihood methods are given for both types of models. In the next section, Bayesian approaches will be discussed.

2.3.1. *Test of homogeneity*

The investigation of homogeneity is a crucial part of the meta-analysis. The fixed effects model assumes that the K study-specific summary statistics share a common mean θ. A statistical test for the homogeneity of study means is equivalent to testing

$$\begin{aligned} &\mathrm{H}_0 : \theta = \theta_1 = \theta_2 = \cdots = \theta_K\,, \\ &\mathrm{H}_1 : \text{At least two } \theta_i\, s \text{ different}\,. \end{aligned}$$

The test statistic

$$Q_w = \sum_i^k W_i(Y_i - \hat{\theta})^2 \tag{4}$$

will asymptotically follow χ^2_{k-1} under H_0 for large sample sizes. The overall treatment effect θ, is estimated as a weighted average, that is

$$\hat{\theta} = \sum W_i Y_i \Big/ \sum W_i \quad \text{and} \quad W_i = 1/s_i^2 \,.$$

If Q_w is greater than the $100(1-\alpha)$ percentile of the χ^2 distribution, the hypothesis of equal means, H_0, would be rejected at the $100(1-\alpha)$ level. If H_0 is rejected, the meta-analyst may conclude that the study means arose from two or more distinct populations and proceed by either attempting to identify covariates that stratify studies into the homogeneous populations or adopting a random-effects model. If H_0 cannot be rejected, it would be concluded that the K studies share a common mean, θ.

Tests of homogeneity have low power against the alternative $Var(\theta_i) > 0$. Note that not rejecting H_0 is equivalent to asserting that the between-study variation is small. The results of simulation by Hardy show that the power of homogeneity test depends on the number of included studies, the total information (i.e. total weight or inverse variance) available and the distributions among the different studies.[13] In practice, if the studies are homogeneous, then the choice between the fixed- and random-effects model is not important, as the models will yield similar results. The use of the random-effects model is not considered to be a defensible solution to the problem of heterogeneity. The random-effects model is generally "conservative". That is, in most situations, use of the random-effects model will lead to wider confidence inference and a low chance to call a difference "statistically significant".

2.3.2. *Parameter estimation*

For fixed-effects model, when s_i^2 is assumed known, $\log(L(\theta|y, s^2)) \propto \sum_i \left(\frac{(Y_i-\theta)^2}{s_i^2}\right)$, which leads to the maximum likelihood estimator (MLE)

$$\hat{\theta}_{\text{MLE}} = \frac{\sum_{i=1}^{k} W_i Y_i}{\sum_{i=1}^{k} W_i} \quad \text{with} \quad W_i = \frac{1}{s_i^2} \,. \tag{5}$$

Standard inferences about θ are available using the fact that

$$\hat{\theta}_{\text{MLE}} \sim N\left(\theta \left(\sum_i w_i\right)^{-1}\right).$$

For random-effects model, if τ^2 is known, the MLE of θ is given by

$$\hat{\theta}(\tau)_{\text{MLE}} = \frac{\sum_{i=1}^k w_i(\tau)Y_i}{\sum_{i=1}^k w_i(\tau)} \quad \text{with} \quad W_i(\tau) = \frac{1}{s_i^2 + \tau^2}\,. \tag{6}$$

However, in the more realistic case of unknown τ^2, restricted maximum likelihood (RMLE) can be employed as a method for estimating variance components in a general linear model. Using the marginal distribution for y, the log-likelihood to be maximized is

$$\log(L(\theta, \tau^2|s^2y) \propto \sum_i \left\{\log(s_i^2 + \tau^2) + \frac{(Y_i - \hat{\theta}_R)^2}{s_i^2 + \tau^2}\right\}$$
$$+ \log\left(\sum (s_i^2 + \tau^2)^{-1}\right).$$

The REML of τ^2 is the solution of

$$\tau_R^2 = \frac{\sum_i w_i^2(\hat{\tau})\left(\frac{k}{k-1}(Y_i - \hat{\theta}_R)^2 - s_i^2\right)}{\sum_i w_i^2(\hat{\tau})}\,.$$

The estimator for the population mean is then calculated as

$$\hat{\theta}_R = \frac{\sum_i^k w_i(\hat{\tau}_R)Y_i}{\sum_i^k w_i(\hat{\tau}_R)}\,, \quad w_i(\hat{\tau}_R) = \frac{1}{s_i^2 + \hat{\tau}_R^2}\,,$$

and inferences are made using $\hat{\theta}_R \sim N(\theta, (\sum_i w_i(\hat{\tau}_R))^{-1})$.

By equating the homogeneity test, Q_w, to its corresponding expected value, DerSimonian and Laird proposed a non-iterative (method of moments) estimator of τ^2 as

$$\tau^2 = \max\left\{0,\ \frac{Q - (k-1)}{\sum w_i - \frac{\sum w_i^2}{\sum w_i}}\right\}.$$

This leads to

$$\hat{\theta}_{DL} = \frac{\sum_i w_i(\hat{\tau}_{DL})Y_i}{\sum_i w_i(\hat{\tau}_{Dl})} \quad \text{with} \quad w_i(\hat{\tau}_{Dl}) = \frac{1}{s_i^2 + \hat{\tau}_{DL}^2}\,.$$

$\hat{\theta}_{DL}$ is also denoted Cochran's semi-weighted estimator of θ and can be easily programmed using most software packages.

A third estimator of τ^2 and θ is to adopt a fully Bayesian approach, which reflect the uncertainty in the estimates of hyperparameters. This will be discussed in detail in the next section.

2.4. *Classical approaches for meta-analysis*

Many methods of meta-analysis have been proposed. Here we focus on the classic approaches based on two kinds of measures, discrete outcome and continuous outcome.

2.4.1. *Measures based on a discrete outcome*

For measures based on discrete outcome, we primary discuss the methods involve the data in the form of 2×2 table, which is widely used in the meta-analysis of clinical trials, cohort studies and case-control studies. Suppose the arrangement of data and table notation is still as shown in Table 2.

2.4.1.1. Mantel-Haenszel method

The Mantel-Haenzel method is a well-known approach for pooling data across strata. Since each study included in meta-analysis could be regarded as a stratum, Mantel-Haenzel method is appropriate for analyzing data for a meta-analysis. The method is based on the assumption of fixed-effects model, and the pooled measure is expressed as a combination of stratum-specific measures. Mantel-Haenzel method can be used when the measure of effect is a ratio measure, typically an odds ratio.[14] In meta-analysis, the pooled estimate using Mantel-Haenzel method is the weighted average of the maximum-likelihood estimate of the odds ratios in each study, using the inverse of study level variances as weights.

The odds ratio for the ith study $OR_i = \frac{a_i d_i}{b_i c_i}$.

The weight for the ith study $w_i = \frac{b_i c_i}{T_i}$.

The pooled estimate of odds ratio is

$$OR_{MH} = \frac{\sum(w_i OR_i)}{\sum w_i} = \frac{\sum(a_i d_i/T_i)}{\sum(b_i c_i/T_i)}\,. \tag{7}$$

The variance of the $\ln OR_{MH}$ is equal to

$$Var(\ln OR_{MH}) = \frac{\sum F}{2\sum R^2} + \frac{\sum G}{2\sum R \sum S} + \frac{\sum H}{2\sum S^2}\,,$$

with

$$F = \frac{a_i d_i(a_i + d_i)}{T_i^2}\,,$$

$$G = \frac{a_i d_i(b_i + c_i) + b_i c_i(a_i + d_i)}{T_i^2}\,,$$

$$H = \frac{b_i c_i (b_i + c_i)}{T_i^2},$$

$$R = \frac{a_i d_i}{T_i}, \quad S = \frac{b_i c_i}{T_i}.$$

The 95% confidence interval for pooled odds ratio is equal to

$$\exp\left(\ln OR_{MH} \pm 1.96\sqrt{Var(\ln OR_{MH})}\right). \tag{8}$$

The Q statistics for homogeneity test is given by

$$\begin{aligned} Q &= \sum w_i(\ln OR_{MH} - \ln OR_i)^2 \\ &= \sum w_i[\ln(OR_i)]^2 - \frac{[\sum w_i \ln(OR_i)]^2}{\sum w_i}. \end{aligned} \tag{9}$$

Under the null hypothesis of homogeneity, Q has an approximate χ^2_{k-1} distribution.

The test based on Mantel-Haenszel χ^2 has optimal statistical properties, being the uniformly most powerful test. But application of the method requires that data to complete a 2×2 table of outcome by treatment groups for each study are available.

2.4.1.2. Peto method

The Peto method is a modification of Mantel-Haenszel method. It is based on the fixed-effects model and the effect measure of interest is odds ratio.[15] Peto method uses a score statistics and Fisher information statistics from conditional likelihood for study-specific effects to estimate pooled effects. The computation involved in Peto method is relatively simple compared to Mantel-Haenszel method. Peto method has been extensively used, especially in clinical trials.

Let O_i and E_i be the observed and expected number of events in the treatment group for ith study, respectively, where $E_i = \frac{n_{1i} m_{1i}}{T_i}$.

The pooled estimate of odds ratio is equal to

$$OR_p = \exp\left(\frac{\sum(O_i - E_i)}{\sum V_i}\right), \tag{10}$$

where $V_i = \frac{n_{1i} m_{1i} n_{2i} m_{2i}}{T_i^2(T_i - 1)}$ is the variance of the difference $O_i - E_i$.

The 95% confidence interval for pooled odds ratio is

$$\exp\left(\ln OR_p \pm \frac{1.96}{\sqrt{\sum V_i}}\right) = \exp\left(\frac{\sum(O_i - E_i) \pm 1.96\sqrt{\sum V_i}}{\sum V_i}\right). \tag{11}$$

Table 4. Data from seven randomized trials of the effectiveness of aspirin after myocardial infarction and the results of meta-analysis (Peto method).

	Aspirin		Placebo						
Study	No. deaths	No. patient	No. deaths	No. patient	E_i	$O_i - E_i$	V_i	OR_i	$(O_i - E_i)^2/v_i$
1	49	615	67	624	5i.6	−8.6	26.3	0.720	2.8
2	44	758	64	771	53.5	−9.5	25.1	0.681	3.6
3	102	832	126	850	112.8	−10.4	49.3	0.803	2.4
4	32	317	38	309	35.4	−3.4	15.5	0.801	0.7
5	85	810	52	406	91.3	−6.3	27.1	0.798	1.5
6	246	2267	219	2257	233.0	13.0	104.3	1.133	1.6
7	1570	8587	1720	8600	1643.8	−73.8	665.1	0.895	8.2
Total						−99.4	912.7		20.8

Source: Fleiss and Gross.[16]

The homogeneity test, Q, is given by

$$Q = \sum \frac{(O_i - E_i)^2}{V_i} - \frac{(\sum(O_i - E_i))^2}{\sum V_i}. \tag{12}$$

Under the null hypothesis of homogeneity, Q has an approximate χ^2_{k-1} distribution.

Although Peto method is widely used, it has been demonstrated to be potentially biased when the true common odds ratio is far from unity or when there are large unbalances between the numbers of death and survival or exposed and non-exposed. In this situation, Mantel-Haenszel may be preferred.

Example 1. Table 4 shows data from seven randomized clinical trials of the effect of aspirin in preventing death after myocardial infarction.[16] The Peto method is used to estimate a summary odds ratio and its 95% confidence interval for these data is as follows:

2.4.1.2.1. Homogeneity test

Calculate $E_i, V_i, O_i - E_i$, and $(O_i - E_i)^2/V_i$, and the results are show in Table 4.

$$Q = \sum \frac{(O_i - E_i)^2}{V_i} - \frac{(\sum(O_i - E_i))^2}{\sum V_i} = 20.8 - \frac{(-99.4)^2}{912.7} = 9.97.$$

Here, $df = 6$, $\chi^2_{(0.05,6)} = 12.6 > 9.97$, $P > 0.05$, the null hypothesis of homogeneous odds ratio would not be rejected at 5 percent level, so that the fixed-effects model may be appropriate to be adopted for pooling the odds ratio.

2.4.1.2.2. Calculate the pooled estimate of odds ratio and its 95% confidence interval

$$OR_p = \exp\left(\frac{\sum(O_i - E_i)}{\sum V_i}\right) = \exp\left(\frac{-99.4}{912.7}\right) = 0.90$$

$$\exp\left(\frac{\sum(O_i - E_i) \pm 1.96\sqrt{\sum V_i}}{\sum V_i}\right) = \exp\left(\frac{-99.4 \pm 1.96\sqrt{912.7}}{912.7}\right)$$
$$= (0.84, 0.96)\,.$$

2.4.1.2.3. Graphical presentation of the results

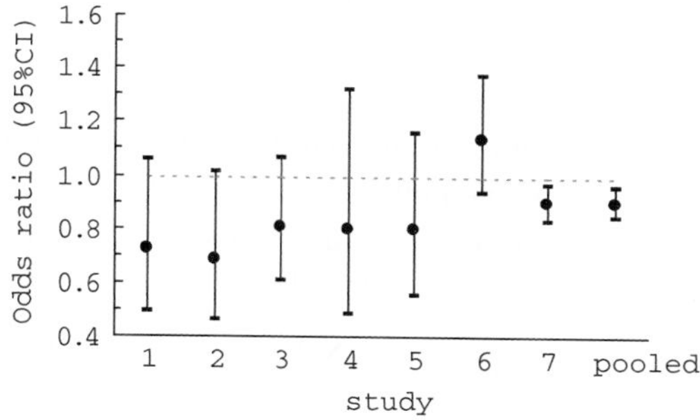

Fig. 1. The odds ratios of seven studies and their 95% confidence interval, and pooled odds ratio and its 95% confidence interval.

2.4.1.3. Fleiss method

When data to complete a 2×2 table is not available, the Peto method could not be adopted unless those studies are excluded. Sometimes the individual study may report the proportions having the characteristic under study, the Fleiss method can be used as alternative the Peto method based on fixed-effect model. For a clinical trial or cohort study, let p_{1i} and p_{2i} be the mortality rate or incidence rate for treated (exposed) and control group, respectively. For a case-control study, let p_{1i} and p_{2i} be the exposure rate for case and control group, respectively. Fleiss draws the formula of pooling the log odds ratio when p_{1i} and p_{2i} are given in the included study in meta-analysis.[16]

The effect for ith study, denoted by y_i, is the logarithm of the odds ratio:

$$y_i = \ln(OR_i) = \ln(p_{1i}(1-p_{2i})/p_{2i}(1-p_{1i})).$$

The variance and weight of y_i are given by

$$Var(y_i) = \frac{1}{n_{1i}p_{1i}(1-p_{1i})} + \frac{1}{n_{2i}p_{2i}(1-p_{2i})}, \quad w_i = \frac{1}{Var(y_i)}.$$

The pooled estimate of odds ratio is equal to

$$OR_F = \exp(\bar{y}) = \exp\left(\sum w_i y_i \Big/ \sum w_i\right). \tag{13}$$

The 95% confidence interval for summary odds ratio is given by

$$\exp\left(\bar{y} \pm 1.96 \Big/ \sqrt{\sum w_i}\right). \tag{14}$$

The Q statistic for homogeneity test is

$$Q = \sum w_i(y_i - \bar{y})^2 = \sum w_i y_i^2 - \frac{(\sum w_i y_i)^2}{\sum w_i}. \tag{15}$$

Example 1 (continued). The Fleiss method is used to estimate a pooled odds ratio and its 95% confidence interval for data in Example 1 in Table 5.

First, calculate the observed effect $y_i = \ln(OR_i)$, variance v_i weight w_i and $w_i y_i$, $w_i y_i^2$ for each individual study, results shown in Table 5.

The Q statistic for homogeneity test is

$$Q = \sum w_i(y_i - \bar{y})^2 = \sum w_i y_i^2 - \frac{(\sum w_i y_i)^2}{\sum w_i}$$
$$= 20.7230 - \frac{(-99.0609)^2}{910.5604} = 9.946.$$

Table 5. Results of meta-analysis for the effectiveness of aspirin after myocardial infarction (Fleiss method).

Study	$y_i = \ln(OR_i)$	v_i	$w_i = 1/v_i$	$w_i y_i$	$w_i y_i^2$
1	−0.3289	0.0389	25.710	−8.4560	2.7812
2	−0.3845	0.0412	24.291	−9.3411	3.5921
3	−0.2196	0.0205	48.801	−10.7148	2.3526
4	−0.2222	0.0648	15.440	−3.4312	0.7625
5	−0.2255	0.0352	28.409	−6.4054	1.4442
6	0.1246	0.0096	103.985	12.9604	1.6153
7	−0.1110	0.0015	663.923	−73.6728	8.1752
Total			910.559	−99.0609	20.7230

$df = 6$, $\chi^2_{(0.05,6)} = 12.6 > 9.95$, $P > 0.05$, H_0 would not be rejected, so the fixed-effects model may be appropriate.

Then the pooled estimate of odds ratio is equal to

$$OR_F = \exp\left(\sum w_i y_i \Big/ \sum w_i\right)$$
$$= \exp(99.0609/910.5604) = \exp(-0.1088) = 0.90\,.$$

The 95% confidence interval for pooled odds ratio is given by

$$\exp\left(\sum w_i y_i \Big/ \sum w_i \pm 1.96 \Big/ \sqrt{\sum w_i}\right)$$
$$= \exp(-0.1088 \pm 1.96/\sqrt{910.5604})$$
$$= (0.84, 0.96).$$

Note that, results of Fleiss method are the same as those of Peto method. If complete 2×2 tables are available for all included studies, Peto method is simpler than Fleiss method, but the latter can be used only for those proportions reported.

2.4.1.4. General variance-based method

When the effect size is measured as a rate difference, the general variance-based method would be applied to estimation of the pooled rate difference. The general variance-based method is also used to estimate the pooled risk ratio, rate ratio and odds ratio.[12] The general variance-based method is also based on the fixed-effect model.

2.4.1.4.1. Effect size is measured as a rate difference

The rate different for ith study is $RD_i = \frac{a_i}{n_{1i}} - \frac{c_i}{n_{2i}}$.

The variance and weight of rate difference are $Var(RD_i) = \frac{n_{1i}n_{2i}}{m_{1i}m_{2i}T_i}$, $w_i = 1/Var(RD_i)$.

The pooled estimate of rate difference is

$$RD_{GV} = \frac{\sum(w_i RD_i)}{\sum w_i}\,. \tag{16}$$

The 95% confidence interval of pooled estimate of rate difference is equal to

$$RD_{GV} \pm 1.96 \Big/ \sqrt{\sum w_i}\,. \tag{17}$$

2.4.1.4.2. Effect size is measured as an incidence density ratio or as a risk ratio

The relative risk for ith study is $RR_i = \frac{a_i}{n_{1i}} / \frac{c_i}{n_{2i}}$.

The variance and weight of relative risk are $Var(RR_i) = \frac{n_{2i}T_i}{m_{1i}m_{2i}n_{1i}}$, $w_i = 1/Var(RR_i)$.

The pooled estimate of relative risk is

$$RR_{GV} = \exp\left(\frac{\sum(w_i \ln(RR_i))}{\sum w_i}\right). \tag{18}$$

The 95% confidence interval of pooled estimate of relative risk is equal to

$$\exp\left(\ln(RR_{GV}) \pm 1.96 \Big/ \sqrt{\sum w_i}\right). \tag{19}$$

When each study in meta-analysis just presents the relative risk and its 95% confidence interval, wherever a complete 2×2 table is unavailable, general variance-based method could also be applied to estimate the pooled effect using Eqs. (18) and (19). The formula for estimating variance from the 95% confidence interval is

$$Var(RR_i) = \left(\frac{\ln(RR_i/RR_l)}{1.96}\right)^2 = \left(\frac{\ln(RR_u/RR_i)}{1.96}\right)^2, \tag{20}$$

where RR_u and RR_l are the upper and lower bound of the 95% confidence interval for ith study.

2.4.1.4.3. Effect size is measured as odds ratio

The pooled estimate of odds ratio is

$$OR_{GV} = \exp\left(\frac{\sum(w_i \ln(OR_i))}{\sum w_i}\right). \tag{21}$$

The 95% confidence interval of pooled estimate of odds ratio is equal to

$$\exp\left(\ln(OR_{GV}) \pm 1.96 \Big/ \sqrt{\sum w_i}\right), \tag{22}$$

where

$$w_i = [Var(\ln(OR)_i)]^{-1} = \left(\frac{1}{a_i} + \frac{1}{b_i} + \frac{1}{c_i} + \frac{1}{d_i}\right)^{-1}. \tag{23}$$

Note that when pooling the effect, relative risk and odds ratio should be transform to logarithmic scale in order to be approximately normally distributed, whereas the rate difference could be computed directly.

2.4.1.5. Meta analysis method for rare events

Most of the aforementioned statistical methods used in meta analysis rely on the large-sample approximation to the point estimator from individual study. Such an approximation may be unreliable and lead to invalid conclusions if the event rate is too low relative to the sample size for individual study. This low event rate often occurs in studying rare adverse event associated with a treatment or medication. When the events of interest is very rare, the typical approach is to apply continuity corrections to studies without any event or simply exclude them before conducting the standard analysis.[58,59] Instead of subjectively handling the zero event studies, there are two general classes of methods.

Firstly, when the number of studies is not small, Mantel-Haenszel method often performs well even with rare events.[60] As with the general variance-based method, the Mantel-Haenszel method estimates the fixed effect by weighted average of point estimators from individual studies. Depending on the types of outcomes, different weighting schemes are employed and summarized in Table 6.

Secondly, when the number of studies is moderate or small, one may need to perform the "exact" meta analysis, whose validity does not depend on the sample size and number of studies.[61] To this end, we may select a set of coverage levels $0 < \eta_1 < \cdots < \eta_J < 1$, and construct the exact one-sided η_j level confidence intervals, $I_i(\eta_j) = [a_{ij}, \infty), j = 1, 2, \ldots, J$ for the parameter of interest which could be odds ratio, risk ratio or risk difference for study $i = 1, \ldots, n$. There are multiple methods for constructing the exact confidence interval in individual studies. For example, the exact

Table 6. Mantel-Haenszel method.

Outcome	$\hat{\theta}_i$	w_i
Odds Ratio	$\frac{a_i d_i}{b_i c_i}$	$\frac{b_i c_i}{T_i}$
Risk Ratio	$\frac{a_i n_{2i}}{c_i n_{1i}}$	$\frac{c_i n_{1i}}{T_i}$
Risk Difference	$\frac{a_i}{n_{1i}} - \frac{c_i}{n_{2i}}$	$\frac{n_{1i} n_{2i}}{T_i}$

confidence interval for the odds ratio can be constructed by inverting the famous Fisher's exact test. The one-sided $(1-\alpha/2)$confidence interval for θ then can be constructed as

$$\{\theta | T(\theta) \geq d\},$$

where

$$T(\theta) = \sum_{j=1}^{J}\sum_{i=1}^{K} \frac{w_i}{\eta_j(1-\eta_j)} I(\theta \geq a_{ij})$$

$w_i, i = 1, \ldots, K$ are study specific weights selected by users and the cut-off value d is selected to satisfy

$$P\left\{\sum_{j=1}^{J}\sum_{i=1}^{K} \frac{w_i}{\eta_j(1-\eta_j)} I(B_i \geq \eta_j) < d\right\} \leq \frac{\alpha}{2},$$

where $\{B_1, \ldots, B_K\}$ follow independent uniform distribution. The resulting confidence interval for θ is in the form of $[a, \infty)$. Similarly, we may also construct the one-sided $(1-\alpha/2)$ confidence interval of θ in the form of $(-\infty, b]$. It follows that $[a, b]$ is the $(1-\alpha)$ confidence interval for the parameter of interest. The point estimator can be obtained by increasing α and thus shrinking the confidence interval of θ into a single point.

Example 2. Table 7 shows data from 48 randomized clinical trials studying whether rosiglitazone increases the risk of myocardial infraction.[61,62] There are ten studies that have no myocardial infraction events and thus excluded from the original meta analysis for odds ratio.[62] We choose risk difference between two groups as the parameter of interest to utilize the information from all studies. The point estimator of risk difference is 0.183% with an exact 95% confidence interval of $(-0.08, 0.38)\%$. Here $0 < \eta_1 < \cdots < \eta_J < 1$ are 20 equally spaced levels from 0.1 to 0.95. For each study, the one-sided confidence interval is constructed using mid-p-value method. The 95% confidence interval based on the Mantel-Haenszel method is (0.02, 0.42)% after excluding 10 studies with no myocardial infarction events. This confidence interval may not be reliable due to low event rate which results in a substantial proportion of studies with no myocardial infarction events being excluded from the analysis. Those excluded studies contain information favoring zero risk difference between Rosiglitazone and control groups.

Table 7. Data from 48 randomized trials of the side effect on myocardial infarction of Rosiglitazone.

	Rosiglitazone		Control	
Study	No. MI	No. patients	No. MI	No. patients
1	2	357	0	176
2	2	391	1	207
3	1	774	1	185
4	0	213	1	109
5	1	232	0	116
6	0	43	1	47
7	1	121	0	124
8	5	110	2	114
9	1	382	0	384
10	1	284	0	135
11	0	294	1	302
12	2	563	0	142
13	2	278	1	279
14	2	418	0	212
15	2	395	1	198
16	1	203	1	106
17	1	104	2	99
18	2	212	0	107
19	3	138	1	139
20	0	196	0	96
21	0	122	1	120
22	0	175	1	173
23	1	56	0	58
24	1	39	0	38
25	0	561	2	276
26	2	116	3	111
27	1	148	0	143
28	1	231	0	242
29	1	89	0	88
30	1	168	0	172
31	0	116	0	61
32	1	1172	0	377
33	0	706	0	325
34	1	204	2	185
35	1	288	0	280
36	1	254	0	272
37	1	314	0	154
38	0	162	0	160
39	1	442	0	112
40	1	394	0	124
41	15	2635	9	2634
42	27	1456	41	2895

(*Continued*)

Table 7. (*Continued*)

Study	Rosiglitazone		Control	
	No. MI	No. patients	No. MI	No. patients
43	0	101	0	51
44	0	232	0	115
45	0	70	0	75
46	0	25	0	24
47	0	196	0	195
48	0	676	0	225

2.4.1.6. DerSimonian-Laird method

The approaches we previously described are all based on the fixed-effect model. When the studies included in meta-analysis lack of homogeneity, the random-effects model may be appropriate to combine the effect size. Formulas of applying the DerSimonian-Laird method summarizing studies in the case where effects are measured as odds ratios are given as follows[17]:

$$OR_{DL} = \exp\left(\frac{\sum w_i^* \ln(OR_i)}{\sum w_i^*}\right). \tag{24}$$

The 95% confidence interval of pooled estimate of odds ratio is equal to

$$\exp\left(\ln OR_D L \pm 1.96 \Big/ \sqrt{\sum w_i^*}\right), \tag{25}$$

where w_i^* is the weighting factor for the ith study, is estimated as

$$w_i^* = \frac{1}{D + (1/w_i)}\,. \tag{26}$$

D is derived from the homogeneity test statistic, Q, in Eq. (15). As described previously about the moment estimate of inter-study variance τ^2 in model choice and homogeneity test, we have

$$D = \frac{Q - (k-1)\sum w_i}{(\sum w_i)^2 - \sum w_i^2} \quad \text{and} \quad D = 0 \text{ if } Q < k-1\,, \tag{27}$$

where k is the number of included studies.

Example 1 (continued). In the example of meta-analysis of seven clinical trials in which aspirin was used to prevent death after myocardial infarction, we have calculated the pooled effect sized using the approaches based on fixed-effects model. The results of homogeneity test is, $Q = 10.8$, and

Table 8. Results of meta-analysis for the effectiveness of aspirin after myocardial infarction (DerSimonian-Laird method).

Study	$y_i = \ln(OR_i)$	w_i	w_i^2	w_i^*	$w_i^* y_i$
1	−0.3289	25.710	660.995	20.605	−6.777
2	−0.3845	24.291	590.060	19.683	−7.569
3	−0.2196	48.801	2381.509	33.191	−7.287
4	−0.2222	15.441	238.410	13.441	−2.987
5	−0.2255	28.409	807.093	22.303	−5.029
6	0.1246	103.985	10812.969	51.937	6.473
7	−0.1110	663.923	440794.250	89.738	−9.958
Total		910.560	456285.285	250.898	−33.133

$df = 6$, $\chi^2_{(0.05,6)} = 12.6 > 10.8$, $P > 0.05$, the null hypothesis was not rejected. In order to evaluate the dependence of the conclusions of the analysis on the model assumption, now we calculate the pooled effect using random-effects model.

$$D = \frac{(Q-(k-1))\sum w_i}{(\sum w_i)^2 - \sum w_i^2} = \frac{(9.946-(7-1)) \times 910.560}{910.560^2 - 456285.285} = 0.00964$$

Each w_i^* for individual study is calculated using Eq. (26), results shown in Table 8.

The pooled estimate of odds ratio and its 95% confidence interval are

$$OR_{DL} = \exp\left(\frac{\sum w_i^* \ln(OR_i)}{\sum w_i^*}\right) = \exp\left(\frac{-33.133}{250.898}\right) = \exp(-0.132) = 0.88$$

$$= \exp\left(\ln OR_{DL} \pm 1.96 \Big/ \sqrt{\sum w_i^*}\right.$$

$$= \exp\left(-0.1321 \pm 1.96 \Big/ \sqrt{250.898}\right) = (0.77, 0.99).$$

Now, if we compare the results of fixed-effects and random-effects model, the pooled point estimate of odds ratio, 0.88 and 0.90, respectively, is almost the same. The length of the 95% confidence interval based on random-effects model is 0.22 (0.99–0.77), which is greater than that based on fixed-effects model, 0.12 (0.96–0.84). So the result of random-effects model is potentially more conservative. But the two methods yield the same conclusion, that is, in general, aspirin make the risk of death after myocardial infarction decrease by nearly 10%.

2.4.1.7. Variations of DerSimonian-Laird method

It is well known that DerSimonian-Laird method tends to produce confidence interval whose empirical coverage level is lower than the nominal level since it ignores the variability in estimating the inter-study variability, i.e., the common variance of the random effect. The under-coverage may become severe when either the number of studies or the sample size for individual study is small. There are a couple of simple remedies.[63,64,65,66] We will illustrate them using odds ratio as the summary measure for the treatment effect.

2.4.1.7.1. Variance-based Method[66]

The point estimator can be obtained as the variance-based estimator under fixed effect model albeit our assumptions of random effect model, i.e.,

$$\exp\left(\frac{\sum (w_i \ln(OR_i))}{\sum w_i}\right),$$

where

$$w_i = [Var(\ln(OR)_i)]^{-1} = \left(\frac{1}{a_i} + \frac{1}{b_i} + \frac{1}{c_i} + \frac{1}{d_i}\right)^{-1}.$$

The 95% confidence interval of pooled estimate of odds ratio is

$$\exp\left(\ln OR_{DL} \pm 1.96\sqrt{\left(\sum_{i=1}^{K} w_i\right)^{-2}\left(\sum_{i=1}^{K} w_i^2(w_i^{-1} + D)\right)}\right),$$

where D is the moment estimate of inter-study variance, τ^2, given in (27). This method may not be the most efficient in terms of the width of the 95% confidence interval. However the confidence interval in general has better coverage level than that based on DerSimonian-Laird method. Furthermore, the simulation studies also demonstrate that the above confidence interval tends to be more robust to the publication bias than the standard DeSimonian-Laird interval.

2.4.1.7.2. Nonparametric method

More robust confidence interval for θ, which is the center of distribution for treatment effect in different studies, can be constructed by inverting a nonparametric statistical test.[67] To this end, let the test statistics be

$$T(\theta) = \sum_{i=1}^{K} [2I(OR_i \leq \theta) - 1] \left| \Phi\left(\frac{\ln\theta - \ln(OR_i)}{\sigma_i}\right) - \frac{1}{2} \right|,$$

where $\Phi(\cdot)$ is the cumulative distribution function for standard normal distribution and

$$\sigma_i = \sqrt{\frac{1}{a_i} + \frac{1}{b_i} + \frac{1}{c_i} + \frac{1}{d_i}}.$$

When θ is the true parameter, the distribution of $T(\theta)$ can be approximated by the conditional distribution of

$$B_\theta = \sum_{i=1}^{K} \xi_i \left| \Phi\left(\frac{\ln\theta - \ln(OR_i)}{\sigma_i}\right) - \frac{1}{2} \right|$$

given the observed data, where $\{\xi_1, \xi_2, \ldots, \xi_K\}$ are independent Bernoulli random variables with a success probability of 0.5. This conditional distribution can be approximated by Monte-Carlo method in practice and used to test the hypothesis $\theta < a$ ($\theta > b$). In the end, the 95% confidence interval of θ is $[c, d]$, where c and d are chosen to satisfy $P\{B_c \leq T(c)\} = P\{B_d \geq T(d)\} = 0.025$. The confidence interval based on the nonparametric method is very robust and has satisfactory coverage level even when the number of studies is as small as four or five.

Example 1 (continued). In the example of meta-analysis of seven clinical trials in which aspirin was used to prevent the death after myocardial infarction, we have calculated the pooled effect sized using the DerSimonian-Laird method and the 95% confidence interval is [0.77, 0.99]. Using the inverse variance method, the point estimator is 0.90 and the 95% confidence interval is [0.77, 1.06], which is slightly wider than that based DerSimonian-Laird method. The 95% confidence interval based on the nonparametric method is [0.68, 1.03], which is very similar to that based on inverse variance method. Note that while the confidence interval based on DerSimonian-Laird excludes one, those based on inverse-variance as well as nonparametric methods include one, suggesting there is no adequate evidence for the protective effect of aspirin at the significance level of 0.05.

2.4.2. *Measures based on a continuous scale*

When the effect size in the studies included in a meta-analysis is measured on a continuous scale, we primarily focus on the estimates of pooled mean difference and standardized mean difference.[10,12]

Suppose the n_{1i} and n_{2i} are the sample sizes, x_{1i} and x_{2i} are the means, of treatment and control group, respectively. The mean difference $y_i = \bar{x}_{1i} - \bar{x}_{2i}$, with standard error, s_i, calculated as

$$s_i^2 = s_{pi}^2 \left(\frac{1}{n_{1i}} + \frac{1}{n_{2i}} \right), \quad \text{where} \quad s_{pi}^2 = \frac{(n_{1i}-1)s_{1i}^2 + (n_{2i}-1)s_{2i}^2}{n_{1i}+n_{2i}-2}.$$

2.4.2.1. Fixed-Effect model

2.4.2.1.1. Effect size is measured on the same scale

The pooled measure of size effect (mean difference) is $y_s = \frac{\sum w_i y_i}{\sum w_i}$, where $w_i = \frac{1}{s_i^2}$.

The Q statistic for homogeneity test is given by

$$Q = \sum w_i (y_s - y_i)^2 = \sum w_i y_i^2 - \frac{(\sum w_i y_i)^2}{\sum w_i}.$$

The 95% confidence interval of summary measure of effect size is $y_s \pm 1.96/\sqrt{\sum w_i}$.

Example 2. Table 9 presents data about the change in Kurtzke Disability Status Scale at two years in four randomized trials of the effect of azathioprine treatment in multiple sclerosis. The summary estimate of mean difference is given as follows:

Table 9. A meta-analysis for Change in Kurzke Disability Status Scale at two years in four randomized trials of the effect of azathioprine treatment in multiple sclerosis.

	Treated			Control								
Study	x_{1i}	s_{1i}	n_{1i}	x_{2i}	s_{2i}	n_{2i}	y_i	y_i^2	s_i^2	w_I	$w_i y_i$	$w_i y_i^2$
1	0.30	1.26	162	0.42	1.28	175	−0.12	0.0144	0.019	52.632	−6.316	0.758
2	0.17	0.90	15	0.83	0.98	20	−0.66	0.4356	0.105	9.524	−6.286	4.149
3	0.20	1.10	30	0.45	1.12	32	−0.25	0.0625	0.080	12.500	−3.125	0.781
4	0.17	1.38	27	0.42	1.36	25	−0.25	0.0289	0.145	6.897	−1.724	0.431
Total								0.5414		81.553	−7.451	6.119

Source: Yudkin *et al.* (1991). *Lancet* **338**: 1051–1055 and Petitti.[12]

2.4.2.1.1.1. Homogeneity test

$$Q = \sum w_i y_i^2 - \frac{(\sum w_i y_i)^2)}{\sum w_i} = 6.119 - \frac{(-17.451)^2}{81.553} = 2.385.$$

Here, $df = 3$, $\chi^2_{(0.05,3)} = 7.28 > 2.385$, $p > 0.05$ therefore, the null hypothesis that the studies are homogeneous is not rejected, and it is appropriate to use fixed-effects model to estimate the pooled weight mean.

2.4.2.1.1.2. Calculating the pooled effect size and its 95% confidence interval

$$y_s = \frac{\sum w_i y_i}{\sum w_i} = \frac{-17.451}{81.553} = -0.197\,,$$

$$y_s \pm 1.96 \Big/ \sqrt{\sum w_i} = -0.197 \pm (1.96/\sqrt{81.553}) = (-0.414, 0.02)\,.$$

The results of meta-analysis suggest, the pooled mean difference of the Kutzke Disability Scale for the effect of azathioprine treatment in multiple sclerosis is −0.197, but the results are statistically non-significant (95% confidence interval covers zero). Based on these results, we still cannot draw the conclusion that azathioprine is beneficial for multiple sclerosis.

2.4.2.1.2. Effect size is measured on different scale

When studies used different scales to measure effect, the standardized mean difference is calculated as the estimate of effect size. Let

$$d_i = \frac{\bar{x}_{1i} - \bar{x}_{2i}}{s_{pi}}\,,$$

then the pooled estimate of effect size is

$$d_s = \frac{\sum w_i d_i}{\sum w_i}\,, \tag{28}$$

where w_i is the weight assigned to each study. This weighted estimator of the effect size was shown by Hedges to be asymptotically efficient when sample sizes in the two groups are both greater than 10 and the effect sizes are less than 1.5.[18] When the sample sizes are about equal in the two groups and both greater than 10, the weight of each study can be estimated as follows:

$$w_i = \frac{2N_i}{8 + d_i^2}\,. \tag{29}$$

The 95% confidence interval for the pooled estimate of effect size is

$$d_s \pm 1.96/\sqrt{w_i}\,. \tag{30}$$

The Q statistic for homogeneity test is given by

$$Q = \sum w_i (d_s - d_i)^2 = \sum w_i d_i^2 - \frac{(\sum w_i d_i)^2}{(\sum w_i)} . \tag{31}$$

2.4.2.2. Random-effects model

If H_0 of homogeneity is rejected, which means that the between-study variance is relatively large, a random-effect model should be used.

The calculation of effect size is the same, that is, $d_i = \frac{\bar{x}_{1i} - \bar{x}_{2i}}{s_{pi}}$.

The pooled estimate of effect size and variance are

$$\bar{d} = \frac{\sum w_i d_i}{\sum w_i} ,$$

$$s_d^2 = \frac{\sum w_i (d_i - \bar{d})^2}{\sum w_i} = \frac{\sum w_i d_i^2}{\sum w_i} - \bar{d}^2 , \tag{32}$$

where, $w_i = N_i = n_{1i} + n_{2i}$.

The random-effect model assumes $d_i = \delta_i + e_i$, with

$$\bar{\delta} = \bar{d} , \quad \bar{e} = 0 \quad \text{and} \quad s_i^2 = \frac{4k}{\sum w_i} \left(1 + \frac{\bar{d}^2}{8} \right). \tag{33}$$

(1) If $s_d^2 > s_e^2$, $s_\delta^2 = s_d^2 - s_e^2$, and the 95% confidence interval of pooled effect size is

$$\bar{d} \pm 1.96 s_\delta . \tag{34}$$

(2) If $s_d^2 \leq s_e^2$, $s_\delta^2 = 0$, and random-effects model is actually fixed-effect model, that is

$$d_i = \delta + e_i .$$

The standard error for $\bar{d}$ is

$$s_{\bar{d}} = \frac{s_e}{\sqrt{k}} . \tag{35}$$

Then the 95% confidence interval of pooled effect size is

$$\bar{d} \pm 1.96 s_{\bar{d}} . \tag{36}$$

In random-effect model, the statistic for homogeneity test is given by

$$x^2 = \frac{k s_d^2}{s_e^2} . \tag{37}$$

Under the null hypothesis of homogeneity, the statistic follows an approximate x_{k-1}^2 distribution.

Table 10. Data from meta-analysis of the effect of aminophylline treatment in severe acute asthma.

Study	$N_i(w_i)$	s_{pi}	d_i	$w_i d_i$	$w_i d_i^2$
1	20	0.76	−0.43	−8.6	3.698
2	50	320.00	−0.04	−2.00	0.08
3	48	0.65	−0.84	−40.32	33.869
4	24	0.42	−1.67	−40.08	66.934
5	29	0.22	−1.03	−29.87	30.766
6	20	17.00	−2.41	−48.2	116.162
7	23	0.62	−0.08	−1.84	0.147
8	13	110.00	0.26	3.38	0.879
9	23	2.10	2.93	67.39	197.453
10	51	6.30	0.51	26.01	13.265
11	61	0.50	0.72	43.92	31.622
12	66	0.67	0.03	1.98	0.059
13	40	0.58	−0.02	−0.8	0.016
Total	468			−29.03	494.95

Source: Littenberg (1988). *JAMA*. **259**: 1678–1684 Petitti.[12]

Example 3. Table 10 presents data from a meta-analysis of the effect of aminophylline in severe acute asthma. The 13 studies included in the meta-analysis reported different measures on pulmonary function. A standardized mean difference should be used as common metric. The pooled estimate of effect size and 95% confidence interval are calculated as follows:

2.4.2.2.1. Homogeneity test

$$s_d^2 = \frac{\sum w_i(d_i - \bar{d})^2}{\sum w_i} = \frac{\sum w_i d_i^2}{\sum w_i} - \left(\frac{\sum w_i d_i}{\sum w_i}\right)^2$$

$$= \frac{494.95}{468} - \frac{(-29.03)^2}{468^2} = 1.054,$$

$$\bar{d} = \frac{\sum w_i d_i}{\sum w_i} = \frac{-29.03}{468} - 0.062\,,$$

$$s_e^2 = \frac{4k}{\sum w_i}\left(1 + \frac{\bar{d}^2}{8}\right) = \frac{4 \times 13}{468}\left[1 + \frac{(-0.062)^2}{8}\right] = 0.111\,,$$

$$x^2 = \frac{ks_d^2}{s_e^2} = \frac{13 \times (1.054)^2}{0.111} = 130.107\,.$$

$df = 12$, $x^2_{(0.05,12)} = 21.03$, $p < 0.05$, the null hypothesis of homogeneity is rejected, which means between-study variance is relatively large, and random-effects model should be adopted.

2.4.2.2.2. Calculating the summary effect size and its 95% confidence interval

$$s_\delta^2 = s_d^2 - s_e^2 = 1.054 - 0.111 = 0.94\,,$$

$$\bar{d} = \frac{\sum w_i d_i}{\sum w_i} = \frac{-29.03}{468} = -0.062\,,$$

$$\bar{d} \pm 1.96 s_\delta = -0.062 \pm (1.96 \times \sqrt{0.94}) = (-1.962, 1.838)\,.$$

The results of meta-analysis suggest that the effect of aminophylline treatment in severe acute asthma is statistically non-significant (95% confidence interval covers zero). In fact, the heterogeneity between studies is greatly large in the example, the smallest effect size is −0.02, whereas the largest is 2.93. It is necessary to explore the source of heterogeneity before meta-analysis, and assess the source of biases and confounding. If the combinability of studies is poor, meta-analysis should be abandoned. The process above is just a typical example for computation.

3. Bayesian Methods in Random-Effects Models for Meta-Analysis

The methods discussed above are basically frequentist procedures. There have been considerable discussions in the literature on the relative merits of fixed- and random-effects model. In practice, when combining the effect, the choice between fixed- and random-effects models is determined by the results of statistical tests of homogeneity (Q statistic). But the power of statistical tests of homogeneity is low. The results of random-effects model may be more "conservative", which leads to somewhat wider confidence intervals than the fixed-effects model. Little is known about the approach describing the random effects quantitatively. The appropriate treatment for small studies and extreme results included in meta-analysis is still unresolved in classic methods. Furthermore, the uncertainty of the parameters, such as the pooled effect size and variance, is not taken into account to use current approaches for meta-analysis.

Bayesian methods for meta-analysis give several options to deal with these problems and have been well-developed in the past decades. Under the

Bayesian framework for random-effect model in meta-analysis, the parameter is an unknown random variable that has a specific distribution. The posterior distribution of parameter is derived from prior distribution and sample information available.

DuMouchel gave a fully Bayesian analysis of the hierarchical model with a complete conjugate prior structure.[19] Carlin developed and implemented a fully Bayesian approach to meta-analysis for 2×2 tables, in which uncertainty about effects in comparable studies is represented by an exchangeable prior distribution.[20]

However, a Bayesian analysis requires integration of each of the conditional posterior distributions. Unfortunately, such integration cannot be performed in closed form in most situations. Approximate solution can be obtained through asymptotic or numerical techniques. With the great progress in Bayesian computational tools, especially the rapid development of Markov Chain Monte Carlo (MCMC) method, it is effective to deal with the problems that could not be resolved by classical meta-analysis method. Gibbs sampling is a recently developed simulation tool for Bayesian inferences, obtaining the simulated joint posterior distribution from the full conditional distributions of parameters.[21,22]

In this section, the Bayesian approaches are introduced, especially the hierarchical model under a full Bayesian framework and the Gibbs sampling in random-effects model for meta-analysis.

3.1. *Bayesian meta-analysis for DuMouchel's model*

Suppose there are K individual studies included in the meta-analysis, and the effect for each study is $Y_1, Y_2, \ldots, Y_K$. The random-effects model is

$$Y_i = \mu_i + \varepsilon_i\,, \quad \varepsilon_i \sim N(0, \sigma_i^2)\,,$$
$$\mu_i = \mu + e_i\,, \quad e_i \sim N(0, \tau^2)\,,$$

with $\{\varepsilon_i, i = 1, \ldots, K\}$ and $\{e_i, i = 1, \ldots, K\}$ are independent. Let $\boldsymbol{Y} = (Y_1, \ldots, Y_K)'$, $\mathbf{1} = (1, \ldots, 1)'$, $\boldsymbol{m} = (\mu_1, \ldots, \mu_k)'$, $\boldsymbol{\varepsilon} = (\varepsilon_1, \ldots, \varepsilon_k)'$, $\boldsymbol{e} = (e_1, \ldots, e_k)'$, $\Sigma = \text{diag}(\sigma_1^2, \ldots, \sigma_k^2)$ and I the $K \times K$ identity matrix, then the random-effect model in matrix form as $Y|m \sim N(m, \sum)$, $m \sim N(1\mu, \tau^2 I)$.

Under the full Bayesian framework, we have the model

$$Y|m\,,\ \sigma^2 \sim N(m, \sigma^2 C)\,,$$
$$\sigma^2 \sim x^2(df_\sigma)\,,$$

$$m|\mu,\, \tau^2 \sim N(1\mu, \tau^2 H)\,,$$
$$\mu|\tau^2 \sim N(0, D \to \infty)\,,$$
$$\tau^{-2} \sim x^2(df_\tau)\,.$$

Here, σ^2, τ^2 and μ are hyperparameters, and **C** and **H** are assumed as known $K \times K$ covariance matrices with unknown scale factor σ^2 and τ^2, respectively. The degrees of freedom df_σ and df_τ for inverse-χ^2 prior distributions allow incorporation of how well known **C** and **H** are, respectively. The prior distribution for μ is the standard diffused and independent of τ^2. In fact, as noted by DuMouchel, these particular prior distributions are chosen for convenience, so that the posterior distribution of **m** given Y is a mixture of multivariate student-t distribution, each with degrees of freedom $df_\sigma + df_\tau + K - 1$. For computational convenience, however, he suggests using a multivariate normal approximation to the posterior, which can then be completely described through the posterior mean and covariance matrices.

Reparameterize the variance parameters as ϕ, let $\phi = \tau^2/\sigma^2$,

$$W(\phi) = (\phi\mathbf{H} + \mathbf{C})^{-1}\,,$$

$$\beta(Y,\phi) = [1'W(\phi)1]^{-1}1'W(\phi)Y\,,$$

$$S(Y,\phi) = [Y - 1\beta(Y,\phi)]'W(\phi)[Y - 1\beta(Y,\phi)]\,,$$

$$\gamma(Y,\phi) = \frac{df_\tau + df_\sigma/\phi + S(Y,\phi)}{df_\sigma + df_\tau + K - 3}\,.$$

The posterior estimate $E(\mu|Y)$ of μ is then given by integrating what is essentially the Weighted Least Squares estimator of μ over the posterior density of ϕ, $f(\phi|Y)$

$$E(\mu|Y) = \int E(\mu|\phi, Y) f(\phi|Y) d\phi\,.$$

Similarly,

$$Var(\mu|Y) = \int \{\gamma(Y,\phi)[1'W(\phi)1]^{-1} + [\beta(Y,\phi) - E(\mu|Y)]$$
$$\times [\beta(Y,\phi) - E(\mu|Y)]'\} f(\phi|Y) d\phi\,.$$

The approximate 95% credible interval for μ using $E(\mu|Y)$ and $Var(\mu|Y)$ and the normal distribution, will be

$$E(\mu|Y) \pm 1.96\sqrt{Var(\mu|Y)}\,.$$

Posterior mean of σ^2 are obtained using

$$E(\sigma^2|Y) = \int \gamma(Y, \phi) f(\phi|Y) d\phi \,.$$

3.2. *Bayesian meta-analysis for Carlin's model*

Carlin adopts a Bayesian approach to meta-analysis for 2×2 tables, in which an exchangeable prior distribution is used. A hierarchical normal model assumes that

$$Y_i|\mu_i\,,\ \sigma_i^2 \sim N(\mu_i, \sigma_i^2)\,, \tag{38}$$

$$\mu_i|\mu\,,\ \tau^2 \sim N(\mu, \tau^2)\,, \tag{39}$$

where σ_i represents the corresponding estimated standard error, which is assumed known without error. μ_i is interpreted as the "true effect" in ith study, which has an exchangeable normal prior, and also it means effects are independently and identically distributed conditional on the values of unknown hyperparameters μ and τ^2. Here, τ^2 is between-study variance. Assume the prior distributions of μ and τ^2 are non-informative or locally uniform prior. Under the framework of Bayesian, the posterior distributions of quantities of interest, conditional on the variance hyperparameter, have closed form solutions. Let $B_i = \tau^2/(\tau^2 + \sigma_i^2)$, then we have

$$\hat{\mu} = E(\mu|Y, \tau^2) = \frac{\sum B_i Y_i}{\sum B_i}\,, \tag{40}$$

$$Var(\mu|Y, \tau^2) = \frac{\tau^2}{\sum B_i}\,. \tag{41}$$

The posterior mean and variance for the individuals μ_i, conditional on both μ and τ^2, for each i, are

$$E(\mu_i|Y, \mu, \tau^2) = B_i Y_i + (1 - B_i)\mu\,, \tag{42}$$

$$Var(\mu_i|Y, \mu, \tau^2) = B_i \sigma_i^2\,. \tag{43}$$

Note that, B_i is usually referred to as the shrinkage factor for the ith study. The larger the inter-study variation, τ^2, is the smaller the shrinkage B_i of the observed study effects. Because $0 \leq B_i \leq 1$, the mean is compromised between the average treatment effect μ and the observed study summary statistics, Y_i. When $\sigma_i^2 = 0$, shrinkage is maximized to $B_i = 1$ so that $\mu_1 = \mu_2 = \cdots = \mu_k = \mu$ and the random-effects model reduces to the fixed-effects model.

Integrating Eqs. (42) and (43) over the posterior distribution of μ conditional on τ^2 we have

$$\begin{aligned} E(\mu_i|Y,\tau^2) &= \int E(\mu_i|Y,\mu,\tau^2) f(\mu|Y,\tau^2) d\mu \\ &= B_i Y_i + (1-B_i)\hat{\mu}_\tau^2 , \end{aligned} \tag{44}$$

$$Var(\mu_i|Y,\tau^2) = B_i\sigma_i^2 + (1-B_i)^2 \frac{\tau^2}{\sum B_i} . \tag{45}$$

The marginal likelihood function

$$f(Y|\tau^2) = \left(\frac{IIB_i}{(\tau^2)^{k-1}\sum B_i}\right)^{1/2} \exp\left\{-\frac{1}{2\tau^2}\left[\sum B_i Y_i^2 - \frac{(\sum B_i Y_i)^2}{\sum B_i}\right]\right\}$$

can be obtained by integrating μ out of the full likelihood. The posterior density for τ^2 is then

$$f(\tau^2|Y) = f(Y|\tau^2) f(\tau^2) ,$$

where $f(\tau^2)$ is the prior density of τ^2. Carlin used Monte Carlo procedure to compute posterior density of estimates of interest, τ^2, τ and μ_i.

3.3. *Gibbs sampling in random-effects model for meta-analysis*

Gibbs sampling is a procedure for numerical integration of complex functions that has come from its origins in statistical mechanics, through image processing into modern statistics. It is based on a simple, although computationally demanding, idea. All unknown quantities are given some initial values. The technique then involves successively sampling from the conditional distribution of each variable in turn, given the current value of all the other variables. These "full conditional" distributions are often of fairly standard form. It can be shown that under broad conditions eventually one will be sampling from the correct posterior distributions of the unknown parameters. There has been much literature on this topic recently, both on methodology and applications.

The key feature of Gibbs sampling is, given a joint posterior density $\mathbf{P}(\boldsymbol{\theta}|\mathbf{X})$, K univariate full conditional densities (the distribution of each individual component of $\boldsymbol{\theta}$ conditional on known values of the data $\mathbf{X}$ and all other components) can be written down in close form.

Now we derive the full conditional distributions for parameters in Gibbs sampling based on random-effects model for meta-analysis. Consider the typical Bayesian hierarchical model as previouly described in Eqs. (38) and (39), that is

$$\begin{aligned}
&\text{Level I}: Y_i|\mu_i,\ \sigma_i^2 \sim N(\mu_i, \sigma_i^2)\,,\\
&\text{Level II}: \mu_i|\mu,\ \tau^2 \sim N(\mu, \tau^2)\,,\\
&\text{Level III}: \mu|(a,b) \sim N(a,b)\,, \quad \tau^2|(c,d) \sim IG(c,d)\,.
\end{aligned}$$

For computational convenience, the prior distributions for hyperparameters μ and τ^2 are generally normal distribution and inverse Gamma distribution, respectively. Under the full Bayesian framework, all full conditional distributions are easily estimated using Gibbs sampling. Samples from the marginal posterior distributions of interest are simulated using the following full conditional distributions:

$$\begin{aligned}
&\mu_i|Y_1,\ldots Y_k,\mu_j \neq i,\mu\,,\\
&\qquad \tau_\mu^2 \sim N\left(Y_i\left(\frac{\tau^2}{\sigma_i^2+\tau^2}\right)+\mu\left(\frac{\sigma_i^2}{\sigma_i^2+\tau^2}\right),\ \frac{\sigma_i^2\tau^2}{\sigma_i^2+\tau^2}\right).
\end{aligned} \tag{46}$$

$$\begin{aligned}
&\mu|Y_1,\ldots,Y_k,\ldots,\mu_k\,,\\
&\tau^2 \sim N\left(\sum_{i=1}^{K}\mu_i\left(\frac{Kb}{\tau^2+Kb}\right)+a\left(\frac{\tau^2}{\tau^2+Kb}\right),\frac{\tau^2}{\tau^2+Kb}\right),
\end{aligned} \tag{47}$$

$$\begin{aligned}
&\tau^2|Y_1,\ldots,Y_k,\mu_1,\ldots,\mu_k\,,\\
&\qquad \mu \sim IG\left(\frac{1}{2}K+c,\ \frac{1}{2}\sum_{i=1}^{K}(\mu_i-\mu)^2+d\right).
\end{aligned} \tag{48}$$

The processes involved in Gibbs sampling are: (i) μ_i, μ, and τ^2 are given some initial values; (ii) Gibbs sampling values are obtained in turn, from the conditional distributions in Eqs. (46), (47) and (48); (iii) update the Gibbs sampling values successively for t iterations. For each run a "burn-in" of m iterations is followed by a further t-m iterations during which the posterior marginal density of parameters, μ_i, μ, and τ^2 are computed; (iv) check the convergence of Gibbs sampling.

Note that, given the prior and conditional distribution, Gibbs sampling is easy to be carried out. When deriving the full conditional distributions, the prior and likelihood are conjugate in the model we discussed above. In some situations, it may be reasonable to assume that the prior of μ and τ^2 are non-informative prior, and the form of full conditional distribution is simpler.

WinBUGS is a program that carries out Bayesian inference for complex statistical analysis via MCMC simulation technique.[23] Using WinBUGS software, Gibbs sampling is easily implemented for many common models and distributions. The WinBUGS language allows the model to be specified by way of construction of a directed graphical model. The summary statistics for the variable, which calculate from the posterior distributions of parameters of interest, are given in the output. The software also produces the plots of the kernel density estimate, dynamic trace for sampling, and autocorrelation function for parameters.

3.4. *An example of Gibbs sampling for meta-analysis*

Table 11 gives the results of 16 case-control studies about the role of hepatitis B virus (HBV) infection, hepatitis C virus (HCV) infection, and dual infection in the patients with primary hepatocellular carcinoma (PHC) in Chinese.

The classic approaches for meta-analysis are not suitable for estimating quantitatively the risk of HBV, HCV and dual infection for PHC. As shown in Table 11, extreme values (zero) are observed for dual infection in the control groups in several studies, due to the quite low population-based dual infection rate. Classic approaches could not deal with the extreme values unless 0.5 is used to substitute zero or the studies containing zero are excluded, and it may potentially lead to biasness. Several special methods for handling rare events have been presented in the previous section. However, those approaches neglect the uncertainty of the parameter of interest, i.e. based on the fixed effect model ignoring the inter-study variance. To fit the random effect model, the flexible Bayesian approach is appropriate. Here, Gibbs sampling is adopted via the WinBUGS software to obtain pooled estimate of parameters by directly fitting three logistic models using the data available in 16 studies.

Arrangement of data and table notation for each individual study is shown in Table 12.

For each individual study, the odds ratio (OR), logarithm of OR, and variance for logarithm of OR, are given using following formula (here 00 denotes non-infection, 10 denotes HBV infection, 01 denotes HCV

Table 11. The data of 16 case-control studies for HBV, HCV and dual infection in PHC.

	Statue of HBV, HCV Infection													
		HBV Infection				HCV Infection				Dual Infection				
Study No.	Non-Infection ca/co	ca/co $Var(\mathrm{Y}^{10})$	OR^{10}		Y^{10}	ca/co	OR^{01}	Y^{01*}	$Var(\mathrm{Y}^{01})$	ca/co $Var(\mathrm{Y}^{11})$	OR^{11}		Y^{11} ca/co	Total
1	42/198	77/40	9.08	2.21	0.07	6/8	3.54	1.26	0.32	15/1	70.71	4.26	1.10	140/247
2	33/101	102/10	31.22	3.44	0.15	3/3	3.06	1.12	0.71	14/1	42.85	3.76	1.11	152/115
3	34/81	43/8	12.81	2.55	0.19	4/3	3.18	1.16	0.63	11/0*	52.41	3.96	2.13	92/92
4	20/70	49/16	10.72	2.37	0.15	0/1*	1.75	0.56	3.06	8/0*	56.00	4.03	2.19	77/87
5	21/36	28/24	2.00	0.69	0.15	8/10	1.37	0.32	0.30	14/1	24.00	3.18	1.15	71/71
6	20/62	64/31	6.40	1.86	0.11	7/7	3.10	1.13	0.35	9/0*	55.80	4.02	2.18	100/100
7	9/75	50/21	19.84	2.99	0.19	11/3	30.56	3.42	0.55	30/1	250.00	5.52	1.16	100/100
8	35/122	53/20	9.24	2.22	0.11	3/1	10.46	2.35	1.37	5/1	17.43	2.86	1.24	96/144
9	9/123	51/14	49.79	3.91	0.21	4/2	27.33	3.31	0.87	6/1	82.00	4.41	1.29	70/140
10	22/278	232/73	40.16	3.69	0.07	49/8	77.40	4.35	0.19	58/2	366.45	5.90	0.57	361/361
11	5/57	87/45	22.04	3.09	0.25	6/3	22.80	3.13	0.72	11/4	31.35	3.45	0.56	109/109
12	7/109	45/16	43.79	3.78	0.24	3/1	46.71	3.84	1.49	9/2	70.07	4.25	0.76	61/128
13	11/179	80/26	50.07	3.91	0.15	3/1	48.82	3.89	1.43	10/2	81.36	4.40	0.70	104/208
14	13/105	79/105	6.08	1.80	0.11	3/4	6.06	1.80	0.67	15/6	20.19	3.01	0.32	110/220
15	15/120	100/27	29.63	3.39	0.12	23/2	92.00	4.52	0.62	12/1	96.00	4.56	1.16	150/150
16	10/138	23/10	31.74	3.46	0.25	4/4	13.80	2.62	0.61	1/0*	27.60	3.32	3.11	38/152

Source: Zhou Xuyu (1999). Postgraduate Dissertation of Sun Yat-Sen University of Medical Science.
ca: Case; co: Control.
*: The data of the included study contain extreme value, zero.

Table 12. Arrangement of data and table notation for 16 case-control studies.

	Non Infection	HBV Infection	HCV Infection	Dual Infection	Total
Case	a_i	c_i	e_i	g_i	m_i
Control	b_i	d_i	f_i	h_i	n_i

infection, and 11 denotes dual infection). The results are also shown in Table 11.

$$OR_i^{10} = \frac{c_i \times b_i}{d_i \times a_i}, \quad Y_i^{10} = \ln OR_i^{10}, \quad Var(Y_i^{10}) = \frac{1}{a_i} + \frac{1}{b_i} + \frac{1}{c_i} + \frac{1}{d_i},$$

$$OR_i^{10} = \frac{e_i \times b_i}{f_i \times a_i}, \quad Y_i^{01} = \ln OR_i^{01}, \quad Var(Y_i^{01}) = \frac{1}{a_i} + \frac{1}{b_i} + \frac{1}{e_i} + \frac{1}{f_i},$$

$$OR_i^{11} = \frac{g_i \times b_i}{h_i \times a_i}, \quad Y_i^{11} = \ln OR_i^{11}, \quad Var(Y_i^{11}) = \frac{1}{a_i} + \frac{1}{b_i} + \frac{1}{g_i} + \frac{1}{h_i}.$$

Three logistic models are introduced for HBV, HCV, and dual infection. Take HBV infection for example. Let r_i^{00} and r_i^{10} denote the number of infection in the control and case group in ith study, arising from n_i^{00} and n_i^{10} subjects which are assumed to have probability of p_i^{00} and p_i^{10} of HBV infection, respectively. β_i^{10} is defined as

$$\beta_i^{10} = \text{logit}(p_i^{10}) - \text{logit}(p_i^{00}) = \ln\left(\frac{p_i^{10}}{1 - p_i^{10}}\right) - \ln\left(\frac{p_i^{00}}{1 - p_i^{00}}\right).$$

β_i^{10} is the true effect for ith individual study, that is, posterior mean of Y_i^{10}. The prior distribution of β_i^{10} is $N(\mu^{10}, (\sigma_\mu^{10})^2)$. μ^{10} is the pooled effect size of interest, and $(\tau^{10})^2$ is the variance of inter-study. Thus, the full model can be written as

$$\begin{array}{lll}
\text{HBV infection} & \text{HCV infection} & \text{Dual infection} \\
r_i^{00} \sim B(p_i^{00}, n_i^{00}) & r_i^{00} \sim B(p_i^{00}, n_i^{00}) & r_i^{00} \sim B(p_i^{00}, n_i^{00}) \\
r_i^{10} \sim B(p_i^{10}, n_i^{10}) & r_i^{01} \sim B(p_i^{01}, n_i^{01}) & r_i^{11} \sim B(p_i^{11}, n_i^{11})
\end{array}$$

$$\begin{array}{lll}
\text{logit}(p_i^{00}) = \alpha_i^{10} & \text{logit}(p_i^{00}) = \alpha_i^{01} & \text{logit}(p_i^{00}) = \alpha_i^{11} \\
\text{logit}(p_i^{10}) = \alpha_i^{10} + \beta_i^{10} & \text{logit}(p_i^{01}) = \alpha_i^{01} + \beta_i^{01} & \text{logit}(p_i^{11}) = \alpha_i^{11} + \beta_i^{11} \\
\beta_i^{10} \sim N(\mu^{10}, (\tau^{10})^2) & \beta_i^{01} \sim N(\mu^{01}, (\tau^{01})^2) & \beta_i^{11} \sim N(\mu^{11}, (\tau^{11})^2).
\end{array}$$

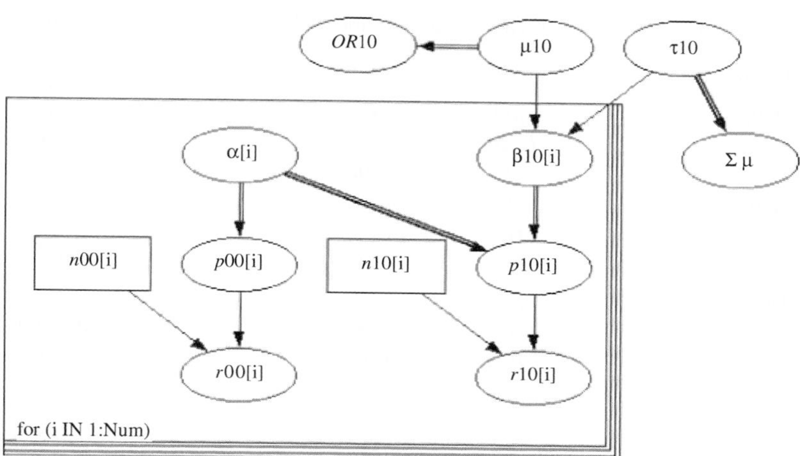

Fig. 2. Directed graphic model for HBV infection in WinBUGS.

Take HBV infection for example. The prior distribution of hyperparameters μ^{10} and $(\tau^{10})^2$ are "non-informative", $\mu^{10} \sim N(0.0, 10^6)$, $(\sigma_\mu^{10})^2 \sim IG(10^{-3}, 10^{-3})$. The prior of parameter α_i^{10} are also "non-informative", $\alpha_i^{10} \sim N(0, 10^{-5})$.

In the WinBUGS, we can describe above models intuitively by the way of construction of directed graphical models, in which nodes in the graph represent the data and parameters of the model (See Fig. 2).

From the conditional independence conditions expressed in the graph, the joint distribution takes the form (ignoring n_i^{00}, n_i^{10}, and using the fact that p_i^{00}, p_i^{10} can be expressed in terms of α_i, β_i^{10})

$$p(r^{00}, r^{10}, \mu^{10}, \tau^{10}, \beta, \alpha) \propto \Pi_i[p(r_i^{00}|\alpha_i, \beta_i^{10})p(r_i^{01}|\alpha_i, \beta_i^{10}) \times p(\alpha_i)p(\beta_i^{00}|\mu^{10}, \tau^{10})p(\mu^{10})p(\tau^{10})\,.$$

First 5000 iterations were used as a "burn in" in order to reduce the effect of initial value of parameters. Then running another 20,000 iterations and the summary statistics of posterior distribution for parameters were estimated. The main results of Gibbs sampling were seen in Table 13, which contains the means, standard deviations, and 95% confidence intervals from the posterior distribution of parameters, μ^{10}, τ^2 and OR. WinBUGS also gives the posterior distributions of "true effect" for each study, β_i^{10}, β_i^{01} and β_i^{11}.

The trace, kernel density and autocorrelation plots for summary effects, μ^{10}, μ^{01}, μ^{11}, in WinBUGS were presented in Figs. 3–5. The dynamic traces

Table 13. The results of Gibbs sampling for HBV, HCV and dual infection.

Status of Infection	Parameter	Mean	SD	95%CI
HBV Infection	μ^{10}	2.862	0.250	2.371–3.360
	OR^{10}	18.050	4.668	10.710–28.800
	τ^{10}	0.892	0.209	0.565–1.380
HCV Infection	μ^{01}	2.489	0.410	1.663–3.297
	OR^{01}	13.110	5.712	5.276–27.020
	τ^{01}	1.344	0.359	0.785–2.191
Dual Infection	μ^{11}	4.489	0.308	3.901–5.120
	OR^{11}	93.540	31.530	49.440–167.300
	μ^{11}	0.487	0.366	0.033–1.320

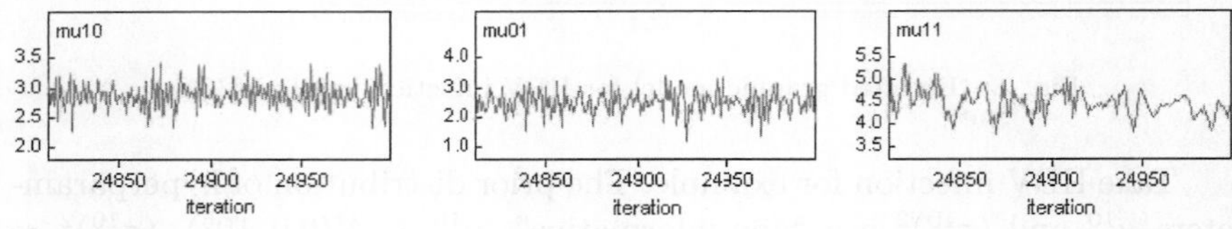

Fig. 3. The trace of Gibbs sampling for parameters μ^{10}, μ^{01}, μ^{11}.

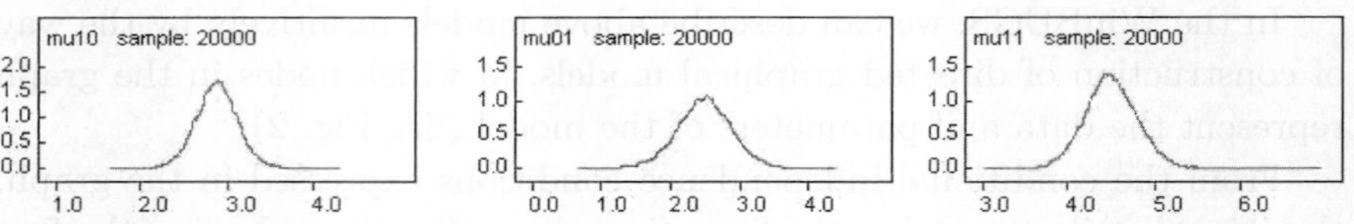

Fig. 4. The kernel density of Gibbs sampling for parameters μ^{10}, μ^{01}, μ^{11}.

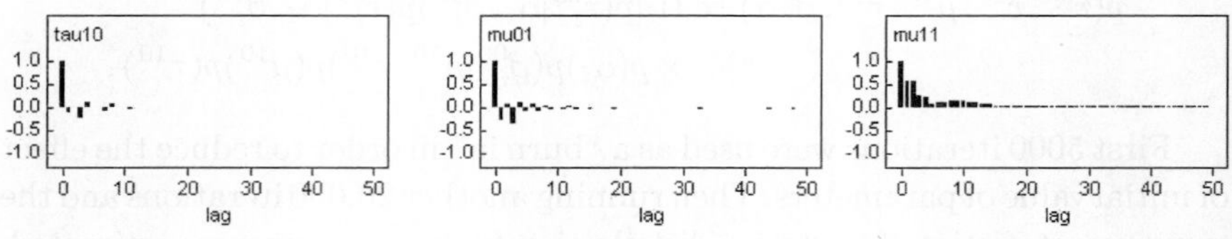

Fig. 5. The autocorrelation of Gibbs sampling for parameters μ^{10}, μ^{01}, μ^{11}.

showed that the Gibbs sampling tends to balance, the plots of kernel density estimate are smooth, and the autocorrelation of sampling is low.

For comparison, the classical DerSimonian-Laird random-effects model is used to estimate the pooled effect. For those studies in which the number

Table 14. The results of meta-analysis using DerSimonian-Laird method.

Parameter	HBV Infection	HCV Infection	Dual Infection
μ	2.815	2.423	4.026
95%CI	$2.359 \sim 3.270$	$1.639 \sim 3.208$	$3.553 \sim 4.500$
τ^2	0.711	1.816	0

of dual infection in control group is zero, 0.5 is substituted in order to calculate the OR. Results are shown in Table 14.

The results in Tables 13 and 14 show that, for HBV, HCV infection, point estimations and 95% confidence intervals of summary effects for parameters μ^{10} and μ^{01} from Gibbs sampling and classical method are similar. But for dual infection, the number of dual infection in control group is quite small in most of 16 case-control studies, and four of them even contain zero. The pooled estimation of μ^{11} is 4.489 (95%CI is 3.901–5.120) via Gibbs sampling, and μ^{11} is 4.026 (95%CI is 3.553–4.500) using classical method, so the difference is relatively large. Moreover, the pooled estimation of between-study variance, $(\sigma_{\mu}^{11})^2$, is zero, when using DerSimonian-Larid method, which means the between-study variance could not be identified for dual infection and result in bias obviously.

In fact, when the data in meta-analysis contain many extreme values, the pooled estimation of true effect and variance is unreliable using classic methods, which are basically based on approximately normalization with large samples.

Gibbs sampling, almost the standard tool for Bayesian method, can flexibly deal with a large of complex models that the classical approaches may find difficult to handle. The key to Gibbs sampling is to obtain the joint posterior distribution from the full conditional distributions of parameters using MCMC method, given the prior distribution and likelihood function. When the full conditional distribution is not given in a close form, Metropolis-Hastings method may be adopted.

Gibbs sampling can be effectively implemented using WinBUGS software, as demonstrated in the example. Furthermore, one can quite easily adjust for specific covariance that may influence the treatment effect by fitting a new model under full Bayesian framework in WinBUGS. For the choice of prior distribution, *student-t* distribution as a population prior may be reasonable and proper in some situations.

3.5. *Empirical Bayes method*

In additional to the Frequentist and Bayes approaches for meta analysis, a good compromise of the two is the so-called empirical Bayes methods. Especially Efron proposed a meta-analysis method based on an empirical Bayes framework for combining likelihoods from multiple studies.[68] Specifically, suppose that $L_k(\theta), k = 1, \ldots, K$ is the likelihood function for the parameter of interest in the *k-th* study. The likelihood function can be generated using any suitable methods and may not have a closed form. For example, the likelihood function could be either a profile likelihood function free from the nuisance parameter or a confidence distribution of the targeted parameter.[69] The distribution of θ is assumed to be from an exponential family:

$$g(\theta|\eta) = \exp\{\eta' t(\theta) - \varphi(\theta)\} g_0(\theta),$$

where η is an unknown parameter vector and $t(\theta)$ is the sufficient vector depending on θ. In practice, one often set $t(\theta) = (\theta, \theta^2)'$ or $(\theta, \theta^2, \theta^3)'$. A convenient choice for the carrier density is $g_0(\theta) = K^{-1} \sum_{i=1}^{K} L_i(\theta)$. The unknown parameter vector η can be estimated by numerically maximizing the likelihood function

$$L(\eta) = \prod_{i=1}^{K} \int g(\theta|\eta) L_i(\theta) d\theta.$$

The variance covariance matrix of the resulting MLE can be estimated by inverting the observed information matrix of $\log\{L(\eta)\}$. Alternatively, one may use the automatic resampling method such as jack-knife method to estimate the variance-covariance matrix. Lastly, one may make statistical inference on any summary measure of the distribution for θ. For example, one may estimate the mean of θ as $\int \theta g(\theta|\hat{\eta}) d\theta$, where $\hat{\eta}$ is the MLE of η. The variance estimator of the point estimator can be obtained by delta-method and the corresponding 95% confidence interval can be constructed. The method is fairly flexible in that as long as one can construct the likelihood from an individual study for the parameter of interest, one can implement the proposed procedure. In the presence of nuisance parameter, the likelihood can be profile likelihood, marginal likelihood or simply induced from the confidence distribution for the parameter of interest.

4. Meta-analysis of Diagnostic Tests

Studies of the diagnostic accuracy of a test conducted at different centers often produce estimates of the sensitivity and specificity of a test that vary greatly. These differences may be due to random sampling variation and differences in the cutoff points of diagnostic test. In order to get summary results of diagnostic tests for different centers, meta-analysis of diagnostic tests is necessary.

The steps in conducting a meta-analysis of diagnostic tests are as follows:

(i) *Determine the objective and scope of meta-analysis*
In order to get the diagnostic accuracy, we must determine the test of interest, the disease of interest and reference standard by which it is measured, and the clinical question and context.

(ii) *Retrieve the relevant literatures and judge the validity of the literatures*
Extract and sort data of primary studies, and assess the eligibility and the quality of retrieved studies for inclusion in the analysis by two or more reader. Analyze the situations that come from different primary studies and get differences of diagnostic accuracy. The situations include as follows: If the reference standard is acceptable as a good representation of the true presence or absence of the disease of interest; if between the test and the reference standard are read independently each other; whether verification by the reference standard is done for all patients who had the test or a stratified random sample of them; if the design of primary studies is correct; how much the cutoff point is; whether the prevalence of population who accept the test is similar to etc.[26] The first author should consider the results from all readers overall.

(iii) *Estimation of a summary diagnostic accuracy of a test*
There are several statistical methods to calculate a summary diagnostic accuracy of a test. In this section, we will introduce *summary receiver operating characteristic* (SROC for short). In the last part of this section, we will introduce briefly the other methods to calculate a summary diagnostic accuracy of a test.

While the goal of meta-analysis for diagnostic tests and the corresponding protocol development are similar in principal to the meta-analysis for clinical trials mentioned earlier, there are some specific issues. First, the performance of a diagnostic test is determined by the sensitivity and the specificity. Meta-analysis for diagnostic tests has two simultaneous endpoints. Secondly, because of the need to balance both sensitivity and specificity, the usual meta-analysis for rates, such as weighted average of sensitivity and specificity separately will miss the essential non-linear

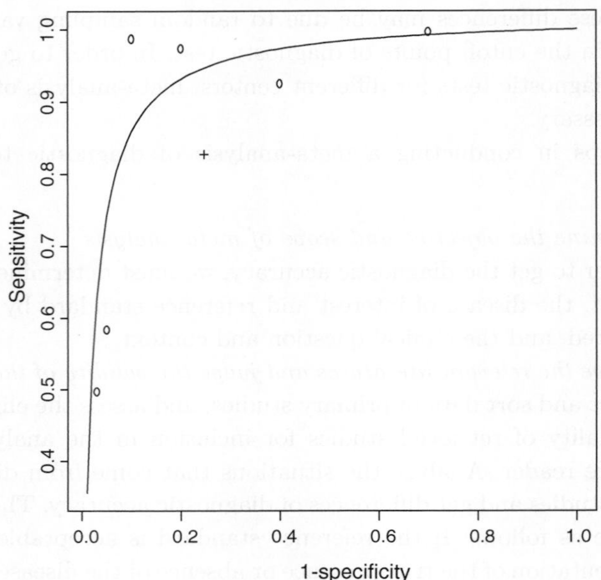

Fig. 6. Mean sensitivity and specificity cannot summarize results of diagnostic test in meta analysis.

relationship between sensitivity and specificity. Figure 6 (for this section) illustrates why the average sensitivity and specificity will not work for meta-analysis of a diagnostic test. Here, the six points are the observed means for sensitivity and specificity from six studies. The solid line is the corresponding ROC curve. When we take the average of sensitivity and specificity without considering their inter-relationship, we have the average point in "+", which is not on the ROC curve.[27−30] This figure demonstrated that using traditional meta-analysis on sensitivity and specificity separately results in the summary characteristics that do not belong to the test.

The mathematical reason for this difficulty is because of the non-linear relationship between sensitivity and specificity. Any transformation that reasonably related 1-specificity in a linear form to sensitivity will help to simplify the meta-analysis of diagnostic tests. One of these approaches is the SROC.

4.1. *SROC analysis*

In order to evaluate the diagnostic accuracy of a test, at first we must be aware of the true presence or absence of the disease of interest. The standard

Table 15. A diagnostic test results for 2 × 2 table.

	Gold Standard		
Test Results	Case	Control	Total
Positive	a(TP)	b(FP)	$a+b$
Negative	c(FN)	d(TN)	$c+d$
Total	$a+c$	$b+d$	$a+b+c+d=N$

which identifies an individual as disease (case) or non-disease (control) is the reference standard or gold standard. Gold standards which are used in medical research include biopsy, autopsy, surgery exploration, follow-up and so on. Although a gold standard need not be perfect, it should be more credible than the diagnostic test of interest and it should be independent from the diagnostic test. For the individuals which are determined case or control by gold standard, the results which are determined by a diagnostic test are labeled as positive or negative respectively. The data can be presented as the form of fourfold table. Among them there are two true results, that is, case is diagnosed as positive (true positive, TP) and control is diagnosed as negative (true negative, TN). There are two false results, that is, case is diagnosed as negative (false negative, FN) and control is diagnosed as positive (false positive, FP) (see Table 15).

The true positive rate (TPR), i.e. sensitivity, is the probability that a test result is positive in patients with disease of interest, namely:

$$TPR = a/(a+c)\,, \tag{49}$$

$(1 - TPR) = c/(a+c)$ is called false negative rate.

The false positive rate (FPR) which equals to (1-specificity), is the probability that a test result is positive in patients without the disease of interest, namely:

$$FPR = b/(b+d)\,, \tag{50}$$

$(1 - FPR) = d/(b+d)$ is true negative rate or specificity.

4.1.1. *SROC linear regression model*

For TPR and FPR, we use logit translation, namely:

$$\text{logit}(TPR) = \ln[TPR/(1-TPR)]\,, \tag{51}$$

$$\text{logit}(FPR) = \ln[FPR/(1-FPR)]\,, \tag{52}$$

let

$$D = \text{logit}(TPR) - \text{logit}(FPR)\,, \tag{53}$$

$$S = \text{logit}(TPR) + \text{logit}(FPR)\,. \tag{54}$$

Through the formula (53), we can get:

$$\begin{aligned} D &= \ln \frac{TPR/(1-TPR)}{FPR/(1-FPR)} \\ &= \ln \frac{\text{true positive rate} \times \text{false negative rate}}{\text{false positive rate} \times \text{true negative rate}} = \ln OR\,. \end{aligned} \tag{55}$$

Through the formula (54), we can get:

$$\begin{aligned} S &= \ln \frac{TPR \times FPR}{(1-TPR)(1-FPR)} \\ &= \frac{\text{true positive rate} \times \text{false positive rate}}{\text{true negative rate} \times \text{false negative rate}}\,. \end{aligned} \tag{56}$$

Let D be dependent variable and S be independent variable. In order to make *SROC curve* into a linear in (S, D) plane, we establish an *SROC* linear regression model as:

$$\hat{D} = A + B \times S\,, \tag{57}$$

where D is a log odds ratio [see formula (55)], representing the odds of a positive test result among people with the disease relative to the odds of a positive test result among people without the disease. D value can reflect the distinguishing ability of a diagnostic test. S is a measure of threshold for classifying a test as positive, which has a value of 0 when a sensitivity equals specificity [see formula (56)]. It becomes positive, i.e. $S > 0$, when a threshold is used that increases sensitivity (and decreases specificity) and becomes negative, i.e. $S > 0$, when a threshold is used that decreases sensitivity (and increases specificity). A is the intercept of the linear model and a log odds ratio when sensitivity equals specificity ($S = 0$). B is the regression coefficient and examines the extent to which the odds ratio (D) is dependent on the threshold (S) used. If the regression coefficient (B) is near zero and not statistically significant, test accuracy for each primary study can be summarized by a common odds ratio given by the intercept A.

4.1.2. *Solving the parameter of SROC linear regression model*

Unweighted least squares linear regression, weighted least squares linear regression, and robust method can be used to solve the parameters of SROC linear regression model (57).

4.1.2.1. Conventional least squares methods

This method can be introduced in a general statistical textbook. The parameter A and B are solved by making minimum of the square sum of the difference between observed value and fitted value (i.e. residual). The disadvantage of the method is not paying more attention to larger study, it does not consider the sample size of primary studies.

4.1.2.2. Weighted least squares method

In order to give more weight to studies of larger sample size, weighted least squares method can be used, weighting each observation using the reciprocal of the variance of log odds ratio (ln OR). The parameter A and B are solved by making minimum of the square sum of weighted residual. Let a, b, c, and d be the number of true positive, false positive, false negative, and true negative respectively (see Table 14). The weight can be calculated by

$$W = [\,Var(D)]^{-1} = (1/a + 1/b + 1/c + 1/d)^{-1}\,. \tag{58}$$

To deal with the 0 of denominator, if a cell of cross-classification of test and gold standard value is 0 among a, b, c, d, we add 0.5 to each cell of the primary study. The observation values of the study become $(a + 0.5)$, $(b + 0.5)$, $(c + 0.5)$, and $(d + 0.5)$.

Weighted method is inappropriate if one assumes that individual primary studies are all measuring the same underlying test accuracy. So, Moses, Shapiro and Littenberg suggested a robust modeling technique of SROC in 1993.[25]

4.1.2.3. Robust method

D plotted against S, coordinate points (S, D) of primary studies are plotted. According to the value of S value, we order the scatters (S, D) pairs and divide the points into 3 approximately equal groups. The total of studies divide 3 and round it, we can get the number of scatter points for left or right side. For example, 10 scatter points are divided, left or right side is round $(10/3) = 3$ respectively. Find the medians of S and D among the left and right side respectively and label them. Link the labeled scatter point

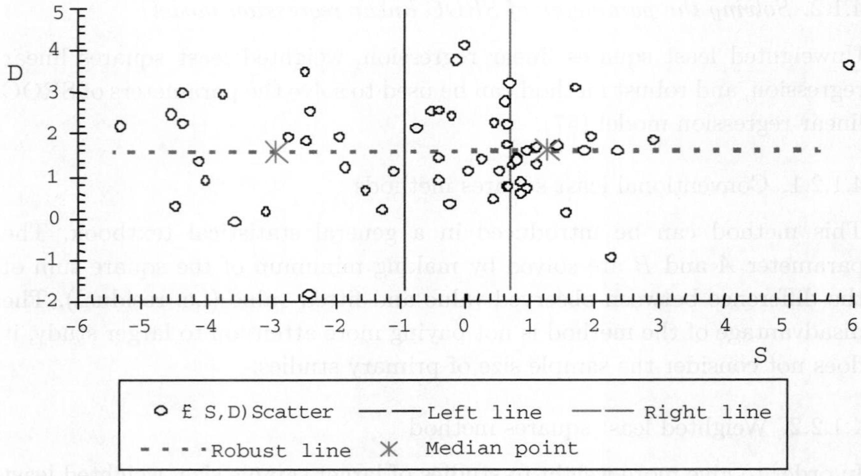

Fig. 7. Solving the parameter of SROC curve using robust method.

into a line. The slope of the line is regression coefficient B. The intercept A is derived by positioning the line so that half of the points lie above and half below it. Let (S_1, D_1) and (S_2, D_2) represent two points which are on the line and far from each other (for example, the two median points of S and D among left or right side respectively). Using the following formula, we can calculate the regression parameters A and B.

$$A = \frac{D_1S_2 - D_2S_1}{S_2 - S_1}, \quad B = \frac{D_2 - D_1}{S_2 - S_1}. \tag{59}$$

Solving the parameter of SROC curve using robust method can be seen in Fig. 7. This figure is plotted using the S and D in Table 16. The regression coefficient of the line is 0.0011. The line approximately parallels the abscissa.

4.1.3. *Establishing SROC curve regression model*

Both regression parameters A and B are solved using above methods. We can establish the SROC curve regression model as follows:

$$TPR = \left[1 + e^{-A/(1-B)}\left(\frac{1 - FPR}{FPR}\right)^{(1+B)/(1-B)}\right]^{-1}, \tag{60}$$

where TPR represents true positive rate and FPR represents false positive rate.

Table 16. The data of Pap test from 59 primary studies.

Studies i	TP a	FP b	FN c	TN d	Sensitivity TPR	1-specificity FPR	Weight W	D	S
1	8	3	23	84	0.258	0.034	1.947	2.276	−4.388
2	31	3	43	14	0.419	0.176	2.173	1.213	−1.868
3	70	12	121	25	0.66	0.324	6.855	0.187	−1.281
4	65	10	6	6	0.915	0.625	2.229	1.872	2.893
5	20	3	19	4	0.513	0.429	1.458	0.339	−0.236
6	35	92	20	156	0.636	0.371	10.433	1.088	0.032
7	39	8	111	270	0.260	0.029	6.122	2.473	−4.565
8	567	117	140	157	0.802	0.427	41.976	1.693	1.105
9	25	37	11	18	0.694	0.673	4.684	0.100	1.542
10	38	28	17	37	0.691	0.431	6.762	1.083	0.526
11	45	35	15	48	0.750	0.422	7.231	1.414	0.783
12	71	87	10	306	0.877	0.221	7.761	3.218	0.702
13	4.5	0.5	36.5	5.5	0.110	0.083	0.411	0.305	−4.491
14	2	2	3	21	0.400	0.087	0.724	1.946	−2.757
15	5	9	3	182	0.625	0.047	1.539	3.518	−2.496
16	38	21	7	62	0.844	0.253	4.293	2.774	0.609
17	4	2	16	31	0.200	0.061	1.184	1.355	−4.127
18	87	13	12	9	0.879	0.591	3.535	1.613	2.349
19	15	3	65	15	0.188	0.167	2.074	0.143	−3.076
20	41	1	61	29	0.402	0.033	0.930	2.970	−3.765
21	76	12	11	12	0.874	0.500	3.694	1.933	1.933
22	10	4	48	174	0.172	0.022	2.655	2.204	−5.341
23	28	11	28	77	0.500	0.125	5.704	1.946	−1.946
24	3.5	0.5	5.5	1.5	0.389	0.250	0.319	0.647	−1.551
25	79	26	13	182	0.859	0.125	7.489	3.750	−0.141
26	61	20	27	35	0.693	0.364	7.576	1.375	0.255
27	62	20	16	49	0.795	0.290	6.710	2.251	0.458
28	284	31	68	68	0.807	0.313	15.340	2.215	0.644
29	66	25	20	44	0.767	0.362	7.820	1.759	0.629
30	40	43	12	47	0.769	0.478	6.542	1.293	1.115
31	11	1	1	2	0.917	0.333	0.386	3.091	1.705
32	23	50	10	44	0.697	0.532	5.370	0.705	0.961
33	65	13	42	13	0.607	0.500	5.180	0.437	0.437
34	1269	928	264	1084	0.828	0.461	152.068	1.725	1.415
35	223	22	74	83	0.751	0.210	13.245	2.431	−0.225
36	154	30	20	237	0.885	0.112	10.633	4.108	−0.026
37	6	2	12	81	0.333	0.024	1.312	3.008	−4.394
38	7	4	3	4	0.700	0.500	1.024	0.847	0.847
39	12	5	11	60	0.522	0.077	2.558	2.572	−2.398
40	348	41	212	103	0.621	0.285	23.987	1.417	−0.426

(*Continued*)

Table 16. (*Continued*)

Studies i	TP a	FP b	FN c	TN d	Sensitivity TPR	1-specificity FPR	Weight W	D	S
41	8	4	11	34	0.421	0.105	2.019	1.822	−2.459
42	12.5	2.5	6.5	0.5	0.658	0.833	0.380	−0.956	2.263
43	95	9	2	1	0.979	0.900	0.617	1.664	6.058
44	40	18	20	19	0.667	0.486	5.459	0.747	0.639
45	71	13	20	18	0.780	0.419	5.087	1.592	0.942
46	1204	186	455	241	0.726	0.436	79.655	1.232	0.714
47	6	20	51	27	0.105	0.426	3.659	−1.840	−2.440
48	35	9	12	12	0.745	0.429	3.264	1.358	0.783
49	10	31	5	32	0.667	0.492	2.751	0.725	0.661
50	3	5	3	15	0.500	0.250	1.071	1.099	−1.099
51	118	40	44	183	0.728	0.179	16.216	2.507	−0.534
52	13	3	82	17	0.137	0.150	2.078	−0.107	−3.576
53	38	14	13	62	0.745	0.184	5.241	2.561	−0.415
54	14	25	67	291	0.173	0.079	7.705	0.889	−4.020
55	12	14	6	12	0.667	0.538	2.471	0.539	0.847
56	238	52	2	16	0.992	0.765	1.707	3.600	5.958
57	111	44	20	39	0.847	0.530	9.313	1.593	1.834
58	491	165	250	701	0.663	0.191	73.944	2.122	−0.772
59	48	16	38	31	0.558	0.340	7.047	0.895	−0.428

For a general ROC analysis, the area under ROC cure is taken as the diagnostic accuracy of a test. For SROC analysis, we can take TPR^* as the diagnostic accuracy of a test. TPR^* is the sensitivity taken by SROC curve of Eq. (60) and line equation

$$TPR + FPR = 1\,. \tag{61}$$

It reflects the extent to which SROC curve approach the top left corner. The larger the value of TPR^* is, the higher the diagnostic accuracy of a test is. $TPR + FPR = 1$ is a line through both the top left corner (1, 0) and the bottom right corner (0, 1). For the line, sensitivity equals specificity, namely $S = 0$.

Using $S = 0$ and formula (54), we have

$$S = \text{logit}(TPR) + \text{logit}(FPR) = 0$$

or

$$\text{logit}\ FPR = -\text{logit}\ TPR\,. \tag{62}$$

Substituting formula (62) into formula (53), we have

$$D = \text{logit}(TPR) - \text{logit}(FPR) = 2\ \text{logit}(TPR) = A + B \cdot S = A\,,$$

and

$$\text{logit}(TPR) = A/2\,, \tag{63}$$

and

$$TPR = (1 + e^{-A/2})^{-1}\,. \tag{64}$$

In order not to be confused with general TPR, we take the diagnostic accuracy of a test of SROC curve as

$$TPR^* = (1 + e^{-A/2})^{-1}\,.$$

Its standard error can be calculated by

$$SE(TPR^*) = \frac{SE(\hat{A})}{8[\cosh(A/4)]^2}\,, \tag{65}$$

where $SE(\hat{A})$ is the standard error of the intercept A of linear regression model. Cosh(.) is the hyperbolic cosine function.

To compare the diagnostic accuracy between 2 independent groups, if the numbers of the primary studies are large enough (more than 10), we can use Z statistic, namely

$$Z = \frac{TPR_1^* - TPR_2^*}{\sqrt{SE^2(TPR_1^*) + SE^2(TPR_2^*)}}\,, \tag{66}$$

where Z is a quantile from the standard normal distribution. Both TPR_1^* and TPR_2^* are the diagnostic accuracy of compared SROC curves. $SE(TPR_1^*)$ or $SE(TPR_2^*)$ are the standard error of TPR_1^* or TPR_2^*, respectively.

If the regression coefficient of a SROC curve has $B = 0$, for the FPR of each primary study, the confidence interval of the TPR can be taken as:

$$\left(\left[1 + e^{-A_L}\left(\frac{1 - FPR}{FPR}\right)\right]^{-1},\ \left[1 + e^{-A_U}\left(\frac{1 - FPR}{FPR}\right)\right]^{-1}\right), \tag{67}$$

where A_L and A_U are the lower and upper confidence intervals of the intercept A respectively.

4.1.4. *Analysis using an example*

The Pap test involves the collection, preparation, and examination of exfoliated cervical cells. It is quick, noninvasive, and relatively inexpensive. These properties make the test appealing for cervical precancer. Currently some doctors use it as a screening test and as a follow-up test for women. Because the accuracy of the test is affected by a doctor's understanding of the natural history of cervical cancer, morbidity of cervical cancer, and the number of samplings of cell, the diagnostic accuracy of test has been reported to have wide variation. The value of the sensitivity and the specificity ranges from 11% to 99% and from 14% to 97% respectively. The method of SROC analysis is illustrated using the data of 59 primary studies reported by Fahey, Irwig and Macaskill.[26]

Example 5. In the Data of Fahey, Irwigand and Macaskil, the number of true positive (TP, a), false positive (FP, b), false negative (FN, c), true negative (TN, d) is not presented, but the number of with disease, the number of without disease, sensitivity, (1-specificity) were given. For this method, according to the known data we calculate a, b, c, d (see Table 15). Because there were 0s in b of 13th and 24th and d of 42nd of primary studies, to avoid 0 of denominator, 0.5 was added to a, b, c, d of the 3 studies (see Table 16).

In the 1st study, the weight was calculated using formula (58),

$$W_1 = \left(\frac{1}{8} + \frac{1}{3} + \frac{1}{23} + \frac{1}{84}\right)^{-1} = 1.947\,.$$

The true positive rate is calculated by formula (49), i.e. $TPR = 8/(8+23) = 0.2581$. The false positive rate is calculated by formula (50), i.e. $FPR = 3/(3+84) = 0.0345$. D and S are calculated by formula (55) and (56) respectively, i.e. $D = \ln\frac{0.2581(1-0.0345)}{0.0345(1-0.2581)} = 2.276$, $S = \ln\frac{0.2581\times 0.0345}{(1-0.2581)(1-0.0345)} = -4.388$ and so on.

Using an above weight, the weighted least square linear regression model is established taking D as the dependent variable, and S as an independent variable. The residual standard deviation of the weighted model is 2.430. Intercept is $A = 1.720$ and its standard error is $SE(A) = 0.100$. The result of t test is $t = 17.227$ and $P \leq 0.001$. Using $A \pm t_{0.05,58} SE(A)$, the 95% confidence interval of A is 1.520–1.920. The results suggest that the difference between A and 0 has statistical significance under 0.05 test level.

The regression coefficient is $B = -0.015$ and its standard error is $SE(B) = 0.070$. The result of t test is $t = -0.215$, $P \leq 0.830$. The results suggest that the difference between B and 0 has no statistical significance under 0.05 test level.

The odds ratio is $\exp(A) = \exp(1.720) = 5.585$. It suggests the odds of positive test in the abnormal group is larger than in the normal group.

According to formula (64) and (65), we can get the diagnostic accuracy of the test $TPR^* = 0.703$ is and its standard error is $SE(TPR^*) = 0.010$.

The general least square linear regression model is established taking D as dependent variable and S as independent variable. The residual standard deviation of the model is 1.1144. Intercept is $A = 1.590$ and its standard error is $SE(A) = 0.151$. The result of t test is $t = 10.522$ and $P \leq 0.001$. Using $A \pm t_{0.05,58}SE(A)$, the 95% confidence interval of A is 1.288–1.892. The results suggest that the difference between A and 0 has statistical significance under 0.05 test level.

Regression coefficient is $B = -0.020$ and its standard error is $SE(B) = 0.063$. The result of t test is $t = 0.319$, $P \leq 0.751$. The results suggest that the difference between B and 0 has no statistical significance under 0.05 test level.

The odds ratio is $\exp(A) = \exp(1.590) = 4.904$. It suggests the odds of positive test in the abnormal group is larger than in the normal group.

According to formula (64) and (65), we can get the diagnostic accuracy of the test is $TPR^* = 0.689$ and its standard error is $SE(TPR^*) = 0.016$.

D plotted against S, coordinate points (S, D) of 59 primary studies are plotted. According to the value of S value, we order the scatters (S, D) pairs and divide the points by 3 approximately equal groups. The 59 studies were divided into 3 groups. The number of scatter points for left or right side is round $(59/3) = 20$. The medians of S and D among left side are $(S_1, D_1) = (-2.916, 1.588)$ and among right side are $(S_2, D_2) = (1.265, 1.593)$. The intercept A and regression coefficient B are $A = 1.5914$ and $B = 0.0011$ respectively obtained by formula (59). So, the linear regression model is

$$\hat{D} = 1.5914 + 0.0011S\,.$$

To make half the points lie above and half below the line, we need to move the line up and down. In this situation, the regression parameter is 0.0011 constantly and the intercept A is derived by positioning the line. In fact, this means that the number of positive sign equals negative sign of residual which is from the difference between observed value and predicted value. Through changed the A value many times, we got the line which scatter points lie above equals below approximately and the intercept is

Table 17. The diagnostic accuracy and related result from 3 methods.

Methods	A	$SE(A)$	$95\%CL$	B	$SE(B)$	$95\%CL$	TPR^*	SE (TPR^*)	Odds Ratio
Weighted	1.720	0.100	$1.520 \sim 1.920$	−0.015	0.070	$-0.155 \sim 0.125$	0.703	0.010	5.585
Unweighted	1.590	0.151	$1.288 \sim 1.892$	0.020	0.063	$-1.241 \sim 1.281$	0.689	0.016	4.904
Robust	1.591	—	—	0.001	—	—	0.689	—	4.911

$A = 1.5914$, the odds ratio is $\exp(A) = \exp(1.5914) = 4.9106$, and the diagnostic accuracy is $TPR^* = 0.6891$.

The results obtained from the weighted linear regression, general linear regression, robust regression are presented in Table 17.

Substituting A, B of 3 methods into formula (60), we obtained the SROC curves of weighted, unweighted and robust method respectively. They are as follows:

$$TPR_{\text{weighted}} = \left[1 + e^{-1.694}\left(\frac{1 - FPR}{FPR}\right)^{0.970}\right]^{-1},$$

$$TPR_{\text{unweighted}} = \left[1 + e^{-1.623}\left(\frac{1 - FPR}{FPR}\right)^{1.041}\right]^{-1},$$

$$TPR_{\text{robust}} = \left[1 + e^{-1.593}\left(\frac{1 - FPR}{FPR}\right)^{1.002}\right]^{-1}.$$

To obtain the smooth SROC curve, let FPR from 0.002 to 0.998 (it is also possible to setup other value) and increase in arithmetic series 0.002. According to the above SROC curve equations TPR is calculated. 499 SROC coordinate points were obtained. Using the above coordinate points obtained and point (0, 0), (1, 1) we can plot the smooth SROC curve. Figure 8 presents smooth SROC curve and SROC coordinate points of the 59 primary studies from Table 16.

From Fig. 8, it is suggested that the area under curve of weighted method is larger. Of unweightd method and of robust method are similar. These results are consistent with the diagnostic accuracy TPR^* and odds ratio in Table 17.

If the association between weighted and unweighted method is ignored and assuming TPR^* obtained by 2 methods is approximately normal distribution, the formula (66) can be used to test the difference between 2 TPR^* s. The result of test is $Z = 0.7132$, $P = 0.4757$ for two-side test.

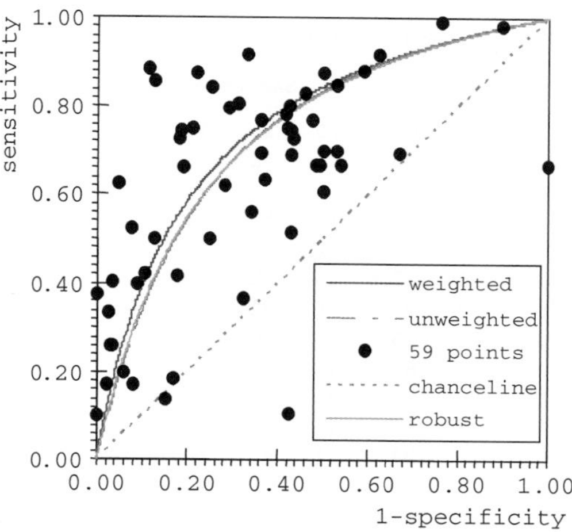

Fig. 8. SROC curves of 3 methods and the scatter points of 59 primary studies.

This suggests that the TPR^* difference between weighted and unweighted method has no statistical significance.

4.1.5. *The SAS code of solving SROC curves parameter*

SAS code 1. SROC analysis of weighted, unweighted and robust method.[31]

SAS Code

```
OPTIONS LS=76 PS=MAX NODATE;
%LET N=59;              /*the number of primary studies N= ***********/
%LET A_ROB=1.5914;      /* changed robust intercept A_ROB= ***********/
DATA SROC;  RETAIN I 0;
INPUT TP FN FP TN@@;
I+1; N_RL=ROUND(&N/3);
W=1/ (1/TP+1/FN+1/FP+1/TN); TPR=TP/(TP+FN);FPR=FP/(FP+TN);
         D=LOG(TPR/(1-TPR))-LOG(FPR/(1-FPR));
         S=LOG(TPR/(1-TPR))+LOG(FPR/(1-FPR));
CARDS;
8    23   3    84   76   11   12   12   8    11   4    34
31   43   3    14   10   48   4    174  12.5 6.5  2.5  0.5
70   121  12   25   28   28   11   77   95   2    9    1
65   6    10   6    3.5  5.5  0.5  1.5  40   20   18   19
20   19   3    4    79   13   26   182  71   20   13   18
35   20   92   156  61   27   20   35   1204 455  186  241
39   111  8    270  62   16   20   49   6    51   20   27
567  140  117  157  284  68   31   68   35   12   9    12
```

(*Continued*)

SAS code 1. (*Continued*).

```
25   11   37   18   66   20   25   44   10   5   31   32
38   17   28   37   40   12   43   47   3   3   5   15
45   15   35   48   11   1   1   2   118   44   40   183
71   10   87   306  23   10   50   44   13   82   3   17
4.5  36.5 0.5  5.5  65   42   13   13   38   13   14   62
2    3    2    21   1269 264  928  1084 14   67   25   291
5    3    9    182  223  74   22   83   12   6   14   12
38   7    21   62   154  20   30   237  238  2   52   16
4    16   2    31   6    12   2    81   111  20   44   39
87   12   13   9    7    3    4    4    491  250  165  701
15   65   3    15   12   11   5    60   48   38   16   31
41   61   1    29   348  212  41   103
;
TITLE 'to calculate sensitivity, 1-specificity, weight, D, S using
TP,FN,FP,TN ' ;
 PROC PRINT;RUN;
 TITLE 'weighted regression model?W=1/(VAR(LN(OR)))';
PROC REG DATA=SROC OUTEST=W OUTSEB SIMPLE;
MODEL D=S;  WEIGHT W;
DATA W1;         SET W;
PROC TRANSPOSE DATA=W PREFIX=AW OUT=WW;
DATA XX1;         SET WW;          OR_SROC=EXP(AW1);
A_L=AW1-AW2*TINV(1-0.05/2,&N-1); A_U=AW1+AW2*TINV(1-0.05/2,&N-1);
TPR_S_W=1/(1+EXP(-AW1/2)); SE_TPR_W=AW2/(8*(COSH(AW1/4))**2);
IF _NAME_^='INTERCEP' THEN DO; A_L=.; A_U=.;
OR_SROC=.; TPR_S_W=.; SE_TPR_W=.; END;
DATA XXX1; SET XX1; IF _NAME_^='INTERCEP' THEN DELETE; PROC PRINT;
PROC REG DATA=SROC OUTEST=NW OUTSEB SIMPLE;
MODEL D=S;
TITLE '******unweighted general linear regression model *********';
DATA NW1;        SET NW;
PROC TRANSPOSE DATA=NW PREFIX=A OUT=WW;
DATA XX2 ;             SET WW;   OR_SROC=EXP(A1);
A_L=A1-A2*TINV(1-0.05/2,&N-1);A_U=A1+A2*TINV(1-0.05/2,&N-1);
 TPR_STAR=1/(1+EXP(-A1/2)); SE_TPR=A2/(8*(COSH(A1/4))**2);
IF _NAME_^='INTERCEP' THEN DO; A_L=.; A_U=.;
 OR_SROC=.; TPR_STAR=.; SE_TPR=.; END;
DATA XXX2; SET XX2;IF _NAME_^='INTERCEP' THEN DELETE; PROC PRINT;
  DATA XXX; MERGE XXX1 XXX2;
  KEEP TPR_S_W TPR_STAR SE_TPR_W SE_TPR Z_SROC P_SROC;
     Z_SROC=(TPR_S_W-TPR_STAR)/(SE_TPR_W**2+SE_TPR**2)**0.5;
P_SROC=2*(1-PROBNORM(Z_SROC)); PROC PRINT;
TITLE 'compare the TPR_STAR between unweighted and weighted regression
 model ';
```

SAS code 1. (*Continued*).

```
Number  SAS Code
63   DATA SROCS; SET SROC;PROC SORT; BY S;
64   DATA BS1;     KEEP II S D; SET SROCS;
65   II+1;       IF II>N_RL THEN DELETE ;
66   PROC UNIVARIATE DATA=BS1 NOPRINT; VAR S; OUTPUT OUT=A1 MEDIAN=S1;
67   PROC UNIVARIATE DATA=BS1 NOPRINT; VAR D; OUTPUT OUT=A2 MEDIAN=D1;
68   DATA BS2;     KEEP II S D; SET SROCS;
69   II+1;       IF II<=&N-N_RL THEN DELETE ;
70   PROC UNIVARIATE DATA=BS2 NOPRINT; VAR S; OUTPUT OUT=A3 MEDIAN=S2;
71   PROC UNIVARIATE DATA=BS2 NOPRINT; VAR D; OUTPUT OUT=A4 MEDIAN=D2;
72     DATA AA; MERGE A1 A2 A3 A4;
73   A_ROBUST=(D1*S2- D2*S1)/(S2-S1); B_ROBUST=(D2-D1)/(S2-S1);
74    OR_ROB=EXP(&A_ROB); TPR_ROB=1/(1+EXP(-&A_ROB/2)); PROC PRINT;
75   TITLE '*****ROBUST REGRESSION METHOD*******************';
76     DATA AAA;    KEEP B_ROBUST A_ROBUST;    SET AA;
77   DO J=1 TO &N;    B_ROBUST=B_ROBUST; A_ROBUST=A_ROBUST; OUTPUT;END;
78   DATA AAAA;    KEEP A_ROBUST B_ROBUST COUNT0-COUNT2;
79   MERGE SROC AAA;
80   Y_HAT=&A_ROB+B_ROBUST*S;
81   SIGN=D-Y_HAT;
82   IF SIGN>0 THEN COUNT1+1;    IF SIGN=0 THEN COUNT0+1;
      IF SIGN<0 THEN COUNT2+1;
83   TITLE 'COUNT1 and COUNT2 are the number of scatter lie above or below
     respectively, COUNT0 is the number of scatter on the line';
          PROC PRINT; RUN;
```

SAS code 1 can solve the regression parameter A and B of SROC curve in S, D plane using the above weighted method, unweighted method, and robust method. The common odds ratio and TPR^* which reflect the diagnostic accuracy of the test are also calculated using the parameters obtained above.

For similar data in Table 17, you need to change the number of primary studies n in 02nd row of SAS code 1, and the number of true positive (TP), false negative (FN), false positive (FP), true negative (TN) from 11th to 30th row.

To obtain the exact intercept of robust regression, according to the request of precision of intercept of robust regression (e.g. decimal digits), the value of 3rd row after "A_ROB=" must be changed again and again after running the SAS code. After each running, the number of scatter points lying above line (COUNT1) and lying below line (COUNT2) must be observed. If COUNT1 = COUNT2, running SAS is end, the intercept A is the intercept of robust regression.

The file of SROC is obtained using the row from 04th to 33rd which include the value of variables of TP, FN, FP, TN, sensitivity, 1-specificity, weight, D and S. The parameter and related value of weighted regression model are obtained through the rows from 34th to 44th. The parameter and related value of unweighted regression model are obtained through the rows from 45th to 55th. The result comparing the diagnostic accuracy TPR^* s between weighted and unweighted methods is gained through the rows from 56th to 60th. The parameter and related value are obtained through the rows from 61st to 83rd.

4.1.6. *Other practical issues of SROC analysis*

TPR^* in ROC analysis is often an important summary statistic for meta-analysis. While it is useful, it may not always be relevant clinically. For example, if all previous studies had false positive rates less than 20%, while the false positive rate of TPR^* is in 30%, TPR^* becomes irrelevant because it is out of the clinical range of practical uses. In such a case, a backward translation of mean D and mean S into ROC curve can provide a more informative summary statistics. This summary point is simply expressed as

$$\overline{TPR} = \frac{\exp\{(\bar{S} + \bar{D})/2\}}{1 + \exp\{(\bar{S} + \bar{D})/2\}}$$

and

$$\overline{FPR} = \frac{\exp\{(\bar{S} - \bar{D})/2\}}{1 + \exp\{(\bar{S} - \bar{D})/2\}},$$

which is always on the SROC curve. Another relevant alternative summary statistics for SROC is the area under the curve (AUC). Just like we use AUC of a ROC curve to compare diagnostic tests, the AUC of SROC does not depend on the selected threshold that TPR^* used. It is particularly useful when two SROC curves cross each other. More useful is the conditional AUC when the upper limit of false positive rates is given. For example, we are only interested in the performance of diagnostic tests when its specificity is above 85%. This corresponds to the AUC of SROC in the section of FPR being less than 15%.

One advantage of SROC is to relate non-linear relationship between TPR and FPR to linear regression S and D. While formula (66) compares two TPR^* points as an approach to compare two diagnostic tests, it did not take advantage of linear relationships between S and D fully. Alternatives include the use of analysis of covariance in the regression step of S and D.

By adding an additional covariate X to indicate different diagnostic modalities, linear modal theory can be used to test statistical significance of different modalities. In addition, we can add other covariates, such as the year of publication and the design of the studies, into the linear model to assess the effects of other uncontrollable factors on the diagnostic utilities. When meta-analysis includes multi-modality studies, i.e. among studies that one patient being evaluated by several diagnostic techniques, a random-effects model of individual study can be built into the linear model to control for correlated results reported in these papers. Several examples of using these generalized linear models can be found in literature.

In meta-analysis, if each individual accepts several diagnostic tests, in order to dispel the correlation among several diagnostic tests, the random-effect model can be established. Some researchers suggest using generalized linear model to control the correlation.[32–34]

4.2. *Other methods of estimating log odds ratio of diagnostic test*

Both Mantel-Haenszel method and exact-based logit method[35] can be used to calculate the log odds ratio of diagnostic test.

4.2.1. *Mantel-Haenszel method*

Assume there are h primary studies of diagnostic test and the symbol a_i, b_i, c_i, d_i, and n_i represent true positive, false positive, false negative, true negative and the total number from ith study ($i = 1, 2, \ldots, h$) respectively. Adjusted odds ratios of Mantel-Haenszel method OR_{MH} is expressed as:

$$OR_{MH} = \sum_{i=1}^{h}\left(\frac{a_i d_i}{n_i}\right) \Big/ \sum_{i=1}^{h}\left(\frac{b_i c_i}{n_i}\right). \tag{68}$$

Using the formula

$$X_{MH}^2 = \sum_{i=1}^{h}\left(\frac{a_i d_i - b_i c_i}{n_i}\right)^2 \Big/ \sum_{i=1}^{h}\left(\frac{(a_i+b_i)(c_i+d_i)(a_i+c_i)(b_i+d_i)}{(n_i-1)n_i^2}\right) \tag{69}$$

performs the test of statistical significance. $100(1-\alpha)\%$ confidence interval of the adjusted odds ratios of Mantel-Haenszel OR_{MH} is

$$\left(OR_{MH}^{1-U_{1-\alpha/2}/\sqrt{X_{MH}^2}}, OR_{MH}^{1+U_{1-\alpha/2}/\sqrt{X_{MH}^2}}\right). \tag{70}$$

$U_{1-\alpha/2}$ is a quantile from the standard normal distribution under test level α, $U_{1-\alpha/2}$ of 95% confidence interval is $U_{1-\alpha/2} = 1.96$.

4.2.2. *Exact-based logit confidence interval*

The method was proposed by Woof in 1955, so it was named Woof method. The odds ratio OR_L can be expressed as:

$$OR_L = \exp\left[\left(\sum_{i=1}^{h}(w_i \ln OR_i)\right) \Big/ \sum_{i=1}^{h} w_i\right]. \tag{71}$$

The $100(1-\alpha)\%$ confidence interval is

$$\left(OR_L \exp\left[-U_{1-\alpha/2} \Big/ \sqrt{\sum_{i=1}^{h} w_i}\right], \; OR_L \exp\left[U_{1-\alpha/2} \Big/ \sqrt{\sum_{i=1}^{h} w_i}\right]\right), \tag{72}$$

where OR_i is the odds ratio of ith study

$$w_i = Var(\ln OR_L))^{-1} = (1/a_i + 1/b_i + 1/c_i + 1/d_i)^{-1}.$$

If there are 0 in any cell of a study, a small value, e.g. 0.5, is added to each cell of the study.

To test if the odds ratio of the primary studies is homogeneity, the Breslow-Day test of homogeneity can be used. The Breslow-Day statistic is expressed as:

$$Q_{BD} = \sum_{i=1}^{h} [a_i - E(a_i|OR_{MH})]^2 / Var(a_i|OR_{MH}), \tag{73}$$

where E and Var represent expected value and variance respectively. Statistic Q_{BD} is an approximate chi-squared statistic with freedom degree $df = h - 1$.

4.2.3. *An example*

Use the file of SROC (data see Example 5) of the SAS code 1 from 01st to 31st and the SAS code 2, the odds ratio of the diagnostic test is estimated by Mantel-Haenszel method and Exact-based logit method. In the SAS code 2, the code of row from 1 to 3 is used to transform the SROC file into the required data format. The code of row from 5 to 6 are used to calculate the crude odds ratio. The code of row from 8 to 9 is used to

SAS code 2. Calculated odds ratio using Mantel-Haenszel method and logit method.

Number	SAS Code
1	`DATA C;              SET SROC;`
2	`A=1 ; B=1; F=TP;OUTPUT;      A=1 ; B=2; F=FN;OUTPUT;`
3	`A=2 ; B=1; F=FP;OUTPUT;      A=2 ; B=2; F=TN;OUTPUT;`
4	`TITLE 'CRUDE ODDS RATIO';`
5	`PROC FREQ DATA=C ;           WEIGHT F;`
6	`TABLES A*B/ALL RISKDIFF RELRISK NOPRINT;`
7	`TITLE 'MANTEL-HAENSZEL ODDS RATIO and LOGIT ODDS RATIO';`
8	`PROC FREQ DATA=C ;           WEIGHT F;`
9	`TABLES I*A*B/ALL RISKDIFF RELRISK NOPRINT ;RUN;`

calculate the adjusted odds ratios of Mantel-Haenszel method and odds ratio of exact-based logit method.

The FREQ procedure in the rows from 4 to 6 calculates the summary from Mantel-Haenszel statistics of 59 studies. The results are $\chi^2_{MH} = 2829.032$, $df = 1$, $P \leq 0.001$. The crude odds ratio of Mantel-Haenszel method is 5.542, and 95% confidence interval is (5.203, 5.903). The crude odds ratio of logit method is 5.542, and 95% confidence interval is (5.193, 5.915).

The FREQ procedure in the rows from 7 to 9 calculates the summary Mantel-Haenszel statistics of 59 studies. The results are $\chi^2_{MH} = 2231.929$, $df = 1$, $P \leq 0.001$. The adjusted odds ratio of Mantel-Haenszel method is $OR_{MH} = 5.573$, and 95% confidence interval is (5.189, 5.984). The adjusted odds ratio of logit method is $OR_L = 5.557$, 95% confidence interval is (5.137, 6.010).

These results are similar to the odds ratio of weighted regression model. Breslow-Day test of homogeneity is performed for the data. We have $Q_{BD} = 394.286$, $df = 58$, $P \leq 0.001$. These suggest the difference among 59 primary studies has statistical significance.

The above results of analysis suggest that the diagnostic accuracy of Pap test is similar to those obtained by several methods. TPR^* is about 0.7, the odds ratio of positive diagnostic result is about 5. These suggest that the test plays an important role in cervical precancer, but these results suggest that the diagnostic accuracy of the test is not high.

The methods above assumed that the gold standard is perfect. If the gold standard is imperfect, the diagnostic accuracy of the test must be adjusted. Walter *et al.* proposed the method estimating the SROC curves of test with imperfect reference standards in 1999.[29]

Although someone proposed the meta-analysis method of diagnostic test using the area under curve (AUC), how to use both AUC and the data of sensitivity and specificity need to be studied further.

5. Meta-analysis for Linkage Studies

Recently, linkage studies are rapidly becoming numerous. At the same time, conflicting claims of linkage arise in genome wide scans. Serious discussion regarding how to control false positives or spurious linkages has begun. Meta-analysis can quantitatively synthesize results from multiple independent studies into a pooled measure of the overall effect of genetic linkage. But because there may exist too many differences between linkage studies, such as different ascertainment of pedigrees, different disease definition, different genetic markers or different statistical techniques, a common effect size is difficult to be found and extracted. And so the general meta-analysis methods are difficult to apply directly. Here we introduce some meta-analysis methods that are appropriate for linkage studies.

5.1. *Meta-Analysis of P Values*

5.1.1. *Statistical method*

Assume that there are m independent studies assessing linkage of a disease or trait to a maker. Let P_i denote the P value associated with the ith study $(i = 1, 2, \ldots, n)$, then n independent P values can be combined into a single test of significance.

$$X^2 = -2\sum_{i=1}^{n} \ln(P_i)\,. \tag{74}$$

If the null hypothesis is true, i.e. if there are no genes underlying the trait near the marker locus, this quantity has a χ^2 distribution with two degrees of freedom as proposed by Fisher in 1954. Alternatively, a weight may be assigned to each individual study indicating its importance. Assigning a weight v_i to the ith study, and form the product

$$P_w = P_1^{v_1} P_2^{v_2} \cdots P_n^{v_n}\,. \tag{75}$$

The validity of the omnibus null hypothesis is tested using the cumulative distribution of P_w, $\text{Prob}(P_w \le q) = \sum_{k=1}^{n}(q^{1/v_k})/a_k$, where $a_k = \Pi_{i=1,i\neq k}^{n}(v_k - v_i)/v_k$. A simple choice for the weight is $v_k = \frac{1}{n_k}/\sum_i \frac{1}{n_i}$, where n_i is the number of sib-pairs used in the ith study (in sib-pair tests).[36] One may assign a different level of importance to each individual study based on the presumption that some designs are more powerful than others. For example, if 1000 random sib-pairs are needed for a power of 80%, and the same power could be achieved by using 40 ED sib-pairs or 200 affected sib-pairs, then all three studies would have equal weights for importance, although their sample size are considerably different.

If all studies we want to summarize have identical genotyped markers and same linkage analysis method being used, then one can apply Fisher's method to combine P value directly. Since in gene mapping studies, genetic markers are used only as references to infer the location of the putative disease gene at the chromosome or infer whether a disease gene is located at a specific region of the genome, different studies may use different genetic markers, although their objectives are same. Moreover, they may use a different linkage analysis method. If we want to synthesize this kind of studies, we must firstly extract a single P value for the region from each study. We will take the summarization of 4 practical studies concerning linkage of BMI with markers in the human OB gene region as an example illustrating some techniques in the following paragraph.

5.1.2. *The extraction of P value*

(i) For study with a single marker, no correction needs to be applied. For example, Borecki *et al.*[37] used only one marker in the area of the human OB gene. This one marker was KELL, located at 7q33. Four hundred sibling pairs were included and the Haseman-Elston procedure was used to yield a p value of 4.8×10^{-6}. It could be used directly.
(ii) If a separate P value for each of several markers is reported in a chromosome region, we could convert each P value to a corresponding (standard normal) Z-score by means of the inverse standard normal distribution function $Z = \Phi^{-1}(1 - P)$. The correlation between any two of them is equal to the correlation of corresponding IBD status between them. For example, the correlation between Z_i and Z_j is $r_{ij} = (1 - 2\theta_{ij})^2$, where θ denotes recombination fraction. θ_{ij} can be determined according to the distance between ith and jth markers. One centimorgan (cM) or 1 million base pairs (bp) is approximately equal to θ of 0.01. We could use statistic $S_k = \sum_{i=1}^{k} Z_i$ to summarize the information of all markers, the variance of the sum is the sum of variances plus twice the sum of the covariances for all component, that is $Var(S_k) = k + 2\sum_{i<j} r_{ij}$. So statistic $T = \frac{S_k}{\sqrt{Var(S_k)}}$ distributed

Table 18. Proportion of alleles IBD in OB markers for concordant (obese-obese) sib-pairs.

Marker	n	$\bar{\pi}$	t	P	P^*	$Z_i = \Phi^{-1}(1 - P_i^*)$
D7S651	66	0.57	1.98	0.03	0.025970	1.943627
D7S692	59	0.52	0.68	NS	0.249605	0.675734
D7S677	46	0.49	−0.29	NS	0.386574	0.288260
D7S680	57	0.59	2.47	0.008	0.008292	2.395791
D7S514	53	0.59	2.44	0.009	0.009066	2.362904
D7S530	65	0.59	2.96	0.002	0.002155	2.854504
D7S640	57	0.55	0.99	NS	0.163216	0.981324
D7S509	56	0.54	1.01	NS	0.158459	1.00081
Total						12.50295

P is the P value reported in the original literature.
P^* is the P value recovered according to t value and degree of freedom $(n-1)$.

as standard normal, and it can be used to derive a single P value for the study.

Example 6. Clement *et al.*[38] evaluated linkage to BMI dichotomized as "greater than 35" or "less than or equal to 35" with 8 markers ranging from D7S651 to D7S509 using sib-pair method. A part of results are displayed in Table 18.

The distances (cM) between every two adjacent markers in Table 18 are 13, 3, 7, 0, 2, 5, 5 respectively. We can get $\sum_{i<j} r_{ij} = 16.3756$, $Var(S_k) = 8 + 2 \times 16.3756 = 40.7512$. The calculation of Z_i is showed in Table 18. Statistic T can be calculated as

$$T = \frac{S_k}{\sqrt{Var(S_k)}} = \frac{12.50295}{\sqrt{40.7515}} = 1.958585\,, \quad P = 0.0251\,.$$

(iii) If a single P value was provided from a multipoint procedure, then Lander-Kruglyak correction could be applied to get a corrected P value,

$$P^* = 1 - \exp(-\mu(T))\,, \tag{76}$$

where $\mu(T) = [C + 2\rho\, GT^2]\alpha(T)$; $T = \Phi^{-1}(1-P)$ is a standard normal Z-score corresponding to cumulative probability $1-P$; C is the number of chromosome; G is the genome length measured in Morgans; $\alpha(T) = P$ is the pointwise significance; ρ is the crossing over rate between the genotypes being compared.

Example 7. Duggirala *et al.*[39] examined the linkage of BMI to markers spanning a 211 cM (D7S531 to D7S483) using a multipoint procedure, and resulted in a combined P value of 0.003.

In this example, $C = 1$(one chromosome used for the study), $\rho = 2$ (for sib-pair tests), $\alpha(T) = 0.003$, $T = \Phi^{-1}(1 - 0.003) = 2.747765$,

$$\mu(T) = (1 + 2 \times 2 \times 2.11 \times 2.747765^2) \times 0.003 = 0.194171\,,$$

$$P^* = 0.1765\,.$$

(iv) Sometimes researchers may use multiple cutoff points or multiple criteria to define the affected or unaffected in one study. If the analysis methods they have used are one-side sib-pair tests, the process of extracting a single P value is similar to that of (ii). Notice that here the multiple criteria of classification are of concern but not the multiple markers. The estimation of correlation is different, for example, the correlation between Z_i and Z_j is calculated as $r_{ij} = \sqrt{\frac{\min(n_i,n_j)}{\max(n_i,n_j)}}$, where n_i, n_j are the number of sib-pairs having been used in ith and jth classification respectively.

In Example 8, Reed combined the marker information into haplotypes and conducted their analysis by looking at sharing of haplotypes rather than alleles. This aspect of their analysis simplifies the extraction of a single P value since significance is assessed only for IBD sharing at the single haplotype rather than at each individual locus, so the P values need not be corrected with Lander-Kruglyak method. With the data in Table 2, we get $\sum_{i<j} r_{ij} = 1.983509$, $Var(S_k) = 3 + 2 \times 1.983509 = 6.967017$. The calculation of Z_i are displayed in column 6 of Table 17. Then the statistic

$$T = \frac{S_k}{\sqrt{Var(S_k)}} = \frac{2.63178}{\sqrt{6.967017}} = 0.997071\,, \quad P = 0.1594\,.$$

Example 8. Reed *et al.*[40] examined linkage of BMI to 8 markers contained in and surrounding the interval D7S1873 through D7S1875 using two methods (sib-pair analysis and TDT). Three cutoff points were used to define obese and linkage analysis respectively. The main results are displayed in Tables 19 and 20.

If a study used a two-sided TDT (Table 18), we could convert the chi-squares to Z-scores by taking their square root, just like the column 6 in Table 20. The correlation among the Z's can again be estimated as the square root of the proportion of subjects in a subset divided by the number of subjects in the larger set. For example, the estimated correlation between

Table 19. Mean proportion of the OB gene haplotypes (D7S1873-D7S1875) identical by descent for obese-obese sib-pairs.

Obese Cutoff	Pairs(n)	Proportion of IBD	t	P	$Z_i = \Phi^{-1}(1 - P_i^*)$
≥ 30	213	0.51 ± 0.33	0.24	0.4038	0.243524
≥ 35	135	0.50 ± 0.35	0.03	0.4333	0.167979
≥ 40	59	0.60 ± 0.33	2.28	0.0132	2.220277
Total	2.63178				

Proportion of IBD is expressed as mean±SD.

Table 20. Transmission disequilibrium of a haplotype (D7S504-D7S1875) flanking the OB locus.

BMI of Sibling	1–5 Transmitted/ Not Transmitted	%Transmitted	χ_1^2	P	$Z_i = \sqrt{\chi_1^2}$
≥ 30	71/50	58.7	3.64	0.056	1.907878
≥ 35	60/39	60.6	4.45	0.035	2.109502
≥ 40	46/24	65.7	6.91	0.009	2.628688

the Z-score in subjects with a BMI ≥ 40 and the Z-score for subjects with a BMI ≥ 30 is $\sqrt{70/121} = 0.761$. If there are m Z-scores, then statistic $Q = ZR^{-1}Z'$ has a chi-square distribution with the degree of freedom equal to $m-1$. Where $Z = (Z_1, Z_2, \ldots, Zm)$ and R is the correlation matrix. With the data in Table 20, we get $Z = (1.907878\ 2.109502\ 2.628688)$

$$Q = ZR^{-1}Z' = Z \begin{pmatrix} 1 & 0.904530 & 0.760600 \\ 0.904530 & 1 & 0.84875 \\ 0.760600 & 0.840875 & 1 \end{pmatrix} Z' = 6.944753$$

$P = 0.0310$.

(v) If a study has performed more than one test with the same data, just like Example 3, we still have two p values after combination, one from sib-pair test and one from TDT. If the correlation between these two tests could be determined, then one could combine these into a single P value. However, it is not immediately apparent how to estimate this correlation. Allison *et al.* (1998) propose several alternatives[41]: First, one could, on some *a priori* grounds of preference, choose one test over another. For example, one might argue that because all of the other studies are using a sib-pair approach rather than TDT it would be more appropriate to combine sib-pair data

Table 21. The results of overall meta-analysis and sensitivity analysis.

Reference		P Value	χ^2 (P Value)[a]	χ^2 (P Value)[b]
Borecki *et al.* (1994)[37]		4.8×10^{-6}	14.51(0.0244)	$17.79(6.7893 \times 10^{-3})$
Clement *et al.* (1996)[38]		0.0251	$31.64(1.9165 \times 10^{-5})$	$34.91(4.4856 \times 10^{-6})$
Dugirala *et al.* (1996)[39]		0.1765	$35.54(3.3919 \times 10^{-6})$	$38.81(7.7944 \times 10^{-7})$
Reed *et al.* (1996)[40]	Sibpair	0.1594	$35.33(3.7152 \times 10^{-6})$	
	TDT	0.0310		$35.33(3.7152 \times 10^{-6})$
Overall			$39.01(4.90 \times 10^{-6})$	$42.28(1.20 \times 10^{-6})$

a: Using Reed *et al.*[40] sib-pair test result.
b: Using Reed *et al.*[40] TDT result.

rather than the TDT data and be consistent with the others. Second, one could multiply the lowest P value by two (the number of test) as a form of Bonferroni correction. However, this is overly conservative because it does not take the correlation between the two tests into account. Third, one could estimate the correlation via simulation. Fourth, one could conduct the overall meta-analysis with the results of each test.

The results of meta-analysis for the above four studies are displayed in the last row of 4th and 5th columns in Table 4. When using Reed *et al.*[40] sib-pair test result, the overall $P = 4.9047 \times 10^{-6}$ (d.f. = 8); when using TDT result, the overall $P = 1.1999 \times 10^{-6}$ (d.f = 8). Besides these, we also have conducted sensitivity analysis. In this example, the sensitivity analysis means that each study result was removed from the analysis, and the chi-square statistic with 6 d.f. (from the remaining study results) was computed. The corresponding P values are given in first 5 rows of 4th and 5th columns in Table 21. This table shows that Borecki *et al.*[37] study has a great influence on the overall P value. But even excluding this study, the remaining results still provide a significant value ($P < 0.05$). So this study suggests that there is evidence for linkage of BMI to somewhere in the OB region. Note that this meta-analysis is only an example; we have not collected all of possible literature.

5.2. *The Meta-analysis for Genome Search*

The Genome Search Meta-analysis method (GSMA) uses a non-parametric ranking procedure to identify genetic regions that show consistently increased sharing statistics or lod scores among several genome screens.[42, 43] This method splits the whole chromosomes into bins of approximately equal length and ranks these bins according to the lod scores, Z-statistics or P values with the most significant result having the highest rank within each genome screen. Then the ranks for each bin are summed across screens. For any bin, the null hypothesis is that no susceptibility loci exist within the bin, and the ranks are assigned randomly. For m studies and n bins, the probability that the sum of ranks (X_i) is equal to a value R is given by

$$P\left(\sum_{i=1}^{m} X_i = R\right) = \begin{cases} 0 & R < m \\ \dfrac{1}{n^m}\sum_{k=0}^{d}(-1)^k \begin{pmatrix} R-kn-1 \\ m-1 \end{pmatrix} \times \begin{pmatrix} m \\ k \end{pmatrix} & m \leq R \leq mn \\ 0 & R > mn\,, \end{cases} \tag{77}$$

where d is the integer part of $(R-m)/n$. From this distribution, we can calculate the probability that a summed rank of R or greater within a bin under the null hypothesis.

The choice of bin width has several constraints: The bin width must be appropriate for all chromosomes, with at least two bins on the smallest chromosome, and at least one marker should be genotyped within each bin. To ensure the independence of lod score or P value for adjacent markers, Wise *et al.* proposed to use 30 cM as the width of each bin.

Since some literatures may report only the most significant results, the information for some bins is lost. This will not bias the results of the GSMA, provided a strict lod score or P value cut-off has been used and all chromosomes have been genotyped. If ranks can be assigned to the top bins, the remaining bins could be given equal ranks of $(120 - x + 1)/2$. If different genome search contributes differently to the meta-analysis, a weight may be assigned to each screen, such as $\log(N)$, where N is the number of pedigrees or sib pairs in each study. Although the above probability distribution for the summed ranks under null hypothesis will no longer hold, the P-value can be generated through simulation of the weighted ranks.

5.3. *Conclusion*

The major forte of Fisher's combining P value method are its simplicity in calculation and its flexibility in pooling results from studies which may examine slightly different hypotheses or use different outcome measures. However, it also has many drawbacks; sometimes its result is difficult to explain because only one highly significant P value from a single study may determine the significance of the Fisher test statistic; it cannot be used to make inferences about the average effect size or the consistency of results across studies. But in practice, published results from heterogeneous studies are likely to report P values only. When nothing else is available, combining P values can provide an overall assessment of linkage.

GSMA allows systematic integration of data from several genome screens. The major strength of the GSMA is its application to a diversity of study designs, it is not restricted by different phenotype definitions, family structures, markers, or analysis methods across studies. Wise *et al.*[42,43] have applied this method to four genome screens in multiple sclerosis and across 11 screens from autoimmune disorders, which showed that the GSMA is a valuable data exploration tool to obtain an overview of the genome search results within and across disease phenotypes.

To ensure the quality of meta-analysis, the pre-analysis process is very important, we must set strict literature inclusion standard according to professional knowledge, and collect literatures through multiple ways to reduce as much publication bias as we can.

6. Bias in Meta-Analysis

6.1. *Source of bias*

Meta-analysis should be viewed as an observational study of the evidence. In epidemiology, bias may be defined as any trend in the collection, analysis, interpretation, publication or review of data that can lead to conclusions that are systematically different from the truth. Bias often causes conflicting results of meta-analysis and threaten its internal validity and reliability. In each step of meta-analysis, like locating and selecting studies for inclusion in meta-analysis, or extracting accurate study data, bias may be introduced. As noted by Felson, there are at least three types of bias involved in meta-analysis: sampling bias, selection bias and within study bias.[44]

6.1.1. *Sampling bias*

The validity of a meta-analysis depends on complete sampling of all the studies performed on a particular topic. Any incomplete sampling is potential to bias. Sampling bias arise when retrieving the relevant studies, which consists of:

(1) Studies with significant results are more likely to get published than studies without significant results, leading to *publication bias*.

(2) In the process of retrieving published studies using computerized database, *indexing bias* and *search bias* may occurr. The former is defined as biased indexing of published studies, which means indexing error or indexing variability. Indexing bias is not under the meta-analysts control. Search bias is another type of sampling bias due to inadequate or incomplete search. Index bias or search bias can lead to failure to capture all indexed studies in a database.
(3) Relying heavily on references published in other articles or in review of literature may cause *reference bias* or *citation bias* into a meta-analysis.
(4) *Multiple publications bias* occurs when studies whose results are published in a series of articles are more likely to be sampled than those published only once. *Multiple publications bias* can induce meta-analyst confusion when the publications do not have the same first author or when one publication does not refer to the prior one. *Multiply used subjects bias* can occur when the same subjects are reported in two separate studies when they are actually a part of only one study.
(5) The included studies in meta-analysis based exclusively on reports in English may lead to *English language bias.*

In practice, to reduce or avoid sampling bias requires that the meta-analyst embarking on a database search choose appropriate index terms and conduct the search with a systematic strategy.

6.1.2. *Selection bias*

Selection bias occurs when eligible studies are chosen in a meta-analysis, according to the criteria of inclusion and exclusion. In this process, two types of bias may be introduced, one is *inclusion criteria bias*, and the other is *selector bias.* If the inclusion criteria is developed by an investigator familiar with the area under study, the criteria can be influenced by knowledge of the results of the set of potential studies, and this would cause bias. *Inclusion criteria bias* is difficult to avoid since a good knowledge of a topic is a prerequisite to develop an inclusion criteria. In *selector bias*, inclusion criteria have been set, although they may not be so specific as to dictate which studies are included or excluded from the meta-analysis. This leaves the meta-analyst selector free to choose studies, a choice which is susceptible to bias.

Selection bias of studies is probably the central reason for discrepant results in meta-analyses. For example, in 1992, two meta-analyses published in BMJ (*British Medical Journal*) and *Lancet*, respectively. Both compared low molecular weight heparins and standard heparin in the prevention of thrombosis after surgery, but the conclusions were widely divergent.[45,46] One concluded that "low molecular weight heparins seem to have a higher benefit to risk ratio than unfractionated heparin in preventing perioperative thrombosis", whereas the other considered that "there is at present no convincing evidence that in general surgery patients low molecular weight heparins, compared with standard heparin, general a clinically important improvement in the benefit to risk ratio". Egger pointed out that the conflicting results of two meta-analyses were mainly related to the selection of studies.[47] Nurmohamed *et al.*[46] based their analysis on a subgroup of trials that they considered possess the highest methodological strength, while Leizorovicz *et al.*[45] included all trials in their analysis. Many other elements, for example, language restrictions or use of unpublished material — could contribute to conflicting conclusions.

Criteria for including studies in a meta-analysis may be influenced by knowledge of the results of the set of potential studies and lead to inclusion bias.

One important way to avoid selection bias is to create extremely specific and clear study inclusion criteria, so that the selector has little chance to inject bias into the selection decision. Blind method is also suggested to limit selector bias. The most common is to blind the methods and results of studies to make it hard for the meta-analyst selector to determine the inclusion of a study through results. In this method, there are often two selectors who work independently. Any disagreement in study selection is solved by a joint meeting or by a third selector. This process certainly decreases the chance of selector bias, but it does not eliminate it.

Another way of handling the selection bias is to include all studies that meet basic entry criteria then perform sensitivity analyses with regard to the different possible entry criteria. Any conclusions from a meta-analysis that are highly sensitive to altering the entry criteria should be treated with caution.

6.1.3. *Within study biases*

After studies are selected for a meta-analysis, data should be accurately extracted from the study. There are several opportunities for bias, the most likely bias is *extractor bias*, which can create systematically biased results. There may be considerable inter- and intra-observer variability in extracting data from studies. To minimize *extractor bias*, an extraction sheet should lay out specific rules for data extraction with clarity.

Meta-analyst bias may affect the scoring of studies for quality. If study results are weighted for quality in the analysis, *a bias in scoring study quality* may have a real impact in meta-analysis results. Giving rigid rules on how to measure the quality of trials may help lessen observer variability and mitigate bias.

The primary study paper included in the meta-analysis itself may not accurately report the study's result. For example, the study has several outcomes which were measured, but the only results reported are those which reach statistical significance, and this can introduce a *reporting bias*. Unfortunately, the prevalence of *reporting bias* is unknown, but it is a widespread problem which could serve to substantially bias meta-analysis results.

6.2. *Publication bias*

Publication bias is usually used to refer to the greater likelihood of research with statistically significant results to be submitted and published compared with non-significant and null results. More generally, publication bias is the systematic error in a statistical inference by conditioning on the achievement of publication status. Publication bias occurs because published studies are not representative of all studies that have ever been done.

6.2.1. *The causes and consequence of publication bias*

Publication bias has long been recognized and much discussed. Publication bias can originate from three sources: The authors, the sponsors of the study, and the editor or reviewers of the journal to which the paper is submitted. First, authors may be less likely submit papers if the results are not significant. Second, the editors of the journal may favor publication of positive results. Finally, the sponsor may play an important role in generating publication bias, especially if it is a pharmaceutical company funded study. The implication is that the pharmaceutical industry discourages the publication of studies which have negative findings. In addition, multicenter studies are more likely to be published than studies from a single center.

Existence of a bias in favor of publication of statistically significant results is well documented. Easterbrook *et al.*[48] carried out a retrospective study of 285 research projects that had been approved by the Central Oxford Research Ethics Committee between 1984 and 1987. They found

154 studies had statistically significant results and 131 did not. Of the 154 studies with statistically significant results, 60.4% had been published, whereas only 34.4% of the studies that did not have statistically significant results had been published. Using logistic regression and adjusting for relevant covariates, they found that studies with statistically significant results were more likely to have been published and/or presented than those with non-significant results (OR = 3.56, 95%CI 1.82–6.99).[48]

Publication bias may seriously distort the findings of a meta-analysis, and certainly threaten the validity and reliability of results. For example, in a meta-analysis about the effect of an alkylating agent alone comparing with combination chemotherapy on survival in patients with advanced ovarian cancer, Simer found that the conclusion based on the published studies is different from that based on studies registered in the International Cancer Research Data Bank. The pooled results from published trials showed significant efficacy, while data from prospectively registered trials (both published and unpublished) showed no significant advantage of combination chemotherapy over single agent treatment.[49]

6.2.2. *Methods of detecting and correcting for publication bias*

Although searching for relevant unpublished studies is important and may sometimes alleviate publication bias, identifying such studies may be difficult. Hence we need methods to assess the magnitude of publication bias in a meta-analysis, based on the data in the available studies. In fact, various methods have been devised to attempt to detect and correct publication bias, but none of the available methods is entirely satisfactory for dealing with this problem. Here, commonly used methods are described as following.

(1) Funnel Plot

Funnel Plot, or, funnel graph, is the frequently used method for detecting the publication bias. The basic idea is that if the point estimates from individual studies are plotted against the inverse of the variances, or another surrogate for sample size, the points visualized together should produce a funnel shape, so they are scattered around the true value of the point estimate with the scattering narrowing as the standard errors decrease.[50] That is, in such a plot, the effect size of studies is plotted against study sample size. If there is no publication bias, the plot would resemble an inverted funnel with a wide dispersion of results among studies of small

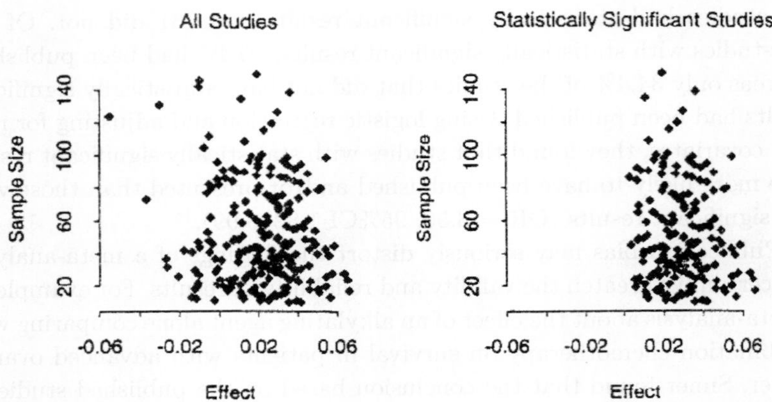

Fig. 9. Two funnel plots based on simulated data. The left plot displays absence of publication, and the right displays the presence of publication bias.
Source: Normand (1999) *Stat. Med.* **18**: 339.

size and a narrower range of study results for large studies. If the plot shows an asymmetrical and skewed shape, publication bias may present. This usually takes the form of a gap in the wide part of the funnel, which indicates the absence of small studies showing no benefit or harm. Figure 9 demonstrates two funnel plots based on simulated data. The left plot displays the simulated summaries for all the studies, which means absence of publication bias. The right plot displays the simulated summaries for studies that are statistically significant at the 0.05 level, which suggests the presence of publication bias.

In fact, the funnel plot is a graphical test for any type of bias that is associated with sample size. The publication bias and sampling bias are more likely to affect smaller studies than large trials and may thus lead to funnel plot asymmetry. Another source of asymmetry arises from differences in the methodological quality. Smaller studies are, on average, conducted and analyzed with less methodological rigor than larger studies, and trials of lower quality tend to show larger effects. Other factor, such as heterogeneity in treatment effect between low and high risk groups can also lead to asymmetry in the funnel plot.

The major advantage of funnel plot is that it is easy to perform which only requires published data. But the method is practically limited to meta-analysis with large enough numbers of studies to allow one to visualize (as opposed to fantasize) a funnel shape to the data. The symmetry of funnel plot is defined informally. So, if the number of studies included in a meta-analysis is small, it is difficult to detect the symmetry of funnel plot through visual examination.

(2) Egger's linear regression method[51]

Egger proposed a linear regression model to measure funnel plot asymmetry. It is a formal test for asymmetry in funnel plot. The standard deviate y_i, ($y_i = t_i/s_i$, t_i is the effect size, s_i is standard error for study i) is regressed on precision $x_i(x_i = 1/s_i)$, then the significance of intercept differing from zero (at $\alpha < 0.1$) is tested. That is, $y_i = a + bx_i$. The points from a homogeneous set of trials, not distorted by publication bias (or other bias), will thus scatter about a line that runs through the origin at standard normal deviate zero ($a = 0$), with the slope b indicating the size and direction of effect. This situation corresponds to a symmetry funnel plot [Fig. 10(a)]. If it is asymmetric, with smaller studies showing effects that differ systematically from larger studies, the regression line will not pass through the origin [Fig. 10(b)]. The intercept a provides a measure of asymmetry — the larger it deviate from zero the more the asymmetric.

Egger examined whether the regression method predicts discordance of results when meta-analyses were compared to large trials.[51] They found in the eight pairs of meta-analysis and large trial, there were four concordant and four discordant pairs. In all case discordant cases, meta-analyses show larger effects. Funnel plot asymmetry was present in three out of four discordant pair but none of concordant pairs. They also found, in 14 (38%)

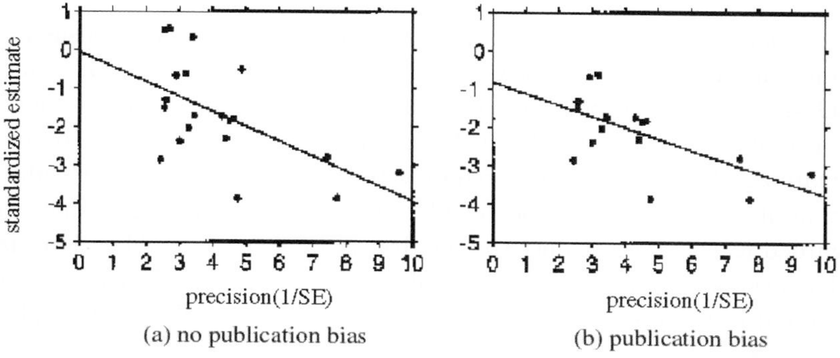

Fig. 10. Example of the Egger's regression method using a simulated meta-analysis. *Source*: Macaskill (2001). *Stat. Med.* **20**: 644.

journal meta-analysis (from four famous medical journals) and 5 (13%) Cochrane reviews, funnel plot asymmetry indicating that there was bias.

But the statistical properties of Egger's linear regression method are not described, and the test may itself be biased. This method violates the usual assumptions of simple linear regression. There is measurement error in the independent variable because the standard errors were estimated from the observed data, and is therefore subject to sampling error. This results in a biased estimate of the regression slope.

(3) Begg's rank correlation test[52]

Begg's method uses Kendall's tau to test for correlation between the standardized treatment effect t_i^*, and the variance of the treatment effect (v_i), where

$$t_i^* = (t_i - \bar{t})/\sqrt{v_i^*}\,,$$

$$\bar{t} = \sum(t_j/v_j)\Big/\sum(1/v_j) \quad \text{and} \quad v_i^* = v_i - 1\Big/\sum(1/v_j)\,.$$

Alternatively, the test can be based on the correlation between t_i^* and the sample size for each study (n_i). Treatment effects are standardized to obtain a set of estimates that can be assumed to be independent and identically distributed under the null hypothesis of no publication bias.

The rank correlation test has been described as a direct statistical analogue of the funnel plot. But the power of the test varies along with the unknown characteristics in meta-analysis. Even though the result is not significant, publication bias cannot be ruled out in small meta-analyses.

(4) Fail-safe number[53]

Rosenthal's "fail-safe number" (N_{FS}), is the number of unpublished null studies needed to remove the significance from the finding of a meta-analysis. The method involves computing the standardized normal deviate Z, associated with each published study and then calculating a combined deviate Z_s. The values of N_{FS} required to bring the new overall P-value to any desired level can then be calculated, an implausibly high value being regarded as evidence against the file-drawer hypothesis (publication bias). It has been suggested that N_{FS} should be presented for all meta-analyses, as an aid in the assessment of the degree of confidence that can be placed in the results.

However, plausibility of existence of certain number of unpublished studies is judged subjectively. Furthermore, this method assumes published and unpublished studies are of similar sizes. Even in similar sized studies, this method will be misleading if the average effect of unpublished studies is in opposite direction to published studies.[54]

Besides the methods describes above, another kind of methods pursues truncated sampling model to deal with publication bias, where it is assumed that statistically non-significant results do not get published. Hedges developed a model of the selection process involving a step function relating the P-value to the probability of selection in the context of a random-effects model. The model permits the estimation of a weight function representing selection along with the means and variances of effects. Dear and Begg's semi-parametric method is quite similar to that of Hedgess model, in which the selection publication is modeled also using a weight function on two-sided P-value scale.[55] The difference is that Hedge's pre-specifying the region of the P-value scale within which the weight function is assumed to be constant. Gleser proposed two general models that revisit Rosenthal's attempts to explore the number of unpublished studies and introduce several frequentist methods for interval estimates.[56] These methods take advantage of the fact that under the null hypothesis of interest, P-values from experiments testing this H_0 have a common known distribution which is independent of each experiment's design, sample size, and concomitant variables. But these methods are not widely accepted and are not recommended.

Recently, source augmentation method has been developed for detecting and correcting the publication bias. Givens used a Bayesian model to augment observed data by simulating the outcomes for missing studies, thereby creating a "complete" data for meta-analysis.[57] The author described how the random-effects model may be extended to account for publication bias, assuming that in addition to the n observed studies there are further m studies that are not observed. The number m and relative risks found from these studies are unknown and must be estimated, and uncertainties about these estimates are reflected in the final meta-analysis inference by treating them as parameters in a Bayesian analysis.

In fact, none of the available methods is entirely satisfactory for dealing with the publication bias so far. Thus, we should consider other ways to avoid publication bias. First, results of large studies most closely approximate the average results of all studies, whether published or unpublished. Furthermore, large studies, even with null results, are almost always published. Therefore, the meta-analyst can test the pooled results of studies to see if they approach the overall pooled result. Second, a meta-analyst can also attempt to obtain data from unpublished studies, an endeavor recommended. Nonetheless, finding those studies can be very difficult. Finally, one important solution to publication bias may be the establishment a clinical trial registries, a movement to register all initiated studies has begun among those in clinical trials field but not yet among those conducting observational studies.

References

1. Glass, G. V. (1976). Primary, secondary and meta-analysis of research. *Education Research* **5**: 3–8.
2. Huque, M. F. (1988). Experiences with meta-analysis in NDA submissions. *Proceedings of the Biopharmaceutical Section of the American Statistical Association* **2**: 28–33.
3. Sackett, D. L., Richardson, W. S., Rosenberg, W. M. *et al.* (2000). *Evidence-based Medicine*: *How to practice and teach EBM*, 2nd edn., Churchill Livingstone, London.
4. Egger, M. and Smith, G. D. (1997). Meta-analysis: potentials and promise. *British Medical Journal* **315**: 1371–1374.
5. Beecher, H. K. (1955). The powerful placebo. *Journal of the American Medical Association* **159**: 1602–1606.
6. Jones, D. R. (1995). Meta-analysis: Weighing the evidence. *Stat. Med.* **14**: 137–139.
7. Stampfer, M. J., Goldhaber, S. Z. and Yusuf, S. (1982). Effects of intravenous streptokinase on acute myocardial infarction: Pooled results from randomized trials. *New England Journal of Medicine* **307**: 1180–1182.
8. Egger, M. and Smith, G. D. (1997). Meta-analysis: Principles and procedures. *British Medical Journal* **315**: 1533–1537.
9. Boyd, N. D., Martin, L. J. and Noffel, M. (1993). A meta-analysis of studies of dietary fat and breast cancer. *British Journal of Cancer* **68**: 627–636.
10. Normand, S. L. (1999). Tutorial in biostatistics. Meta-analysis: Formulating, evaluating, combining, and reporting. *Stat. Med.* **18**: 321–359.
11. Hedges, L. V. and Olkin, I. (1985). *Statistical Methods for Meta-Analysis*, Academic Press, Orlando.
12. Petitti, D. B. (2000). *Meta-Analysis, Decision Analysis, and Cost-Effectiveness Analysis*: *Methods for Quantitative Synthesis in Medicine*, 2nd edn., Oxford University Press, New York.
13. Hardy, R. J. and Thompson, S. G. (1998). Detecting and describing heterogeneity in meta-analysis. *Stat. Med.* **17**: 841–856.
14. Robinn, J., Greenland, S. and Breslow, N. E. (1986). A general estimator for the variance of the Mantel-Haenszel odds ratio. *The American Journal of Epidemiology* **124**: 719–723.
15. Yusuf, S., Peto, R., Lewis, J. *et al.* (1985). β-blockade during and after myocardial infartion: An overview of the randomized trials. *Progress in Cardiovascular Diseases* **27**: 335–371.

16. Feiss, J. L. and Gross, A. J. (1991). Meta-analysis in epidemiology, with special reference to studies of the association between exposure to environmental tobacco smoke and lung cancer: A critique. *Journal of Clinical Epidemiology* **44**: 127–139.
17. DerSimonian, R. and Laird, N. (1986). Meta-analysis in clinical trials. *Controlled Clinical Trials* **7**: 177–188.
18. Hedges, L. V. (1982). Estimation of effect size from a series of independent experiments. *Psychology Bulletin* **92**: 490–492.
19. DuMouchel, W. (1990). Bayesian meta analysis, in *Statistical Methodology in the Pharmaceutical Sciences*, ed. D. Berry Marcel Dekker, New York, 509–529.
20. Carlin, J. B. (1992). Meta-analysis for 2 × 2 tables: A Bayesian approach. *Stat Med.* **11**: 141–158.
21. Smith, A. F. M. and Roberts, G. O. (1993). Bayesian computation via the Gibbs sampler and related Markov chain Monte Carlo methods. *Journal of the Royal Statistical Society* **B55**: 3–23.
22. Gelfand, A. E., Hills, S. E., Racine-Poom, A. *et al.* (1990). Illustration of Bayesian inference in normal data models using Gibbs sampling. *Journal of the American Statistical Association* **85**: 972–985.
23. Spiegelhalter, D., Thomas, A., Best, N. *et al.* (1996). *WinBUGS User Manual (Version 1.1.1)*. MRC Biostatistics Unit, Institute of Public Health, Cambridge.
24. Irwig, L., Tosteson, A. N. A., Gatsonis, C. *et al.* (1994). Guideline for meta-analysis evaluating diagnostic tests. *Annals of International Medicine* **120**(8): 667–676.
25. Moses, L. E., Shapiro, D. and Littenberg, B. (1993). Combining independent studies of a diagnostic test into a summary ROC curve: Data-analytic approaches and some addition considerations. *Stat Med.* **12**: 1293–1316.
26. Fahey, M. T., Irwig, L. and Macaskill, P. (1995). Meta-analysis of Pap test accuracy. *The American Journal of Epidemiology* **141**: 680–689.
27. Kinkel, K., Hricak, H., Lu, Y. *et al.* (2000). US charaterization of ovarian masses, a meta-analysis. *Radiology* **217**: 803–811.
28. Kinkel, K., Kaji, Y., Yu, K. K. *et al.* (1999). Radiologic staging in patients with endometrial cancer: A meta analysis. *Radiology* **212**(3): 711–718.
29. Walter, S. D., Irwig, L. and Glasziou, P. P. (1999). Meta analysis of diagnostic tests with imperfect reference standards. *Journal of Clinical Epidemiology* **52**(10): 943–951.
30. Frei, K. A., Kinkel, K., Bonel, H. M. *et al.* (2000). Endometrial cancer: Frequency of myometrial invasion per grade and incremental value of pre-operative MRI in specialist referral: Meta- and Bayesian-analysis. *Radiology* **216**(2): 444–449.
31. Yu, C. H. (2000). The methods of ROC analysis and applications in medical research. Doctoral Dissertation of Fourth Military Medical University, 111–122.
32. Eleftherios, C. V. (1998). Meta-analysis of studies of the diagnostic accuracy of laboratory tests. *Pathology and Laboratory Medicine* **122**: 675–685.

33. Kester, A. D. and Buntinx, F. (2000). Meta-analysis of ROC curves. *Medical Decision Making* **20**(4): 430–439.
34. Vamvakas, E. C. (1998). Meta-analysis of studies of the diagnostic accuracy of laboratory tests: A review of the concepts and methods [see comments]. *Archives of Pathology and Laboratory Medicine* **122**(8): 675–686.
35. SAS Institute Inc (1996). *SAS/STAT Software: Changes and Enhancements through Release 6.11*, SAS Institute Inc., Cary, NC, 221–230.
36. Gu, c., Province, M., Todorov, A. *et al.* (1998). Meta-analysis methodology for combining non-parametric sibpair linkage results: Genetic homogeneity and identical markers. *Genetic Epidemiology* **15**: 609–626.
37. Borecki, I. B., Perusse, L. *et al.* (1994). An exploratory investigation of genetic linkage with body composition and fatness phenotypes: The Quebec family study. *Obesity Research* **2**: 213–219.
38. Clement, K., Garner, C., Hager, J. *et al.* (1996). Indication for linkage of the human OB gene region with extreme obesity. *Diabetes* **45**: 687–690.
39. Duggirala, R., Michael, P. and Mitchell, B. D. (1996). Quantitative variation in obesity-related traits and insulin precursors linked to the OB gene region on human chromosome 7. *American Journal of Human Genetics* **59**: 694–703.
40. Reed, D. R., Ding, Y., Xu, W. *et al.* (1996). Extreme obesity may be linked to markers flanking the human OB gene. *Diabetes* **45**: 691–694.
41. Allison, D. B. and Heo, M. (1998). Meta-analysis of linkage data under worst-case conditions: A demonstration using the human OB region. *Genetics* **148**: 859–865.
42. Wise, L. H., Lanchbury, J. S. and Lewis, C, M. (1999). Meta-analysis of genome searches. *Annals of Human Genetics* **63**(3): 263–272.
43. Wise, L. H. and Lewis, C. M. (1999). A method for meta-analysis of genome searches: Application to simulated data. *Genetic Epidemiology* **17**(suppl 1): 767–771.
44. Felson, D. (1992). Bias in meta-analytic research. *Journal of Clinical Epidemiology* **45**: 885–892.
45. Leizorovicz, A., Haugh, M. C., Chapuis, F. R. *et al.* (1992). Low molecular weight heparin in prevention of perioperative thrombosis. *British Medical Journal* **305**: 913–920.
46. Nurmohamed, M. T., Rosendaal, F. R. and Bueller, H. R. (1992). Low-molecular-weight heparin versus standard heparin in general and orthopaedic surgery: A meta-analysis. *Lancet* **340**: 162–156.
47. Egger, M. and Smith, D. G. (1998). Meta-analysis: Bias in location and selection of studies. *British Medical Journal* **316**: 61–66.
48. Easterbrook, P. J., Berlin, J. A., Gopalan, R. *et al.* (1991). Publication bias in clinical reaserch. *Lancet* **337**: 867–872.
49. Simes, J. R. (1986). Publication bias: The case for an international registry of trials. *Journal Clinical Oncology*, 1529–1541.
50. Light, R. J. and Pillemer, D. B. (1984). Quantitative procedures. *Summing Up: The Science of Reviewing Research.* Harvard University Press, Cambridge, MA.

51. Egger, M., Smith, G. D., Schneidet, M. *et al.* (1997). Bias in meta-analysis detected by a simple, graphical test. *British Medical Journal* **315**: 629–634.
52. Begg, C. B. and Mazumdar, M. (1994). Operating characteristics of a rank correlation test for publication bias. *Biometrics* **50**: 1088–1099.
53. Rosenthal, R. (1979). The "file drawer problem" and tolerance for null results. *Psychology Bulletin* **86**: 638–641.
54. Thornton, A. and Lee, P. (2000). Publication bias in meta-analysis: Its causes and consequences. *Journal of Clinical Epidemiology* **53**: 207–216.
55. Dear, K. B. G. and Begg, C. B. (1992). An approach for assessing publication bias prior to performing a meta-analysis. *Statistical Sciences* **7**: 237–245.
56. Gleser, L. J. and Olkin, I. (1996). Model for estimating the number of unpublished studies. *Stat. Med.* **15**: 2493–2507.
57. Givens, G. H., Smith, D. D. and Tweedie, R. L. (1997). Publication bias in meta-analysis: A Bayesian data-augmentation approach to account for issues exemplified in the passive smoking debate. *Statistical Sciences* **12**: 221–250.
58. Sweeting, M., Sutton, A., Lambert, P. (2004). What to add to nothing? Use and avoidance of continuity corrections in meta-analysis of sparse data. *Stat Med.* **23**: 1351–1375.
59. Bradurn, M., Deeks, J., Berlin, J. Russell, L. (2007). Much ado about nothing: a comparison of the performance of meta-analytical methods with rare events. *Stat. Med.* **26**: 53–77.
60. Robins, J., Breslow, N., Greeland, S. (1986). Estimators of the Mantel-Haenszel variance consistent in both sparse data and large strata models. *Biometrics* **42**: 311–323.
61. Tian, L., Cai, T., Pfeffer, M., Piankov, N., Cremieux, P., Wei, L. J. (2009). Exact and efficient inference procedure for meta-analysis and its application to the analysis of independent 2 by 2 tables with all available data but without artificial continuity correction. *Biostat.* **10**: 275–281.
62. Nissen, S., Wolski, K. Effect of Rosiglitazone on the risk of myocardial infarction and death from cardiovascular causes, *N Engl J Med.* **256**: 2457–2471.
63. Brockwell, S. and Gordon, I. (2001). A comparison of statistical methods for meta-analysis. *Stat Med.* **20**: 825–840.
64. Brockwell, S., and Gordon, I. (2007). A simple method for inference on an overall effect in meta-analysis. *Stat. Med.* **26**: 4531–4543.
65. Noma, H. (2011). Confidence intervals for random-effects meta-analysis based on Bartlett-type correction. *Stat. Med.* **30**: 3304–3312.
66. Henmi, M., Copas, J. (2010). Confidence intervals for random effects meta-analysis and robustness to publication bias. *Stat. Med.* **29**: 2969–2983.
67. Wang, R., Tian, L., Cai, T. and Wei, L. J. (2010). Nonparametric inference procedure for percentiles of the random effects distribution in meta-analysis. *Ann. App. Stat.* **4**: 520–532.
68. Efron, B. (1996). Empirical Bayes methods for combining likelihoods. *J Amer Statis Assoc.* **91**: 538–550.
69. Singh, K., Xie, M., Strawderman, W. (2005). Combining information from independent sources through confidence distributions. *Ann. Stat.* **33**: 159–183.

About the Authors

Xuyu Zhou is Vice Director of the Institute for Medical Information at Sun Yat-Sen University, People's Republic of China. She was a visiting scholar at Yale University, and obtained a master degree of biostatistics at the School of Public Health, Sun Yat-Sen University, People's Republic of China. She is a Committee Member of the Chinese Society of Medical Information, and an Editorial board member of "Evidence-based Medicine" journal. She has published 12 books, and about 30 papers. Her research interests include meta-analysis, clinical epidemiology, and information literacy education.

JiQian Fang received the "National Teaching Master" award in 2009, and "Outstanding Contribution to Preventive Medicine" award in 2010 from the Chinese Central Government. He is the leading professor in research and education of Medical statistics in China. Ji-Qian Fang was born in Shanghai 1939, earned his Bachelor of Science in 1961 from the Department of Mathematics, Fu Dan University and Ph.D in 1985 from the Program of Biostatistics, University of California at Berkeley. His Ph.D thesis studied multi-state survival analysis for life phenomena under the guidance of Professor Chin-Long Chiang. From 1985–1990, Dr. Fang was a Professor and Director, Department of Biostatistics and Biomathematics, Beijing Medical University. Since 1991, he has been the Director and Chair Professor, Department of Medical Statistics, Sun Yat-Sen University, People's Republic of China. Professor Fang was a visiting professor of University of Kent, UK in 1987 and Australian National University in 1990, as well as an adjunct professor at Chinese University of Hong Kong, since 1993. He is the secretary for the Group China of International Biometric Society and vice president of Chinese Association of Health Informatics. Professor Fang has supervised many post graduate students and post-doctorate fellows in medical statistics. His research projects widely cover various fields, including "Stochastic Models of Life Phenomena", "Gating Dynamics of Ion Channels", "Statistical Methods for Data on Quality of Life", "Health and Air Pollution", "Analysis of DNA Finger Printing", and "Linkage Analysis between Complex Trait and Multiple Genes" etc. These projects were sponsored by either the National Foundation of China or international organizations, such as the World Health Organization and European Commission. He is the chief editor of the textbook *Health Statistics* in Chinese (5, 6, 7-th ed.), and the co-editor of the monograph *Advanced Medical Statistics* in Chinese and English respectively (1st and 2nd Ed.).

Yu Chuanhua, Professor of Biostatistics and Doctoral Advisor is Deputy Dean at the School of Public Health, Wuhan University. He was a visiting scholar at the Department of Biostatistics, University of Washington (Seattle), postdoctoral fellow at Department of Medical Statistics, Sun Yat-Sen University. He got his Ph.D at Department of Health Statistics, Fourth Military Medical University; Master and undergraduate degree at School of Public Health, Tongji Medical University. He is a member of the Teaching Guidance Committee in Ministry of Education (Medical Humanities Quality); Committee Member of Chinese Health Information Society; Vice President of Health Statistics and Information Institute of Hubei Province; Editorial board of "Chinese Journal of Health Statistics", "Public Health and Preventive Medicine". He has published 30 books (including 8 chief editors) and more than 90 papers. His main research interests include the global burden of disease, diagnostic test evaluation, health services evaluation, and data mining and software development.

Zongli Xu works as a Staff Scientist at the National Institute of Health. Xu received a Ph.D. degree in statistical genetics at Sun Yat-Sen University, Guangzhou, China, in 2002. Xu's research involves both methodology and application studies in genetic epidemiology. Much of his methodological work is to develop bioinformatics methods and software tools to facilitate genetic epidemiology study. His applied work is mainly focused on human carcinogenesis. For the last few years, his emphasis has been on the role of epigenetics in cancer development.

Lu Tian obtained his Bachelor degree in Mathematics from Nankai University (1995); Master degree in Applied Mathematics from Nankai University (1998); Doctor of Science degree in Biostatistics from Harvard University (2002). His graduate study was supported by Howard Hughes Fellowship. He was awarded the Robert B. Reed Award for Excellence in Biostatistics at Harvard University. He worked at the Department of Preventive Medicine, Northwestern University (2004–2008) as Assistant Professor. He is currently Associate Professor at the Department of Health Research and Policy, Stanford University. He has rich experience in conducting statistical methodological research, planning large epidemiological studies, running data management for randomized clinical trials and conducting applied data analysis. His current research interest is in developing statistical methods in semiparametric regression modeling, survival analysis and high throughput data analysis.

Ying Lu, Ph.D., is a Professor of Biostatistics, Department of Health Research and Policy, Stanford University and Director of the Palo Alto VA Cooperative Studies Program Coordinating Center at Palo Alto Veterans Affairs Health Care System. He received his Bachelor of Science degree in Mathematics from Fudan University 1982, Master of Science degree in Applied Mathematics from Shanghai Jiao Tong University 1984, both in Shanghai, China, and Ph.D. in Biostatistics from the University of California, Berkeley, 1990, California, USA. After graduation, he worked as an assistant professor at the University Miami School of Medicine 1990–94, assistant, associate and full professor at the University of California, San Francisco, from 1994–2009, and professor in biostatistics at the Stanford University. Dr. Lu's research focuses on biostatistics methodology development and application to address clinical questions, in particular, in medical diagnosis, clinical trial design, and medical decision making. He is a fellow of American Statistical Association (2011) and president elect of the International Chinese Statistical Association 2013. Further information can be found from http://med.stanford.edu/profiles/Ying_Lu/.

CHAPTER 10

STATISTICAL MODELS AND METHODS IN INFECTIOUS DISEASES

HULIN WU

Department of Biostatistics and Computational Biology
University of Rochester School of Medicine and Dentistry
601 Elmwood Avenue, Box 630
Rochester, New York 14642, USA
Hulin_Wu@urmc.rochester.edu

SHOUJUN ZHAO

Department of Surgery Laurel Heights,
Suite 265 3333 California Street,
San Francisco, CA 94143, USA

1. Introduction

1.1. *Infectious diseases*

Infectious diseases are the illnesses caused by a specific infectious agent or its toxic products. Most of the agents are microorganisms, like bacteria, virus, parasites, etc. The transmission of the agent from an infected person, animal, or reservoir to a susceptible host, results in the infectious diseases of human, either directly or indirectly through an intermediate plant or animal host, vector, or the inanimate environment. For example, influenza, hepatitis, AIDS are caused by virus; dysentery, typhoid by bacteria; and schistosomiasis, filariasis by parasites.[1] Infectious diseases are also called communicable diseases.

Infectious disease was a great threat to human beings in the past. In this new century, understanding and controlling the spread of infections is still vitally important to public health. The challenging problems in studies of infectious diseases include: (i) how to evaluate the epidemics of an infectious disease in a population; (ii) how to understand the pathogenesis of infections and transmissions; (iii) if intervention measures such as drugs and therapies, and prevention measures such as education program and vaccines are developed, how to evaluate their effectiveness. Mathematics and statistics have played a central role in all these three aspects in the past decades. To accurately evaluate and project the epidemics of an infectious disease would help to determine the health care needs which is useful for the public health department or government to prepare and allocate the resources to fight the disease. It also signals a message on how serious a particular infectious disease is and draws public attention to the danger of the disease.

1.2. *Mathematical and statistical challenges from infectious diseases*

The application of mathematical methods to infectious diseases dates back to Daniel Bernoulli's paper in 1760[2] in which he used a mathematical model to evaluate the impact of smallpox on life expectancy. More analytical work has been done by Hamer[3] and Ross,[4] who tried to understand the mechanisms of disease transmission early of last century. Kermack and McKendrick[5] studied the mass action principle and threshold theorem originally proposed by Hamer and Ross respectively. The well-known chain binomial models of disease spread may be traced back to En'ko,[6] and a stochastic counterpart of chain binomial models was introduced by Greenwood.[7]

Throughout the last century, theory and quantitative techniques have been developed to study both the dynamics of disease within individuals and the transmission of infections through populations. Mathematics and statistics have played an important role in the studies of infectious diseases. In particular, over the last two decades, there has been a great deal of work on HIV/AIDS. Both mathematics and statistics have played and will continue to play an important role in epidemic studies as well as intervention and prevention studies of infectious diseases. A recent brief review on these methods can be found in Farrington,[8] Heesterbeek and Roberts,[9] and Gani.[10]

1.3. *Outline*

Many mathematicians and statisticians have responded to the challenges from infectious diseases in the past two centuries, and continue to meet the new challenges in this millennium.

In this chapter, we will first introduce the back-calculation method for a projection of epidemics proposed recently for estimating epidemics of AIDS, followed by models for natural history of infectious diseases. Deterministic and stochastic models as well as their recent developments are presented in Sec. 2. In Sec. 3, we introduce viral dynamic models which are heavily studied for understanding pathogenesis of HIV, HBV, and HCV infection during the last decade. We briefly review the mathematical and statistical methods for evaluation of intervention and prevention measures in infectious diseases in Sec. 4. We conclude the chapter with a brief summary.

2. Epidemic Models

2.1. *Estimation and projection of epidemics — Back-calculation*

Estimation and projection of epidemics, such as disease incidence and prevalence, are very important for intervention and prevention of infectious diseases. It is also critical for a government to make decisions and to prepare public health needs. Back-calculation or back-projection method has received tremendous attention in estimating and projecting AIDS epidemics in the past 15 years. In this section, we briefly introduce the back-calculation method and its applications.

Back-calculation is a method for estimating past infection rates of an infectious disease by working backward from observed disease incidence using knowledge of the incubation period between infection and disease. Although it can be used for any infectious disease in theory, it was first proposed to study AIDS epidemics by Brookmeyer and Gail.[11,12] It has since been widely used in AIDS epidemics.

The basic idea is to use the convolution equation of the expected cumulative number of disease cases diagnosed by time t, $A(t)$, the infection rate $g(s)$ at time s, and the incubation period distribution $F(t)$, i.e.

$$A(t) = \int_0^t g(s) \cdot F(t-s)ds\,. \tag{1}$$

If the disease cases $A(t)$ are known (may be obtained from case reports) and the incubation period distribution $F(t)$ can be estimated from epidemiological studies, the infection rate $g(s)$ then can be estimated by deconvolution of Eq. (1). If the infection rate $g(s)$ and incubation period distribution $F(t)$ are known, the disease cases can be estimated or projected using the convolution Eq. (1).

We introduce the back-calculation using a discrete-time formulation since it is more realistic. We assume that we have n non-overlapping time interval, (T_{j-1}, T_j), $j = 1, \ldots, n$; let Y_j be the number of disease cases diagnosed in the jth interval; denote f_{ij} as the probability of developing disease in time interval j given infection in interval i, or $f_{ij} = F(T_{j-i+1})$

$-F(T_{j-i})$ where $F(T_0) = 0$; let g_i denote the expected number of new infections in time interval i (infection rate). The discrete-time statistical convolution equation can be written as

$$\mathrm{E}(Y_j) = \sum_{i=1}^{j} g_i f_{ij}\,, \quad j = 1, \ldots, n\,. \tag{2}$$

Usually Y_j is assumed to follow a Poisson distribution. A Poisson regression analysis may be used to estimate parameters g_i while we regard f_{ij} as known covariates. The generalized linear model algorithms in the standard statistical packages such SAS or Splus can be used to fit the model. However, a difficulty with this is that the number of parameters equal the number of data points. This may result in an unstable estimate of g_i. To resolve this problem, one may model $g(s)$ parametrically or nonparametrically. The parametric models include damped exponential model, log-logistic model, logistic (prevalence) model, and piecewise constant step function model. For nonparametric modeling methods, smoothing spline, kernel method, and series-based splines can be used. More details can be found in the book (Chapter 8) by Brookmeyer and Gail.[13]

If we model g_i as a parametric function, say, $g_i = g(i, \boldsymbol{\beta})$, where $\boldsymbol{\beta}$ is a vector of parameters, the maximum likelihood method may be used to estimate the parameter vector $\boldsymbol{\beta}$ or the infection rate function $g_i = g(i, \boldsymbol{\beta})$. Assume that Y_j follows a nonhomogeneous Poisson process, the log-likelihood function of Y_j can be written as

$$L(\boldsymbol{Y}|\boldsymbol{\beta}) = \sum_{j=1}^{n} \left[Y_j \log \left(\sum_{i=1}^{j} g(i, \boldsymbol{\beta}) f_{ij} \right) - \sum_{i=1}^{j} g(i, \boldsymbol{\beta}) f_{ij} - \log Y_j! \right]. \tag{3}$$

The maximum likelihood estimate of $\boldsymbol{\beta}$ is obtained by maximizing $L(\boldsymbol{Y}|\boldsymbol{\beta})$ with respect of $\boldsymbol{\beta}$ using general numerical approaches such as the Newton-Raphson method or EM algorithm.[16] The variance of the estimate can be obtained using Fisher information or bootstrap method. As long as the infection rate function $g(i, \boldsymbol{\beta})$ is estimated, the number of infections and future disease cases can be estimated and projected.

The cumulative number of infections from time T_0 to time T_k can be estimated by

$$\hat{G}(T_k) = \int_{T_0}^{T_k} g(s, \hat{\boldsymbol{\beta}}) ds \quad \text{(continuous time)} \tag{4}$$

$$= \sum_{i=0}^{k} g(i, \hat{\boldsymbol{\beta}}) \qquad \text{(discrete time)} \tag{5}$$

The variance of this estimate can be obtained by the delta method or by bootstrap method. Also note that the infection prevalence is defined to be the number of infected individuals who are alive. Thus, the estimate of the infection prevalence is $\hat{G}(T_k) - D(T_k)$, where $D(T_k)$ is the cumulative number of deaths during the same time interval.

The projection of disease incidence in a future time interval $[T_{l-1}, T_l)$ is obtained by projecting forward the number of individuals infected prior to the current time T_n, i.e.

$$\hat{A}(T_l) - \hat{A}(T_{l-1})$$

$$= \int_{T_0}^{T_n} g(s, \hat{\boldsymbol{\beta}})[F(T_l - s) - F(T_{l-1} - s)]ds \quad \text{(continuous time)} \qquad (6)$$

$$= \sum_{i=0}^{n} g(i, \hat{\boldsymbol{\beta}}) f_{il} \quad \text{(discrete time)}. \qquad (7)$$

However, this estimate is a lower bound since it only considers the infected individuals prior to time T_n. To make an adjustment, the infections during time T_n and T_l need to be considered, that is, the following term needs to be added to the above projection,

$$\int_{T_n}^{T_l} g(s, \boldsymbol{\beta})[F(T_l - s) - F(T_{l-1} - s)]ds$$

in continuous time or

$$\sum_{i=n}^{l} g(i, \boldsymbol{\beta}) f_{il}$$

in discrete time. However, the future infection rate $g(s, \boldsymbol{\beta})$ or $g(i, \boldsymbol{\beta})$ is unknown. A guess or extrapolation of current infection rate is usually used.

A brief introduction on back-calculation can be found in Bacchetti[16] and a detailed description can be found in Brookmeyer and Gail.[13] Note that the above methods for projection of disease incidence or infection prevalence should be used with caution. There are many sources of uncertainty in back-calculation methods. The first is the uncertainty in the incubation period distribution. The estimate of the incubation period distribution may be subject to errors and uncertainty of the designed epidemiological studies. The sensitivity analysis is usually used to evaluate these uncertainties. More details on the incubation period distribution can be found in the book (Chapter 4) by Brookmeyer and Gail.[13] The projection is also sensitive to the assumption of infection rate models, especially for the unknown future infection rates. Thus, the model of $g(s)$ needs to be chosen with care. Another problem is the reported disease incidence data. Different countries have different reporting systems for infectious diseases. Some of them may not be reliable. Reporting delay or underreporting occurs frequently. Some formal methods have been developed to account for the reporting uncertainty, see Harris[14] and Lawless and Sun.[15] Also note that the effect of immigration and emigration from one community (country) to another community (country) is not considered in above projection models. In summary, the back-calculation method only provides a rough (a lower bound) estimate or prediction for the disease incidence or infection prevalence.

2.2. *Model the natural history*

The natural history of a disease is the evolution of a disease in the absence of medical intervention. Today, however, most diseases are treated after they are diagnosed. The term "clinical course" is usually used to describe the natural history of a disease that has been affected by intervention. A broader definition of the term "natural history" may also include clinical course.

The endpoints of a natural history study may be dichotomous outcomes (such as death, relapse of a tumor or acquisition of AIDS following HIV infection, etc.), time-to-event (such as time to a clinical outcome occurs), or a repeated biomarker (such as CD4+ cell counts or HIV RNA copies in AIDS patients). To study the relationship between these endpoints and prognostic factors, standard statistical methods may be used. For example, logistic regression or tree-structured regression methods (see related chapter of this book) may be used to study dichotomous outcome endpoints. These methods are pretty standard, we omit the details here. To study the survival endpoints, a Kaplan-Meier curve or a product-limit estimator (life table) is widely used to describe the natural history. The popular proportional hazards model or Cox regression model can be used to study the relationship between the survival endpoints and prognostic factors. Since neither the time of HIV infection nor the AIDS incidence can be observed exactly, the doubly censored or interval censored data need to be considered in this case. This problem motivated the development of new methods, see De Gruttola and Lagakos,[17] Kim *et al.*,,[18] Jewell *et al.*,[19] Jewell[20] and Sun.[21] The detailed survival analysis methods can be found in Chapter[28] of this book or in other textbooks. For repeated measurement endpoints, statistical methods for longitudinal data have been developed in the past two decades. A good survey of these methods can be found in the book by Diggle *et al.*,[22] and others. Modeling biomarkers of HIV/AIDS such as CD4+ cell counts and HIV RNA copies (viral load) have been paid special attention in the last decade. Many new models and methods have been developed. In the following, we briefly introduce several new models and methods, but refer the readers to the original papers for details. Standard longitudinal data analysis methods can also be found in related chapter of this book.

In the early stage of HIV/AIDS research, CD4+ T cell count is the most important biomarker to study natural history of HIV infection and evaluate the treatment effects. Recently HIV RNA copies (viral load) became the new focus in HIV/AIDS research. But the methodology in modeling CD4+ T cell counts can be adopted to model viral load with minor modifications.

De Gruttola, Lange and Dafni *et al.*[23] proposed a linear mixed-effect model with errors-in-variables to model CD4+ T cell trajectory, i.e.

$$\boldsymbol{y}_i = \boldsymbol{X}_i\boldsymbol{a} + \boldsymbol{Z}_i\boldsymbol{\beta}_i + \boldsymbol{\varepsilon}_i\,, \quad i = 1, \ldots, n\,, \tag{8}$$

where design matrices $\boldsymbol{X}_i$ and $\boldsymbol{Z}_i$ are subject to measurement error since they depend on observed time measurements, $\boldsymbol{a}$ is population parameter, and $\boldsymbol{\beta}_i$ is subject-specific random effects with an i.i.d. normal distribution and is independent from $\boldsymbol{\varepsilon}_i$ which also follows an i.i.d. normal distribution. Taylor *et al.*[24] considered a linear mixed-effect model with within-subject covariance specified as an OU stochastic process, i.e.

$$\boldsymbol{y}_i = \boldsymbol{X}_i\boldsymbol{a} + \boldsymbol{Z}_i\boldsymbol{\beta}_i + \boldsymbol{W}_i + \boldsymbol{\varepsilon}_i\,, \quad i = 1, \ldots, n\,, \tag{9}$$

where $\boldsymbol{W}_i$ is an OU process. They claimed that this model tracked CD4+ T cell data better compared to standard linear mixed-effect models.

To better track the nonlinearity of CD4+ T cells, some nonparametric and semiparametric models have been proposed. For example, Zeger and Diggle[25] introduced a semiparametric model,

$$Y_{ij} = \boldsymbol{x}_{ij}\boldsymbol{\beta} + \mu(t_{ij}) + \varepsilon_i(t_{ij})\,, \tag{10}$$

where $\boldsymbol{x}_{ij}$ is a covariate matrix (prognostic factors) and $\mu(t_{ij})$ is an unknown smooth function of t. They proposed a back-fitting algorithm to fit the model, i.e. estimating $\boldsymbol{\beta}$ and fitting $\mu(t_{ij})$ (using kernel or other nonparametric regression methods) iteratively. See Zeger and Diggle[25] for details.

Nonparametric mixed-effects models have been proposed to model CD4+ T cell courses.[26,27] The basic idea is to decompose a population (cohort) of CD4+ T cell curves into two parts, a population effect and a subject-specific random effect, $y_i(t) = f(t) + h_i(t) + \varepsilon_i(t)$, where $f(t)$ and $h_i(t)$ denote the population curve and the subject-specific random effect curve respectively, and both of them are assumed to be smooth functions of t. Cubic B-spline method was proposed to fit $f(t)$ and $h_i(t)$. Let $B(t)$ be a vector of a cubic B-spline basis. Assume $f(t) = \alpha B(t)$ and $h_i(t) = \gamma_i B(t)$, then the CD4+ T cell model can be written as

$$y_i(t) = \alpha B(t) + \gamma_i B(t) + \varepsilon_i(t) \,. \tag{11}$$

This is a standard linear mixed-effects model by treating $B(t)$ as covariates, and α and γ_i as fixed and random effects respectively. The existing statistical packages such as SAS procedure MIXED or Splus lme function can be used to fit this model. Standard inference procedures for linear mixed-effects models are also available. Similarly, Wang and Taylor[28] also proposed a piecewise cubic polynomial model for CD4+ T cell changes and used the model to conduct inferences such as treatment comparisons.

Recently more flexible models such as functional linear models or varying-coefficient models[29–32] have been proposed. The model can be written as

$$Y_i(t_{ij}) = \boldsymbol{X}_i^T(t_{ij})\boldsymbol{\beta}(t_{ij}) + \boldsymbol{e}_i(t_{ij}) \,, \tag{12}$$

where $\boldsymbol{\beta}(t_{ij})$ is a time-varying coefficient vector which is assumed to be a smooth function of t. Fan and Zhang[29,30] proposed a two-step procedure to fit the model. That is, for fixed time t, fit a standard linear regression model to obtain the raw estimates of $\boldsymbol{\beta}(t_{ij})$, and then smooth the raw estimates using one of the existing smoothing techniques. Hoover *et al.* and Wu *et al.*[31,32] proposed smoothing spline and local polynomials methods.

Hierarchical Bayes models have been introduced by Lange *et al.*[33] to model CD4+ T cell counts. This model is similar to a mixed-effects model, but in Bayes framework. De Gruttola and Tu[34] and Tsiatis *et al.*[35] also proposed a method for jointly modeling survival endpoints and longitudinal biomarkers. They modeled the longitudinal biomarkers (CD4+ T cell counts) as a linear mixed-effect model and model survival data using a standard Cox model, and then construct a joint log-likelihood function of these two models. Thus, the likelihood-based method can be applied to the models.

Although above models are developed to model CD4+ T cell counts in AIDS research, the methodology is generally applicable to other similar repeatedly measured biomarker data for other infectious diseases. However, in most countries, especially for developed countries such as United States, patients with infectious diseases such as HIV/AIDS are mostly under active treatments. How to model the natural history or clinical course of infectious diseases under effective treatments is a great challenge, since the treatment may affect the changes of biomarkers and disease progression dramatically. Also note that there are many resources of biases and uncertainties in natural history studies. For examples, sampling or selection bias in study subject selection process, follow-up length bias due to study length limitations and long latent period of some infectious diseases such as AIDS, drop-out or missing data bias when the drop-out or missing pattern is not random. Another problem is that the time zero of a natural history may not be well-defined and exactly observed in a study, for instance, the exact time of HIV infection is difficult to obtain for some cohorts. See more discussions in Cnaan.[36] In summary, a careful design of a natural history study is necessary to eliminate or reduce these biases.

2.3. *Deterministic models for epidemic transmission*

A standard deterministic model for epidemic transmission is a compartmental model. For example, a general susceptible-infection-removal (SIR) compartment model can be written as

$$\dot{S} = \mu - \beta SI - d_S S\,, \tag{13}$$

$$\dot{I} = \beta SI - rI - d_I I\,, \tag{14}$$

where S and I represent the proportions of susceptible and infectious subjects in the population, and $\dot{S}$ and $\dot{I}$ denote their derivatives respectively. Parameter μ denotes the birth rate of susceptible subjects per time unit and β represents the infection rate when S and I are randomly interacted (mixed). Parameters d_S and d_I denote the death rates of susceptible and infectious subjects, respectively, and r denotes the recovered (removal) rate of infectious subjects. The basic reproduction ratio is defined as

$$R_0 = \mu\beta/[d_S(r + d_I)]\,.$$

R_0 is an important summary measure of the infectiousness of a disease. This is the mean number of secondary cases generated by a single infective in a totally susceptible population. The higher the value of R_0, the more infectious the disease. If $R_0 \leq 1$, transmission of the infection cannot be sustained and will eventually die out.

If the infection has a latent stage with a proportion of E (during this stage, they are not infectious), a standard SEIR model is

$$\dot{S} = \mu - \beta SI - d_S S\,, \tag{15}$$

$$\dot{E} = \beta SI - \alpha E - d_E E\,, \tag{16}$$
$$\dot{I} = \alpha E - rI - d_I I\,, \tag{17}$$

where α is the transmission rate from latent to infectious, and d_E is the death rate of latently-infected subjects. For some infectious diseases, we may assume that $d_S = d_E = d_I = d$, but this may not be true in general. These compartment models are derived from a principle of mass action and homogeneously mixing pattern.

The age of subjects is another important factor in the epidemics of infectious diseases. The age-structured compartment model may be used to account for age effects. Here is a simple example,

$$\frac{\partial S}{\partial t} + \frac{\partial S}{\partial a} = \mu - \lambda S - d_S S\,, \tag{18}$$

$$\frac{\partial I}{\partial t} + \frac{\partial I}{\partial a} = \lambda S - rI - d_I I\,, \tag{19}$$

$$\frac{\partial R}{\partial t} + \frac{\partial R}{\partial a} = rI - d_R R\,, \tag{20}$$

where a is the age of subjects, R is the proportion of recovered (removal) of subjects in the population. Parameter λ is the so-called force of infection (age-specific hazard rate of infection) which is a function of time t, and can be defined by

$$\lambda(t) = \int_0^\infty k(a')I(t,a')da'\,,$$

where $k(a')$ is a kernel function. The partial differential equation system (18)–(20) can be solved numerically with appropriate initial conditions.

Note that the above models are very general for infectious diseases. But for a particular disease, these models may need to be modified to accommodate the special feature or characteristics of the disease. For example, HIV-infected patients cannot be cured or recovered from infection with current treatments, instead they may progress to AIDS or death. Thus, in the differential equation of infectious population (I), r is the rate of progression to AIDS. An additional equation of AIDS cases, $\dot{A} = rI - d_A A$, may be added.

Hepatitis B virus (HBV) infection is another example of infectious diseases with its transmission to be characterized by a model of five compartments. A community population can be divided into five compartments: (1) susceptible $S(a,t)$; (2) latent period (the time interval from infection to development of infectiousness), $L(a,t)$; (3) temporary HBV carriers, $T(a,t)$; (4) chronic HBV carriers $C(a,t)$; and (5) immune $I(a,t)$.[37,38] Here "a" represents the age and "t" represents the length of follow-up. Among the five stages, compartments 3 and 4 are infectious. In this model, birth rate is considered as a constant; age specific death rates are collected from death notification systems. The immune status is assumed to be life-long and newborns are assumed susceptible. For simplicity of modeling, the rare intrauterine HBV infection,[39,40] the short period of newborn maternal antibody and the sex differences ignored. The model parameters are defined as the following: $\lambda(a,t)$ is the force of infection; α is the rate of transition from latent period to temporary HBV viremia; $\beta(a)$ is the risk of transient viremia progressing to chronic HBV carriage; ε is the rate of transition from temporary HBV viremia to immune per time unit; $\nu(a)$ is the rate of HBV clearance in chronic HBV carriers; $\tau(a)$ is the mortality rate of HBV related diseases; $\mu(a)$ is the age-specific mortality rate of non HBV related diseases; $V_c(a,t)$ is the effectiveness of hepatitis B vaccine immunization. Then the age-structured compartment model for HBV can be written as,

$$\frac{\partial S(a,t)}{\partial a} + \frac{\partial S(a,t)}{\partial t} = [\lambda(a,t) + V_c(a,t) + \mu(a)]S(a,t)\,, \tag{21}$$

$$\frac{\partial L(a,t)}{\partial a} + \frac{\partial L(a,t)}{\partial t} = \lambda(a,t)S(a,t) - [\alpha + \mu(a)]L(a,t)\,, \tag{22}$$

$$\frac{\partial T(a,t)}{\partial a} + \frac{\partial T(a,t)}{\partial t} = \alpha L(a,t) - [\beta(a) + \varepsilon + \mu(a)]T(a,t)\,, \tag{23}$$

$$\frac{\partial C(a,t)}{\partial a} + \frac{\partial C(a,t)}{\partial t} = \beta(a)T(a,t) - [\nu(a) + \tau(a) + \mu(a)]C(a,t)\,, \tag{24}$$

$$\begin{aligned}\frac{\partial I(a,t)}{\partial a} + \frac{\partial I(a,t)}{\partial t} &= V_c(a,t)S(a,t) + \varepsilon T(a,t)\\ &\quad + \nu(a)C(a,t) - \mu(a)I(a,t)\,.\end{aligned} \tag{25}$$

After all the parameters were estimated from the data of epidemiological studies,[41–43] the probabilities or variables, $S(a,t), L(a,t), T(a,t), C(a,t)$ and $I(a,t)$ at age a and time t in the model can be calculated by the integral of the partial differential equations. These estimates can describe the dynamics of HBV transmission in the population at the pre-vaccination period or predict the trend with different vaccination coverage $V_c(a,t)$ in the population. Detailed information about HBV modeling and parameter estimation can be found in references.[44,45]

The deterministic models for other diseases such as Malaria and Helminths can be found in Heesterbeek and Roberts.[9] More details on deterministic compartment models can be found in the books by Bailey,[46] Becker,[47] Anderson and May[48] and Daley and Gani.[49]

2.4. *Stochastic models for epidemic transmission*

2.4.1. *Branching processes*

In the cases in which it is reasonable to assume an unlimited pool of susceptibles, for instance during the initial stage of an epidemic, a branching process can be used to model the spread of infection. Let Y_0 denote an initial number of infectives at generation 0. These Y_0 individuals infect Y_1 individuals as the next generation. In turn, these Y_1 individuals infect Y_2 individuals as the third generation, and so on. Let Z denote the number of infections directly caused by one individual, which is a random variable with a mean of μ, variance σ^2 and a probability density function of $g(z)$. Thus, for each i, $Y_i = Z_1 + \cdots + Z_{Y_{i-1}}$, where Z_j are independent variables with density $g(z)$.

Harris[50] proposed a nonparametric maximum likelihood estimator for μ:

$$\hat{\mu} = \sum_{i=1}^{k} Y_i \Big/ \sum_{i=1}^{k} Y_{i-1} \, .$$

The properties of this estimator are discussed by Keiding.[51] Becker[52] suggested an alternative estimator:

$$\hat{\mu} = \begin{cases} (Y_k/Y_0)^{1/k} & \text{if } Y_k > 0\,, \\ 1 & \text{if } Y_k = 0\,. \end{cases}$$

Note that the expected number of infections caused by one individual, μ, plays the same role as the basic reproduction ratio (R_0) in deterministic models. It can be shown that if $\mu \leq 1$, the process will become extinct with probability one.[50] Inferences for branching processes are usually conditional on extinction and non-extinction. Heyde[53] suggested a Bayesian approach which allows the extinction ($\mu \leq 1$) and non-extinction ($\mu > 1$) to be treated without distinction. Becker[47] gave several applications of branching processes to smallpox epidemics.

2.4.2. *Chain binomial models*

The branching process is unsuitable for the epidemics within small communities such as households. In this context, chain binomial models are more appropriate. The chain binomial model, or refer to the Reed-Frost epidemic model was introduced by the biostatistician Lowell J. Reed and the epidemiologist Wade Hampton Frost around 1930, as a teaching tool at Johns Hopkins University. Although they did not publish their results formally, their model was introduced in later publications.[54, 55]

Consider a fixed number of community (such as household, sexual partners, needle sharing group) with n individuals. At generation k there are X_k susceptibles exposed to Y_k infectives. The distribution of the number of infectives in the next generation, Y_{k+1}, conditional on X_k and Y_k, is binomial:

$$\Pr(Y_{k+1} = z | X_k = x, Y_k = y) = \frac{x!}{z!(x-z)!} p_k^z (1-p_k)^{x-z} ,$$

where p_k is the probability that a susceptible of generation k will acquire infection from one of the y_k infectives. The parameter p_k can be modeled under different assumptions. One assumption due to Reed and Frost[54] is that contacts with infectives occur independently, so that

$$p_k = 1 - (1-\pi)^{y_k} ,$$

where π is the probability of infection for the contact with the infectives. An alternative assumption, due to Greenwood,[7] is that the probability of infection does not depend on the number of infectives that the susceptible is exposed to, then

$$p_k = \begin{cases} \pi & \text{if } y_k > 1 , \\ 0 & \text{otherwise} . \end{cases}$$

Under this assumption, it is usually called the Greenwood chain binomial model. More complicated models for p_k can be developed for complicated transmission mechanisms such as HIV infection. Some other extensions to the Reed-Frost model can be found in Longini and Koopman.[56]

Inference for chain binomial models is usually based on likelihood methods. See Bailey,[46] Becker,[47] Longini and Koopman,[56] Longini *et al.*[57] and Saunders.[58] A brief introduction can be found in Longini.[59] For an updated review, see Becker and Britton.[60]

2.4.3. *Stochastic compartment models*

The stochastic version of the SIR model (13) is useful to capture stochastic features of epidemics in a small population or in the early stage of the epidemics. Consider $S(t)$ and $I(t)$ as the number (rather than the proportion) of susceptibles and infectives respectively. Then the transition probabilities in a short time interval $(t, t+\delta t)$ are

$$\Pr[S(t+\delta t) = S(t) - 1; I(t+\delta t) = I(t) + 1] = \beta S(t) I(t) \delta t\,, \tag{26}$$

$$\Pr[S(t+\delta t) = S(t); I(t+\delta t) = I(t) - 1] = (r + d_I) I(t) \delta t\,, \tag{27}$$

$$\Pr[S(t+\delta t) = S(t) + 1; I(t+\delta t) = I(t)] = \mu \delta t\,, \tag{28}$$

$$\Pr[S(t+\delta t) = S(t) - 1; I(t+\delta t) = I(t)] = d_S S(t) \delta t\,. \tag{29}$$

The solution of this stochastic systems is not straightforward. Monte Carlo methods may be used to solve it.[61–63]

Tan and Hsu[64] proposed a stochastic SEIR model (including a latent stage of infection) for AIDS epidemics. Recently, Wu and Tan[65] suggested a multiple stage stochastic model (the chain multinomial model) for AIDS epidemics in a homosexual population. Here we briefly introduce this model.

Let $S(t), I_r(t)$, and $A(t)$ denote the numbers of susceptible people, people at rth infection stage ($r = 1, 2, \ldots, k$) and people on set of AIDS at time t respectively. Then we are entertaining a $(k+2)$-dimensional discrete stochastic process $\boldsymbol{X}(t) = [S(t), I_1(t), I_2(t), \ldots, I_k(t), A(t)]^T$, where $[\cdot]^T$ denote the transpose of a vector or matrix. To formulate the dynamic model (the chain multinomial model) for this process, let $\alpha_S(t)$ denote the conditional probability of $S \to I_1$ given $\boldsymbol{X}(t)$ during $[t, t+1)$ and give the other notations of the transition probabilities and numbers of various transitions of the HIV epidemic in Table 1.

Table 1. Notation for transitions of the HIV epidemic in homosexual populations during $[t, t+1)$.

Transition	Transition probability	Transition numbers
Immigration $\longrightarrow S$	$\mu_S(t)$	$R_S(t)$
Immigration $\longrightarrow I_r$	$\mu_r(t)$	$R_{I_r}(t)$
$S \longrightarrow I_1$	$\alpha_S(t)$	$F_S(t)$
$I_r \longrightarrow I_{r+1},\ r = 1, 2, \ldots, k-1$	$\alpha_r(t)$	$F_{I_r}(t)$
$I_1 \longrightarrow S$	$\beta_1(t) = 0$	$B_{I_1}(t) = 0$
$I_r \longrightarrow I_{r-1},\ r = 2, 3, \ldots, k$	$\beta_r(t)$	$B_{I_r}(t)$
$A \longrightarrow I_k$	$\beta_{k+1}(t) = 0$	$B_A(t) = 0$
$I_r \longrightarrow A,\ r = 1, 2, \ldots, k$	$\omega_r(t)$	$A_{I_r}(t)$
$S \longrightarrow$ Death	$d_S(t)$	$D_S(t)$
$I_r \longrightarrow$ Death	$d_r(t)$	$D_{I_r}(t)$
$A \longrightarrow$ Death	$d_A(t)$	$D_A(t)$

By using the chain multinomial model, we obtain the following stochastic difference equations:

$$S(t+1) = R_S(t) + S(t) - F_S(t) - D_S(t)\,, \tag{30}$$

$$\begin{aligned} I_r(t+1) &= R_{I_r}(t) + F_{I_{r-1}}(t) + B_{I_{r+1}}(t) + I_r(t) \\ &\quad - [F_{I_r}(t) + B_{I_r} + A_{I_r}(t) + D_{I_r}(t)]\,, \end{aligned} \tag{31}$$

$$A(t+1) = \sum_{r=1}^{k} A_{I_r}(t) + A(t) - D_A(t)\,, \tag{32}$$

where $r = 1, 2, \ldots, k$, and $F_{I_0}(t) = F_S(t)$, $F_{I_k}(t) = 0$. The distributional properties of the quantities in the equations are listed as follows:

- $R_S(t) \sim$ Binomial $[S(t), \mu_S(t)]$, independent of $F_S(t)$ and $D_S(t)$.
- $[F_S(t), D_S(t)] | \boldsymbol{X}(t) \sim$ Multinomial $[S(t); \alpha_S(t), d_S(t)]$.
- $R_{I_r}(t) | I_r(t) \sim$ Binomial $[I_r(t); \mu_r(t)]$, independent of $F_{I_r}(t)$, $B_{I_r}(t)$, $A_{I_r}(t)$ and $D_{I_r}(t)$.
- $[F_{I_1}(t), A_{I_1}(t), D_{I_1}(t)] | \boldsymbol{X}(t) \sim$ Multinomial $[I_1(t); \alpha_1(t), \omega_1(t), d_1(t)]$.
- $[F_{I_r}(t), B_{I_r}(t), A_{I_r}(t), D_{I_r}(t)] | \boldsymbol{X}(t) \sim$ Multinomial $[I_r(t); \alpha_r(t), \beta_r(t), \omega_r(t), d_r(t)]$, for $r = 2, \ldots, k-1$.
- $[B_{I_k}(t), A_{I_k}(t), D_{I_k}(t)] | \boldsymbol{X}(t) \sim$ Multinomial $[I_k(t); \beta_k(t), \omega_k(t), d_k(t)]$.
- $D_A(t) | A(t) \sim$ Binomial $[A(t), d_A(t)]$.

Equations (30)–(32) provide an avenue for computing the probability distributions of $\boldsymbol{X}(t)$. Although the exact probability distributions of $\boldsymbol{X}(t)$ are quite complicated, one may use these equations to derive equations for the means, the variances and higher cumulants of $\boldsymbol{X}(t)$ as well as other results. Wu and Tan[65] also proposed using a state-space model to approximate the above stochastic model, and then Kalman filter can be used for estimation and projections. See Wu and Tan[65] for details.

3. Viral Dynamic Models

Recently great attention has been paid to modeling interaction and dynamics of virus and immune systems at cellular level within a host. It brought up a breakthrough in studying pathogenesis of HIV, HBV and HCV infections. In this section, we briefly introduce the basic models and their extensions, and summarize the important results obtained by applying these models to clinical data. Some statistical methods for parameter estimation will be briefly introduced.

3.1. *HIV dynamics*

Modeling HIV dynamics within a host can be traced back to 1980s.[66–68] In the early stage of HIV modeling, the focus was to understand the mechanism and pathogenesis of HIV infection and antiviral drug action using computer simulations based on the developed models. When the simplified version of the complicated simulation models were successfully applied to the clinical data in the last several years,[69–72] it led to a new understanding of the pathogenesis of HIV infection. Mathematical models and statistical methods played an important role in this breakthrough. Here we briefly introduce the models and the results.

In the seminar papers, Ho *et al.*[69] and Wei *et al.*[70] proposed simple compartment models (one or two compartments) for their clinical data of plasma HIV viral load (the number of RNA copies) in HIV-1-infected patients treated with potent antiviral agents. In Ho *et al.*,[69] a simple one-compartment model, $\frac{d}{dt}V = P - cV$, was proposed, where V denotes the concentration of virus (measured by the number of HIV RNA copies per *ml* plasma), P denotes the production rate of virus, and c denotes the clearance rate of virus. If we assume that the antiviral treatment is perfect, or $P = 0$ after initiation of a potent antiviral treatment, the solution to above ordinary differential equation is $V = V_0 e^{-ct}$, where V_0 is the initial viral concentration. When we have repeated measurements of V on individual patients, we can fit a nonlinear model, $Y(t) = V_0 e^{-ct} + \varepsilon$ or a linear model in a log scale, $Y(t) = \log(V_0) - ct + \varepsilon$, to obtain the parameter estimate of c. The mean life-span or half-life of HIV can be estimated by $1/c$ and $\ln 2/c$ respectively. Ho *et al.*[69] applied this simple method to 20 HIV-infected patients, and they obtained a half-life of HIV (in fact, it is the half-life of productively infected cells) that is 2.1 ± 0.4 days with a range of 1.3 to 3.3 days. Wei *et al.*[70] obtained similar results. This estimated rapid turnover rate of HIV virus (or infected cells) has important implications for HIV therapy and pathogenesis. One of the implications is that the rapid turnover of HIV may generate viral diversity and increase the opportunities for viral escape from antiviral agents. This motivated the idea of the therapy with combination of several antiviral agents (or so-called "cocktail" therapy).

To refine the estimate of viral replication, Perelson *et al.*[71] considered a more complicated compartment model when HIV infected patients are treated with more potent protease inhibitor (PI) antiviral agents. The mechanism of the PI drug antiviral action is to block the replication (generation) of infectious virus. Under the assumption of perfect PI drug treatment, the model can be written as

$$\frac{dT^*}{dt} = kV_I T - \delta T^* ,$$

$$\frac{dV_I}{dt} = -cV_I ,$$

$$\frac{dV_{NI}}{dt} = N\delta T^* - cV_{NI} ,$$

where T represents the concentration of uninfected CD4+ T cells; T^* denotes the concentration of productively infected T cells; V_I denotes the concentration of noninfectious virions; V_{NI} denotes the concentration of noninfectious virions; c denotes the clearance rate of virus; δ denotes the clearance rate of infected cells; k is the infection rate. A closed-form solution to above differential equations under the assumption of constant T (it is reasonable at initial stage of infection) can be obtained:

$$V(t) = V_I(t) + V_{NI}(t) = V_0 \exp(-ct) + \frac{cV_0}{c-\delta} \times \left\{ \frac{c}{c-\delta}[\exp(-\delta t) - \exp(-ct)] - \delta t \exp(-ct) \right\} .$$

When frequent repeated measurement data on $V(t)$ are available, a nonlinear model, $Y(t) = V(t) + \varepsilon$, can be fitted to obtain the estimates of important parameters such as clearance rate of virus (c) and infected cells (δ). Perelson *et al.*[71] applied this method to the data from 5 HIV infected individuals, and obtained a refined estimate of half-life of free HIV that is 0.24 ± 0.06 days (about 6 hours in average) which is much more rapid than the previous estimate in Ho *et al.*[69] and Wei *et al.*[70] The estimated half-life of infected cells is 1.55 ± 0.57 days.

Furthermore, Perelson *et al.*[72] developed a compartment model for the observed biphasic viral load data. They speculated that the first phase is due to viral replication from productively infected cells such as CD4+ T cells, and the second phase as latent or long-lived infected cells such as macrophages or dendritic cells. Based on clinical data, Perelson *et al.*[72] estimated that the half-life of short-lived productively infected cells is about 1.1 ± 0.4 days, for long-lived infected cells is 14.1 ± 7.5 days, and for latently infected cells is 8.5 ± 4.0 days. Using their model and the estimated results, they predicted that it might need 2.3–3.1 years to eliminate the HIV virus by the potent antiviral therapies, although later it was shown that this estimate was too optimistic.

Wu and Ding[73] recently proposed a unified approach for modeling observed HIV dynamic data. First Wu and Ding[73] proposed a comprehensive mathematical model for HIV dynamics considering all the potential cell and virus compartments: (1) uninfected target cells, such as T cells, macrophages, lymphoid mononuclear cells (MNCs), and tissue langerhans cells, which are possible targets of HIV-1 infection; (2) mysterious infected cells, cells other than T cells, such as tissue langerhans cells and microglial cells whose behavior is not completely known so far; (3) long-lived infected cells, such as macrophages, that are chronically infected and long-lived; (4) latently infected cells, infected cells that contain the provirus but are not producing virus immediately, and only start to produce virus when activated; (5) productively infected cells, infected cells which are actively producing virus; (6) infectious virus, virus that are functional and capable of infecting target cells; (7) noninfectious virus, virus that are dysfunctional and cannot infect target cells. We denote the concentration of the variety of these cells and virus by $T, T_m, T_s, T_l, T_p, V_I$, and V_{NI} respectively.

Without the intervention of antiviral treatment, the uninfected target cells may either decrease due to HIV infection or be in an equilibrium state due to the balancing between the regeneration and proliferation of uninfected target cells and HIV infection. Some uninfected target cells (T) are infected by infectious virus (V_I) and may become mysterious infected cells (T_m), long-lived infected cells (T_s), latently infected cells (T_l) or productively infected cells (T_p) with proportions of $\alpha_m kV_I, \alpha_s kV_I, \alpha_l kV_I$, and $\alpha_p kV_I$ respectively, where $\alpha_m + \alpha_s + \alpha_l + \alpha_p = 1$. The latently infected T cells may be stimulated to become productively infected cells with a rate of δ_l. The infected cells, T_m, T_s and T_p, are killed by HIV at the rates of δ_m, δ_s and δ_p respectively after producing an average of N virions per cell during their lifetimes. The infected cells, T_m, T_s and T_l may also die at the rates of μ_m, μ_s and μ_l respectively without producing virus. We assume that the proportion of noninfectious virus produced by infected cells is η without the intervention of protease inhibitor (PI) antiviral drugs. The elimination rates for infectious virus and noninfectious virus are assumed to be the same, say c.

We assume that the antiviral therapy consists of one or more protease inhibitor (PI) drugs and reverse transcriptase inhibitor (RTI) drugs. We model the effect of RTI drugs by reducing the infection rate from k_0 to $(1-\gamma)k_0$, where $0 \leq \gamma \leq 1$. Parameter γ reflects the RTI drug efficacy. If $\gamma = 0$, the RTI drugs have no effect; if $\gamma = 1$, the RTI drugs are perfect and completely block HIV infection. The PI drugs are assumed to be so potent that the production of infectious virions is almost blocked except for a small fraction. To account for some compartments where the PI drugs cannot reach and some persistent virus that the PI drugs cannot completely block the production, we consider an additional virus production term with a constant (average) rate, P, in the model. If only a small fraction of persistent virus can escape from the attack of PI drugs, it may be considered as a Poisson process, and thus also be modeled by a constant production in a deterministic model. Thus after initiation of combination treatment of PI and RTI drugs, the HIV dynamic model can be written as,

$$\begin{aligned}
\frac{d}{dt}T_m &= (1-\gamma)\alpha_m k_0 T V_I - \delta_m T_m - \mu_m T_m \,, \\
\frac{d}{dt}T_s &= (1-\gamma)\alpha_s k_0 T V_I - \delta_s T_s - \mu_s T_s \,, \\
\frac{d}{dt}T_l &= (1-\gamma)\alpha_l k_0 T V_I - \delta_l T_l - \mu_l T_l \,, \\
\frac{d}{dt}T_p &= (1-\gamma)\alpha_p k_0 T V_I + \delta_l T_l - \delta_p T_p \,, \\
\frac{d}{dt}V_I &= (1-\eta)P - cV_I \,, \\
\frac{d}{dt}V_{NI} &= \eta P + N\delta_m T_m + N\delta_s T_s + N\delta_p T_p - cV_{NI} \,.
\end{aligned} \tag{33}$$

where $\alpha_m + \alpha_s + \alpha_l + \alpha_p = 1$. Under the assumption of constant T and perfect treatments, then the system of Eq. (33) can be solved analytically and the final solution for the total virus $V = V_I + V_{NI}$ has a form of (see Appendix in Wu and Ding[73]),

$$\begin{aligned}
V(t) &= P_0 + P_1 e^{-\lambda_1 t} + P_2 e^{-\lambda_2 t} + P_3 e^{-\lambda_3 t} + P_4 e^{-\lambda_4 t} \\
&\quad + (P_5 + P_6 t)e^{-\lambda_5 t} + P_7 e^{-\lambda_6 t} + P_8 e^{-\lambda_7 t} \,,
\end{aligned} \tag{34}$$

where $P_i, i = 0, \ldots, 8$ are functions of model parameters and $\lambda_1 = \delta_p, \lambda_2 = \delta_m + \mu_m, \lambda_3 = \delta_s + \mu_s, \lambda_4 = \delta_l + \mu_l, \lambda_5 = c, \lambda_6 = r$, and $\lambda_7 = c + r$. At time $t = 0$, $V(0) = \sum_{i \neq 6} P_i$. Parameter P_i represents the initial viral production rate, and Parameter λ_i represents the exponential decay rate of virus due to the corresponding compartment. This model is too complicated (too many parameters) to be used in practice. Wu and Ding[73] suggested to use simplified version of the model based on available data. For example, if only the biphasic data are available, a bi-exponential model, $V(t) = P_1 e^{-\delta_p t} + P_2 e^{-\lambda_l t}$ or a one-exponential plus a constant model, $V(t) = P_0 + P_1 e^{-\delta_p t}$ may be used.[73] To fit the model with sparse individual data, Wu *et al.*[74] and Wu and Ding[73] also proposed using nonlinear mixed-effect model approach.[75,76] The two-stage nonlinear mixed-effect model is briefly introduced as follows.

Stage 1. Intra-patient variation in viral load measurement:

$$y_{ij} = \log(V(t_{ij}, \boldsymbol{\beta}_i)) + e_{ij}\,, \quad \boldsymbol{e}_i|\boldsymbol{\beta}_i \sim (\mathbf{0}, \mathbf{R}_\mathrm{i}(\boldsymbol{\beta}_\mathrm{i}, \boldsymbol{\xi}))\,, \tag{35}$$

where y_{ij} is the log-transform of the total viral load measurement for the ith patient and at the jth time point t_{ij}, $i = 1, \ldots, m; j = 1, \ldots, n_i$. The log-transformation of raw data is used to stabilize the variance (it is also more normally distributed). The function $V(t_{ij}, \boldsymbol{\beta}_i)$ is a nonlinear function of treatment time t which may be selected based on the available data and model assumptions. See Wu and Ding[73] for details.

Stage 2. Inter-patient variation:

$$\boldsymbol{\beta}_i = \boldsymbol{\beta} + \boldsymbol{b}_i\,. \tag{36}$$

Population parameters are $\boldsymbol{\beta}$, and random effects are $\boldsymbol{b}_i \sim (\mathbf{0}, \mathbf{D})$.

More detailed inferences regarding the nonlinear mixed-effect model can be found in the books by Davidian and Giltinan[75] and Vonesh and Chinchilli.[76]

A comparison for viral dynamic model-fitting procedures can be found in Ding and Wu.[77] Applications to more adult HIV-1 infected patients and pediatric patients can be found in Wu *et al.*[78] and Luzuriaga *et al.*[79] Recently, Ding and Wu[80] and others have suggested using viral dynamics (decay rates) to evaluate the potency of antiviral therapies. Statistical methods have been proposed to implement this idea by Ding and Wu.[81] Modeling drug resistance can be found in Nowak *et al.*[82] and others. For a good review of viral dynamic modeling and their extensions, see Perelson and Nelson[83] and Nowak and May.[84]

3.2. *Hepatitis virus dynamics*

Following the success of HIV dynamics modeling, similar studies have been done for hepatitis B and C virus (HBV and HCV). For example, Nowak *et al.*[85] proposed a simple compartment model for HBV dynamics. Let X, Y and V be uninfected cells, infected cells and free HBV virus respectively, then a mathematical model for HBV dynamics is

$$\dot{X} = \lambda - \beta X V - d_x X\,, \tag{37}$$

$$\dot{Y} = \beta XV - d_y Y\,, \tag{38}$$

$$\dot{V} = \alpha Y - d_v V\,, \tag{39}$$

where λ is the production rate of susceptible cells. Uninfected cells die at a rate of $d_x X$ and become infected at rate βXV. Infected cells are produced at rate βXV and die at rate $d_y Y$. Free virions are produced from infected cells at rate αY and are removed at rate $d_v V$. Nowak *et al.*[85] assumed that the potent treatment (the reverse transcriptase inhibitor, lamivudine) is perfect, i.e. $\alpha = \beta = 0$. Thus, $V(t) = V_0 \exp(-d_v t)$ and $Y(t) = Y_0 \exp(-d_y t)$. If the treatment is not perfect (more likely in reality), a model for free virion is $V(t) = V_0[1-r+r\exp(-d_v t)]$, where r is an efficacy parameter, which can be estimated from the viral load data. Nowak *et al.*[85] fitted a clinical data to these models, and found that the half-life of HBV free virions is about 1 day, the half-life of infected cells ranges from 10 to 100 days in different patients.

Many researchers have studied HCV dynamics using models similar to HBV under the antiviral treatment with Interferon-α.[86–90] The recent report from Neumann[90] showed that the half-life of HCV free virions was, on average, 2.7 hours, the half-life of infected cells was 1.7 to 70 days. All modeling techniques and statistical methods for HIV dynamics are applicable to both HBV and HCV with minor modifications.

4. Intervention and Prevention

Intervention and prevention measures are critical to stop the epidemic of infectious diseases. To evaluate the effectiveness of the intervention and prevention methods, clinical trials are usually conducted. Since other chapters have addressed the general methods of clinical trials, here we only emphasize some special features of clinical trials for infectious diseases, in particular, AIDS clinical trials.

4.1. *Medical intervention*

The general design of clinical trials can be found in clinical trial textbooks.[91–94] One of the most important issues in clinical trials is the selection of an endpoint which can be used to measure the effectiveness of interventions such as medical treatments.

In general, an endpoint of a clinical trial should possess the following properties: (i) relevant to the treatment effectiveness and easy to interpret; (ii) clinically apparent and easy to diagnose (or measure); (iii) sensitive to treatment differences. An earlier discussion on the choice of an endpoint for AIDS clinical trials can be found in Amato and Lagakos.[95] In the early stage of AIDS clinical trials (before 1994), the time to progression to AIDS or survival (time to death) was used. Since many different types of events or symptoms were defined as AIDS, the endpoints of progression to AIDS are often referred to as "combined endpoints". After reviewing and comparing the clinical data, Neaton *et al.*[96] recommended that the survival, instead of combined endpoints, be a preferred primary endpoint of antiviral trials. However, due to long incubation period of AIDS, the trial requires a long-term follow-up if the survival was used as the endpoint. Recently, surrogate markers such as viral load (HIV RNA copies) or CD4+ cell counts have been proposed and used as endpoints after validation of these markers (it is out of scope of this chapter to discuss how to validate a surrogate marker, see Prentice[97] for details).

The commonly used primary endpoints in recent AIDS clinical trials are viral load based endpoints which include: (i) the magnitude of reduction in viral load (HIV-1 RNA level) from baseline to a prespecified primary follow-up time (e.g. Week 24 or Week 48); (ii) the proportion of patients having viral load below the limit of quantification of the assay being used at the primary follow-up time; (iii) the durability based on the time-to-virologic-failure (the time until plasma viral load becomes detectable again). Marschner *et al.*[98] studied the first endpoint, the magnitude of reduction in viral load, and proposed statistical methods to deal with censored (below detection limit) viral load measurements. They argued that the dichotomous endpoint (the proportion of patients having viral load below the limit of detection) was more straightforward and less subject to bias than the analysis of the magnitude of viral load reduction. Standard methods of analysis for binary data would be appropriate. However, the dichotomous endpoint may lead to a lower power to detect the treatment difference than the endpoint of the actual magnitude of viral load change. By classifying virologic responses as either successes or failures, information is lost regarding the degree of virologic response. However, the endpoint based on the magnitude of viral load change involves complicated censored data problem due to the limit of detection of viral load assays, which may be subject to bias, see Marschner *et al.*[98] and Hughes.[99]

Gilbert *et al.*[100] studied the time-to-virologic-failure endpoints. They recommended the endpoint of time-to-virologic-failure from randomization due to its advantages in flexibility and sample size. They argued that the time-to-failure endpoint is generally more powerful than the binary endpoint, and it is flexible for evaluating covariate effects and for extending the study by prolonging the follow-up period. Also the interpretation of time-to-failure endpoint is more close to clinical practice than that of a binary endpoint, since physicians monitor viral load levels in patients over time for treatment managements.

Other endpoints such as the area under the curve (AUC) of viral load change, time-to-below-detection in viral load, and viral dynamic parameters (viral decay rates) were also suggested, but not widely used in large AIDS clinical trials. For the comparison of some of these endpoints, see Weinberg and Lagakos.[101] To evaluate the short-term potency of antiviral therapies using viral dynamic parameters, see Ding and Wu.[80,81]

Although the general clinical trial design methods can be used in most AIDS clinical studies, some new issues have arised from the complicated treatments for AIDS patients. See De Gruttola *et al.*[102] and Hughes[99] for some discussions on the design issues in AIDS clinical trials. Also note that the computer-assisted design techniques or clinical trial simulations (CTS)[103] may be useful for designing the complicated clinical trials.

Successful medical interventions will result in the change of epidemic patterns.[104–106] How to evaluate the epidemic trends under medical interventions is challenging. In this regards, computer simulations based on the epidemic models with considering treatment effects will be helpful.

Clinical studies on HBV and HCV are currently very active. HBV patients are treated with antiviral agents such as lamivudine and famciclovir,[85] and HCV patients are treated with interferon (IFN) and ribavirin therapy.[90] New anti-HBV and anti-HCV agents are under development, some of them are already in the stage of clinical trials. The methods for studying anti-HIV medical interventions are generally applicable to HBV and HCV.

4.2. *Prevention*

Preventive interventions are widely used to stop or reduce the epidemic of infectious diseases. Prevention measures include “lifestyle” maneuvers such as the change of social behavior to reduce the exposure risk to infectives, and modifications of sexual behavior for sexually transmitted infectious diseases via public education and advertisement. Another effective prevention measure is to prevent the infectious diseases by vaccination. To evaluate the effectiveness of these prevention measures is very challenging in terms of designing and implementing a prevention study due to the high cost and long-term follow-up.

4.2.1. *Prevention trials*

A prevention trial is different from standard randomized clinical trials. The goal of prevention trials for infectious diseases is to evaluate the effectiveness of prevention measures to protect individuals from infections. If the infection rate in a community or population is low for a particular infectious disease, a prevention trial generally needs a large sample size with tens of thousands of subjects. If it takes time for the prevention measures to start to work or for an individual to acquire the infection via exposure to infectives, it may require long duration such as several years of follow-up to evaluate the effectiveness of the prevention programs. Thus, the prevention study is logistically challenging with high cost.

Traditionally an observation study, for example, a cohort or community study, is employed to evaluate the prevention programs (historical control may be used in this case). When prevention measures are taken in a cohort or a community, the infection rate may be evaluated within a prespecified time period, and then compare this rate with a historical infection rate in this cohort or community. This kind of observational studies are subject to several problems such as within-subject variations, measurement errors, confounding factors, and adherence to prevention measures. For example, to evaluate the promotion of condom use and education of safe sexual practices among homosexual men community to prevent HIV infection, not all subjects in the study adhere to condom use during the study, and their sexual behavior may change during the study period (within-subject variation). Also the epidemics of an infectious disease under the prevention may confound with other factors. The causal inferences for epidemiologic associations with corresponding preventive strategies are also subject to measurement errors.

Ideally it is most effective and informative to conduct a randomized and controlled prevention trial to evaluate prevention programs. This would avoid the difficulties in observational studies. The study subjects may be selected from a high risk community of an infectious disease to reduce the sample size and the cost in a randomized prevention trial. For example, homosexual men, IV drug users, or sexual workers are high risk communities that are targeted for prevention from HIV infection. The design, conduct, monitoring, and analysis for randomized prevention trials are similar to standard therapeutic clinical trials. However, in some cases, it may not be ethical and practical to conduct a randomized prevention trial. For example, needle sharing is a confirmed cause of HIV infection among IV drug users and safe sex such as condom use may reduce the risk of sexually transmitted infectious diseases, so education or advertisements to the public promoting those messages is a good prevention measure. However, it is not ethical nor practical to randomize high-risk subjects into groups without access to education or advertisement on needle sharing risk and safe sex. For more discussion on prevention studies, see Prentice[107] and Jacobs.[108]

4.2.2. *Vaccine studies*

Vaccine studies are designed to evaluate different effects of vaccination during different stages of vaccine development. The major purpose of vaccines is to protect the vaccinated person against infection or reduce the severity or risk of disease progression after being infected. Successful vaccination can reduce person-to-person transmission and change the pattern of epidemics of an infectious disease within a population by reducing the infectiousness of an vaccinated person or by preventing individuals from infection. Thus, vaccination is an important intervention tool to the epidemics of infectious diseases and has great contributions to the public health.

It is important to understand the biological background of a vaccine in order to evaluate its efficacy. A vaccine is usually composed of an antigen and an adjuvant. The antigen contains either a piece of or the whole infectious agent in question and is the component of the vaccine that induces the immune response which is specific to the infectious agent. An adjuvant may increase the immunogenicity of the antigen. Thus, active immunization by vaccination does not prevent infection or disease, but the immune responses induced by vaccination interfere with infection or disease. For this reason, the efficacy of a vaccine also depends on the condition of the host's immune system. An important part of vaccine studies is evaluation of immunogenicity of the vaccine which is the ability of the vaccine to produce a measurable immune response in a host.

Three different types of population level effects of vaccination are identified. The indirect effects are the effects or benefits on those people not receiving the vaccine in the targeted population. The total effects in vaccinated individuals are the combination of the indirect effects with the individual-level effects of vaccination. Overall public health effect of the vaccination in the entire population of interest is a weighted average of the indirect effects on the unvaccinated people and the total effects on the vaccinated people. Vaccine studies can be used to evaluate the indirect, total, or overall effects of vaccination in a population. Note that safety is also an important aspect for evaluation of vaccines since vaccination can cause side effects due to the induction of the immune system.

A general definition of vaccine efficacy is the percentage reduction in the attack rate attributable to the vaccine, or

$$VE = \frac{p_u - p_v}{p_u} = 1 - \frac{p_v}{p_u} = 1 - \rho,$$

where p_u and p_v denote the risk of infection in unvaccinated and vaccinated individuals respectively, and $\rho = p_v/p_u$ is the relative risk of infection. Alternatively, the vaccine efficacy can be defined as the relative hazard of infection:

$$VE = 1 - \frac{\lambda_v}{\lambda_u},$$

where $p_u = 1 - \exp(-\lambda_u t), p_v = 1 - \exp(-\lambda_v t)$. Vaccine efficacy can also be defined based on the cumulative incidence rates (attack rates) at the end of a study,

$$VE = 1 - \frac{C_v}{C_u},$$

where $C_v q$ and C_u denote the cumulative incidence (infection) rates for vaccinated and unvaccinated individuals. To define the vaccine efficacy for infectiousness, we need to know the infection rate in exposures to vaccinated individuals (r_v) and unvaccinated individuals (r_u), then,

$$VE = 1 - \frac{r_v}{r_u}.$$

These definitions are used to evaluate vaccine efficacy in vaccine clinical trials and in the field. Vaccine efficacy can be estimated in a cohort study or a clinical trial involving n_v and n_u individuals in vaccinated and unvaccinated cohorts or groups respectively. Assume that r_v and r_u are the number of infection cases from vaccinated and unvaccinated cohorts, respectively, during a prespecified follow-up period, then the vaccine efficacy is estimated as

$$\widehat{VE} = 1 - \frac{r_v/n_v}{r_u/n_u}.$$

The vaccine efficacy can also be similarly estimated by a case-control study using the case-control study methodology. The screening method may also be used to estimate the vaccine efficacy in a population. Let θ denote the proportion of infection cases from vaccinated individuals, and let π as the proportion of the population vaccinated (known). The vaccine efficacy is estimated by

$$\widehat{VE} = 1 - \frac{\theta}{1-\theta}\frac{1-\pi}{\pi}.$$

In the screening method, the vaccination rate π is fixed and known, while θ is estimated. To investigate covariate effects, the generalized linear model such as logistic regression techniques can be used.

Vaccine development and studies can be divided into several phases. Phase 0 is the candidate vaccine development. In this early phase of vaccine development, the focus is the search for antigen candidates. A broad types of vaccine candidates may be investigated. Phase I is safety and immunogenicity testing in animals. In this phase, a study is designed to demonstrate the safety and immunogenicity of the vaccine candidate in animals. The question of whether the vaccine candidate is safe or effective in animals is a primary interest in the study. Usually the sample size of this kind of studies is small (only several animals involved). Thus the exact statistics such as Fisher's exact test are usually used for inferences Phase II is safety and immunogenicity testing in humans. Since infectious agents tend to be host-specific, and immune responses and the adverse reactions to a vaccine candidate may be different between animals and humans, safety and immunogenicity studies in humans are required before large-scale trials. Phase II trials may also try to determine dose levels and vaccination schedules. The sample size of Phase II vaccine trials can be very small or as large as several hundreds. Experimental challenges with infectious agents are usually not ethical in humans. The use of the immune response as a surrogate for protective immunity is still questionable since the correlation between the measurable immune response and the actual protection against infection or disease by the vaccine cannot be confirmed without investigation. Thus, it is a very difficult decision to move the vaccine study from Phase II to a large scale Phase III field efficacy testing. In fact, only a very small proportion of vaccine candidates move to Phase III studies, although sometimes a rare Phase IIb, a small field study, may be conducted.

The primary objective of Phase III field trials is to estimate the protective efficacy of vaccination, rather than to test whether there is an effect. Usually a randomized and double-blinded trial is ideal for a Phase III vaccine trial, but may be limited due to ethical or implemental problems. Since the number of infection cases depends on the exposure to infection and transmission rate (difficult to estimate), the sample size of Phase III trials is usually difficult to determine. A liberal strategy may be taken. Many vaccine trials have been inconclusive due to unpredicted transmission or exposure rate. If efficacy and safety of a vaccine is demonstrated in Phase III trials, the vaccine may be licensed by the responsible agency. However, the postlicensure Phase IV studies are still needed to evaluate: (i) protective efficacy under normal usage; (ii) safety under normal usage; (iii) duration of protection; and (iv) indirect and overall effects. Postlicensure studies are usually nonrandomized observational studies (subject to potential biases). Case-control studies are commonly used. Since Phase III efficacy trials are often too small to detect rare adverse events of vaccination, much larger postlicensure studies are very useful in this case. Thus, the design of a vaccine study depends on the scientific questions of interest and the phase of vaccine development. The corresponding statistical methods need to be selected for different studies.

The design of vaccine studies can be traced to early 19th century.[109] More detailed discussions can be found in Smith and Morrow[110] and Farrington and Miller.[111] Most materials of this section are taken from Halloran[112] and Farrington.[8]

4.2.3. *Mathematical modeling and simulations*

Prevention strategies or measures can be included in the deterministic or stochastic epidemic models of infectious diseases introduced in Sec. 2 of this chapter. Computer simulations may be used to evaluate or project how the pattern of epidemics will be changed by effective prevention strategies. Here we introduce an example of HBV infection with vaccine interventions.

The HBV model (21–25) introduced in Sec. 2 can be used to simulate the hepatitis B transmission dynamics before and after vaccination, so we utilize the models to predict the long-term effectiveness of hepatitis B immunization, and to describe the transmission dynamics of HBV in the population. The HBV carriers in a vaccinated cohort will decrease sharply. If all newborn babies can be immunized, the proportion of HBV carriage for immunized children will decrease to a very low level ($< 1\%$). Following up the immunization program with 100% coverage, the transmission dynamics of HBV carriers can be described by the model (21–25). The majority of HBV carriers will shift gradually from children to the elderly. After the vaccination program has been implemented for 70 years or more, the average HBV carrier rate will decrease to a lower level (Fig. 1).

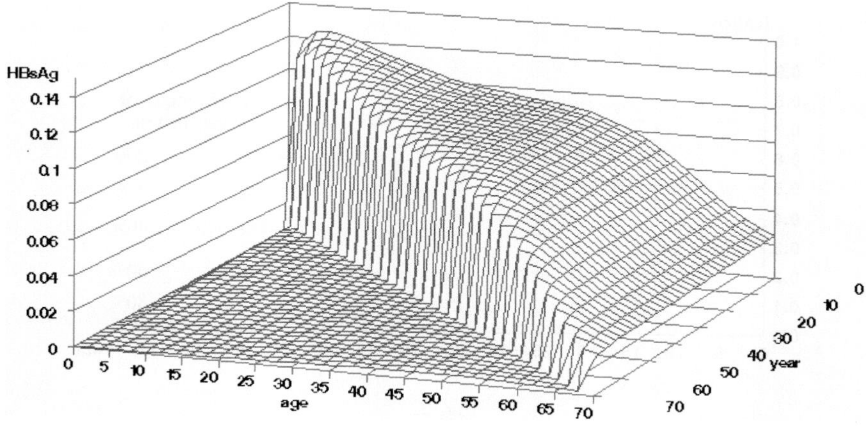

Fig. 1.

In order to evaluate the impact of the vaccination program on future incidence rate of hepatitis B, we can also define two incidence ratios: an acute hepatitis B and a chronic hepatitis B incidence ratio. Both of them can be calculated based on the dynamics of HBV carriers, that is, as a linear function of carrier proportion since vaccination implementation. The incidence ratio of acute hepatitis B, $R_a(a_1, a_2 : t)$ is the number of acute cases in the age range from a_1 to a_2 at time t divided by the corresponding number of acute cases at $t = 0$, the baseline before vaccination. Mathematically,

$$R_a(a_1, a_2 : t) = \int_{a_1}^{a_2} T(a, t)da \bigg/ \int_{a_1}^{a_2} T(a, 0)da\,.$$

The range in the equation has been defined as $a_1 = 10$ and $a_2 = 45$, because the peak of the incidence curve for acute hepatitis B was observed in the age interval of 10 to 45 years old. The incidences in other age groups are at very low levels. The $R_a(a_1, a_2 : t)$ at time t with different vaccination coverage is shown in Fig. 2. It decreases steeply at the beginning of the hepatitis B vaccination program. The higher the vaccination coverage, the steeper the decrease of the ratio. The decrease slows down in a few years after the start of the vaccination program.

The incidence ratio of chronic hepatitis B, $R_c(a_1, a_2 : t)$ is defined as the number of chronic HBV carriers in the age range from a_1 to a_2, at time t divided by the corresponding number of chronic HBV carriers at $t = 0$,

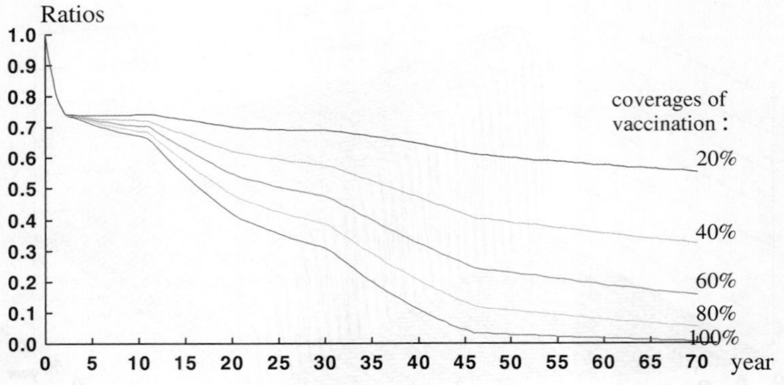

Fig. 2.

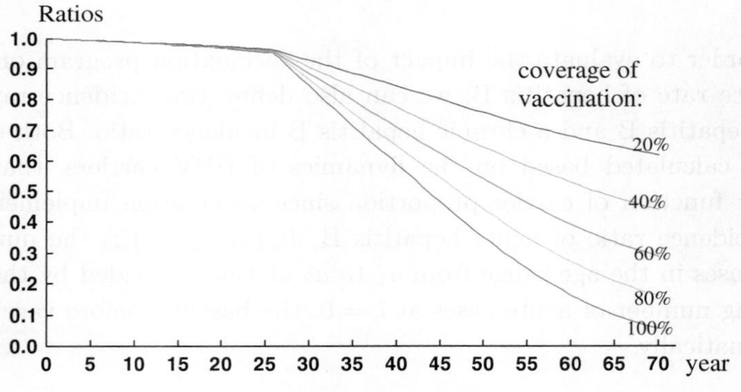

Fig. 3.

the baseline before vaccination. Mathematically

$$R_c(a_1, a_2 : t) = \int_{a_1}^{a_2} C(a,t)da \Big/ \int_{a_1}^{a_2} C(a,0)da\,.$$

In the equation, $a_1 = 25$ and $a_2 = 70$. Most of chronic liver diseases were observed in adults of 25 years and older. The disease incidence in the younger age group was negligible. The $R_c(a_1, a_2 : t)$, at time t with different vaccination coverage, is shown in Fig. 3. It remains almost unchanged at the beginning of the vaccination program, and drops rapidly after 25 years of immunization. Again, the decrease in the ratio is closely related to the vaccination coverage.

5. Summary

Infectious diseases are dangerous and threaten public health as a whole. To evaluate and project the epidemic of an infectious disease is a great challenge to biomathematicians and statisticians. Enormous efforts have been made in the past century. In this chapter, we have briefly reviewed the epidemic models and methods, especially for HIV and hepatitis viruses, the two most active research areas. Mathematics and statistics have contributed to understanding the pathogenesis of infectious diseases, particularly to understanding the mechanisms of HIV, HBV, and HCV infection in recent years via viral dynamics modeling. We have introduced these models and statistical methods. Statistics always plays an important role in evaluating interventions and preventions of any diseases via clinical trials. Motivated by clinical studies, many advanced statistical methods have been developed. For infectious diseases, statistics even plays more critical role in evaluating medical interventions, prevention measures and vaccine efficacy. Apparently, the study of HIV/AIDS has spurred the statistical research in infectious diseases in the past two decades. Brief reviews on statistical issues in HIV research can be found in an special issue of Journal of Royal Statistical Society A (Vol. 161, Part 2, 1998). A good review on the references can be found in Foulkes.[113]

Acknowledgment

The first author was supported by NIAID/NIH grants No. R29 AI43220, RO1 AI45356 and U01 AI38855.

References

1. Last, J. M. (1988). *A Dictionary of Epidemiology*, Oxford University Press, New York, 27.
2. Bernoulli, D. (1760). Essai d'une nouvelle analyse de la mortalite causee par la petite verole et des avantages de l'inoculation pour la prevenir. Memoires de Mathematiques et de Physique, in Histoire de l'Academie Royale des Sciences, Paris, 1–45.
3. Hamer, W. H. (1906). Epidemic disease in England: The evidence of variability and persistency. *Lancet* **ii**: 733–739.
4. Ross, R. (1911). *The Prevention of Malaria*, 2nd edn. John Murray, London.
5. Kermack, W. O. and McKendrick, A. G. (1927). A contribution to the mathematical theory of epidemics. *Proceedings of the Royal Society, Series* **A115**: 700–721.

6. En'ko, P. D. (1889). *The Epidemic Course of Some Infectious Diseases.* Vrach, St Petersburg, **10**: 1008–1010, 1039–1042, 1061–1063 (in Russian).
7. Greenwood, M. (1931). On the statistical measure of infectiousness. *Journal of Hygiene*, Cambridge, **31**: 336–351.
8. Farrington, C. P. (1998). Communicable diseases. In *Encyclopedia of Biostatistics*, Vol. 1, eds. P. Armitage and T. Colton, John Wiley and Sons, New York, 795–815.
9. Heesterbeek, J. A. P. and Roberts, M. G. (1998). Epidemic models, deterministic. In *Encyclopedia of Biostatistics*, Vol. 2, eds. P. Armitage and T. Colton, John Wiley and Sons, New York, 1332–1340.
10. Gani, J. (1998). Epidemic models, stochastic. In *Encyclopedia of Biostatistics*, Vol. 2, eds. P. Armitage and T. Colton, John Wiley and Sons, New York, 1345–1351.
11. Brookmeyer, R. and Gail, M. H. (1986). Minimum size of the acquired immunodeficiency syndrome (AIDS) epidemic in the United States. *Lancet* **2**: 1320–1322.
12. Brookmeyer, R and Gail, M. H. (1988). A method for obtaining short-term projections and lower bounds on the size of the AIDS epidemic. *Journal of the American Statistical Association* **83**: 301–308.
13. Brookmeyer, R. and Gail, M. H. (1994). *Journal of Acquired Immune Deficiency Syndromes Epidemiology*: *A Quantitative Approach.* Oxford University Press, New York.
14. Harris, J. E. (1990). Reporting delays and the incidence of AIDS. *Journal of the American Statistical Association* **85**: 915–924.
15. Lawless, J. and Sun, J. (1992). A comprehensive back-calculation framework for the estimation and prediction of AIDS cases. In *Journal of Acquired Immune Deficiency syndromes Epidemiology*: *Methodological Issues*, eds. N. Jewell, K. Dietz and C. Farewell, Birkhauser, Boston, 81–104.
16. Bacchetti, P. (1998). Back-calculation. In *Encyclopedia of Biostatistics*, Vol. 1, eds. P. Armitage and T. Colton, John Wiley and Sons, New York, 235–242.
17. De Gruttola, V. and Lagakos, S. W. (1989). Analysis of doubly-censored survival data, with application to AIDS. *Biometrics* **45**: 1–11.
18. Kim, M. Y., De Gruttola, V. and Lagakos, S. W. (1993). Analysis of doubly censored data with covariates; with application to AIDS. *Biometrics* **49**: 13–22.
19. Jewell, N. P., Malani, H. M. and Vittinghoff, E. (1994). Nonparametric estimation for a form of doubly censored data, with application to two problems in AIDS. *Journal of the American Statistical Association* **89**: 7–18.
20. Jewell, N. P. (1994). Nonparametric estimation and doubly-censored data: General ideas and applications to AIDS. *Statistics in Medicine* **13**: 2081–2096.
21. Sun, J. (1995). Empirical estimation of a distribution function with truncated and doubly interval-censored data and its application to AIDS studies. *Biometrics* **51**: 290–295.

22. Diggle, P. J, Liang, Ky. and Zeger, S. L. (1994). Analysis of Longitudinal Data, Oxford University Press, New York.
23. De Gruttola, V., Lange, N. and Dafni, U. (1991). Modeling the progression of HIV infection. *Journal of the American Statistical Association* **86**: 569–577.
24. Taylor, J. M. G., Cumberland, W. G. and Sy, J. P. (1994). A stochastic model for analysis of longitudinal AIDS data. *Journal of the American Statistical Association* **89**: 727–736.
25. Zeger, S. L. and Diggle, P. J. (1994). Semi-parametric models for longitudinal data with application to CD4 cell numbers in HIV seroconverters. *Biometrics* **50**: 689–699.
26. Shi, M., Weiss, R. E. and Taylor, J. M. G. (1996). An analysis of paediatric CD4 counts for Acquired Immune Deficiency Syndrome using flexible random curves. *Applied Statistics* **45**: 151–163.
27. Rice, J. A. and Wu, C. O. (2001). Nonparametric mixed effects models for unequally sampled noisy curves. *Biometrics* **57**: 253–259.
28. Wang, Y. and Taylor, J. M. G. (1995). Inference for smooth curves in longitudinal data with application to an AIDS clinical trial. *Statistics in Medicine* **14**: 1205–1218.
29. Fan, J. and Zhang, J. T. (1998). Comments on "smoothing spline models for the analysis of nested and crossed samples of curves" (by B. Brumback and J. A. Rice). *Journal of the American Statistical Association* **93**: 980–983.
30. Fan, J. and Zhang, J. T. (1999). Two-step estimation of functional linear models with application to longitudinal data. *Journal of the Royal Statistical Society, Series* **B62**: 303–322.
31. Hoover, D. R., Rice, J. A., Wu, C. O. and Yang, L. P. (1998). Nonparametric smoothing estimates of time-varying coefficient models with longitudinal data. *Biometrika* **85**: 809–822.
32. Wu, C. O., Chiang, C. T. and Hoover, D. R. (1998). Asymptotic confidence regions for kernel smoothing of a varying-coefficient model with longitudinal data. *Journal of the American Statistical Association* **93**: 1388–1402.
33. Lange, N., Carlin, B. P. and Gelfand, A. E. (1992). Hierarchical Bayes models for the progression of HIV infection using longitudinal CD4 T-cell numbers (with discussion). *Journal of the American Statistical Association* **87**: 615–632.
34. De Gruttola, V. and Tu, X. M. (1994). Modelling progression of CD4-lymphocyte count and its relationship to survival time. *Biometrics* **50**: 1003–1014.
35. Tsiatis, A. A., De Gruttola, V. and Wulfsohn, M. S. (1995). Modeling the relationship of survival to longitudinal data measured with error. Applications to survival and CD4 counts in patients with AIDS. *Journal of the American Statistical Association* **90**: 27–37.
36. Cnaan, A. (1998). Natural history study of prognosis. In *Encyclopedia of Biostatistics*, Vol. 4, eds. P. Armitage and T. Colton, John Wiley and Sons, New York, 2956–2962.

37. Xu, Z. Y. (1991). Impact and control of viral hepatitis in China. In *Viral Hepatitis and Liver Diseases*, eds. F. Blaine Hollinger, Williams and Wilkins, 700–706.
38. Szmuness, W. (1978). Sociodemograghic aspect of the epidemiology of HB. In *Viral Hepatitis.*, eds. G. N. Vyas, S. N. Cohen and R. Schmidt, Franklin Institute Press, Philadelphia, Pennsylvania, 296–320.
39. Tang, S. X. (1991). Study of the mechanisms and influential factors of intrauterine infection of hepatitis B virus. *Chinese Journal of Epidemiology* **12**(6): 325–328.
40. Wang, S. S. (1991). Transplacental transmission of hepatitis B virus. *Chinese Journal of Epidemiology* **12**(1): 33–35.
41. Zhao, S. J., Xu, Z. Y., Ma, J. C. *et al.* (1994). A follow up study of spontaneous clearance rates on hepatitis B surface agent persistent carriers. *Chinese Journal of Preventive Medicine* **29**(6): 378–379.
42. Zhao, S. J. and Xu, Z. Y. (1991). A study of hepatitis B infection force in China. *Chinese Journal of Epidemiology* **14**(suppl.): 70–74.
43. Zhao, S. J., Xu, Z. Y., Cao, H. L. *et al.* (1995). An estimating model of relationship between the infection age of hepatitis B virus and the age-specific chronic carrier rate. *Chinese Journal of Experimental and Clinical Virology* **9**(Suppl.): 101–104.
44. Zhao, S. J. and Xu, Z. Y. (1995). Mathematical simulation of hepatitis B transmission and application in immunization police. In *Proceeding of Epidemiology*, ed. X. W. Zhen, Beijing, **8**: 162–181.
45. Zhao, S., Xu, Z. Y. and Lu, Y. (2000). A mathematical model of hepatitis B virus transmission and its application for vaccination strategy in China. *International Journal of Epidemiology* **29**: 744–752.
46. Bailey, N. T. J. (1975). *The Mathematical Theory of Infectious Diseases and Its Applications*, 2nd edn., Griffin, London.
47. Becker, N. J. (1989). *Analysis of Infectious Disease Data*, Chapman and Hall, London.
48. Anderson, R. M. and May, R. M. (1991). *Infectious Diseases of Humans: Dynamics and Control*, Oxford University Press, Oxford.
49. Daley, D. J. and Gani, J. (1999). *Epidemic Modelling*, Cambridge University Press, Cambridge.
50. Harris, T. E. (1948). Branching processes. *Annals of Mathematical Statistics* **19**: 474–494.
51. Keiding, N. (1975). Estimation theory for branching processes. *Bulletin of the International Statistical Institute* **46**(4): 12–19.
52. Becker, N. (1977). Estimation for discrete time branching processes with applications to epidemics. *Biometrics* **33**: 515–522.
53. Heyde, C. C. (1979). On assessing the potential severity of an outbreak of a rare infectious disease: A Bayesian approach. *Australian Journal of Statistics* **21**: 282–292.
54. Frost, W. H. (1976). Some conceptions of epidemics in general. *American Journal of Epidemiology* **103**: 141–151.

55. Fine, P. (1977). A commentary on the mechanical analogue to the Reed-Frost epidemic model. *American Journal of Epidemiology* **106**: 87–100.
56. Longini, I. and Koopman, J. (1982). Household and community transmission parameters from final distributions of infections in households. *Biometrics* **38**: 115–126.
57. Longini, I., Koopman, J., Haber, M. and Otsonis, G. (1988). Statistical inference for infectious diseases: Risk-specified household and community transmission parameters. *American Journal of Epidemiology* **128**: 845–859.
58. Saunders, I. (1980). An approximate maximum likelihood estimator for chain binomial models. *Australian Journal of Statistics* **22**: 307–316.
59. Longini, I. (1998). Chain binomial model. In *Encyclopedia of Biostatistics*, Vol. 1, eds. P. Armitage and T. Colton, John Wiley and Sons, New York, 593–597.
60. Becker, N. G. and Britton, T. (1999). Statistical studies of infectious disease incidence. *Journal of the Royal Statistical Society, Series* **B61**: 287–307.
61. Bartlett, M. S. (1957). Measles periodicity and community size. *Journal of the Royal Statistical Society, Series* **A120**: 48–70.
62. Bartlett, M. S. (1960). The critical community size for measles in the United States. *Journal of the Royal Statistical Society, Series* **A123**: 37–44.
63. Tan, W. Y. and Wu, H. (1998). Stochastic modeling the dynamics of CD4+ T cell infection by HIV with Monte Carlo studies, *Mathematical Biosciences* **147**: 173–205.
64. Tan, W. Y. and Hsu, H. (1989). Some stochastic models of AIDS spread. *Statistics in Medicine* **8**: 121–136.
65. Wu, H. and Tan, W. Y. (2000). Modeling HIV epidemic: A state-space approach. *Mathematical and Computer Modelling* **32**: 197–215.
66. Merrill, S. (1987). AIDS: Background and the dynamics of the decline of immunocompetence. In *Theoretical Immunology*, Part 2, ed. A. S. Perelson, Addison-Wesley, Redwood City, Calif.
67. Anderson, R. M. and May, R. M. (1989). Complex dynamical behavior in the interaction between HIV and the immune system. In *Cell to Cell Signaling: From Experiments to Theoretical Models*, ed. A. Goldbeter, Academic, New York.
68. Perelson, A. S. (1989). Modeling the interaction of the immune system with HIV. In *Mathematical and Statistical Approaches to Journal of Acquired Immune Deficincy Syndromes Epidemiology* (Lect. Notes Biomath., Vol. 83), ed. C. Castillo-Chavez, Springer-Verlag, New York.
69. Ho, D. D., Neumann, A. U., Perelson, A. S., Chen, W., Leonard, J. M. and Markowitz, M. (1995). Rapid turnover of plasma virions and CD4 lymphocytes in HIV-1 infection. *Nature* **373**: 123–126.
70. Wei, X., Ghosh, S. K., Taylor, M. E., Johnson, V. A., Emini, E. A., Deutsch, P., Lifson, J. D., Bonhoeffer, S., Nowak, M. A., Hahn, B. H., Saag, M. S. and Shaw, G. M. (1995). Viral dynamics in human immunodeficiency virus type 1 infection. *Nature* **373**: 117–122.

71. Perelson, A. S., Neumann, A. U., Markowitz, M., Leonard, J. M. and Ho, D. D. (1996). HIV-1 dynamics *in vivo*: Virion clearance rate, infected cell life-span, and viral generation time. *Science* **271**: 1582–1586.
72. Perelson, A. S., Essunger, P., Cao, Y., Vesanen, M., Hurley, A., Saksela, K., Markowitz, M. and Ho, D. D. (1997). Decay characteristics of HIV-1-infected compartments during combination therapy. *Nature* **387**: 188–191.
73. Wu, H. and Ding, A. (1999). Population HIV-1 dynamics *in vivo*: Applicable models and inferential tools for virological data from AIDS clinical trials. *Biometrics* **55**: 410–418.
74. Wu, H., Ding, A. and De Gruttola, V. (1998). Estimation of HIV dynamic parameters, *Statistics in Medicine* **17**: 2463–2485.
75. Davidian, M. and Giltinan, D. M. (1995). *Nonlinear Models for Repeated Measurement Data*. Chapman and Hall, New York.
76. Vonesh, E. F. and Chinchilli, V. M. (1996). *Linear and Nonlinear Models for the Analysis of Repeated Measurements*, Marcel Dekker, New York.
77. Ding, A. A. and Wu, H. (2000). A comparison study of models and fitting procedures for biphasic viral dynamics in HIV-1 infected patients treated with antiviral therapies. *Biometrics* **56**: 16–23.
78. Wu, H., Kuritzkes, D. R., McClernon, D. R. *et al.* (1999). Characterization of viral dynamics in Human Immunodeficiency Virus Type 1-infected patients treated with combination antiretroviral therapy: Relationships to host factors, cellular restoration and virological endpoints. *Journal of Infectious Diseases* **179**(4): 799–807.
79. Luzuriaga, K., Wu, H., McManus, M. *et al.* (1999). Dynamics of HIV-1 replication in vertically-infected infants. *Journal of Virology* **73**: 362–367.
80. Ding, A. A. and Wu, H. (1999). Relationships between antiviral treatment effects and biphasic viral decay rates in modeling HIV dynamics. *Mathematical Biosciences* **160**: 63–82.
81. Ding, A. A. and Wu, H. (2001). Assessing antiviral potency of anti-HIV therapies *in vivo* by comparing viral decay rates in viral dynamic models. *Biostatistics* **2**: 13–29.
82. Nowak, M. A., Bonhoeffer, S., Shaw, G. M. and May, R. M. (1997). Antiviral drug treatment: Dynamics of resistance in free virus and infected cell populations. *Journal of Theoretical Biology* **184**: 203–217.
83. Perelson, A. S. and Nelson, P. W. (1999). Mathematical Analysis of HIV-1 dynamics *in vivo*. *SIAM Review* **41**(1): 3–44.
84. Nowak, M. A. and May, R. M. (2000). *Virus Dynamics*: *Mathematical Principles of Immunology and Virology*, Oxford University Press.
85. Nowak, M. A., Bonhoeffer, S., Hill, A. M. *et al.* (1996). Viral dynamics in hepatitis B virus infection. *Proceedings of National Academic Sciences* **93**: 4398–4402.
86. Fukumoto, T., Berg, T., Ku, Y. *et al.* (1996). Viral dynamics of hepatitis C early after orthotopic liver transplantation: Evidence for rapid turnover of serum virions. *Hepatology* **24**: 1351–1354.

87. Zeuzem, S., Schmidt, J. M., Lee, J. H. *et al.* (1996). Effect of interferon alfa on the dynamics of hepatitis C virus turn over *in vivo*. *Hepatology* **23**: 366–371.
88. Lam, N. P., Neumann, A. U., Gretch, D. R. *et al.* (1997). Dose-dependent acute clearance of hepatitis C genotype 1 virus with interferon alfa. *Hepatology* **26**: 226–231.
89. Yasui, K., Okanoue, T., Murakami, Y. *et al.* (1998). Dynamics of hepatitis C viremia following interferon-α administration. *The Journal of Infectious Diseases* **177**: 1475–1479.
90. Neumann, A. U., Lam, N. P., Dahari, H. *et al.* (1998). Hepatitis C viral dynamics *in vivo* and the antiviral efficacy of interferon-α therapy. *Science* **282**: 103–107.
91. Friedman, L. M., Furberg, C. D. and DeMets, D. L. (1981). *Fundamentals of Clinical Trials*, John Wright, PSG Inc.
92. Pocock, S. J. (1983). *Clinical Trials on Protocol Approach*, New York, Wiley.
93. Meinert, C. L. (1986). *Clinical Trials, Design, Conduct and Analysis*, Oxford, Oxford University Press.
94. Piantadosi, S. (1997). *Clinical Trials, A Methodologic Perspective*, New York, Wiley.
95. Amato, D. A. and Lagakos, S. W. (1990). Considerations in the selection of end points for AIDS clinical trials. *Journal of Acquired Immune Deficiency Syndromes* **3**(Suppl): S64–S68.
96. Neaton, J. D., Wentworth, D. N., Rhame, F. *et al.* (1994). Methods of studying interventions, Considerations in choice of a clinical endpoint for AIDS clinical trials. *Statistics in Medicine* **13**: 2107–2125.
97. Prentice, R. L. (1989). Surrogate endpoints in clinical trials: Definition and operational criteria. *Statistics in Medicine* **8**: 431–440.
98. Marschner, I. C., Betensky, R. A., De Gruttola, V. *et al.* (1999). Clinical trials using HIV-1 RNA-based primary endpoints: Statistical analysis and potential biases. *Journal of Acquired Immune Deficiency Syndromes and Human Retrovirology* **20**: 220–227.
99. Hughes, M. D. (2000). Analysis and design issues for studies using censored biomarker measurements, with an example of viral load measurements in HIV clinical trials. *Statistics in Medicine* **19**: 3171–3191.
100. Gilbert, P., Ribaudo, H. J., Greenberg, L. *et al.* (2000). Considerations in choosing a primary endpoint that measures durability of virologic suppression in an antiretroviral trial. *Journal of Acquired Immune Deficiency Syndromes* **14**: 1961–1972.
101. Weinberg, J. and Lagakos, S. W. (2001). Efficiency comparisons of rank and permutation tests based on summary statistics computed from repeated measures data. *Statistics in Medicine* **20**: 705–731.
102. De Gruttola, V., Hughes, M. D., Gilbert, P. and Phillips, A. (1998). Trial design in the era of highly effective antiviral drug combinations for HIV infection. *Journal of Acquired Immune Deficiency Syndromes* **12**: S149–S156.

103. Krall, R. L., Engleman, K. H., Ko, H. C. and Peck, C. C. (1998). Clinical trial modeling and simulation–work in progress. *Drug Information Journal* **32**: 971–976.
104. Mocroft, A., Vella, S., Benfield, T. L. *et al.* (1998). Changing patterns of mortality across Europe in patients infected with HIV-1. *Lancet* **352**: 1725–1730.
105. Palella, F. J., Jr, Delaney, K. M., Moorman, A. C. *et al.* (1998). Declining morbidity and mortality among patients with advanced human immunodeficiency virus infection. *New England Journal of Medicine* **338**: 853–860.
106. Vittinghoff, E., Scheer, S., O'Malley, P. *et al.* (1999). Combination antiretroviral therapy and recent declines in AIDS incidence and mortality, *Journal of Infectious Diseases* **179**: 717–720.
107. Prentice, R. L. (1998). Prevention trials. In *Encyclopedia of Biostatistics*, Vol. 4, eds. P. Armitage and T. Colton, John Wiley and Sons, New York, 3494–3499.
108. Jacobs, Jr., D. R. (1998). Preventive medicine. In *Encyclopedia of Biostatistics*, Vol. 4, eds. P. Armitage and T. Colton, John Wiley and Sons, New York, 3500–3502.
109. Greenwood, M. and Yule, U. G. (1915). The statistics of anti-typhoid and anti-cholera inoculations, and the interpretation of such statistics in general. *Proceedings of the Royal Society of Medicine* **8**: 113–194.
110. Smith, P. G. and Morrow, R. N. (1991). *Methods for Field Trials of Interventions Against Tropical Diseases*: *A Toolbox*, Oxford, Oxford University Press.
111. Farrington, P. and Miller, E. (1996). Clinical trials. In *Methods in Molecular Medicine*: *Vaccine Protocols*, eds. A. Robinson, G. Farrar and C. Wiblin, Totowa, Humana Press.
112. Halloran, M. E. (1998). Vaccine studies. In *Encyclopedia of Biostatistics*, Vol. 6, eds. P. Armitage and T. Colton, John Wiley and Sons, New York, 4687–4694.
113. Foulkes, M. A. (1998). Advances in HIV/AIDS statistical methodology over the past decade. *Statistics in Medicine* **17**: 1–25.

About the Authors

Dr. Hulin Wu obtained his Bachelor of Science and Master of Science degrees from Department of Automatic Control, National University of Defense Technology of China in 1984 and 1987 respectively. In 1989, he went to USA, and obtained his Ph.D. in Statistics from Florida State University in 1994. He was a visiting assistant professor at University of Memphis (USA) from 1994–1996. In 1996, he joined the Frontier Science & Technology Research Foundation and Center for Biostatistics in AIDS Research (CBAR) at Harvard School of Public Health as a senior statistician, and he headed the Pharmacology/Dynamic Modeling Section of the Center. He also held an adjunct faculty position at the Biostatistics Department of Harvard University. In 2003, Dr. Wu joined the Department of Biostatistics and Computational Biology, University of Rochester School of Medicine and Dentistry (UR-SMD) as a full professor. He is currently Dean's Professor of Biostatistics and Computational Biology, Professor of Medicine and Public Health Sciences at the UR-SMD. Dr. Wu founded the Division of Biomedical Modeling and Informatics, now expanded and evolved into the new Center for Integrative Bioinformatics and Experimental Mathematics (CIBEM) housing more than 30 multi-disciplinary investigators. He is Director/Co-PI for the NIH-funded Center for Biodefense Immune Modeling (CBIM) since 2005. As PI or Co-PI, Dr. Wu has received a total of more than $28 million funding from NIH to develop computational/mathematical models, statistical methods and bioinformatics tools for infectious diseases.

Shoujun Zhao studied medicine from 1977 to 1982, and obtained his Master degree in Biostatistics at Shanxi Medical College in 1986. He then received his PhD. degree of epidemiology from Shanghai Medical University in 1993, and worked there as an associate professor for three years. Dr Zhao participated in hepatitis A and B studies of Chinese National 8.5 and 9.5 Projects and received the prestigious China National Science and Technology Progress Award in 2000. Dr Zhao finished his post-doctoral training in Department of Radiology at the University of California, San Francisco in 2000. Since then, he has been working as a biostatistics specialist on medical research areas, including clinical trial design, data quality control, large scale medical database management and analysis. His main interests are in the areas of infectious disease transmission model, multivariate statistical mode application and diagnostic statistical methods.

CHAPTER 11

SPECIAL MODELS FOR SAMPLING SURVEY

SUJUAN GAO

Department of Biostatistics,
Indiana University School of Medicine,
410 West 10th Street, Suite 3000, Indianapolis,
IN 46202-2872, USA
Tel: (317)274-0820; sgao@iupui.edu

1. Introduction

Sample surveys have been widely used in everyday life and scientific research, from our attitude towards a specific television program to major economic indices. Sample surveys are broadly classified into two types — descriptive and analytical. In a descriptive survey the objective is simply to obtain information about large groups. For example, the total number of men, women and children living in a certain geographic area may be the objective of a descriptive survey. In an analytical survey, comparisons are made between different subgroups of the population in order to ascertain whether true differences exist among them and to verify hypotheses about the reasons for these differences. Sample surveys in medical research fields are mostly taken for analytical purposes. Early well-known surveys include the survey of the teeth of school children before and after fluoridation of water, of the death rates and causes of death of people who smoke different amounts, and the huge study on the effectiveness of the Salk polio vaccine.

Recent surveys in the medical fields, still analytical in nature, can be further divided into two categories. The first category is large scale surveys with the intent to make inference on a large population. These surveys are designed to derive reliable estimates on various health, nutrition, medical expenditure, etc. on a national level. Examples of surveys of this nature are the National Health and Nutrition Examination Survey (NHAINES), Survey of Asset and Health Dynamics of the Oldest Old (AHEAD), Health and Retirement Survey (HRS), National Long Term Care Survey, to name just a few. These surveys have elaborate sampling frames with oversampling of certain subgroups and extensive questionnaire containing a vast amount of information. They tend not to be disease specific, concerning instead about national trends on the general health of the entire population. The second category of medical surveys are community-based surveys, where a geographically defined catchment area is first defined and the survey is given to individuals selected from a sampling plan within this community only. Community-based surveys are usually focused on a specific disease, advantageous specifically on diseases that require extensive diagnosis, such as dementia and Alzheimer's disease. Community-based surveys offer the advantages of extensiveness on studying specific disease, but may suffer from limitations on the scope of populations they represent.

The basic steps and components of a survey are described in details in classical sample survey books such as Cochran (1977)[5] and Kish (1965).[15] We will review here some terminology central to the development in this chapter.

Population: The aggregate from which the sample is chosen. The population to be sampled (the *sampled population*) should coincide with the population about which information is desired (the *target population*). Sometimes, due to practical constraints, the sampled population is more restricted than the target population. It should be noted that the conclusion drawn from the samples under these situations should only apply to the sampled population. The extent to which the conclusion from the sampled population applies to the target population depends on a lot of additional information.

Sampling plan: The rule by which the samples are selected.

Sampling units: The parts the population is divided into and selection rules are based upon. They must cover the entire population without any overlap. Sometimes the choice of sampling units is obvious, as in a surveys of hospitals where each hospital constitutes a sampling unit. In other situations, there may be many possible choices of sampling units. For example, sampling of individuals in a city can be done by selecting the whole family, or selecting individuals living in a whole city block. The decision on which sampling unit to use is often based on an array of factors such as logistic, economic and convenience.

Sampling frame: The list containing all sampling units so that random selection from the population is accomplished by random sampling from the list. An ideal sampling frame should be complete containing every unit in the population and without any duplicates. The legitimacy of a survey often rests on how well the sampling frame is constructed to represent the population.

Simple random sampling: A method of selecting n units out of N such that every distinct sample has an equal chance of being drawn. Conventional statistical inference and software all apply to simple random sampling.

Stratified random sampling: In stratified random sampling, the population of N units is first divided into non-overlapping subpopulations of $N_1, \ldots, N_S$ units, respectively. These subpopulations are called *strata*. If a simple random sampling is taken within each stratum, the whole procedure is described as stratified random sampling. Stratification may produce a gain in precision in the estimates of characteristics of the whole population by creating relative homogeneity within each stratum.

Sample survey data differ from data collected from conventional observational studies in two fundamental ways. The first is that samples from surveys are usually selected with unequal probability, which if ignored may create a distorted picture of the target population. For example, if a health survey oversamples elderly individuals, the simple frequencies on diseases associated with increasing age are likely to overestimate disease rates in the population. The second difference between survey data and conventional studies is that survey data often present a natural clustering inherited from the sampling design. For example, if all family members in a selected household are interviewed in a survey, the outcomes on social-economical scales, behavior measures and attitudes are likely to be correlated.

A vast body of literature on methods of analyzing survey data exists, see, for example, Skinner, Holt and Smith[28] for review of earlier works in the area. The most used approach for analyzing survey data is the so-called pseudo-likelihood method where the score equation in a general likelihood framework is modified by including appropriate sampling weights. Variance estimation is achieved by taking the sample design into consideration and by using Taylor series linearization. Software packages implementing the pseudo-likelihood approach are also available, e.g. SUDAAN from the Research Triangle Institute[25] and WesVarPC from Westat.[22]

This chapter focuses on several special models used in analyzing survey data from epidemiological studies. First, we discuss the use of special models for estimating prevalence rate of a rare disease from community-based surveys, followed by a discussion about the use of random effect models for small area estimation on both continuous and discrete outcomes. The final section is devoted to capture–recapture models in epidemiology.

2. Models for the Estimation of Disease Prevalence

Disease prevalence is the percentage of individuals with a disease at the study time in a certain population. It describes the disease's effect on the population. Multi-phase samplings are often used in epidemiological studies where a disease is rare and diagnosis of the disease is expensive or difficult. The design has been used interchangeably with "multi-stage" sampling by medical researchers without distinction from multi-phase sampling. However, multi-stage sampling is a standard terminology from sampling theory which usually implies that different sampling units are used at various stages of sampling (for example, city blocks in the first stage, households in the second stage, and individuals in the third stage). We therefore prefer the term multi-phase sampling for the type of study where individuals are the sampling units in all sampling selections.

Two-phase sampling is by far the most often used design of all multiphase studies. In the first phase of the study a large random sample from the targete population is screened with less intensive and expensive screening tests for the disease. Based on the results of the screening tests, subjects are stratified and randomly selected within each stratum for extensive clinical evaluations at the second phase to determine disease status. The sampling plans are usually designed to identify as many diseased subjects as possible for risk factor studies and at the same time allow efficient estimation of disease prevalence for the population. The two-phase sampling design has been used to estimate the prevalence rates of Alzheimer's disease,[1] heart disease[4] and sexually transmitted disease.[31]

Data for our first example comes from the Indianapolis Study of Health and Aging, an on-going longitudinal study of dementia in elderly African Americans aged 65 and over living in Indianapolis, USA. Population-based two-phase surveys were conducted to estimate the prevalence rate of dementia in this population. At the first phase, 2212 individuals were randomly selected from the community and administered screening tests aimed at measuring their cognitive functions. Each individual received a cognitive score which ranged from 0 to 33. Based on the screening scores the subjects were grouped into three performance groups: good, intermediate and poor.

The initial sampling plan was to invite 100% of the subjects from the poor performance group, 50% from the intermediate group, 5% from the good performance group of which 75% should come from those older than 75 years of age. However, due to refusal, death, severe sickness and other reasons, the study had to sample more than the prespecified percentages in all groups except the poor performance group to achieve the targeted number of total clinical evaluations. The following table gives the number of demented subjects diagnosed from each of the sampling stratum by age group.

A weighting type estimator, also referred to as the direct standardization approach, is often used to estimate disease prevalence from a multi-phase sampling study. It assumes that subjects within each stratum are homogeneous and random sampling is used within each stratum. Suppose that in the first phase of the study N individual subjects are sampled by simple random sampling from the target population and information is collected from all N subjects on a set of characteristics X. X can be a vector containing several predictors, such as age, gender, screening scores, etc., that relate to the disease of interest. The N subjects are then divided into S strata, labeled as $I_1, \ldots, I_S$, based on the values of X. The total numbers of subjects in the respective strata are denoted by $N_1, \ldots, N_S$. In the second phase n_s subjects are sampled from the N_s subjects in the sth stratum using stratified random sampling. Disease status is ascertained on the selected n_s subjects only. Let y_{si} represents disease status on the ith subject from the sth stratum, with $y_{si} = 1$ denoting disease and $y_{si} = 0$ for non-disease. The probabilities for second phase sampling can be different for subjects from different strata. However, subjects from the same stratum are assumed to have equal probability of sampling.

The weighting type estimator of prevalence rate for a stratified random sampling is:

$$\hat{p}_{\text{wt}} = \frac{1}{N}\sum_{s=1}^{S}\sum_{i=1}^{n_s}\frac{N_s}{n_s}y_{si} = \sum_{s=1}^{S}\frac{N_s}{N}\hat{p}_s\,, \tag{1}$$

where $\hat{p}_s = \sum_{i=1}^{n_s}\frac{y_{si}}{n_s}$ is the average disease rate from the sth stratum. The variance of the estimator is estimated by

$$\text{var}(\hat{p}_{\text{wt}}) = \sum_{s=1}^{S}\hat{p}_s(1-\hat{p}_s)\frac{N_s^2}{N^2 n_s}\,. \tag{2}$$

Problems in the weighting type estimation approach can occur in groups with no affected individuals or no unaffected individuals ($\hat{p}_s = 0$ or $\hat{p}_s = 1$), or groups where no individual is sampled ($n_s = 0$). Prevalence estimate can be very unstable with possible variance 0 or infinity.

An alternative method of estimating disease prevalence from two-phase surveys is the modeling type estimator. A model is assumed for the population where the finite population is sampled from and smoothed estimates from the model are used to estimate disease prevalence. The modeling type estimator for binary data was first proposed by Roberts *et al.*[26] and used by Beckett *et al.*[1] to estimate the prevalence of Alzheimer's disease from two-phase surveys. The modeling type estimator is preferred in situations where the disease is rare and estimates from strata containing few or zero events are desired.

Let X_{si} be a set of covariates collected at the first phase. Therefore, X_{si} is available for all N subjects. Let $\text{Prob}(y_{si} = 1) = p_{si}$. A logistic regression model is assumed for the disease model:

$$\log \frac{p_{si}}{1 - p_{si}} = X_{si}\beta \,, \tag{3}$$

where β is a $p \times 1$ vector of parameter. If β is known, then the average of the predicted probability of disease from the model is an unbiased estimator of disease prevalence. In practice, one has to estimate β from the sample. A psudo-maximum likelihood estimate $\hat{\beta}$ is obtained using data from the second phase and estimate of disease prevalence is then obtained using the average predicted probabilities of disease on every subject in the population:

$$\hat{p}_{\text{model}} = \frac{1}{N} \sum_{s=1}^{S} \sum_{i=1}^{N_s} \frac{1}{1 + e^{-X_{si}\hat{\beta}}} \,. \tag{4}$$

The estimated variance of the prevalence estimate is

$$\text{var}(\hat{p}_{\text{model}}) = W'QXVX'Q'W \,, \tag{5}$$

where W is an $N \times 1$ vector with elements equal to $\frac{1}{N}$, Q is an $N \times N$ diagonal matrix with elements $\hat{p}_{si}(1 - \hat{p}_{si})$, X is the covariate matrix and V is the estimated variance covariance matrix of the logistic regression parameter β. Note that the above variance estimator assumes that X is fixed. Variance estimators accounting for the variability in X for survey data is given by Graubard and Korn.[9]

Prevalence estimates from the modeling approach can be more efficient than the weighting type estimate if the logistic model fits the data well. The weighting type estimates may mask trends in prevalence rates due to small sample sizes in some groups. Lastly, the weighting type estimator requires the assumption of missing completely at random while the modeling type estimator is unaffected under the missing at random mechanism (using the definitions of Little and Rubin[21]), provided that covariates related to missing data are incorporated in the model.[7]

We return now to the example data in Table 1. Prevalence estimates for the three age groups are desired. Note in age groups 65–74 and 85+, the first two sampling strata produced zero disease case, the weighting type estimator is expected to underestimate the true prevalence in these two age groups. Prevalence estimates for the three age groups using both the weighting type approach and the modeling estimator along with standard error estimates are included in Table 2.

It can be seen from Table 2 that the modeling type estimator yields larger prevalence estimates for two age groups whiles the estimates for age

Table 1. Number of demented subjects diagnosed from the three sampling groups in each age group. Data from the Indianapolis Study of Health and Aging.

Age Group	Performance Group	Number in Population	Number Sampled	Number with Dementia
65–74	1	1133	27	0
	2	77	34	0
	3	97	63	10
75–84	1	523	58	1
	2	69	35	5
	3	112	75	31
85+	1	127	14	0
	2	21	10	0
	3	53	37	18

Table 2. Estimated age-specific prevalence rates of dementia using the weighting method and the modeling method. Data from Indianapolis Study of Health and Aging.

	Weighting		Modeling	
Age Group	Rate	Std Err	Rate	Std Err
65–74	1.18	0.34	1.83	0.37
75–84	9.26	1.66	6.73	0.85
85+	12.83	2.17	17.07	2.31

group 75–84 is smaller than the weighting type estimates. A simulation study conducted by Beckett *et al.*[1] demonstrated that the modeling type estimator can increase the accuracy and efficiency of the rate estimates substantially if the model fits the data well.

In this section we are mainly concerned with estimating disease prevalence which is the mean of a binary variable. It should be noted that similar approaches exist in survey theory to estimate the means of continuous variables. For further details see the section on regression estimator in Cochran.[5]

3. Random Effect Models for Small Area Estimation

The terms "small area" were initially used to denote a small geographical area, such as a county, or a census division. They may also describe a "small domain" which is a small subpopulation such as a specific age-sex-race group of people within a large geographical area. Small area estimation arises usually from secondary analysis of large survey data, where the survey is designed to estimate the characteristics of a large domain. For example, in a national hospital cost survey, the sample selection is designed to estimate mean hospital cost with a desired precision at the national level. However, it may also be of interest to use the survey to derive hospital cost estimates by census region, or by state or county, possibly for the apportionment of government funds, and in regional and city planning. Direct estimates by region, state or county in this case based on only data from the small area are likely to yield unacceptably large standard errors due to the unduly small size of the sample in the area.

Suppose that the population is divided into k small areas, each contains N_i samples. n_i out of N_i units are sampled from the ith area. Y_{ij} denote the jth unit value in the ith small area. For convenience we let the first n_i units in Y_{ij} be sampled, and the remaining $N_i - n_i$ not sampled. In addition, we assume auxiliary information X_{ij} is available on *every* unit in the population. Alternative models can also be formed when X_{ij} is only available on the area-specific level. See Ghosh and Rao[8] for further details. The focus of inference is to estimate the small area mean $\bar{Y}_{i\cdot}$.

A conceptualized example is described here without direct reference to a specific survey or real data set. The example is in the context of a study by Taylor *et al.*[29] published in the *New England Journal of Medicine.* We have modified the setting so that the sampling units are hospitals instead of patients to make the inference straightforward. Taylor *et al.*[29] pointed out that it is important to study hospital cost and outcome and to investigate any differences among various hospitals. Suppose a national survey on hospital cost is conducted. The primary interest of the survey is to estimate the average hospital cost for various primary diagnoses such as hip fracture, stroke, coronary heart disease or congestive heart failure at the national level. Suppose we are also interested in using the survey data to provide average hospital cost estimates for the counties within a region. Suppose in addition, we have information on Medicare claim data for *all hospitals in the region* in the same time period of the survey. Medicare is a federal program that purchases inpatient services, primarily for persons 65 years and older, from various types of hospital. It is reasonable to assume that as the amount of Medicare claims increase, hospital cost is also likely to increase. For this hypothetical example, we will assume that there is no major systematic difference between the hospitals. In a real world situation, the type (teaching or non-teaching), size (numbers of bed) and location (urban or rural) of the hospital are all likely to affect hospital cost, as concluded in the article by Taylor *et al.*[29] A simulated data set for 114 hospitals in 16 small areas is generated using the equation:

$$y_{ij} = -2.0 + 0.2x_{ij} + \mu_i + e_{ij}\,,$$

where $\mu_i \sim N(0, 20)$, and $e_{ij} \sim N(0, 40)$. Thirty-eight hospitals are sampled using simple random sampling. The sampled data is presented in Table 3. For each county (small area), N_i represents the total number of hospitals in that county and n_i is the number of hospitals sampled in the survey. x_{ij} is the Medicare claim amount and y_{ij} is the true hospital cost.

A problem immediately seen with this data set, present also in many small area estimation situation, is that there are two counties without sampled hospital so that direct estimates from samples from those counties are not possible. Another problem is that some counties have a very small numbers of hospital sampled. Hence direct estimates for these counties may be unstable. We will describe three approaches commonly used for estimation from small area.

A synthetic estimator is similar in spirit to the ratio estimator in sample survey.[5] The estimator uses the percentage of $\frac{\bar{X}_i}{\bar{X}_.}$ in the estimate $\hat{\bar{Y}}_.$ of the overall mean as the estimate of the total in the ith area, where $\bar{X}_i = \frac{1}{N_i}\sum_{j=1}^{N_i} x_{ij}$, $\bar{X}_. = \frac{1}{N}\sum_{i=1}^{k} X_i$, and $\hat{\bar{Y}}_. = \frac{1}{n}\sum_{i=1}^{k}\sum_{j=1}^{n_i} y_{ij}$. The synthetic estimator of small area mean is given by:

$$\hat{\bar{Y}}_i(S) = \frac{\bar{X}_i}{\bar{X}_.}\hat{\bar{Y}}_.\,, \tag{6}$$

Table 3. Data from a simple random sample drawn from a synthetic population ($n = 38, N = 114$).

Area No.	N_i	n_i	x_{ij}	y_{ij}	Area No.	N_i	n_i	x_{ij}	y_{ij}
1	1	0	—	—	9	27	10	86.54	12.51
2	6	1	169.99	38.19				101.55	15.27
3	4	2	6.16	7.43	10	5	2	61.34	11.56
			30.09	10.42				102.77	17.62
4	1	0	—	—	11	12	4	61.49	7.02
5	8	2	94.60	20.52				99.77	27.09
			86.34	25.61				52.08	10.39
6	6	2	90.53	22.01				136.46	39.48
			86.34	25.61	12	7	3	92.28	9.53
7	6	2	95.10	22.52				93.73	9.43
			130.45	35.24				62.29	10.89
8	6	1	46.09	8.38	13	4	1	164.14	35.79
9	27	10	89.88	12.44	14	6	2	134.88	35.30
			145.68	26.23				164.94	40.81
			113.54	8.77	15	13	5	64.44	14.92
			114.54	17.98				63.51	9.07
			96.51	23.22				73.10	8.34
			84.58	9.41				109.66	10.35
			139.38	15.61				123.09	29.39
			117.24	34.42	16	2	1	186.16	28.08

The bias of the synthetic estimator is given by:

$$E(\hat{\bar{Y}}_i(S)) - \bar{Y}_i = \bar{X}_i \left(\frac{\bar{Y}_.}{\bar{X}_.} - \frac{\bar{Y}_i}{\bar{X}_i} \right).$$

It can be seen that the bias is not zero unless $\frac{\bar{Y}_.}{\bar{X}_.} = \frac{\bar{Y}_i}{\bar{X}_i}$. Under the assumption that the sample average $\bar{X}_i$ equals to the population average $\bar{X}_.$, the synthetic estimator will only be unbiased if each small area mean $\bar{Y}_i$ equals to the overall mean $\bar{Y}$. Such an assumption can be very strong and can produce biased estimates in situations when the assumption does not hold.

In an effort to reduce or balance the bias of the synthetic estimator a weighted estimator is proposed in the form of

$$\hat{\bar{Y}}_i(SD) = w_i \hat{\bar{Y}}_{1i} + (1 - w_i)\hat{\bar{Y}}_{2i}\,, \tag{7}$$

where $\hat{\bar{Y}}_{1i}$ is the direct estimator from the selected samples, $\hat{\bar{Y}}_{2i}$ is an indirect estimator and w_i is a pre-determined weight ($0 \leq w_i \leq 1$). An optimal weight may be obtained to minimize the mean squared error of $\hat{\hat{Y}}_i(SD)$. See Ghosh and Rao[8] for further details on obtaining the optimal weight. In practice a sample size dependent weight is chosen as $w_i = \frac{n_i N}{n N_i}$, where N and N_i are the total number of units and number of units in each small area in the population, respectively. n and n_i are the total selected sample size and the selected sample size in each small area, respectively. Therefore, the sample size dependent estimator can be written as:

$$\hat{\hat{Y}}_i(SD) = \begin{cases} \hat{\hat{Y}}_i\,, & \text{if } w_i \geq 1\,, \\ w_i\hat{\hat{Y}}_i + (1-w_i)\hat{\hat{Y}}_i(S)\,, & \text{if } w_i < 1\,, \end{cases} \tag{8}$$

where $\hat{\hat{Y}}_i(S)$ is the synthetic estimator.

In a random effect model approach the finite population containing N units is itself assumed to be random samples from an infinite population, the so-called superpopulation. The finite population is further assumed to have the following distribution:

$$y_{ij} = x_{ij}\beta + \nu_i + e_{ij}\,, \quad i = 1, \ldots, k\,, \quad j = 1, \ldots, N_i\,, \tag{9}$$

where x_{ij} is the value of the auxiliary variable, β is the parameter for the auxiliary effect. ν_i and e_{ij} are two independent random variables with

$$E(\nu_i) = 0\,, \quad V(\nu_i) = \sigma_\nu^2\,, \quad E(e_{ij}) = 0\,, \quad V(e_{ij}) = \sigma^2\,.$$

In addition, normality of the two random variables is assumed.

Using matrix notations, and an asterisk for the nonsampled elements, the above random effect model can be written as:

$$\begin{bmatrix} \mathbf{y}_i \\ \mathbf{y}_i^* \end{bmatrix} = \begin{bmatrix} \mathbf{X}_i \\ \mathbf{X}_i^* \end{bmatrix} \beta + \nu_i \begin{bmatrix} \mathbf{1}_i \\ \mathbf{1}_i^* \end{bmatrix} + \begin{bmatrix} \mathbf{e}_i \\ \mathbf{e}_i^* \end{bmatrix}, \tag{10}$$

where $\mathbf{y}_i = (y_{i1}, \ldots, y_{in_i})'$ represents the sampled units, and $\mathbf{y}_i^* = (y_{in_i+1}, \ldots, y_{iN_i})'$ the non-sampled ones. Other vectors in the equation are similarly defined.

The difference between the random effect model for sampling survey and the random effect models in classical statistics textbook is demonstrated by Eq. (10). A component of the outcome variable is unobserved because it is not sampled. Therefore, there are two steps in estimating the means of small areas. The first step involves estimating the parameters in the model, i.e. β, σ_ν^2 and σ^2, using the sampled data only. The second step uses the parameter estimates to predict $\mathbf{y}_i^*$.

Three estimation approaches exist for parameter estimation from the random effect model, namely, the best linear unbiased predictor approach (BLUP), the empirical Bayes approach (EB) and the hierarchical Bayes approach (HB). We will focus on the discussion of the BLUP and be brief on the EB and HB approaches. Interested readers can find a rather thorough review on all three approaches from Ghosh and Rao.[8]

For the estimation of parameters from the random effect model using sampled data only, we start with a more general mixed effect model:

$$\mathbf{y} = \mathbf{X}\boldsymbol{\beta} + \mathbf{Z}\boldsymbol{\nu} + \mathbf{e}\,, \tag{11}$$

where

$$E(\boldsymbol{\nu}) = 0\,, \quad V(\boldsymbol{\nu}) = \mathbf{G}\,, \quad E(\mathbf{e}) = 0\,, \quad V(\mathbf{e}) = \mathbf{R}\,,$$

and $\boldsymbol{\nu}$ and $\mathbf{e}$ are assumed to be independent of each other. Parameter estimates for $\boldsymbol{\beta}$ and $\boldsymbol{\nu}$ are obtained by solving the following equations simultanenously:

$$\begin{aligned} \mathbf{X}'\mathbf{R}^{-1}\mathbf{X}\boldsymbol{\beta} + \mathbf{X}'\mathbf{R}^{-1}\mathbf{Z}\boldsymbol{\nu} &= \mathbf{X}'\mathbf{R}^{-1}\boldsymbol{y} \\ \mathbf{Z}'\mathbf{R}^{-1}\mathbf{X}\boldsymbol{\beta} + (\mathbf{Z}'\mathbf{R}^{-1}\mathbf{Z} + \mathbf{G}^{-1})\boldsymbol{\nu} &= \mathbf{Z}'\mathbf{R}^{-1}\mathbf{y}\,, \end{aligned} \tag{12}$$

which can be expressed alternatively as:

$$\begin{aligned} \hat{\boldsymbol{\beta}} &= (\mathbf{X}'\mathbf{V}^{-1}\mathbf{X})^{-1}\mathbf{X}'\mathbf{V}^{-1}\mathbf{y} \\ \hat{\boldsymbol{\nu}} &= \mathbf{G}\mathbf{Z}\mathbf{V}^{-1}(\mathbf{y} - \mathbf{X}\hat{\boldsymbol{\beta}})\,, \end{aligned} \tag{13}$$

where $\mathbf{V} = \mathbf{Z}\mathbf{G}\mathbf{Z}' + \mathbf{R}$.

With the variance-covariance matrices $\mathbf{G}$ and $\mathbf{R}$ known, it is proved that $\hat{\beta}$ derived above is the best linear unbiased estimator and $\hat{\nu}$ is the best linear unbiased predictor in the measures of mean squared error.

In practice the variance-covariance matrices are unknown and have to be estimated from the data. Estimation of the variance-covariance matrix can be accomplished by using the restricted maximum likelihood (REML) approach proposed by Patterson and Thompson.[23] REML yields unbiased estimates of the variance covariance parameters for balanced designs. Technically, the optimality of the BLUP is lost when one uses estimated variance covariance matrices. However, such an approach coincides with the empirical Bayes approach with normal error assumption. Therefore, the empirical BLUP (EBLUP) and EB lead to identical estimates.

In the HB approach, a prior distribution on the model parameters is specified and the posterior distribution of the parameters of interest is then obtained. Inferences are based on the posterior distribution; in particular, a parameter of interest is estimated by its posterior mean and its precision is measured by its posterior variance.

The EBLUP approach is implemented by various statistical software packages. For example, SAS Proc MIXED derives parameter estimates and prediction using the EBLUP method. To illustrate the various approaches on small area estimation discussed in this section we use the synthetic population in Table 3. In Table 4 we compare the small area estimates of means derived by the synthetic estimator ($\hat{Y}_{\text{SYN}}$), the sample size dependent estimator ($\hat{Y}_{\text{SD}}$) and the empirical BLUP estimator ($\hat{Y}_{\text{EBLUP}}$) to the true small area mean ($\bar{Y}_i$). Note that the true means are available to us because the data is simulated. We also define two criteria for comparing the overall

Table 4. Small area estimates by the synthetic estimator ($\hat{Y}_{\text{SYN}}$), the sample size dependent estimator ($\hat{Y}_{\text{SD}}$) and the empirical best linear unbiased predictor estimator ($\hat{Y}_{\text{EBLUP}}$).

Area No.	N_i	n_i	$\bar{X}_i$	$\bar{Y}_i$	$\hat{Y}_{\text{SYN}}$	$\hat{Y}_{\text{SD}}$	$\hat{Y}_{\text{EBLUP}}$
1	1	0	137.70	32.68	26.93	26.93	28.41
2	6	1	106.18	24.12	20.76	29.48	22.53
3	4	2	23.38	4.64	4.57	8.92	6.67
4	1	0	45.64	4.12	8.93	8.93	8.97
5	8	2	102.08	21.08	19.96	22.05	20.77
6	6	2	77.96	22.53	15.25	23.81	18.21
7	6	2	125.81	28.36	24.60	28.88	28.28
8	6	1	79.80	13.50	15.61	11.99	16.00
9	27	10	104.06	17.33	20.35	17.59	17.60
10	5	2	84.57	13.41	16.54	14.59	16.33
11	12	4	93.84	19.43	18.35	20.99	21.03
12	7	3	85.55	15.12	16.73	9.95	13.85
13	4	1	120.90	23.79	23.64	32.75	25.33
14	6	2	177.58	38.00	34.73	38.06	39.77
15	13	5	94.96	12.92	18.57	14.41	17.31
16	2	1	123.30	21.01	24.11	28.08	22.59
Average relative error %					21.31	25.49	19.59
Average squared error:					13.46	16.98	7.10

performances of the estimators across all small areas.

$$\text{Average relative error} = \frac{1}{16}\sum_{i=1}^{16}\frac{|\hat{Y}_i - \bar{Y}_i|}{\bar{Y}_i},$$

$$\text{Average squared error} = \frac{1}{16}\sum_{i=1}^{16}(\hat{Y}_i - \bar{Y}_i)^2 .$$

These two criteria provide measures on the overall bias and efficiency of the various estimators. The EBLUP estimator is shown to perform the best in having the smallest average relative error and the smallest average squared error. The sample size dependent estimator failed to improve on the performance of the synthetic estimator, perhaps due to the use of a non-optimal weight.

So far we have discussed methods for small area estimation appropriate for a continuous outcome. Small area estimation for discrete outcomes such counts and proportions are often desired as well. Random-effect models can also be applied in these situations.

In the generalized linear model framework, the discrete outcome has its first two moments specified as:

$$E(y_{ij}|\nu_i) = h(x_{ij}\beta + \nu_i) = \mu_{ij}\,, \tag{14}$$

$$V(y_{ij}|\nu_i) = a_i\nu(\mu_{ij})\,, \tag{15}$$

where ν_i is assumed to be normally distributed with mean 0 and variance covariance matrix D.

There are two steps involved in small area estimation from discrete outcome, similar to the continuous variable case. In the first step we estimate the model parameters using the sampled data only. The second step involves prediction using the estimated model parameters and the auxiliary values for the non-sampled units in the population.

Several estimation approaches exist for parameter estimation from the generalized linear mixed model. The first approach is the full likelihood approach which requires the specification of the distributions of the random effects and often requires numerical integration of the likelihood function over the distribution of the random effect variables. To overcome these problems, Breslow and Clayton[3] proposed the penalized quasi-likelihood approach (PQL) where only the first two moments are specified and parameter estimation can be achieved using iterative weighted least square estimation. Raghunathan[24] proposed a quasi-empirical Bayes method for small area estimation on discreate outcomes.

We concentrate on a description of the PQL method, simply because it is implemented in some statistical software packages. For a detailed derivation of the PQL equations see Breslow and Clayton.[3] The PQL method requires iteratively solving the following equations:

$$\hat{\beta} = (\mathbf{X}'\mathbf{V}^{-1}\mathbf{X})^{-1}\mathbf{X}'\mathbf{V}^{-1}\mathbf{Y},$$
$$\hat{\nu} = \mathbf{D}\mathbf{V}^{-1}(\mathbf{Y} - \mathbf{X}\hat{\beta}), \tag{16}$$

where $\mathbf{V} = \mathbf{W}^{-1} + \mathbf{D}$, and $\mathbf{W}$ is a diagonal matrix with the elements:

$$w_{ij} = \frac{\text{var}(y_{ij}|\nu_i)}{g'(\mu_{ij})^2}$$

and $g(\mu_{ij}) = h^{-1}(x_{ij}\beta + \nu_i)$, and

$$Y_{ij} = x_{ij}\beta + \nu_i + (y_{ij} - h(x_{ij}\beta + \nu_i))g'(\mu_{ij}).$$

In the context of the previous example on a hospital survey, suppose we wish to estimate the average cancer-specific remission rate for each county. Such rates can be used in part to assess the quality of a hospital. We use the same setting as in the previous example and assume that the same 38 hospitals are randomly selected. A complete data set on all 114 hospitals is generated using a two-stage model:

$$E(y_{ij}) = m_{ij}\mu_{ij}, \quad \log\frac{\mu_{ij}}{1 - \mu_{ij}} = 0.2x_{ij} + \nu_i,$$

where $\nu_i \sim N(0, 0.9)$.

The synthetic samples are presented in Table 5. We are interested in estimating the average cancer remission rate for each county. In Table 6 we present the estimates of proportions obtained using the PQL method as implemented in the SAS Glimmix macro.[20] These estimates are compared with the direct estimates using data from each small area only. For counties without sampled hospitals, the overall mean is used as the estimate. The average relative error and the average squared error are defined in the same way as in the previous example and are included in the table. Although the PQL estimates show smaller overall bias than the direct estimates, it has a slightly larger average squared error than the direct estimates.

Raghunathan[24] demonstrated the quasi-empirical Bayes method on a data set to estimate county-specific mean number of hospital admission for cancer chemotherapy. A Poisson model for count data was assumed.

Table 5. Data from a simple random sample drawn from a synthetic population ($n = 38, N = 114$).

Area No.	N_i	n_i	$x_{ij} \times 100$	m_{ij}	y_{ij}	Area No.	N_i	n_i	$x_{ij} \times 100$	m_{ij}	y_{ij}
1	1	0	—	—	—	9	27	10	86.54	64	19
2	6	1	169.99	37	1				101.55	9	1
3	4	2	6.16	24	9	10	5	2	61.34	126	26
			30.09	3	1				102.77	10	2
4	1	0	—	—	—	11	12	4	61.49	3	1
5	8	2	94.60	52	26				99.77	57	24
			129.93	47	16				52.08	17	9
6	6	2	90.53	24	15				136.46	5	3
			86.34	22	13	12	7	3	92.28	1067	455
7	6	2	95.10	9	4				93.73	246	114
			130.45	72	37				62.29	8	2
8	6	1	46.09	37	7	13	4	1	164.14	25	6
9	27	10	89.88	3	1	14	6	2	134.88	64	32
			145.68	80	22				164.94	9	4
			113.54	246	58	15	13	5	64.44	94	12
			114.54	8	1				63.51	40	5
			96.51	25	7				73.10	3	0
			84.58	340	73				109.66	57	1
			139.38	390	87				123.09	3	1
			117.24	24	7	16	2	1	186.16	45	19

We want to conclude this section by pointing out that the random effect model approach we described here is a general approach in modeling sampling data in that each small area mean is itself assumed to be random variables following certain distributions. Parameter estimation is always a concern because the estimates directly contribute to the prediction of the non-sampled units. Noted that we might appear biased in choosing to present in more details the techniques that are implemented in computer software packages. The emphasis simply reflects the convenience in deriving estimates for our example data. It does not, however, reflect the superiority of performances of the estimation approaches we presented. In fact many approaches for the discrete outcomes have yet to be compared in a well designed simulation study. Therefore, readers are advised to keep an open mind on estimation techniques when applying random effect models themselves and when more results on comparing various estimation methods are available.

Table 6. Small area estimates of proportions (in %) by raw proportion and by the PQL method. $\bar{Y}_i$ is the true population rate for each small area.

Area No.	N_i	n_i	$\bar{X}_i \times 100$	$\bar{Y}_i$	$\hat{Y}_{\text{raw}}$	$\hat{Y}_{\text{PQL}}$
1	1	0	137.70	30.00	33.55	35.43
2	6	1	106.18	44.30	51.35	48.88
3	4	2	23.38	37.66	37.04	36.70
4	1	0	45.64	40.38	33.55	35.28
5	8	2	102.08	36.93	42.42	41.97
6	6	2	77.96	68.47	60.87	57.74
7	6	2	125.81	47.39	50.62	49.50
8	6	1	79.80	18.16	18.92	21.80
9	27	10	104.06	23.15	23.21	23.28
10	5	2	84.57	21.70	20.59	21.41
11	12	4	93.84	45.78	45.12	44.41
12	7	3	85.55	42.98	43.22	43.17
13	4	1	120.90	20.60	24.00	26.54
14	6	2	177.58	43.70	49.32	48.26
15	13	5	94.96	11.45	9.64	10.85
16	2	1	123.30	42.29	42.22	41.26
Average relative error %					6.89	6.71
Average squared error:					0.0011	0.0013

4. Capture–Recapture Models

The use of capture–recapture models in epidemiology is generally different from the sampling surveys we discussed so far in the previous two sections. Capture–recapture setting usually works with several sampling frames, instead of just one in conventional surveys. Capture–recapture model concentrates on matching individuals identified by different sources rather than sampling selection from one sampling frame. However, capture–recapture model does share a common goal with some sample surveys in that it also focuses on the estimation of the size of a population.

As an alternative to the community survey we introduced in Sec. 2, capture–recapture systems can be thought as multiple surveys on the same population trying to estimate the same quantity. This is especially useful when there does not exist one complete sampling frame from which a conventional sample survey can be established to reliably estimate population characteristics.

Capture–recapture methods have a long history. They were first introduced in the study of fish and wildlife populations before being adopted for other populations. In animal studies, the animals being captured by the first attempt will be marked and returned to wildlife. This allows cross-classify the animals captured by various attempts. Hence the name capture–recapture. Various authors have argued against the use of capture–recapture model for human population on the bases that the various capture attempts of humans are usually not random.[2,11] In epidemiological studies, hospital records, doctors' medical files, and medical prescription lists are examples of various sources to locate individuals with certain diseases. Each of these sources is incomplete by their true nature, and the problem is to estimate those missing from all sources.

The simplest capture–recapture model is the so called two-source model used to estimate the unknown size of the population. The first sample provides the individuals for *marking* and the second sample provides the recapture.

We begin with two source model having sources A and B. Let n_{11}, n_{10}, n_{01} and n_{00} be the numbers of individuals captured by both sources (n_{11}), by source A only (n_{10}), by source B only (n_{01}), and by neither source (n_{00}). Note that n_{00} is unobservable. By estimating n_{00}, the number of cases missing by both sources, we provide an estimate of the number of cases in the population. The layout of a two source capture–recapture setting is illustrated in Table 7.

Four assumptions are implicitly made on capture–recapture analysis:

(1) There is no change to the population during the investigation. Such a population is usually called a *closed* population.
(2) Individuals can be matched from sources A to source B.
(3) In each source each individual has the same chance of being included in the sample.

Table 7. Layout of a two source capture–recapture setting.

		Source B	
		Yes	No
Source A	Yes	n_{11}	n_{10}
	No	n_{01}	n_{00}

(4) The two sources are independent meaning a "Yes" from source A does not affect the chance of a "Yes" from source B.

In epidemiological studies assumptions 1 and 2 can generally be assumed true. However, assumptions 3 and 4 present the biggest problem and have been the subject of debate since the application of capture–recapture model in epidemiological fields. Human subjects are known to be heterogeneous with regard to being "caught" by a specific source. Methods to incorporate covariate in the method are becoming available. Tilling and Sterne[30] gave the latest development including a review of previous work. Assumption 4 is invariably false and is perceived as the biggest weakness on the use of capture–recapture models in epidemiology. Humans are not fish where the chance of being recaptured is truly independent of whether they have been marked. For example, if certain doctors refer their patients to certain hospitals, then hospital records and doctors' records will not be two independent sources. Fienberg[6] approached the interdependence among sources of capture using log-linear model framework. We will focus our presentation using this approach.

Depending on the ways of parametrization, a 2×2 contingency table can be represented by the following log-linear models:

$$\begin{aligned} \log E(n_{11}) &= \mu \\ \log E(n_{01}) &= \mu + \mu_A \\ \log E(n_{10}) &= \mu + \mu_B \\ \log E(n_{00}) &= \mu + \mu_A + \mu_B + \mu_{AB} \,. \end{aligned} \tag{17}$$

The parameters on the right hand side of the above equations represent the logarithm of the number expected for each cell. Notice that there are four parameters in the log-linear models but only three known quantities to use for the estimation. One parameter is unestimatable. The customary solution is to assume $\mu_{AB} = 0$ which is equivalent of assumption 4. Hence n_{00} can be estimated by its expected value under the log-linear models:

$$\hat{n}_{00} = e^{\hat{\mu}+\hat{\mu}_A+\hat{\mu}_B} = e^{\log n_{11} + \log \frac{n_{10}}{n_{11}} + \log \frac{n_{01}}{n_{11}}} = \frac{n_{10}n_{01}}{n_{11}} \,. \tag{18}$$

The estimate of the total sample size is:

$$\hat{N} = n_{11} + n_{10} + n_{01} + \hat{n}_{00} = n_{11} + n_{10} + n_{01} + \frac{n_{10}n_{01}}{n_{11}} \,. \tag{19}$$

An example was taken from Bruno[2] and modified for presentation here. Four sources were used to identify known cases of diabetes among the

Table 8. Capture–recapture models with two sources.[2]

		Source B	
		Yes	No
Source A	Yes	377	1417
	No	115	n_{00}

Table 9. Parameter estimates from a two source log-linear model with the interaction term set to zero.

Parameter	Estimate	Standard Error
μ	5.8201	0.0545
μ_A	−1.0752	0.1082
μ_B	1.4362	0.0606

residents in the area of Casale Nonferrato in Northern Italy. Data are presented in Table 8. Here, we illustrate the example with the first two sources only.

Source A: A list of all patients with a previous diagnosis of insulin-dependent diabetes mellitus (IDDM) or non-insulin dependent mellitus (NIDDM), via diabetes clinic and/or family physicians.

Source B: A list of all patients discharged with a primary or secondary diagnosis of diabetes in all public and private hospitals in the region.

Using the log-linear approach described above, we fit a log-linear model with the PROC GENMOD procedure in SAS with the log-link function. Parameter estimates were displayed in Table 9.

The estimated number of cases missed by both cases is:

$$\hat{n}_{00} = e^{\hat{\mu}+\hat{\mu}_A+\hat{\mu}_B} = 483.54\,.$$

The total number of diabetes estimated from using both sources is 2353. Notice in this example, source A identified 1754 cases of diabetes and source B identified 452 cases, corresponding to 75% and 19% of the estimated total cases by using both sources, respectively. Both sources are seen to be relatively incomplete.

Note in the two source setting, dependency between the two sources cannot be estimated without additional information. If external data is used to estimate the dependency, μ_{AB} in the above log-linear models, estimation of n_{00} may be possible. If we define P(A), P(B) and P(A∩B) be the probability of captured by source A only, by source B only and by both sources, respectively, we can define the dependence between the two sources to be positive if $P(A \cap B) > P(A)*P(B)$, negative if $P(A \cap B) < P(A)*P(B)$. It has been shown that positive dependence of sources tends to underestimate the true population size and negative dependence tends to overestimate.

Extensions to modeling more than two sources are straightforward. In a capture–recapture model with k sources, it is customary to set the highest interaction parameter of order k to be zero. We illustrate the cases of more than two sources with a three-sources analysis.

The layout of a three-source capture–recapture model is presented in Table 10.

We use the saturated model to construct the log-linear models for the three-source analysis.

$$\begin{aligned}
\log E(n_{111}) &= \mu \\
\log E(n_{110}) &= \mu + \mu_C \\
\log E(n_{101}) &= \mu + \mu_B \\
\log E(n_{011}) &= \mu + \mu_A \\
\log E(n_{100}) &= \mu + \mu_B + \mu_C + \mu_{BC} \\
\log E(n_{010}) &= \mu + \mu_A + \mu_C + \mu_{AC}
\end{aligned}$$

Table 10. The layout of a three source (A, B and C) capture–recapture model.

		Source B			
		Yes		No	
		Source C		Source C	
		Yes	No	Yes	No
Source A	Yes	n_{111}	n_{110}	n_{101}	n_{100}
	No	n_{011}	n_{010}	n_{001}	n_{000}

$$\log E(n_{001}) = \mu + \mu_A + \mu_B + \mu_{AB}$$
$$\log E(n_{000}) = \mu + \mu_A + \mu_B + \mu_C + \mu_{AB} + \mu_{BC} + \mu_{AC} + \mu_{ABC} \,. \quad (20)$$

Recall that there are 8 models, 8 parameters and 7 observations (counts). Therefore, one parameter is unestimable. An untestable assumption is made so that inference is possible: $\mu_{ABC} = 0$.

With more than two sources there is the possibility that a model with fewer parameters will fit the model equally well as the saturated model with 7 parameters (μ_{ABC} is set to 0). Statistically, the model with the fewest number of parameters fitting the data is to be chosen to represent the data. This leads us to the discussion of model selection criteria.

Three methods are commonly used for log-linear model selection: the G^2 deviance statistic which is a likelihood ratio statistic comparing a current model to the saturated model, Akaike Information Criterion (AIC) and the Bayesian Information Criterion (BIC).

For the three source model, the G^2 statistic can be expressed as:

$$G^2 = -2 \sum_{i,j,k} n_{ijk} \log \frac{n_{ijk}}{E(n_{ijk})} \,,$$

where $E(n_{ijk})$ is the expected cell counts under the assumed alternative model other than the saturated one. If a model represents the data, then the difference in deviance between the considered model and the saturated model for which $G^2 = 0$ has an approximate χ^2 distribution.

The Akaike's Information Criterion is defined to be:

$$\text{AIC} = G^2 - 2\,(\text{d.f. of the model}) \,.$$

The Bayesian Information Criterion is defined as:

$$\text{BIC} = G^2 - \frac{\log N}{2\pi}(\text{d.f. of the model}) \,,$$

where N is the total number of observed cases. Both AIC and BIC take the number of parameters in the model into consideration. The BIC also considers sample size. Both criteria select the model with the lowest value on the respective criterion.

A three-source example data from LaPorte *et al.*[17] is modified here to illustrate the issues in model selection. Capture–recapture method was used to identify the most accurate and efficient approaches to monitor adolescent injuries. For our example, we consider the issue of accuracy only. We take three sources from the article: 127 identified by student monthly recalls

Table 11. Injuries captured by three sources:[17] A: student recall at either 1 or 4 month; B: medical excuses; C: daily attendance records.

		Medical excuses			
		Yes		No	
		Attendance record		Attendance record	
		Yes	No	Yes	No
Student Recall	Yes	16	39	13	69
	No	0	3	4	n_{000}

Table 12. The values of G^2, AIC and BIC for all seven models on the LaPorte data.[17]

Number	Model	G^2	d.f.	p-value	AIC	BIC	$\hat{n}_{000}$	$\hat{N}$
1	A, B, C	8.1222	3	0.0436	2.1222	2.8509	6	150
2	A, B, C, AB	4.8084	2	0.0903	0.8084	1.2942	15	159
3	A, B, C, AC	7.4284	2	0.0244	3.4284	3.9142	5	149
4	A, B, C, BC	6.3624	2	0.0415	2.3624	2.8482	7	151
5	A, B, C, AB, AC	3.3987	1	0.0652	1.3987	1.6416	*	*
6	A, B, C, AB, BC	1.9983	1	0.1575	−0.0017	0.2412	21	165
7	A, B, C, BC, AC	5.8258	1	0.0158	3.8258	4.0687	5	149

at either 1 month or 4 months, 58 by medical excuses and 33 by daily attendance records. Data is presented in Table 11.

A series of seven possible models were fit by using the SAS system for log-linear model. Table 12 includes the values of three model selection criteria: the G^2, AIC and BIC, and the estimated number of cases missed by all three sources and the estimated total number of injuries from all three sources.

Using the G^2 statistic, three models (models 2, 5 and 6) are not rejected at the 0.05 significance level which means that these models are not significantly different from the saturated model. Model 5 failed to converge in parameter estimates. The likelihood based statistic would have favored model 2 because it is the simplest model not rejected by G^2. In fact, this model was chosen by LaPorte *et al.*[17] in the original paper. This model predicts 15 cases missed by all three sources and total number of injuries is estimated to be 159. However, both AIC and BIC identified model 6 as the optimal model. The number of cases missed by all sources is estimated to be 21 using model 6 and the total number of cases is estimated to be 165.

Notice that the G^2 method is based on large sample theory which assumes that each cell count is reasonably large. When there are small or zero cell counts as in this example, the validity of the test is questionable. In the above example, we would favor the use of model 6 over that of model 2 based on this observation.

Notice also that the conclusion on the validity of each source is very much dependent on which model one has chosen to represent the data. For example, LaPorte *et al.*[17] stated that student recall is the most accurate source of identifying injury with an estimated accuracy of 86% (137/159) using estimates derived from model 2. If the alternative model 6 is chosen, the accuracy rate for student recall will be estimated to be 83% (137/165), although it remains the most accurate of the three sources.

AIC and BIC base their decision on minimization. Therefore, uniqueness of the selected model is generally satisfied. Simulation studies have been conducted to compare AIC, BIC and several modified forms of the two criteria.[12] In general, the two criteria are quite comparable.

To conclude this chapter, we would like to reiterate the need for proper statistical methods in analyzing complex survey data. Many large national survey data are now accessible to the public for secondary data analysis providing medical researchers unique opportunities to study relationship and trend on the national level. However, great care must be exercised in analytical methods if one is to draw proper conclusions. The intention of this chapter is not on a exclusive coverage of general techniques on analyzing sampling data. Instead our focus of this chapter is on "special models" used for sampling data in the field of epidemiology. Readers are referred to Cochran[5] and Kish[15] for the background knowledge on sampling theory, to Skinner, Holt and Smith[28] for more theoretical development on statistical inference on sampling data. Examples of analysis of health survey data can be found in Leclerc *et al.*,[19] Korn and Graubard,[16] Graubard and Korn[9] and LaVange *et al.*[18]

Acknowledgment

The research os supported in part by NIH grant R01 15813.

References

1. Beckett, L. A., Scherr, P. A. and Evans, D. A. (1992). Population prevalence estimates from complex samples. *Journal of Clinical Epidemiology* **45**: 393–402.

2. Brenner, H. (1994). Use and limitations of the capture–recapture method in disease monitoring with two dependent sources. *Epidemiology* **6**: 42–48.
3. Breslow, N. E. and Clayton, D. G. (1993). Approximate inference in generalized linear mixed models. *Journal of the American Statistical Association* **88**: 9–25.
4. Chambless, L. E. and Boyle, K. E. (1985). Maximum likelihood methods for complex sample data: Logistic regression and discrete proportional hazard models. *Communications in Statistics-Theory and Methods* **14**: 1377–1392.
5. Cochran, W. G. (1977). *Sampling Techniques*, John Wiley and Sons, New York.
6. Fienberg, S. E. (1972). The multiple-recapture census for closed populations and incomplete 2^k contingency tables. *Biometrika* **59**: 591–603.
7. Gao, S., Hui, S. L., Hall, K. S. and Hendrie, H. C. Estimating disease prevalence from two-phase surveys with nonresponse at the second phase. *Statistics in Medicine*, in press.
8. Ghosh, M. and Rao, J. N. K. (1994). Small area estimation: An appraisal. *Statistical Science* **9**: 55–93.
9. Graubard, B. I. and Korn, E. L. (1996). Modelling the sampling design in the analysis of health surveys. *Statistical Methods in Medical Research* **5**: 263–281.
10. Graubard, B. I. and Korn, E. L. (1999). Predictive margins with survey data. *Biometrics* **55**: 652–659.
11. Hook, E. B. and Regal, R. R. (1995). Capture–recapture methods in epidemiology: Methods and limitations. *Epidemiologic Reviews* **17**: 243–264.
12. Hook, E. B. and Regal, R. R. (1997). Validity of methods for model selection, weighting for model uncertainty, and small sample adjustment in capture–recapture estimation. *American Journal of Epidemiology* **145**: 1138–1144.
13. Hurvich, C. M and Tsai, C. L. (1995). Model selection for extended Quasi-likelihood models in small samples. *Biometrics* **51**: 1077–1084.
14. International working group for disease monitoring and forecasting (1995). Capture–recapture and multiple-record systems estimation I: History and theoretical development. *American Journal of Epidemiology* **142**: 1047–1058.
15. Kish, L. (1965). *Survey Sampling*, John Wiley and Sons, New York.
16. Korn, E. L. and Graubard, B. I. (1995). Analysis of large health surveys: Accounting for the sampling design. *Journal of Royal Statistical Society* **A158**: 263–295.
17. LaPorte, R. E., Dearwater, S. R., Chang, Y. F. *et al.* (1995). Efficiency and accuracy of disease monitoring systems: Application of capture–recapture methods to injury monitoring. *American Journal of Epidemiology* **142**: 1069–1077.
18. LaVange, L. M., Stearns, S. C., Lafata, J. E., Koch, G. G. and Shah, B. V. (1996). Innovative strategies using SUDAAN for analysis of health surveys with complex samples. *Statistical Methods in Medical Research* **5**: 311–329.
19. Leclerc, A., Luce, D., Lert, F., Chastang, J. F. and Logeay, P. (1988). Correspondence analysis and logistic modelling: Complementary use in the analysis of a health survey among nurses. *Statistics in Medicine* **7**: 983–995.

20. Littell, R. C., Milliken, G. A., Stroup, W. W. and Wolfinger, R. D. (1996). *SAS System for Mixed Models*, SAS Institute Inc., Cary, NC.
21. Little, R. J. A. and Rubin, D. B. (1987). *Statistical Analysis with Missing Data*, John Wiley and Sons, New York.
22. Morganstein, D. and Brick, J. M. (1996). WesVarPC: Software for computing variance estimates from complex designs. *Proceedings of the 1996 Annual Research Conference*, Bureau of Census, 861–866.
23. Patterson, H. D. and Thompson, R. (1971). Recovery of interblock information when block sizes are unequal. *Biometrika* **58**: 545–554.
24. Raghunathan, T. E. (1993). A quasi-empirical Bayes method for small area estimation. *Journal of the American Statistical Association* **88**: 1444–1448.
25. Research Triangle Institute (1993). *Statistical Methods and Mathematical Algorithms Used in SUDAAN*, Research Triangle Park, NC.
26. Roberts, G., Rao, J. N. K. and Kumar, S. (1987). Logistic regression analysis of sample survey data. *Biometrika* **74**: 1–12.
27. Robinson, G. K. (1991). That BLUP is a good thing: The estimation of random effects. *Statistical Science* **6**: 15–51.
28. Skinner, C. J., Holt, D. and Smith, T. M. F. (1989). *Analysis of Complex Surveys*, John Wiley and Sons, New York.
29. Taylor, D. H., Whellan, D. J. and Sloan, F. A. (1999). Effects of admission to a teaching hospital on the cost and quality of care for medicare beneficiaries. *The New England Journal of Medicine* **340(4)**: 293–299.
30. Tilling, K. and Sterne, A. C. (1999). Capture–recapture models including covariate effects. *American Journal of Epidemiology* **149**: 392–400.
31. Warszawski, J., Messiah, A., Lellouch, J., Meyer, L. and Deville, J. C. (1997). Estimating means and percentages in a complex sampling surveys: Application to a French national survey on sexual behaviour. *Statistics in Medicine* **16**: 397–423.

About the Author

Sujuan Gao, Ph.D, is currently an assistant professor at the Division of Biostatistics, Indiana University School of Medicine, Indianapolis, USA. She received her Bachelor of Science in Mathematics from Beijing Normal University, Beijing, China, in 1985 and a Ph.D in Statistics from the University of Southampton, UK, in 1991. She joined the Division of Biostatistics at Indiana University School of Medicine as a post-doc fellow in 1994 and became a faculty member shortly after. Sujuan Gao's research interest includes the analysis of longitudinal data with missing values, the analysis of data collected using complex sampling scheme, the development and application of statistical methods in medical and epidemiological studies.

CHAPTER 12

THE USE OF CAPTURE–RECAPTURE METHODOLOGY IN EPIDEMIOLOGICAL SURVEILLANCE AND ECOLOGICAL SURVEYS

ANNE CHAO[*,†] and T. C. HSIEH

Institute of Statistics
National Tsing Hua University
Hsin-Chu, Taiwan 30043
[*] *Tel: 886-3-571-5131 ext 3161;*
[†] *chao@stat.nthu.edu.tw*

HSIN-CHOU YANG

Institute of Statistical Science,
Academia Sinica
Taipei, Taiwan 115

1. Introduction

Accurate and timely estimates of disease occurrence over time or across geographic area play an important role in disease monitoring and health care planning. Traditional simple random sampling and other probabilistic sampling schemes are not easily applicable to such situations or are prohibitively expensive. Multiple surveillance systems are usually employed to ascertain cases using different resources or efforts. Although some studies manage to identify almost all patients, most epidemiological approaches merging different lists and eliminating duplicate cases are likely to significantly underestimate true occurrence rates.[25,27] That is, the final merged list misses those who are in the target population but were missed by all lists. This chapter discusses the use of capture–recapture models to estimate the number of missed cases under proper assumptions.

The purpose of this chapter is to find out what assumptions or models we can make in order to estimate the number of missed cases and adjust for under-ascertainment with or without considering the relevant covariates in the analysis. This has analogues in the biological and ecological sciences: estimating the number of undetected animals in a closed population considering environmental factors and/or individual covariates. Here a closed population means that there is no addition and loss so that the population size is a constant during the study period. The estimation of population size is a classical problem and has been extensively discussed in the literature.

Biologists and ecologists have long realized that it is almost impossible to determine the size of a population by counting every animal. Most animals cannot be drawn like balls in an urn or numbers on a list, thus special types of sampling schemes have been developed. Capture–recapture sampling has been widely used to adjust for undercount in the biological sciences. The recapture information (i.e., source-overlap information or source intersection) collected by marking or tagging can be used to estimate the number of missed cases under proper assumptions. Therefore, it is not necessary to count every animal in order to obtain an accurate estimate of population size.

In contrast, epidemiologists have attempted to enumerate all relevant cases to obtain the prevalence rates for various diseases. Cases in various lists are usually merged and any duplicate cases are eliminated. The overlap information is thus ignored. This typical approach assumes complete ascertainment and does not correct or adjust for under-ascertainment. As Hook and Regal[25,27] indicated, most prevalence surveys merging several records of lists are likely to miss some cases and thus (the estimate will) be negatively biased. There is relatively little literature in the health sciences on the assessment of the completeness of these types of surveys or on the adjustment for under-ascertainment. Therefore, as commented by LaPorte *et al.*,[37] people know more about the number of animals than the count of diseases. In a similar way that ecologists and biologists count animals, we introduce with proper modifications in this chapter the use of capture–recapture models to count human populations.

We use three real data sets of human study and one data set of animal survey to illustrate the use of the capture–recapture methodology to correct for under-ascertainment of cases in epidemiological surveillance and under-estimation of population size in ecological survey, respectively. The animal survey data represent typical capture–recapture records in biological and ecological studies and thus can be used to compare with epidemiological surveillance data. Ecological models can be similarly applied to analyze human data in many applications. The four examples are briefly described as follows.

1.1. *Example 1. Data on hepatitis A virus (HAV)*

Chao *et al.*[15] documented the details of a large outbreak of the HAV that occurred in and around a college in northern Taiwan from April to July 1995. Cases of students in that college were ascertained by three sources: (1) P-list: records based on a serum test taken by the Institute of Preventive Medicine, Department of Health of Taiwan; 135 cases were identified. (2) Q-list: local hospital records reported by the National Quarantine Service; 122 cases were found. (3) E-list: records collected by epidemiologists; of which there were 126 cases. Merging the three lists by eliminating duplicate records resulted in 271 ascertained cases.

The categorical data are shown in Table 1 where all ascertained cases are classified according to their presence/absence in the three lists. Presence or absence on any list is denoted by 1 and 0, respectively. For three lists, we can use a sequence of three numbers (each is either 0 or 1) to denote the record of each individual. For example, a record (001) describes an individual on the third list only and a record (011) describes an individual on the second and third lists but not on the first list. The three lists are displayed in an order of P, Q and E; this ordering is arbitrary and any legitimate inference procedure should be independent of the ordering of the lists. Those patients who were missed by all lists have the record (000). There are seven observable records and their counts over all ascertained cases are denoted as Z_{001}, Z_{010}, Z_{011}, Z_{100}, Z_{101}, Z_{110} and Z_{111}. From Table 1, there were 63 people listed in the E-list only, 55 people listed in the Q-list only, and 18 people listed in both lists Q and E but not in the

Table 1. Aggregated categorical data on hepatitis A virus. A question mark "?" indicates the number of missed cases in the data.

Hepatitis A List			
P	Q	E	Data
0	0	0	Z_{000} =?
0	0	1	$Z_{001} = 63$
0	1	0	$Z_{010} = 55$
0	1	1	$Z_{011} = 18$
1	0	0	$Z_{100} = 69$
1	0	1	$Z_{101} = 17$
1	1	0	$Z_{110} = 21$
1	1	1	$Z_{111} = 28$

P-list. Similarly, we can interpret the other records. In the P-list, there were 135 cases, which means $Z_{1++} = Z_{100} + Z_{101} + Z_{110} + Z_{111} = 135$. Here, when we add over a sample, the subscript corresponding to that sample is replaced by a "+" sign. Similar relationship holds for the other two lists.

The number of different cases ascertained in at least one of the lists, 271 in this study, is the sum of all observable cell counts. Epidemiologists suspected that the observed number of cases considerably undercounted the true number of infected and an evaluation of the degree of undercount was needed.[15] The purpose was then to estimate the number of missed cases, Z_{000}, or equivalently, to estimate the number of total individuals who were infected in the outbreak. This data set was analyzed.[12] As opposed to many real data sets, this one has the advantage of a known true number of infected because a screen serological check for all students was conducted after the three surveys. In this chapter, we therefore select the HAV data set as an illustrative example to assess the relative merit of various estimation methods.

1.2. *Example 2: Data on neurologic illness (Stratified by diagnostic group)*

Bobo *et al.*[3] reported a comprehensive surveillance system for acute neurologic illness in children from August 1987 to July 1988 in two States of USA. Three surveillance strategies were employed: (1) Hospital surveillance system (H-list): cases were identified based on hospitals discharge records. (2) Provider surveillance system (P-list): cases were reported by pediatricians and neurologists. (3) Study staff surveillance system (S-list): cases collected by the staff members by visiting all participating facilities and checking clinical records of potential cases. For this data set, we only use the available primary diagnostic groups (encephalopathies, infantile spasms, afebrile seizure and complex febrile seizure) as a covariate or stratifying variable. These four groups are referred to as stratum A, B, C and D for convenience. There are other covariates (gender and geographic location), but these information is not available in the literature.

Bobo *et al.*[3] found that substantial difference exists in case ascertainment rates by diagnostic groups. The post-stratified data by diagnostic groups are shown in Table 2. This covariate (diagnostic group) is also referred to as a post-stratifying or stratifying variable. The data structure for each group is similar to that in Example 1. The collapsed data over the four groups are shown in the last column. In the original data, there were

Table 2. Aggregated categorical data on neurologic illness. A question mark "?" indicates the number of missed cases in the data.

List			Diagnostic Group (Stratum)				
H	P	S	A	B	C	D	Total
0	0	0	?	?	?	?	?
0	0	1	11	7	131	103	252
0	1	0	2	1	38	4	45
0	1	1	6	5	31	20	62
1	0	0	6	1	37	26	70
1	0	1	7	2	62	44	115
1	1	0	1	1	14	11	27
1	1	1	2	4	31	11	48

626 ascertained cases. In Table 2 and our analysis in Section 4, we only consider 619 cases with known diagnostic groups. There were 260, 182 and 477 cases, respectively, in H-list, P-list and S-list.

Despite the comprehensive surveillance systems, Bobo *et al.*[3] concluded that there were still some people who could not be identified. They performed capture–recapture adjustment for the data within each stratum and the collapsed data in order to obtain an accurate occurrence rate for various sub-populations defined by the available covariates. Their results showed that the ascertainment rate for the four groups were respectively 82%, 94%, 69% and 91%. The rate was substantially low for the afebrile seizures.

1.3. *Example 3: Drug Data (Stratified by the Length of Time on Drug)*

Wittes[52] presented an ascertainment data set on patients receiving synthetic penicillin called methicillin. Cases were identified by the following four systems: (1) intravenous nurses (100 cases); (2) hospital floor nurses (21 cases); (3) hospitals pharmacists (156 cases) and (4) medication sheets (348 cases). We refer to these four lists as list 1, 2, 3 and 4, respectively. A total of 428 cases were found. Wittes[52] indicated that the length of time a patient was given the drug was related to his/her probability of being recorded. The original data consist of four strata for the time length (1–3 days, 4–6 days, 7–10 days and 11+ days). We combine the last two strata and the data are shown in Table 3. For each stratum, there are 15 observable

Table 3. Aggregated categorical data on drug use. A question mark "?" indicates the number of missed cases in the data.

List				Usage on Drug (Stratum)			
1	2	3	4	1–3 days	4–6 days	7+ days	Total
0	0	0	0	?	?	?	?
0	0	0	1	48	83	66	197
0	0	1	0	18	13	12	43
0	0	1	1	14	33	27	74
0	1	0	0	1	4	1	6
0	1	0	1	1	1	1	3
0	1	1	0	1	0	0	1
0	1	1	1	0	3	1	4
1	0	0	0	8	6	6	20
1	0	0	1	8	16	17	41
1	0	1	0	1	2	5	8
1	0	1	1	1	6	17	24
1	1	0	0	0	0	1	1
1	1	0	1	2	0	2	4
1	1	1	0	0	0	1	1
1	1	1	1	0	0	1	1

presence/absence records and each can be expressed by a sequence of four numbers.

Wittes[52] found that an independent model (see Section 2 for explanation of the model) in each stratum fitted well and obtained an estimate of 544 (s.e. 22.4) for the total number of patient receiving the drug. Dependence was suspected between lists 3 and 4 because the records from the pharmacy were duplicates of the medication sheets. To eliminate this possible dependence, the lists 3 and 4 were combined to form only one list. Then based on this combined list, list 1 and list 2, an estimate of 536 was obtained under independence. Both models provide evidences that a non-negligible number of patients were missed by all four identification sources.

1.4. *Example 4: Deer mice data (with three individual's covariates)*

We use a small animal data set to illustrate covariate analysis. Otis *et al.*[38] reported a capture–recapture experiment of *Peromyscus manicultatus* conducted by V. Ried in Rio Blanco County, Colorado during the summer of 1975. Baited traps were set to catch mice in six consecutive nights. In the trapping, each newly captured mouse was uniquely tagged so that the capture history of each mouse captured in the experiment was known. In addition to capture history data, gender (male or female), age (young, semi-adult or adult) and body weight for each mouse were recorded. Only three semi-adult mice were caught, so they were re-classified as adults in analysis. We list data of individual capture history and three covariates in Table 4. In total, there are 38 distinct mice caught in this experiment.

Unlike the epidemiological data (Examples 1–3) for which there is usually no natural ordering among lists, animal capture–recapture data do have a natural ordering. Biologists often record the number of first-captures and recaptures on each trapping occasion. In these data, the numbers of captures for the six occasions are $(n_1, n_2, n_3, n_4, n_5, n_6) = (15, 20, 16, 19, 25, 25)$. Out of the n_j animals, there are u_j first-captures and m_j recaptures, so that $u_j + m_j = n_j$, with $(u_1, u_2, u_3, u_4, u_5, u_6) = (15, 8, 6, 3, 3, 3)$ and $(m_1, m_2, m_3, m_4, m_5, m_6) = (0, 12, 10, 16, 22, 22)$. Since capture probabilities vary with individual, environmental and/or other auxiliary variables recorded or measured in a capture–recapture study, these covariates are commonly used to model heterogeneous capture probabilities. In these data, gender, age and weight are individual covariates. How to incorporate the available covariates in our modeling and assess the effect of each covariate is a topic not only in animal studies but also in many health-related research fields.

In this chapter, we present the concept and analysis of capture–recapture models and apply them to the above four data sets. Based on these four examples, we show how capture–recapture models can be used to estimate the undercount in epidemiological studies and in biological surveys. In Section 2, the background and motivation of the capture–recapture technique and its adaptation for use in human populations are reviewed. Section 3 summarizes the capture–recapture models when no covariates are available. Section 3.1 reviews the simple two-sample cases because results for any pair of samples provide useful preliminary information. Then the sample coverage approach developed by Chao *et al.*[12] is reviewed in Section 3.2; an application to Example 1 is discussed in Section 3.3. A new R program CARE1 which features sample coverage estimates is introduced in Section 3.4. Section 3.5 reviews ecological models that are useful in human studies; an application to Example 4 without using covariates is presented in Section 3.6 along with an introduction to program CARE-2. Section 4 presents a logistic regression model in which individual covariates (including a stratifying variable) and environmental/occasional variables can be considered. Examples 2, 3 and 4 (all with covariates) are respectively analyzed in Sections 4.2, 4.3 and 4.4. Concluding remarks and relevant discussion are provided in Section 5.

Table 4. Individual capture history and three covariates of 38 mice caught in six occasions. Gender (m: male, f: female); age (y: young, sa: semi-adult, a: adult); and weight (in grams). A question mark "?" indicates the missing covariates for the non-captures.

Occasion						Covariate		
1	2	3	4	5	6	Gender	Age	Weight
0	0	0	0	0	0	?	?	?
0	0	0	0	0	0	?	?	?
:	:	:	:	:	:	:	:	:
1	1	1	1	1	1	m	y	12
1	0	0	1	1	1	f	y	15
1	1	0	0	1	1	m	y	15
1	1	0	1	1	1	m	y	15
1	1	1	1	1	1	m	y	13
1	1	0	1	1	1	m	a	21
1	1	1	1	1	0	m	y	11
1	1	1	0	0	1	m	sa	15
1	1	1	1	1	1	m	y	14
1	1	0	1	1	1	m	y	13
1	1	0	1	1	1	m	y	14
1	1	1	0	1	1	f	a	22
1	1	1	1	1	1	m	y	14
1	0	1	1	1	0	m	y	11
1	0	0	1	0	0	f	y	10
0	1	0	0	1	0	f	a	23
0	1	0	0	0	1	f	y	7
0	1	0	0	0	1	m	y	8
0	1	0	1	0	1	m	a	19
0	1	1	0	1	0	m	y	13
0	1	0	1	0	1	f	y	5
0	1	0	0	0	1	f	a	20
0	1	0	0	1	1	m	y	12
0	0	1	0	0	0	f	y	6
0	0	1	1	1	1	f	a	22
0	0	1	0	1	1	f	y	10
0	0	1	1	1	1	f	y	14
0	0	1	0	1	0	f	a	19
0	0	1	0	0	0	f	a	19
0	0	0	1	0	0	f	a	20
0	0	0	1	1	1	m	sa	16
0	0	0	1	1	0	f	y	11
0	0	0	0	1	0	m	y	14
0	0	0	0	1	0	f	y	11
0	0	0	0	1	0	m	a	24
0	0	0	0	0	1	m	y	9
0	0	0	0	0	1	m	sa	16
0	0	0	0	0	1	f	a	19

2. Background and Motivation of Capture — Recapture

Capture–recapture sampling has been widely used for estimating demographic parameters of animal populations.[44–46] In a typical animal capture–recapture experiment, traps or nets are placed in the study area at several times, often called capture occasions (or trapping samples). At the first occasion, a number of animals are captured. A tag or mark with a unique number or record is attached to each captured animal. These animals are then released back into the population. At each subsequent occasion, animals that are first-captures are similarly marked and the tag numbers of re-captures are recorded. At the end of the experiment, a sequence of samples is obtained and the complete capture history for each captured animal is known.

Why is marking or tagging necessary in animal studies? Clearly, many animals look the same and individuals cannot be distinguished by sight. Marking or tagging is used to distinguish captured individuals so that the recapture information (overlap information) by marking or tagging can be used to estimate the number of missed animals in the experiment. Marks include banding and tagging, paint brushing, toe clipping, ear clipping and in some species individual animals can be identified. Intuitively, if the proportion of newly captured animals in the later capture occasions is high, we know that the population size is much higher than the number of distinct captures. On the other hand, if there is a low proportion of newly captured animals, then we are likely to have caught most of the animals and the population size is close to the number of captured animals.

According to Seber,[44] the original idea of two-sample capture–recapture technique can be traced back to Laplace, who implemented it to estimate the population size of France. The interesting history of Laplace's survey conducted in 1802 was described in Cochran.[17] The earliest applications to ecology include Petersen's and Dahl's work on fish populations and Lincoln's use of band returns to estimate waterfowl in 1930. More sophisticated statistical theory and inference procedures have been proposed since Darroch's paper,[21] in which the mathematical framework of this topic was founded. Seber,[44–46] Pollock,[40] Schwarz and Seber,[43] Chao[6,7] and Chao and Huggins[8,9] provided comprehensive reviews on the methodologies and applications.

The capture–recapture technique has been applied to human populations under the term "multiple-record system" (Sekar and Deming;[47] Fienberg;[23] Wittes and Sidel[50]; Wittes[51]; IWGDMF[34,35]). The special

Table 5. Comparison of capture–recapture applied to human and animal populations.

Human Populations (Multiple-List System)	Animal Populations (Capture–Recapture Sampling)
Similarities:	
Lists, sources, records	Trapping samples or occasions
Identification numbers and/or names	Marks or tags
Ascertainment probability	Capture probability
Differences:	
Usually only 2 to 5 lists	Any t number of samples or occasions ($t \geq 2$)
No natural time ordering among lists	Natural time ordering in samples or occasions
Different ascertainment methods (Usually no behavioral response)	Identical trapping methods (Behavioral response often exists)
Some Shared Models:	
Ecological models[7, 38, 40, 44, 49]	
Log-linear models[18, 23, 34, 35]	
Sample coverage method[11, 12]	
Logistic regression models[1, 32, 33, 54]	

two-sample cases are often referred to as the "dual-system" or "dual-record system". For ascertainment data, if each list is regarded as a trapping sample and identification numbers, names and other characteristics are used as tags or marks, then this framework is similar to a capture–recapture setup for wildlife estimation. Comparisons of the applications to human and animal populations are listed in Table 5.

The earliest references to the application of the capture–recapture techniques to health science include the pioneering paper by Sekar and Deming[47] for two samples, Wittes and Sidel[50] for three samples, Wittes[51] for four samples, Wittes *et al.*[52] and Fienberg[23] for five samples. Hook and Regal[25] also suggested the use of capture–recapture models even for apparently exhaustive surveys. In recent years, there has been growing interest in the use of this technique in various disciplines, e.g., software reliability (see Briand *et al.*[4]). Hook and Regal,[27] IWGDMF[34, 35] and Chao[6] provided overviews of the applications of the capture–recapture models specifically to epidemiological data. However, some critical comments and concerns about the use of capture–recapture models in analyzing ascertainment data have been expressed by several authors (Schouten *et al.*[42]; Kiemeney *et al.*[36]; Desenclos and Hubert[22]; Papoz *et al.*[39]; Cormack[19]). For some of the concerns, Chao *et al.*[12] provided relevant discussions from a statistical point of view.

As shown in Table 5, there are some principal differences between wildlife and human applications. Researchers for wildlife and human populations have developed models and methodologies along separate lines. In Table 5, we list the approaches that are applicable to both populations. We will address approaches that we suggest to use in Sections 3 and 4 after the introduction of notational conventions.

Throughout this paper, we use the following notational conventions:

- The true unknown population size (i.e., the number of individuals in the target population) is N and all individuals can be conceptually indexed by $1, 2, \ldots, N$.
- There are t lists (samples, records, or sources) and they are indexed by $1, 2, \ldots, t$.
- There are M identified individuals, that is, M equals to the sum of all observable cell counts.
- Denote $Z_{s_1 s_2 \ldots s_t}$ as the number of individuals with record $s_1, s_2, \ldots, s_t$, where $s_j = 0$ denotes absence in list j and $s_j = 1$ denotes presence in list j.
- Denote n_j, $j = 1, 2, \ldots, t$ as the number of individuals identified in the jth list.
- Denote P_{ij} as the capture or ascertainment probability of the ith individual in the jth list.

Basic assumptions are:

- All individuals act independently.
- Interpretation or definition for the characteristic of the target population should be consistent for all data sources.
- Closure assumption: the size of the population is approximately a constant during the study period.
- Ascertainable assumption: any individual must have a positive probability to be ascertained by any source; any un-ascertainment is purely due to a small chance rather than impossibility. When a random sample is feasible in a dual-system, some special types of structures zeros are permitted; see Section 6.1 of Chao *et al.*[12]
- For all sources, identification marks are correctly recorded and matched.

Traditional statistical approach further assumes that the samples are independent. In animal studies, this traditional assumption is in terms of an even more restrictive "equal-catchability" assumption, i.e., in each fixed trapping sample all animals have the same capture probability.

(Equal catchability assumption implies independence among samples but the reverse is not true.) Dependence or unequal catchabilities may be caused by the following two sources:

(1) Local dependence (also called local list dependence) within each individual/stratum: conditional on any individual, the presence/absence in one source has a direct causal effect on this individual's probability of inclusion in other sources. In animal populations, local dependence arises mainly from a behavioral response to capture due to identical trapping method. Animals may become trap-happy, and have an increased probability of subsequent capture, if baited traps are used whereas they may become trap-shy, and have a decreased probability of subsequent capture, if mist nets or ear clipping are used. Local dependence within each individual/stratum may also arise for human populations. For example, the probability of going to a hospital for treatment for any individual depends on his/her result on the serum test of the HAV, leading to dependence between the ascertainment of the serum sample and that of the hospital sample.
(2) Heterogeneity among individuals: even if the two lists are independent within an individual/stratum, the ascertainment of the two sources may become dependent if the capture probabilities are heterogeneous among individuals/strata. Hook and Regal[26] presented an interesting epidemiological example. For many populations, capture or ascertainment probability may vary with age, gender, location, activity, diagnostic symptom, severity of illness or other individual characteristics. For example, in animal populations, some females tend to be less likely to be captured in all trapping occasions, leading to dependence among samples. In human populations, severe cases are more ascertainable in all lists than less severe cases, also leading to positive dependence.

These two types of dependencies are usually confounded and cannot be easily disentangled in a data analysis. Lack of independence leads to a bias (called "correlation bias") for the usual estimator which assumes independence. See Section 3.1 for details. When only two lists are available, the data are insufficient for estimating dependence unless additional covariates are available. All existing methods unavoidably encounter this problem and adopt the independence assumption. Therefore, when there are no available covariates, at least three lists are required to model dependence between samples.

3. Models Without Covariates

A number of capture–recapture models have been proposed to estimate population size for animal survey and human data. Chao[7] reviewed three categories of models: ecological models, log-linear models and sample-coverage approach. For epidemiological data without any covariates, we will mainly in this chapter discuss the sample coverage approach (in Section 3.2) and ecological models (in Section 3.5). The reader is referred to Chao *et al.*[12] for the log-linear model approach. However, no matter which model is applied, analysis of any pair of samples (or lists) provides useful preliminary information. So we first review two-sample capture–recapture models.

3.1. *Two-sample models*

As described in Section 2, the earliest idea of the two-sample capture–recapture technique was applied to estimate human population size. Petersen and Lincoln's work represents a landmark in the historical development of capture–recapture models. The Petersen-Lincoln estimator in animal populations (or the dual-system estimator in human populations) has been widely used to estimate population size in two-sample closed capture–recapture experiments.

Assume the size of a population is N. A first sample of n_1 animals is captured, marked and released back to the population. Thus the marked rate in the population is n_1/N. A second sample of n_2 animals is subsequently drawn and there are m_2 previously marked. Equating the proportion of the marked rate in the population to the marked rate in the second sample suggests that $m_2/n_2 \approx n_1/N$, which yields the following Petersen estimator (or the Petersen-Lincoln estimator) for the population size:

$$\hat{N} = n_1 n_2 / m_2. \tag{1a}$$

Based on a hypergeometric model (in which n_1 and n_2 are regarded as fixed), Chapman[16] derived the following estimator to adjust the bias that arises mainly due to a small value of m_2:

$$\tilde{N} = (n_1 + 1)(n_2 + 1)/(m_2 + 1) - 1. \tag{1b}$$

Under the same model, both estimators have approximately the same variance given by

$$\text{Var}\tilde{N} \approx (n_1 + 1)(n_2 + 1)(n_1 - m_2)(n_2 - m_2)/[(m_2 + 1)^2(m_2 + 2)]. \tag{1c}$$

Since the Petersen and Chapman estimates are typically skewed, a log-transformation has been used to obtain a confidence interval for population size.[5] For example, for the Chapman estimator, we assume that $\log(\tilde{N}-M)$ follows a normal distribution (where M denotes the number of animals caught in the experiment), implying the 95% confidence interval for the Chapman estimator with an estimated variance given in Equation (1c) can be constructed as follows:

$$[M+(\tilde{N}-M)/C, M+(\tilde{N}-M)\times C], \tag{1d}$$

where

$$C=\exp\left\{1.96\sqrt{\log\left[1+\frac{var\tilde{N}}{(\tilde{N}-M)^2}\right]}\right\}.$$

The lower bound of this interval is always greater than the number of different animals actually captured in all occasions. The confidence interval can be applied to not only the Chapman estimator but also any other population size estimators discussed in this chapter.

A critical assumption for the validity of the Petersen and Chapman estimators is that the two samples are independent. In animal studies, a more restrictive assumption is the "equal-catchability assumption", i.e., in each fixed sample all animals have the same probability of being caught. Seber[44] thoroughly discussed the validity of the Petersen-Lincoln estimator using various models. An intuitive concept of "independence" between samples based on 2×2 categorical data formed by capture/non-capture in each of the two samples is provided by Chao *et al.*[10]

As described in Section 2, local list dependence and unequal catchabilities are two sources of dependences that lead to bias for the Petersen and Chapman's estimators. For example, if the two samples are positively correlated (because animals exhibit a trap-happy behavioral response or if individual heterogeneity exists and is consistent over sampling occasions), then the animals captured in the first sample are more easily caught in the second sample. Thus the recapture rate (m_2/n_2) in the second sample tends to be larger than the true proportion of marked animals in the population n_1/N. Then it is expected that $m_2/n_2 > n_1/N$, which yields $N > n_1n_2/m_2 = \hat{N}$. As a result, the Petersen estimator tends to underestimate the true size. Conversely, it tends to overestimate when two samples are negatively correlated. Similar arguments and conclusions are also valid for more than two capture occasions. In Section 3.2, a general measure of "dependence" will be defined to quantify the correlation bias in some dependent models and to theoretically understand the bias. The bias direction has an important implication: if the Petersen or Chapman estimates for any two samples are relatively high (low) compared to other pairwise estimates, then it indicates the two samples are negatively (positively) dependent. Thus, models which incorporate dependence among samples should be considered.

3.2. *Sample coverage approach (for 3–5 lists)*

This approach was proposed by Chao and Tsay[11] for the three-list case. The extension to a general case is presented in Tsay and Chao.[48] Details and relevant software are reviewed in Chao *et al.*[12] The approach aims to provide a measure to quantify the overlap information and also to propose parameters to quantify sources of dependence.

Dependence is modeled by parameters called the "coefficient of covariation" (CCV). Define $X_{ij} = I$ [the ith individual is captured in Sample j], $i = 1, 2, \ldots, N$ and $j = 1, 2, \ldots, t$, where $I[\cdot]$ denotes an indicator function. Thus the capture probability of the ith individual in Sample j is $E(X_{ij})$, and the probability of being caught in both Samples j and k is $E(X_{ij}X_{ik})$.

We define a dependence measure, the coefficient of covariation (CCV), between Sample j and Sample k as

$$\begin{aligned}\gamma_{jk} &= \frac{N\sum_{i=1}^{N} E(X_{ij}X_{ik})}{[\sum_{i=1}^{N} E(X_{ij})][\sum_{i=1}^{N} E(X_{ik})]} - 1 \\ &= \frac{1}{N}\sum_{i=1}^{N} \frac{E[(X_{ij}-\mu_j)(X_{ik}-\mu_k)]}{\mu_j\mu_k}, \end{aligned} \tag{2a}$$

where $\mu_j = \sum_{i=1}^{N} P_{ij}/N = E(n_j)/N$ denotes the average probability of being listed in the jth sample. Similarly, we can define CCV for more than two samples. For example, the CCV measure for three samples j, k and m, is defined as

$$\gamma_{jkm} = \frac{1}{N}\sum_{i=1}^{N} \frac{E[(X_{ij}-\mu_j)(X_{ik}-\mu_k)(X_{im}-\mu_m)]}{\mu_j\mu_k\mu_m}.$$

To better understand the CCV parameters, consider the special case that there is no local list dependence. Let the two sets of probabilities, $\{P_{ij};\ i = 1, 2, \ldots, N\}$ and $\{P_{ik};\ i = 1, 2, \ldots, N\}$, denote the capture probabilities for N individuals in samples j and k, respectively, i.e., $E(X_{ij}) = P_{ij}$, and $E(X_{ik}) = P_{ik}$. In this special case, we have $E(X_{ij}X_{ik}) = P_{ij}P_{ik}$, and the

CCV reduces to

$$\gamma_{jk} = \frac{1}{N}\sum_{i=1}^{N}\frac{(P_{ij}-\mu_j)(P_{ik}-\mu_k)}{\mu_j\mu_k} = \frac{1}{N}\frac{\sum_{i=1}^{N}P_{ij}P_{ik}}{\mu_j\mu_k} - 1, \qquad (2b)$$

$$\gamma_{jkm} = \frac{1}{N}\sum_{i=1}^{N}\frac{(P_{ij}-\mu_j)(P_{ik}-\mu_k)(P_{im}-\mu_m)}{\mu_j\mu_k\mu_m}. \qquad (2c)$$

The magnitude of γ_{jk} measures the degree of dependence between samples j and k. The two heterogeneous samples are independent if and only if $\gamma_{jk}=0$, i.e., $N^{-1}\sum_{i=1}^{N} P_{ij}P_{ik} = \mu_j\mu_k$, which means that the covariance between the two sets of probabilities is zero. Thus if only one set of probabilities is homogeneous, then it suffice to assure independence provided no local dependence exists.

Two samples are positively (negatively) dependent if $\gamma_{jk} > 0 (\gamma_{jk} < 0)$, which is equivalent to $N^{-1}\sum_{i=1}^{N} P_{ij}\ P_{ik} > \mu_j\mu_k\ (N^{-1}\sum_{i=1}^{N}\ P_{ij}P_{ik} < \mu_j\mu_k)$, that is, the average probability of jointly being listed in the two samples is greater (less) than that in the independent case. The CCV can be similarly defined for more than two sets of heterogeneous probabilities.

The relative bias of the Petersen estimator (bias divided by the estimate) for Sample j and Sample k is approximately $-\gamma_{jk}$.[10,11] That is, the correlation bias is approximately equal to

$$\text{Correlation bias } = E(\hat{N}) - N \approx -\gamma_{jk}E(\hat{N})$$

This explains the direction of the correlation bias for Petersen's estimator. That is, the Petersen estimator overestimates when two samples are negatively correlated, whereas it underestimates when two samples are positively correlated, as stated in Section 3.1. The value of CCV also quantifies the correlation bias.

The sample coverage is used as a measure of overlap fraction of the available lists. While the mathematical formula for the sample coverage is complicated, its estimator is intuitively understandable. In the following, we only consider the three-list case. The estimated sample coverage can be written as[11]

$$\hat{C} = 1 - \frac{1}{3}\left(\frac{Z_{100}}{n_1} + \frac{Z_{010}}{n_2} + \frac{Z_{001}}{n_3}\right)$$

$$= \frac{1}{3}\left[\left(1-\frac{Z_{100}}{n_1}\right) + \left(1-\frac{Z_{010}}{n_2}\right) + \left(1-\frac{Z_{001}}{n_3}\right)\right],$$

which is the average (over three lists) of the fraction of cases found more than once. Note that Z_{100}, Z_{010} and Z_{001} are the numbers of individuals listed only in one sample. Hence this estimator is the complement of the averaged fraction of singletons. Obviously, singletons cannot contain any overlapping information. Define

$$D = \frac{1}{3}[(M - Z_{100}) + (M - Z_{010}) + (M - Z_{001})]$$
$$= M - \frac{1}{3}(Z_{100} + Z_{010} + Z_{001}).$$

Here $(Z_{100} + Z_{100} + Z_{100})/3$ represents the average of the non-overlapped cases and recall that M denotes the total number of identified cases. Thus D can be interpreted as the average of the overlapped cases. The sample coverage estimation procedures for the three-list case are summarized in the following:

1. When the three sources are independent, a simple population size estimator is derived as:

$$\hat{N}_0 = D/\hat{C}. \tag{3}$$

   It can also be intuitively thought of as ratio of overlapped cases to overlap fraction.
2. When dependence exists and the overlap information is large enough (how large it should be will be discussed further below), we take into account the dependence by adjusting the above simple estimator $\hat{N}_0$ based on a function of two-sample CCV's. The resulting estimator has the following explicit form:

$$\hat{N} = \left[\frac{Z_{+11} + Z_{1+1} + Z_{11+}}{3\hat{C}}\right] \div \left\{1 - \frac{1}{3\hat{C}}\left[\frac{(Z_{1+0} + Z_{+10})Z_{11+}}{n_1 n_2} + \frac{(Z_{10+} + Z_{+01})Z_{1+1}}{n_1 n_3} + \frac{(Z_{0+1} + Z_{01+})Z_{+11}}{n_2 n_3}\right]\right\}. \tag{4}$$

3. For relatively low sample coverage data, we feel the data do not contain sufficient information to accurately estimate the population size. In this case, the following "one-step" estimator $\hat{N}_1$ is suggested: (The estimator

is called "one-step" because it is obtained by one iterative step from the aforementioned adjustment formula.)

$$\hat{N}_1 = \frac{D}{\hat{C}} + \frac{1}{3\hat{C}}[(Z_{1+0} + Z_{+10})\hat{\gamma}_{12} + (Z_{10+} + Z_{+01})\hat{\gamma}_{13} + (Z_{01+} + Z_{0+1})\hat{\gamma}_{23}], \tag{5}$$

where CCV estimates are

$$\hat{\gamma}_{12} = \hat{N}'\frac{Z_{11+}}{n_1n_2} - 1, \quad \hat{\gamma}_{13} = \hat{N}'\frac{Z_{1+1}}{n_1n_3} - 1, \quad \hat{\gamma}_{23} = \hat{N}'\frac{Z_{+11}}{n_2n_3} - 1, \tag{6}$$

and

$$\begin{aligned}\hat{N}' = \frac{D}{\hat{C}} + \frac{1}{3\hat{C}}\bigg[&(Z_{1+0} + Z_{+10})\left(\frac{D}{\hat{C}}\cdot\frac{Z_{11+}}{n_1n_2} - 1\right)\\ &+ (Z_{10+} + Z_{+01})\left(\frac{D}{\hat{C}}\cdot\frac{Z_{1+1}}{n_1n_3} - 1\right)\\ &+ (Z_{01+} + Z_{0+1})\left(\frac{D}{\hat{C}}\cdot\frac{Z_{+11}}{n_2n_3} - 1\right)\bigg].\end{aligned}$$

This one-step estimator can be regarded as a lower (upper) bound for positively (negatively) dependent samples. Hook and Regal[29,30] noted that most data sets used in epidemiological applications tend to have a net positive dependence. Thus the one-step estimator is often used as a lower bound.

The above three population size estimators ($\hat{N}_0$, $\hat{N}$, $\hat{N}_1$) will be simply referred to as sample coverage estimators if there is no confusion with the coverage estimator $\hat{C}$. A bootstrap resampling method[11] was proposed to obtain estimated standard errors for the above three estimators and to construct confidence intervals using a log-transformation.[5] A relatively low overlap fraction means that there are many singletons. In this case, the undercount cannot be measured accurately due to insufficient overlap. Consequently, a large standard error is usually associated with the estimator $\hat{N}$ in Equation (4). How large should the overlap information be? Chao *et al.*[12] suggested that the estimated sample coverage $\hat{C}$ should be at least 55%. A practical data-dependent guideline can be determined from the estimated bootstrap s.e. associated with the estimator $\hat{N}$. If the estimated bootstrap standard error becomes unacceptable (say, it exceeds one-third of the population size estimate), then only the lower or upper bound in Equation (5) is recommended. The estimation procedure for the general t-sample case is parallel to that for the 3-sample case as discussed above.[12,48]

Table 6. Analysis results for the HAV data.

(1) Estimates for pair of lists:

Lists	Petersen Estimate (s.e.)	Chapman estimate (s.e.)
(P, Q)	336 (29)	334 (29)
(P, E)	378 (36)	374 (36)
(Q, E)	334 (30)	331 (30)

(2) Sample coverage approach

	D	$\hat{C}$	$\hat{\gamma}_{12}$	$\hat{\gamma}_{13}$	$\hat{\gamma}_{23}$	$\hat{\gamma}_{123}$	Estimate (s.e.)
$\hat{N}_0$: Eq. (3)	208.7	0.513	0.21	0.08	0.22	0.73	407 (28)
$\hat{N}$: Eq. (4)	208.7	0.513	1.89	1.57	1.91	6.35	971 (925)
$\hat{N}_1$: Eq. (5)	208.7	0.513	0.51	0.34	0.52	1.11	508 (40)

3.3. *Example 1 — HAV data (Three lists)*

Table 6 shows the results for analyzing the HAV data using CARE1 written in R language (see Section 3.4 for introduction) mainly based on sample coverage approach. The first part of the table presents Petersen's estimate based on any pair of lists. Although Petersen's estimator is valid only under the restrictive independence assumption, they are practically useful as a preliminary analysis. It has been suggested[24, 25] that estimates based on any two lists can be used to detect possible dependence. A substantially higher (lower) estimate signifies possible negative (positive) dependence for those two samples. For the HAV data, Petersen's estimates are in the range of 330 to 380. The narrow range of these estimates would not indicate the possible direction of dependence at this stage.

The second part of Table 6 contains the sample coverage approach. The sample coverage is estimated to be $\hat{C} = 51.3\%$, and the average of the overlapped cases is equal to $D = 208.67$. If we ignore the possible dependence between samples, an estimate based on Equation (3) is $\hat{N}_0 = D/\hat{C} = 208.67/0.513 = 407$, which is slightly higher than the estimate of 388 based on the independent log-linear model (see Chao *et al.*[12] for the log-linear model analysis). The estimator given in Equation (4) is $\hat{N} = 971$, but a large estimated bootstrap s.e. (925) renders the estimate useless. The estimated s.e. was calculated by using a bootstrap method based on 1000 replications. We feel these data with a relatively low sample coverage estimate of 51% do not contain enough information to correct for undercount. The proposed one-step estimator in Equation (5) is $\hat{N}_1 = 508$

with an estimated s.e. of 40 using 1000 bootstrap replications. The same bootstrap replications produce a 95% confidence interval of (442, 600) using a log-transformation. We remark that the estimated s.e. might vary from trial to trial because replications vary in the bootstrap procedures.

It follows from Equation (6) that the CCV measures depend on the value of N. The CCV estimates in Table 6 based on the three estimates of N show that any two samples are positively dependent. As a result, the estimate $\hat{N}_1 = 508$ can only serve as a lower bound. Also, the estimates assuming independence based on two samples should have a negative bias. However, we cannot distinguish which type of dependence (local dependence or heterogeneity) is the main cause of the bias.

In December 1995, the National Quarantine Service of Taiwan conducted a screen serum test for the HAV antibody for all students of the college at which the outbreak of the HAV occurred.[15] After suitable adjustments, they concluded that the final figure of the number infected was about 545. Thus this example presents a very valuable data set with the advantage of a known true parameter. Our estimator $\hat{N}_1$ does provide a satisfactory lower bound. This example shows the need for undercount correction and also the usefulness of the capture–recapture method in estimating the number of missed cases.

3.4. *Introducing* `CARE1` *with Example 1*

The R package `CARE1`, the first part of the program `CARE` (Capture–Recapture) in http://chao.stat,nthu.edu.tw/softwareCE.html, can be used to analyze epidemiological data via sample coverage approach.[12] Based on the input of records from several incomplete lists (or samples) of individuals, the R package `CARE1` provides output of population size estimate and related statistics. The maximum number of lists is 5. Note this section is mainly written as a User's Guide to `CARE1`. For self-contained purposes, a small portion of the material in this section overlaps with that of other sections.

The original version of `CARE1`[12] must be run in an S-plus environment which is not readily accessible for many users. We now change the programming language to R which can be freely downloaded from the internet. We use a real example to demonstrate how to run `CARE1`.

Consider the `HAV` data set in which all the ascertained hepatitis A virus (HAV) cases were classified according to their presence/absence in the three lists or sources; see Chao *et al.*[12] for details. The data set may be viewed using the following functions in CARE1:

```
> library(CARE1)
> data(HAV)
> HAV
   001 010 011 100 101 110 111
1  63  55  18  69  17   21  28
> estN.n(HAV)
      n1 n2 n3
[1,] 135122126
```

The above shows that the HAV data set contains seven possible "capture histories" or "ascertainment records" based on three sources: (001), (010), (011), (100), (101), (110) and (111), and function estN.n() outputs the number of individuals listed in the three sources are respectively 135, 122 and 126.

It has been suggested[24,25] that the Petersen and Chapman estimates based on any pair of lists can be used as preliminary analysis to detect possible dependence among lists. If these estimates for two samples are relatively high (low) compared to other pairwise estimates, then it indicates the two samples are negatively (positively) dependent. The Petersen and Chapman estimates along with their s.e.'s and the 95% confidence intervals of population size are given by the function estN.pair().

```
> round(estN.pair(HAV))
    Petersen Chapman se cil ciu
pa12     336         334 29 289 403
pa13     378         374 36 319 461
pa23     334         331 30 285 404
```

However, for the HAV data set, the Petersen and Chapman estimates for three pairs of lists are in the range of 330 to 380. The narrow range of these estimates would not indicate the possible direction of dependence at this stage.

Now, consider the sample coverage approach by using the function estN.stat().

```
> estN.stat(HAV)

    M       D     C^
1 271 208.667 0.513
```

Here $M = 271$ is the number of individuals ascertained in at least one list, $D = 208.667$ is the average of the overlapped cases, and C^ = 0.513 denotes the sample coverage estimate.

The function estN() computes three estimators of population size via sample coverage.

```
> round(estN(z, method="Indep", se=TRUE, nboot=1000))
    est se cil ciu
est 407 28 363 472

> round(estN(z, method="HSC", se=TRUE, nboot=1000))
    est se cil ciu
est 971 925 369 5290

> round(estN(z, method="LSC", se=TRUE, nboot=1000))
    est se cil ciu
est 508 40 442 600
```

The function with parameter method="Indep" outputs the population size estimator $\hat{N}_0$ that ignores the possible dependence between samples (Equation (9) in Chao *et al.*[12] or Equation (3) in this chapter). Here the output shows that $\hat{N}_0 = 407$ with a bootstrap s.e. 28 based on 1000 bootstrap replications (nboot=1000 in the function input; the user can modify this number simply replacing 1000 by any other positive numbers). The 95% confidence interval lower (cil) limit is 363 and the upper limit (ciu) is 472. You can change the setting se=TRUE to se=FALSE, then the bootstrap s.e. and confidence intervals will not be computed.

The function with method="HSC" outputs the population size estimator $\hat{N}$ for the cases with a relatively high sample coverage (a rough (or an empirical) guideline is C^ $\geq$ 55%). See Equation (12)[12] or Equation (4) in this chapter). Here we have for the HAV data that $\hat{N} = 971$, but a large estimated bootstrap s.e. (925) renders the estimate useless. It is then concluded that these data with a relatively low sample coverage estimate of 51% do not contain enough information to correct for undercount. See the preceding paragraph for the description of nboot=1000 and se=TRUE.

The function with method="LSC" outputs the one-step population size estimator $\hat{N}_1$ for relatively low sample coverage (a rough (or an empirical) guideline is C_hat < 55%) cases. (See Equation (13)[12] or Equation (5) in this chapter. For the HAV data, the one-step estimator is $\hat{N}_1 = 508$ with an estimated s.e. of 40. The 95% confidence interval lower (cil) limit is 442 and the upper limit (ciu) is 600. See the aforementioned explanations for the description of `nboot=1000` and `se=TRUE`.

`CARE1` also outputs the estimated mean ascertainment probabilities u1,u2,u3 and the coefficients of covariation (CCV, Equation (6)[12]) `r12,r13, r23,r123`. The CCV are parameters that are used to show the direction and magnitude of dependence among samples. All these depend on the value of N. Thus the estimators would be different in the three estimated methods. These estimates are computed by the function `estN.para()` in the package.

```
> round(estN.para(z, estN(z, method = "Indep")),2)
      u1    u2   u3  r12  r13  r23 r123
est 0.33 0.30 0.31 0.21 0.08 0.22 0.73

> round(estN.para(z, estN(z, method = "HSC")),2)
      u1   u2   u3  r12  r13  r23 r123
est 0.14 0.13 0.13 1.89 1.57 1.91 6.35

> round(estN.para(z, estN(z, method = "LSC")),2)
      u1   u2   u3  r12  r13  r23 r123
est 0.27 0.24 0.25 0.51 0.34 0.52 1.11
```

The output shows that for each population estimate, the estimated mean ascertainment probabilities, `u1`, `u2`, and `u3` have no apparent difference. The CCV estimates, `r12`, `r13` and `r23`, based on the three estimates of N show that any two samples are positively dependent. As a result, the estimate $\hat{N}_1 = 508$ can only serve as a lower bound.

`CARE1` features a quick analysis function, `CARE1.print()`, which calculates all output as shown below. This following output is the same as the first and the third parts of the output given in Chao *et al.*.[12] The second part, log-linear model approach, is omitted in this package. The reader is referred to the above paper for details.

```
> CARE1.print(HAV)
Number of identified cases in each list:
       n1        n2      n3
      135       122     126

ESTIMATES BASED ON ANY PAIR OF SAMPLES:
           Petersen      Chapman      se        cil       ciu
```

```
pair(1,2)       336         334       29       289       403
pair(1,3)       378         374       36       319       461
pair(2,3)       334         331       30       285       404
```

Note1: Refer to Seber(Pages 59 and 60)[44] for Petersen estimator and Chapman estimators as well as s.e formula.

Note2: A log-transformation is used is used to obtain the confidence interval so that the lower limit is always greater than the number of ascertained. Refer to Chao[5] for the construction of the confidence interval.

```
SAMPLE COVERAGE APPROACH:
          M          D       C^    est     se    cil     ciu
Nhat-0 271    208.667   0.513   407     28    363     472
Nhat   271    208.667   0.513   971    925    369    5290
Nhat-1 271    208.667   0.513   508     40    442     600

PARAMETER ESTIMATES:
         u1      u2      u3       r12    r13     r23     r123
Nhat-0 0.33   0.30    0.31     0.21   0.08    0.22    0.73
Nhat   0.14   0.13    0.13     1.89   1.57    1.91    6.35
Nhat-1 0.27   0.24    0.25     0.51   0.34    0.52    1.11
```

DEFINITIONS for the sample coverage approach:

M: number of individuals ascertained in at least one list.

D: the average of the number of individuals listed in the combination of any two lists omitting the other one; see Equation (8).[12]

C^: sample coverage estimate, see Equation (7).[12]

est: population size estimate.

se: estimated standard error of the population size estimation based on bootstrap replications.

cil: 95% confidence interval lower limit(using a log-transformation).

ciu: 95% confidence interval upper limit(using a log-transformation).

Nhat-0: Population size estimate for independent model; see Equation (9).[12]
Nhat: Population size estimate for sufficiently high sample coverage cases; see Equation (12).[12]

Nhat-1: One-step population size estimate for low sample coverage cases; see Equation (13).[12] This estimator is suggested for use when the estimated se of Nhat is relatively large.
u1,u2,u3: estimated mean probabilities.
r12,r13,r23,r123 etc.: estimated coefficient of covariation(CCV).

3.5. *Ecological models*

The most commonly used ecological models were proposed by Pollock (e.g. see Pollock[40]; Otis *et al.*[38]; White[49]). This approach specifies various forms of capture probabilities based on empirical investigations of animal ecology. Pollock considered a sequence of models to relax the equal catchability assumption, and these models were reviewed[40] and fully discussed in Otis *et al.*[38] and White.[49] Three sources of variation in capture probability are considered: (i) model $\mathbf{M}_{\mathrm{t}}$, which allows capture probabilities to vary by time; (ii) model $\mathbf{M}_{\mathrm{b}}$, which allows behavioral responses to capture; and (iii) model $\mathbf{M}_{\mathrm{h}}$, which allows heterogeneous capture probabilities. Various combinations of the above three variations (i.e., models $\mathbf{M}_{\mathrm{tb}}$, $\mathbf{M}_{\mathrm{th}}$, $\mathbf{M}_{\mathrm{bh}}$ and $\mathbf{M}_{\mathrm{tbh}}$) and the model M_0, in which no variation exists, are also considered.

Let P_{ij} be the conditional probability of capturing the ith animal in the jth sample given the capture history of samples $1, 2, \ldots, j-1$. A multiplicative form for the most general model is

$$P_{ij} = \begin{cases} p_i e_j & \text{until first capture,} \\ \phi p_i e_j & \text{for any recapture,} \end{cases} \tag{7}$$

where $0 < p_i e_j$, $\phi p_i e_j < 1$. Thus the parameters $\{e_1, e_2, \ldots, e_t\}$, $\{p_1, p_2, \ldots, p_N\}$ and ϕ are used, respectively, to model the time effects, individual heterogeneity and the behavioral response to capture. In this model, the recapture probabilities are assumed to be proportional to the initial capture probabilities. All sub-models of this general model are formulated in Table 7.

For models incorporating behavioral response, which induces local dependence among samples, the capture probability in a sample depends on whether the animal was captured in the "previous" samples. Hence the ordering of the trapping samples is involved and estimators do depend on the ordering of samples. Since there is usually no ordering among human lists or the ordering may vary with individuals, models with behavioral response are rarely adopted in modeling local dependence for humans. However, for animal data, the behavioral response model is useful as empirical

Table 7. Ecological models without covariates in CARE-2.

Model	Assumption	Restriction in model $\mathbf{M}_{\mathrm{tbh}}$
$\mathbf{M}_{\mathrm{tbh}}$	$P_{ij} = \begin{cases} p_i e_j & \text{until first capture} \\ \phi\, p_i e_j & \text{for any recapture} \end{cases}$	
$\mathbf{M}_{\mathrm{bh}}$	$P_{ij} = \begin{cases} p_i & \text{until first capture} \\ \phi\, p_i & \text{for any recapture} \end{cases}$	set $e_j = 1$
$\mathbf{M}_{\mathrm{tb}}$	$P_{ij} = \begin{cases} e_j & \text{until first capture} \\ \phi\, e_j & \text{for any recapture} \end{cases}$	set $p_i = 1$
$\mathbf{M}_{\mathrm{th}}$	$P_{ij} = p_i e_j$	set $\phi = 1$
$\mathbf{M}_{\mathrm{h}}$	$P_{ij} = p_i$	set $e_j = 1$, $\phi = 1$
$\mathbf{M}_{\mathrm{b}}$	$P_{ij} = \begin{cases} p & \text{until first capture} \\ \phi\, p & \text{for any recapture} \end{cases}$	set $p_i = p$, $e_j = 1$
$\mathbf{M}_t$	$P_{ij} = e_j$	set $p_i = 1$, $\phi = 1$
$\mathbf{M}_0$	$P_{ij} = p$	set $p_i = p$, $e_j = 1$, $\phi = 1$

P_{ij} denotes the capture probability of the ith individual on the jth occasion
p_i: heterogeneity effect of the ith individual, $i = 1, 2, \ldots, N$;
e_j: time or occasional effect of the jth occasion, $j = 1, 2, \ldots, t$;
ϕ: behavioral response effect.

studies have provided evidence that mice, voles and other mammals often exhibit trap response to capture, especially the first capture.

Heterogeneous model which allows different capture probabilities among animals are potentially useful in health science. Most estimators for such a heterogeneous model require that the number of trapping occasions should be at least five (Otis *et al.*,[38] p. 34; Chao *et al.*,[12]). Thus, we specifically use Example 4 (with six lists) to illustrate the use of ecological models.

3.6. *Introducing* CARE-2 *with Example 4*

Program CARE-2 (http://chao.stat.nthu.edu.tw/softwareCE.html) calculates population size estimates for various closed capture–recapture models. See CARE-2 User's Guide by Chao and Yang[13] for details about the models and estimators featured in CARE-2. The program consists of two parts: one part, written in C Language, deals with models without covariates and the other part, written in GAUSS language, deals with models with covariates. The latter part will be introduced in Section 4.

Using the six-occasion capture–recapture data in Table 4 (but covariates are not considered) in CARE-2, the following output is shown in the Output

Table 8. Partial CARE-2 output of deer mice data analysis (without using covariates).

(1) Basic Data Information:

```
-----------------------------------------------
   Data filename : c:\program files\CARE-2\data\example1.dat
   Total # of distinct animals : 38
   Number of capture occasions : 6
   Bootstrap replications : 1000
-----------------------------------------------
```

(2) Summary Statistics:

i	u[i]	m[i]	n[i]	M[i]	ft[i]	f1[i]
1	15	0	15	0	9	15
2	8	12	20	15	6	11
3	6	10	16	23	7	14
4	3	16	19	29	6	11
5	3	22	25	32	6	8
6	3	22	25	35	4	9
7				38		

ft[i]: # of individuals that were captured exactly i times on occasions 1, 2, ..., t.
f1[i]: # of individuals that were captured exactly once on occasions 1, 2, ..., i.

(3) Estimation Results:

Model	Estimate	Boot_s.e.	Asy_s.e.	Phi	CV	95% CI (log-transf.)	95% CI (percentile)
Mb(UMLE)	40.8	6.91	3.05	1.79		(38.18, 81.43)	(38.00, 51.98)
Mh(SC1)	43.5	3.81	3.72		0.50	(39.64, 56.78)	(39.65, 50.94)
Mh(SC2)	42.4	3.52	3.40		0.48	(39.09, 55.48)	(38.73, 49.29)
Mth(SC1)	43.6	3.97	3.77		0.51	(39.62, 57.57)	(39.70, 51.76)
Mth(SC2)	42.5	3.41	3.45		0.49	(39.18, 54.85)	(38.90, 48.89)
Mth(EE)	40.3	2.20	----		0.51	(38.48, 49.14)	(38.00, 44.26)
Mbh(SC)	50.5	23.43	----		0.60	(39.13, 176.57)	(38.89, 125.72)
Mbh(EE)	43.5	4.44	----	1.68	0.40	(39.36, 60.04)	(38.00, 51.33)
Mtbh(EE)	44.2	4.58	----	1.89	0.36	(39.72, 60.60)	(38.10, 53.58)

SC: sample coverage approach

EE: estimating equation approach

UMLE: unconditional maximum likelihood estimate

95% CI are based on the bootstrap s.e.

window after execution. The output contains three parts: (1) basic data information; (2) summary statistics; and (3) results of estimation.

The first part of the output in Table 8 shows basic information including the data filename, the number of distinct animals caught in the experiment (38 in this case), the number of trapping occasions (6 in this case) and the number of bootstrap replications (1000 in this case) which is used for assessing bootstrap s.e. The summary statistics are listed in the second part of the output. The third part shows estimation results. For these data, Otis *et al.*[38] (p. 32) indicated that the most suitable model for these data was model $\mathbf{M}_b$. Based on the usual unconditional maximum likelihood estimator (UMLE), which is denoted by Mb(UMLE) in Table 8, the estimated population size in model $\mathbf{M}_b$ is 41 with bootstrap s.e. of 6.9 and asymptotic s.e. of 3.1. The 95% confidence intervals are (38.2, 81.4) and (38.0,

52.0) for log-transformation and percentile methods respectively based on the bootstrap procedure. The proportion constant between the re-capture probability and first-recapture probability (ϕ in Table 7 or Phi in Table 8) is estimated to be 1.79, suggesting animals became trap-happy after their first capture.

Chao and Huggins[9] suggested considering further general models $\mathbf{M}_{\mathrm{bh}}$ and $\mathbf{M}_{\mathrm{tbh}}$ by use of estimating equation (EE) approach. The two models produce close estimates, as shown by the two estimates Mbh(EE) and Mtbh(EE) in Table 8. So it is reasonable to adopt the most general model $\mathbf{M}_{\mathrm{tbh}}$ and conclude that the population size is about 44 (standard error 4.6). The data based on model $\mathbf{M}_{\mathrm{tbh}}$ show strong trap-happy behavior (Phi $= 1.89$ in Table 8), a low degree of heterogeneity (the CV estimate is 0.36, where CV denotes the coefficient of variation of $\{p_1, p_2, \ldots, p_N)$, and slight time-varying effects as the relative time effects are estimated to be $(\bar{p}e_1, \ldots, \bar{p}e_6) = (0.34, 0.32, 0.26, 0.26, 0.33, 0.33)$, where $\bar{p}$ denotes the average of p_i's. These time effects are not shown in the output; refer to Chao *et al.*[14] for calculation formula. The 95% confidence interval using a log-transformation under model $\mathbf{M}_{\mathrm{tbh}}$ is 40 to 61. Usually, a simpler model yields an estimator with smaller variance but larger bias whereas a general model using the same estimation method yields an estimator with lower bias but larger variance. For interval estimation, a simpler model produces narrow confidence interval with possibly poor coverage probability whereas a more general model produces wide interval with more satisfactory coverage probability. However, different estimation methods are used here for models $\mathbf{M}_{\mathrm{b}}$ and $\mathbf{M}_{\mathrm{tbh}}$. Thus the resulting confidence intervals are not comparable.

4. Models with Covariates

For epidemiological data, individual's covariates include age, gender, race, geographic area, marital groups, diagnostic group, time of onset, severity of diseases and many other explanatory variables. For animal studies, individual's covariates include age, gender, body weight, wing length and others; environmental covariates include temperature, rainfall, number of traps and others. The covariate variables are usually classified as either discrete (categorical type) or continuous (numerical type).

As discussed earlier, traditional approach depends on a crucial assumption of "equal-ascertainment" or "equal-catchability". Heterogeneity in ascertainment/capture probabilities induces dependence among samples, which causes correlation bias in the usual estimator. One approach to assessing heterogeneity is based on the assumption that heterogeneity can be largely explained by some relevant observable covariates. If covariates are discrete, Sekar and Deming[47] were the first to suggest post-stratification to reduce the bias due to heterogeneity. That is, if the population can be divided into several homogeneous sub-populations defined by relevant covariates, then a stratified analysis can be performed. That is, model is fitted to the data within each stratum, then all population size estimates are added to obtain an overall estimate (e.g., Wittes[51]; IWGDMF,[34,35]).

Pollock, Hines and Nichols[41] were the first to use a logistic regression model to include continuous covariates in the analysis. In this approach, covariates are used to model heterogeneous capture probabilities via a logistic regression model. They developed an estimation procedure based on the full likelihood. However, the covariates for the un-captured animals were not observable. Therefore, they had to make some assumption about the covariates for the un-captured animals. Huggins[32,33] and Alho[1] avoided this difficult by using a likelihood conditional on the captured animals so that the covariates of the un-captured are not needed. Alho *et al.*[2] applied this logistic regression approach to the 1990 census and the Post-Enumeration Survey of the United States. Yip *et al.*[54] extended this logistic regression to allow random removals in the experiments.

4.1. *Logistic regression models in* CARE-2

In program CARE-2, we distinguish covariates as two types: individual covariates and occasional covariates as in Huggins,[32,33] as described earlier. Suppose for each individual, there are s individual covariates. Let the individual covariates for the ith animal be denoted as $\boldsymbol{W}_i' = (W_{i1}, W_{i2}, \ldots, W_{is})$ and $\boldsymbol{\beta}' = (\beta_1, \beta_2, \ldots, \beta_s)$ denotes the effects of these covariates. It is necessary to assume that the individual covariates are constant across the t capture occasions in the experiment, as they cannot be measured on an occasion if the individual is not captured. If heterogeneity is fully explained by individuals' covariates, then the heterogeneity effect can be expressed conveniently as $\boldsymbol{\beta}'\boldsymbol{W}_i = \beta_1 W_{i1} + \beta_2 W_{i2} + \cdots + \beta_s W_{is}$.

Assume that there are b known occasional or time covariates: $\{R_{11}, R_{12}, \ldots, R_{1t}\}, \{R_{21}, R_{22}, \ldots, R_{2t}\}, \ldots, \{R_{b1}, R_{b2}, \ldots, R_{bt}\}$. For example, $\{R_{11}, R_{12}, \ldots, R_{1t}\}$ may represent the temperature on each occasion, and $\{R_{b1}, R_{b2}, \ldots, R_{bt}\}$ may represent the capture effort on each occasion. Let $r' = (r_1, r_2, \ldots, r_b)$ denote the effects of the occasional covariates. Define $\boldsymbol{R}_j' = \{R_{1j}, R_{2j}, \ldots, R_{bj}\}$, then the occasional effect for the jth occasion can be expressed as $\boldsymbol{r}'\boldsymbol{R}_j = r_1 R_{1j} + r_2 R_{2j} + \cdots + r_b R_{bj}$.

Table 9. Logistic regression models with covariates in CARE-2.

Model	Assumption	Restriction in model $\mathbf{M}^*_{\text{tbh}}$
$\mathbf{M}^*_{\text{tbh}}$	$\text{logit}(P_{ij}) = a + c_j + vY_{ij} + \boldsymbol{\beta}'\boldsymbol{W}_i + \boldsymbol{r}'\boldsymbol{R}_j$	
$\mathbf{M}^*_{\text{bh}}$	$\text{logit}(P_{ij}) = a + vY_{ij} + \boldsymbol{\beta}'\boldsymbol{W}_i$	set $c_j = 0$, $\boldsymbol{r} = \mathbf{0}$
$\mathbf{M}^*_{tb}$	$\text{logit}(P_{ij}) = a + c_j + vY_{ij} + \boldsymbol{r}'\boldsymbol{R}_j$	set $\boldsymbol{\beta} = \mathbf{0}$
$\mathbf{M}^*_{th}$	$\text{logit}(P_{ij}) = a + c_j + \boldsymbol{\beta}'\boldsymbol{W}_i + \boldsymbol{r}'\boldsymbol{R}_j$	set $v = 0$
$\mathbf{M}^*_{h}$	$\text{logit}(P_{ij}) = a + \boldsymbol{\beta}'\boldsymbol{W}_i$	set $c_j = 0$, $\boldsymbol{r} = \mathbf{0}$, $v = 0$
$\mathbf{M}^*_{\text{b}}$	$\text{logit}(P_{ij}) = a + vY_{ij}$	set $\boldsymbol{\beta} = \mathbf{0}$, $c_j = 0$, $\boldsymbol{r} = \mathbf{0}$
$\mathbf{M}^*_{t}$	$\text{logit}(P_{ij}) = a + c_j + \boldsymbol{r}'\boldsymbol{R}_j$	set $\boldsymbol{\beta} = \mathbf{0}$, $v = 0$
$\mathbf{M}^*_{0}$	$\text{logit}(P_{ij}) = a$	set $\boldsymbol{\beta} = \mathbf{0}$, $c_j = 0$, $\boldsymbol{r} = \mathbf{0}$, $v = 0$

P_{ij}: capture probability of the ith animal on the jth occasion;
a: baseline intercept;
c_j: unknown time or occasional effect of the jth occasion, $j = 1, 2, \ldots, t$;
v: behavioral response effect;
$\boldsymbol{\beta}' = (\beta_1, \beta_2, \ldots, \beta_s)$: heterogeneity effect of the known individual covariates;
$\boldsymbol{r}' = (r_1, r_2, \ldots, r_b)$: effects of the known occasional or time covariates.

Define $Y_{ij} = 1$ if the ith animal has been captured at least once before the jth occasion, and $Y_{ij} = 0$ otherwise. The general logistic regression model, denoted by $\mathbf{M}^*_{\text{tbh}}$, incorporating time effects, behavioral response effect and heterogeneous covariates considered in CARE-2[33] is

$$\text{logit}(P_{ij}) = a + c_j + vY_{ij} + \boldsymbol{\beta}'\boldsymbol{W}_i + \boldsymbol{r}'\boldsymbol{R}_j, \tag{8}$$

where a denotes the baseline intercept, $\{c_1, c_2, \ldots, c_{t-1}\}$ represents the unknown occasional or time effect ($c_t \equiv 0$ is used for the reference group), v denotes the behavioral response effect, $\boldsymbol{\beta}' = (\beta_1, \beta_2, \ldots, \beta_s)$ denotes the heterogeneity effect of the known individual covariates, $r' = (r_1, r_2, \ldots, r_b)$ denotes the effects of the known occasional or time covariates. Table 9 summarizes all sub-models.

In assessing the effect of each individual covariate, one coefficient is associated with a continuous covariate. For a discrete covariate with k categories, we need to construct $k-1$ dummy indicators to specify the effect of each category by selecting one category as a reference group with zero effect. Thus, the effect of this covariate is described by $k-1$ beta coefficients. For example, if the first covariate is discrete with $k > 2$ categories, then the corresponding beta is a vector $(\beta_{1(1)}, \beta_{1(2)}, \ldots, \beta_{1(k-1)})$. The coefficient $\beta_{n(l)}$ denotes the effect of the lth group relative to the reference group for the nth covariate. See Section 4.2 for an example.

The interpretation of the coefficient of any β is based on the fact that when $\beta > 0$, the larger the covariate is, the larger the capture probability is, while if $\beta < 0$ then the larger the covariate is, the smaller the capture probability is. Similar interpretation pertains to the coefficient of any occasional covariate. The parameter v represents the effect of a recapture, which implies that $v > 0$ corresponds to a case of trap-happy and $v < 0$ corresponds to a case of trap-shy.

The parameters in the logistic regression models in Equation (8) are estimated by a conditional ML method based on the captured individuals.[32, 33] Typically numerical iterative procedures are required to obtain parameter estimates. The default of the maximum number of iterations in CARE-2 is 500. Model selection can be performed using Akaike information criterion (AIC) which is defined as $-2\log L + 2m$, where L denotes the likelihood computed at the conditional MLE and m denotes the number of parameters in the model. A model is selected if AIC is the smallest among all models considered. After the coefficients of the logistic regression are obtained, the population size is estimated by the Horvitz-Thompson[31] estimator, which is $\hat{N}_{HT} = \sum_{i=1}^{M} \{1 - \prod_{j=1}^{t}(1 - \hat{P}_{ij})\}^{-1}$, where $\hat{P}_{ij}$ is the estimated capture probability evaluated at the conditional MLE and M denotes the number of distinct individuals caught in the sample. The variance of the resulting estimator can be estimated by an asymptotic variance formula derived in Huggins.[32, 33] Below two examples are used for CARE-2 to illustrate the estimation and model selection.

4.2. *Stratified neurologic illness data* (*Example 2, three lists*)

We first analyze the data by using stratified analysis (Example 2, data are given in Table 2). Within each stratum, various models are applied to the data and the results are shown in Table 10. We also present the un-stratified results (i.e., using the collapsed data over strata) in the last column. Fro the two-sample results, except for the first stratum, the estimate based on the H-list and P-list is much lower than the other two Petersen's estimates, implying positive dependence exists between the two lists. This finding is further confirmed by the CCV estimates (not reported) in the sample coverage approach.

The sample coverage estimate under independence for un-stratified data ($\hat{N}_0$, in Equation (3)) gives an estimate of 762 (s.e. 21) which is close to the stratified results (757 with s.e. 21). However, these estimates are suspected to be underestimates as there is significantly positive dependence exists for

Table 10. Various estimates of the population size for neurologic illness data. (Standard error is in the parenthesis).

	Diagnostic Group (Stratum)					
Model/Method	A	B	C	D	Stratified	Un-stratified
Petersen's estimate:						
(H, P)	59 (16)	18 (3)	365 (34)	192 (24)	634 (45)	631 (46)
(H, S)	46 (7)	24 (3)	395 (19)	298 (21)	763 (29)	761 (29)
(P, S)	36 (5)	22 (2)	469 (34)	264 (23)	791 (41)	789 (41)
Sample coverage:						
$\hat{N}_0$: Eq. (3)	43 (5)	23 (2)	436 (17)	255 (10)	757 (21)	762 (21)
$\hat{N}$: Eq. (4)	42 (20)	24 (15)	524 (68)	218 (15)	808 (74)	812 (65)
$\hat{N}_1$: Eq. (5)	42 (7)	23 (3)	468 (29)	239 (16)	772 (34)	782 (32)
Logistic regression model:						
Model M_{th}^* in Eq. (9) with covariate and list effects, the Horvitz-Thompson estimate: 765 (s.e. 22), deviance = 38.8 (d.f. 22, P-value = 0.015), indicating inadequate fit.						

the H-list and P-list. Bobo *et al.*[3] suggested fitting a log-linear model with the interaction term between H-list and P-list to the collapsed data, and obtained an estimate of 787.

We can regard the stratum as an individual covariate in the logistic regression model. Since there is no natural ordering among the three lists, models with behavioral response effect are not meaningful. We only consider a model with stratum effects and occasional (or list) effects. The stratifying variable is regarded as a categorical covariate. As described in Section 4.1, for a covariate with k strata ($k = 4$ in this case), we need to construct $k-1$ dummy indicators to specify the effect of each stratum. That is, for the ith individual define the dummy variable $W_{i1(s)} = I$ (the ith individual is in the sth stratum), $s = 1, 2, \ldots, k-1$, a logistic regression model M_{th}^* can be expressed as

$$\text{logit}(P_{ij}) = a + c_j + \beta_{1(1)} W_{i1(1)} + \beta_{1(2)} W_{i1(2)} + \cdots + \beta_{1(k-1)} W_{i1(k-1)}. \tag{9}$$

In this model, the parameters are

a: baseline intercept,

$(c_1, c_2, \ldots, c_{t-1})$: occasional or list effects, $(c_t = 0)$.

$(\beta_{1(1)}, \beta_{1(2)}, \ldots, \beta_{1(k-1)})$: stratum effect, $\beta_{1(s)}$ denotes the effect of the sth stratum, $s = 1, 2, \ldots, k-1$. $(\beta_{1(k)} = 0.)$

Under model (9), an analogous population size estimate of 765 (s.e. 22) is obtained by a logistic regression model incorporating the stratifying variable and the list effects. However, the deviance statistic of the logistic regression model is 38.8 with 22 degrees of freedom (P-value $= 0.015$), indicating inadequate fit. So the logistic regression model (9) and its all-submodels cannot be applied to these data.

Back to the sample coverage approach, the coverage $\hat{C} = 65.2\%$ for collapsed data, and $\hat{C} = (67.3\%, 79.8\%, 63.2\%, 68.4\%)$ for each stratum, indicating relatively high coverages. So our population size estimate $\hat{N}$ for relative high coverage in Equation (4) is applicable. The sample coverage estimates $\hat{N}$ for both un-stratified and stratified data match well. Recall that the purpose of stratification is mainly to reduce the dependence due to heterogeneity. The overall dependencies are considered and adjusted in the sample coverage estimators $\hat{N}$. Therefore, the closeness of the stratified and un-stratified results is expected. (As will be seen in Section 4.3, post-stratification is not warranted because insufficient overlap may arise in some strata, leading to an unstable stratified result.) For this data set, the estimator $\hat{N}$ that can take account of two types of dependencies in each stratum has acceptable precision. Both stratified and un-stratified estimates can be recommended since they result in comparable variation using 1000 bootstrap replications. The latter estimate is 812 with an estimated bootstrap s.e. of 65, which yields a 95% confidence interval of (720, 988). The former yields a slightly lower estimate of 808 with a higher s.e. of 74, which implies a 95% confidence interval of (709, 1015).

4.3. *Stratified drug data (Example 3, four lists)*

Table 11 shows the analysis results for the drug data (Example 3, data are given in Table 3). Estimates based on various models are presented for each stratum and for the collapsed data. Except for the stratum of 4–6 days, the Petersen estimates based on the lists 1 and 2 are lower than the others and thus positive dependence is expected. The CCV estimate (not shown) for the total data reveals that positive dependence also exists between the lists 1 and 3. Wittes (1974) suspected that positive dependence may arise between list-3 and list-4, but the CCV estimate only shows very weak dependence.

Wittes[54] fitted an independent log-near model to the data in each stratum and obtained a stratified estimate of 544 (s.e. 22.4). She also obtained an un-stratified estimate under an independent model is 524 (s.e. 18). The sample coverage estimator under independence model gives an un-stratified

Table 11. Various estimates of the total number of patients for drug data.(Standard error is in the parenthesis).

Model/Method	Usage on Drugs (Stratum) 1–3 days	4–6 days	7+ days	Stratified	Un-stratified
Petersen's estimate:					
(1, 2)	50 (14)	278# (183)	80 (16)	408 (184)	300 (71)
(1, 3)	350 (112)	214 (49)	133 (15)	697 (123)	459 (54)
(1, 4)	135 (22)	194 (18)	178 (12)	507 (31)	497 (28)
(2, 3)	175 (49)	152 (42)	171 (47)	498 (80)	468 (112)
(2, 4)	123 (28)	284 (69)	211 (43)	618 (86)	609 (99)
(3, 4)	173 (27)	193 (12)	184 (11)	550 (32)	527 (25)
Sample coverage:					
$\hat{N}_0$: Eq. (3)	151 (22)	226 (23)	178 (10)	555 (33)	541 (26)
$\hat{N}$: Eq. (4)	170 (575)	286 (63)	185 (26)	641 (579)	635 (93)
$\hat{N}_1$: Eq. (5)	157 (32)	247 (28)	182 (17)	586 (46)	579 (44)
Logistic regression model:					
Model $\mathbf{M}_{th}^*$ in Eq. (9) with covariate and list effects, the Horvitz-Thompson estimate: 539 (s.e. 21), deviance = 39.81 (d.f. 39, P-value = 0.43), indicating adequate fit. See the text for the fitted parameters and interpretations.					

#Petersen's estimate does not exist due to there are no overlapped cases; Chapman's estimator is calculated instead (see Seber,,[44] p. 59 and 60)

estimate of 541 (s.e. 26) and stratified estimate of 555 (s.e. 33). The logistic regression model $\mathbf{M}_{\text{th}}^*$ in Equation (9) which takes account of the stratifying variable and list effects provides proper fit to the data because the deviance is 39.81 with 39 degrees of freedom (P-value = 0.43). Under model $\mathbf{M}_{\text{th}}^*$, the fitted intercept is 1.04. The coefficient, $\beta_{1(1)} = -0.86$ (s.e. 0.22) and $\beta_{1(2)} = -0.47$ (s.e. 0.18) are the stratum effects for time length "1–3 days" and "4–6 days", respectively; the stratum effect of time length "7+ days" is set to be 0. The results demonstrate that the shorter the time length of drug use, the lower the ascertainment probability. For the unknown list effect, $c_1 = -2.13$ (s.e. 0.16), $c_2 = -3.87$ (s.e. 0.25) and $c_3 = -1.54$ (s.e. 0.14); c_4 is set to be 0. Model (9) gives a population size 539 (s.e. 21) and the 95% confidence interval of (505, 587).

In the first stratum, the relatively large bootstrap s.e. of the sample coverage estimator $\hat{N}$ indicates that data information cannot provide a reliable estimate and thus only a reasonable lower bound can be obtained. Consequently, the stratified estimate based on $\hat{N}$ is not recommended for use. For the collapsed data, the coverage $\hat{C} = 66.8\%$, indicating a relatively high coverage the precision is acceptable, showing the collapsed data are sufficient to incorporate both types of dependencies. We obtain an estimate $\hat{N} = 635$ with an estimated s.e. of 93 based on 1000 bootstrap replications (see Table 11). A 95% confidence interval of the size can be constructed as (520, 895). The sample coverage approach for un-stratified data produces estimator much higher than the estimate from a logistic regression model (9). As described in Section 1.3, local dependence was suspected between lists 3 and 4 because the records from the pharmacy were duplicates of the medication sheets. Although the logistic type of regression model can be used to assess the effect of any type of covariates (both discrete and continuous), it does not take account of any local dependence and heterogeneity is entirely explained by covariates. But the sample coverage approach can take local dependence into account. Therefore, there are relative merits for the sample coverage estimator $\hat{N}$ and the logistic regression model.

4.4. *Deer mice data* (*Example 4, six occasions*)

We now apply the logistic regression model in Equation (8) and sub-models in Table 9 to the mice data (Example 4, data are given in Table 4). In addition to the data of six capture occasions (time effect) and three individual's covariates (individual heterogeneity), behavioral response arose by the natural time ordering of capture occasions can also be considered.[38,53] As to individual heterogeneity, there are two categorical variables: gender (male and female) and age (adult and young; semi-adult is classified as adult). Since there are only two categories for each of these two variables, we only need one effect for each. For the first covariate gender, let $W_{i1} = I$ (the ith mouse is male) and its corresponding effect be $\beta_{1(1)}$. For the second covariate age, let $W_{i2} = I$ (the ith mouse is adult) its corresponding effect be $\beta_{2(1)}$. The variable weight is a continuous variable W_{i3} = weight, and its effect is denoted by β_3. Then a logistic regression model $\mathbf{M}^*_{\text{tbh}}$ can be written as follows:

$$\text{logit}(P_{ij}) = a + c_j + vY_{ij} + \beta_{1(1)}W_{i1} + \beta_{2(1)}W_{i2} + \beta_3 W_{i3}, \qquad (10)$$

where c_j and Y_{ij} are defined in Equation (8). Under this model or any sub-model, the capture probability for each capture record can be determined and thus the conditional likelihood can be formulated. Then the maximum likelihood estimates of the parameters a, v, $(c_1, c_2, \ldots, c_{t-1})$ and $(\beta_1, \beta_2, \ldots, \beta_{k-1})$ are searched by numerical iteration. Table 12 shows the fitting and estimation results for the logistic regression model and all

Table 12. The CARE-2 output of covariate analysis for deer mice data (example 4). $\mathrm{M}^*_{\mathrm{bh}}$ is selected based on the AIC and the fitted model is shown in bold. Deviance = 4.43 with d.f. 5 when compared with $\mathrm{M}^*_{\mathrm{tbh}}$, P-value = 0.49, indicating adequate fit.

=== The Fit & Estimation of all models ===

Model	Estimate	S.E.	MIN(-LL)	AIC	95% CI	Status
M*0	38.47	0.72	157.27	316.54	(38.06, 42.04)	Converge
M*t	38.40	0.66	152.42	316.84	(38.04, 41.80)	Converge
M*b	42.25	3.76	150.43	304.87	(38.96, 56.86)	Converge
M*h	39.85	1.72	144.87	297.75	(38.39, 46.67)	Converge
M*tb	46.48	12.65	148.18	310.36	(39.02, 108.74)	Converge
M*th	39.66	1.61	139.55	297.10	(38.34, 46.20)	Converge
M*bh	**47.15**	**7.17**	**139.54**	**289.09**	**(40.35, 73.52)**	**Converge**
M*tbh	47.13	10.08	137.33	294.66	(39.59, 90.50)	Converge

=== The MLEs of Regression Coefficients ===

*** Model M*0 ***

	a
MLE	0.08
S.E.	0.13

*** Model M*t ***

	a	c_1	c_2	c_3	c_4	c_5
MLE	0.62	-1.07	-0.54	-0.96	-0.64	0.00
S.E.	0.24	0.42	0.42	0.42	0.42	0.17

*** Model M*b ***

	a	v
MLE	-0.76	1.22
S.E.	0.34	0.38

*** Model M*h ***

	a	beta1(1)	beta2(1)	beta3
MLE	-1.95	0.81	-1.90	0.16
S.E.	0.71	0.31	0.57	0.06

*** Model M*tb ***

	a	v	c_1	c_2	c_3	c_4	c_5
MLE	-1.16	1.72	0.42	0.31	-0.45	-0.37	0.12
S.E.	1.09	0.98	0.80	0.57	0.49	0.45	0.42

*** Model M*th ***

	a	beta1(1)	beta2(1)	beta3	c_1	c_2	c_3	c_4	c_5
MLE	-1.43	0.84	-1.98	0.16	-1.18	-0.59	-1.06	-0.70	0.00
S.E.	0.74	0.32	0.58	0.06	0.44	0.43	0.44	0.43	0.19

***** Model M*bh *****

	a	v	beta1(1)	beta2(1)	beta3
MLE	**-2.91**	**1.18**	**0.92**	**-1.88**	**0.16**
S.E.	**0.87**	**0.40**	**0.35**	**0.63**	**0.06**

*** Model M*tbh ***

	a	v	beta1(1)	beta2(1)	beta3	c_1	c_2	c_3	c_4	c_5
MLE	-2.76	1.21	0.94	-1.92	0.16	-0.11	0.02	-0.71	-0.50	0.08
S.E.	1.30	0.74	0.36	0.64	0.06	0.87	0.80	0.60	0.56	0.57

sub-models. For each model, the corresponding estimated population size (number under the heading Estimate in Table 12), its s.e. (under the heading S.E.), negative value of the minimum log-likelihood under the heading MIN(-LL), the Akaike information criterion (AIC) and 95% confidence interval (Chao, 1987) are calculated and a "Status" indicates whether the iterative procedures were converged or not.

We use AIC as a criterion for model selection and find that the models considering behavioral response perform better than the models without considering behavioral response. Among behavioral response models, the $\mathbf{M}^*_{\mathrm{bh}}$ has the minimum AIC, 289.1. The results suggest that capture probabilities of mice is affected by behavioral response and individual heterogeneity but not for time occasion effect. Insignificant time effects can be observed from that c_j approaches to zero in model $\mathbf{M}^*_{\mathrm{tbh}}$. From the values of AIC, we select model $\mathbf{M}^*_{\mathrm{bh}}$ because AIC of this model is the smallest among all models. If we compare this model with the most general $\mathbf{M}^*_{\mathrm{tbh}}$, then the deviance is 4.43 (d.f. =5) P-value $= 0.49$, indicating adequate fit.

Under model $\mathbf{M}^*_{\mathrm{bh}}$, the fitted intercept is -2.91, the behavioral response effect is 1.18 (s.e. 0.4) for re-capture (the first capture effect is set to be 0, so recaptures have higher probabilities). The behavioral response effect is significantly larger than 0, implicating that baited traps made mice trap-happy. The coefficient, $\beta_{1(1)} = 0.92$ (s.e. 0.35), is the effect for male; the female is set to be 0, so males have larger probabilities. The second coefficient, $\beta_{2(1)} = -1.88$ (s.e. 0.63), is the effect for adult; the young effect is set to be 0, so young have larger capture probabilities. The last coefficient in the output, $\beta_3 = 0.16$ (s.e. 0.06) is the effect for a unit change of body weight. This implies the heavier the weight, the larger the capture probability. Then from the summary of model fitting the estimated population size under the selected model $\mathbf{M}^*_{\mathrm{bh}}$ is 47.2 (s.e. 7.17) with a 95% confidence interval of (40.4, 73.5). If behavioral response or individual heterogeneity was ignored improperly and a reduced model $\mathbf{M}^*_{\mathrm{h}}$ or $\mathbf{M}^*_{\mathrm{b}}$ was used then the population size will be underestimated. Although we use animal data as an illustrative example, such analysis can be readily applied to analyze epidemiological data. If there is no natural ordering among lists, then all models with behavioral response can be omitted in the analysis.

5. Remarks and Discussion

Capture–recapture models provide a potentially useful method for assessing the extent of incomplete ascertainment in epidemiological studies but there are assumptions and limitations to this approach. We have reviewed three methods (ecological models, sample coverage approach and logistic regression analysis) and applied them to three epidemiological data sets and one animal data set with/without covariates. The four data analyses have demonstrated the usefulness of the capture–recapture analysis.

Basic assumptions must be checked to validate the implementation of the capture–recapture method. Hook and Regal[28, 30] presented 17 recommendations for the use of the capture–recapture method in epidemiology. We also urge the readers to check the assumptions listed in Section 2 before capture–recapture analysis.

We have shown that for some data sets (e.g., the HAV data and the first stratum of the drug data), insufficient overlap information usually results in an imprecise estimate. This implies that a serious limitation of the capture–recapture methods is that sufficiently high overlapping information is required to produce reliable population size estimates and to model dependence among samples. Coull and Agresti[20] also indicated that the likelihood functions under some models for sparse information might become flat and the resulting estimates are likely to become unstable. In such cases, we feel that a precise lower bound as provided by the sample coverage approach, Equation (5), is of more practical use than an imprecise point estimate.

Almost all methods discussed in this chapter require extensive numerical iterations or calculations to obtain estimators and standard errors. Therefore, user-friendly software is essential for applications. We have demonstrated two parts of program CARE (for capture–recapture): CARE1 and CARE-2. The program CARE and user guides are online available and can be downloaded freely from the first author's website at http://chao.stat.nthu.edu.tw/softwareCE.html.

Acknowledgments

Research for Anne Chao was supported by the National Science Council of Taiwan under Contract/grant number 97-2118-M007-003-MY3.

References

1. Alho, J. M. (1990) Logistic regression in capture–recapture models. *Biometrics* 1990, **46**: 623–635.
2. Alho, J. M., Mulry, M. H., Wurdeman, K., and Kim, J. (1993). Estimating heterogeneity in the probabilities of enumeration for dual-system estimation. *Journal of the American Statistical Association*, **88**: 1130–1136.

3. Bobo, J. K., Thapa, P. B., Anderson, J. A., and Gale, J. L. (1994). Acute encephalopathy and seizure rates in children under age two years in Oregon and Washington state. *American Journal of Epidemiology*, **140**: 27–38.
4. Briand, L. C., El Emam, K., Freimut, B. G., and Laitenberger, O. (2000). A comprehensive evaluation of capture–recapture models for estimating software defect content. *Software Engineering, IEEE Transactions on*, **26**: 518–540.
5. Chao, A. (1987). Estimating the population size for capture–recapture data with unequal catchability. *Biometrics*, **43**: 783–791.
6. Chao, A. (1998). Capture–recapture. In *Encyclopedia of Biostatistics*, eds. P. Armitage and T. Colton, Wiley, New York, 482–486.
7. Chao, A. (2001). An overview of closed capture–recapture models. *Journal of Agricultural, Biological, and Environmental Statistic*, **6**: 158–175.
8. Chao, A., and Huggins, R. M. (2005a). Classical closed-population capture–recapture models. In *The Handbook of Capture–Recapture Methods*, eds. S. Amstrup, T. McDonald and B. Manly, Princeton University Press, 22–35.
9. Chao, A., and Huggins, R. M. (2005b). Modern closed-population capture–recapture models. In *The Handbook of Capture–Recapture Methods*, eds. S. Amstrup, T. McDonald and B. Manly, Princeton University Press, 58–87.
10. Chao, A., Pan, H. Y., and Chiang, S. C. (2008). The Petersen–Lincoln Estimator and its Extension to Estimate the Size of a Shared Population. *Biometrical Journal*, **50**: 957–970.
11. Chao, A., and Tsay, P. K. (1998). A sample coverage approach to multiple-system estimation with application to census undercount. *Journal of the American Statistical Association*, **93**: 283–293.
12. Chao, A., Tsay, P. K., Lin, S. H., Shau, W. Y., and Chao, D. Y. (2001a). The applications of capturerecapture models to epidemiological data. *Statistics in Medicine*, **20**: 3123–3157.
13. Chao, A., and Yang, H.-C. (2003). Program CARE-2 (Capture–Recapture, Part. 2). *Program and User's Guide published at* http://chao.stat.nthu.edu.tw/softwareCE.html.
14. Chao, A., Yip, P. S. F., Lee, S. M., and Chu, W. (2001b). Population size estimation based on estimating functions for closed capture–recapture models. *Journal of Statistical Planning and Inference*, **92**: 213–232.
15. Chao, D., Shau, W., Lu, C., Chen, K., Chu, C., Shu, H., and Horng, C. (1997). A large outbreak of hepatitis A in a college school in Taiwan: associated with contaminated food and water dissemination. *Epidemiology Bulletin*, Department of Health, Executive Yuan, Taiwan Government.
16. Chapman, D. G. (1951). Some properties of the hypergeometric distribution with applications to zoological censuses. *University of California Publications in Statistics*, **1**: 131–160.
17. Cochran, W. G. (1978). Laplace's ratio estimators. In *Contributions to Survey Sampling and Applied Statistics*, ed A. David, Academic Press, New York, 3–10.
18. Cormack, R. M. (1989). Loglinear models for capture–recapture. *Biometrics*, **45**: 395–413.

19. Cormack, R. M. (1999)_Problems with using capture–recapture in epidemiology: An example of a measles epidemic. *Journal of Clinical Epidemiology* 1999, **52**: 909–914.
20. Coull, B. A., Agresti, A. (1999) The use of mixed logit models to reflect heterogeneity in capture–recapture studies. *Biometrics,* **55**: 294–301.
21. Darroch, J. (1958). The multiple-recapture census: I. Estimation of a closed population. *Biometrika*, **45:** 343–359.
22. Desenclos, J. C., and Hubert, B. (1994). Limitations to the universal use of capture–recapture methods. *International Journal of Epidemiology*, **23**: 1322.
23. Fienberg, S. E. (1972). The multiple recapture census for closed populations and incomplete 2^k contingency tables. *Biometrika*, **59**: 591–603.
24. Fienberg, S. E., Johnson, M. S., and Junker, B. W. (1999). Classical multilevel and Bayesian approaches to population size estimation using multiple lists. *Journal of the Royal Statistical Society* **A162:** 383–405.
25. Hook, E. B., and Regal, R. R. (1992). The value of capture–recapture methods even for apparent exhaustive surveys. *American Journal of Epidemiology*, **135**: 1060–1067.
26. Hook, E. B., and Regal, R. R. (1993). Effect of variation in probability of ascertainment by sources ("variable catchability") upon "capture–recapture" estimates of prevalence. *American Journal of Epidemiology*, **137**: 1148–1166.
27. Hook, E. B., and Regal, R. R. (1995). Capture–recapture methods in epidemiology: methods and limitations. *Epidemiologic Reviews*, **17**: 243–264.
28. Hook, E. B., and Regal, R. R. (1999). Recommendations for presentation and evaluation of capture–recapture estimates in epidemiology. *Journal of Clinical Epidemiology*, **52**: 917–926.
29. Hook, E. B., and Regal, R. R. (2000a). Accuracy of alternative approaches to capture–recapture estimates of disease frequency: internal validity analysis of data from five sources. *American Journal of Epidemiology,***152**: 771–779.
30. Hook, E. B., and Regal, R. R. (2000b). On the need for a 16th and 17th recommendations for capture–recapture analysis. *Journal of Clinical Epidemiology*, **53**: 1275–1277.
31. Horvitz, D. G., and Thompson, D. (1952). A generalization of sampling without replacement from a finite universe. *Journal of the American Statistical Association*, **47**: 663–685.
32. Huggins, R. (1989). On the statistical analysis of capture experiments. *Biometrika*, **76**: 133–140.
33. Huggins, R. (1991). Some practical aspects of a conditional likelihood approach to capture experiments. *Biometrics*, **47**: 725–732.
34. International Working Group for Disease Monitoring and Forecasting (IWGDMF) (1995a). Capture–recapture and multiple-record systems estimation II: Applications in human diseases. *American Journal of Epidemiology*, **142**: 1059–1068.
35. International Working Group for Disease Monitoring and Forecasting (IWGDMF) (1995b). Capture–recapture and multiple-record systems estimation. I: History and theoretical development. *American Journal of Epidemiology*, **142**: 1047–1058.

36. Kiemeney, L. A. L. M., Schouten, L. J., and Straatman, H. (1994). Ascertainment corrected rates (Letter to Editor). *International Journal of Epidemiology*, **23**:203–204.
37. LaPorte, R. E., Mccarty, D. J., Tull, E. S., and Tajima, N. (1992). Counting birds, bees, and NCDs. *Lancet*, **339**: 494.
38. Otis, D. L., Burnham, K. P., White, G. C., and Anderson, D. R. (1978). Statistical inference from capture data on closed animal populations. *Wildlife Monographs*, **62**: 1–135.
39. Papoz, L., Balkau, B., and Lellouch, J. (1996). Case counting in epidemiology: limitations of methods based on multiple data sources. *International Journal of Epidemiology*, **25**: 474–477.
40. Pollock, K. H. (1991). Modeling capture, recapture, and removal statistics for estimation of demographic parameters for fish and wildlife populations: past, present, and future. *Journal of the American Statistical Association*, **86**: 225–238.
41. Pollock, K. H., Hines, J. E., and Nichols, J. D. (1984). The use of auxiliary variables in capture–recapture and removal experiments. *Biometrics*, **40**: 329–340.
42. Schouten, L. J., Straatman, H., Kiemeney, L. A. L. M., Gimbrere, C. H. F., and Verbeek, A. L. M. (1994). The capture–recapture method for estimation of cancer registry completeness: a useful tool? *International Journal of Epidemiology*, **23**: 1111–1116.
43. Schwarz, C. J., and Seber, G. A. F. (1999). A review of estimating animal abundance III. *Statistical Science*, **14**: 427–456.
44. Seber, G. A. F. (1982). *The estimation of animal abundance* (2 ed.): Griffin, London.
45. Seber, G. A. F. (1986). A review of estimating animal abundance. *Biometrics*, **42**: 267–292.
46. Seber, G. A. F. (1992). A review of estimating animal abundance II. *International Statistical Review*, **60**: 129–166.
47. Sekar, C. C., and Deming, W. E. (1949). On a method of estimating birth and death rates and the extent of registration. *Journal of the American Statistical Association*, **44**: 101–115.
48. Tsay, P., and Chao, A. (2001). Population size estimation for capture–recapture models with applications to epidemiological data. *Journal of Applied Statistics*, **28**: 25–36.
49. White, G. C. (1982). *Capture–recapture and removal methods for sampling closed populations*: Los Alamos National Lab, LA-8787-NERP, Los Alamos, New Mexico, USA.
50. Wittes, J., and Sidel, V. W. (1968). A generalization of the simple capture–recapture model with applications to epidemiological research. *Journal of Chronic Diseases*, **21**: 287–301.
51. Wittes, J. T. (1974). Applications of a multinomial capture–recapture model to epidemiological data. *Journal of the American Statistical Association*, **69**: 93–97.

52. Wittes, J. T., Colton, T., and Sidel, V. W. (1974). Capture–recapture methods for assessing the completeness of case ascertainment when using multiple information sources. *Journal of Chronic Diseases*, **27**: 25.
53. Yang, H. C., and Chao, A. (2005). Modeling animals' behavioral response by Markov chain models for capture–recapture experiments. *Biometrics*, **61**: 1010–1017.
54. Yip, P. S. F., Wan, E. C. Y., and Chan, K. (2001). A unified approach for estimating population size in capture–recapture studies with arbitrary removals. *Journal of Agricultural, Biological, and Environmental Statistics*, **6**: 183–194.

About the Authors

Anne Chao is currently Tsing Hua Distinguished Chair Professor, Institute of Statistics, National Tsing Hua University, Taiwan where she has taught since 1978. She received her PhD in Statistics from the University of Wisconsin-Madison in 1977. Her main research areas include statistical inferences and methodologies for biodiversity measures and ecological/ environmental survey data. Recent interests focus on developing a unified mathematical/statistical framework and appropriate software for genetic, taxonomic and functional diversities. A full list of 100 publications in the above research areas is given on the website http://chao.stat.nthu.edu.tw/ (There are over 4200 citations of her work in SCI journals.)

T. C. Hsieh is currently a PhD candidate at the Institute of Statistics, National Tsing Hua University, Taiwan, under the supervision of Anne Chao. His research interests include conservation biology, population genetics and epidemiology. He is now working on quantifying and integrating biodiversity measures, and on developing related statistical software including the R statistical package CARE1 (which was developed for implementing the methodology of this chapter) and iNEXT-online.

Hsin-Chou Yang received his Ph.D. from Institute of Statistics, National Tsing Hua University in Taiwan at 2002 under the supervision of Anne Chao. He worked as a Postdoctoral Fellow in Institute of Biomedical Sciences, Academia Sinica from 2002 to 2006. He became an Assistant Research Fellow in Institute of Statistical Science, Academia Sinica in 2006 and was promoted as an Associate Research Fellow in 2011. He is also an Adjunct

Associate Professor in School of Public Health, National Defense Medical Center. He is a member of editorial boards of four international journals and has reviewed papers for 25 international journals. His major research interests are statistical genomics, genetic epidemiology, bioinformatics, and ecological statistics.

CHAPTER 13

STATISTICAL METHODS IN THE EFFECTIVE EVALUATION OF MASS SCREENING FOR DISEASES

QING LIU

Department of Cancer Prevention
Sun Yat-Sen University Cancer Center,
651 Dongfeng Road East, Guangzhou 510060, P.R. China
liuqing@sysucc.org.cn

Mass screening is important in detecting disease earlier for chronic disease control. The purpose of screening is to detect disease in an early stage, in expectation of better treatment effect, the improvement of patients' prognosis and the reduction of disability or death. Mass screening may achieve its objective of early detection in two approaches: one is to encourage patients to visit the doctor when early signs and symptoms of disease appear; second is to supply a regular physical test to detect disease in an asymptomatic stage.

1. Basic Concept of Mass Screening for Disease

The American Commission on Chronic Illness gave a definition of screening in 1957[1]: "The presumptive identification of unrecognized disease or defect by the application of tests, examinations, or other procedures which can be applied rapidly. Screening tests sort out apparently well persons who probably have a disease from those who probably do not. A screening test is not intended to be diagnostic. Persons with positive or suspicious findings must be referred to their physicians for diagnosis and necessary treatment." This definition emphasized two points. Firstly, the potential disease states identified by mass screening include two subgroups: one is the state in the high risk of disease and another is the state of disease unrecognized by patients themselves. A person in the first group may not be ill but he may have disease with a high probability, such as people with multiple intestinal polyps, oesophageal epithelial dysplasia and metaplasia. People in the second group have suffered from the disease but not recognized it, such as patients with small liver cancer found by α-fetoprotein (AFP). Secondly, the screening procedure itself does not diagnose illness. Those who test positive are sent for further evaluation by a subsequent diagnostic test or procedure to determine whether they do have the disease.

In 1968, the World Health Organization (WHO)[2] suggested some governing principles and pre-requisites of mass screening:

(1) Disease is a serious health problem. It means a high morbidity, mortality and social burden.
(2) Early detection of disease may improve the prognosis, reduce proportion of disability and death of patients. It means that there are the effective treatments of early stage disease.
(3) The natural history of disease is well known and the screening test is able to detect disease in preclinical phase.
(4) There is an effective screening test meaning the test is sensitive, specific, high predictive value and safe.
(5) The screening program is acceptable to the population, simple and inexpensive, has high compliance rate and low complication and pain.
(6) There is a proper procedure of further diagnosis and follow-up.

Simply speaking, the success of a screening program depends on how many lives are saved. By the exact statistical statement, screening is effective only if the mortality rate of the disease in screened population is lower than that of in unscreened population. It may exist by the difference of the mortality rates or by the relative rates. The methods of statistical analysis for screening data are similar to that for general epidemiological study. The life-year savings of a disease is also a common index for screening assessment and especially useful in the cost-effectiveness evaluation. Mass screening does not only reduce the mortality rate of disease but sometimes also reduces the incidence rate and the medication cost of disease. However, the quantitative assessment on this aspect of screening is much more difficult than death reduction.

The cost must be considered in the assessment of screening. The direct cost includes charges of screening test, further diagnostic procedure and follow-up for positive result. The indirect cost includes expense of time and work, management and organization of program, etc. The evaluation of the psychological and biological impact of screening, such as the anxiety for positive results, risk of complication, harm and pain brought on by screening test is much more complicated but must be taken into consideration.

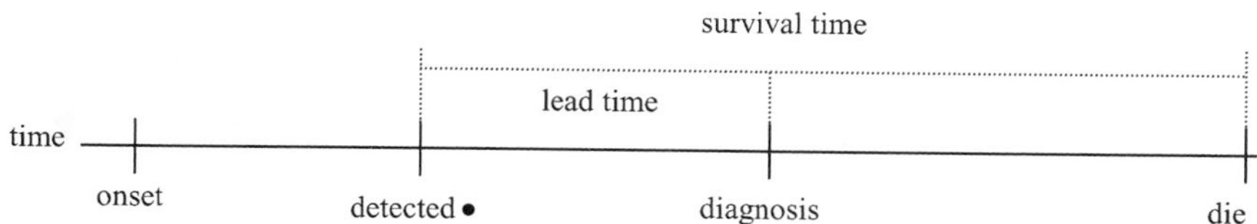

Fig. 1. Illustration of lead time bias.

The assessment of screening is very complicated and difficult. The current method of assessment for screening still needs to be improved. In the beginning, one hopes to compare the survival time of the cases detected by screening and the cases diagnosed in clinic. If the survival time of the cases detected by screening is longer than that of the cases diagnosed in the clinic, the screening is said to be effective. However, this comparison suffers from many biases. Firstly, the screening population is not a random sample of the general population. They may be different in some important demographic characteristics from the general population where the cases come, such as occupation, life status and education, etc. Secondly, longer survival time in the cases detected by screening may be caused by earlier diagnostic time rather than the prolonged life. This is called lead time bias.[3] As shown in Fig. 1, we suppose the survival time of patients are not changed no matter if it is detected by screening or diagnosed in clinic. The average longer survival time may be due to the screening advancing the diagnostic time. The lead time in an uncontrolled clinical trial appears to increase survival time although the natural history of the disease and the time of death are unchanged, whereas, patients stay longer in disease phase and suffer more from pain and anxiety. Finally, the probability that a disease will be detected by screening is directly proportional to the length of its preclinical detectable phase, which is inversely related to its rate of disease progression. Individuals with rapidly progressive disease — those with short preclinical phases — are more likely than average to die of their disease and are less likely to be identified by screening. Therefore, long survival time may not be the effect of screening nor the selective effects of screening procedure on cases. This is called length bias.[4] The screening tends to detect disease subsets with long preclinical phase, less aggressive progression and perhaps better inherent prognosis.

As shown in Fig. 2, for Cases 1 and 2, the disease is less aggressively progressive, detected by screening and has a better prognosis. For Cases 3 and 4, disease progresses rapidly, misses the opportunity of screening detection

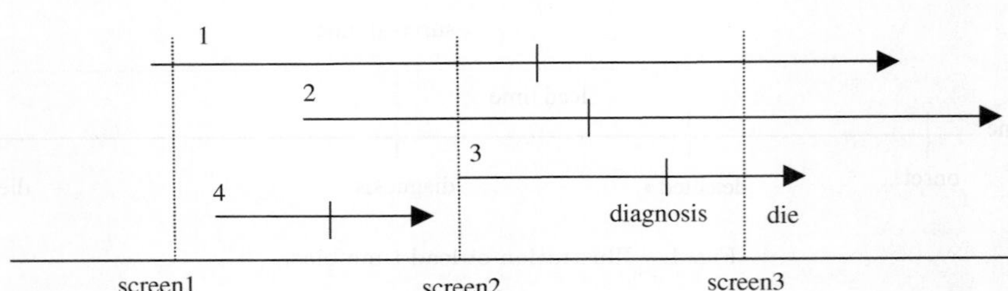

Fig. 2. Illustration of length bias.

and has a poor prognosis. In the comparison of survival time of patients detected by screening and detected clinically, these biases must be adjusted. This adjustment is very difficult, depends on the full perception of natural history of the disease and needs a very complex counting process.

Early diagnostic rate is one of the indices for assessment in the pilot period of a screening program. However, this index only suggests that the screening may be effective but has not been proven. If there is no effective treatment for detected patients, early detection of disease will not improve the prognosis of patients and reduce the death or disability caused by disease. Only when there is the effective treatment for disease in early stage and not for later stage, does the early detection of disease have special meaning.

Obviously, the comparison of survival rates of patients detected by screening and detected in clinic is not an ideal method of screening assessment. Early diagnostic rate of disease is also not a good index and only an indirect index. An ideal assessment of screening is to compare the mortality rates of the disease and death rates in screening population and control population in a randomized controlled population-based design. The mortality rates of the disease and death rates are crucial in the assessment of screening effects. The comparison of mortality rates is not interfered with by lead time bias and length bias. The results of the comparison reflect the true effectiveness of screening. For example, in the Health Insurance Plan (HIP)[5] in New York, the women aged 40 to 64 who participated of the plan are randomly separated into two groups, one group accepts yearly physical checks and mammography, another group receives a routine medical care service. Four repeat screening tests were given to the first group in total. In the first 5 years, the mortality rates of breast cancer in screening group reduced about 40%. After 14 years follow-up, there is still a 20% of mortality reduction of breast cancer (Table 1). The results from a randomized

Table 1. Cumulative deaths of breast cancer in screening population and control in HIP.

Years from first screens to diagnosis	Cases of breast cancer	Deaths from breast cancer according to follow-up years			
		5 years	7 years	10 years	14 years
5 years					
Screening group	306	39	71	95	118
Control group	300	63	106	133	153
Difference of rates (%)		38.1	33.0	28.6	22.9
7 years					
Screening group	425	39	81	123	165
Control group	443	63	124	174	212
Difference of rates (%)		38.1	34.7	29.3	22.2
10 years					
Screening group	600	39	81	146	218
Control group	604	63	124	192	262
Difference of rates (%)		38.1	34.7	24.0	16.8

Table 2. The mortality analysis of breast cancer between screening population and control.

Age	Groups	Deaths	Screening population	*RR* (95%CI)
40–49	Screen	28	19844	0.92(0.52–1.60)
	Control	24	15604	
50–59	Screen	45	23485	0.60(0.40–0.90)
	Control	54	16805	
60–69	Screen	52	23412	0.65(0.44–0.95)
	Control	58	16269	
70–74	Screen	35	10339	0.77(0.47–1.27)
	Control	31	7307	
Total	Screen	160	77080	0.69(0.55–0.88)*
	Control	171	55985	

*Adjusting for age.

control clinical trial of breast cancer screening in Sweden,[6] also proved that the screening of breast cancer may effectively reduce the deaths caused by the disease (Table 2).

It is shown in Tables 1 and 2 that the methods of statistical analysis are similar to those in the treatment of traditional epidemiological data. Mantel-Haenszel stratified analysis was used to estimate the relative risks and confidence interval of disease mortality. The methods of hypothesis testing are also same.

If a randomized control clinical trial is not feasible, a population-based cohort study is the next choice. For example, a study in England compares the mortality rates of the disease between the screening area and the non-screening area. This kind of design requires a relatively high participation rate in screening population. It means a good compliance. For comparison, the demographic characteristics of populations in different areas need to be adjusted.

The randomized control clinical trial or other observational design only evaluates a single screening scheme. The usage of them is limited because it cannot estimate the extra effects of a screening scheme applied in different populations with different age distributions and different prevalence rates of disease, or the extra effects of different screening schemes, such as different frequency and different test. In practice, people cannot carry out a randomized control clinical trial for every screening scheme to evaluate its effects. In this situation, the mathematical model of natural history of disease based on the current data from a RCT or other observational studies may complement this limitation. The prevalence rate of disease on every screening and the incidence rates in the screening interval are estimated based on a stochastic model and the effects of different screening policies are evaluated.

The screening programs for a variety of diseases have been implemented in many countries. The practice proves that the mortality rates of some diseases, such as breast cancer, cervical cancer, hypertension and diabetes may be reduced by screening. The question is which one in different screening test and different schemes detect disease earlier, with higher efficacy and higher cost-effectiveness. Two important parameters decide the effect of screening. One is the sensitivity of the screening test. Another is the distribution of sojourn time in preclinical detectable phase (PCDP). A high sensitivity, or low false negative rate of screening test means a strong power to detect disease. A long sojourn time of preclinical detectable phase means more chance to be detected by screening and in an early stage of disease. A short sojourn time of preclincial detectable phase gives little chance to be detected by screening. That means that the proportion of cases detected by screening is low, the effect of screening is poor and the screening may be not feasible. If the sojourn time of preclinical detectable phase is long, the interval between screens may be designed longer. When the distribution of preclinical detectable phase is known, the lead time bias may be

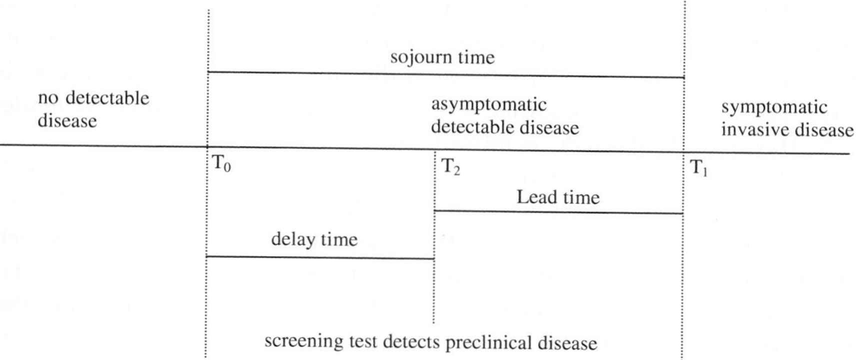

Fig. 3. Schema for the progression of a disease with the intervention of an early detection.

estimated for the assessment of screening. Therefore, the core of analysis of screening data and optimization of screening schemes is to estimate these two parameters.

We assume that the disease progresses in the manner shown in Fig. 3. An individual enters the preclinical detectable phase of the disease, detectable by the screening modality in question, at time T_0, and would begin to manifest symptoms, i.e. the disease would become clinically apparent, at time T_1, if no intervention were to take place. For this individual, the "sojourn time" is defined as $T_1 - T_0$. Suppose now that the individual is screened at time $T_2(T_0 < T_2 < T_1)$ and is diagnosed in the preclinical state. For this individual, the "lead time", the interval by which diagnosis is brought forward, is defined as $T_1 - T_2$. The probability that the screening test correctly identifies an individual as being in the preclinical detectable phase is termed the "sensitivity" of the test; the "false-negative rate" is one minus the sensitivity.

2. One-stage Models of the Natural History of Disease for Screening

The data from screening process consist of: (1) prevalent cases diagnosed in preclinical detectable state during the screening; (2) incidence cases diagnosed clinically in the interval of two screenings or both before and after screening. The purpose of a natural history model of screening for a disease is to express these prevalence and incidence rates in terms of the false-negative rate and of the sojourn-time distribution. General models have been developed[7,8] to describe the effect of screening on the disease process in order to identify those parameters which determine the expected benefit. Estimation of parameters of interest is difficult with these general models since the number of unknowns is large. Here firstly the simplified model (NE Day and SD Walter)[9] is introduced.

In the absence of screening, the incidence of clinical disease at age t will be denoted by $I(t)$. For the screening modality in question, $f(y)$ will denote the probability density function of the length of the interval y during which the disease is preclinical but detectable, i.e. the sojourn time. For simplicity, we assume $f(y)$ to be independent of t. The function $J(t)$ will denote the incidence of the preclinical state, i.e. the rate at which individuals enter it. The "false-negative rate", i.e. the probability that an individual in the preclinical state is screened negative, will be denoted by β; thus $1-\beta$ is the "sensitivity". We assume that β is independent of both the lead time and the sojourn time.

The functions $I(t)$ and $J(t)$ are related through $f(y)$ by the equation

$$I(t) = \int_0^t J(s)f(t-s)ds \,. \tag{1}$$

Suppose that the population is screened at t_1. Then for $t > t_1$ the incidence is made up of two components, individuals with short sojourn time who entered the preclinical state after t_1, and individuals with a longer sojourn time falsely screened negative at t_1. Thus, after one screen, the incidence, $I_1(t)$ is given by

$$I_1(t) = \beta \int_0^{t_1} J(s)f(t-s)ds + \int_{t_1}^t J(s)f(t-s)ds \,. \tag{2}$$

Similarly, if screens occur at times $t_1, t_2, \ldots, t_n$, then the incidence $I_n(t)$ after the nth screen is given by

$$I_n(t) = \sum_{i=0}^{n} \beta^{n-i} \int_{t_i}^{t_{i+1}} J(s)f(t-s)ds \,, \tag{3}$$

where $t_0 = 0$ and $t_{n+1} = t$. We make an assumption that $J(t)$ is uniform for an individual over the duration of the study. For cancer, the screening interval usually is 1 or 2 years, in this interval the assumption of uniform incidence rate of preclinical state may hold approximately.

$$I_n(t) = J \sum_{i=0}^{n} \beta^{n-i} \int_{t-t_{i+1}}^{t-t_i} f(y)dy \,. \tag{4}$$

The prevalence, P_1 observed at a first screen at time t_1, is given by

$$P_1 = (1-\beta)\int_0^{t_1} J(s)\int_{t_1-s}^{\infty} f(y)dyds\,. \tag{5}$$

That is, for each time $s < t_1$, those individuals entering the preclinical state at time s will be prevalent cases at time t_1 if their sojourn time is greater than $t_1 - s$. On reversing the order of integration and setting $J(s)$ as constant, this expression becomes

$$P_1 = (1-\beta)J\left(\int_0^{t_1} yf(y)dy + \int_{t_1}^{\infty} f(y)dy\right) \tag{6}$$

If there are n previous screens, at times $t_1, \ldots, t_n$. Summation over the n intervals, gives the following expression for the total prevalence P_n at the nth screen at time t_n:

$$P_n = (1-\beta)J\sum_{i=1}^{n} \beta^{n-i}\int_{t_n-t_i}^{\infty} \min\{y-(t_n-t_i), t_i - t_{i-1}\}f(y)dy\,. \tag{7}$$

If the interval between screens is constant, i.e. if $t_{i+1} - t_i = \Delta$, $i = 1, 2, \ldots, n-1$. Above expressions may be further simplified. For incidence rates,

$$I_n(t) = J\sum_{i=0}^{n-1} \beta^{n-i}\int_{t-t_n+(n-i-1)\Delta}^{t-t_n+(n-i)\Delta} f(y)dy + J\beta^n\int_0^{t-t_n} f(y)dy\,. \tag{8}$$

For the prevalence rates,

$$P_n = (1-\beta)J\sum_{i=1}^{n} \beta^{n-i}\int_{(n-i)\Delta}^{\infty} \min\{y-(n-i)\Delta, \Delta\}f(y)dy\,. \tag{9}$$

We consider first the idealized situation where a total population is screened at regular intervals, each individual being screened with the same inter-screening interval Δ. The constant incidence rates are assumed known from a pre-existing disease registry. At the ith screen ($i = 1, \ldots, n$) one knows r_i, the number of cases of preclinical disease found, and n_i, the number screened; and between screen i and screen $i+1$ one knows the total c_i of cases diagnosed outside screening from a total of y_i person-years at risk. The probability q_i of a case developing between screen i and screen $i+1$ outside screening is given by

$$q_i = 1 - \exp\left\{-\int_{t_i}^{t_{i+1}} I_i(y)dy\right\}, \tag{10}$$

Which can be well approximated by

$$q_i = \int_{t_i}^{t_{i+1}} I_i(t)dt\,.$$

The cases at screen i can be taken to have a Poisson distribution with parameter n_iP_i and the cases emerging outside screening between screens i and $i+1$ can be taken to have a Poisson distribution with parameter y_iq_i. Then the likelihood function is

$$L = \prod_{i=0}^{n-1} \frac{n_iP_i}{r_i!} e^{-n_iP_i} \prod_{i=1}^{n} \frac{y_iq_i}{c_i!} e^{-y_iq_i}\,. \tag{11}$$

Based on likelihood function, the maximum likelihood values of parameters may be estimated.

Three different forms for $f(y)$ may be considered: a step function with arbitrary probabilities defined over short time intervals, a lognormal and an exponential. Here, we only discuss the exponential distribution as an example for the application since it not only gives simpler expressions for the quantities of interest but also fits the data better.

2.1. *Example*

Breast cancer screening by the Health Insurance Plan of Greater New York (the HIP study).[5]

The data we have used are summarized in Tables 3 and 4. There were 4 screens at yearly interval and the cases arising between screens were

Table 3. Prevalence rates of breast cancer in the first 5 years of the HIP study.

Years since start of study	No. of women screened	No of prevalent breast cancer cases		Prevalence (‰)
		Observed	Expected	
0	20166	55	59.5	2.73
1	15936	32	25.8	2.01
2	13679	17	20.4	1.24
3	11971	23	17.7	1.92

Table 4. Incidence rates of breast cancer in the first 5 years of the HIP study.

Years since start of study	No of previous negative screens	Women-months of follow-up	No of prevalent breast cancer cases		Annual incidence (‰)
			Observed	Expected	
0–1	1	240277	13	14.9	0.65
1–2	1	81337	7	9.0	1.03
2–3	1	38370	1	5.3	0.31
3–4	1	30942	3	4.7	1.16
4–5	1	26701	5	4.3	2.25
1–2	2	190474	8	9.6	0.50
2–3	2	52934	5	5.5	1.13
3–4	2	19036	2	2.6	1.26
4–5	2	12626	4	1.9	3.80
2–3	3	163642	10	8.1	0.73
3–4	3	45964	5	4.7	1.31
4–5	3	13151	2	1.8	1.82
3–4	4	145118	10	7.0	0.84
4–5	4	89371	10	9.2	1.34

identified. We use the data from the first 5 years of follow-up after the start of screening.

We assume that the distribution of sojourn time of preclinical phase is an exponential.

$$f(y) = \lambda \exp(-\lambda y)\,, \quad y \geq 0\,.$$

With this assumption, for $t > t_n$, the incidence rate of screening interval is

$$I_n(t) = J - J\exp(-\lambda t)\{\exp(\lambda t_n) - \sum_{i=1}^{n-1} \beta^{n-i}[\exp(\lambda t_{i+1}) - \exp(\lambda t_i)] - \beta^n \exp(\lambda t_i)\}\,. \quad (12)$$

The q_j are then given, for $j = 1, \ldots, n$ by the integrals of (12) from t_j to $t_j + 1$, so

$$q_j = J(t_{j+1} - t_j) - J\lambda^{-1}[\exp(-\lambda t_j) - \exp(\lambda t_{j+1})] \times \left\{\exp(\lambda t_j) - \sum_{i=1}^{j-1} \beta^{j-i}[\exp(\lambda t_{i+1}) - \exp(\lambda t_i)] - \beta^j \exp(\lambda t_1)\right\}. \quad (13)$$

If the screens are equally spaced, q_j reduces to

$$q_j = J\Delta - J\lambda^{-1}[1 - \exp(-\lambda\Delta)] \times \left\{1 - [\exp(\lambda\Delta) - 1]\sum_{i=1}^{j-1}\beta^i \exp(-i\lambda\Delta) + \beta^j \exp[-(j-1)\lambda\Delta]\right\}. \quad (14)$$

The expression for P_j, from (9) reduces to

$$P_j = (1-\beta)J\lambda^{-1}\sum_{i=1}^{j}\beta^{j-1}\{\exp[-\lambda(t_j - t_i)] - \exp[-\lambda(t_j - t_{i-1})]\}, \quad (15)$$

which for equal spaced intervals becomes

$$P_j = (1-\beta)J\lambda^{-1}[1 - \exp(-\lambda\Delta)]\sum_{i=0}^{j-1}\beta^i \exp(-i\lambda\Delta). \quad (16)$$

Since the example is a screening at an equal spaced interval, the expression (14) and (16) are used to develop the maximum likelihood function. Then it is relatively straightforward to compute the log likelihood as a function of λ and β. The results are: $\beta = 0.18$, $\lambda = 0.585$. According to the exponential distribution, the average sojourn time equals 1.71. Also shown in Table 4 are the expected numbers of cases based on the best-fitting exponential distribution, with an overall χ^2 goodness-of-fit test. The fit is clearly good.

3. Two-Stage Models of the Natural History of Disease for Screening

The models of natural history of the disease introduced before are based on a progressive disease model. The progressive disease model assumes individuals are in a healthy state until they enter the preclinical disease state and all individuals in this state eventually emerge with clinical symptoms if untreated. The key assumption of this model is that preclinical disease, if left untreated, would ultimately surface clinically. This assumption is true for a part of invasive diseases, such as breast cancer. When the mammography may detect the malignant tumor in the breast, the tumor must progress until patient feels the symptom or sign and goes to visit physician. Similar cases are the chest radiography for lung cancer and α-fetoprotein (AFP) test for liver cancer. However, it is not always true for some other cancers or diseases. For example, the Pap smear for screening of

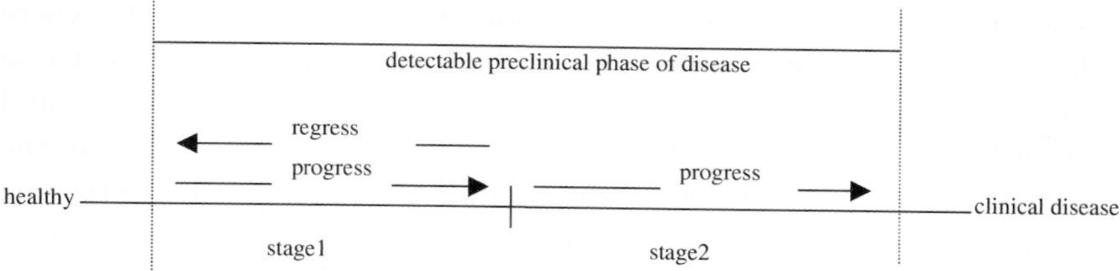

Fig. 4. Schematic illustration of two stage model for preclinical period of disease.

cervical cancer may detect the heavy epithelial dysplasia and metaplasia, and carcinoma *in situ*; the gastroscopy for screening of stomach cancer may detect the gastric mucous dysplasia and metaplasia; the enteroscopy for screening of colon cancer may detect multiple intestinal polyps; etc. These non-invasive lesions may progress to invasive disease but also may persist or revert to normal automatically. However, once a lesion becomes invasive, it almost never regresses without treatment and it is assumed all invasive lesions arise from a preinvasive lesion. According to this situation, a two-stage model for the analysis of cancer screening data has been suggested.[10] The two-stage model is illustrated schematically in Fig. 4.

We define the random variable X to be the duration of time a progressive lesion spends in the preclinical stage 1 and Y the duration of time a progressive lesion spends in the preclinical stage 2. The cumulative distribution function of the joint sojourn times (X, Y) is called $F(x, y)$ with density $f(x, y)$. Then the cumulative distribution function of the total preclinical duration $(X + Y)$ of progressive lesions is given by

$$F_T(t) = \int_0^t \int_0^s f(s - y, y) dy ds \,. \tag{17}$$

F_T is the distribution function of the total preclinical duration for progressive lesions only.

3.1. *The likelihood for the interval (clinical incident) cases*

Suppose the hazard function of clinical disease in the absence of screening is given by i and a steady state is assumed, before time t, the screening history of the jth individual in this risk set had a history of n_{ij} previous negative screens at time $H_{ij} = \{t_{ij1}, t_{ij2}, \ldots, t_{ijn_i}\}$. These times are given in reverse chronological order so that t_{ij1} refers to the time since the most recent screen and t_{ijn_i} refers to the time of first screens. By convention, $j = 1, \ldots, M_{1i}$ refers to the cases. Then the hazard of clinical disease at age

t is given a screening history H_{ij} is approximately $I_\rho(H_{ij}; F_T, \beta)$, where $\rho(H_{ij}; F_T, \beta)$ is the probability that an individual who is destined to be clinically incident at age t in the absence of screening intervention, would have tested negative at prior times H_{ij} if the individual was in fact in the screening program. Then, the conditional likelihood of that the screening history H_{i0} corresponds to the interval case and the other screening histories among R_i screening subjects is

$$L_{1i} = \frac{\rho(H_{i0}; F_T, \beta)}{\sum_{j=1}^{R_i} \rho(H_{ij}; F_T, \beta)} . \tag{18}$$

It is shown that the constant I cancels out in (18). Suppose M_{1i} incident cases are clinically diagnosed at age a_i and there are an additional N_{1i} individuals at risk at a_i; that is, in addition to the cases there are N_{1i} individual in the cohort still at risk of being diagnosed with clinical disease at age a_i. Suppose the jth individual in this risk set had a history of n_{ij} previous negative screens at time H_{ij}, where $R_{1i} = M_{1i} + N_{1i}$ is the size of the risk set. Then the partial likelihood contribution of incident cases at age a_i is

$$L_{1i} = \frac{\prod_{j=1}^{M_{1i}} \rho(H_{ij}; F_T, \beta)}{\sum_l \prod_{j \in sl} \rho(H_{ij}; F_T, \beta)} , \tag{19}$$

where S_l is the subsets consisting of M_{2i} individuals from the R_{2i} screened at age a_i,

$$l = 1, 2, \ldots, \binom{R_{1i}}{M_{1i}} .$$

Suppose an interval case could have entered between the kth and $(k-1)$th most recent screen, and then the probability of falsely screened negative on all $k-1$ subsequent screens is

$$\rho(H_{ij}; F_T, \beta) = \sum_{k=1}^{n_{ij}+1} \beta^{k-1} [F_T(t_{ijk}) - F_T(t_{ijk-1})] , \tag{20}$$

with the conventions $F_T(t_{ijn_{ij}+1}) = 1, \quad F_T(t_{ij0}) = 0$.

3.2. *Likelihood for screen-detected stage 2 prevalent cases*

The prevalence (probability) of stage 2 screen-detected disease at age t conditional on a screening history H_{ij} is

$$[(1-\beta) I \mu_2] \rho(H_{ij}; F_{B2}, \beta) , \tag{21}$$

where $\mu_2 = \int y f(x,y) dx dy$ is the mean duration in stage 2. The first factor in brackets is the prevalence of screen-detected stage 2 disease unconditional on any screening history. The second factor $\rho(H_{ij}; F_{B2}, \beta)$ is the probability that an individual who is destined to be in stage 2 at age t in the absence of screening intervention, would have tested negative at prior times H_{ij} if the individual was in a screening program. F_{B2} is the backward recurrence distribution function. The backward recurrence time is the amount of time that a screen-detected lesion spent in the preclinical stage (stage 1 plus the time spent in stage 2 up to detection. The backward recurrence density is

$$f_{B2}(t) = \frac{\int_0^t \int_{t-x}^{\infty} f(x,y) dy dx}{\mu_2} . \qquad (22)$$

This expression is derived by first noting the probability of being in stage 2 is $I_{\mu 2}$ and second, in order to have been in the preclinical phase for duration t and currently in stage 2 one must be in stage 1 for duration x and stage 2 for at least $t - x$, $0 < x < t$. It is defined $F_{B2}(t_{ijn_{ij}+1}) = 1$ and

$$F_{B2}(t_{ijo}) = 0 .$$

$$L_{2i} = \frac{\rho(H_{i0}; F_{B2}, \beta)}{\sum_{j=1}^{R_i} \rho(H_{ij}; F_{B2}, \beta)} . \qquad (23)$$

Similarly, suppose M_{2i} screen-detected stage 2 cases are detected at age a_i and an additional N_{2i} individuals also are screened at age a_i and are negative. Then the partial likelihood contribution of the screen-detected cases at a_i is

$$L_{1i} = \frac{\prod_{j=1}^{M_{1i}} \rho(H_{ij}; F_{B2}, \beta)}{\sum_l \prod_{j \in sl} \rho(H_{ij}; F_{B2}, \beta)} , \qquad (24)$$

where meaning of s_l and l as same as before. If the screening times are randomly assigned, that is, the R_{2i} individuals who are screened at age a_i are a random sample of all individuals R_{1i} at risk at age a_i. Suppose the incident cases have C_l strata and prevalent cases screen-detected have C_2 strata, the partial likelihood is then the product of factors for the contributions from incident cases and contributions from screen-detected cases.

$$L = \prod_{i=1}^{c_1} L_{1i} \prod_{i=1}^{c_2} L_{2i} . \qquad (25)$$

3.3. *The joint sojourn distribution of two stage model*

3.3.1. *The independent model*

The simplest model assumes that the sojourn times for the two stages X and Y are independent with cumulative distribution functions $F_1(x)$ and $F_2(y)$ and densities $f_1(x)$ and $f_2(y)$, respectively. The distribution function for the total sojourn time is

$$F_T(t) = \int_0^t f_1(x)F_2(1-x)dx\,. \tag{26}$$

The backward recurrence cumulative distribution function is

$$F_{B2}(t) = \frac{1}{\mu_2}\int_0^t [1-F_2(y)]F_1(t-y)dy\,. \tag{27}$$

For the two-stage independent model, with exponential sojourn distributions $[F_1(t) = 1 - e^{-\lambda_1 t}$, and $F_2(t) = 1 - e^{-\lambda_2 t}]$, both the total sojourn (F_T) and backward recurrence (F_{B2}) cumulative distribution functions are identical and given by

$$F_T(t) = F_{B2}(t) = \begin{cases} 1 + \dfrac{\lambda_2 e^{-\lambda_1 t} - \lambda_1 e^{-\lambda_2 t}}{\lambda_1 - \lambda_2}\,, & \lambda_1 \neq \lambda_2 \\ 1 - e^{-\lambda t}(1+\lambda t)\,, & \lambda_1 = \lambda_2 = \lambda\,. \end{cases} \tag{28}$$

3.3.2. *Limiting dependent models*

For many diseases, the second stage (the preclinical invasive stage) is short relative to the first (the noninvasive stage). It is useful to consider the limiting behavior of $F_T(t)$ and $F_{B2}(t)$ as $\mu_2 \to 0$ with F_1 fixed. These limiting expressions could then be substituted into expression of likelihood. For example, consider the complete positive dependent exponential model, the relationship of X and Y may express as

$$\begin{gathered} Y = \lambda_1 X/\lambda_2\,, \\ F_T(t) = 1 - e^{-ut}\,, \\ F_{B2}(t) = 1 - \left[e^{-ut} + \frac{\lambda_2}{\lambda_1}(e^{-ut} - e^{-\lambda_1 t})\right], \end{gathered} \tag{29}$$

where $u = \lambda_1\lambda_2/(\lambda_1+\lambda_2)$. Under this model the limiting backward recurrence distribution is

$$\lim_{\mu_2 \to 0} F_{B2}(t) = 1 - e^{-\lambda_1 t}(1+\lambda_1 t)\,. \tag{30}$$

For this limiting situation, $F_1(t) = 1 - e^{-\lambda_1 t}$ is substituted into expression (19) for total sojourn distribution while the cumulative distribution function in expression (30) is substituted into expression (24) for the backward recurrence distribution.

Brookmeyer and Day applied the two-stage model to the analysis of data from a case-control study. Data is from the case-control study of the Northeast Scotland Cervical Cancer Screening Program.[11] The program was started in 1960 when women were asked to come for an initial Pap smear. Records on all subsequent Pap tests were kept. The definition of a positive Pap test is given in MacGregor *et al.*[11] When a woman had a positive Pap test she was biopsied and/or treated. Thus, the natural history of the disease was interrupted at the time of the first positive Pap test. A case-control study was conducted and consisted of 85 women who were diagnosed with invasive squamous carcinoma of the cervix between 1968 and 1982. Of these 85 cases, 35 were clinically incident (interval cases) and 50 were screen-detected with preclinical invasive disease (stage 2). Each interval case was matched by year of birth to five controls who were healthy at the time of the case's diagnosis. Each stage 2 screen-detected case was matched by year of birth to a control who screened negative within 6 months of the date at which the case was screen-detected. The screening histories of all cases and controls were ascertained; these histories consisted of the number and timing of previous negative screens (prior to diagnosis date of the case).

The two-stage model was fitted to the data and results showed in Table 5.

The independent model gave two estimated values of λ, one is big and one is small. The author thought the development of preclinical invasive disease is very rapid so that he chose the big one as $\lambda 2$. The maximized

Table 5. Conditional likelihood analysis for independent (model 1) and limiting dependent (model 2) two-stage exponential models.

Maximum likelihood estimates	Model 1	Model 2
β	0.025	0.001
λ	0.003, 0.247*	0.013*
Proportion with < 5 years total sojourn	0.18	0.55
Proportion with < 10 years total sojourn	0.33	0.70
Maximum log-likelihood	−120.54	−119.35

*In time units of months.

log-likelihood was slightly higher with the dependent model and it suggested the limiting dependent model is better. Both the independent and limiting dependent analysis suggested a small false negative rate. However, there was some discrepancy in the estimates of the sojourn distribution. As expected, the value of λ is big in the limiting dependent model suggesting the shorter sojourn duration than the independent model.

4. Multiple Stages Markov model for the Natural History of Disease Screening

The two-stage model suggested by Brookmeyer and Day presented the concept of regression of disease development in preclinical phase. It describes the disease progression better and is of an important significance in evaluation and prediction of effect of screening for the disease in the different stages. But the two-stage model of Brookmeyer and Day does not fully describe the transition of disease in different stages. The parameter of the model may only be used to estimate the total sojourn time in preclinical phase. The structure of the model and the parameter estimation are relatively complex. The history of a disease may look like a transition process of ones discrete healthy status. For example, in a certain period, the healthy status of an individual may change from healthy to potential illness. Later may progress further to clinical disease. The transition of status may be in a single direction or even double direction. Therefore, a stochastic process model is very convenient and reasonable to describe the transition of disease status and the sojourn time in each stage. If the future status only depends on the current status and is independent to all status before, that is called the Markov property. We may use Markov process or Markov chain to describe the disease progression when it is of this property.

We assume that the single stage model and two-stage model of natural history of disease are illustrated in Fig. 5.

4.1. *Time homogeneous Markov chain model*

Duffy and Chen[12] suggested to describe the natural history of the disease for screening by the Markov process model. A Markov process with the following instantaneous transition matrix:

$$\begin{matrix} 0 \\ 1 \\ 2 \end{matrix} \begin{bmatrix} -\lambda_1 & \lambda_1 & 0 \\ 0 & -\lambda_2 & \lambda_2 \\ 0 & 0 & 0 \end{bmatrix}.$$

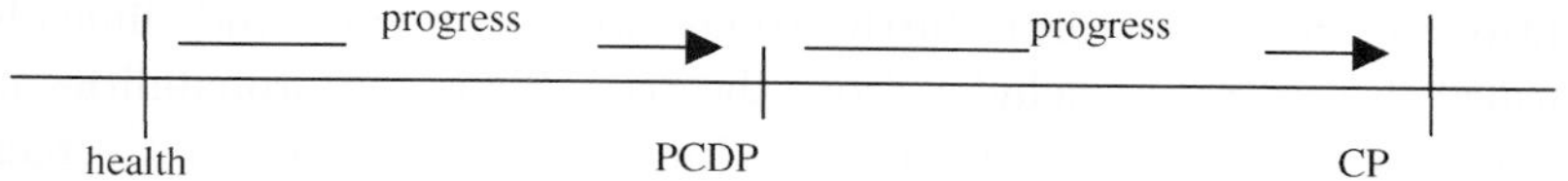

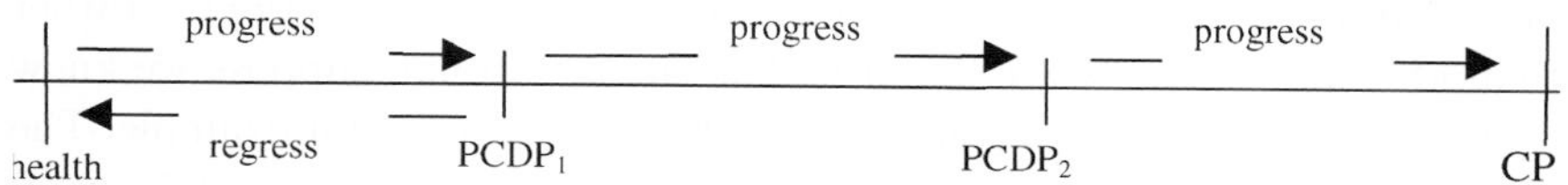

Fig. 5. Schematic illustration of state transition of disease screened.

Here 0 is the "no disease state", 1 is "preclinical but detectable disease" and 2 is "clinical disease". Implicit in this model is the assumption that diseases are "born" into the preclinical state with an exponential distribution of time to birth with

$$P(\text{Time to birth} \leq t) = \int_0^t \lambda_1 e^{-\lambda_1 x} dx = 1 - e^{-\lambda_1 t} . \tag{31}$$

Time remaining in the preclinical phase conditional on being in the phase at time $t = 0$, is also assumed exponentially distributed with

$$\begin{aligned} P(\text{Time to transition to clinical state} \leq t) &= \int_0^t \lambda_2 e^{-\lambda_2 x} dx \\ &= 1 - e^{-\lambda_2 t} . \end{aligned} \tag{32}$$

Based on the solution of (dI-Q) to obtain the eigenvalues and eigenvectors, the transition probabilities for time t may be obtained:

$$P(t) = \begin{bmatrix} e^{-\lambda_1 t} & \dfrac{\lambda_1(e^{-\lambda_2 t} - e^{-\lambda_1 t})}{(\lambda_1 - \lambda_2)} & 1 + \dfrac{\lambda_2 e^{-\lambda_1 t} - \lambda_1 e^{-\lambda_2 t}}{(\lambda_1 - \lambda_2)} \\ 0 & e^{-\lambda_2 t} & 1 - e^{-\lambda_2 t} \\ 0 & 0 & 1 \end{bmatrix} . \tag{33}$$

This can also readily be obtained from the exponential distribution properties.

The transition probabilities in Eq. (33) are unconditional probabilities. There are two complications, however, which necessitate the replacement of some with conditional or compound probabilities. First, those found to be free of disease or to have preclinical disease at first screen are not from an entire cohort followed from birth; women with a previous and clinically confirmed disease were excluded from the trial. Thus the probabilities of being free of disease and of having preclinical disease at the first screen should be conditional on having no clinical disease between birth and first screen. Also, the time of entering the clinical phase is known exactly. Their probabilities should therefore be of becoming clinical at the time t_i rather than at some time between 0 and t_i. For one individual, suppose we know that the exact time the person becomes clinical is 5 years, for example. The probability of clinical disease at exactly five years is P(clinical at 5 years) $= P$(not clinical up to $5 - \Delta t$ years) $\times\, P$(become clinical in the interval $(5-\Delta t, 5)$). Since the model does not allow the possibility of instantaneous transition from no disease to clinical state, and since we wish to explicitly allow for the probability of both rapid and slow progression through preclinical phase, we use our limit of accuracy, in this case one month, and further approximate the correct probability as P(clinical at 5 years) $= P$(not clinical up to $5 - \Delta t$ years) P(become clinical in the interval $(5 - \Delta t, 5)$).

As 1 month = 0.08 years, approximately,

$$P = P_{00}(t_i - 0.08)P_{02}(0.08) + P_{01}(t_i - 0.08)P_{12}(0.08)\,.$$

Therefore, the probabilities of being free of disease at first and second screen, P_1 and P_2, were calculated as

$$P_1 = \frac{e^{\lambda_1 t}}{e^{-\lambda_1 t} + \frac{\lambda_1(e^{-\lambda_2 t} - e^{-\lambda_1 t})}{\lambda_1 - \lambda_2}} \tag{34}$$

$$P_2 = e^{-\lambda_1 t} \tag{35}$$

The probabilities of having preclinical disease at first and second sceeen, P_3 and P_4 and the probability of clinical disease at time t_i ($I = 1, 2, \ldots, t$) are

$$P_3 = 1 - P_1\,,$$

$$P_4 = \frac{\lambda_1(e^{\lambda_2 t} - e^{\lambda_1 t})}{\lambda_1 - \lambda_2} \tag{36}$$

$$P_{5i} = e^{-\lambda_1(t_i - 0.08)}\left(1 + \frac{\lambda_2 e^{-\lambda_1 0.08} - \lambda_1 e^{-\lambda_2 0.08}}{\lambda_1 - \lambda_2}\right)$$
$$+ \frac{\lambda_1(e^{-\lambda_2(t_i - 0.08)} - e^{-\lambda_1(t_i - 0.08)})(1 - e^{-\lambda_2 0.08})}{\lambda_1 - \lambda_2}\,. \tag{37}$$

The total likelihood function is

$$L = \prod_{l-1}^{n} (P_1^{1-\delta} P_3^{\delta})(P_2^{1-\delta} P_4^{\delta}) P_{5i} \,. \tag{38}$$

δ is the index variable of screening results. If the result of screening test is negative, $\delta = 0$, otherwise, $\delta = 1$. The solution of the likelihood function is complicate, it must be iteratively maximized by a non-standard program. For simplicity, Duffy and Chen equate observed numbers of different types of observation to expected numbers and estimate the parameters by non-linear least squares. Thus, the least squares approximations to maximum likelihood estimates were obtained by a procedure similar to the method of moments. Then the non-linear procedure (NLIN) in SAS[13] may be used to estimate the parameters.

4.1.1. *Example*

A randomized trial was conducted in women aged 40–74 in two counties, Kopparberg and Ostergotland, in Sweden[14] to assess the effect on breast cancer mortality of screening by single-view mammography. The data from two screens were used in the example. The number of invited women at first and second screens was 5410 and 4823. Among those subjects, only 4383 and 3494, respectively, were actually screened. Of those who attended the second screen, 3347 had attended the first screen and 147 had not. Therefore following are the transition histories:

(1) 4383 women were screened at the first screen and 52 cancers were detected. There are 4331 (4383-52) women with transition history (72, 0-0), that is transition from no disease to no disease in 72 years (the average age at baseline was 72).
(2) The 52 cases detected at first screen have transition history (72, 0-1).
(3) 3494 women attended the second screen and 35 cancers were detected, all among the 3347 women who had attended the first screen. Thus 3312 (3347-35) have subsequent transition history (74.72, 0-0).
(4) The 35 cases detected at the second screen have subsequent history (2.75, 0-1).
(5) The 147 women who missed the first screen but attended the second screen have transition history (74.75, 0-0).
(6) There are 10 interval cancers between the first and second screens. Thus, of the above 4331, there are 10 with subsequent transition history (time to interval cancer, 0-2).

Table 6. The estimated sojourn time in PCDP of breast cancer.

λ_1	λ_2	$SE(\lambda_2)$	Mean sojourn time	95%CI
0.0052	0.43	0.014	2.3	$2.1 \sim 2.5$

(7) There are 68 cases diagnosed clinically after the last screen, which is either the first screen (10 cases) or second (58 cases), depending on whether the subject attended the second screen. These have subsequent history (time to surface to clinical stage, 0-2).

The results of analysis are showed in Table 6.

4.1.2. *Estimation of sensitivity*

Day shows that under the constant incidence assumption, in a time interval T after a negative screen one would expect K new cases, where

$$K = J(1-s)\int_0^T (1-F(t)dt) + J\int_0^T F(t)dt\,. \tag{39}$$

J is the annual (constant) incidence rate, S is the sensitivity and F is the comulative distribution function of the sojourn time. The first component in the formula for K is the number of cases missed at the screen and the second is the number of new cases "born" since the screen. This suggests as a formula for an estimate of sensitivity

$$\hat{S} \approx 1 - \frac{1-\hat{K}/J}{1-\frac{1}{T}\int_0^T f(t)dt}\,, \tag{40}$$

where K is the observed number of new cases. Using the proposed three-state Markov model, the corresponding expected number K of cases in time T after a negative screen at time t_i is

$$K = N(1-S)\int_0^{t_1} \lambda_1 e^{-\lambda_1 t}\int_{t_1-t}^{t_1+T-t} \lambda_2 e^{-\lambda_2 u}dudt$$

$$+N\int_{t_1}^{t_1+T} \lambda_1 e^{-\lambda_1 t}\int_0^{t_1+T-t} \lambda_2 e^{-\lambda_2 u}dudt\,, \tag{41}$$

where N is the number screened at time t_1. After some integration and algebra, this given an estimate of sensitivity

$$\hat{S} = 1 - \frac{\hat{K}(\lambda_2-\lambda_1)/N - a}{b}\,, \tag{42}$$

where

$$a = (\lambda_2 - \lambda_1)e^{-\lambda_1 t_1}(1 - e^{-\lambda_1 T}) - \lambda_1 e^{-\lambda_2 T} e^{-\lambda_1 t_1}(e^{-(\lambda_2 - \lambda_1)T} - 1)$$

and

$$b = \lambda_1(e^{-\lambda_1 t_1} - e^{-\lambda_2 t_1})(1 - e^{-\lambda_2 T}).$$

Thus, the same data as in the Markov model are used to estimate sensitivity, but in a second stage of estimation.

4.2. *Non homogeneous Markov model with covariables*

In the description of disease progression, the transition of disease states may be interfered by a lot of important factors. For example, some risk factors in living environment may decide the probability of transition from healthy state to ill state. A stochastic model of transition of disease states in the consideration of these factors will be benefit to identify the population with high risk of disease. This population is more appropriate to implement of screening program and is expected to get higher effectiveness. Another case is that the clinical disease characters decide the probability of transition from preclinical state to clinical state. The inclusion of these variables may strengthen the identification power of stochastic model for different types of diseases and the precise of estimation for the sojourn time in preclinical detectable phase. Therefore, the purpose of developing a stochastic model describes the transition probability of healthy state of an individual not only by populational transition but also by the consideration of individual characters, such as age, gender, disease history, etc. To consider the individual variability, a regression combination of the variables of individual characters may be used to describe the transition probability and it is called as the non-homogeneous Markov model with covariables.

4.2.1. *Non-homogeneous time discrete Markov chain model*

J. Q. Fang and W. Q. Zhou[15,16] suggested a parameterized non-homogeneous Markov chain model in the analysis of screening data for disease. They assumed that the disease process is like in Fig. 5. The state space $S = \{0, 1, 2, 3\}$. The transition probability from state I to state j is defined as

$$P_{ij}(\tau, t) = P\{X(t) = j | X(\tau) = i\}. \tag{43}$$

In general screening practice, the screens were given in a fixed interval and the time intervals may only differ in several days. This error may be neglected. Then the time t may be assumed as a fixed unit, such as year or month. Among the Eq. (46), τ and t belong to screening time set $T \equiv \{ttt\}$. Based on the professional knowledge, it is assumed that the state of individual may just transfer one step in one interval. Suppose the one step transition matrix during the time from t to $t + I$ is

$$P(t) = \begin{bmatrix} p_{00}(t) & p_{01}(t) & 0 & 0 \\ p_{10}(t) & p_{11}(t) & p_{12}(t) & 0 \\ 0 & 0 & p_{22}(t) & p_{23}(t) \\ 0 & 0 & 0 & 1 \end{bmatrix} \quad i, j = 0, 1, 2, 3 . \tag{44}$$

Among expression (44)

$$P_{01}(t) = \alpha_{01} \cdot /\text{È}(t) \,, \quad P_{00}(t) = 1 - P_{01}(t) \,,$$

$$P_{10}(t) = \alpha_{10} \cdot (1 - \theta(t)) \,, \quad P_{12}(t) = \alpha_{12} \cdot /\text{È}(t) \,,$$

$$P_{22}(t) = 1 - P_{10}(t) - P_{12}(t) \,, \tag{45}$$

$$P_{23}(t) = \alpha_{23} \cdot /\text{È}(t) \,, \; P_{22}(t) = 1 - P_{23}(t) \,,$$

$$\theta(t) = 1 - \exp(-\beta' Z(t)) \,, \quad \beta = (\beta_1, \beta_2, \ldots, \beta_p)' \,. \tag{46}$$

Here the proportional factor α and vector β are the unknown parameters to be estimated. The transition matrix of m steps during the time from t to $t + m$ is

$$A_m(t) = \prod_{\substack{k=0 \\ t+k \in T}}^{m-1} P(t + k) \,. \tag{47}$$

Suppose there is only one step discriminant error in the state 0, 1, 2, 3, $s \in S$, $P\{s + i|s\} = 1 - \gamma$, here γ is the false negative rate. Therefore, the discriminant vectors are

$$B(0) = (1 - \gamma, \gamma, 0, 0)' \,, \quad B(1) = (0, 1 - \gamma, \gamma, 0)'$$

$$B(2) = (0, 0, 1 - \gamma, \gamma)' \,, \quad B(3) = (0, 0, 0, 1 - \gamma)' \,. \tag{48}$$

The maximum likelihood function is

$$L = \prod_{k=1}^{N} \prod_{j=1}^{q_k - 1} B'(s_{kj}) Am_{kj}(t_{kj}) B(s_{k,j+1}) \,. \tag{49}$$

The hypothesis test of parameters may use the likelihood ratio test. The statistic is

$$G = 2(\ln L(\hat{\alpha}, \hat{\beta}) - \ln L\alpha_0, \beta_0)\,. \tag{50}$$

When the sample size is big enough and H_0 is true, the statistic G follows the chi-square distribution and the degree of freedom is the number of estimating parameters.

4.2.2. *Non-homogeneous time continuous Markov process model*

J. Q. Fang and J. H. Mao[15, 16] suggested a time continuous Markov process model. They assumed that the transition power from state i to state j is

$$\begin{aligned} \lambda_{ij}(t) \cdot dt = P\{X(t+dt) = j|X(t) = i\} = P_{ij}(t, t+dt)\,, \\ t \in [0, \infty)\,, \quad i, j \in S\,. \end{aligned} \tag{51}$$

They also assumed that the transition power of two stage model for disease screening was related with p covariables. The model is

$$\begin{cases} \lambda_{01}(t) = A_0 + A_1 Z_1(t) + \cdots + A_p Z_p(t)\,, \\ \lambda_{10}(t) = B_0 + B_1 Z_1(t) + \cdots + B_p Z_p(t)\,, \\ \lambda_{12}(t) = C_0 + C_1 Z_1(t) + \cdots + C_p Z_p(t)\,, \\ \lambda_{23}(t) = D_0 + D_1 Z_1(t) + \cdots + D_p Z_p(t)\,. \end{cases} \tag{52}$$

Among the expression (52) A_i, C_i, D_i, $(I = 1, 2, \ldots, p)$ are the estimating parameters. The one step transition probability and stay probability are

$$P_{00}(\tau, t) = \sum_{i \neq j}^{1,2} \frac{\rho_i + \lambda_{10} + \lambda_{12}}{\rho_i - \rho_j} e^{\rho_i(t-\tau)}\,, \quad P_{11}(\tau, t) = \sum_{i \neq j}^{1,2} \frac{\rho_i + \lambda_{01}}{\rho_i - \rho_j} e^{\rho_i(t-\tau)}\,,$$

$$P_{01}(\tau, t) = \sum_{i \neq j}^{1,2} \frac{\lambda_{01}}{\rho_i - \rho_j} e^{\rho_i(t-\tau)}\,, \quad P_{10}(\tau, t) = \sum_{t \neq j}^{1,2} \frac{\lambda_{10}}{\rho_i - \rho_j} e^{\rho_i(t-\tau)}\,,$$

$$P_{12}(\tau, t) = \sum_{i \neq j}^{1,2} \frac{\rho_i + \lambda_{01}}{\rho_i - \rho_j} \cdot \frac{\lambda_{12}}{\rho_i + \lambda_{23}} (e^{\rho_i(t-\tau)} - e^{-\lambda_{23}(t-\tau)})\,,$$

$$P_{23}(\tau, t) = 1 - e^{-\lambda_{23}(t-\tau)}\,, \quad P_{22}(\tau, t) = e^{-\lambda_{23}(t-\tau)}\,. \tag{53}$$

Among them, $\lambda_{ij} \equiv \lambda_{ij}(t)$, $i \to j \in S$ and

$$\rho_1 = \frac{\lambda_{01} - \lambda_{10} - \lambda_{12} + \sqrt{(\lambda_{10} + \lambda_{12} - \lambda_{01})^2 + 4\lambda_{01}\lambda_{10}}}{2},$$

$$\rho_2 = \frac{\lambda_{01} - \lambda_{10} - \lambda_{12} + \sqrt{(\lambda_{10} + \lambda_{12} - \lambda_{01})^2 + 4\lambda_{01}\lambda_{10}}}{2}.$$

The multiple step transition probability is

$$P_{02}(\tau, t) = \int_{\tau}^{t} P_{01}(\tau, \xi) \cdot P_{12}(\xi, t) d\xi,$$

$$P_{03}(\tau, t) = \int_{\tau}^{t} P_{02}(\tau, \xi) \cdot P_{23}(\xi, t) d\xi,$$

$$P_{13}(\tau, t) = \int_{\tau}^{t} P_{12}(\tau, \xi) \cdot P_{23}(\xi, t) d\xi. \tag{54}$$

During the screening process, the total sample of screening population is N and individual i is observed staying in state $s \in S$ and with covariables $Z_j(t)$ at screening time t_i. Therefore, the likelihood model for parameter estimation is

$$L = \prod_{i=1}^{N} \prod_{k=1}^{m_i - 1} P_{s(t_{ik})s(t_{ik+1})}(t_{ik}, t_{ik+1}). \tag{55}$$

The estimation of parameters may use the maximum likelihood method and the hypothesis testing may use likelihood ratio test.

4.2.3. *Example*

The stochastic model of natural history of disease for nasopharyngeal carcinoma (NPC) screening is used as the example to introduce the development of non-homogeneous Markov model with covariables. The natural history of NPC is showed in Fig. 6.

Three states were assumed in the progress of NPC: health, PCDP of NPC and clinical phase of NPC. When the individual transfers from health to PCDP of NPC, gender, age, antibody level and variability characters of Epstein Barr virus (EBV) are the covariables deciding the transition power. According to the natural history of NPC, the transition probability matrix

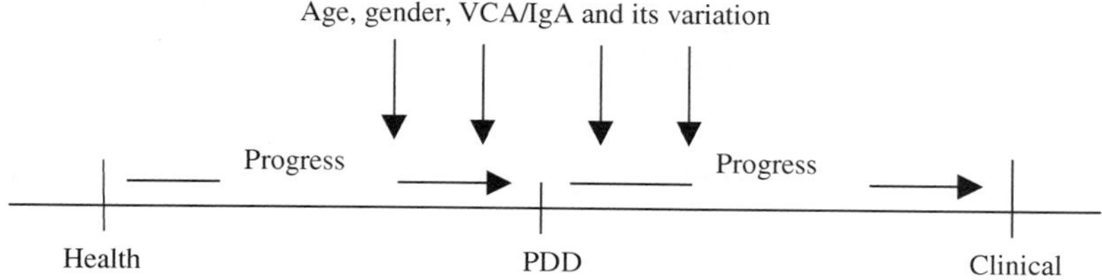

Fig. 6. Natural history model of NPC.

of Markov chain is

$$P(i,j) = \begin{bmatrix} p_{11} & P_{12} & 0 \\ 0 & p_{22} & p_{23} \\ 0 & 0 & 1 \end{bmatrix} \quad i,j = 0,1,2,3\,,$$

where 1 is state of health, 2 is state of PCDP of NPC and 3 is state of clinical phase of NPC.

Since there is no reverse transition between the states, the $p_{21} = 0$, $p_{32} = 0$ and $p_{32} = 0$. This assumption is reasonable for the progressive diseases, such as malignant tumor. The state 3 is the absorbable state. It is also assumed that the transition between states is no jump. That means $p_{13} = 0$. Suppose θ is the parameter of transition intension. The transition probabilities are

$$P_{12}(t) = \alpha_{12}\theta(t)\,, \quad P_{11}(t) = 1 - P_{12}(t)\,,$$

$$P_{23}(t) = \alpha_{23}\theta(t)\,, \quad P_{22}(t) = 1 - P_{23}(t)\,, \tag{56}$$

$$\theta(t) = 1 - e^{-\beta X(t)}\,, \tag{57}$$

$$\beta = \{\beta_0, \beta_1, \beta_2, \beta_3, \beta_4\} \quad 0 \le \beta \le \infty\,,$$

$$X(t) = \{x_1, x_2(t), x_3(t), x_4(t)\}\,.$$

Among them, X_1 is gender (1 = woman, 2 = man) and does not change with time. X_2 is age at the time of screen. X_3 is the titer of antibody of EBV(VCA/IgA), 1 = negative, 2 = 1:5 1:10, 3 = 1:20 1:40, 4 = 1:80+. X_4 is the characteristics of variation of VCA/IgA, 1 = negative, 2 = low level of positive antibody, 3 = persistent high level, 4 = increasing level, 5 = both positive of VCA/IgA and EA/IgA. The age and level of antibody of EBV are covariables with time.

It is assumed that the maximum times of transition during a fixed screening interval is m. An individual stays in state i at the time t and transfers to state j during a fixed interval (for example 1 year) m. The matrix of m step transition probability is

$$A_m(t) = \prod_{\substack{k=0 \\ t+k\in T}}^{m-1} P(t+k)\,. \tag{58}$$

In order to estimate the false negative rate, it is assumed that the one step missing discriminant may happen only and suppose $s \in S = 1, 2, 3$. $P(\text{state} = s+1|\text{diagnosis} = s) = \gamma \cdot \gamma$ is the false negative rate and the diagnostic vector is

$$B(1) = (1-\gamma, \gamma, 0)\,,$$
$$B(2) = (0, 1-\gamma, \gamma)\,,$$
$$B(3) = (0, 0, 1)\,.$$

Suppose N individuals are screened, individual $k = 1, 2, \ldots, N$ participates q_k screens and then the likelihood function is

$$L = \prod_{k=1}^{N} \prod_{j=1}^{q_k-1} B'(s_{kj}) Am_{kj}(t_{kj}) B(s_{k,j+1})\,. \tag{59}$$

A mass screening for nasopharyngeal carcinoma was carried out in Guangzhou, Zhongshan and Sihui.[17] 2970 cases with positive results of for VCA/IgA and 3 cases of NPC among them were found in Guangzhou. All the cases with positive VCA/IgA and 214 controls with negative VCA/IgA were followed up and 35 NPC were found during a 7-year period. 2988 cases with positive VCA/IgA and 34 cases of NPC were found in the first screen in Zhongshan. All cases with positive VCA/IgA and 2068 controls with negative VCA/IgA were followed up and 40 cases of NPC were found during a 7-year period. 1297 cases with positive VCA/IgA and 13 cases of NPC were found in the first screen in Sihui. 19 cases of NPC were found during a 7-year follow-up for the cases with positive VCA/IgA.

A Markov model with time dependent covariables was developed and the results showed in Table 7.

5. The Simulation and Optimization of Screening Policy

Based on the parameters of natural history of disease and screening implement, the disease process and the effects of screening intervention may

Table 7. Estimated values of parameters in natural history model of NPC and hypothesis test.

Parameters	Values	Likelihood test	P value
α_{12}	0.001908		
α_{23}	0.2051		
β_0	−0.4163		
β_1 (gender)	0.1651	10.7338	< 0.00005
β_2 (age)	0.00002217	0.0194	> 0.9
β_3 (VCA/IgA)	0.1553	34.2804	< 0.0001
β_4 (variation of VCA/IgA)	0.1879	25.1728	< 0.0001
γ (false negative rate)	0.0002		
M (Maxi. transitions)	2		

be simulated and the cost-effectiveness may be evaluated. There are two purposes of analysis and assessment of screening data. One is to estimate the parameters of screening, including the attendance rate, cost, the characteristics of screening test (sensitivity and specificity) natural history of disease (the sojourn time in preclinical detectable phase PCDP), the impact of screening on the mortality and prevalence of disease, etc. Based on these parameters, one may make a conclusion if the mass screening is efficacious. Another point is to choose an optimized screening policy. It refers to choosing the population in eligible age group, frequency of screening and the interval between subsequent screening test, the combination of screening test and sequential diagnostic procedures. An optimized screening policy is expected to yield benefits maximum health given limited resources. The choice of a screening policy should preferably be based on the balance between expected health effects and costs. The development of natural history model of disease serves for first purpose and the simulation of disease process and screening serves for second one. The fundament of simulation for disease process is the technique of Monte Carlo. Based on the known and hypothetic parameters, a screening process for disease in a large population is simulated by computer and the simulated effects of screening policy are evaluated. A variety of screening policies are simulated repeatedly and the optimized policies of screening are identified for the consideration of policy decision-maker.

Knox[18] first used the macro-simulation method to evaluate the health effects of screening for cervical cancer in England. He assumed that the duration of the interval between the point at which the disease first becomes detectable and the point at which it becomes incurable is a constant (A).

The duration of the interval between incurability and death is B. The sensitivity of screening test is S. The interval between subsequent screens is I. The disease incidence rates in different age groups are P. Now a mass screening program was carried out starting in age B in a 100,000 population. In the population, the disease onsets in a speed of P. It is assumed that the disease is curable if it is detected by screening and the life may be saved. The disease is incurable if it is diagnosed in the hospital and the life lost is the mortality rate (D) of disease. If the main concern were to save life year rather than lives, the life year lost ($Y = De_x^0$ taken from the current life-table) and as another compromise, the weighted index ($\text{Id} = D\sqrt{e_x Y^{-1}}$), that is long survivals are not weighted in proportion to their length. The health effects of different screening policy are demonstrated in Fig. 7. The dash line is the original Id caused by the disease. Each test, after an interval of B, produces a deep cut in the mortality, proportional in depth to the sensitivity of the test. The cut persists for a period A, and ends. Closely set tests involve some waste because of overlap, but later tests cut by the same proportion into the cases missed by earlier tests. The interval of first screen and second screen is wider than A so that the Id returns to the original line when the health effects of early detection of screening on the disease

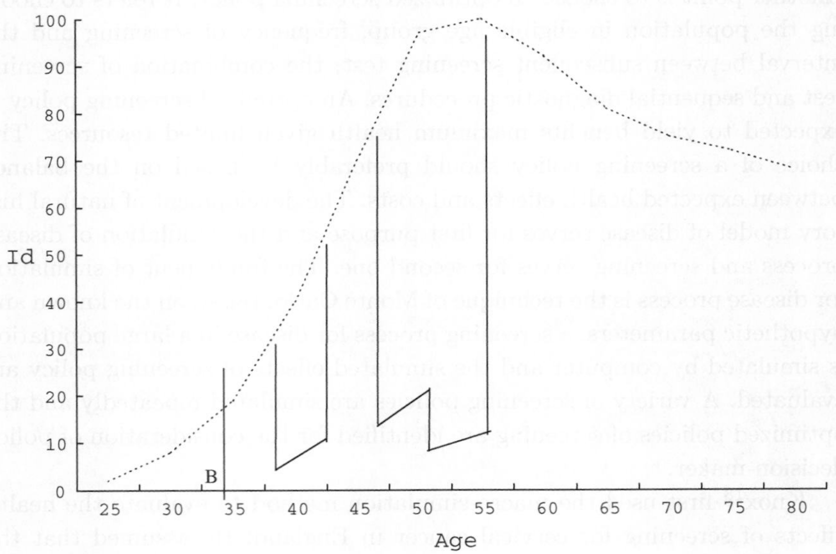

Fig. 7. Illustration of simulated effects of screening for disease.

mortality disappear. The interval of second screen and third one is shorter than A, so that Id goes down again before it returns to original value. The sensitivity of screening test decides the depth of cut. A high sensitivity means the cut is close to the horizontal axis and a good health effect of screening. However, the expense of high sensitivity is a low specificity and a high false positive rate when the power of screening test is fixed. That means an increase in amount of follow-up diagnostic work and the total cost of screening.

Knox simulated the cost-effectiveness of mass screening for cervical cancer in England by a simplified macro-simulation model. It is shown in Fig. 7 that the maximum health benefit maybe obtained when screening is started just before the steep increase of disease incidence rate and more frequently screening in the age with high mortality rate of disease. It can be seen by simulation that a very wide range of results can be obtained from different deployments of the same resource, the range itself depending upon the natural history. For example, Knox assumed that the natural history distribution centered upon a mean interval of 6-year for cervical cancer, a 5-year spacing of tests beginning at age 35 gives something like 30 times the benefit of a one-year spacing beginning at age 20 and ending at age 29. The health effects of different screening policies can be roughly compared by macro-simulation model with relatively simple calculation and the optimized scheme can be suggested. However, the parameters in macro-simulation are only assumed as constants and the average disease process and health effects of screening in the whole population are simulated. The variability of individuals is ignored. It is known that the sojourn time of preclinical detectable phase is a variable with a certain distribution. The sensitivity and specificity of screening tests depend on the individual characteristics of disease. And the disease process may change in different individuals. Therefore the macro-simulation can not consider the variations between individuals and evaluate the cost-effectiveness of different screening policies precisely.

Habbema[19] developed a micro-simulation model of the screening process by the assistance of computer. The disease process and the impact of screening intervention of every individual in a population of 100,000 were simulated by the method of Monte Carlo. This simulation model divided into two parts: the disease part and the screening part. The disease part generates a large number of life histories. Together, the life histories constitute the target population that will be screened in the screening part. The stochastic model underlying the simulation of the population is specified by the input of the program. The input related to the population (e.g. the life table), the epidemiology of the disease (e.g. age-specific incidence) and the disease process. Important aspects of the disease process include disease states into which preclinical and clinical disease is subdivided, the duration of preclinical disease, the probability that preclinical disease will regress spontaneously, etc. The output of disease part consists of the simulated life histories. All types of epidemiological data are computed from the aggregation of life histories: incidence of clinical disease, the prevalence of the disease states, the mortality, and survival figures. The input of the screening part consists of assumptions on the screening process (properties of the screening test, prognosis after early detection) and of a specification of the screening policy. The output of the screening part consists of the simulated screening results (e.g. the number of cases detected, number of cases missed, mortality among screen-detected cases) and of the simulated effects of screening (e.g. the number of lives/life years saved, and the number of unnecessarily treated persons). Habbema applied this model to the evaluation of screening for breast cancer and colorectal cancer.

Here the structure of micro-simulation model is introduced by an example of screening for nasopharyngeal carcinoma.[20] The basic structure of model for disease process and screening process of NPC is illustrated in Fig. 8.

The main biomarker of NPC risk is the antibody level of Epstein Barr virus (VCA/IgA). In order to simplify, the positive rate of VCA/IgA is

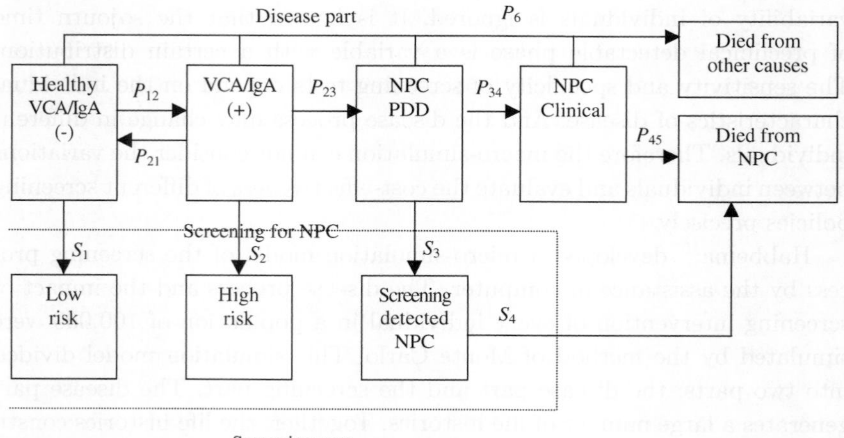

Fig. 8. Structure of the disease model for NPC and stages used in model.

assumed as a constant, e.g. instantaneous transition rate λ. It is supposed that the distribution of λ depended upon the time is an exponential distribution and then the accumulated distribution probability at certain time can be estimated, e.g. transition probability (P_{12}). It is assumed that a part of population with positive VCA/IgA may become negative and the transition probability is P_{21}. It is reasonable that the progression of nasopharyngeal carcinoma is irreversible. Therefore, the preclinical cases should progress to clinical without the intervention of medication. It means the incidence of preclinical NPC is same as the incidence of clinical NPC. The transition probabilities from normal population with negative VCA/IgA to preclinical NPC are the incidence rates (I_{0i}) of NPC in different age groups with negative VCA/IgA. The incidence rates among the population with positive VCA/IgA are $I_{1i} = I_{0i} \times RR_{EB}$ (the relative risk of positive VCA/IgA). These are the instantaneous transition probabilities. The transition probabilities (P_{13} and P_{23}) can be estimated if the distribution functions are assumed. If there is no intervention of screening, the preclinical NPC cases enter the clinical phase according to the distribution probability (P_{34}) of sojourn time in preclinical detectable phase. And then these cases will die according to survival rate (P_{45}) of clinical cases of NPC. All individuals may die from other cause in every stages depended upon the age-specific mortality rates (P_6). Finally, the death age of every individual are simulated. That is the disease part of the model without the intervention of screening. The output of disease part includes the simulated life history of every individual and other disease index such as incidence rate, prevalence rates in different disease stages, mortality rate, etc. The simulated results are compared to the actual figures. Some adjustment of parameters should be done to make simulation model close to realistic population.

In the screening part, the simulated population goes through the screening intervention according to the different policies of screening. For example, the population is divided into the low and the high risk groups according the level of VCA/IgA and are screened in different frequencies. The early detected cases will be checked by further diagnostic procedure. Therefore, the simulated population will enter these three states according to the sensitivity and specificity of screening tests. The transition probability (S_4) from screening detected NPC to death is estimated depending upon the survival rate of preclinical NPC cases. In theory, $S_4 < P_{45}$. It means that the early detection may save the life of NPC cases. The simulated results of screening part are also the death age (d) of every individual. The total effect of screening is the life year saving ($Y = \sum(D-d)$). The total

Table 8. Simulated effects of screening in different policies.

VCA/IgA		VCA/IgA ≥ 1:5		VCA/IgA ≥ 1:20		VCA/IgA ≥ 1:80	
(−)	(+)	Life year saving	Cost per life year	Life year saving	Cost per life year	Life year saving	Cost per life year
1	1	5848	7210.30	6212	6787.53	5620	7503.04
3	1	5716	3243.40	5227	3268.65	4603	3617.20
3	2	4606	3788.55	4562	3697.57	4547	3653.35
3	3	4025	3738.33	4171	3607.44	3696	4070.09
5	1	4921	2605.28	4542	2523.95	3759	2967.23
5	2	4376	2772.54	4051	2809.80	3340	3336.29
5	3	4100	2871.37	3758	3005.80	3208	3466.84
5	4	3804	3053.20	3697	3046.84	3343	3326.62
5	5	3591	2679.13	3282	2930.68	3239	2969.72

cost (C) of screening can be estimated according to the simulated screening process including physical check, test of VCA/IgA, further diagnostic procedure and the organization of screening program. The cost-effectiveness index of screening is the average cost per life year saving $= C/Y$. The lower the cost-effectiveness index, the more the total life year saving, the more the health benefit screening has.

The simulated results of different screening schemes for NPC are listed in Table 8. It is showed that the cost-effectiveness is the best when the positive value of VCA/IgA sets on 1:20. A lower value increases the false positive rate and the cost for further diagnosis. A higher value increases the missing rate and the cost-effectiveness index since the less life saving obtains. The cost is the lowest and the total life year saving is median when the interval between screens is every year for population with positive VCA/IgA and every 5 years for population with negative VCA/IgA. That may be considered as the optimized screening scheme for NPC.

From the results of simulation, it is showed that the cost-effectiveness index of the poorest scheme is four times higher than that of the best one. The importance of simulation study for the assessment of screening cannot be overemphasized.

References

1. United States Commission on Chronic Illness (1957). *Chronic illness in the United States*, Vol. 1, Cambridge, MA:harvard University Press, MA, 267.

2. Wilson, J. and Jungner, G. (1968). Principles and practices of screening for disease. *Public Health Paper 34*, World Health Organization, Geneva, 26–39.
3. Shapiro, S., Goldberg, J. D. and Hutchinson, G. B. (1974). Lead-time in breast cancer screening detection and implication for periodicity of screening. *The American Journal of Epidemiology* **100**: 357–360.
4. Zelen, M. and Feinleib, M. (1969). On the theory of screening for chronic diseases. *Biometrika* **56**: 601–614.
5. Shapiro, S., Venet, W., Strax, P. *et al.* (1982). Ten- to fourteen-year effect of screening on breast cancer mortality. *Journal of National Cancer Institute* **69**: 249–255.
6. Tabar, L., Fagerberg, G., Duffy, S. W. *et al.* (1989). The Swedish two county trial of mamographic screening for breast cancer: Recent results and calculation of benefit. *Journal of Epidemiology Community Health* **43**: 107–114.
7. Albert, A., Gertman, P. M. and Liu, S. (1978). Screening for the early dectection of cancer: II. The impact of screening on the natural history of the disease. *Mathematical Biosciences* **40**: 61–109.
8. Eddy, D. (1980). *Screening for Cancer: Theory, Analysis and Design*, Englewood Cliffs, Prentice-Hall, New Jersey.
9. Day, N. E. and Walter, S. D. (1984). Simplified models of screening for chronic disease: Estimation procedures from mass screening programmes. *Biometrics* **40**: 1–14.
10. Brookmeyer, R. and Day, N. E. (1987). Two-stage models for the analysis of cacner screening data. *Biometrics* **43**: 657–669.
11. MacGregor, J. E., Moss, S., Parkin, D. M. *et al.* (1985). A case-control study of cervical cancer screening in Northeaset Scotland. *British Medical Journal* **290**: 1543–1546.
12. Duffy, S. W., Chen, H. H., Tabar, L. *et al.* (1995). Estimation of mean sojourn time in breast cancer screening using a markov chain model of both entry to and exit from the preclinical detectable phase. *Statistics in Medicine* **14**: 1531–1543.
13. SAS Institute Inc. (1989). SAS/STAT Users Guide, Version6, Volume 2, Cary NC: SAS Institute Inc.
14. Tabar, L., Fagerberg, G., Duffy, S. W. *et al.* (1992). Update of the Swedish two-county program of mammographic screening for breast cancer. *Radiologic Clinics of North America* **30**: 187–210.
15. Fang, J. Q., Wu, C. B., Mao, J. H. *et al.* (1995). Two stage model of tumor sojourn time(I)-non-homogeneous Markov Model. *Applied Probability and Statistics* **11**(2): 205–212.
16. Fang, J. Q. and Wu, C. B. (1995). Two stage model of tumor sojourn time(II) — Counting process and Bootstrap method. *Applied Probability and Statistics* **11**(2): 213–222.
17. Liu, Q., Fang, J. Q., Hu, M. X. *et al.* (1997). Stochastic model of natural history of nasopharyngeal carcinoma. *Chinese Journal of Health Statistics* **14**(4): 12.
18. Knox, E. G. (1976). Ages and frequences for cervical cancer screening. *British Journal of Cancer* **34**: 444–452.

19. Habbema, J. D. F., Van Oortmarssen, G. J., Lubbe, J. T. N. *et al.* (1984). The MISCAN simulation program for the evaluation of screening for disease. *Computation Methods and Programs Biomedicine* **20**: 79–93.
20. Liu, Q. (1995). Simulation study of effect evaluation of screening for tumor. *Chinese Journal of Tumor* **17**: 182.

About the Author

Qing Liu, Professor in cancer epidemiology, graduated in prevention medicine from Guangdong Medical and Pharmacological College in 1982, and obtained his Masters degree in medical statistics at Sun Yat-Sen University of Medical Sciences in 1985. He attained his Ph.D in medical statistics at Sun Yat-Sen University of Medical Sciences in 1996. Dr. Liu worked in the Department of analytic epidemiology in IARC as a fellow from 1990–1991. From 1985–2004, he worked in the department of medical statistics, School of Public Health, Sun Yat-Sen University as teacher, associate professor and full professor. He has also worked in the department of epidemiology, Cancer Center, Sun Yat-Sen University since 2004. His research interests include cancer epidemiology and statistics, including epidemiological study of lung cancer, breast cancer and nasopharyngeal carcinoma, screening for breast cancer and nasopharyngeal carcinoma, effect evaluation and scheme optimization of screening.

Section 2

Statistics in Clinical Trials

CHAPTER 14

STATISTICS IN BIOPHARMACEUTICAL RESEARCH AND DEVELOPMENT

SHEIN-CHUNG CHOW

2424 Erwin Road Ste 1102
11068 Hock Plaza
Durham, NC 27705, USA
sheinchung.chow@duke.edu

ANNPEY PONG

Principal Scientist of Biostatistics and
Research Decision Science
Merck Research Laboratories,
126 E. Lincoln Avenue
RY34 A240, Rahway, NJ 07065, USA
annpey.pong@merck.com

1. Pharmaceutical Research and Development

In the process of research and development of a pharmaceutical entity, statistics are necessarily applied at various critical stages of the process to meet regulatory requirements for the effectiveness, safety, identity, strength, quality, purity, stability, and reproducibility of the pharmaceutical entity under investigation. A pharmaceutical entity could be a drug product, a biological product, a medical device, or a combination of a drug product, a biological product and a medical device. The critical stages of the process of pharmaceutical research and development include pre-IND (Investigational New Drug Application), IND, NDA (New Drug Application) and post-NDA. The role of statistics at these critical stages is briefly described below.

At the very early stage of pre-IND, pharmaceutical scientists may have to screen thousands of potential compounds in order to identify a few promising compounds. An appropriate use of statistics with efficient screening and/or optimal designs will assist pharmaceutical scientists to cost effectively identify the promising compounds within a relatively short period of time. As indicated by the United States Food and Drug Administration (FDA), an IND should contain information regarding chemistry, manufacturing, and controls (CMC) of the drug substance and drug product to ensure the identity, strength, quality, and purity of the investigational drug. In addition, the sponsors are required to provide adequate information regarding pharmacological studies for absorption, distribution, metabolism, and excretion (ADME) and acute, subacute, and chronic toxicological studies and reproductive tests in various animal species to support that the investigational drug is reasonably safe to be evaluated in clinical trials in humans. At this stage, statistics are usually applied to (i) validate a developed analytical method, (ii) establish drug expiration dating period through stability studies, and (iii) assess toxicity through animal studies. Statistics are required to meet standards of accuracy and reliability.

Before the drug can be approved, the FDA requires that substantial evidence of the effectiveness and safety of the drug be provided in the Technical Section of Statistics of an NDA submission. Since the validity of statistical inference regarding the effectiveness and safety of the drug is always a concern, it is suggested that a careful review be performed to ensure an accurate and reliable assessment of the drug product. In addition, in order to have a fair assessment of the efficacy and safety of the investigational drug, the FDA also establishes advisory committees, each consisting of clinical experts, pharmacological experts, statistical experts, and one advocate (not employed by the FDA) in designated drug classes and specialties, to provide a second but independent review of the submission. The responsibility of the statistical expert is not only to ensure that a valid design is used but also to evaluate whether statistical methods used are appropriate for addressing the scientific and medical questions regarding the effectiveness and safety of the drug.

After the drug is approved, the FDA also requires that the drug product be tested for its identity, strength, quality, purity, and stability before it can be released for use. For this purpose, the current Good Manufacturing Practice (cGMP) is necessarily implemented to (i) validate the manufacturing process, (ii) monitor the performance of the manufacturing process, and (iii) provide quality assurance of the final product. At each stage of the manufacturing process, the FDA requires that sampling plans, acceptance criteria, and valid statistical analyses be performed for the intended tests such as potency, content uniformity, and dissolution (USP/NF, 2000). For each test, sampling plan, acceptance criteria, and valid statistical analysis are crucial for determining whether the drug product pass the test based on the results from a representative sample.

In this chapter, we will not only introduce some key statistical concepts commonly encountered in pharmaceutical research and development, but also provide a comprehensive review of some important topics such as assay validation, stability design and analysis, bioavailability/bioequivalence, QT/QTc studies, global clinical development, statistics in diagnostic imaging, and statistical principles for good clinical practice. Detailed information regarding the application of statistics at various critical stages during the process of pharmaceutical research and development can be found in Chow (2000).

2. Key Statistical Concepts

Key statistical concepts in the design and analysis of studies that are commonly conducted at various stages of pharmaceutical research and development are described below.

2.1. *Bias and variability*

For approval of a drug product, regulatory agencies usually require that the results of the studies conducted at various stages of drug research and development must be accurate and reliable to provide a valid and fair assessment of the treatment effect. The accuracy and reliability are usually referred to as the closeness and the degree of the closeness of the results to the true value (i.e., true treatment effect). Any deviation from the true value is considered a bias, which may be due to selection, observation, and statistical procedures. Pharmaceutical scientists should make any attempts to avoid bias whenever possible to ensure that the collected data are accurate. The reliability of a study is an assessment of the precision of the study, which measures the degree of the closeness of the results to the true value. The reliability reflects the ability to repeat or reproduce similar outcomes in the targeted population. The higher precision a study is, the more likely the results would be reproducible. The precision of a study can be characterized by the variability incurred during the conduct of the study.

In practice, since studies are usually planned, designed, executed, analyzed, and reported by a team consisting of pharmaceutical scientists from different disciplines, bias and variability inevitably occurs. It is then suggested that possible sources of bias and variability be identified at the planning stage of the study not only to reduce the bias but also to minimize the variability.

2.2. *Type I/II error, significance level, and power*

In statistical analysis, two different kinds of mistakes are commonly encountered when performing hypotheses testing. As an example, consider the example of pharmaceutical application. Suppose that a pharmaceutical company is interested in demonstrating that a newly developed drug is efficacious. The null hypothesis is often chosen as that the drug is inefficacious versus the alternative hypothesis of that the drug is efficacious. The objective is to reject the null hypothesis and conclude the alternative hypothesis that the drug is efficacious. Under the null hypothesis, a type I error is made if we conclude that the drug is efficacious when in fact it is not. This error is also known as consumer's risk. The acceptable level of probability of committing type I error is known as the significance level. If the probability of observing type I error based on the data is less than the significance level, we conclude that a statistically significant result is observed. The probability of observing type I error is usually referred to as p-value of the test. Similarly, a type II error is committed if we conclude that the drug is inefficacious when in fact it is. This error is referred to as the producer's risk. The power is defined as the probability of correctly concluding that the drug is efficacious when in fact it is. For assessment of drug effectiveness and safety, a sufficient sample size is often selected to have a desired power with a pre-specified significance level. The purpose is to control both type I error (significance level) and type II error (1-power).

2.3. *Confounding and interaction*

In pharmaceutical research and development, there are many sources of variation, which have impact on the evaluation of the treatment. If these variations are not identified and properly controlled, then they may be mixed up with the treatment effect for which the studies are intended to demonstrate. In this case, the treatment effect is confounded with the effects due to these variations. Statistical interaction is to investigate whether the joint contribution of two or more factors is the same as the sum of the contributions from each factor when considered alone. If an interaction between factors exists, an overall assessment cannot be made. In practice, it is suggested that possible confounding factors be identified and properly controlled at the planning stage of the studies. When significant interactions among factors are observed, subgroup analyses may be necessary for a careful evaluation of the treatment effect.

2.4. *Randomization*

Statistical inference on a parameter of interest of a population under study is usually derived under the probability structure of the parameter. The probability structure depends upon the randomization method employed in sampling. The failure of the randomization will have a negative impact on the validity of the probability structure. Consequently, the validity, accuracy, and reliability of the resulting statistical inference of the parameter are questionable. Therefore, it is suggested that randomization be performed using appropriate randomization method under a valid randomization model according the study design to ensure the validity, accuracy, and reliability of the derived statistical inference. Details regarding various randomization models and methods that are commonly employed in clinical research can be found in Chow and Liu (1998, 2003).

2.5. *Sample size determination/justification*

One of the major objectives of most studies during drug research and development is to determine whether the drug is effective and safe. During the planning stage of a study, the following questions are of particular interest to the pharmaceutical scientists: (i) how many subjects are needed in order to have a desired power for detecting a meaningful difference, (ii) what is the trade off if only a small number of subjects are available for the study due to limited budget and/or some scientific considerations. To address these questions, a statistical evaluation for sample size determination/justification is often employed. Sample size determination is usually referred to the calculation of sample size for some desired statistical properties such as power or precision, while sample size justification is to provide statistical justification for a selected sample size, which is often a small number.

For a given study, sample size can be determined/justified based on some criteria on type I error (a desired precision) or type II error (a desired power). The disadvantage for sample size determination/justification based on the criteria of precision is that it may have a small chance of detecting a true difference. As a result, sample size determination/justification based on the criteria of power becomes the most commonly used method. Sample size is selected to have a desired power for detection of a meaningful difference at a pre-specified level of significance.

In practice, however, it is not uncommon to observe discrepancies among study objective (hypotheses), study design, statistical analysis (test statistic) and sample size calculation. These inconsistencies often result in (i) wrong test for right hypotheses, (ii) right test for wrong hypotheses, (iii) wrong test for wrong hypotheses, or (iv) right test for right hypotheses with insufficient power. Therefore, before the sample size can be determined, it is suggested that the following be carefully considered; (i) the study objective or the hypotheses of interest be clearly stated, (ii) a valid design with appropriate statistical tests be used, and (iii) sample size be determined based on the test for the hypotheses of interest.

Note that procedures for sample size calculation based on a pre-study power analysis for comparing means, proportions, time-to-event data, and variabilities can be found in Chow, Shao and Wang (2003, 2007).

2.6. *Statistical difference and scientific difference*

A statistical difference is defined as a difference that is unlikely to occur by chance alone, while a scientific difference is referred to as a difference that is considered to be of scientific importance. A statistical difference is also referred to as a statistically significant difference. The difference between the concepts of statistical difference and scientific difference is that statistical difference involves chance (probability), while scientific difference does not. When we claim there is a statistical difference, the difference is reproducible with a high probability.

When conducting a study, basically, there are four possible outcomes. The result may show that (i) the difference is both statistically and scientifically significant, (ii) there is a statistically significant difference yet the difference is not scientifically significant, (iii) the difference is of scientifically significant yet it is not statistically significant, and (iv) the difference is neither statistically significant nor scientifically significant.

If the difference is both statistically and scientifically significant or it is neither statistically or scientifically significant, then there is no confusion. However, in many cases, a statistically significant difference does not agree with the scientifically significant difference. This inconsistence has created confusion/arguments among pharmaceutical scientists and biostatisticians. The inconsistence may be due to large variability and/or insufficient sample size.

2.7. *One-sided test versus two-sided test*

For evaluation of drug product, the null hypothesis of interest is often the one of no difference. The alternative hypothesis is usually the one that there is a difference. Statistical test for this setting is called a two-sided test. In some cases, the pharmaceutical scientist may test the null hypothesis of no difference against the alternative hypothesis that the drug is superior to the placebo. Statistical test for this setting is known as one-sided test.

For a given study, if a two-sided test is employed at the significance level of 5%, then the level of proof required is one out of 40. In other words, at the 5% level of significance, there is 2.5% chance (or one out of 40) that we may reject the null hypothesis of no difference in the positive direction and conclude the drug is effective at one side. On the other hand, if a one-sided test is used, the level of proof required is one out of 20. It turns out that one-sided test allows more ineffective drugs to be approved because of chance as compared to the two-sided test. It should be noted that when testing at the 5% level of significance with 80% power, the sample size required increases by 27% for a two-sided test as compared to a one-sided test. As a result, there is a substantial cost saving if a one-sided test is used.

However, there is no universal agreement among the regulatory, academia, and the pharmaceutical industry as to whether a one-sided test or a two-sided test should be used. The FDA tends to oppose the use of a one-sided test though several pharmaceutical companies on the Drug Efficacy Study Implementation (DESI) drugs at the Administrative Hearing have challenged this position. Dubey (1991) pointed out that several viewpoints that favor the use of one-sided test were discussed in an administrative hearing. These points indicated that one-sided test is appropriate in the following situations of (i) where there is truly only concern with outcomes in one tail and (ii) where it is completely inconceivable that the results could go in the opposite direction.

2.8. *Non-inferiority versus equivalence*

In clinical investigation, unlike testing for equality (i.e., no treatment difference), the purpose of testing for non-inferiority is to show that the test treatment is not inferior to or at least as effective as a standard therapy or an active agent. Situations where it is applicable (i) the test treatment is less toxic, (ii) the test treatment is easier to administer, (iii) the test treatment is less expensive, and (iv) the test treatment has other clinical benefits. The null hypothesis is one of that the test treatment is inferior to the standard therapy, while the alternative hypothesis is that the test treatment is at least as effective as the standard of care therapy. One of the most controversial issues in non-inferiority trials is probably the selection of non-inferiority margin. A different choice of non-inferiority margin may affect the method of analyzing clinical data and consequently may alter the conclusion of the clinical study.

On the other hand, the purpose of testing for equivalence is to show that the test treatment can reach the same therapeutic effect as that of a standard therapy (or an active agent) or they are therapeutically equivalent. In practice, testing for equivalence consists of (1) testing for therapeutic equivalence between a test treatment and a standard therapy or an active control agent and (2) testing for bioequivalence between an innovator drug product and its generic copies. The null hypothesis is one of that the test treatment is not equivalent to the standard therapy, while the alternative hypothesis is that the test treatment is equivalent to the standard of care therapy.

Testing for non-inferiority include testing for equivalence and testing for superiority. In other words, we may test for equivalence or test for superiority once the non-inferiority has been established. Thus, non-inferiority does not imply equivalence. It should be noted that testing for non-inferiority/superiority is often employed based on a one-sided test procedure at the 5% level of significance, which is equivalent to one of a two-sided test procedure at the 10% level of significance. Thus, it is suggested that a one-sided test procedure at the 2.5% level of significance, which is equivalent to a two-sided test procedure at the 5% level of significance should be used for testing non-inferiority.

2.9. *Good statistics practice*

Good Statistics Practice (GSP) is defined as a set of statistical principles for the best pharmaceutical practices in design and analysis of studies conducted at various stages of drug research and development (Chow, 1997). The purpose of GSP is not only to minimize bias but also to minimize variability that may occur before, during, and after the conduct of the studies. More importantly, GSP provides a valid and fair assessment of the drug product under study. The concept of GSP can be seen in many guidelines and guidance that issued by the FDA and the International Conference on Harmonization (ICH) at various stages of drug research and development. These guidelines and guidances include Good Laboratory Practice (GLP), Good Clinical Practice (GCP), current Good Manufacturing Practice (cGMP), and Good Regulatory Practice (GRP). Another example of GSP is the guideline on *Statistical Principles in Clinical Trials* issued by the ICH (1997). As a result, GSP can not only provide accuracy and reliability of the results derived from the studies but also assure the validity and integrity of the studies.

The implementation of GSP in pharmaceutical research and development is a teamwork, which requires mutual communication, confidence, respect, and cooperation between statistician, pharmaceutical scientists in the related areas, and regulatory agents. The implementation of GSP involves some key factors that have an impact on the success of GSP. These factors include (i) regulatory requirements for statistics, (ii) the dissemination of the concept of statistics, (iii) an appropriate use of statistics, (iv) an effective communication and flexibility, (v) statistical training. These factors are briefly described below.

In the pharmaceutical development and approval process, regulatory requirements for statistics are the key to the implementation of GSP. They not only enforce the use of statistics but also establish standards for statistical evaluation of the drug products under investigation. An unbiased statistical evaluation helps pharmaceutical scientists and regulatory agents in determining (i) whether the drug product has the claimed effectiveness and safety for the intended disease, and (ii) whether the drug product possesses good drug characteristics such as the proper identity, strength, quality, purity, and stability.

In addition to regulatory requirements, it is always helpful to disseminate the concept of statistical principles described above whenever possible. It is important for pharmaceutical scientists and regulatory agents to recognize that (i) a valid statistical inference is necessary to provide a fair assessment with certain assurance regarding the uncertainty of the drug product under investigation, (ii) an invalid design and analysis may result in a misleading or wrong conclusion about the drug product, (iii) a larger sample size is often required to increase statistical power and precision of the studies. The dissemination of the concept of statistics is critical to establish the pharmaceutical scientists and regulatory agents' brief in statistics for scientific excellence.

One of the commonly encountered problems in drug research and development is the misuse or sometimes the abuse of statistics in some studies.

The misuse or abuse of statistics is critical which may result in either having the right question with the wrong answer or having the right answer for the wrong question. For example, for a given study, suppose that a right set of hypotheses (the right question) is established to reflect the study objective. A misused statistical test may provide a misleading or wrong answer to the right question. On the other hand, in many clinical trials, point hypotheses for equality (the wrong question) are often wrongly used for establishment of equivalency. In this case, we have right answer (for equality) for the wrong question. As a result, it is recommended that appropriate statistical methods be chosen to reflect the design, which should be able to address the scientific or medical questions regarding the intended study objectives for implementation of GSP.

Communication and flexibility are important factors to the success of GSP. Inefficient communication between statisticians and pharmaceutical scientists or regulatory agents may result in a misunderstanding of the intended study objectives and consequently an invalid design and/or inappropriate statistical methods. Thus, effective communications among statisticians, pharmaceutical scientists and regulatory agents is essential for the implementation of GSP. In addition, in many studies, the assumption of a statistical design or model may not be met due to the nature of drug product under investigation, experimental environment, and/or other causes related/unrelated to the studies. In this case, the traditional approach of doing everything by the book does not help. In practice, since the concerns from a pharmaceutical scientist or the regulatory agent may translate into a constraint for a valid statistical design and appropriate statistical analysis, it is suggested that a flexible and yet innovative solution be developed under the constraints for the implementation of GSP.

Since regulatory requirements for the drug development and approval process vary from drug to drug and country to country, various designs and/or statistical methods are often required for a valid assessment of a drug product. Therefore, it is suggested that statistical continued/advanced education and training programs be routinely held for both statisticians and non-statisticians including pharmaceutical scientists and regulatory agents. The purpose of such continued/advanced education and/or training program is threefold. First, it enhances communications within the statistical community. Statisticians can certainly benefit from such a training and/or educational program by acquiring more practical experience and knowledge. In addition, it provides the opportunity to share/exchange information, ideas and/or concepts regarding drug development between professional societies. Finally, it identifies critical practical and/or regulatory issues that are commonly encountered in drug development and regulatory approval process. A panel discussion from different disciplines may result in some consensus to resolve the issues, which helps in establishing standards of statistical principles for implementation of GSP.

3. Pharmaceutical Validation

3.1. *Assay validation*

When a new pharmaceutical compound is discovered, the FDA requires that an analytical method or test procedure for determination of the active ingredients of the compound be developed and validated before it can be applied to animal and/or human subjects. The cGMP requires that test methods, which are used for assessing compliance of pharmaceutical products with established specifications, must meet proper standards of accuracy and reliability. The USP/NF defines the validation of analytical methods as the process by which it is established, in laboratory studies, that performance characteristics of the methods meet the requirement for the intended analytical application.

The analytical application may be referred to as a drug potency which is usually based on gas chromatography (GC) or high performance liquid chromatography (HPLC) for potency and stability studies, immunoassays such as radioimmunoassay (RIA) for the *in vitro* activity of an antibody or antigen, or a biological assay for the *in vivo* activity such as median effective dose (ED_{50}). The performance characteristics include accuracy, precision, limit of detection (LOD), limit of quantitation (LOQ), selectivity (or specificity), linearity, range, and ruggedness, which are useful measures for assessment of accuracy and reliability of the assay results. Among these performance characteristics, accuracy, precision, and ruggedness are considered the primary parameters for the validation of an analytical method.

For the validation of an analytical method, whether the analytical method can generate true values is often of great concern. To address this question, one may measure how close the assay result obtained by the analytical method is to the true value. This performance characteristic is referred to as the accuracy of the assay result. In practice, one may consider the analytical method to be validated in terms of accuracy if the mean value is within $\pm 15\%$ of the actual value, except at LOQ, where it should not deviate by more than 20% (Shah, *et al.*, 1992). In addition, the precision, which is defined as the degree of agreement among individual assay results when the assay method is applied repeatedly to multiple sampling of a homogenous sample can be measured based on measurement error of the assay. Similarly, Shah *et al.* (1992) indicated that one may claim that the analytical method is validated if the precision around the mean value does not exceed a 15% coefficient of variation (CV), except for LOQ, where it should not exceed 20% CV.

In many cases, different analysts and different laboratories under different operating circumstances such as different instruments, different lots of reagents, different elapse time, or different assay temperatures may perform a specific analytical method. Assay ruggedness is often used to assess the influence of uncontrollable factors or the degree of reproducibility on assay performance. One may conclude that the analytical method is validated in terms of reproducibility if its assay ruggedness is within 15% of the mean value.

Accuracy is typically assessed using multiple testing by linear regression. Precision can be assessed by testing the null hypothesis that the variability is less than an acceptable limit. Typical approaches for assessing assay ruggedness include the one-way nested random effects model and the two-way crossed-classification mixed model. For the assessment of assay ruggedness, it should be noted; however, that the classical analysis of variance method may produce negative estimates for the variance components and that the sum of best estimates of variance components may not be the best estimate of the total variability. In these situations, methods proposed by Chow and Shao (1988) and Chow and Tse (1991) are useful. In practice, the validation of an analytical method can be carried out by the following steps: First, it is important to develop a prospective protocol which clearly states the validation design, sampling procedure, acceptance criteria for the performance characteristics to be evaluated, and how the validation is to be carried out. Second, collect the data and document the experiment, including any violations from the protocol that may occur. The data should be audited to assure their quality. The collected data are then analyzed based on appropriate statistical methods. Appropriate statistical methods are referred to as those methods, which can reflect the validation design and meet the study objective. Finally, we can then draw a conclusion regarding whether the analytical method is validated based on the statistical inference drawn about the accuracy, precision, and ruggedness of the assay results.

3.2. *Process validation*

The objective of the validation of a manufacturing process is to ensure that the manufacturing process does what it purports to do. A validated process assures that the final product has a high probability of meeting the standards for identity, strength, quality, purity, and stability of the drug product. A manufacturing process is a continuous process, which usually involves a number of critical stages. For example, for the manufacturing of tablets, the process may include initial blending, mill, primary blending, final blending, compression, and coating stages. At each critical stage, some problems may occur. For example, the ingredients may not be uniformly mixed at the primary blending stage; the segregation may occur at the final blending stage, and the weight of tablets may not be suitably controlled during the compression stage. In practice, therefore, it is important to evaluate the performance of the manufacturing at each critical stage by testing in process and/or processed materials for potency, dosage uniformity, dissolution, and disintegration according to sampling plans and acceptance criteria stated in the USP/NF. These tests are usually referred to as the USP tests. For sampling plans of USP tests, the USP/NF requires that representative samples be drawn from the container.

A manufacturing process is considered to pass the USP/NF tests if each critical stage of the manufacturing process and the final product meet the required USP/NF specifications for the identity, strength, quality, and purity of the drug product. A manufacturing process is considered validated if at least three validation batches (or lots) pass all required USP/NF tests. Since manufacturing procedures vary from drug product to drug product and/or from site to site during the development of a validation protocol of manufacturing process, it is important to discuss the issues such as (i) critical stages, (ii) equipment to be used at each critical stage, (iii) possible problems, (iv) USP tests to be performed, (v) sampling plans, (vi) testing plans, (vii) acceptance criteria, (viii) pertinent information, (ix) test or specification to be used as reference, and (x) validation summary with project scientists to acquire a good understanding of the manufacturing process.

Process validation usually refers to as the establishment of documented evidence that a process does what it purports to do. Basically, there are four different types of manufacturing process validations in the pharmaceutical industry: prospective, concurrent, retrospective, and re-validation. Prospective validation establishes documented evidence that a process does what it purports to do based on a pre-planned protocol. Prospective validation is usually performed in the situations where (i) historical data are not available or sufficient and in-process and end-product testing data are not adequate, (ii) new equipment or components are used, (iii) a new product is reformulated from an existing product, or there are significant modifications or changes in the manufacturing process, and (iv) the manufacturing process is transferred from development laboratory to full-scale production. Retrospective validation provides documented evidence based on review and analysis of historical information, which is useful when there is a stable process with a larger historical database. One of the objectives of the retrospective validation is to support the confidence of the process. Concurrent validation evaluates the process based on information generated during actual implementation of the process. In some situations where (i) a step of the process is modified, (ii) the product is made infrequently, and (iii) a new raw material must be introduced, a concurrent validation is recommended. In practice, a well-established manufacturing process may need to be revalidated when there are changes in critical components (e.g., raw materials), changes/replacement of equipment, changes in facility/plant (e.g., location or size), and a significant increase and/or decrease in batch size.

For a validated process, there is no guarantee that if the test is performed again it will have a high probability of meeting the specification. Thus, it is of interest to conduct some in-house acceptance limits (specifications), which guarantee that future batches produced by the process will pass the USP test with a high probability. A common approach to process validation is to obtain a single sample and test the attributes of interest to see whether the USP/NF specifications are met. Bergum (1990) proposed constructing acceptance limits that guarantee that future samples from a batch will meet a given product specification a given percentage of times. The idea is to consider a multiple stage test. If the criteria for the first stage are met, the test is passed. If the criteria for the first stage are not met, then additional stages of testing are done. If the criteria at any stages are met, the test is passed. Acceptance limits for a validation sample are them constructed based on sample mean and standard deviation of the test results to assure that a future sample will have at least a certain chance of passing a multiple stage test. More details can be found in Chow and Liu (1995).

4. Stability Studies

4.1. *Drug shelf-life*

For every drug product in the marketplace, the FDA requires that an expiration dating period (or shelf-life) must be indicated on the immediate container label. The shelf-life is defined as the time interval at which the characteristics of a drug product (e.g., strength) will remain within the approved specifications after manufacture. Along this line, Shao and Chow (2001b) studied several statistical procedures for estimation of drug shelf-life. Before a shelf-life of a drug product can be granted by the FDA, the manufacturers (drug companies) need to demonstrate that the average drug characteristics can meet the approved specifications during the claimed shelf-life period through a stability study.

For determination of the shelf life of a drug product, both the FDA stability guideline and the stability guideline issued by the ICH requires that a long term stability study be conducted to characterize the degradation of the drug product over a time period under appropriate storage conditions. Both the FDA and ICH stability guidelines suggest that stability testing be performed at 3-month intervals during the first year, 6-month intervals during the second year, and annually thereafter. The degradation curve can then be used to establish an expiration dating period or shelf life applicable to all future batches of the drug product.

For a single batch, the FDA stability guideline indicates that an acceptable approach for drug products that are expected to decrease with time is to determine the time at which the 95% one-sided lower confidence bound for the mean degradation curve intersects the acceptable lower product specification limit, e.g., as specified in the USP/NF (FDA, 2000). More details regarding design and analysis of stability studies can be found in Chow (2007).

4.2. *Statistical model*

Consider the case where the drug characteristic is expected to decrease with time. The other case can be treated similarly. Assume that drug characteristic decreases over time linearly (i.e., the degradation curve is a straight line). In this case, the slope of the straight line is considered as the rate of stability loss of the product. Let X_j be the jth sampling (testing) time point (i.e., 0 months, 3 months, etc.) and Y_{ij} be the corresponding testing result of the ith batch ($j = l, \ldots, n$; $i = l, \ldots, k$). Then

$$Y_{ij} = \alpha_i + \beta_i X_j + e_{ij} \tag{1}$$

where e_{ij} are assumed to be independent and identically distributed (i.i.d.) random errors with mean 0 and variance σ_e^2. The total number of observations is $N = kn$. The α_i (intercepts) and β_i (slopes) vary randomly from batch to batch. It is assumed that α_i ($i = l, \ldots, k$) are i.i.d. with mean a and variance σ_a^2, and that β_i $(i = l, \ldots, k)$ are i.i.d. with mean b and variance σ_b^2. The e_{ij}, α_i, and β_i are mutually independent.

If $\sigma_a^2 = 0$ (i.e., β_i are equal), then the above model has a common intercept. Similarly, if $\sigma_b^2 = 0$ (i.e., β_i are equal), then the above model has a common slope. If both $\sigma_a^2 = 0$ and $\sigma_b^2 = 0$, then there is no batch-to-batch variation and the above model reduces to a simple linear regression. Under the above model, Chow and Shao (1989) proposed several statistical tests for batch-to-batch variation.

4.3. *Statistical methods*

4.3.1. *Fixed batches approach*

If there is no batch-to-batch variation, a commonly used method for fitting the above model is the ordinary least squares (OLS) and a 95% lower confidence bound for E(Y) = a + bξ, the expected drug characteristic at time ξ, can be obtained as

$$\hat{a} + \hat{b}\xi - t_{0.95}S(\xi),$$

where $\hat{a}$ and $\hat{b}$ are the OLS estimators of a and b, respectively, $t_{0.95}$ is the one-sided 95th percentile of the t distribution with $N-2$ degrees of freedom, and

$$S^2(\xi) = MSE\left\{\frac{1}{N} + \frac{(\xi - \bar{X})^2}{k\sum_{j=1}^{n}(X_j - \bar{X})^2}\right\},$$

where

$$\bar{X} = \frac{1}{n}\sum_{j=1}^{n} X_j$$

and

$$MSE = \frac{1}{N-2}\sum_{i=1}^{k}\sum_{j=1}^{n}(Y_{ij} - \hat{a} - \hat{b}X_j)^2.$$

The estimated shelf-life can be obtained by solving the following equation

$$\eta = \hat{a} + \hat{b}\xi - t_{0.95}S(\xi),$$

where η is a given approved lower specification limit.

When there is a batch-to-batch variation (i.e., there are different intercepts and different slopes), the FDA recommends the minimum approach be used for estimation of the shelf-life of a drug product. The minimum approach considers the minimum of the estimated shelf-lives of the individual batches. The minimum approach, however, has received considerable criticisms because it lacks of statistical justification. As an alternative, Ruberg and Hsu (1992) proposed an approach using the concept of multiple comparisons to derive some criteria for pooling batches with the worst batch. The idea is to pool the batches that have slopes similar to the worst degradation rate with respect to a pre-determined similarity (equivalence) limit.

4.3.2. *Random batches approach*

As indicated in the FDA guideline, the batches used in long-term stability studies for establishment of drug shelf-life should constitute a random sample from the population of future production batches. In addition, all estimated shelf-lives should be applicable to all future batches. As a result, statistical methods based on random effects model seem more appropriate. Several methods for determination of drug shelf-life with random batches have been considered. See, for example, Chow and Shao (1989, 1991), Murphy and Weisman (1990), Chow (1992), and Shao and Chow (1994). Under the assumption that batch is a random variable, stability data can be described by a linear regression model with random coefficients. Consider the following model

$$\boldsymbol{Y}_{ij} = \boldsymbol{X}'_{ij}\beta_i + e_{ij}$$

where Y_{ij} is the jth assay result (percent of label claim) for the ith batch, $\boldsymbol{X}_{ij}$ is a pxl vector of the jth value of the regressor for the ith batch and $\boldsymbol{X}'_{ij}$ is its transpose, β_i is a pxl vector of random effects for the ith batch, and e_{ij} is the random error in observing Y_{ij}. Note that $\boldsymbol{X}'_{ij}\beta_i$ is the mean drug characteristic for the ith batch at $\boldsymbol{X}_{ij}$ (conditional on β_i). The primary assumptions for the model are similar to those for model (1). Since $\boldsymbol{X}_{ij}$ is usually chosen to be $\mathbf{x}_j$ for all i, where $\mathbf{x}_j$ is a pxl vector of nonrandom covariate which could be of the form $(1, \mathrm{t}_j, \mathrm{t}_j\mathrm{w}_j)$' or $(1, \mathrm{t}_j, \mathrm{w}_j, \mathrm{t}_j\mathrm{w}_j)$', where t_j is the jth time point and w_j is the jth value of qxl vector of nonrandom covariate (e.g., package type and dosage strength). Denote $\mathbf{x}_j = \mathbf{x}(t_j, w_j)$, where $\mathbf{x}$(t,w) is a known function of t and w. If there is no batch-to-batch variation, the average drug characteristic at time t is $\mathbf{x}(\mathrm{t})'\beta$ and the true shelf-life is equal to

$$\bar{t}_{true} = \inf\{t : x(t)'\beta \leq \eta\},$$

which is an unknown but non-random quantity. The shelf-life is then given by

$$\hat{t} = \inf\{t : L(t) \leq \eta\},$$

where

$$L(t) = x(t)'\bar{b} - t_{\alpha,nk-p}\left[\frac{x(t)'(\boldsymbol{X}'\boldsymbol{X})^{-1}x(t)}{k(nk-p)}SSR\right]^{1/2}$$

where SSR is the usual sum of squared residuals from the ordinary least squares regression.

When there is batch-to-batch variation, t_{true} is random since β_i is random. Chow and Shao (1991) and Shao and Chow (1994) proposed considering an (1-α)x100% lower confidence bound of the εth quantile of t_{true} as the labeled shelf-life, where ε is a given small positive constant. That is,

$$P\{t_{label} \leq t_\varepsilon\} \geq 1 - \alpha,$$

where t_ε satisfies

$$P\{t_{true} \leq t_\varepsilon\} = \varepsilon.$$

It follows that

$$t_\varepsilon = \inf\{t\colon \boldsymbol{x}(t)'\beta - \eta = z_\varepsilon \sigma(\mathrm{t})\}$$

where $z_\varepsilon = \Phi^{-1}(1-\varepsilon)$ and $\sigma(t)$ is the standard deviation of $\mathbf{x}(\mathrm{t})'\beta_i$. As a result, the shelf-life is given by

$$\hat{t} = \inf\{t : x(t)'\bar{b} \leq \bar{\eta}(\mathrm{t})\},$$

where

$$\bar{\eta}(t) = \eta + c_K(\varepsilon, \alpha) z_\varepsilon \sqrt{v(t)},$$

$$c_K(\varepsilon, \alpha) = \frac{1}{\sqrt{k}z_\varepsilon} t_{\alpha, K-1, \sqrt{k}z_\varepsilon},$$

$$v(t) = \frac{1}{k-1}\boldsymbol{x}(t)'(\boldsymbol{X}'\boldsymbol{X})^{-1}\boldsymbol{X}'\boldsymbol{S}\boldsymbol{X}(\boldsymbol{X}'\boldsymbol{X})^{-1}\boldsymbol{x}(t).$$

Note that $t_{\alpha,k-1,\sqrt{k}z_\varepsilon}$ is the αth upper quantile of the noncentral t distribution with $k-1$ degrees of freedom and non-centrality parameter $\sqrt{k}z_\varepsilon$.

4.4. *Two-phase shelf-life estimation*

Unlike most drug products, some drug products are required to be stored at several temperatures such as −20°C, 5°C and 25°C (room temperature) in order to maintain stability until use (Mellon, 1991). The drug products of this kind are usually referred to as frozen drug products. Unlike the usual drug products, a typical shelf life statement for frozen drug products usually consists of multiple phases with different storage temperatures. For example, a commonly adopted shelf life statement for frozen products could be either (i) 24 months at −20°C followed by 2 weeks at 5°C or two days at 25°C or (ii) 24 months at −20°C followed by 2 weeks at 5°C and one days at 25°C. As a result, the drug shelf life is determined based on a two-phase stability study. The first phase stability study is to determine drug shelf-life under frozen storage condition such as −20°C, while the second phase stability study is to estimate drug shelf-life under refrigerated or ambient conditions. A first phase stability study is usually referred to as a frozen study and a second phase stability study is known as a thawed study.

Since the stability study of a frozen drug product consists of frozen and thawed studies, the determination of the shelf-life involves a two-phase linear regression. The frozen study is usually conducted similar to a regular long term stability study except the drug is stored at frozen condition. In other words, stability testing will be normally conducted at 3-month intervals during the first year, 6-month intervals during the second year, and annually thereafter. Stability testing for the thawed study is conducted followed the stability testing for the frozen study, which may be performed at 2-day intervals up to two weeks. It should be noted that the stability at the second phase (i.e., thawed study) might depend upon the stability at the first phase (i.e., frozen study). In other words, an estimated shelf-life from the thawed study followed stability testing at 3-month of the frozen study may be longer than that obtained from the thawed study followed the frozen study at 6-month. For simplicity, Mellon (1991) suggested that stability from the frozen study and the thawed study be analyzed separately to obtain a combined shelf life for the drug product. As an alternative, Shao and Chow (2001a) consider the following method for determination of drug shelf lives for the two phases based on a similar concept proposed by Chow and Shao (1991) and Shao and Chow (1994).

For the first phase shelf-life, we have stability data

$$Y_{ik} = \alpha + \beta t_i + \varepsilon_{ik},$$

where $i = 1, \ldots, I \geq 2$ (typically $t_i = 0, 3, 6, 9, 12, 18$ months), $k = 1, \ldots, K_i \geq 1$, α and β are unknown parameters, and ε_{ik},'s are i.i.d. random errors with mean 0 and variance $\sigma_1^2 > 0$. The total number of data for the first phase is $n_1 = \sum_i K_i$ ($= IK$ if $K_i = K$ for all i).

At time t_i, $K_{ij} > I$ second phase stability data are collected at time intervals t_{ij}, $j = 1, \ldots, J \geq 2$. The total number of data for the second phase is $n_2 = \sum_i \sum_j K_{ij}$ ($= IJK$ if $K_{ij} = K$ for all i and j). Data from two phases are independent. Typically, $t_{ij} = t_i + s_j$, where $s_j = 1, 2, 3$ days, etc.

Let α(t) and β(t) be the intercept and slope of the second phase degradation line at time t. Since the degradation lines for the two phases intersect,

$$\alpha(t) = \alpha + \beta t.$$

Then, at time t_i, i =1,. . ., I, we have stability data

$$Y_{ijk} = \alpha + \beta t_i + \beta(t_i)s_j + e_{ijk},$$

where β(t) is an unknown function of t and e_{ijk}'s are i.i.d. random errors with mean 0 and variance $\sigma_{2i}^2 > 0$. We assume that β(t) is a polynomial in t. Typically,

$$\beta(t) = \beta_0 \quad \text{Common slope model,}$$
$$\beta(t) = \beta_0 + \beta_1 t \quad \text{Linear trend model,}$$

or

$$\beta(t) = \beta_0 + \beta_1 t + \beta_2 t^2 \quad \text{Quadratic trend model.}$$

In general,

$$\beta(t) = \sum_{h=0}^{H} \beta_h t^h$$

where β_h's are unknown parameters and $H + 1 < \sum_j K_{ij}$ for all i, and $H < I$.

4.4.1. *First phase shelf-life*

The first phase shelf-life can be determined based on the first phase data $\{Y_{ik}\}$ as the time point at which the lower product specification limit intersects the 95% lower confidence bound of the mean degradation curve (FDA,

1993; ICH, 1993). Let $\hat{\alpha}$ and $\hat{\beta}$ be the least squares estimators of α and β, based on the first phase data, and let

$$L(t) = \hat{\alpha} + \hat{\beta}t - t_{0.05;n_1-2}\sqrt{v(t)}$$

be the 95% lower confidence bound for $\alpha + \beta t$, where $t_{.05;n_1-2}$ is the upper 0.05 quantile of the t-distribution with $n_1 - 2$ degrees of freedom,

$$v(t) = \hat{\sigma}_1^2 \frac{nt^2 - (2\sum_{i,k} t_i)t + \sum_{i,k} t_i^2}{n\sum_{i,k} t_i^2 - (\sum_{i,k} t_i)^2},$$

and

$$\hat{\sigma}_1^2 = \frac{1}{n_1 - 2} \sum_{i,k} (Y_{ik} - \hat{\alpha} - \hat{\beta}t_i)^2$$

is the usual error variance estimator based on residuals. Suppose that the lower limit for the drug characteristic is η (we assume that $\alpha + \beta t$ decreases as t increases). Then the first phase shelf-life is the first solution of L(t) $= \eta$, i.e.,

$$\hat{t} = \inf\{t : L(t) \leq \eta\}.$$

Note that the first phase shelf-life is constructed so that

$$P\{\hat{t} \leq \text{ the true first phase shelf-life}\} = 95\%,$$

assuming that e_{ik}'s are normally distributed. Without the normality assumption, result approximately holds for large n_l. We now consider the second phase shelf-life which is described below.

4.4.2. *The case of equal second phase slopes*

To introduce the idea, we first consider the simple case where the slopes of the second phase degradation lines are the same. When $\beta(t) \equiv \beta_0$, the common slope β_0 can be estimated by the least squares estimator based on the second phase data:

$$\hat{\beta}_0 = \frac{\sum_{i,j,k} (s_j - \bar{s})Y_{ijk}}{\sum_{i,j,k} (s_j - \bar{s})^2},$$

where s_j is the second phase time intervals and $\bar{s}$ is the average of s_j's. The variance of $\hat{\beta}_0$ is

$$V(\hat{\beta}_0) = \frac{\sigma_2^2}{\sum_{i,j,k} (s_j - \bar{s})^2},$$

which can be estimated by

$$\hat{V}(\hat{\beta}_0) = \frac{\hat{\sigma}_2^2}{\sum_{i,j,k}(s_j - \bar{s})^2},$$

where

$$\hat{\sigma}_2^2 = \frac{1}{n_2 - 2}\sum_{i,j,k}(Y_{ijk} - (\hat{\alpha} + \hat{\beta}t_i) - \hat{\beta}_0 s_j)^2.$$

For fixed t and s, let

$$v(t,s) = v(t) + \hat{V}(\hat{\beta}_0)s^2$$

and

$$L(t,s) = \hat{\alpha} + \hat{\beta}t + \hat{\beta}_0 s - t_{0.05;n_1+n_2-4}\sqrt{v(t,s)}.$$

For any fixed t less than the first phase true shelf-life, i.e., t satisfying $\alpha + \beta t > \eta$, the second phase shelf-life can be estimated as

$$\hat{s}(t) = \inf\{s \geq 0 : L(t,s) \leq \eta\}$$

(if $L(t,s) < \eta$ for all s, then $\hat{s}(t) = 0$). That is, if the drug product is taken out of the first phase storage condition at time t, then the estimated second phase shelf-life is$\hat{s}(t)$.

The justification for $\hat{s}(t)$ is that for any t satisfying $\alpha + \beta t > \eta$,

$$P\{\hat{s}(t) \leq \text{ the true second phase shelf-life}\} = 95\%$$

assuming that e_{ik}'s and e_{ijk}'s are normally distributed. Without the normality assumption, the above result approximately holds for large n_1, and n_2.

In practice the time at which the drug product is taken out of the first phase storage condition is unknown. In such a case we may apply the following method to assess the second phase shelf-life. Select a set of time intervals $t_l < \hat{t}, l = 1, \ldots, L$, and construct a table (or a figure) for $(t_l, \hat{s}(t_i))$, $l = 1, \ldots, L$. If a drug product is taken out of the first phase storage condition at time t_o which is between t_l and t_{l+1}, then its second phase shelf-life is $\hat{s}(t_{l+1})$. However, a single shelf-life label may be required. We propose the following method.

4.4.3. *Determination of a single two-phase shelf-life label*

In most cases, $L(\hat{t}, s)$ is less than η for all s, i.e., $\hat{s}(\hat{t}) = 0$. Hence, we propose to select a $\hat{t}_1 < \hat{t}$ such that $\hat{s}(\hat{t}) > 0$ and use $\hat{t}_1 + \hat{s}(\hat{t}_1)$ as the two phase shelf-life label. The justification for this two-phase shelf-life label is:

1. If the drug product is stored under the first phase storage condition until time $\hat{t}_1$, then

$$P\{\hat{t}_1 \leq \text{ the true first phase shelf-life}\} \geq 95\%$$

   since $\hat{t}_1 < \hat{t}$.
2. If the drug product is taken out of the first phase storage condition at time $\hat{t}_1 < \hat{t}$, then its estimated second phase shelf-life is $\hat{s}(\hat{t})$, and

$$\begin{aligned} P\{\hat{s}(\hat{t}_1) &\leq \text{the true second phase shelf-life at time } t_0\} \\ &\geq P\{\hat{s}(\hat{t}_0) \leq \text{ the true second phase shelf-life at time } t_0\} \\ &\geq 95\% \end{aligned}$$

However, this two-phase shelf-life label is very conservative if t_0 is much less than $\hat{t}_1$.

A general rule of choosing $\hat{t}_1$ is that $\hat{t}_1$ should be close to $\hat{t}$ while $\hat{s}(\hat{t})$ is reasonably large. For example, if the units of the first and second phase shelf lives are month and day, respectively, and if $\hat{t} = 24.5$, then we can choose $\hat{t}_1 = 24$; if $\hat{t} = 24$, then we choose $\hat{t}_1 = 23$. A table of $(t_l, \hat{s}(t_l)), l = 1, \ldots, L$, will be useful for the selection of $\hat{t}_1$.

4.4.4. *The general case of unequal second phase slopes*

In general, the slope of the second phase degradation line varies with time. Let $\bar{Y}_i$ be the average of Y_{ijk}'s with a fixed i, $Z_{ijk} = Y_{ijk} - \bar{Y}_i$, and $X_{hij} = (s_j - \bar{s})t_i^h$. Then the least squares estimator of $(\beta_0, \ldots, \beta_H)$, denoted by $(\hat{\beta}_0, \ldots, \hat{\beta}_H)$, is the least squares estimator of the following linear regression model:

$$Z_{ijk} = \sum_{h=0}^{H} \beta_h X_{hij} + error.$$

Let

$$\hat{\beta}(t) = \sum_{h=0}^{H} \hat{\beta}_h t^h$$

and

$$\hat{V}(\hat{\beta}(t)) = \hat{\sigma}_2^2 1'(\mathbf{X}'\mathbf{X})^{-1}1,$$

where $1' = (1, t, t^2 \ldots t^H)$, $\mathbf{X}$ is the design matrix and

$$\hat{\sigma}_2^2 = \frac{1}{n_2 - (H+2)} \sum_{i,j,k} \left(Z_{ijk} - \sum_{h=0}^{H} \hat{\beta}_h X_{hij} \right)^2 .$$

The second phase shelf-life and the two-phase shelf-life label can be determined in the same way as described in the previous section with

$$L(t, s) = \hat{\alpha} + \hat{\beta}t + \hat{\beta}(t)s - t_{0.05; n_1+n_2-(H+4)} \sqrt{v(t, s)}$$

and

$$v(t, s) = v(t) + \hat{V}(\hat{\beta}(t))s^2.$$

For the proposed method for two-phase shelf-life estimation, assume that the assay variabilities are the same across different phases. Detailed information regarding two-phase shelf-life estimation can be found in Shao and Chow (2001a) and Chow and Shao (2002). In practice, the assay variability may vary from phase to phase. In this case, the proposed method is necessarily modified for determination of the expiration dating period of the drug product.

In practice, it is of interest to determine the allocation of sample size at each phase. For a fixed total of sample size, it is of interest to examine the relative efficiency for estimation of shelf lives using either more sampling time points in the first phase or less sampling time points in the second phase or less sampling time points in the first phase and more sampling time points in the second phase. The allocation of sampling time points at each phase then becomes an interesting research topic for two-phase shelf-life estimation. In addition, since the degradation at the second phase is highly correlated with the degradation at the first phase, it may be of interest to examine such correlation for future design planning.

4.5. *Practical issues*

4.5.1. *Matrixing and bracketing designs*

For a new drug product, stability studies are necessarily conducted not only to characterize the degradation of the compound over time but also to determine the expiration dating period (shelf-life). The estimated shelf-life should be applicable for all strengths and packages of the drug product. However, accelerated stability testing is required for 6 months and long-term stability testing is required for the length of shelf-life. The cost of the stability studies could be substantial. As a result, it is of interest to adopt a design where only a fraction of the total number of samples are tested but at the same still maintain the validity, accuracy and precision of the estimated shelf-life. For this consideration, matrixing and bracketing designs have become increasingly popular in drug research and development for stability. As indicated in the ICH stability guideline, bracketing design is defined as the design of a stability schedule so that at any time point only the samples on the extremes, for example, of container size and/or dosage strengths, are tested (ICH, 1994). Matrix design is a design where only a fraction of the total number of samples is tested at any specified sampling point (ICH, 1994; Nordbrock, 2000). The matrixing design and bracketing design were evaluated by Pong and Raghavarao (2000).

Lin (1994) indicated that a matrixing design might be applicable to strength if there is no change in proportion of active ingredients, container size, and immediate sampling time points. The application of a matrixing design to situations such as closure systems, orientation of container during storage, packaging form, manufacturing process, and batch size should be evaluated carefully. It is discouraged to apply a matrixing design to sampling times at two endpoints (i.e., the initial and the last) and at any time points beyond the desired expiration date. If the drug product is sensitive to temperature, humidity, and light, the matrixing design should be avoided.

4.5.2. *Bias and interval estimation of shelf-life*

As indicated in the FDA stability guideline, the estimated shelf-life of a drug shelf-life can be obtained at the time point at which the 95% one-sided lower confidence limit for the mean degradation curve intersects the acceptable lower specification limit. In practice, it is of interest to study the biasedness of the estimated shelf-life. If the bias is positive, the estimated shelf-life overestimates the true shelf-life. On the other hand, if there is a downward bias, the estimated shelf-life is said to underestimate the true shelf-life. In the interest of the safety of the drug product, the FDA might prefer a conservative approach, which is to underestimate rather than overestimate the true shelf-life. Sun, Chow, Li, and Chen (1999) studied distribution properties of the estimated shelf-life proposed by Chow and Shao (1991) and Shao and Chow (1994) for both cases with and without batch-to-batch variation. The result indicate that when there is no batch-to-batch variation (i.e., $\sigma_a^2 = \sigma_b^2 = 0$), there is a downward bias which is given by

$$\frac{t_\alpha \sigma_e}{b^2}\left[\frac{b^2}{n} + \frac{(b\bar{X} + a - \eta)^2}{\sum_{j=1}^{n}(X_j - \bar{X})^2}\right]^{1/2},$$

where t_α is the (1-α)th quantile of the t distribution with $k-1$ degrees of freedom.

4.5.3. *Shelf-life estimation with multiple active components*

For the study of drug stability, the FDA guideline requires that all drug characteristics be evaluated. In most drug products, we obtain an estimated drug shelf-life based primarily on the study of the stability of the strength of the active ingredient. However, some drug products may contain more than one active ingredient. For example, Premarin (conjugated estrogens, USP) contains three active ingredients: estrone, equilin, and 17a-dihydroequilin.The specification limits for each component are different. To ensure identity, strength, quality, and purity, it is suggested that each component be evaluated separately for determination of drug shelf-life. In this case, although a similar concept can be applied, the method suggested in the FDA stability guideline is necessarily modified. It should be noted that the assay values observed from each component might not add up to a fixed total, which is due to the possible assay variability for each component. The modified model should be able to account for these sources of variation. Pong and Raghavarao (2001) proposed a statistical method for estimation of drug shelf-life for drug products with two components. The distributions of shelf-life for two components were evaluated by Pong and Raghavarao (2002) under different designs.

4.5.4. *Stability analysis with discrete responses*

For solid oral dosage forms such as tablets and capsules, the FDA stability guideline indicates that following characteristics should be studied in stability studies: (i) tablets — appearance, friability, hardness, color, odor, moisture, strength, and dissolution, and (ii) capsules — strength, moisture, color, appearance, shape brittleness and dissolution. Some of these characteristics are measured based on discrete rating scale. As a result, the usual methods for stability analysis may not be appropriate. Chow and Shao (2003) proposed some statistical methods for estimation of drug shelf-life based on discrete responses following the concept as described in the FDA stability guideline. However, it may be of interest to consider a mixture of a continuous response variable (e.g., strength) and a discrete response variable (e.g., color or hardness) for estimation of drug shelf-life. This requires further research.

5. Bioavailability and Bioequivalence

5.1. *Introduction*

In pharmaceutical research and development, *in vivo* bioequivalence testing is usually considered a surrogate for assessment of clinical efficacy and safety. This is based on the so-called *Fundamental Bioequivalence Assumption* that when two formulations of the same drug product or two drug products (e.g., a brand-name drug and its generic copy) are equivalent in the rate and extent of drug absorption, it is assumed that they will reach the same therapeutic effect or they are therapeutically equivalent (Chow and Liu, 2000, 2008). Pharmacokinetic (PK) responses such as area under the blood or plasma concentration-time curve (AUC) and maximum concentration ($C_{\max}$,) are usually considered to assess the rate and extent of drug absorption. The current regulation of the FDA requires that the evidence of bioequivalence in average bioavailabilities in terms of some primary PK responses such as AUC and C_{max}, between the two formulations of the same drug product or the two drug products be provided (FDA, 1992, 2000b). This type of bioequivalence is usually referred to as average bioequivalence (ABE). Under current ABE criterion, however, it is not clear whether we are able to demonstrate that the absorption profiles of a brand-name drug and its generic copies are similar; consequently, it is not clear whether the brand name drug and its generic copies will have the same therapeutic effect in terms of efficacy and safety and hence can be used interchangeably.

In medical community, as more generic drug products become available in the marketplace, it is of great concern whether a number of generic drug products of the same brand-name drug can be used safely and interchangeably. Basically drug interchangeability can be classified as drug prescribability or drug switchability. Drug prescribability is defined as the physician's choice for prescribing an appropriate drug product for his/her new patients between a brand-name drug product and a number of generic drug products of the brand-name drug product, which have been shown to be bioequivalent to the brand-name drug product. The underlying assumption of drug prescribability is that the brand-name drug product and its generic copies can be used interchangeably in terms of the efficacy and safety of the drug product. Under current practice, the FDA only requires evidence of equivalence in average bioavailabilities be provided, the bioequivalence assessment does not take into account equivalence in variability of bioavailability. A relatively large intrasubject variability of a test drug product (e.g., a generic drug product) as compared to that of the reference drug product (e.g., its brand-name drug product) may present a safety concern. To overcome this disadvantage, in addition to providing evidence of ABE, it is recommended that bioequivalence in variability of bioavailabilities between drug products be established. This type of bioequivalence is called *population bioequivalence* (PBE). In practice, although PBE is often considered for assessment of drug prescribability, it does not fully address drug switchability due to possible existence of the subject-by-formulation interaction.

Drug switchability is related to the switch from a drug product (e.g., a brand-name drug product) to an alternative drug product (e.g., a generic copy of the brand-name drug product) within the same subject whose concentration of the drug product has been titrated to a steady, efficacious, and safe level. As a result, drug switchability is considered more critical than drug prescribability in the study of drug interchangeability for patients who have been on medication for a while. To assure drug switchability, it is recommended that bioequivalence be assessed within individual subjects. This type of bioequivalence is known as *individual bioequivalence* (IBE). The concept of IBE has attracted FDA's attention since introduced by Anderson and Hauck (1990), which has led to a significant change in regulatory consideration for assessment of bioequivalence (see, e.g., FDA, 2001, 2003). In what follows, we will focus on the review of guidance on *Statistical Approaches to Establishing Bioequivalence,* which was recently issued by the FDA (FDA, 2001).

5.2. *Limitations of average bioequivalence*

Under current FDA regulation, two formulations of the same drug or two drug products are said to be bioequivalent if the ratio of means of the primary PK responses such as AUC and $C_{\max}$ between the two formulations of the same drug or the two drug products is within (80%, 125%) with 90% assurance (FDA, 1992, 2003). A generic drug product can serve as the substitute of its brand-name drug product if it has been shown to be bioequivalent to the brand-name drug. The FDA, however, does not indicate that a generic drug can be substituted by another generic drug even though both of the generic drugs have been shown to be bioequivalent to the same brand-name drug. Bioequivalence among generic copies of the same brand-name drug is not required. As more generic drugs become available in the marketplace, it is very likely that a patient may switch from one generic drug to another. Therefore, an interesting question to the physicians and the patients is whether the brand-name drug and its generic copies can be used safely and interchangeably.

Chen (1997) pointed out that current ABE approach for bioequivalence assessment has limitations for addressing drug interchangeability especially for drug switchability. These limitations include (i) ABE focuses only on the comparison of population average between the test and reference drug products, (ii) ABE does not provide independent estimated of the intra-subject variances of the drug products under study, and (iii) ABE ignores the subject-by-formulation interaction, which may have an impact on drug switchability. As a result, Chen (1997) suggested that current regulation of ABE be switched to the approach of PBE and IBE to overcome these disadvantages.

Chow and Liu (1997) proposed to perform a meta-analysis for an overview of ABE. The proposed meta-analysis provides an assessment of bioequivalence among generic copies of a brand-name drug that can be used as a tool to monitoring the performance of the approved generic copies of the brand-name drug. In addition, it provides more accurate estimates of intersubject and intrasubject variabilities of the drug product.

Note that for assessment of bioequivalence for highly variable drug products, Haidar *et al.* (2008) suggested that a scaled average bioequivalence (SABE) criterion be used in order to account for reference products with huge variability.

5.3. *Drug interchangeability*

As indicated earlier, drug interchangeability can be classified as drug prescribability or drug switchability. It is recommended that PBE and IBE be used to assess drug prescribability and drug switchability, respectively. More specifically, the FDA guidance recommends that PBE be applied to new formulations, additional strength, or new dosage forms in NDAs (new drug applications), while IBE should be considered for ANDA (abbreviated new drug application) or AADA (abbreviated antibiotic drug application) for generic drugs. In what follows, we will only focus on the concept, decision rule, and statistical method of IBE for assessment of drug interchangeability.

The individual bioequivalence is motivated by the 75/75 rule which claims bioequivalence if at least 75% of individual subject ratios (i.e., relative individual bioavailability of the generic drug product to the innovator drug product) are within (75%, 125%) limits. Along this line, Anderson and Hauck (1990) first proposed the concept of testing for individual equivalence ratios (TIER). The idea is to test individual bioequivalence based on the dichotomization of continuous PK metrics by calculating the p value for at least the observed number of subjects who fall within bioequivalence limits with the minimum proportion of the population in which the two drug products must be equivalent in order to claim individual bioequivalence.

It should be noted that no universal definition of IBE exists which is uniformly accepted by researchers from the regulatory agency, the academia and the pharmaceutical industry. For example, IBE may be established based on the comparison between distributions within each subject or it could be based on the distribution of the difference or ratio within each subject (Liu and Chow, 1997). In addition to average bioavailability and variability of bioavailability, we may also consider assessment for the variability due to the subject by formulation interaction. In this case, IBE can be assessed by means of a union-intersection test approach, which concludes IBE if and only if all of the hypotheses are rejected at a prespecified level of significance. Most current methods for assessment of IBE, however, are derived from the distribution of either difference or ratio within each subject. Under this setting, IBE can be classified as probability-based and moment-based according to different criteria for bioequivalence (e.g., Anderson and Hauck, 1990; Esinhart and Chinchilli, 1994; Sheiner, 1992; Schall and Luus, 1993; Holder and Hsuan, 1993).

To address drug switchability, the FDA proposed the following aggregated, scaled moment based one-sided criterion:

$$IBC = \frac{(\mu_T - \mu_R)^2 + \sigma_D^2 + (\sigma_{WT}^2 - \sigma_{WR}^2)}{\max(\sigma_{WR}^2, \sigma_{W0}^2)} \leq \theta_I,$$

where σ_{WT}^2 and σ_{WR}^2 are the within subject variances for the test drug product and the reference drug product, respectively, σ_D^2 is the variance due to subject-by-formulation interaction, σ_{W0}^2 is a constant which can be adjusted to control the probability of passing IBE, and θ_I is the bioequivalence limit. The FDA 2001 guidance suggests that θ_I be chosen as follows

$$\theta_I = \frac{(\ln 1.25)^2 + \varepsilon_I}{\sigma_{W0}^2},$$

where ε_I is the variance allowance factor which can be adjusted for control sample size. As indicated in the FDA 2001 guidance, ε_I may be fixed between 0.04 and 0.05. For the determination of σ^2_{W0}, the FDA 2001 guidance recommends the use of individual difference ratio (IDR), which is defined as

$$\begin{aligned} IDR &= \left[\frac{E(T-R)^2}{E(R-R')^2}\right]^{1/2} \\ &= \left[\frac{(\mu_T-\mu_R)^2+\sigma^2_D+(\sigma^2_{WT}+\sigma^2_{WR})}{2\sigma^2_{WR}}\right]^{1/2} \\ &= \left[\frac{IBC}{2}+2\right]^{1/2}. \end{aligned}$$

Therefore, assuming that the maximum allowable IDR is 1.25, substitution of $(\ln 1.25)^2/\sigma^2_{W0}$for IBC without adjustment of the variance term approximately yields $\sigma_{W0} = 0.2$.

The FDA 2001 guidance suggests that a mixed effects model in conjunction with the restricted maximum likelihood (REML) method be used to estimate variance components of σ^2_D, σ^2_{WT} and σ^2_{WR}. An intuitive statistical test can then be obtained by simply replacing the unknown parameters with their corresponding estimates. However, exact statistical properties of the resultant test are unknown. The FDA 2001 guidance recommends that the small sample method proposed by Hyslop, Hsuan and Holder (2000) be used to obtain the confidence interval or confidence bound of the test. If the upper 95% confidence bound is less than θ_I, we conclude IBE.

5.4. *A review of the FDA guidance on population/individual bioequivalence*

As indicated earlier, the FDA 2001 guidance on *Statistical Approaches to Establishing Bioequivalence* is intended to address drug interchangeability. As a result, the guidance for assessment of PBE and IBE has a significant impact on pharmaceutical research and development. In what follows, we provide a comprehensive review of the FDA 2001 guidance on population and individual bioequivalence from both scientific/statistical and practical points of view. Without loss of generality, we will only focus on IBE.

5.4.1. *Aggregated criteria versus disaggregated criteria*

The FDA 2001 guidance recommends aggregated criteria as described earlier for assessment of IBE. The IBE criterion takes into account for average of bioavailability, variability of bioavailability, and the variability due to subject-by-formulation interaction. Under the proposed aggregated criteria, however, it is not clear whether IBE criterion is superior to ABE criterion for assessment of drug interchangeability. In other words, it is not clear whether or not IBE implies ABE under aggregate criteria. Hence, the question of particular interest to pharmaceutical scientists is that *whether the proposed aggregated criterion can really address drug interchangeability?*

Liu and Chow (1997) suggested disaggregated criteria be implemented for assessment of drug interchangeability. The concept of disaggregated criteria for assessment of IBE is described below. In addition to ABE, we may consider the following hypotheses testing for equivalence in variability of bioavailabilities, and variability due to subject-by-formulation interaction:

$$H_0\colon \sigma^2_{WT}/\sigma^2_{WR} \geq \Delta_v$$
$$vs\ H_a\colon \sigma^2_{WT}/\sigma^2_{WR} < \Delta_v$$

and

$$H_0\colon \sigma^2_D \geq \Delta_s$$
$$vs\ H_a\colon \sigma^2_D < \Delta_s$$

where Δ_v is bioequivalence limit for the ratio of intrasubject variabilities and Δ_s is an acceptable limit for variability due to subject-by-formulation interaction. We conclude IBE if both 100(1-α)% upper confidence limit for $\sigma^2_{WT}/\sigma^2_{WR}$ is less than Δ_v and 100(1-α)% upper confidence limit for σ^2_D is less than Δ_s. Under the above disaggregated criteria, it is clear that IBE implies ABE.

In practice, it is of interest to examine the relative merits and disadvantages between the FDA recommended aggregated criteria and the disaggregated criteria described above for assessment of drug interchangeability. In addition, it is also of interest to compare the aggregated and disaggregated criteria of IBE with the current ABE criterion in terms of the consistencies and inconsistencies in concluding bioequivalence for regulatory approval.

5.4.2. *Masking effect*

The goal for evaluation of bioequivalence is to assess the similarity of the distributions of the PK metrics obtained either from the population or from individuals in the population. However, under the aggregated criteria, different combinations of values for the components of the aggregated criterion can yield the same value. In other words, bioequivalence can be reached by two totally different distributions of PK metrics. This is another artifact of the aggregated criteria. For example, at the 1996 Advisory Committee meeting, it was reported that the data sets from the FDA's files showed that a 14% increase in the average (ABE only allow 80% to 125%) is offset by a 48% decrease in the variability and the test passes IBE but fails ABE.

5.4.3. *Power and sample size determination*

For the proposed aggregated criterion, it is desirable to have sufficient statistical power to declare IBE if the value of the aggregated criterion is small. On the other hand, we would not want to declare IBE if the value is large. In other words, a desirable property for assessment of bioequivalence is that the power function of the statistical procedure is a monotone decreasing function. However, since different combinations of values of the components in the aggregated criteria may reach the same value, the power function for any statistical procedure based on the proposed aggregated criteria is not a monotone decreasing function. The experience for implementing the aggregated criteria in regulatory approval of generic drugs is lacking.

Another major concern is how the proposed criteria for IBE will affect the sample size determination based on power analysis. Unlike ABE, there exists no closed form for the power function of the proposed statistical procedure for IBE. As a result, the sample size may be determined through a Monte Carlo simulation study. Chow and Shao (2002) provided formulas (based on normal approximation) for sample size calculation for assessment of PBE and IBE under a 2×4 replicated crossover design. Sample sizes calculated from the formulas were shown to be consistent with those obtained from simulation studies.

5.4.4. *Two-stage test procedure*

To apply the proposed criteria for assessment of IBE, the FDA 2001 guidance suggests the constant scale be used if the observed estimator of σ_{TR} or σ_{WR} is smaller than σ_{T0} or σ_{W0}. However, statistically, the observed estimator of σ_{TR} or σ_{WR} being smaller than σ_{T0} or σ_{W0} does not mean that σ_{TR} or σ_{WR} is smaller than σ_{T0} or σ_{W0}. A test on the null hypothesis that σ_{TR} or σ_{WR} is smaller than σ_{T0} or σ_{W0} is necessarily performed. As a result, the proposed statistical procedure for assessment of IBE becomes a two-stage test procedure. It is then recommended that the overall type I error rate and the calculation of power be adjusted accordingly.

5.4.5. *Study design*

The FDA 2001 guidance recommends a 2×4 replicated designs, i.e., (TRTR, RTRT) be used for assessment of IBE without any scientific and/or statistical justification. As an alternative to the 2×4 replicated design, the FDA 2001 guidance indicates that a 2×3 replicated crossover design, i.e., (TRT, RTR) may be considered. Several questions are raised. First, it is not clear whether the two replicated crossover designs the optimal design (in terms of power) among all 2×4 and 2×3 replicated crossover designs with respect to the aggregated criterion? Second, it is not clear what the relative efficiency of the two designs is if the total number of observations is fixed. Third, it is not clear how these two designs compare to other 2×4 and 2×3 replicated designs such as (TRRT, RTTR) and (TTRR, RRTT) designs and (TRR, RTT) and (TTR, RRT) designs. Finally, it may be of interest to study the relative merits and disadvantages of these two designs as compared to other designs such as Latin square designs and four sequence and four period designs.

Other issues regarding the proposed replicated designs include (i) it will take longer time to complete, (ii) subject's compliance may be a concern, (iii) it is likely to have a higher dropout rate and missing values especially in 2×4 designs, and (iv) there are little literature on statistical methods dealing with dropouts and missing values in a replicated crossover design setting.

Note that the FDA 2001 guidance provides detailed statistical procedures for assessment of PBE and IBE under the recommended 2×4 replicated design. However, no details regarding statistical procedures for assessment of PBE and IBE under the alternative 2×3 replicated design are given. Chow, Shao and Wang (2003) and Chow, Shao, and Wang (2002) provided detailed statistical procedures for assessment of PBE and IBE, respectively. In addition, Chow and Shao (2002) pointed out that the statistical procedure for assessment of PBE under the recommended 2×4 replicated design as described in the FDA 2001 guidance was inappropriate due to the violation of the primary assumption of independence.

5.4.6. *Outlier detection*

The procedure suggested for detection of outliers is not appropriate for the standard 2×2, the 2×3 or the 2×4 replicated crossover designs because the observed PK metrics from the same subject are correlated. For a valid statistical assessment, the procedures proposed by Chow and Tse (1990) and

Liu and Weng (1992) should be used. These proposed statistical procedures for outlier detection in bioequivalence studies were derived under crossover designs, which incorporate the correlations within the same subject. The FDA 2001 guidance provides little or no discussion regarding the treatment of identified outliers.

6. QT/QTc Studies with Recording Replicates

6.1. *Background*

As indicated by Tsong and Zhang (2008), delay in cardiac repolarization creates an electrophysiological environment that may set off cardiac arrhythmias, particularly a polymorphic ventricular tachycardia. This condition can degenerate into ventricular fibrillation, leading to sudden cardiac death. The QT interval represents the duration of ventricular depolarization and subsequent repolarization and is typically measured on a 12-lead surface ECG from the beginning of the QRS complex to the end of the T wave (see Figure 1). The RR interval, which is the distance between two consecutive R waves, is the inverse of the heart rate. In pharmaceutical research and development, drug induced prolongation of the QT interval has been used as an indicator of possible cardiac safety problems. QT interval is often used to indirectly assess the delay cardiac repolarization, which can pre-dispose to the development of life threatening cardiac arrhythmias such as torsade depointes (Moss, 1993). QTc interval is referred to the

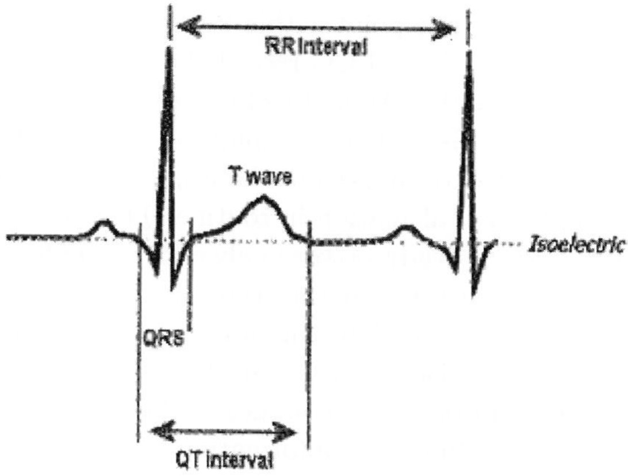

Fig. 1. QT and RR intervals of the surface electrocardiogram.

QT interval corrected by heart rate. In clinical practice, it is recognized that the prolongation of the QT/QTc interval is related to increase risk of cardiotoxicity such as a life threatening arrhythmia (Temple 2003). Thus it is suggested that a careful evaluation of potential QT/QTc prolongation be assessed for potential drug-induced cardiotoxicity.

For development of a new pharmaceutical entity, most regulatory agencies such as the United States Food and Drug Administration (FDA) require the evaluation of pro-arrhythmic potential (see, e.g., CPMP, 1997; FDA/TPD, 2003). In recent years, after several drugs were removed from the market because of deaths due to ventricular tachycardia resulting from drug-induced QT prolongation (Khongphatthanayothin *et al.*, 1998; Lasser *et al.*, 2002; Pratt *et al.*, 1994; Wysowski *et al.*, 2001), the ICH issued a guideline on the evaluation of QT/QTc interval prolongation and proarrhythmic potential for non-antiarrhythmic drugs (ICH E14, 2005) and requests all sponsors submitting new drug applications to conduct at least one thorough QT (TQT) study, normally early in clinical development with some information about the pharmacokinetics of the drug. The ICH E14 guideline also provides the basic recommendations on the regulatory requirements on the assessment of drug-induced prolongation of the QT interval. The ICH E14 guideline calls for a placebo-controlled study in normal healthy volunteers with a positive control to assess cardiotoxicity by examining QT/QTc prolongation. Under a valid study design (e.g., a parallel-group design or a crossover design), ECG's will be collected at baseline and at several time points post-treatment for each subject. Malik and Camm (2001) recommend that it would be worthwhile to consider 3 to 5 replicate ECGs at each time point within 2 to 5 minute period. Replicate ECGs are then defined as single ECG recorded within several minutes of a nominal time (PhRMA, 2003). Along this line, Strieter, *et al* (2003) studied the effect of replicate ECGs on QT variability in health subjects. In practice, it is then of interest to investigate the impact of recording replicates on power and sample size calculation in routine QT studies.

In clinical trials, a pre-study power analysis for sample size calculation is usually performed to ensure that the study will achieve a desired power (or the probability of correctly detecting a clinically meaningful difference if such a difference truly exists). For QT studies, the following information is necessarily obtained prior to the conduct of the pre-study power analysis for sample size calculation. The information includes (i) the variability associated with the primary study endpoint such as the QT intervals (or the QT interval endpoint change from baseline); (ii) the maximal difference in QT interval between treatment groups; and (iii) the number of time points where QT measurements are taken. Under the above assumptions, the procedures as described in Longford (1993) and Chow *et al.* (2003) can then be applied for sample size calculation under the study design (e.g., a parallel-group design or a crossover design). Although QT/QTc studies involve multiple time points, the simplified case with only one time point is considered. The argument is that considering one time point, though conservative, is reasonable for sample size determination purpose. This is particularly true if we focus on the time point where the maximal QT difference between treatments is expected.

The ICH E14 guidance recommends a *thorough* QT/QTc study to decide whether the drug induces QT/QTc prolongation as is evidenced if the upper bound of the 95% confidence interval of the mean drug effect on QTc exceeds 10 ms. Statistical Methods for thorough QT/QTc study have been proposed by Patterson *et al.* (2005) under linear mixed model and Eaton *et al* (2006) using a confidence interval approach. Hosmane and Locke (2005) examined the power in thorough QT/QTc studies via a simulation study. For a review of statistical design and analysis in QT/QTc studies, see Patterson *et al.* (2005). The testing method proposed in Patterson *et al.* (2005) was essentially an intersection-union method which is typically conservative. To address this issue, Eaton *et al.* (2006) constructed a confidence interval, via delta-method, for a parameter which sufficiently approximates the parameter of interest. However, this method technically assumes that mean QT/QTc differences between drug and placebo are positive at all time intervals which is too restrictive and unverifiable in reality. Furthermore, when applying to a function (although smooth) which is presumably close to a non-smooth function (i.e., maximum function), the delta-method may yield a confidence interval whose actual coverage considerably differ from the nominal one, particularly when the sample size is moderate in size. To address these restrictions, Cheng *et al.* (2008) proposed a new testing method based on the maximum of correlated normal random variables.

6.2. *Study designs and models*

As indicated by Zhang and Machado (2008), for a typical thorough QT, a randomized four-treatment group design is usually considered. The four treatment arms are (i) drug with therapeutic dose, (ii) drug with supratherapeutic dose, (iii) positive control, and (iv) placebo. A typical study design for thorough QT studies could be either a parallel-group design or a crossover design. In this section, simple statistical models under a parallel-group design and a crossover design are briefly outlined below.

Under a parallel-group design, qualified subjects will be randomly assigned to receive either treatment A or treatment B. ECG's will be collected at baseline and at several time points post-treatment. Subjects will fast at least 3 hours and rest at least 10 minutes prior to the scheduled ECG measurements. Identical lead-placement and same ECG machine will be used for all measurements. As recommended by Malik and Camm (2001), 3 to 5 recording replicate ECGs at each time point will be obtained within 2 to 5 minute period.

Let y_{ijk} be the QT interval observed from the kth recording replicate of the jth subject who receives treatment i, where $i = 1, 2$, $j = 1, \ldots, n$, and $k = 1, \ldots, m$. Consider the following model

$$y_{ijk} = \mu_i + e_{ij} + \varepsilon_{ijk}, \tag{2}$$

where e_{ij} are independent and identically distributed as normal random variables with mean 0 and variance σ_S^2 (between subject or inter-subject variability) and ε_{ijk} are independent and identically distributed as normal random variables with mean 0 and variance σ_e^2 (within subject or intra-subject variability or measurement error variance). Thus, we have $Var(y_{ijk}) = \sigma_S^2 + \sigma_e^2$.

Under a crossover design, qualified subjects will be randomly assigned to receive one of the two sequences of test treatments under study. In other words, subjects who are randomly assigned to sequence 1 will receive treatment 1 first and then be crossovered to receive treatment 2 after a sufficient period of washout. Let y_{ijkl} be the QT interval observed from the kth recording replicate of the jth subject in the lth sequence who receives the ith treatment, where $i = 1, 2$, $j = 1, \ldots, n, k = 1, \ldots, m$, and $l = 1, 2$. We consider the following model

$$y_{ijkl} = \mu_i + \beta_{il} + e_{ijl} + \varepsilon_{ijkl}, \tag{3}$$

Where β_{il} are independent and identically distributed normal random period effects (period uniquely determined by sequence l and treatment i) with mean 0 and variance σ_p^2, e_{ijl} are independent and identically distributed normal subject random effects with mean 0 and variance σ_S^2, and ε_{ijkl} are independent and identically distributed normal random errors with mean 0 and varianceσ_e^2. Thus, $Var(y_{ijkl}) = \sigma_p^2 + \sigma_S^2 + \sigma_e^2$.

To ensure a valid comparison between the parallel design and the crossover design, we assume that μ_i, σ_S^2, and σ_e^2 are the same as those given in (2) and (3) and consider an extra variability σ_p^2, which is due to the random period effect for the crossover design

6.3. *Power and sample size calculation*

Under models (2) and (3), Chow, Cheng, and Cosmatos (2008) derived formulas for sample size calculation and examined the relationship between a crossover design and a parallel group design for QT studies with recording replicates. The power analysis for sample size calculations under a parallel group design and a crossover design are described in the subsequent subsections.

6.3.1. *Parallel group design*

Under the parallel-group design as described in the previous section, to evaluate the impact of recording replicates on power and sample size calculation, for simplicity, we will only consider one time point post treatment. The results for recording replicates at several post-treatment intervals can be similarly obtained. Under model (2), consider sample mean of QT intervals of the jth subject who receives the ith treatment then $Var(\bar{y}_{ij\cdot}) = \sigma_S^2 + \sigma_e^2/m$. The hypotheses of interest regarding treatment difference in QT interval are given by

$$H_0\colon \mu_1 - \mu_2 \geq 10 \textit{ versus } H_a : \mu_1 - \mu_2 < 10. \tag{4}$$

Under the null hypothesis of no treatment difference, the following statistic can be derived

$$T = \frac{\bar{y}_{1\cdot\cdot} - \bar{y}_{2\cdot\cdot} - 10}{\sqrt{\frac{2}{n}\left(\hat{\sigma}_S^2 + \frac{\hat{\sigma}_e^2}{m}\right)}},$$

where

$$\hat{\sigma}_e^2 = \frac{1}{2n(m-1)} \sum_{i=1}^{2} \sum_{j=1}^{n} \sum_{k=1}^{m} (y_{ijk} - \bar{y}_{ij\cdot})^2,$$

and

$$\hat{\sigma}_S^2 = \frac{1}{2(n-1)} \sum_{i=1}^{2} \sum_{j=1}^{n} (\bar{y}_{ij\cdot} - \bar{y}_{i\cdot\cdot})^2 - \frac{1}{2nm(m-1)} \sum_{i=1}^{2} \sum_{j=1}^{n} \sum_{k=1}^{m} (y_{ijk} - \bar{y}_{ij\cdot})^2.$$

Under the null hypothesis in (4), T has a central t-distribution with $2n-2$ degrees of freedom. Let $\sigma^2 = Var(y_{ijk}) = \sigma_S^2 + \sigma_e^2$ and $\rho = \sigma_S^2/(\sigma_S^2 + \sigma_e^2)$, then under a given alternative that $H_a : \mu_1 - \mu_2 = d < 10$ in (4), the power of the test can be approximated as follows

$$1-\beta \approx \Phi\left(-z_\alpha + \frac{\delta}{\sqrt{\frac{2}{n}\left(\rho + \frac{1-\rho}{m}\right)}}\right), \tag{5}$$

where $\delta = (10 - d)/\sigma$ is the relative effect size and Φ is the cumulative distribution of a standard normal. To achieve the desired power of $1-\beta$ at the α level of significance, the sample size needed per treatment is

$$n = \frac{2(z_\alpha + z_\beta)^2}{\delta^2}\left(\rho + \frac{1-\rho}{m}\right). \tag{6}$$

6.3.2. *Crossover design*

Under a crossover model (3), it can be verified that $\bar{y}_{i\cdots}$ is an unbiased estimator of μ_i with variance $\frac{\sigma_p^2}{2} + \frac{\sigma_s^2}{2n} + \frac{\sigma_e^2}{2nm}$ Thus, we used the following test statistic to test the hypotheses in (4)

$$T = \frac{\bar{y}_{1\cdots} - \bar{y}_{2\cdots} - 10}{\sqrt{\hat{\sigma}_p^2 + \frac{1}{n}\left(\hat{\sigma}_S^2 + \frac{\hat{\sigma}_e^2}{m}\right)}},$$

where

$$\hat{\sigma}_e^2 = \frac{1}{4n(m-1)}\sum_{i=1}^{2}\sum_{j=1}^{n}\sum_{k=1}^{K}\sum_{l=1}^{2}(y_{ijkl} - \bar{y}_{ij\cdot l})^2,$$

and

$$\hat{\sigma}_S^2 = \frac{1}{4(n-1)}\sum_{i=1}^{2}\sum_{j=1}^{n}\sum_{l=1}^{2}(\bar{y}_{ij\cdot l} - \bar{y}_{i\cdot\cdot l})^2$$

$$- \frac{1}{4nm(m-1)}\sum_{i=1}^{2}\sum_{j=1}^{n}\sum_{k=1}^{m}\sum_{l=1}^{2}(y_{ijkl} - \bar{y}_{ij\cdot l})^2,$$

and

$$\hat{\sigma}_p^2 = \frac{1}{2}\sum_{i=1}^{2}\sum_{l=1}^{2}(\bar{y}_{i\cdot\cdot l} - \bar{y}_{\cdots\cdot})^2 - \frac{1}{4n(n-1)}\sum_{i=1}^{2}\sum_{j=1}^{n}\sum_{l=1}^{2}(y_{ij\cdot l} - \bar{y}_{i\cdot\cdot l})^2.$$

Under the null hypothesis in (4), T has a central t-distribution with 2n-4 degrees of freedom. Let σ^2 and ρ be defined as in the previous section, and

$\gamma = \sigma_p^2/\sigma^2$, then $Var(y_{ijkl}) = \sigma^2/(1+\gamma)$. Under a given alternative that $\mu_1 - \mu_2 = d < 10$ in (4), the power of the test can be approximated as follows

$$1 - \beta \approx \Phi\left(-z_\alpha + \frac{\delta}{\sqrt{\gamma + \frac{1}{n}(\rho + \frac{1-\rho}{m})}}\right), \tag{7}$$

where $\delta = (10 - d)/\sigma$. To achieve the desired power of $1 - \beta$ at the α level of significance, the sample size needed per treatment group is given by

$$n = \frac{(z_\alpha + z_\beta)^2}{\delta^2 - \gamma(z_\alpha + z_\beta)^2}\left(\rho + \frac{1-\rho}{m}\right). \tag{8}$$

6.3.3. *Remarks*

Let n_{old} be the sample size with $m = 1$ (i.e., there is single measure for each subject). Then, we have $n = \rho n_{old} + (1-\rho)n_{old}/m$. Thus, sample size (with recording replicates) required for achieving the desired power is a weighted average of n_{old} and n_{old}/m. Note that this relationship holds under both a parallel and a crossover design. Table 1 provides sample sizes required under a chosen design (either parallel or crossover) for achieving the same power with single recording ($m = 1$), three recording replicates ($m = 3$), and five recording replicates ($m = 5$).

Table 1. Sample size for achieving the same power with m recording replicates.

ρ	m		
	1	3	5
1.0	n	1.00 n	1.00 n
0.9	n	0.93 n	0.92 n
0.8	n	0.86 n	0.84 n
0.7	n	0.80 n	0.76 n
0.6	n	0.73 n	0.68 n
0.5	n	0.66 n	0.60 n
0.4	n	0.60 n	0.52 n
0.3	n	0.53 n	0.44 n
0.2	n	0.46 n	0.36 n
0.1	n	0.40 n	0.28 n
0.0	n	0.33 n	0.20 n

Source: Chow *et al.* (2007).

Table 2. Sample sizes required under a parallel-group design.

	Power = 80%					Power = 90%				
	ρ					ρ				
(m, δ)	0.2	0.4	0.6	0.8	1.0	0.2	0.4	0.6	0.8	1.0
(3, 0.3)	81	105	128	151	174	109	140	171	202	233
(3, 0.4)	46	59	72	85	98	61	79	96	114	131
(3, 0.5)	29	38	46	54	63	39	50	64	73	84
(5, 0.3)	63	91	119	147	174	84	121	159	196	233
(5, 0.4)	35	51	67	82	98	47	68	89	110	131
(5, 0.5)	23	33	43	53	63	30	44	57	71	84

Source: Chow *et al.* (2007).

Note that if ρ closes to 0, then these repeated measures can be treated as independent replicates. As it can be seen from the above, if $\rho \approx 0$, then $n \approx n_{old}/m$. In other words, sample size is indeed reduced when the correlation coefficient between recording replicates is close to 0 (in this case, the recording replicates are almost independent). Table 2 shows the sample size reduction for different values of ρ under the parallel design. However, in practice, ρ is expected to be close to 1. In this case, we have $n \approx n_{old}$. In other words, there is not much gain for considering recording replicates in the study.

In practice it is of interest to know whether the use of a crossover design can further reduce the sample size when other parameters such as d, σ^2, and ρ, remain the same. Comparing formulas (6) and (8), we conclude that the sample size reduction by using a crossover design depends upon the parameter $\gamma = \sigma_p^2/\sigma^2$, which is a measure of the relative magnitude of period variability with respect to the within period subject marginal variability. Let $\theta = \gamma/(z_\alpha + z_\beta)^2$, then by (6) and (8) the sample size n_{cross} under the crossover design and the sample size $n_{parallel}$ under the parallel group design satisfy $n_{cross} = n_{parallel}/2(1 - \theta)$. When the random period effect is negligible, that is, $\gamma \approx 0$ and hence $\theta \approx 0$, then we have $n_{cross} = n_{parallel}/2$. This indicates that the use of a crossover design could further reduce the sample size by half as compared to a parallel group design when the random period effect is negligible (based on the comparison of the above formula and the formula given in (6)). However, when the random period effect is not small, the use of a crossover design may not result in sample size reduction. Table 3 shows the sample size under different values of γ. It is seen that the possibility of sample size reduction under a crossover design depends upon whether the carryover effect of the QT

Table 3. Sample sizes required under a crossover design with $\rho = 0.8$

	Power = 80%					Power = 90%				
	γ					γ				
(m, δ)	0.000	0.001	0.002	0.003	0.004	0.000	0.001	0.002	0.003	0.004
(3, 0.3)	76	83	92	102	116	101	115	132	156	190
(3, 0.4)	43	45	47	50	53	57	61	66	71	77
(3, 0.5)	27	28	29	30	31	36	38	40	42	44
(5, 0.3)	73	80	89	99	113	98	111	128	151	184
(5, 0.4)	41	43	46	48	51	55	59	64	69	75
(5, 0.5)	26	27	28	29	30	35	37	39	40	42

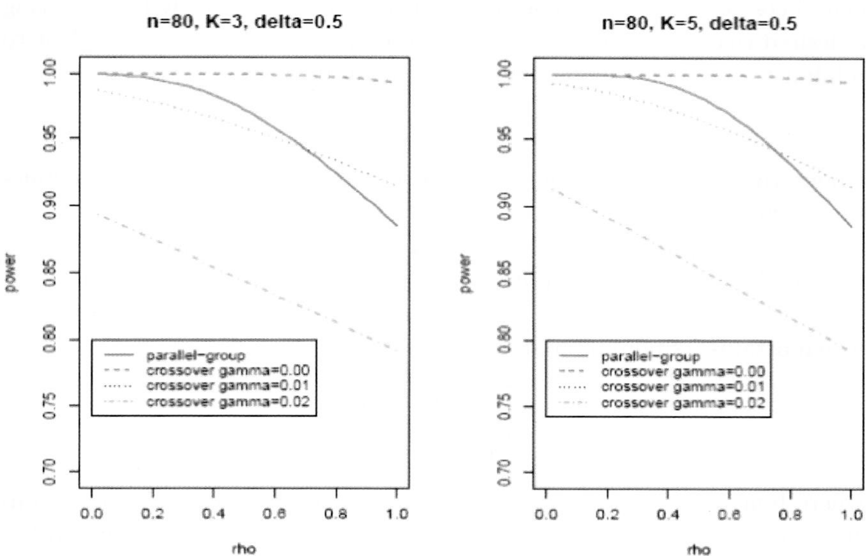

Fig. 2. Power comparison under parallel-group and crossover designs.

intervals could be avoided. As a result, it is suggested that a sufficient length of washout period be applied between dosing periods to wear off the residual (or carryover) effect from one dosing period to another. For a fixed sample size, the possibility of power increase by crossover design also depends on parameter γ. Figure 2 shows that crossover design results in power increase when γ is close to 0 but may result in considerable power loss when γ is not close to 0.

6.4. *Optimization for sample size allocation*

For optimization of the allocation of n (the number of subjects) and m (the number of recording replicates) in routine QT studies with recording replicates, we may consider two approaches, namely, the fixed power approach and the fixed budget approach. The fixed power approach is to find optimal allocation of n and m for achieving a desired (fixed) power in the way that the total budget is minimized. For the fixed budget approach, the purpose is to find optimal allocation of n and m for achieving maximum power.

In this section, for simplicity, we will only describe the solution under a parallel-group design. The results under a crossover design can be similarly obtained. Let C_1 be the cost for recruiting a subject and C_2 be the associated cost for each QT recording replicate. To find n and K for achieving a desired (fixed) power of $1-\beta$ under the minimal budget is equivalent to minimize $C = nC_1 + nmC_2$ under the constraint of

$$2(z_\alpha + z_\beta)^2(\rho m + 1 - \rho) - nm\delta^2 = 0.$$

Under the given constraint, the total cost can be expressed as a function of m

$$C(K) = \frac{2(z_\alpha + z_\beta)^2}{\delta^2}\left(\rho C_2 m + \frac{(1-\rho)C_1}{m} + \rho C_1 + (1-\rho)C_2\right),$$

which attains its minimum at

$$m = \left[\sqrt{\frac{C_1(1-\rho)}{C_2\rho}}\right] + 1,$$

where function $[t]$ denotes the integer part of t. In practice, we may consider choosing the m value among $m = 1, 3$, and 5 that will result in the smallest C.

When the total budget is fixed, say, $nC_1 + nmC_2 = C_0$, where C_0 is a known constant, the power function (5) becomes a function of m only

$$H(m) = \Phi\left(-z_\alpha + \frac{\delta}{\sqrt{\frac{2(C_1+C_2m)}{C_0}\left(\rho + \frac{1-\rho}{m}\right)}}\right),$$

whose maximal value also occurs at $K = [\sqrt{\frac{C_1(1-\rho)}{C_2\rho}}] + 1$.

Note that for any fixed ρ, both the fixed power approach (for achieving a desired power but minimizing the total budget) and the fixed budget approach (for achieving the minimal power under a fixed total budget) result in the same optimal choice of m the number of replicates), which is given by $m = [\sqrt{\frac{C_1(1-\rho)}{C_2\rho}}] + 1$.

6.5. *Test for QT/QTc prolongation*

In the previous sections, we focus on statistical tests for mean QT/QTc difference between treatment groups for a given time interval under a parallel group design and a crossover design. As an alternative, Cheng *et al.* (2008) proposed to test the maximum of QT/QTc differences between treatment groups across all time interval for detection of potential QT/QTc prolongation. Their proposed method under a parallel group design and a crossover design are described below.

6.5.1. *Parallel design*

Under model (2), define $\delta_k = \mu_{1k} - \mu_{2k}$ and $\theta = \max_{1\leq k\leq m}\delta_k$, then a thorough QT/QTc study is equivalent to test the following hypotheses

$$H_0\colon \theta \geq 10 \textit{ versus } H_a : \theta < 10. \tag{9}$$

Suppose the non-inferiority in QTc prolongation can be claimed via a 95% confidence upper bound based on a statistic U, then according to the ICH E14 guidance this means that $U + z_{0.05}SE(U) < 10$, or equivalently, $(U - 10)/SE(U) < -z_{0.05}$, which rejects H_0 (9) at the 5% level of significance . Here SE(U) denotes the estimated standard error of U. Define $W_k = \bar{y}_{1\cdot k} - \bar{y}_{2\cdot k}$, where $\bar{y}_{i\cdot k}$ is the sample mean for the ith treatment at the kth time interval, and $W = (W_1, \ldots, W_m)'$. Cheng *et al.* (2008) proved the following asymptotic result.

Theorem 1. *Let* $T = \max_{1\leq k\leq m} W_k$, *and* θ *is defined in* (9), *then*

$$\sqrt{n}(T - \theta) \to_d N(0, 2(\sigma_1^2 + \sigma^2)),$$

where $\to_d$ *means convergence in distribution.*

Proof: The random vector W is normally distributed with mean $\delta = (\delta_1, \ldots, \delta_m)'$ and variance $\Sigma = (\tau_{kl}) = \frac{2\sigma_1^2}{n}U_m + \frac{2\sigma^2}{n}I_m$, where U is the $m \times m$ matrix of one's and I_m is the $m \times m$ identity matrix. By Afonja (1972), the moment generating function of T is

$$M_T(t) = \sum_{k=1}^{m} e^{\delta_k t + (\sigma_1^2+\sigma^2)\frac{t^2}{n}}\Phi_{m-1}(d_k; R_{-k}),$$

where

$$d_k = \{d_{kl}\}_{l \neq k}, d_{kl} = \frac{(\delta_l - \delta_k)}{2\sigma}\sqrt{n} - \frac{\sigma t}{\sqrt{n}},$$

and $\Phi_{m-1}(d_k; R_{-k})$ is the survival function of an m − 1 dimensional mean 0 normal random vector whose variance is the correlation matrix of W_{-k}, the random vector formed by removing the kth component of W. Then the moment generating function of $\sqrt{n}(T - \theta)$ is

$$\begin{aligned} M_{\sqrt{n}(T-\theta)}(t) &= e^{-t\sqrt{n}} \sum_{k=1}^{m} e^{\delta_k t\sqrt{n} + (\sigma_1^2+\sigma^2)t^2} \Phi_{m-1}(d_k; R_{-k}) \\ &= e^{-t\sqrt{n}} \sum_{k=1}^{m} e^{\delta_k t\sqrt{n} + (\sigma_1^2+\sigma^2)t^2} I(\delta_k = \theta)(1 + o(1)) \\ &= e^{(\sigma_1^2+\sigma^2)t^2}(1 + o(1)), \end{aligned}$$

which implies the claim. By Theorem 1, an asymptotic α level test rejects H_0 in (9) if and only if

$$\frac{T - 10}{\sqrt{2(\hat{\sigma}_1^2 + \hat{\sigma}^2)/n}} < -z_\alpha, \tag{10}$$

where

$$\hat{\sigma}_1^2 + \hat{\sigma}^2 = \sum_{i=1}^{2}\sum_{k=1}^{m}(y_{ijk} - \bar{y}_{i\cdot k})^2/(2m(n-1)).$$

When the number of patients n for each treatment is small, the normal approximation of distribution of T as suggested in Theorem 1 may not work well. Thus, Cheng *et al.* (2008) proposed a small sample correction of the distribution of T. Let $a_k = \{a_{kl}\}$, where $a_{kl} = \sqrt{n}(\delta_l - \delta_k)/2\sigma$ for $k \neq l$ and $a_{kk} = -\infty$. Let k_0 be such that $\delta_{k_0} = \max_{1 \leq k \leq m} \delta_k = \theta$, then by Afonja (1972),

$$\begin{aligned} E(T) &= \sum_{k=1}^{m} \delta_k \int_{a_k}^{\infty} \phi_m(z, R_k) + \sum_{k=1}^{m} \sqrt{\frac{2(\sigma_1^2 + \sigma^2)}{n}} \int_{a_k}^{\infty} z_k \phi_m(z, R_k) \\ &= \theta \int_{a_{k_0}}^{\infty} z_k \phi_m(z, R_{k_0}) + o(\frac{1}{\sqrt{n}}) \\ &= \theta\rho + o\left(\frac{1}{\sqrt{n}}\right), \end{aligned}$$

thus

$$E(T) \approx \theta\rho, \rho = \int_{a_{k_0}}^{\infty} \phi_m(z, R_{k_0}). \tag{11}$$

Similarly since

$$E(T^2) = \sum_{k=1}^{m} \delta_k^2 \int_{a_k}^{\infty} \phi_m(z, R_k) + \sum_{k=1}^{m} \sqrt{\frac{2(\sigma_1^2 + \sigma^2)}{n}} \int_{a_k}^{\infty} z_k \phi_m(z, R_k),$$

$$+ \sum_{k=1}^{m} \frac{2(\sigma_1^2 + \sigma^2)}{n} \int_{a_k}^{\infty} z_k^2 \phi_m(z, R_k)$$

$$= \theta^2 \int_{a_{k_0}}^{\infty} \phi_m(z, R_{k_0}) + \frac{2(\sigma_1^2 + \sigma^2)}{n} \int_{a_{k_0}}^{\infty} z_{k_0}^2 \phi_m(z, R_{k_0}) + o(\frac{1}{\sqrt{n}}),$$

we have

$$Var(T) \approx \frac{2(\sigma_1^2 + \sigma^2)}{n}\gamma, \quad \gamma = \int_{a_{k_0}}^{\infty} z_{k_0}^2(z, R_{k_0}). \tag{12}$$

Now by replacing in (11) and (12) k_0, a_{k_0}, σ_1^2, and σ^2 with their obvious estimators, we get $\hat{\rho}$ and $\hat{\gamma}$. Then a small sample corrected level α test rejects H_0 in (6.10) if and only if

$$\frac{T - 10\hat{\rho}}{\sqrt{2(\hat{\sigma}_1^2 + \hat{\sigma})\hat{\gamma}/n}} < -z_\alpha. \tag{13}$$

6.5.2. *Crossover design*

Let y_{ijkl} be the average QTc responses (possibly adjusted for baseline) over the recording replicates at the lth time interval of the kth treating period for the jth subjects in the ith sequence, $i = 1, 2$, $j = 1, \ldots, n, k = 1, 2$, and $l = 1, \ldots, m$. Under a crossover design, treatment index u is a function of (i, k), hence denoted as $u = d(i, k)$. Consider the following model

$$y_{ijkl} = \mu + \alpha_k + \beta_{ul} + a_{ij} + b_{ijk} + \varepsilon_{ijkl}, \tag{14}$$

where μ is the overall mean, α_k is the period effect, β_{ul} is the treatment effect at lth time interval, a_{ij} is the subject random effect, b_{ijk} is the period random effect nested in the jth subject in the ith sequence, and ε_{ijkl} is the random error. We assume that $a_{ij} \sim N(0, \sigma_2^2), b_{ijk} \sim N(0, \sigma_1^2), \varepsilon_{ijkl} \sim N(0, \sigma^2), a_{ij}, b_{ijk}$, and $\varepsilon_{ijkl}s$' are independent. Under model (14), the treatment effect at the lth time interval is $\delta_l = \beta_{1l} - \beta_{2l}$. Let $\theta = \max_{1 \le l \le m} \delta_l$, then the hypotheses of QTc prolongation in a thorough QT/QTc study under the crossover design is the same as (9).

Define $W_l = (\bar{y}_{1\cdot 1l} - \bar{y}_{1\cdot 2l} + \bar{y}_{2\cdot 2l} - \bar{y}_{2\cdot 1l})/2, l = 1, \ldots, m$, then it is straightforward to show that $W = (W_1, \ldots, W_m)'$ has the same distribution as described earlier A test similar to the one derived in the previous section can therefore be constructed.

6.6. *Recent development*

To discuss some statistical issues that are commonly encountered in thorough QT studies, Tsong and Zhang (2008) put together a special issue on *Statistical Issues in Design and Analysis* at the *Journal of Biopharmaceutical Statistics* (JBS, 18, No. 3, pp. 405–594). These recent development are briefly summarized below.

In an ongoing effort to try to understand the variability of QT/QTc data and determine how that variability would affect the design, analysis, and conclusions drawn from data collected in thorough QT/QTc studies, five PhRMA companies performed a retrospective analysis of placebo and non-drug resting ECG data (Agin *et al.* 2008). Based on the variability observed in the placebo and non-drug data, and on the power simulations, the PhRMA QT Statistics Expert Team suggested raising the upper confidence bound to define a negative QT/QTc study from 7.5 msec to at least 10 msec in the final version of the ICH E14 guideline. On the other hand, Ma *et al.* (2008) examined the performances of several approaches (including individual QT corrections and model-based QT analysis methods) to the analysis of QT changes based on QTc data obtained from a pharmaceutical company. Their simulation results suggested that the mixed effects modeling approach is more powerful than other methods which are commonly used in QT studies.

In their article, Zhang and Machado (2008) attempt to address some statistical issues including study design, primary statistical analysis, assay sensitivity analysis, and sample size calculation for a thorough QT study from regulatory perspectives. Chow, Cheng, and Cosmatos (2008) discussed the strategy of using replicate ECG recordings at each time point to improve the power in the assessment of the drug-induced QT/QTc prolongation. Zhang *et al.* (2008), on the other hand, discussed the design strategy of assessing the maximum QTc changes using the bootstrap approach. Along this line, Cheng *et al.* (2008) proposed an asymptotic test based on the maximum differences under both parallel-group and crossover designs.

Wang *et al.* (2009) investigated the statistical properties of QT_C intervals using individual based correction (IBC), population based correction (PBC), and fixed correction (FC) methods under both linear and log-linear regression models for the QT-RR relationship where RR is the time elapsing between two consecutive heart beats. Based on a simulation study, Wang *et al.* (2009) suggested that in the analysis of QT intervals using PBC or FC methods, RR interval may be included as a covariate in the model to adjust for the remaining correlation of QTc interval with RR interval. This approach will not only reduce the within-subject variability, but also increase the statistical power for assessment of QT/QTc prolongation.

For assessment of QT/QTc prolongation, Zhang (2008) proposed two approaches, namely, a multiple local tests approach and a global average test. Zhang (2008) indicated that the type I error rate needs to be adjusted for the multiple local tests procedure, while no type I error rate adjustment is needed for the global average test. Tsong *et al.* (2008) indicated that the approaches proposed by Zhang are testing seemingly different hypotheses (the two sets of hypotheses are nested). Because of the property of the nested hypotheses, Tsong *et al.* (2008) suggested that Zhang's proposed methods may be applied to the same study data for assay validation tests.

Tian and Natarajan (2008) raised concerns on the impact of baseline measurement on the change from baseline in QTc intervals. In their article, they evaluated the effect of baseline on the change from baseline using the placebo data from several thorough QT studies. Tsong *et al.* (2008) pointed out that current QT-concentration methods might result in a biased underestimate of the maximum prolongation of the QTc interval.

6.7. *Concluding remarks*

Although the ICH E14 guideline provides the basic recommendations on the regulatory requirements on the assessment of drug-induced prolongations of the QT interval, details in measurements and statistics under various study designs (e.g., time-matched design with recording replicates) are yet fully developed. For the thorough QT studies using replicate ECG recordings, one of the controversial issues is that whether a recording replicate is truly a replicate. Another controversial issue relates to the validity of matched-time points approach. In other words, is it clinically/statistically justifiable? In addition, the control of inter- and intra-subject variabilities in the assessment of QT/QTc prolongation is another issue of practical interest to the clinical scientists and biostatistician.

Under a parallel group design, the possibility that the sample size can be reduced depends upon the parameter ρ, the correlation between the QT recording replicates. As indicated earlier, when ρ closes to 0, these recording repeats can be viewed as (almost) independent replicates. As a result, $n \approx n_{old}/m$. When ρ is close to 1, we have $n \approx n_{old}$. Thus, there is not much gain for considering recording replicates in the study. On the other hand, assuming that all other parameters remain the same, the possibility of further reducing the sample size by a crossover design depends upon the parameter γ, which is a measure of the magnitude of the relative period effect. When analyzing QT intervals with recording replicates, we may consider change from baseline. It is, however, not clear which baseline should be used when there are also recording replicates at baseline. Strieter *et al.* (2003) proposed the use of the so-called time-matched change from baseline, which is defined as measurement at a time point on the post-baseline day minus measurement at same time point on the baseline. The statistical properties of this approach, however, are not clear. In practice, it may be of interest to investigate relative merits and disadvantages among the approaches using (i) the most recent recording replicates, (ii) the mean recording replicates, or (iii) time-matched recording replicates as the baseline. This requires further research.

As in discussed in the previous section, the test procedure based on maximum of correlated normal random variables proposed by Cheng *et al.* (2008). Although the tests were derived under a balanced design without covariates, they can be easily generalized to allow for unbalance between the two treatment groups and adjustment of important covariates such as baseline QTc measures and/or heart rates. Note that the method by Cheng *et al.* (2008) did not assume any specific form for the variance structure of the model. This implies that our proposed method with still be valid when covariance structures other than compound symmetric, for example, an AR(1) structure, is more appropriate, or when heteroscedasticity is suspected. It should be noted that the hypotheses in (4) represents only one of the possible interpretations of QTc prolongation evidence. Other definition is worth consideration. For example, under a parallel-group design, define

$$\vartheta = \max_{1\leq k\leq m} \mu_{1k} - \max_{1\leq k\leq m} \mu_{2k},$$

then we could propose testing the following hypotheses

$$H_0 : \vartheta \geq 10 \quad \textit{versus} \quad H_a : \vartheta < 10.$$

The above hypotheses are relevant in an active-controlled QT/QTc study where the maximal prolongation of the two drugs occurs at different time intervals where a globe comparison rather than a time-matched comparison is desired. The method by Cheng *et al.* (2008) can be easily modified to test the above hypotheses.

7. Global Clinical Development

7.1. *Introduction*

For approval of a drug product, the United States Food and Drug Administration (FDA) requires that at least two adequate and well-controlled clinical trials be conducted in order to provide substantial evidence of the effectiveness and safety of the drug product. The characteristics of an adequate and well-controlled clinical trial include a valid design and appropriate statistical tests for data analysis. A valid statistical design cannot only minimize bias and variability that may associate with the trial, but also help to address the scientific/medical questions and/or hypotheses of the trial. An appropriate statistical test can provide a fair and unbiased assessment of the effectiveness and safety of the study drug with certain assurance. When conducting a clinical trial, it may be desirable to have the study done at a single study site if (i) the study site can provide an adequate number of relatively homogenous patients that represent the targeted patient population under study and (ii) the study site has sufficient capacity, resources, and supporting staff to sponsor the study. The advantage of a single site study is that it provides consistent assessment for efficacy and safety in a similar medical environment. However, a single site study has some limitations and hence may not be feasible in many clinical trials, especially when the intended clinical trials are for relatively rare chronic diseases and the clinical endpoints for the intended clinical trials are relatively rare (Goldberg and Kury, 1990). As an alternative, a multi-center trial is usually considered. A multi-center study is a study conducted at more than one distinct center where the data collected from these centers are intended to be analyzed as a whole. Unlike a single site study, a multi-center trial is much more complicated. Although, in practice, multi-center trials do expedite the patient recruitment process, some practical issues in design and analysis need to be carefully considered. These design and analysis issues include the selection of centers, the randomization of treatments, the use of a central laboratory for laboratory evaluation, and the existence of treatment-by-center interaction (Chow and Liu, 1998). Note that the

FDA indicates that an a priori division of a single multi-center trial into two studies is acceptable to the FDA for establishing the reproducibility of drug efficacy to new drug application (NDA) approval. However, a multi-center trial does not address the question whether the clinical results can be generalized to different patient population (e.g., different race or same race with different culture) with similar patient characteristics. For this purpose, a multinational multi-center trial is usually considered. A multi-national trial is a trial conducted at more than one distinct country where the data collected from these countries are intended to be analyzed as a whole.

In recent years, multi-national (multi-regional or global) trials have become increasingly common in clinical development. In addition to the interest of generalizability, the purpose of multi-national or multi-regional trials is multifold. First, a multi-regional (multi-national) trial makes the study drug available to patients from different regions (or countries) which will be beneficial to the region or country especially when no other alternative therapies are available at that region or country. Second, a multi-regional (multi-national) trial provides physicians from different regions (countries) the opportunity to obtain experience on medical practice of the study drug through the trial. In addition, a multi-regional (multi-national) trial may be used as a pivotal trial to fulfill with regulatory requirement of drug registration at some regions (or countries). Finally, a multi-regional (multi-national) trial provides an overall assessment of the performance of the study drug across regions or countries under study.

7.2. *Multi-regional, (multi-national) multi-center trials*

7.2.1. *Multi-center trials*

In a multi-center trial, an identical study protocol is used at each center. A multi-center trial is a trial with a center or site as a natural blocking or stratified variable that provides replications of clinical results. As a result, a multi-center trial should permit an overall estimation of the treatment effect for the targeted patient population across various centers. As was indicated earlier, a multi-center trial with a number of center is often conducted to expedite the patient recruitment process. Although these centers follow the same study protocol, some design and analysis issues need to be carefully considered when planning a multi-center trial. These design and analysis issues include the selection of centers, the randomization of treatment, the use of a central laboratory for laboratory evaluation, and the evaluation of treatment-by-center interaction. These issues are briefly outlined below.

Site Selection — In multi-center trials, the selection of centers is important to constitute a representative sample for the targeted patient population. In practice, the centers are usually selected based on convenience and availability. When planning a multi-center trial with a fixed sample size, it is important to determine the allocation of the centers and the number of patients in each center. For comparative clinical trials, it is not desirable to have too few patients in each center because the comparison between treatments is usually made between patients within centers. A rule-of-thumb is that the number of patients in each center should not be less than the number of centers for a reliable evaluation of the effectiveness and safety of the study drug. For example, if the intended clinical trial calls for 100 patients, the selection of not more than 10 sites may be preferable. Some statistical justification in provided in the next section. Although a multi-center trial has its advantages, it also suffers from some difficulties in site selection. For example, if the enrollment is too slow, the sponsor may wish to (i) terminate the inefficient study sites, (ii) increase the enrollments for the most aggressive sites, or (iii) open new sites during the course of the trial. Each action may introduce potential biases to the study. In addition, the sponsor may ship unused portions of the study drugs from the terminated sites to the newly opened sites for cost-effectiveness consideration. This can certainly increasing the chance of mixing up the randomization schedules and consequently decrease the reliability of the study.

Randomization of Treatments — In multi-center trials, we usually select investigators first and then select patients at each selected investigator's site. At each selected investigator's site, the investigator will usually enroll qualified patients sequentially. A qualified patient is referred to as a patient who meets the inclusion and exclusion criteria and has signed the informed consent form. The primary concern is that neither the selection of investigators nor the recruitment of patients is random. In practice, although the selection of investigators and patients at the selected sites is not random, patients are assigned to treatment groups at random. The collected clinical data are then analyzed as if they were obtained under the assumption that the sample is randomly selected from a homogenous patient population. This process is referred to as the invoked population model and currently widely accepted in clinical research. As a result, randomization is usually performed by study sites in multi-center trials. Note that Lachin (1988) provides a comprehensive summary of the randomization basis for statistical tests under various models. To provide a valid statistical evaluation of the effectiveness and safety of the study drug, randomization is important to ensure that patients selected from the intended patient population constitute a representative sample of the intended patient population. Statistical inference can then be drawn based on some probability distribution assumption of the intended patient population. The probability distribution assumption depends on the method of randomization under a randomization model. A study without randomization will result in the violation of the probability distribution assumption, and consequently no accurate and reliable statistical inference on the study drug can be drawn. It should be noted that in multi-center trials, a large number of study sites may increase the chance of making error in randomization schedules.

Central Laboratory — As indicated earlier, a multi-center trial is usually conducted to enroll enough patients within a desired time frame. In this case, a concern may be whether the laboratory tests should be performed by local laboratories or by a central laboratory. The relative advantages and drawbacks between the use of a central laboratory and local laboratories include (i) the combinability of data, (ii) timely access to laboratory data, (iii) laboratory data management, and (iv) cost. A central laboratory provides combinable data with unique normal ranges, while local laboratories may produce uncombinable data due to different equipment, analysts and normal ranges. As a result, laboratory data obtained from a central laboratory are more accurate and reliable compared with those obtained from local laboratories. In multi-center trials, it is not uncommon that laboratory tests are performed by local laboratories. In this case, it is suggested that laboratory test results be standardized according to the investigator's normal ranges or local laboratories normal ranges before analysis (see, e.g., Chung-Stein, 1996). Note that before the data from different laboratories can be combined for analysis, it may be of interest to evaluate the repeatability (within-laboratory variability) and reproducibility (between-site variability) of the results which can be done by sending to each laboratory identical samples that represent a wide range of possible values and analyze using the method of analysis of variance.

Treatment-by-center Interaction — For a multi-center trial, the FDA guideline suggests that individual center results should be presented. In addition, the FDA suggests tests for homogeneity across centers (i.e., for detecting treatment-by-center interaction) be done. The significant level used to declare the significance of a given test for a treatment-by-center interaction should be considered in light of the sample size involved. Any extreme or opposite results among centers should be noted and discussed. For the presentation of the data, demographic, baseline, and post-baseline data as well as efficacy data should be presented by center, even though the combined analysis may be the primary one. Gail and Simon (1985) classify the nature of interaction as either quantitative or qualitative. A quantitative interaction between treatment and center indicates that the treatment differences are in the same direction across centers but the magnitude differs from center to center, while a qualitative interaction reveals that substantial treatment differences occur in different directions in different centers. If there is no evidence of treatment-by-center interaction, the data can be pooled for analysis across centers. The analysis with combined data provides an overall estimate of the treatment effect across centers. In practice, however, if there are a large number of centers, we may observe significant treatment-by-center interaction, either quantitative or qualitative. In addition, a multi-center trial with too many centers may end up with a major imbalances among centers, in that some centers may have a few patients and others a large number of patients. If there are too many small centers with a few patients in each center, we may consider the following two approaches. The first approach is to combine these small centers to form a new center based on their geographical locations or some criteria pre-specified in the protocol. The data can then be by treating the created center as a regular center. Another approach is to randomly assign the patients in these small centers to those larger centers and re-analyze the data. This approach is valid under the assumption that each patient in a small center has an equal chance of being treated at a large center.

7.2.2. *Multi-national, multi-center trials*

As indicated earlier, a multinational trial is a trial conducted at more than one distinct country where the data collected from these countries are intended to be analyzed as a whole. Within each country, the trial in fact is a multi-center trial. As a result, a multinational trial can be viewed as a trial consists of a number of multi-center trials conducted at different countries under the same study protocol. In practice, it is a concern whether a multinational trial can maintain the integrity of the trial due to the complexity which includes difficulties that are already common in multi-center trials within each country as described in the previous section.

To maintain the integrity of the trial and to achieve the desired accuracy and reliability for an overall assessment of the effectiveness and safety of the study drug, it is important to identify all possible causes of bias and variability. These possible causes of bias and variability could be classified into four categories of (i) expected and controllable, (ii) expected but uncontrollable, (iii) unexpected but controllable, and (iv) unexpected and uncontrollable. In general, these biases and variabilities are mostly due to confounding and differences in culture, medical culture/practice, standards, and regulatory, which will be discussed below.

Confounding — In a multi-center trial, qualified patients within a particular country (e.g., China or Japan) tend to be of the same race which may be different than those patients who are from other countries (e.g., the United States of America and Germany). An immediate concern is what if there is a potential confounding effect between treatment and race. If the confounding effect between treatment and race does exist, it is difficult to evaluate whether the observed treatment difference is due to treatment or race. In addition, the use of concomitant medication is also a concern especially when the multinational trial involves the third countries. This is because the quality, efficacy and safety of the concomitant medications may be a concern. Most of these concomitant medications may or may not be approved by regulatory agencies from other countries. The potential drug-to-drug interaction may contaminate the true treatment effect of the study drug. This is very commonly for those patients from Chinese countries in Asian pacific region who are likely to take traditional Chinese medicines (TCM) (or herbal medicines) during the conduct of the trial even they are told not to. These confounding effects present great challenges to clinical researchers and biostatisticians as well.

Culture — When planning a multinational trial, it is very important to understand and appreciate culture differences from different countries. These culture differences may have an impact on the conduct of the trial. For example, before a multinational trial can be conducted, most regulatory agencies require that the study protocol be submitted to an institutional review board (IRB) for review and approval. The purpose of IRB review is not only to assess the potential risk of the intended trial for patient protection but also to ensure the validity and integrity of the intended trial. Different countries, however, may assess the potential risk differently due the difference in culture. In addition, patients are required to sign an informed consent form before they can be enrolled into the study. It is investigator's responsibility to explain the potential risk/benefit of the study drug to the patients before they sign the informed consent form. However, in some countries such as China, most patients are unlikely and unwilling to sign an informed consent form if they were told that the study medication is a test drug rather than a new drug under investigation. It is a traditional Chinese culture not to take a test drug. Patients are likely to try a new drug. As a result, we may have a problem to obtain signed informed consent forms from patients. For good clinical practice, it is unethical to tell patients that they will be taking a new drug rather than a test drug under investigation. Therefore, it is suggested that a well-designed educational program be implemented by the health authority to eliminate the difficulties caused by the difference in culture.

Medical Culture/Practice — In multinational trials, one of the primary concerns is whether the collected clinical data can be combined for assessment of the effectiveness and safety of the study drug. Although critical information can be captured by a set of standard case report forms (CRF), it is very likely that we may capture different information due to differences in (i) the translation of the CRF in different languages, (ii) the understanding of medical personnel, and (iii) medical culture/practice. At different countries, there is certainly a need to translate the CRF to their respective languages so that patients, clinical monitors, and investigators have same knowledge regarding what information the trial is intended to capture. This is important especially for those countries in which English is not a popular language. A poorly translated CRF may mislead patients to provide inaccurate or even wrong information of little value to the intended trial. In many cases, differences in medical culture and/or practice may result in a very different diagnosis of a similar symptom; consequently, the interpretation or assessment of the efficacy and safety parameters may be different. This is always true for reporting of adverse events (AE). For example, an observed rare but severe AE in one country may be coded differently at a different country if the observed AE is commonly seen in the medical community of the particular country. As a result, AE coding may be different from one country to another which provides a challenge for having a fair and unbiased assessment of safety across different countries. As described earlier in the previous section, it is likely that a local laboratory will be used for laboratory tests in multinational trials. It is expected that different laboratories in different countries will have different laboratory normal ranges due to differences in medical culture and/or practice. In the interest of combining laboratory data for an overall assessment of safety, it is suggested that the laboratory data be standardized according to respective laboratory normal ranges before pooling for analysis.

Regulatory Requirement — For drug research and development, most regulatory agencies have similar but slightly different regulations to assure the drug product has the claimed efficacy and safety. In addition, many regulations and guidelines/guidances were also imposed to assure that the approved drug product meets standards for identity, strength, quality, purity, and stability as specified in the pharmacopeia at the respective countries such as the United States Pharmacopeia (USP) in the United States of America and Chinese Pharmacopeia (CP) in the People's Republic of China. It should be noted that the standards for assay development/validation and test procedures, sampling plans, and acceptance criteria for potency, content uniformity, dissolution, and disintegration may differ from one country to another. These differences may result in a potential treatment-by-country interaction. Consequently, it is difficult to combine the collected clinical data for an overall assessment of the efficacy and safety of the study drug.

Drug Management — Drug management is a great challenge in multinational trials. Randomization schedules are usually generalized by country with a stratification factor (if desirable) and an appropriate block size for treatment balance. The generalized randomization schedules will then be forwarded to drug management for packaging and shipment. The complication is not the randomization or drug packaging but the shipment to the study sites. In many cases, the study drug may not be available in some countries and need to be imported from other countries. Different countries have different regulations for importing investigational drugs. It may takes weeks or months for the processing. If the duration of the intended trial is over a few years, the sponsor may have to take drug expiration dating period into account to make sure that the study drug will not be expired prior to the end of the study. Another consideration for drug management is to make sure that sufficient drugs will be supplied during the conduct of the study. Any unused drugs need to be returned or disposed depending on specific regulations of individual countries. One solution, which is probably the most cost-effective, is to consider the so-called interactive voice randomization system (IVRS) for randomization and drug management. The IVRS to ship sufficient drugs to specific sites on time in a more cost-effective.

7.3. *Selection of the number of sites*

In clinical trials, multiple sites are necessarily considered because one single study site may not have enough resource and/or capacity to handle all of the subjects enter the study. In addition, multiple sites will expedite patient enrollment. In practice, it is not desirable to have too few subjects in each study site. On the other hand, too many study sites may increase the chance of observing so-called treatment-by-interaction, which makes overall inference on treatment effect impossible. Thus, at the planning stage of a clinical trial, how many study sites should be used in order for achieving optimal statistical properties for a given sample size is a commonly asked question.

The question regarding how many study sites should be used is, in fact, a two-stage sampling problem. One first selects a number of study sites and, for each sampled study site, one then selects a number of patients. Shao and Chow (1993) propose statistical testing procedures in a two-stage sampling problem with large within-class sample sizes. In addition, they derived a two-stage sampling plan by minimizing the expected squared volume (or the generalized variance) of the confidence region related to the test. Some results for a two-stage sampling plan are described in the subsequent subsections.

7.3.1. *Two-stage sampling*

For a given clinical trial comparing K treatment groups, we first draw a random sample of n study sites. For each sampled study site, we then recruit M_k subjects, $k = 1, \ldots, K$. Denote by X_{ijk} random variable for the jth subject from the kth treatment group in the ith study site, $i(\text{site}) = 1, \ldots, n, j(\text{subject}) = 1, \ldots, M_k$, and $k(\text{treatment}) = 1, \ldots, K$ and

$$X_i = (X_{ijk}, j = 1, \ldots, M_k, k = 1, \ldots, K).$$

Then, X_i is a random $(\sum_k M_k)$ vector and $X_1, \ldots, X_n$ are independent and identically distributed. For each i, the components of X_i have the same distribution if they are from the treatment group. Thus, the means and the variances of X_{ijk}, denoted by μ_k and σ_k^2 respectively, are unknown but depend on k only. In the second-stage sampling, for each selected study site, we recruit a simple random sample of m_k subjects without replacement who will receive the kth treatment, where $1 \leq m_k \leq M_k$ and $k = 1, \ldots, K$. The total number of subjects recruited from each selected study site is $\sum_k m_k$

and the total number of subjects in the clinical trial is $(\sum_k m_k)n$. Now, the question is how to select n and m_k.

Denote x_{ijk} clinical response observed from the jth subject in the ith study site who receives the kth treatment group, where $i = 1, \ldots, n, j = 1, \ldots, m_k$, and $k = 1, \ldots, K$. Also, let $\bar{x}_k$ and $\hat{\sigma}_k^2$ be the sample mean and sample variance from the kth treatment group, respectively, where

$$\bar{x}_k = \frac{1}{nm_k} \sum_{i=1}^{n} \sum_{j=1}^{m_k} x_{ijk},$$

and

$$\hat{\sigma}_k^2 = \frac{1}{nm_k - 1} \sum_{i=1}^{n} \sum_{j=1}^{m_k} (x_{ijk} - \bar{x}_k)^2.$$

Thus, we have $E(\bar{x}_k) = \mu_k$ and

$$Var(\bar{x}_k) = \frac{1}{nm_k} \sigma_k^2 \left[1 + (m_k - 1)\rho_k\right],$$

where ρ_k is the correlation coefficient between x_{ijk} and $x_{ij'k}$ with $j \neq j'$. In many pharmaceutical problems, $\rho_k = 0$ and hence

$$Var(\bar{x}_k) = \frac{1}{nm_k} \sigma_k^2. \tag{15}$$

Under (15),

$$s_k^2 = \hat{\sigma}_k^2 / nm_k \tag{16}$$

is an unbiased estimator of $Var(\bar{x}_k)$. In the case where $\rho_k \neq 0$, the variance estimator in (16) is not valid. For each fixed k,

$$\bar{x}_{ik} = \frac{1}{m_k} \sum_{j=1}^{m_k} x_{ijk}, i = 1, \ldots, n,$$

are independent and identically distributed. Therefore,

$$Var(\bar{x}_k) = \frac{1}{n} Var(\bar{x}_{ik}), i = 1, \ldots, n.$$

An unbiased estimator of $Var(\bar{x}_k)$ is the sample variance of $\{\bar{x}_{ik}, i = 1, \ldots, n\}$:

$$s_k^2 = \frac{1}{n(n-1)} \sum_{i=1}^{n} (\bar{x}_{ik} - \bar{x}_k)^2, \tag{17}$$

which we can use to replace the estimator in (16) when $\rho \neq 0$. Note that the estimator in (16) is more efficient than that in (17) when $\rho_k = 0$, and (16) and (17) are equivalent when $m_k = 1$.

Assume that nm_k is large so that approximate $100 \times (1-\alpha)\%$ lower and upper confidence bounds for μ_k are given by

$$L_k = \bar{x}_k - z_\alpha s_k \quad \text{and} \quad U_k = \bar{x}_k + z_\alpha s_k, \tag{18}$$

respectively, where z_α is the $(1-\alpha)$th quantile of the standard normal distribution. An approximate $100 \times (1-\alpha)\%$ joint confidence region for the vector $\mu = (\mu_1, \ldots, \mu_K)$ is

$$\left\{ \mu : \sum_k [(\bar{x}_k - \mu_k)/s_k]^2 \leq \chi^2_\alpha(K) \right\}, \tag{19}$$

where $\chi^2_\alpha(K)$ is the $(1-\alpha)$th quantile of the chi-square distribution with K degrees of freedom.

7.3.2. *Testing procedure*

Shao and Chow (1993) proposed a testing procedure in a two-stage sampling problem with large within-class (i.e., within treatment in our case) sample sizes and derived a two-stage sampling plan by minimizing the expected squared volume (or the generalized variance) of the confidence region related to the test assuming that there is an increasing order of mean across treatment groups, that is

$$\mu_1 < \mu_2 < \cdot s < \mu_K, \tag{20}$$

where $\mu_k' s$ satisfy

$$a_k < \mu_k < b_k, \quad k = 1, \ldots, K, \tag{21}$$

at which (a_k, b_k) are in-house acceptance limits or release targets used for quality assurance of the manufactured products. The basis for construction of $a_k' s$ and $b_k' s$ is information obtained from previously studies. Note that if we choose the $a_k' s$ and $b_k' s$ so that $b_k \leq a_{k+1}$, $k = 1, \ldots, K-1$, then (21) implies (20). Since the $\mu_k' s$ are unknown, we need to make a decision based on $x_{ijk}' s$. Let H_0 denote the null hypothesis that (20) (or (21)) does not hold and H_a, the alternative hypothesis that (20) (or (21)) is true. Then our problem becomes a statistical testing problem of H_0 versus H_a. The form of the null hypothesis, however, is so complicated that there is no simple testing procedure available in the literature. When we test (21), we can express H_0 as

$$H_0\colon \mu_k < a_k \quad \text{or} \quad \mu_k > b_k \quad \text{for at least one } k. \tag{22}$$

In the special case of $K = 1$, we may adopt the two one-sided α level tests approach in the assessment of bioequivalence (see, e.g., Westlake, 1976; Hauck and Anderson, 1984; Schuirmann, 1987). That is, we reject H_0: $\mu_1 < a_1$ or $\mu_1 > b_1$ if and only if

$$a_1 < L_1 \quad \text{or} \quad U_1 < b_1,$$

where L_1 and U_1 are given in (18). Generalizing this idea to the case of $K \geq 3$, Shao and Chow (1993) proposed the following testing procedure for (21): H_0 in (22) is rejected if and only if

$$a_k < L_k \quad \text{and} \quad U_k < b_k, \quad k = 1, \ldots, K, \tag{23}$$

where L_k and U_k are given in (18). A geometric interpretation of this test procedure is that we reject H_0 whenever

$$C \subset R, \tag{24}$$

where $C = (L_1, U_1) \times \cdot s \times (L_K, U_K)$ and $R = (a_1, b_1) \times \cdot s \times (a_K, b_K)$. Since $(L_k, U_k)'s$ are independent, C is actually a confidence region for μ with an approximate level $(1 - \alpha)^K$. It can be shown that

$$\sup_{H_0} \lim_{nm_k \to \infty, k=1,\ldots,K} P(C \subset R | H_0) = \alpha. \tag{25}$$

For example, when $K = 1$, the left-hand side of (8.11) is greater than or equal to

$$\lim_{nm_1 \to \infty} P(a_1 < L_1 \quad \text{and} \quad U_1 < b_1) \geq \alpha - \lim_{nm_1 \to \infty} P(U_1 < b_1 | \mu_1 = a_1)$$

$$= \alpha - \lim_{nm_1 \to \infty} \Phi\left(z_\alpha - \frac{b_1 - a_1}{s_1} \right) = \alpha,$$

since $s_1 \to 0$. Hence (25) holds. We now turn to the test of H_0 that (20) does not hold. Let $\delta_k = \mu_{k+1} - \mu_k, k = 1, \ldots, K - 1$. Then we can express H_0 as

$$H_0\colon \delta_k < 0 \quad \text{for at least one } k. \tag{26}$$

Note that (26) is a special case of (22) with $a_k = 0$ and $b_k = \infty$. Hence we can test (26) based on a procedure similar to (23): we reject H_0 in (26) if and only if

$$0 < \bar{x}_{k+1} - \bar{x}_k - z_\alpha [s_{k+1}^2 + s_k^2]^{1/2}, \quad k = 1, \ldots, K - 1. \tag{27}$$

7.3.3. *Optimal selection*

As indicated above, although we are able to control the type I error rate, we are unable to control the other type of error rate that is

$$P(H_0 \text{ is not rejected } |H_a) = P(C \not\subset R|H_a),$$

where C and R are given in (24). One way to reduce this statistical error is to minimize the *size* of the region C. The K-dimensional volume of C is

$$v = (U_1 - L_1) \cdot s(U_K - L_K) = (2z_\alpha)^K (s_1 \cdot ss_K).$$

Since we cannot minimize v by selecting sample sizes before the samples are drawn, we propose to select n and m_k by minimizing the expected squared volume

$$ESV = E(v^2) = (2z_\alpha)^{2K} (\sigma_1^2 \sigma_2^2 \cdot s\sigma_K^2) \frac{1}{n^K (m_1 m_2 \cdot s m_K)}, \tag{28}$$

under the constraint that study site can handle only a limited number of subjects. Motivation for this approach is also the fact that the ESV in (28) is proportional to the generalized variance, which is the K-dimensional volume of the confidence region defined by (19) and is a measure of the asymptotic relative efficiency (see, e.g., Serfling, 1980); hence, minimizing the ESV is equivalent to minimizing the generalized variance.

From (28), minimizing ESV is equivalent to minimizing the function

$$J(n, m_1, \ldots, m_K) = \frac{1}{n^K (m_1 m_2 \cdot s m_K)}.$$

Note that although the $\sigma_k' s$ affect the ESV, they do not affect the selection of sample sizes according to the criterion of minimizing the ESV.

Let c_0 denote the cost of each subject. The total cost is then $c_0 n(\sum_k m_k)$ and the cost constraint is

$$c_0 n \left(\sum_k m_k \right) \leq c,$$

where c is a given upper limit for the total cost. Suppose that a given study site can handle only N subjects owing to limited availability of resources. The resources constraint is then

$$n \left(\sum_k m_k \right) \leq N.$$

When there is no cost constraint (e.g., resources constraint), we simply take $C = \infty (N = \infty)$. Let L be the integer part of $\min(N, c/c_0)$. We then minimize $J(n, m_1, \ldots, m_K)$ subject to $n(\sum_k m_k) \le L, 1 \le m_k \le M_k$, and $n, m_k's$ are integers, $k = 1, \ldots, K$. Consider the problem of minimizing the function $J(n, m_1, \ldots, m_K)$ over the region

$$A = \left\{ (n, m_1, \ldots, m_K) : 1 \le m_k \le M_k, k = 1, \ldots, K, n\left(\sum_k m_k\right) \le L \right\}.$$

Clearly, the derivative of the function J does not vanish on the set

$$A_0 = \left\{ (n, m_1, \ldots, m_K) : 1 \le m_k \le M_k, k = 1, \ldots, K, n\left(\sum_k m_k\right) \le L \right\}.$$

Hence, the minimum of J is on the set

$$A_1 = \left\{ (n, m_1, \ldots, m_K) : 1 \le m_k \le M_k, k = 1, \ldots, K, n\left(\sum_k m_k\right) = L \right\}.$$

On the set A_1, $n = L/(\sum_k m_k)$ and

$$J(n, m_1, \ldots, m_K) = J_1(m_1, \ldots, m_K) = L^{-K} m/w,$$

where $m = \sum_k m_k$ and $w = m_1 \ldots m_K$. Then

$$\frac{\partial J_1}{\partial m_k} = L^{-K}\left(\frac{Km^{K-1}}{w} - \frac{m^K}{m_k w}\right), \quad k = 1, \ldots, K.$$

Setting

$$\frac{\partial J_1}{\partial m_k} = 0, \quad k = 1, \ldots, K,$$

We obtain that

$$m_k = m/K, k = 1, \ldots, K,$$

That is J has a minimum on A_1 as long as $m_1 = m_2 = \cdot s = m_K$. If there is an integer m^* such that $1 \le m^* \le M_k$ for all k and L/Km^* is an integer, then J has a minimum at $m_1 = \cdot s = m_k = m^*$ and $n = L/Km^*$. If L/Km^* is not an integer for all possible m^*, then we should select an m^* in the set $\{1, 2, \ldots, \min(M_1, M_2, \ldots, M_K)\}$ such that $Km^*[L/Km^*]$ is as large as possible. Thus, a solution is given by

$$m_1 = m_2 = \cdot s = m_K = m^*, \tag{29}$$

$$n = [L/Km^*], \tag{30}$$

where $[L/Km^*]$ is the integer part of L/Km^* and we choose m^* from the set of integers $\{1, 2, \ldots, \min(M_1, M_2, \ldots, M_K)\}$ such that

$$Km^*[L/Km^*] \text{ is as large as possible.} \tag{31}$$

In particular, if there is an integer $m^* \leq \min(M_1, \ldots, M_K)$ such that L/Km^* is an integer, then $m_1 = \cdot s = m_K = m^*$ and $n = L/Km^*$ is a solution. There may be several sampling plans that satisfy (29)–(31).

A sampling plan that satisfies (29)–(31) is optimal in terms of the ESV only. We would have to use other criteria to choose a sampling plan when there are several plans that satisfy As an example, consider the situation where $K = 4, M_1 = 2, M_2 = 4, M_3 = 6, M_4 = 8$ and $L = 100$. Since $\min(M_1, M_2, M_3, M_4) = 2$, possible values of m^* are 1 and 2. For $m^* = 2$, $Km^* = 4 \times 2 = 8$, the largest n we can take is 12, which gives the total sample size $96 < L$. Similarly, for $m^* = 1$, $Km^* = 4$, the largest n we can use is 25, which gives the total sample size $100 = L$. Hence $m^* = 1$ and $n = 25$ is the unique plan that satisfies (29)–(31). To compare this plan with other sampling plans, consider the single-stage sampling plan with $m_k = M_k$ for all k and $n = 5$ (which also gives the total sample size 100). A simple calculation shows that the ESV of the single-stage sampling plan over the $ESV$of the plan that satisfies (29)–(31) is 162.8%. Therefore, the single-stage sampling plan is not efficient. Note that the sampling plan that takes $\{m_k\}$ in proportion to $\{M_k\}$ produces the same ESV as the single-stage sampling.

In case of $\rho_k \neq 0$, although the testing procedures described above are valid regardless of whether $\rho_k = 0$ (assuming we use the variance estimator (17)), the sampling plan given by (29)–(31) is not necessarily good when $\rho_k \neq 0$. In fact, when $\rho_k \neq 0$ the optimal sampling plan, if it exists, depends on the $\rho_k's$ and, therefore, the problem may be unsolvable since $\rho_k's$ are unknown. This difficulty is not a serious concern for many problems in the pharmaceutical industry, since $\rho_k = 0$ for all k is a reasonable assumption. Furthermore, in many cases $\rho_k \neq 0$ but is relatively small. We then expect that the sampling plan given by (29)–(31) is nearly optimal.

7.4. *Sample size calculation and allocation*

7.4.1. *Some background*

As indicated by Uesaka (2009), the primary objective of a multi-regional bridging trial is to show the efficacy of a drug in all participating regions while also evaluating the possibility of applying the overall trial results to each region. To apply the overall results to a specific region, the results in that region should be consistent with either the overall results or the results from other regions. A typical approach is to show consistency among regions by demonstrating that there exists no treatment-by-region interaction. Recently, the Ministry of Health, Labor and Welfare (MHLW) of Japan published a guidance on *Basic Principles on Global Clinical Trials* that outlines the basic concepts for planning and implementation the multiregional trials in a Q&A format. In this guidance, special consideration was placed on the determination of the number of Japanese subjects required in a multi-regional trial. As indicated, the selected sample size should be able to establish the consistency of treatment effects between the Japanese group and the entire group.

To establish the consistency of the treatment effects between the Japanese group and the entire group, it is suggested that the selected size should satisfy

$$P\left(\frac{D_J}{D_{All}} > \rho\right) \geq 1-\gamma, \tag{32}$$

where D_J and D_{All} are the treatment effects for the Japanese group and the entire group, respectively. Along this line, Quan *et al.* (2009) derived closed form formulas for the sample size calculation/allocation for normal, binary and survival endpoints. As an example, the formula for continuous endpoint assuming that $D_J = D_{NJ} = D_{All} = D$, where D_{NJ} is the treatment effect for the non-Japanese subjects, is given below.

$$N_J \geq \frac{z_{1-\gamma}^2 N}{(z_{1-\alpha/2}+z_{1-\beta})^2(1-\rho)^2 + z_{1-\gamma}^2(2\rho-\rho^2)}, \tag{33}$$

where N and N_J are the sample size for the entire group and the Japanese group. Note that the MHLW of Japan recommends that ρ should be chosen to be either 0.5 or greater and γ should be chosen to be either 0.8 or greater in (32). As an example, if we choose $\rho = 0.5, \gamma = 0.8, \alpha = 0.05$, and $\beta = 0.9$, then $N_J/N = 0.224$. In other words, the sample size for the Japanese group has to be at least 22.4% of the overall sample size for the multi-regional trial.

In practice, $1-\rho$ is often considered a non-inferiority margin. If ρ is chosen to be greater than 0.5, the Japanese sample size will increase substantially. It should be noted that the sample size formulas given in Quan *et al.* (2009) are derived under the assumption that there are no difference in treatment effects for the Japanese group and non-Japanese group. In practice, it is expected that there is a difference in treatment effect due to ethnic difference. Thus, the formulas for sample size calculation/allocation derived by Quan *et al.* (2009) are necessarily modified in order to take into consideration of the effect due to ethnic difference.

As an alternative, Kawai *et al.* (2008) proposed an approach to rationalize partitioning the total sample size among the regions so that a high probability of observing a consistent trend under the assumed treatment effect across regions can be derived, if the treatment effect is positive and uniform across regions in a multi-regional trial. Uesaka (2009) proposed new statistical criteria for testing consistency between regional and overall results, which do not require impractical sample sizes and discussed several methods of sample size allocation to regions. Basically, three rules of sample size allocation in multi-regional clinical trials are discussed. These rules include (i) allocating equal size to all regions, (ii) minimizing total sample size, and (iii) minimizing the sample size of a specific region. It should be noted that the sample size of a multi-regional trial may become very large when one wishes to ensure consistent results between region of interest and the other regions or between the regional results and the overall results regardless which rules of sample size allocation is used.

7.4.2. *Proposals of statistical guidance — Asian perspective*

As indicated earlier, based on MHLW guidance, several methods for determination of sample size at specific region have been proposed (see, e.g., Quan *et al.*, 2009; Uesaka, 2009). In addition, Ko *et al.* (2010) focus on a specific region and establish four statistical criteria for consistency between the region of interest and overall results. More specifically, two criteria are to assess whether the treatment effect in the region of interest is as large as that of the other regions or of the regions overall, while the other two criteria are to assess the consistency of the treatment effect of the specific region with other regions or the regions overall.

The global drug development plays an important role in a scientific manner to pharmaceutical research. However, the statistical work to draw a statistical inference with regard to translational medicine research is still in a preliminary stage. To provide a comprehensive understanding of statistical design and methodology that are commonly employed in global drug development, under the support of the Bureau of Pharmaceutical Affairs, Department of Health, Taiwan, National Health Research Institutes and Formosa Cancer Foundation organized one symposium on "Current

Advanced Statistical Issues in Clinical Trials — Flexibility and Globalization" held on November 21, 2008, and a closed-door meeting on "Designs of Clinical Trials in New Drug Developments" held on November 22, 2008 in Taipei, Taiwan. As a result, a proposal of statistical guidance to multi-regional trials was developed. This proposal is briefly described below. We first give a definition of so-called *Asian region*.

Definition of the Asian region — When planning a multi-regional trial, the definition of the Asian region is very critical, since there are many regional countries in Asia. According to the ICH E5 guideline, the ethnic factors are classified into the following two categories: intrinsic and extrinsic factors (ICH, 1997). Intrinsic ethnic factors are factors that define and identify the population in the new region and maybe influence the ability to extrapolate clinical data between regions. They are more genetic and physiologic in nature, e.g., genetic polymorphism, age, gender, etc. On the other hand, extrinsic ethnic factors are factors associated with the environment and culture. Extrinsic ethnic factors are more social and cultural in nature, e.g., medical practice, diet, and practices in clinical trials and conduct.

For example, the increasing evidence that genetic determinants may mediate variability among persons in response to a drug implies that the patients' responses to therapeutics may vary among racial and ethnic groups. In other words, after the intake of identical doses of a given agent, some ethnic groups may have clinically significant side effects, whereas others may show no therapeutic response. An example of such a situation can be seen in the study by Caraco (2004). Caraco pointed out that some of this diversity in rates of response can be ascribed to differences in the rate of drug metabolism, particularly by the cytochrome P-450 superfamily of enzymes. While 10 isoforms of cytochrome P-450 are responsible for the oxidative metabolism of most drugs, the effect of genetic polymorphisms on catalytic activity is most prominent for 3 isoforms—CYP2C9, CYP2C19, and CYP2D6. Among these three, CYP2D6 has been most extensively studied and is involved in the metabolism of about 100 drugs, including β-blockers, antiarrhythmic, antidepressant, neuroleptic, and opioid agents. Several studies revealed that some patients are classified as having "poor metabolism" of certain drugs owing to the lack of CYP2D6 activity. On the other hand, patients having some enzyme activity are classified into three subgroups: those with "normal" activity (or extensive metabolism), those with reduced activity (intermediate metabolism), and those with markedly enhanced activity (ultrarapid metabolism). Most importantly, the distribution of CYP2D6 phenotypes varies with race. However, the frequency of the phenotype associated with poor metabolism is 1% in both the Chinese and Japanese populations. Another study also showed that there exist no ethnic differences in CYP2C19 among Chinese, Japanese and Korean populations (Myrand *et al.* (2008)). Considering genetic polymorphism, the International HapMap Project also shows that the Chinese and Japanese genome look alike. All of these may reasonably support that countries of China, Hong Kong, Japan, Korea, and Taiwan can be regarding as an *Asian region.*

On the other hand, the frequency of HLA alleles is associated Stevens-Johnson syndrome (Chung *et al.*, 2004). However, the prevalence rates of HLA-B*1502 for Chinese, Japanese, and Korean populations are respectively 1.9–7.1%, <0.3%, and 0.2% (see, e.g., Ueta *et al.* (2007). That is, there exist differences within Asian populations in this regard. Consequently, the definition of a region may possibly vary from disease to disease. In fact, all differences and similarities in both intrinsic and extrinsic ethnical factors should be considered for the definition of the *Asian Region.*

Within the Asian region, each country may consider accepting all the data derived from other countries in the "Asian region." For example, Taiwan accepts all Asian data. A study by Lin *et al.* (2001) found that the so-called *Taiwanese*, accounting for 91% of the total population in Taiwan, are comprised of Minnan and Hakka people who are closely related to the southern Han, and are clustered with other southern Asian populations such as Thai and Malaysian in terms of HLA typing. Those who are the descendants of northern Han are separated from the southern Asian cluster, and form a cluster with the other northern Asian populations such as Korean and Japanese. The Taiwanese regulatory authority, therefore, accepts data from trials conducted in Taiwan as well as in other Asian countries, if those trials meet Taiwanese regulatory standards and were conducted in compliance with GCP requirements.

Bridging the results to the Asian region — The aim of a multi-regional trial is to show the efficacy of a drug in various global regions, and concurrently to evaluate the possibility of applying the overall trial results to each region. Therefore, how to bridging the results of the multi-regional trial to the "Asian region" is another important issue. As indicated earlier, the Japanese Ministry of Health, Labor and Welfare (MHLW) has published the *Basic Principles on Global Clinical Trials* guidance to promote Japan's participation in global development and international clinical study recently. Special consideration was placed on the establishment of the consistency of treatment effects between the Japanese group and the entire group. The same consistency criterion can also be used to examine whether the overall results from the multi-regional trial can be applied to the Asian region.

Let D_{Asia} be the observed treatment effect for the Asian region and D_{All} the observed treatment effect from all regions. Given that the overall result is significant at α level, we will judge whether the treatment is effective in the Asian region by the following criterion:

$$D_{Asia} \geq \rho D_{All} \quad \text{for some } 0 < \rho < 1. \tag{34}$$

Other consistency criteria can be found in Uesaka (2009) and Ko *et al.* (2010). Selection of the magnitude, ρ, of consistency trend may be critical. All differences in ethnic factors between the Asian region and other regions should be taken into account. The Japanese MHLW suggests that ρ be 0.5 or greater. However, the determination of ρ will be and should be different from product to product, and from therapeutic area to therapeutic area. For example, in a multi-regional liver cancer trial, the Asian region can definitely require a larger value of ρ, since it will contribute more subjects than other regions.

In addition to the consistency criterion in (34), the following criteria suggested by Uesaka (2009) and Ko *et al.* (2010) can also be used:

$$\begin{aligned} &D_{Asia} \geq \rho D_C && \text{for some } 0 < \rho < 1; \\ &\rho \leq D_{Asia}/D_{All} \leq 1/\rho && \text{for some } 0 < \rho < 1; \\ &\rho \leq D_{Asia}/D_C \leq 1/\rho && \text{for some } 0 < \rho < 1; \end{aligned}$$

where D_C denotes the observed treatment effect from regions other than the Asian region. The first criterion is to assess whether the treatment effect in the Asian region is as large as that of the other regions, while the last two criteria are to assess the consistency of the treatment effect of the Asian region with overall regions or other regions.

Sample size for multi-regional trials — When planning a multi-regional trial, it is suggested that the study objectives should be clearly stated in the study protocol. Once the study objectives are confirmed, a valid study design can be chosen and the primary clinical endpoints can be determined accordingly. Based on the primary clinical endpoint, sample size required for achieving a desired power can then be calculated. Recent approaches for sample size determination in multi-regional trials developed by Kawai *et al.* (2008), Quan *et al.* (2009), and Ko *et al.* (2010) are all based on the assumption that the effect size is uniform across regions. For example, assume that we focus on the multi-regional trial for comparing a test product and a placebo control based on a continuous efficacy endpoint. Let X and Y be some efficacy responses for patients receiving the test product and the placebo control respectively. For convention, both X and Y are normally distributed with variance σ^2. We assume that σ^2 is known, although it can generally be estimated. Let μ_T and μ_P be the population means of the test and placebo, respectively, and let $\Delta = \mu_T - \mu_P$. Assume that effect size (Δ/σ) is uniform across regions. The hypothesis of testing for the overall treatment effect is given as

$$H_0 : \Delta \leq 0 \quad \text{versus} \quad H_a : \Delta > 0.$$

Let N denote the total sample size for each group planned for detecting an expected treatment difference $\Delta = \delta$ at the desired significance level α and with power $1 - \beta$. Thus,

$$N = 2\sigma^2\{(z_{1-\alpha} + z_{1-\beta})/\delta\}^2,$$

where $z_{1-\alpha}$ is the $(1-\alpha)$th percentile of the standard normal distribution. Once N is determined, special consideration should be placed on the determination of the number of subjects from the Asian region in the multi-regional trial. The selected sample size should be able to establish the consistency of treatment effects between the Asian region and the regions overall. To establish the consistency of treatment effects between the Asian region and the entire group, it is suggested that the selected sample size should satisfy that the assurance probability of the consistency criterion in (34), given that $\Delta = \delta$ and the overall result is significant at α level, is maintained at a desired level, say 80%. That is,

$$P_\delta(D_{Asia} \geq \rho D_{All} | Z > z_{1-\alpha}) > 1 - \gamma \tag{35}$$

for some pre-specified $0 < \gamma \leq 0.2$. Here Z represents the overall test statistic.

Ko *et al.* (2010) calculated the sample size required for the Asian region based on (35). For $\beta = 0.1$, $\alpha = 0.025$, and $\rho = 0.5$, the sample size for the Asian region has to be around 30% of the overall sample size to maintain the assurance probability of (35) at 80% level. On the other hand, by considering a two-sided test, Quan H. *et al.* (2009) derived closed form formulas for the sample size calculation for normal, binary and survival endpoints based on the consistency criterion (34). For examples, if we choose

$\rho = 0.5$, $\gamma = 0.2$, $\alpha = 0.025$, and $\beta = 0.9$, then the Asian sample size has to be at least 22.4% of the overall sample size for the multi-regional trial.

It should be noted that the sample size determination given in Kawai *et al.* (2008), Quan *et al.* (2009), and Ko *et al.* (2010) are all derived under the assumption that the effect size is uniform across regions. In practice, it might be expected that there is a difference in treatment effect due to ethnic difference. Thus, the sample size calculation derived by Kawai *et al.* (2008), Quan *et al.* (2009), and Ko *et al.* (2010) may not be of practical use. More specifically, some other assumptions addressing the ethnic difference should be explored. For example, we may consider the following assumptions that (i) Δ is the same but σ^2 is different across regions, (ii) Δ is different but σ^2 is the same across regions, and (iii) Δ and $\sigma^2$are both different across regions.

Statistical methods for the sample size determination in multi-regional trials should be developed based on the above assumptions.

Remarks — A multi-regional trial may incorporate subjects from many countries around the world under the same protocol. After showing the overall efficacy of a drug in all global regions, we can simultaneously evaluate the possibility of applying the overall trial results to each region and consequently support registration in each region. Tsou *et al.* (2011) proposed the statistical guidance to multi-regional trials. In Tsou *et al.*'s proposal, both the MHLW guidance and the 11th Q&A for the ICH E5 guideline can serve as a framework on how to demonstrate the efficacy of a drug in all participating regions while also evaluating the possibility of applying the overall trial results to each region by conducting a multi-regional trial. Most importantly, the consistency criterion presented in the Japanese guideline can be used to apply the overall results from the multi-regional trial to the Asian region.

In Tsou *et al.*'s proposal, the sample size calculation for multi-regional trials should take the possibility of ethnic differences into account. When planning a multi-regional trial, the regions involved are expected to participate in the global development as early as possible. Therefore, the ethnic differences might be able to be detected at any stage of early drug development. On the other hand, the analyses on the Asian data in the multi-regional trial may not have enough statistical power. Thus, the number of subjects required for the Asian region in the multi-regional trial should be large enough to establish the consistency of treatment effects between the Asian region and the regions overall. Also note that the sample size required in (35) is for the entire Asian region with similar ethnicity. Each country in the Asian region may contribute different size of subjects to the multi-regional trial. However for the evaluation of consistency, each country may consider accepting all the data derived from other countries in the Asian region.

Multi-regional trials might have benefits on decreasing Asian patients' exposures on unapproved drugs, reducing drug lag, and increasing available treatment options. From the beginning of 21st century, the trend for simultaneous clinical development in Asian countries being undertaken simultaneously with clinical trials conducted in Europe and the United States has been speedily rising. In particular, Taiwan, Korea, Hong-Kong, and Singapore have already had much experience in planning and conducting the multi-regional trials. It should be noted that conducting multi-regional trials may require more management skills due to various cultures, languages, religions, and medical practices. This kind of cross-cultural management may be challenging.

7.5. *Statistical methods for bridging studies*

In recent years, the influence of ethnic factors on clinical outcomes for evaluation of efficacy and safety of study medications under investigation has attracted much attention from regulatory authorities, especially when the sponsor is interested in bringing an approved drug product from the original region (e.g., the United States of America or European Union) to a new region (e.g., Asian Pacific Region). To determine if clinical data generated from the original region are acceptable in the new region, the International Conference on Harmonization (ICH) issued a guideline on Ethnic Factors in the Acceptability of Foreign Clinical Data (ICH, 1997). The purpose of this guideline is not only to permit adequate evaluation of the influence of ethnic factors, but also to minimize duplication of clinical studies in the new region (ICH, 1997). This guideline is known as ICH E5 guideline.

As indicated in the ICH E5 guideline, a bridging study is defined as a study performed in the new region to provide pharmacokinetic (PK), pharmacodynamic (PD), or clinical data on efficacy, safety, dosage, and dose regimen in the new region that will allow extrapolation of the foreign clinical data to the population in the new region. The ICH E5 guideline suggests the regulatory authority of the new region to assess the ability to extrapolate foreign data based on the bridging data package, which consists of (i) information including PK data and any preliminary PD and dose-response data from the complete clinical data package (CCDP) that is relevant to the population of the new region and if needed, (ii) bridging study to extrapolate the foreign efficacy data and/or safety data to the new region. The ICH E5 guideline indicates that bridging studies may not be necessary if the study medicines are insensitive to ethnic factors. For medicines characterized as insensitive to ethnic factors, the type of bridging studies (if needed) will depend upon experience with the drug class and upon the likelihood that extrinsic ethnic factors could affect the medicine's safety, efficacy, and dose-response. On the other hand, for medicines that are ethnically sensitive, bridging study is usually needed since the populations in two regions are different. In the ICH E5 guideline, however, no criteria for assessment of the sensitivity to ethnic factors for determining whether a bridging study is needed are provided. Moreover, when a bridging study is conducted, the ICH guideline indicates that the study is readily interpreted as capable of bridging the foreign data if it shows that dose-response, safety, and efficacy in the new region are similar to those in the original region. However, the ICH does not clearly define the similarity.

Shih (2001) interpreted it as consistency among study centers by treating the new region as a new center of multicenter clinical trials. Under this definition, Shih (2001) proposed a method for assessment of consistency to determine whether the study is capable of bridging the foreign data to the new region. Alternatively, Shao and Chow (2002) proposed the concepts of reproducibility and generalizability probabilities for assessment of bridging studies. If the influence of the ethnic factors is negligible, then we may consider the reproducibility probability to determine whether the clinical results observed in the original region are reproducible in the new region. If there is a notable ethnic difference, the generalizability probability can be assessed to determine whether the clinical results in the original region can be generalized in a similar but slightly different patient population due to the difference in ethnic factors. In addition, Chow, Shao and Hu (2002) proposed to assess bridging studies based on the concept of population (or individual) bioequivalence. Along this line, Hung, (2003) and Hung, *et al.* (2003) considered the assessment of similarity based on testing for non-inferiority between a bridging study conducted in the new region as compared to the previous conducted in the original region. This leads to the argument regarding the selection of non-inferiority margin (Chow and Shao, 2006). Note that other methods such as the use of Bayesian approach have also been proposed in literature (see, e.g., Liu, Hsueh, and Hsiao, 2002).

7.5.1. *Test for consistency*

For assessment of similarity between a bridging study conducted in a new region and studies conducted in the original region, Shih (2001) considered all of the studies conducted in the original region as a multi-center trial and proposed to test consistency among study centers by treating the new region as a new center of a multi-center trial.

Suppose there are K reference studies in the CCDP. Let T_i denotes the standardized treatment group difference, i.e.,

$$T_i = \frac{\bar{x}_{T_i} - \bar{x}_{C_i}}{s_i\sqrt{\frac{1}{m_{T_i}} + \frac{1}{m_{C_i}}}},$$

where $\bar{x}_{T_i}(\bar{x}_{C_i})$ is the sample mean of $m_{T_i}(m_{C_i})$ observations in the treatment (control) group, and s_i is the pooled sample standard deviation. Shih (2001) considered the following predictive probability for testing consistency

$$p(T|T_i, i = 1, \ldots, K) = \left(\frac{2\pi(K+1)}{K}\right)^{-K/2} \exp\left[-K(T - \bar{T})^2/2(K+1)\right]. \tag{36}$$

7.5.2. *Test for reproducibility and generalizability*

On the other hand, when the ethnic difference is negligible, Shao and Chow (2002) suggested assessing reproducibility probability for similarity between clinical results from a bridging study and studies conducted in the CCPD. Let x be a clinical response of interest in the original region. Let y be similar to x but is a response in a clinical bridging study conducted in the new region. Suppose the hypotheses of interest are

$$H_0 : \mu_1 = \mu_0 \ vs \ H_a : \mu_1 \neq \mu_0.$$

We reject H_0 at the 5% level of significance if and only if $|T| > t_{n-2}$, where t_{n-2} is the (1-$\alpha/2$)th percentile of the t distribution with $n-2$ degrees of freedom, $n = n_1 + n_2$

$$T = \frac{\bar{y} - \bar{x}}{\sqrt{\frac{(n_1-1)s_1^2+(n_0-1)s_0^2}{n-2}}\sqrt{\frac{1}{n_1} + \frac{1}{n_0}}},$$

and $\bar{x}, \bar{y}, s_0^2$,and s_1^2 are sample means and variances for the original region and the new region, respectively. Thus, the power of T is given by

$$p(\theta) = P(|T| > t_{n-2}) = 1 - \Im_{n-2}(t_{n-2}|\theta) + \Im_{n-2}(-t_{n-2}|\theta),$$

where

$$\theta = \frac{\mu_1 - \mu_0}{\sigma\sqrt{\frac{1}{n_1} + \frac{1}{n_0}}},$$

and $\Im_{n-2}(\cdot|\theta)$ denotes the cumulative distribution function of the non-central t distribution with $n - 2$ degrees of freedom and the non-centrality parameter θ. Replacing θ in the power function with its estimate $T(x)$, the estimated power

$$\hat{p} = P(T(x)) = 1 - \Im_{n-2}(t_{n-2}|T(x)) + \Im_{n-2}(-t_{n-2}|T(x)) \qquad (37)$$

is defined as a reproducibility probability for a future clinical trial with the same patient population. Note that when the ethnic difference is notable, Shao and Chow (2002) recommended assessing so-called generalizability probability for similarity between clinical results from a bridging study and studies conducted in the CCPD.

7.5.3. *Test for similarity*

Using the criterion for assessment of population (individual) bioequivalence, Chow, Shao, and Hu (2002) proposed the following measure of similarity between x and y:

$$\theta = \frac{E(x-y)^2 - E(x-x')^2}{E(x-x')^2/2},$$

where x' is an independent replicate of x and y, x, and x' are assumed to be independent. Since a small value of θ indicates that the difference between x and y is small (relative to the difference between x and x'), similarity between the new region and the original region can be claimed if and only if $\theta < \theta_U$, where θ_U is a similarity limit. Thus, the problem of assessing similarity become a problem of testing the following hypotheses

$$H_0 : \theta \geq \theta_U \ vs \ H_a : \theta < \theta_U.$$

Let $k = 0$ indicate the original region and $k =$ 1indicate the new region. Suppose that there are m_k study centers and n_k responses in each center for a given variable of interest. For simplicity, we only consider the balanced case where centers in a given region have the same number of observations. Let z_{ijk} be the ith observation from the jth center of region k, b_{jk} be the between-center random effect, and e_{ijk} be the within center measurement error. Assume that

$$z_{ijk} = \mu_k + b_{jk} + e_{ijk}, i = 1, \ldots, n_k, j = 1, \ldots, m_k, k = 0, 1,$$

where μ_k is the population mean in region k, $b_{jk} \sim N(0, \sigma_{Bk}^2), e_{ijk} \sim N(0, \sigma_{Wk}^2)$, and $\{b_{jk}\}$ and $\{e_{ijk}\}$ are independent. Under the above model, the criterion for similarity becomes

$$\theta = \frac{(\mu_0 - \mu_1)^2 + \sigma_{T1}^2 - \sigma_{T0}^2}{\sigma_{T0}^2}, \tag{38}$$

where $\sigma_{Tk}^2 = \sigma_{Bk}^2 + \sigma_{Wk}^2$ is the total variance (between center variance plus within center variance) in region k. The above hypotheses are equivalent to

$$H_0 : \varsigma \geq 0 \; vs \; H_a : \varsigma < 0,$$

where $\varsigma = (\mu_0 - \mu_1)^2 + \sigma_{T_1}^2 - (1 + \theta_U)\sigma_{T_0}^2$.

7.6. *Concluding remarks*

In multi-national (multi-regional) multi-center trials, it is important to maintain the integrity of the trial by minimizing or controlling all possible sources (both expected and unexpected) of bias, variability, and/or confounding effects that may occur during the conduct of the trial. For this purpose, it is strongly recommended that a steering committee which consists of key individuals across countries be established. The purpose of this committee is multifold. It monitors the performance of the trial to maintain the integrity of the trial. It provides scientific/medical advice to medical community from different countries for consistent assessment of the study drug. In addition, it helps to resolve any issues/problems that may encounter during the conduct of the study. The function of the committee should be independent of the sponsor to maintain the integrity of the trial. Note that analysis of a multinational trial is different from that of a meta-analysis of independent clinical trials at different countries. The analysis of multinational trials combines data observed from each country; the data are generated based on the methods prospectively specified in the same study protocol with the same method of randomization and probably at the same time. In contrast, a meta-analysis combines data retrospectively observed from a number of independent clinical trials involving different countries, which may be conducted under different study protocols with different randomization schemes at different times. In either case, the treatment-by-country interaction for multinational trials or treatment-by-country for meta-analysis must be carefully evaluated before pooling the data for analysis.

In addition to the controversial issues regarding (i) the selection of the optimal number of study sites, (ii) sample size calculation and allocation of specific region, and (iii) statistical methods for bridging studies described above, another controversial issue which has a direct impact on the quality and validity of the conduct of multi-regional clinical trials is the possible lost-in-translation due to ethnic difference among regions. Translation in language is referred to possible lost in translation of inform consent form and/or case report forms in multi-national (multi-regional or global) clinical trials. Lost in translation is commonly encountered due to not only difference in language, but also differences in perception, culture, medical practices, and etc. A typical approach for assessment of the possible lost in translation is to first translate the inform consent form and/or the case report forms by an experienced expert in the subject area and then perform a back-translation by a different experienced but independent expert in the subject area. The back-translated version is then compared with the original version for consistency. This can be done through the conduct of a small scale of pilot study. Qualified subjects from the target patient population will be randomly assigned to receive either the original version or the back-translated version. The responses will be collected and analyzed for comparison. If the back-translated version passes the test for consistency as compared to the original version, we then conclude that there is no evidence of lost-in-translation in the translated version and hence the translated version is considered validated. The translated version can then be used in the intended multi-national clinical trial.

8. Statistics in Diagnostic Imaging

The techniques for evaluation of the performance of diagnostic medical products are very different from therapeutic pharmaceuticals and non-diagnostic devices. However, medical imaging drugs are generally governed by the same regulations as other drug and biological products. Because of the medical imaging drugs have special characteristics that do not reflect from other drug and biological products. The purpose of this section will focus on the different considerations for designs in diagnostic studies.

8.1. *Introduction*

Medical imaging drug products are drugs used with medical imaging methods (such as radiography, computed tomography [CT], ultrasonography [US], and magnetic resonance imaging [MRI]) to provide information on anatomy, physiology and pathology. The term "images" can be used as films, likenesses or other renderings of the body, body parts, organ systems, body functions, or tissues. For example, an image of the heart obtained with a diagnostic radiopharmaceutical or ultrasound contrast agent may in some cases refer to a set of images acquired from different views of the heart. Similarly, an image obtained with an MRI contrast agent may refer to a set of images acquired with different pulse sequences and interpluse delay times. In other words, medical imaging uses advanced technology to "see" the structure and function of the living body. The intentions of a medical imaging drug have two-fold: (i) delineate nonanatomic structures such as tumors or abscesses (ii) detect disease or pathology within an anatomic structure. Therefore, the indications for medical imaging drugs may fall within the following general categories. However, they need not be mutually exclusive.

a. Structure delineation — normal or abnormal
b. Functional, physiological, or biochemical assessment
c. Disease or pathology detection or assessment
d. Diagnostic or therapeutic patient management

The details of drug regulations are shown in the draft guidance to INDs, NDAs, biologics license applications (BLAs), ANDAs, and supplements to NDAs or BLAs for the medical imaging drug and biological products. This guidance was issued by FDA for industry entitled *Development Medical Imaging Drugs and Biologics* (FDA 2000a). For premarket review of regulation and labeling for imaging drugs and devicies is shown in FDA 2009 guidance for industry: *New Contrast Imaging Indication Considerations for Devices and Approved Drug and Biological product.*

Images are usually created from computerized acquisition of digital Signals. The medical imaging drugs can be classified into contrast drug products and diagnostic radiopharmaceuticals.

8.1.1. *Contrast drug product*

Contrast drug products are used to increase the relative difference of signal intensities and to provide the additional information in combination with an imaging device beyond by the device alone. In other words, imaging with the contrast drug product should add value when compared to imaging without the contrast drug product. The most common used contrast drug products that are in combination with medical imaging devices are shown as follows:

Modality	Contrast Drug Products
X-Ray and CT	Iodine agents (photon scattering)
MRI	Gadolinium, dysprosium, helium
Ultrasound	Liposomes, microbubbles
Suspensions	Nuclear Tc-99rn, TI-201, indium, samarium

8.1.2. *Diagnostic Radiopharmaceuticals*

Radiopharmaceuticals are used for a wide variety of diagnostic, monitoring, and therapeutic purposes. Diagnostic Radiopharmaceuticals are used to image or otherwise identify an internal structure or disease process. In other words, diagnostic Radiopharmaceuticals are radioactive drugs that contain a radioactive nuclide that may be linked to a legend and carrier. These products are used in planar imaging, single photon emission computed tomography (SPECT), positron emission tomography (PET), or with other radiation detection probes.

8.2. *Design of blinded-reader studies*

In order to demonstrate efficacy of a medical imaging drug, readers who are both independent and blinded should perform evaluation of images. These independent, blinded image evaluations are intended to limit possible bias that could be introduced into the images evaluation by non- independent or unblinded readers. This evaluation is conducted in controlled setting with minimal clinical information provided to the reader. The definitions of "independent" and "blinded" are shown below.

The independent readers are defined as those who have not participated studies and who are not affiliated with the sponsor or with institutions at which the studies were conducted. The meaning of blinding differs from the common way the term used in therapeutic clinical trials. Blinding in this sense is a critical aspect of clinical trials of medical imaging agents. "Blinded readers" are those who are unaware (1) of treatment identity used to obtain a given image and (2) of patient-specific clinical information or study protocol. For example, blinded readers should not have the knowledge about which images were obtained prior to drug administration and which were obtained after drug administration, although this may be apparent upon viewing the images. In addition, blinded readers should not know the patients' final diagnoses and may have limited or no knowledge of the results of other diagnostic tests that were performed on the patients. In some cases, blinded readers should not be familiar with the inclusion and exclusion criteria for patient selection that were specified in the protocol.

8.2.1. *Assessing reader agreement*

As indicated in the draft guidance (FDA, 2000a), at least two independent, blinded readers (and preferably three or more) are recommended for each study that is intended to demonstrate efficacy. The purpose is to provide a better basis for the findings in the studies. Therefore, the determination of inter-reader agreement and variability is the typical design issue to blinded read studies.

According to the guidance, the consistency among readers should be measured quantitatively. The most commonly used statistical test to assess the inter-reader agreement is the κ (kappa) statistic. The Cohen's kappa coefficient, introduced by Cohen (1960), is a measure of inter-reader agreement in terms of count data.

For a 2×2 table,

$$\kappa = \frac{P_0 - P_e}{1 - P_e},$$

where

$$P_0 = \sum_i p_{ii} \quad \text{poportion of observed agreement}$$

$$P_e = \sum_i p_{i.}p_{.i} \quad \text{poportion ofexpected agreement}$$

It assumes that two response variables are two independent ratings of the n subjects. It should be noted that the kappa coefficient equals +1 when there is complete agreement of the readers. When the observed agreement exceeds chance agreement, kappa is positive. Also, the magnitude of kappa statistics reflects the strength of agreement. In a very unusual practice, kappa could be negative when the observed agreement is less than chance agreement.

The total range of kappa is between −1 and 1. The asymptotic variance of simple kappa coefficient can be estimated by the following, according to Fleiss at al. (1969):

$$Var(\kappa) = \frac{A + B + C}{(1 - P_e)^2 n},$$

where

$$A = \sum_i p_{ii}[1 - (p_{i\cdot} + p_{\cdot i})(1 - \hat{\kappa})]^2$$

$$B = (1 - \hat{\kappa})^2 \sum\sum_{i \neq j} p_{ij}(p_{i\cdot} + p_{\cdot i})^2$$

and

$$C = [\hat{\kappa} - P_e(1 - \hat{\kappa})]^2.$$

For measuring the inter-reader agreement in continuous data, Snedecor and Cochran proposed the intra-class correlation in 1967.

8.2.2. *Diagnostic accuracy*

To determine how well a diagnostic imaging agent can distinguish disease subjects and non-diseased subjects, the outcome may often be classified into one of the four groups depending on (i) whether disease is present and (ii) the results of the diagnostic test of interest (positive or negative). The terms "positive" and "negative" concern some particular disease status, which must be specified clearly. The categories can be defined in any meaningful way to the problem. For example, patients could be classified as having one or more tumors (positive) or no tumor (negative), malignant (positive) or benign/no tumor (negative).

It should be noted that the disease is often determined with a "truth" standard or "gold" standard. A "truth" standard or "gold" standard is an independent method of measuring the same variable being measured by the investigational drug that is known or believed to give the truth state of a patient or true value of a measurement. In other words, "truth" standards are used to demonstrate that the results obtained with the medical imaging drug are valid and reliable. For example, for a MRI contrast agent intended to visualize the number of lesions in liver or determine whether a mass is malignant, the truth standard might include results from the pathology or long-term clinical outcomes. In diagnostic imaging studies, "truth" or "gold" standard are usually called as standard of reference (SOR). There are a number of possible choices of SOR in an imaging trail. These are:

a. Histopathology
b. Therapeutic response
c. Clinical outcome
d. Another valid imaging procedure (validated against a valid gold standard)
e. Autopsy

The typical outcome table (2×2) in the evaluation of a diagnostic test is shown below

		Disease Status	
		Present	Absent
Diagnostic Test	Positive	a (TP)	b (FP)
	Negative	c (FN)	d (TN)

where TP, FP, FN, TN represent the true positive, false positive, false negative, and true negative, respectively. After completing a well-defined classification based on the disease status and diagnostic test of interest, the efficacy of imaging agent can be expressed as the diagnostic performance of the agent.

The simplest measure of diagnostic decision is the fraction of cases for which the physician is correct, which is often called "accuracy". In other words, the accuracy is defined as the proportion of cases, considering both positive and negative test results, for which the test results are correct. It also can be expressed in mathematics as following:

$$Accuracy = \frac{a+d}{a+b+c+d}$$

However, accuracy is of limited usefulness as an index of diagnostic performance because two diagnostic modalities can yield equal accuracies but perform differently with respect to the types of decisions. Also, it can be affected by the disease prevalence strongly. Due to the limitation of the accuracy index, the sensitivity and specificity are used in the evaluation scheme.

$$Sensitivity = \frac{Number\ of\ TP\ decisions}{Number\ of\ actually\ positive\ cases} = \frac{a}{a+c}$$

$$Specificity = \frac{Number\ of\ TN\ decisions}{Number\ of\ actually\ negative\ cases} = \frac{d}{b+d}$$

In effect, sensitivity and specificity represents two kinds of accuracy: the first is for actually positive cases and the second is for actually negative cases. However, very often a single pair of sensitivity and specificity measurements may provide a possibly misleading and even hazardous oversimplification of accuracy (Zweig *et al.* 1993). It should be noted that the method for evaluating and comparing sensitivity and specificity for diagnostic tests is based on:

Assumption 1: Diagnostic tests are independent given the disease status; and
Assumption 2: The gold standard is error free.

These two assumptions are not always valid. Several statistical methods have been considered, such as Qu and Hadgu (1998), Baker (1990), and Baker *et al.* (1998).

8.3. *Statistical analysis*

Most of the imaging trials are designed to provide dichotomous or ordered categorical outcomes. Therefore, the statistical tests for proportions and rates are commonly used, and the methods based on ranks are often applied to ordinal data. The analyses based on odds ratios and the Mantel-Haenszel procedures are useful for data analysis. In -addition, the use of model-based techniques, such as logistic regression models for binomial data, proportional odds models for ordinal data, and log-linear models for normal outcome variables are usually applied.

The diagnostic validity can be assessed in many ways. For example, the pre- and post-images can be compared to the gold standard, and the sensitivity and specificity of the pre-image compared to the post-image. Similarly, the same approaches can be used for two different active agents. The common methods used to test for differences in diagnosis are the McNemar test and Stwart-Maxwell test. The confidence intervals for sensitivity and specificity, and other measures can be also provided in the analysis.

The Receiver Operating Characteristic (ROC) analyses are becoming increasing important. Not only because it is recommended in the FDA draft guidance (2000a), but also its advantage over more traditional measures of diagnostic performance (Metz 1986). In next section, the ROC analysis is discussed in details.

8.3.1. *Receiver operating characteristic* (*ROC*) *analyses*

In the use of most diagnostic test, test data do not necessarily fall into one of two obviously defined categories. Imaging studies usually require some confidence threshold be established in the mind of the decision maker. For example, if an image suggests the possibility of disease, how strong the suspicion is in order for the image to be called positive? Therefore, the decision maker chooses between positive and negative diagnosis by comparing his/her confidence concerning with an arbitrary confidence threshold. Figure 3 is an example of the model that underlies ROC analysis. The bell-shaped curves represent the probability density distributions of a decision maker's confidence in a positive diagnosis that arise from actually positive patients and actually negative, patients.

The true positive fraction (TPF) is represented by the area under the left-hand distribution to the threshold. Similarly, the false positive fraction (FPF) is represented by the area under the left-hand distribution to the

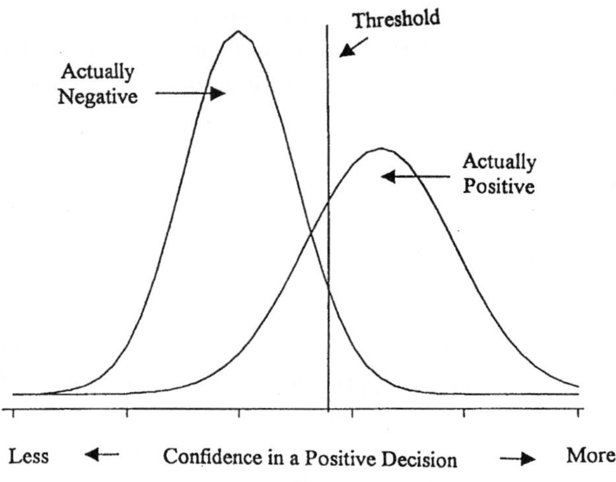

Fig. 3. Model of ROC Analysis.

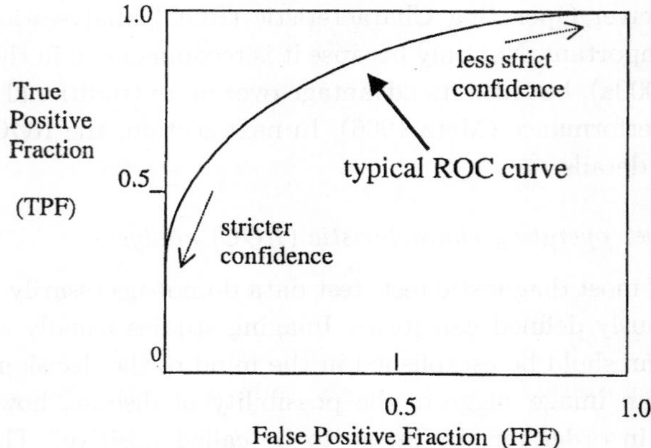

Fig. 4. Typical ROC curve.

threshold. These imply that the sensitivity and specificity vary inversely as the confidence threshold is changed. In other words, TPF and FPF will increase or decrease together as the confidence threshold is changed.

If we change the decision threshold several times, we will obtain several different pairs of TPF and FPF. These pairs can be plotted as points on a graph, such as that in Figure 4. This curve is called the ROC curve for diagnostic test. Then, we may conclude that better performance is indicated by an ROC curve that is higher to the left in the ROC space.

A practical technique for generating response data that can be used to plot a ROC curve is called the *rating method.* This method requires the decision maker select a value from a continuous scale, such as

a. Definitely negative
b. Probably negative
c. Questionable
d. Probably positive
e. Definitely positive

The advantages of the ROC curves are the following: it is simple and graphical. Also, it is independent of prevalence and it provides a direct visual comparison between tests on a common scale. However, the drawbacks of the ROC curves are the decision thresholds and the numbers of subjects are usually not displayed on the graph. In addition, the appropriate software is not widely available.

The ROC curve provides more information than just a single sensitivity and specificity pair to describe the accuracy of a diagnostic test. The curve depicts sensitivity and specificity levels over the entire range of decision thresholds. However, it would be helpful if the performance of a diagnostic test could be assessed by a single number. One such measurement that can be derived from the ROC curve is the area under the curve (AUC). If a diagnostic test that discriminates almost perfect, then its ROC curve passes near the upper left corner. This makes an AUC approaching 1. On the other hand, if the curve of a test that discriminates almost randomly, then the curve would lie near the 45-degree diagonal line. This would turn an AUC close to 0.5. The AUC range is between 0.5 and 1.

The AUC is calculated by summing the area of the trapezoids formed between the graph and the horizontal axis. This nonparametric method of calculation makes no assumptions regarding the underlying distributions of the diseased and non- diseased status. The meaning of AUC has been proved mathematically to be the probability that a random pair of positive/diseased and negative/non-diseased individuals would be identified correctly by the diagnostic test (Green and Swets, 1966). Also, it had been shown that the statistical properties of the Mann-Whitney-Wilcoxon statistics could be used to predict the statistical properties of AUC (Hanley and McNeil, 1982). For comparing corrected ROC curves, Delong *et al.* (1998) suggested a nonparametric approach for comparing the AUCs. For the parametric approach, Swets and Pickett (1982) proposed a more exact method using the maximum likelihood estimation to estimate the AUC and its standard error. A comparison of non-parametric and binomial parametric areas can be found in Center and Schwartz (1985).

9. Statistical Principles for Good Clinical Practice

For approval of a drug product, the FDA requires that substantial evidence of the effectiveness and safety of the drug product be provided through the conduct of two adequate and well-controlled clinical studies. To assist the sponsors in preparation of final clinical reports for regulatory submission and review, the FDA developed guidelines for the format and content of a clinical report in 1988. In addition, in 1994, the Committee for Proprietary Medicinal Products (CPMP) Working Party on Efficacy on Medicinal Products of the European Community issued a similar guideline entitled *A Note for Guidance on Biostatistical Methodology in Clinical*

Trials in Applications for Marketing Authorizations for Medicinal Products. At the same time, the ICH also signed off on the step 4 final draft of the *Structure and Content of Clinical Study Reports* and recommended its adoption to the three regulatory authorities of the United States, European Community, and Japan. The ICH guidelines require that some critical statistical issues be addressed in the final clinical report. These critical issues include baseline comparability, adjustments for covariates, dropouts or missing values, interim analyses and data monitoring, multicenter studies, multiplicity, efficacy subsets, active control trials, and subgroup analyses, which are briefly described below (see also, Pong and Chow, 1997; Chow 2011).

9.1. *Baseline comparability*

Baseline measurements are those collected during the baseline periods as defined in the protocol. Baseline usually refers to at randomization and prior to treatment. Sometimes, measurements obtained at screening are used as baselines. Basically, the objectives for analysis of baseline data are three-fold. First, the analysis of baseline data is to provide a description of patient characteristics of the targeted population to which statistical inference is made. In addition, the analysis of baseline data provided useful information regarding whether the patients enrolled in the study are a representative sample of the targeted population according to the inclusion and exclusion criteria of the trial. Second, since baseline data measure the initial patient disease status, they can serve as reference values for the assessment of the primary efficacy and safety clinical endpoints evaluated after the administration of the treatment. Finally, the comparability between treatment groups can be assessed based on baseline data to determine potential covariates for statistical evaluations of treatment effects. The ICH guideline requires that baseline data on demographic variables such as age, gender, or race and some disease factors such as specific entry criteria, duration, stage and severity of disease and other clinical classifications and subgroups in common usage or of known prognostic significance be collected and presented.

The commonly employed statistical tests for baseline comparability are Cochran-Mantel-Henzsel test for categorical data and analysis of variance for continuous variables. Preliminary investigation of baseline comparability helps identifying possible confounding and interaction effects between treatment and baseline characteristics.

9.2. *Adjustments for covariates*

For assessment of the efficacy and safety of a drug product, it is not uncommon that the primary clinical endpoints are affected by some factors (or covariates) such as demographic variables, patient characteristics, concomitant medications, and medical history. If these covariates are known to have an impact on the clinical outcomes, one may consider stratified randomization. In practice, however, one may collect information on some covariates, which may influential and yet unknown at the planning stage of the trial. In this case, if patients are randomly assigned to receive treatments, the estimated treatment effect is asymptotically free of the accidental bias induced by these covariates. If the covariate were balanced, then the difference in simple treatment averages would be an unbiased estimate for the treatment effect. On the other hand, if the covariate is not balanced, then the difference in simple average between treatment groups will be biased for estimation of the treatment effect. In this case, it is suggested that the covariates be included in the statistical model such as an analysis of variance (or covariance) model for an unbiased estimate of the treatment effect. In the case where covariates are balanced between the treatment groups, it is still necessary to adjust for covariates for clinical endpoints in order to obtain valid inference of the treatment effect if the covariates are statistically significantly correlated with the clinical endpoints.

The ICH guidelines require that selection of and adjustments for demographic or baseline measurements, concomitant therapy, or any other covariate or prognostic factor should be explained. In addition, methods of adjustments, results of analyses, and supportive information should be included in the detailed documentation of statistical methods.

9.3. *Dropouts or missing values*

In clinical research, there are many possible causes for the occurrence of dropouts and missing values. These possible causes include the duration of the study, the nature of the disease, the efficacy and adverse effects of the drug under study, intercurrent illness, accidents, patient refusal or moving, or other administrative reasons. The ICH guidelines suggest that the reasons for the dropouts, the time to dropout, and the proportion of dropouts among treatment groups be analyzed to examine the effects of dropouts for evaluation of the efficacy and safety of the study drug. Little and Rubin (1987) classified missing values into three different types based on the possible causes. If the causes of missing values are independent of the observed responses, then the missing values are said to be completely random. On the other hand, if the causes of missing values are dependent on the observed responses but are independent of the scheduled but unobserved responses, then missing values are said to be random. The missing values are said to be informative if the causes of missing values are dependent upon the scheduled but unobserved measurements.

If missing mechanism is either completely random or random, then statistical inference derived from the likelihood approaches based on patients who complete the study is still valid. 'However, the inference is not as efficient as it supposes to be. If the missing values were informative, then the inference based on the completers would be biased. As a result, it is suggested that despite the difficulty, the possible effects of dropouts and missing values on magnitude and direction of bias be expressed as fully as possible.

9.4. *Interim analysis and data monitoring*

Interim analysis and data monitoring are commonly employed for clinical trials in treatment of life-threatening disease or severely debilitating illness with long-term follow-up and endpoints such as mortality or irreversible morbidity. Interim analyses based on the data monitoring can be classified into formal interim analysis and administrative analysis. The aim of a formal interim analysis is to determine whether a decision for early termination can be reached before the planned study completion due to compelling evidence of beneficial effectiveness or harmful side effects. The administrative interim analysis is usually carried out without any intentions of early termination because of the results of the interim analysis results. Since interim analyses, either formally or informally, can introduce bias and/or increase type I error, the ICH guidelines require that all interim analyses, formal or informal, pre-planned or ad hoc, by any study participant, sponsor staff member, or data monitoring group should be described in full, even if the treatment groups were not identified. Data monitoring without code-breaking should also be described, even if this kind of monitoring is considered to cause no increase in type I error.

9.5. *Multicenter studies*

A multicenter trial is often conducted to expedite the patient recruitment process. The objective of the analysis of clinical data from a multicenter trial is two-fold. It is not only to investigate whether a consistent treatment effect can be observed across centers but also to provide an estimate of the overall treatment effect. Nevins (1988) proposed a set of four conditions under which evidence from a single multicenter trial would provide sufficient statistical evidence of efficacy.

Although all of the centers in multicenter trials follow the same protocol, many practical issues are likely to occur. For example, some centers may be too small for a reliable interpretation of the results, while some centers may be too big which dominate the results. In addition, there may be a significant treatment-by-center interaction. As a result, a statistical test for homogeneity across centers is necessarily performed for detection of possible quantitative or qualitative treatment-by-center interaction. Gail and Simon (1985) indicated that the existence of a quantitative interaction between treatment and center dose not invalidate the analysis by pooling data across centers. However, if a qualitative interaction between treatment and center is observed, an overall or average summary statistic may be misleading and hence considered inadequate. In this case, treatment effect should be carefully evaluated by center.

9.6. *Multiplicity*

In clinical trials, multiplicity may occur depending upon the objective of the intended trial, the nature of the design, and statistical analysis. The causes of multiplicity are mainly due to the formulation of statistical hypotheses and the experiment-wise false positive rates in subsequent analyses of the data. The ICH guidelines require that the overall type I error rate be adjusted to reflect multiplicity. Basically, multiplicity in clinical trials can be classified as repeated interim analyses, multiple comparisons, multiple endpoints, and subgroup analyses.

In the interest of an overall type I error rate, the commonly employed approach is probably the application of the Bonferroni technique. The concept of Bonferroni's technique is to adjust p values for control of experiment-wise type I error rate for pairwise comparisons. Bonferroni's method does not require that the structure of the correlation among comparisons be specified. In addition, it allows an unequal number of patients in each treatment group. Bonferroni's method works well when the number of treatment groups is small. When the number of treatment groups increases, however, Bonferroni's adjustment for p values becomes very conservative and may lack adequate power for the alternative in which most or all efficacy endpoints are improved. In this situation, as an alternative, one may consider a modified procedure proposed by Hochberg (1988). Hochberg's procedure is shown to be more powerful because it only requires one p value smaller than α to declare one statistically significant comparison.

9.7. *Efficacy subsets*

In clinical trials, despite the fact that there is a thoughtful study protocol, deviation from the protocol may be encountered during the course of the trial. In addition, it is very likely that patients will withdraw from the study prematurely before the completion of the trial due to various reasons. Patients who complete the study might miss some scheduled visits. As a result, which patients should be included in the analysis for a valid and unbiased assessment of the efficacy and safety of the treatment is a legitimate question to ask.

To provide a fair and unbiased assessment of the treatment effect, the ICH guideline suggests that the primary analysis for the demonstration of the efficacy and safety of the drug product should be conducted based on the intention-to-treat sample. In addition to the intention-to-treat sample, some subsets of the intention-to-treat sample may be constructed for efficacy analysis. These subsets are usually referred to efficacy subsets. These efficacy subsets include (i) patients with any efficacy observations or with a certain minimum number of observations, (ii) patients who complete the study, (iii) patients with an observation during a particular time window, and (iv) patients with a specified degree of compliance. The ICH guidelines require that efficacy subsets be analyzed to examine the effects of dropping patients with available data from analyses because of poor compliance, missed visits, ineligibility, or any other reasons. Any substantial differences resulting from the analyses of the intention-to-treat sample and the efficacy subsets should be the subject of explicit discussion.

9.8. *Active control trials*

An active control trial is often considered an alternative to placebo control study for evaluation of the effectiveness and safety of a test drug with very ill patients or patients with severe or life-threatening diseases based on ethical considerations. The primary objective of an active control trial could be to establish the efficacy of the test drug, to show that the test drug is equivalent to an active control agent, or to demonstrate that the test drug is superior to the active control agent. Pledger and Hall (1986) pointed out that active control trials offer no direct evidence of effectiveness of the test drug. The only trial that will yield direct evidence of effectiveness of the test drug is a placebo-controlled trial, which compares the test drug with a placebo. Temple (1983) indicated that if we cannot be very certain that the active control agent in a study would have beaten a placebo group, the fundamental assumption of the active control study cannot be made and that design must be considered inappropriate.

ICH guidelines indicated that if an active control study is intended to show equivalence between the test drug and an active control, the analysis should show the confidence interval for the comparison between the two agents for critical endpoints and the relation of that interval to the pre-specified degree of inferiority that would be consider unacceptable.

Note that in the 2010 FDA draft guidance defines two non-inferiority margins, namely M_1 and M_2, where M_1 is defined as the entire effect of the active control assumed to be present in the non-inferiority study and M_2 is referred to as the largest clinically acceptable difference (degree of inferiority) of the test drug compared to the active control. As indicated in the 2010 FDA draft guidance, M_1 is based on (i) the treatment effect estimated from the historical experience with the active control drug, (ii) assessment of the likelihood that the current effect of the active control is similar to the past effect (the constancy assumption), and (iii) assessment of the quality of the non-inferiority trial, particularly looking for defects that could reduce a difference between the active control and the new drug. On the other hand, M_2 is a clinical judgment which is never be greater than M_1, even if for active control drugs with small effects, a clinical judgment might argue that a larger difference is not clinically important. Ruling out a difference between the active control and test drug that is larger than M_1 is a critical finding that supports the conclusion of effectiveness.

9.9. *Adaptive design methods in clinical trials*

In recent years, the use of adaptive design methods has become very popular due to its flexibility and efficiency for identifying any possible signal or trend of clinical benefits (preferably the optimal clinical benefits) with limited resources available (see, e.g., Chow and Chang, 2006; Pong and Chow, 2010). In its recent draft guidance, the FDA defines an adaptive design clinical study as a study that includes a prospectively planned opportunity for modification of one or more specified aspects of the study design and hypotheses based on analysis of data (usually interim data) from subjects in the study. The FDA emphasizes that one of the major characteristics of an adaptive design is the prospectively planned opportunity. Changes should be made based on analysis of data (usually interim data).

On the other hand, Chow, Chang and Pong (2005) provided a broader definition of an adaptive design. They define an adaptive design of a clinical trial as a design that allows adaptations or modifications to some aspects (e.g., trial procedures and/or statistical methods) of the trial after its initiation without undermining the validity and integrity of the trial. Trial procedures are referred to as the eligibility criteria, study dose, treatment duration, study endpoints, laboratory testing procedures, diagnostic procedures, criteria for evaluability, and assessment of clinical responses. Statistical methods include randomization scheme, study design selection, study objectives/hypotheses, sample size calculation, data monitoring and interim analysis, statistical analysis plan, and/or methods for data analysis.

Depending upon the types of adaptation or modification made, commonly employed adaptive design methods in clinical trials include, but are not limited to: (i) a group sequential design, (ii) a sample size re-estimation (or an N-adjustable) design, (iii) an adaptive seamless (e.g., phase I/II or phase II/III) design, (iv) a drop-the-loser (or pick-the-winner) design, (v) an adaptive randomization design, (vi) an adaptive dose finding (escalation) design, (vii) a biomarker-adaptive design, (viii) an adaptive treatment-switching design, (ix) an adaptive-hypotheses design, and (x) any combinations of the above (see also, Chow and Chang, 2006; Pong and Chow, 2010).

In its draft guidance, the FDA classifies adaptive designs into categories of well-understood and less well-understood designs. For those less well-understood adaptive designs such as adaptive dose finding designs and two-stage phase I/II (or phase II/III) seamless adaptive designs, statistical methods are not well established and hence should be used with caution. In practice, misuse of adaptive design methods in clinical trials is a concern to both clinical scientists and regulatory agencies. It is suggested that the escalating momentum for the use of adaptive design methods in clinical trials be slowed in order to allow time for development of appropriate statistical methodologies.

References

1. Afonja, B. (1972). The moments of the maximum of correlated normal and t-variate. *Journal of the Royal Statistical Society*, B, **34**, 251–262.
2. Agin, M.A., Aronstein, W.S., Ferber, G., Geraldes, M.C., Locke, C., and Sager, P. (2008). QT/QTc prolongation in placebo-treated subjects: A

PhRMA collaborative data analysis. *Journal of Biopharmaceutical Statistics*, **18**, 408–426.

3. Anderson, S. and Hauck, W.W. (1990). Consideration of individual bioequivalence. *Journal of Pharmacokinetics and Biopharmaceutics*, **18**, 259–273.
4. Baker S.G., Cannor R.J., and Kessler L.G. (1998). The partial testing design: a less costly way to test equivalence for sensitivity and specificity. *Statistics in Medicine,* **17**, 2219–2232.
5. Baker, S.G. (1990). A simple EM algorithm for capture-recapture data with categorical covariates. *Biometrics,* **46**, 1193–1200.
6. Bergum, J.S. (1990). Constructing acceptance limits for multiple stage tests. *Drug Dev. Ind. Pharm.*, **16**, 2153–2166.
7. Caraco, Y. (2004). Genes and the response to drugs. *The New England Journal of Medicine*, **351**, 2867–2869.
8. Center, R.M. and Schwartz J.S. (1985). An evaluation of methods for estimating the area under the receiver operating characteristics (ROC) curve. *Medical Decision Making*, **5**, 149–156.
9. Chen, M.L. (1997). Individual bioequivalence — a regulatory update. *Journal of Biopharmaceutical Statistics*, **7**, 5–11.
10. Cheng, B., Chow, S.C., Burt, D. and Cosmatos, D. (2008). Statistical assessment of QT/QTc prolongation based on maximum of correlated normal random variables. *Journal of Biopharmaceutical Statistics*, **18**, 494–501.
11. Chow, S.C. (1992). Statistical design and analysis of stability studies. Presented at the 48th Conference on Applied Statistics, Atlantic City, N.J., December 1992.
12. Chow, S.C. (1997). Good statistics practice in the drug development and regulatory approval process. *Drug Information Journal*, **31**, 1157–1166.
13. Chow, S.C. (2000). *Encyclopedia of Biopharmaceutical Statistics.* Marcel Dekker, Inc., New York, New York.
14. Chow, S.C. (2007). *Statistical Design and Analysis of Stability Studies.* Taylor & Francis, New York, New York.
15. Chow, S.C. (2011). *Controversial Statistical Issues in Clinical Trials.* Chapman and Hall/CRC Press, Taylor & Francis, New York, New York.
16. Chow, S.C. and Chang, M. (2006). *Adaptive Design Methods in Clinical Trials.* Chapman and Hall/CRC Press, Taylor and Francis, New York, New York.
17. Chow, S.C., Chang, M., and Pong, A. (2005). Statistical consideration of adaptive methods in clinical development. *Journal of Biopharmaceutical Statistics*, **15**, 575–591.
18. Chow, S.C., Cheng, B., and Cosmatos, D. (2008). On power and sample size calculation for QT studies with recording replicates at given time point. *Journal of Biopharmaceutical Statistics*, **18**, 483–493.
19. Chow, S.C. and Liu, J.P. (1995). *Statistical Design and Analysis in Pharmaceutical Science*, Marcel Dekker, Inc., New York, New York.
20. Chow, S.C. and Liu, J.P. (1997). Meta-analysis for bioequivalence review. *Journal of Biopharmaceutical Statistics*, **7**, 97–111.

21. Chow, S.C. and Liu, J.P. (1998). *Design and Analysis of Clinical Trials*, Wiley, New York.
22. Chow, S.C. and Liu, J.P. (2003). *Design and Analysis of Clinical Trials — Revised and Expanded*, Second Edition, John Wiley & Sons, New York, New York.
23. Chow, S.C. and Liu, J.P. (2000). *Design and Analysis of Bioavailability and Bioequivalence*, Marcel Dekker, Inc., New York, New York.
24. Chow, S.C. and Liu, J.P. (2008). *Design and Analysis of Bioavailability and Bioequivalence Studies — Revised and Expanded*, Third Edition, Taylor & Francis, New York, New York.
25. Chow, S.C., and Shao, J. (1988). A new procedure for estimation of variance components. *Statistics & Probability Letters*, **6**, 349–355.
26. Chow, S.C., and Shao, J. (1989). Test for batch-to-batch variation in stability analysis. *Statistics in Medicine*, **8**, 883–890.
27. Chow, S.C. and Shao, J. (1991). Estimating drug shelf-life with random batches. *Biometrics*, **47**, 1071–1079.
28. Chow, S.C. and Shao, J. (2002). *Statistics in Drug Research — Methodologies and Recent Development*. Marcel Dekker, Inc., New York, New York.
29. Chow, S.C. and Shao, J. (2003). Stability analysis with discrete response. *Journal of Biopharmaceutical Statistics*. **13**, 451–462.
30. Chow, S.C, and Shao, J. (2006). On non-inferiority margin and statistical tests in active control trials. *Statistics in Medicine*, **25**, 1101–1113.
31. Chow, S.C., Shao, J., and Hu, Y.P. (2002). Assessing sensitivity and similarity in bridging studies. *Journal of Biopharmaceutical Statistics*, **12**, 385–400.
32. Chow, S.C., Shao, J., and Wang, H. (2002). Individual bioequivalence testing under 2 × 3 designs. *Statistics in Medicine*, **21**, 629–648.
33. Chow, S.C., Shao, J., and Wang, H. (2003). Statistical tests for population bioequivalence. *Statistica Sinica*, **13**, 539–554.
34. Chow, S.C., Shao, J., and Wang, H. (2003). *Sample Size Calculation in Clinical Research*. Marcel Dekker, Inc., New York, New York.
35. Chow, S.C., Shao, J. and Wang, H. (2007). *Sample Size Calculation in Clinical Research*. Second Edition, Taylor & Francis, New York, New York.
36. Chow, S.C., and Tse, S.K. (1991). On variance estimation in assay validation. *Statistics in Medicine*, **10**, 1543–1553.
37. Chung, W.H., Hung, S.I., Hong, H.S., Hsih, M.S., Yang, L.C., Ho, H.C., Wu, J.Y., and Chen, Y.T. (2004). Medical genetics: A marker for Stevens-Johnson syndrome. *Nature*, **428** (6982), 486.
38. Chung-Stein, C. (1996). Summarizing laboratory data with different reference ranges in multi-center clinical trials. *Drug Information Journal*, **26**, 77–84.
39. Cohen, J. (1960). A coefficient of agreement for nominal scales. *Educational and Psychological Measurement*, **20**, 37–46.
40. CPMP (1997). Points to consider: The assessment of the potential for QT interval prolongation by non-cardiovascular products. Available at: www.coresearch.biz/regulations/cpmp.pdf.

41. DeLong E.R. and DeLong D.M. (1988). Comparing the areas under two or more correlated receiver operating characteristic curves: A nonparametric approach. *Biometrics,* **44**, 837–845.
42. Dubey, S.D. (1991). Some thoughts on the one-sided and two-sided test. *Journal of Biopharmaceutical Statistics*, **1**, 139–150.
43. Eaton, M. L., Muirhead, R. J., Mancuso, J. Y., and Kolluri, S. (2006). A confidence interval for the maximal mean QT interval change caused by drug effect. *Drug Information Journal*, **40**, 267–271.
44. Esinhart, J.D. and Chinchilli, V.M. (1994). Extension to the use of tolerance intervals for assessment of individual bioequivalence. *Journal of Biopharmaceutical Statistics*, **4**, 39–52.
45. FDA (1992). Guidance on *Statistical Procedures for Bioequivalence Studies Using a Standard Two- Treatment Crossover Design*, Division of Bioequivalence, Office of Generic Drugs, Center for Drug Evaluation and Research, Food and Drug Administration, Rockville, Maryland.
46. FDA (1993). Guideline for *Submitting Documentation for the Stability of Human Drugs and Biologics.* Center for Drugs and Biologics, Office of Drug Research and Review, Food and Drug Administration, Rockville, Maryland, U.S.A.
47. FDA (2000a). Draft Guidance on *Developing Medical Imaging Drugs and Biologics. Division of Medical Imaging and Radiopharmaceutical Drug Product*, Center for Drug Evaluation and Research and Center for Biologics Evaluation and Research, Food and Drug Administration, Rockville, Maryland.
48. FDA (2000b). Guidance for industry: *Bioavailability and Bioequivalence Studies for Orally Administrated Drug Products — General Considerations.* Office of Generic Drugs, Center for Drug Evaluation and Research, Food and Drug Administration, Rockville, Maryland.
49. FDA (2009). Guidance for industry: *New Contrast Imaging Indication Considerations for Devices and Approved Drug and Biological Product.* Office of Generic Drugs, Center for Drug Evaluation and Research, Food and Drug Administration, Rockville, Maryland.
50. FDA (2001). Guidance for industry: *Statistical Approaches to Establishing Bioequivalence.* Office of Generic Drugs, Center for Drug Evaluation and Research, Food and Drug Administration, Rockville, Maryland.
51. FDA (2003). Guidance on *Bioavailability and Bioequivalence Studies for Orally Administrated Drug Products — General Considerations*, Center for Drug Evaluation and Research, the US Food and Drug Administration, Rockville, Maryland, USA.
52. FDA (2010a). *Guidance for Industry — Non-Inferiority Clinical Trials.* Center for Drug Evaluation and Research, Center for Biologics Evaluation and Research, the United States Food and Drug Administration, Siler Spring, Maryland.
53. FDA (2010b). *Draft Guidance for Industry — Adaptive Design Clinical Trials for Drugs and Biologics.* The United States Food and Drug Administration, Rockville, Maryland, USA.

54. FDA/TPD (2003). Preliminary concept paper: *The clinical evaluation of QT/QTc interval prolongation and proarrythmic potential for non-arrythmic drug products.* Released on November 15, 2002. Revised on February 6, 2003.
55. Fleiss, J.L., Cohen, J., and Everitt, B.S. (1969). Large-sample standard errors of kappa and weighted kappa. *Psychological Bulletin,* **72**, 323–327.
56. Gail, M. and Simon, R. (1985). Testing for qualitative interactions between treatments and patient subsets. *Biometrics*, **41**, 361–372.
57. Goldberg, J.D. and Kury, K.J. (1990). Design and Analysis of Multicenter Trials. In *Statistical Methodology in the Pharmaceutical Industry*, ed. by Berry, D., Marcel Dekker, New York, New York, 201–237.
58. Green, D.M. and Swets, J.A. (1966). *Signal Detection Theory and Psychophysics.* New York: John Wiley.
59. Haidar, S.H., Davit, B., Chen, M.L., Conner, D., Lee, L., Li, Q.H., Lionberger, R., Makhlouf, F., Patel, D., Schuirmann, D.J. and Yu, L.X. (2008). Bioequivalence approaches for highly variable drugs and drug products. *Pharmaceutical Research*, **25**, 237–241.
60. Hanley, J.A. and McNeil, B.J. (1982). The meaning and use of the area under a receiver operating characteristic (ROC) curve. *Diagnostic Radiology.* Vol. **143**, 29–36.
61. Hauck, W. W. and Anderson, S. (1984). A new statistical procedure for testing equivalence in two-group comparative bioavailability trials. *Journal of Pharmacokinetics and Biopharmaceutics,* **12**, 83–91.
62. Hochberg, Y. (1988). A sharper Bonferroni's procedure for multiple test of significance. *Biometrika,* **75**, 800–803.
63. Hyslop, T., Hsuan, F., and Holder, D.J. (2000). A small-sample confidence interval approach to assess individual bioequivalence. *Statistics in Medicine*, **19**, 2885–2897.
64. Holder, D.J. and Hsuan, F. (1993). Moment-based criteria for determining bioequivalence. *Biometrika*, **80**, 835–846.
65. Hosmane, B. and Locke, C. (2005). A simulation study of power in thorough QT/QTc studies and a normal approximation for planning purposes. *Drug Information Journal*, **39**, 447–455.
66. Hung, H.M.J. (2003). Statistical issues with design and analysis of bridging clinical trial. Presented at the 2003 Symposium on Statistical Methodology for Evaluation of Bridging Evidence, Taipei, Taiwan.
67. Hung, H.M.J., Wang, S.J., Tsong, Y., Lawrence, J., and O'Neil, R.T. (2003). Some fundamental issues with non-inferiority testing in active controlled trials. *Statistics in Medicine*, **22**, 213–225.
68. ICH (1993). *Stability Testing of New Drug Substances and Products.* Tripartite International Conference on Harmonization Guideline.
69. ICH (1994). ICH QIA. Guideline for Industry. *Stability Testing Guideline of New Drug Substances and Products.* Sep. 1994.
70. ICH (1997). E5 Guideline on Ethnic Factors in the Acceptability of Foreign Data. The U.S. Federal Register, Vol. **83**, 31790–31796.

71. ICH (1998). E9 Guideline for *Statistical Principles for Clinical Trials*. Tripartite International Conference on Harmonization Guideline, http://www/ich.org/LOB/media/MEDIA485.pdf
72. ICH (2005). ICH E14 Guidance on *The Clinical Evaluation of QT/QTc Interval Prolongation and Proarrythmic Potential for Non-Antiarrythmic Drugs*. Geneva, Switzerland: International Conference on Harmonisation, May 2005.
73. Kawai, N, Stein, C, Komiyama O, and Li, Y. (2008). An approach to rationalize partitioning sample size into individual regions in a multiregional trial. *Drug Information Journal*, **42**, 139–147.
74. Khongphatthanayothin, A., Lane, J., Thomas, D., Yen, L., Chang, D., and Bubolz, B. (1998). Effects of cisapride on QT interval in children. *Journal of Pediatrics*, **133**, 51–56.
75. Ko, F.S., Tsou, H.H., Liu, J.P., and Hsiao, C.F. (2010). Sample size determination for a specific region in a multi-regional trial. *Journal of Biopharmaceutical Statistics*, **20**, 870–875.
76. Lachin, J.M. (1988). Statistical properties of randomization in clinical trials. *Controlled Clinical Trials*, **9**, 289–311.
77. Lasser, K.E., Allen, P.D., Woolhandler, S.J., Himmelstein, D.U., Wolfe, S.M., and Bor, D.H. (2002). Timing of new black box warnings and withdrawals for prescription medications. *The Journal of American Medical Association*, **287**, 2215–2220.
78. Lin, M., Chu C.C., Chang, S.L. *et al.* (2001). The origin of Minnan and Hakka, the so-called "Taiwanese", inferred by HLA study. *Tissue Antigen*, **57**, 192–199.
79. Lin, T.Y. D. (1994). Applicability of matrixing and bracketing approach to stability study design. Presented at the 4th ICSA Applied Statistics Symposium, Rockville, Maryland.
80. Little, R.J.A. and Rubin, D.B. (1987). *Statistical Analysis with Missing Values*. John Wiley & Sons, New York, New York.
81. Liu, J.P. and Chow, S.C. (1997). Some thoughts on individual bioequivalence, *Journal of Biopharmaceutical Statistics*, **7**, 41–48.
82. Liu, J.P., Hsueh, H.M., and Hsiao, C.F. (2002). Bayesian approach to evaluation of the bridging studies. *Journal of Biopharmaceutical Statistics*, **12**, 401–408.
83. Liu, J.P., and Weng, C.S. (1992). Detection of outlying data in bioavailability/bioequivalence studies, *Statistics in Medicine*, **10**, 1375–1389.
84. Longford, N. T. (1993). *Random Coefficient Models*. Oxford University Press Inc., New York, New York.
85. Ma, H., Smith, B., and Dmitrienko, A. (2008). Statistical analysis methods for QT/QTc prolongation. *Journal of Biopharmaceutical Statistics*, **18**, 553–563.
86. Malik, M. and Camm, A. J. (2001). Evaluation of drug-induced QT interval prolongation. *Drug Safety*, **24**, 323–351.

87. Mellon, J.1. (1991). Design and analysis aspects of drug stability studies when the product is stored at several temperatures. Presented at the 12th Annual Midwest Statistical Workshop, Muncie, Indiana.
88. Metz, C.E. (1986). ROC methodology in radiologic imaging. *Investigative Radiology*, **21**, 720–733.
89. Moss, A. J. (1993). Measurement of the QT interval and the risk associated with QT interval prolongation. *American Journal of Cardiology*, **72**, 23B–25B.
90. Murphy, J.R. and Weisman, D. (1990). Using random slopes for estimating shelf-life. *Proceedings of the Biopharmaceutical Section of the American Statistical Association*, 196–203.
91. Myrand, S.P., Sekiguchi, K., Man, M.Z., Lin, X., Tzeng, R.Y., Teng, C.H., Hee, B., Garrett, M., Kikkawa, H., Lin, C.Y., Eddy, S.M., Dostalik, J., Mount, J., Azuma, J., Fujio, Y., Jang, I.J., Shin, S.G., Bleavins, M.R., Williams, J.A., Paulauskis, J.D., Wilner, K.D. (2008). Pharmacokinetics/genotype associations for major cytochrome P450 enzymes in native and first- and third-generation Japanese populations: Comparison with Korean, Chinese, and Caucasian populations. *Clinical Pharmacology & Therapeutics*, **84**(3), 347–361
92. Nevins, S.E. (1988). Assessment of evidence from a single multicenter trial. *Proceedings of the Biopharmaceutical Section of the American Statistical Association*, 43–45.
93. Nordbrock, E. (2000). Stability matrix design. In *Encyclopedia of Biopharmaceutical Statistics*. Ed. S. Chow, Marcel Dekker, Inc., New York, New York.
94. Patterson, S., Agin, M., Anziano, R. *et al.* (2005). Investigating drug-induced QT and QTc prolongation in the clinic: A review of statistical design and analysis considerations: Report from the Pharmaceutical Research and Manufacturers of America QT Statistics Expert Team. *Drug Information Journal*, **39**, 243–266.
95. PhRMA (2003). Investigating drug-induced QT and QTc prolongation in the clinic: Statistical design and analysis considerations. Report from the Pharmaceutical Research and Manufacturers of America QT Statistics Expert Team, August 14, 2003.
96. Pledger, G.W. and Hall, D. (1986). Active control trials: Do they address the efficacy issue? *Proceedings of the Biopharmaceutical Section of the American Statistical Association*, 1–7.
97. Pong, A. and Chow, S.C. (1997). Statistical/practical issues in clinical trials. *Drug Information Journal*, **31**, 1167–1174.
98. Pong, A. and Chow, S.C. (Ed) (2010). *Adaptive Design in Pharmaceutical Research and Development.* Taylor & Francis, New York, New York.
99. Pong, A. and Raghavarao, D. (2000). Comparison of bracketing and matrixing designs for a two-year stability study, *Journal of Biopharmaceutical Statistics*, **10**, 217–228.
100. Pong, A. and Raghavarao, D. (2001). Shelf life estimation for drug products with two components. *Proceedings of the Biopharmaceutical Section of the American Statistical Association*, Alexandria, VA.

101. Pong, A. and Raghavarao, D. (2002). Comparing distributions of drug shelf lives for two components under different designs, *Journal of Biopharmaceutical Statistics*, **12**, 277–293.
102. Pratt, C.M., Hertz, R.P. Ellis, B.E., Crowell, S.P., Louv, W., and Moye, L. (1994). Risk of developing life-threatening ventricular arrhythmia associated with tefenadine in comparison with over-the-counter antihistamines, ibuprofen and clemastine. *American Journal of Cadiology*, **73**, 346–352.
103. Qu, Y. and Hadgu A. (1998). A model for evaluating sensitivity and specificity for correlated diagnostic tests in efficacy studies with an imperfect test. *Journal of the American Statistical Association*, **93**, 920–928.
104. Quan, H., Zhao, P.L., Zhang, J., Roessner, M., and Aizawa, K. (2009). Sample size considerations for Japanese patients based on MHLW guidance. *Pharmaceutical Statistics*, **9**, 100–112.
105. Ruberg, S. and Hsu, J. (1992). Multiple comparison procedures for pooling batches in stability studies. *Technometrics*, **34**, 465–472.
106. Schall, R. and Luus, R.E. (1993). On population and individual bioequivalence. *Statistics in Medicine*, **12**, 1109–1124.
107. Schuirmann, D. J. (1987). A comparison of the two one-sided tests procedure and the power approach for assessing the equivalence of average bioavailability. *Journal of Pharmacokinetics and Biopharmaceutics*, **15**, 657–680.
108. Serfling, R. J. (1980). *Approximation Theorems of Mathematical Statistics*, Wiley, New York.
109. Shah, V.P., Midha, K.K., Dighe. S., McGilveray, I.J., Skelly, J.P., Yacobi, A., Layoff, T., Viswanathan, C.T., Cook, C.E., McDowall, R.D., Pittman, K.A. and Spector, S (1992). Analytical methods validation: Bioavailability, bioequivalence and pharmaceutical studies. *Pharmaceutical Research,* **9**, 588–592.
110. Shao, J. and Chow, S.C. (1993). Two-stage sampling with pharmaceutical applications. *Statistics in Medicine*, **12**, 1999–2008.
111. Shao, J. and Chow, S.C. (1994). Statistical inference in stability analysis. *Biometrics*, **50**, 753–763.
112. Shao, J. and Chow S.C. (2001a). Two-phase shelf-life estimation. *Statistics in Medicine*, **20**, 1239–1248.
113. Shao, J. and Chow S.C. (2001b). Drug shelf life estimation. *Statistica Sinica*, 11, 737–745.
114. Shao, J. and Chow, S.C. (2002). Reproducibility probability in clinical trials. *Statistics in Medicine*, **21**, 1727–1742.
115. Sheiner, L.B. (1992). Bioequivalence revisited. *Statistics in Medicine*, **11**, 1777–1788.
116. Shih, W.J. (2001). Clinical trials for drug registrations in Asian Pacific countries: Proposal for a new paradiam from a statistical perspective. *Controlled Clinical Trials*, **22**, 357–366.
117. Snedecor, G.W. and Cochran, W.G. (1967). *Statistical Methods*, sixth edition. Ames, Iowa: The Iowa State University Press.
118. Strieter, D., Wu, W., and Agin, M. (2003). Assessing the effects of replicate ECGs on QT variability in healthy subjects. Presented at Midwest Biopharmaceutical Workshop, May 21, 2003.

119. Sun, Y., Chow, S.C., Li, G., and Chen, K.W. (1999). Assessing distributions of estimated drug shelf lives in stability analysis. *Biometrics*, **55**, 896–899.
120. Swets, J.A. and Pickett, R.M. (1982). *Evaluation of Diagnostic System.* New York: Academic Press.
121. Temple, R. (1983). Difficulties in evaluating positive control trials. *Proceedings of the Biopharmacentical Section of the American Statistical Association*, 1–7.
122. Temple, R. (2003). Overview of the concept paper, history of the QT/TDP concern; regulatory implications of QT prolongation. Presentations at Drug Information Agency/FDA Workshop. Available at: www.diahome.org.
123. Tian, H. and Natarajan, J. (2008). Effect of baseline measurement on the change from baseline in QTc intervals. *Journal of Biopharmaceutical Statistics*, 18, 542–552.
124. Tsong, Y. and Zhang, J. (2008). Guest editors' notes on statistical issues in design and analysis of thorough QTc studies. *Journal of Biopharmaceutical Statistics*, **18**, 405–407.
125. Tsong, Y., Zhong, J., and Chen, W.J. (2008). Validation testing in thorough QT/QTc clinical trials. *Journal of Biopharmaceutical Statistics*, **18**, 529–541.
126. Tsou, H.H., Chow, S.C., Wang, S.J., Hung, H.M., Lan, K.K., Liu, J.P., Wang, M., Chen, H.D., Ho, L.T., Hsiung, C.A., and Hsiao, C.F. (2011). Proposal of statistical consideration to evaluation of results for a specific region in multi-regional trials — Asian perspective. *Pharmaceutical Statistics*, 9, 201–206.
127. Uesaka, H. (2009). Sample size allocation to regions in multiregional trial. *Journal of Biopharmaceutical Statistics*, **19**, 580–594.
128. Ueta, M., Sotozono, C., Tokunaga, K., Yabe, T., and Kinoshita, S. (2007). Strong association between HLA-A*0206 and Stevens-Johnson syndrome in the Japanese. *American Journal of Ophthalmology*, **143**(2), 367–368.
129. USP/NF (2000). The United States Pharmacopeia 24 and the National Formulary 19. United States Pharmacopeia Convention, Inc., Rockville, Maryland, U.S.A.
130. Wang, X., Wu, Y., and Zhou, H. (2009). Outcome- and auxiliary-dependent subsampling and its statistical inference. *Journal of Biopharmaceutical Statistics*, **19**, 1132–1150.
131. Westlake, W. J. (1976). Symmetrical confidence intervals for bioequivalence trials. *Biometrics*, **32**, 741–744.
132. Wysowski, D.K., Corken, A., Gallo-Torres, H., Talarico, L., and Rodriguez, E.M. (2001). Postmarketing reports of QT prolongation and ventricular arrhythmia in association with cisapride and Food and Drug Administration regulatory actions. *American Journal of Gastroenterology*, **96**, 1698–1703.

133. Zhang, J. (2008). Testing for positive control activity in a thorough QTc study. *Journal of Biopharmaceutical Statistics*, **18**, 517–528.
134. Zhang, L., Dmitrienko, A., and Luta, G. (2008). Sample size calculations in thorough QT studies. *Journal of Biopharmaceutical Statistics*, **18**, 468–482.
135. Zhang, J. and Machado, S.G. (2008). Statistical issues including design and sample size calculation in thorough QT/QTc studies. *Journal of Biopharmaceutical Statistics*, **18**, 451–467.
136. Zweig M.1i. and Campbell G. (1993). Receiver-operating characteristic (ROC) plots: A fundamental evaluation tool in clinical medicine. *Clinical Chemistry*, **39**(4), 561–577.

About the Authors

Shein-Chung Chow, Ph.D. is currently a Professor at the Department of Biostatistics and Bioinformatics, Duke University School of Medicine, Durham, North Carolina and the Founding Director of Global Clinical Trial and Research Center, Tianjin, China. Dr. Chow also held various positions in the pharmaceutical industry. He is the Editor-in-Chief of the *Journal of Biopharmaceutical Statistics* and the *Biostatistics Book Series* published by Chapman and Hall/CRC Press of Taylor & Francis Group. He was elected Fellow of the American Statistical Association in 1995 and an elected member of the ISI (International Statistical Institute) in 1999. He was the recipient of the DIA Outstanding Service Award (1996), International Chinese Statistical Association (ICSA) Extraordinary Achievement Award (1996), and Chapter Service Recognition Award of the American Statistical Association (1998). Dr. Chow was appointed Scientific Advisor to the Department of Health, Taiwan in 1999–2001 and 2006–2008. Dr. Chow was President of the ICSA in 1997. Dr. Chow is the author or co-author of over 230 methodology papers and over 22 books. He received his Bachelor of Science in Mathematics from National Taiwan University, Taiwan, and his Ph.D. in Statistics from the University of Wisconsin, Madison, Wisconsin, USA.

Annpey Pong is currently a principal scientist at the Department of Biostatistics and Research Decision Sciences, Merck Research Laboratories, Rahway, New Jersey. Dr. Pong has 20 years working experiences in the pharmaceutical industry. Dr. Pong is the Book Review Editor and Associate Editor of the *Journal of Biopharmaceutical Statistics*, co-author of the book "Handbook of Adaptive Designs in Pharmaceutical and Clinical

Development", and the author or co-author of over 30 papers in the field of pharmaceutical research. Dr. Pong received his Bachelor of Science in Mathematics from Providence University, Taiwan, two Master of Science degrees in Biostatistics and Mathematics from University of Michigan, Ann Arbor, and Eastern Michigan University, Ypsilanti, respectively, and a Ph.D. in Statistics from Temple University, Philadelphia, Pennsylvania, USA.

CHAPTER 15

STATISTICS IN PHARMACOLOGY AND PRE-CLINICAL STUDIES

TZE LEUNG LAI

Department of Statistics, Stanford University,
Room 127, Sequoia Hall, 390 Serra Mall,
Stanford, CA 94305-4065, USA
lait@stat.stanford.edu

MEI-CHIUNG SHIN[*,†]

[*]*VA Cooperative Studies Program,*
701-B N Shoreline Blvd, Mountain View,
CA 94043, USA

[†]*Department of Health Research and Policy,*
Stanford University, Stanford,
CA 94305, USA

GUANGRUI ZHU

Allergan, Inc
P.O. Box 19534 Irvine,
CA 92623 USA

1. Introduction

Pharmacology[1] is the science dealing with interactions between living systems and molecules, especially chemicals introduced from outside the system. This broad definition includes clinical pharmacology, whose objective is to prevent, diagnose and treat diseases with drugs, and the pathogenesis of diseases due to chemicals in the environment. A drug is defined in[1] as a small molecule that, when introduced into the body, alters the body's function. The component of a cell or organism that interacts with a drug and initiates the chain of biochemical events leading to the drug's therapeutic and toxic effects is called a *receptor*. The receptor concept has become the central focus of investigation of *pharmacodynamics* — the study of drug effects and their mechanisms of action. The relation between the dose of a drug and its clinically observed effects can be quite complex. In carefully controlled *in vitro* systems, however, the relation between the concentration of a drug at the site(s) of action and its effects can often be described by relatively simple mathematical models.

How a drug dose produces its effects involves not only pharmacodynamics but also *pharmacokinetics*. The latter is concerned with the concentration-time curve that is associated with the following "history" of a single adminstration of a drug:

(i) absorption phase of the drug into the body — transfer of the drug from its site of administration (via oral, or inhalational, or intravenous, or other route) into the bloodstream,
(ii) distribution phase — distribution of the drug to different compartments of the body, including receptor binding sites in the target tissue, and resulting in rapid decline in plasma concentration,
(iii) elimination phase — excretion of chemically unchanged drug or elimination via metabolism that converts the drug into one or more metabolites (e.g. at the liver).

Section 2 presents an overview of the basic principles, models and statistical methods in pharmacokinetics and pharmacodynamics. An active area of research in the field is pharmacometrics and Sec. 2 also gives some recent trends in this area. Particular attention will be directed to population pharmacokinetics and its interactions with several branches of modern statistics, including nonlinear mixed effects models, hierarchical and empirical Bayes methods, and generalized linear mixed effects models.

Section 2 also discusses the role of pharmacokinetic and pharmacodynamic studies in drug development. Specifically they are used to determine the *dosage regimen* of the drug (i.e. how much and how often it should be taken). These studies are initially performed *in vitro* and then on animals to come up with rough guesses of a region of dosage regimens in which clinical studies on human subjects are to be performed. The *in vitro* and animal studies are called *pre-clinical* and precede the clinical studies that are classified as Phase I studies (on healthy volunteers) and Phases II and III clinical trials (on patients).

Other statistical applications in pharmacology and pre-clinical studies include bioequivalence and bioavailability (treated in Sec. 3), assay development and validation (summarized in Sec. 4), drug discovery (reviewed in Sec. 5) and toxicology (treated in Chapter 13).

2. Pharmacokinetics and Pharmacodynamics

Drug administration can be divided into two phases, a pharmacokinetic (PK) phase in which the kinetics of drug absorption, distribution, and elimination translate into drug concentration-time relationships in the body, and a pharmacodynamic (PD) phase in which the drug concentration at the site(s) of action leads to the response/effects produced. Knowledge of both phases is important for the design of a dosage regimen to achieve the therapeutic objective. Since both the desired response and toxicity of the drug are functions of the drug concentration at the site(s) of action, the therapeutic objective can be achieved only when the drug concentration lies within a "therapeutic window," outside which the therapy is either ineffective or has unacceptable toxicity. Drug concentrations, however, can rarely be measured directly at the sites of action and are typically measured at the plasma, which is a more accessible site. An optimal dosage regimen can therefore be defined as one that maintains the plasma concentration of a drug within the therapeutic window. This can be achieved for many drugs by giving an initial dose to yield a plasma concentration within the therapeutic window and then maintaining the concentration within this window by periodic doses to replace the drug lost over time.

2.1. *PK/PD models*

Many PK and PD models have been developed in clinical pharmacology. The monographs[1–5] give a comprehensive introduction to these models and their applications. The PK models can be roughly classified as "mechanistic" or "empirical," while mechanistic models can be classified as "physiologic" or "compartmental." In physiologic models, the body is viewed in physiologic terms, making use of *a priori* knowledge of physiology, anatomy and biochemistry. Although the tissues or organs differ from one another, they share many qualitative features. As an illustrative example, consider how anatomy affects elimination. First "clearance" CL is defined as the rate of elimination divided by the concentration of the drug. If the organs of elimination are in parallel, then CL is the sum of the CL_i over the elimination organs i. On the other hand, if the organs of elimination are in series (working sequentially one after another), then CL is proportional to $1 - \Pi(1 - E_i)$, where E_i is the extraction ratio of the drug at organ i. In particular, since the gut-liver system is in series for portal circulation whereas the portal and arterial systems into the liver are in parallel, it follows that

$$\mathrm{CL} = Q_H\{f_{HP}[1 - (1 - E_{\mathrm{gut}})(1 - E_{\mathrm{liver}})] + (1 - f_{HP})E_{\mathrm{gut}}\}\,, \quad (1)$$

where f_{HP} is the fraction of total hepatic blood flow Q_H that enters the liver via the hepatic portal vein.

In compartmental models, the body is viewed in terms of kinetic compartments between which the drug distributes and from which elimination occurs. The kinetics is often described by a linear system of ordinary differential equations, which have explicit solutions involving exponential functions. On the other hand, the rate constants of a compartmental model may be functions of the concentration of the drug itself or another metabolite/interacting drug, leading to a system of nonlinear differential equations that have to be solved numerically. Empirical PK models are typically poly-exponential models of the form $\Sigma \alpha_i e^{-\lambda_i t}$. It is well known that different compartmental models may imply the same poly-exponential models, leading to identifiability difficulties with compartmental models in empirical work.[7,8]

A basic goal of PD models is to describe and quantify the steady-state relationship of drug concentration (C) at an effector site to the drug effect (E). The simplest PD model for one drug is the so-called "Emax model" defined by

$$E = e_{\max} C/(C + c_{50})\,, \quad (2)$$

where $e_{\max}$ is the maximum effect that the drug can produce and c_{50} is the concentration that yields 50% of $e_{\max}$. Note that this equation is the same as the Langmuir model in thermodynamics or the Michaelis–Mantern model in enzyme kinetics, in which the equilibrium state of ligand binding reactions is given by

$$B = \nu F/(\alpha + F)\,, \quad (3)$$

where B and F are the concentrations of the bound and free ligand, respectively, ν is the capacity of the binding site and $1/\alpha$ is the affinity constant. In fact, assuming that E is proportional to B, Eq. (2) follows from Eq. (3). A variant of Eq. (2) to incorporate the baseline effect e_0 is

$$E = e_0 + e_{\max} C/(C + c_{50})\,. \quad (4)$$

When the effect decreases response, $e_0 = e_{\max}$ and Eq. (4) has the form

$$E = e_0 - e_0 C/(C + c_{50}) = e_0 c_{50}/(C + c_{50})\,.$$

A convenient surrogate for the drug concentration at an effector site, which is difficult to measure directly, is dose (D). In empirical work, the Emax model is often reformulated as

$$E = e_0 + e_{\max} D/(D + \mathrm{ED}_{50})\,. \tag{5}$$

A more general form of Eq. (2) is

$$E = bX/(X + a)\,. \tag{6}$$

For $b = e_{\max}$, $a = 1$ and $X = (C/c_{50})^{\gamma}$ with $\gamma > 0$, Eq. (6) is called the "Sigmoid-Emax model." While the special case $\gamma = 1$ of such models reduces to Eq. (2), the inclusion of γ gives an additional adjustable parameter in fitting the model from data.

A general Emax model for two drugs, with concentrations C and C^*, incorporating both competitive and noncompetitive interactions is of the form

$$E = e_{\max} \left\{ \frac{(C/c_{50}) + \alpha(C^*/c^*_{50}) + \beta(C/c_{50})(C^*/c^*_{50})}{1 + (C/c_{50}) + (C^*/c^*_{50}) + \delta(C/c_{50})(C^*/c^*_{50})} \right\}, \tag{7}$$

where $0 \le \alpha \le 1$, $0 \le \delta \le 1$, and $\beta \ge 0$ with $\beta = 0$ if $\delta = 0$. In particular, for $\delta = 1$ and $\beta = 1 + \alpha$, the right hand side of Eq. (7) can be written as a sum of $(C/c_{50})/\{1 + (C/c_{50})\}$ and $\alpha(C^*/c^*_{50})/\{1 + (C^*/c^*_{50})\}$, yielding additive effects of the two drugs. The case $\beta = \delta = 0$ gives a "competitive interaction model," which can be written as a linear combination of two terms of the form in Eq. (6) with $b = e_{\max}$ and $(X, a) = (C/c_{50}, 1 + C^*/c^*_{50})$ or $(C^*/c^*_{50}, 1 + C/c_{50})$. The case $\beta > \delta > 0$ shows synergism between the two drugs, while $\delta > \max(\beta, 0)$ shows antagonism. In particular, the case $\beta = 0$ and $\delta = 1$ gives a "non-competitive antagonism model," which can be written as a linear combination of two terms of the form in Eq. (6) with $b = e_{\max}$ and

$$(X, a) = (C/c_{50}, 1 + C^*/c^*_{50} + CC^*/c_{50}c^*_{50}) \quad \text{or}$$

$$(C^*/c^*_{50}, 1 + C/c_{50} + CC^*/c_{50}c^*_{50})\,.$$

Non-competitive antagonism can be explained by using receptor theory as follows. A drug interacts with two sites, one of which activates a receptor which may still interact with a second drug to form another non-activated receptor.

2.2. *PK parameters and their nonparametric estimates*

Several physiologic (e.g. maturation of organs in infants) and pathologic (e.g. kidney failure, heart failure) processes require dosage adjustments in individual patients to modify specific PK parameters. Two basic parameters in this connection are **clearance** (a measure of the ability of the body to eliminate the drug) and **volume of distribution** (a measure of the apparent space in the body available to contain the drug).

Drug clearance principles are similar to clearance concepts in renal physiology, in which creatinine or urea clearance is defined as the rate of elimination of the compound in the urine relative to the plasma concentration. Thus clearance CL of a drug is the rate of elimination by all routes relative to the concentration C of the drug in a biologic fluid:

$$\text{CL} = \text{Rate of elimination}/C\,. \tag{8}$$

The commonly used biologic fluid in Eq. (8) is plasma, for which CL is, strictly speaking, "plasma clearance." When C is C_b (blood concentration) or C_u (unbound or free drug concentration), then Eq. (8) gives "blood clearance" or "clearance based on unbound drug concentration," respectively. In healthy subjects, the clearance of amikacin is 91 ml/min, with 98% of the drug excreted in the urine unchanged. This means that the kidney is able to remove this drug from approximately 89 ml of plasma per minute. Propranolol is cleared at the rate of 840 ml/min, almost exclusively by the liver. This means that the liver is able to remove this drug from 840 ml of plasma per minute. For most drugs, clearance is constant over the plasma or blood concentration range in clinical settings, so the rate of elimination of the drug is proportional to its concentration C, in view of Eq. (8).

Clearance is perhaps the most important PK parameter to be considered in defining a rational drug dosage regimen. In most cases, the clinician would like to maintain steady-state drug concentrations C_{ss} within a known therapeutic window. Steady state will be achieved when the dosing rate (rate of active drug entering the systemic circulation) equals the rate of drug elimination. Therefore,

$$\text{Dosing rate} = \text{CL} \times C_{ss}\,. \tag{9}$$

The two major sites of drug elimination are the kidneys and the liver. Clearance of unchanged drug in the urine represents renal clearance. Within the liver, drug elimination occurs via biotransformation of the drug to one or more metabolites, or excretion of unchanged drug into the bile, or both. When no other organs are involved in elimination of the drug,

$\mathrm{CL} = \mathrm{CL}_{\mathrm{renal}} + \mathrm{CL}_{\mathrm{liver}}$ since the liver and kidneys work in parallel. The rate of elimination of a drug by a single organ can be defined in terms of the blood flow entering and exiting from the organ and the concentration of drug in the blood. The rate of presentation of the drug to the organ is the product of blood flow (Q) and entering drug concentration (C_i), while the rate of exit of drug from the organ is the product of blood flow and exiting drug concentration (C_o). The difference between these rates at steady state is the rate of drug elimination:

$$\text{Rate of elimination} = Q \times C_i - Q \times C_o\,. \tag{10}$$

Dividing Eq. (10) by the concentration C_i of the drug entering the organ yields

$$\mathrm{CL}_{\mathrm{organ}} = \frac{Q \times C_i - Q \times C_o}{C_i} = Q \times \frac{C_i - C_o}{C_i}\,. \tag{11}$$

The expression $(C_i - C_o)/C_i$ is called the extraction ratio (ER) of the drug.

Bioavailability is the fraction of unchanged drug reaching the systemic circulation after its administration by any route. For an intravenous dose of the drug, bioavailability is 1. For a drug administered orally, bioavailability may be less than 1 since the drug may be incompletely absorbed, or metabolized in the gut, the portal blood or the liver prior to entry into the systemic circulation. If a drug is metabolized in the liver or excreted in bile, some of the active drug absorbed from the gastrointestinal tract will be inactivated by hepatic processes before the drug can reach the general circulation and be distributed to its sites of action. If the metabolizing or biliary excreting capacity of the liver is great, the so-called "first-pass effect" on the extent of availability will be substantial. The systemic bioavailability (F) of a drug that is completely absorbed and eliminated only by metabolism in the liver is given by

$$F = 1 - \mathrm{ER}\,, \tag{12}$$

where $\mathrm{ER} = \mathrm{CL}_{\mathrm{liver}}/Q_{\mathrm{liver}}$ is the hypatic extraction ratio.

The **AUC** (area under the plasma or blood concentration-time curve) is a commonly used measure of the extent of absorption or availability of the drug absorbed in the body. It is usually calculated using the trapezoidal rule based on the blood or plasma concentrations obtained at various blood sampling times. Yeh and Kwan[8] considered spline and Lagrange interpolation schemes in lieu of the linear interpolation implied by the trapezoidal rule and compared these methods. Let $C_0, C_1, \ldots, C_k$ be the plasma or blood concentrations obtained at times $0, t_1, \ldots, t_k$, respectively. The AUC from time 0 to t_k, denoted by AUC_{0,t_k}, can be obtained via the trapezoidal rule as

$$\mathrm{AUC}_{0,t_k} = \sum_{i=1}^{k} (t_i - t_{i-1})(C_i + C_{i-1})/2\,. \tag{13}$$

Typically t_k should be chosen so that C_k does not fall below the so-called "limit of quantitation" (LOQ) that will be defined in Sec. 4. In principle, the AUC should be calculated from 0 to ∞ (not just to the time of the last blood sample), and the portion of the remaining area from t_k to ∞ can be large. An estimate of AUC ($= \mathrm{AUC}_{0,\infty}$) is

$$\mathrm{AUC} = \mathrm{AUC}_{0,t_k} + C_k e^{-\lambda t_k}/\lambda\,, \tag{14}$$

where λ, called the *elimination rate constant* is estimated from the elimination phase of the graph of log-concentration versus time by linear regression, assuming that it is linear so that λ corresponds to the slope of the fitted regression line; (see Ref. 2, Chapter 3 and Appendix A). The United States Food and Drug Administration (FDA) regulations require that sampling be continued through at least 3 half-lives of the active drug ingredient, measured in blood or urine, so that the remaining area beyond time t_k is only a small proportion of AUC_{0,t_k}.

The AUC also provides a simple relationship between the volume of distribution and dose. The volume of distribution (V) is defined as

$$V = \text{Amount of drug in body}/C\,, \tag{15}$$

where C is the concentration of the drug in blood or plasma, depending on the fluid measured. It reflects the apparent space available in both the general circulation and the tissue of distribution. It does not represent a real volume but should be regarded as the size of the pool of blood fluids that would be required if the drug were distributed equally throughout all parts of the body. From mass balance and steady state considerations, V is related to clearance via $\mathrm{CL} = \lambda V$, where λ is the elimination rate constant in Eq. (14). Moreover, $F \times \mathrm{Dose} = \mathrm{CL} \times \mathrm{AUC}$ (= total amount eliminated), where F is the systematic bioavailability in Eq. (12).[2] Hence,

$$V = \mathrm{CL}/\lambda = (F \times \mathrm{Dose})/(\lambda \times \mathrm{AUC})\,. \tag{16}$$

Besides CL, V, and AUC (measuring bioavailability), another PK variable, called the **elimination half-life** and denoted by $t_{1/2}$, has to be considered when designing drug dosage regimens. It is given by

$$\mathrm{t}_{1/2} = (\ell n2)/\lambda = 0.693\ V/\mathrm{CL} \tag{17}$$

and corresponds to the time taken for the concentration to drop to half of its initial level, assuming a one-compartment model for the drug's elimination phase in the body, as is usually done in designing drug dosage regimens.

In view of Eq. (17), $\mathrm{t}_{1/2}$ can be estimated by $(\ell n2)/\hat{\lambda}$, where $\hat{\lambda}$ is an estimate of the elimination rate constant described after Eq. (14). When $F = 1$, we can estimate CL by $\widehat{\mathrm{CL}} = \mathrm{Dose}/\mathrm{AUC}$. Without assuming F to be 1, we have to replace Dose above by $\hat{F} \times \mathrm{Dose}$, where $\hat{F}$ is an estimate of F. Once CL has been estimated, we can estimate V by $\widehat{\mathrm{CL}}/\hat{\lambda}$. To estimate F, we need additional data following an intravenous dose D^*, yielding AUC^* and whose F^* can be assumed to be 1. Then F can be estimated from the original (extravascular) dose D and AUC by

$$\hat{F} = \min\left\{\frac{\mathrm{AUC}/D}{\mathrm{AUC}^*/D^*}, 1\right\}.$$

The above PK parameters are considered in a single dose trial. In practice, drugs are most commonly prescribed to be taken at fixed and equal time intervals, each of width τ. The maximum, minimum, and average concentration of the drug in steady state, denoted by $C_{ss,\max}$, $C_{ss,\min}$ and $C_{ss,av}$, respectively, are considered in conjunction with the steady-state volume of distribution and AUC during a dosing interval in steady state. See Chapter 7 of Rowland and Tozer,[2] which also shows how to develop a dosage regimen from knowledge of these PK parameters and the therapeutic window of a drug. Data obtained on multiple dosing can be used to estimate the PK parameters of a drug as follows. The most useful information derived from a multiple dosing study is the ratio of clearance to availability. It is obtained from

$$\frac{\mathrm{CL}}{F} = \frac{(\mathrm{Dose}/\tau)}{C_{ss,av}}, \tag{18}$$

where $C_{ss,av}$ is determined from the area under the plasma concentration-time curve within a dosing interval at steady state divided by τ. Occasionally, the drug is given as a multiple intravenous regimen, in which case the ratio $(\mathrm{Dose}/\tau)/C_{ss,av}$ is simply clearance, since $F = 1$. The accuracy of the clearance estimate depends on the number of plasma concentrations measured in the dosing interval and on the ratio of $\tau/\mathrm{t}_{1/2}$. The estimate can be improved by using several dosing intervals in steady state. Equation (18) is also useful for determining the relative availability of a drug administered extravascularly, between two treatments (e.g. dosage forms) A and B. Assuming that clearance remains unchanged, we have

$$\text{Relative availability} = \frac{(C_{ss,av})_B}{(C_{ss,av})_A} \cdot \frac{(\text{Dose}/\tau)_A}{(\text{Dose}/\tau)_B} . \tag{19}$$

2.3. *Parametric and population PK/PD models*

The nonparametric estimates of PK parameters described above assume that the blood (or urine) samples are collected frequently through at least 3 half-lives of the active ingredient, so that the curve between successive times t_k and t_{k+1} is well approximated by the line joining its values at these two points. When the experiment does not meet such conditions, the nonparametric estimates of AUC, CL and $t_{1/2}$ become unreliable and there are no satisfactory ways to evaluate the bias and standard error of such estimate. In this case it is preferable to use a parametric approach, based on the commonly used one-compartment model

$$y_j = \frac{Dk_a}{V(k_a - k_e)}(e^{-k_e t_j} - e^{-k_a t_j}) + \epsilon_j , \quad 1 \le j \le n , \tag{20}$$

in which y_j is the concentration at time t_j after the administration of a single oral dose D. Here V, k_a, k_e are the volume of distribution, absorption rate constant and elimination rate constant, respectively. Note that model (20) has the form of a bi-exponential model $\alpha_1 e^{-\lambda_1 t} + \alpha_2 e^{-\lambda_2 t}$ with $\alpha_1 = \alpha_2$.

Lai[7] gives a review of the literature on fitting the poly-exponential regression model $y_j = \beta + \sum_{k=1}^{k} \alpha_k e^{-\lambda_k t_j} + \epsilon_j$, in which the errors ϵ_j are assumed to be independent with zero means and

(i) $\text{var}(\epsilon_j) = \sigma^2$ (constant variance error models), or
(ii) $\text{var}(\epsilon_j) = f_\theta^2(t_j)\sigma^2$ (constant coefficient of variation error models), or
(iii) $\text{var}(\epsilon_j) = f_\theta(t_j)\sigma^2$ (Poisson-type error models),

where $\theta = (\lambda_1, \ldots, \lambda_k; \alpha_1, \ldots, \alpha_k, \beta)$ and $f_\theta(t) = \beta + \sum \alpha_k e^{-\lambda_k t}$. We can estimate θ by weighted least squares, i.e. by minimizing

$$S(\theta) = \sum_{j=1}^{n} w_j [y_j - f_\theta(t_j)]^2 . \tag{21}$$

For fixed $\lambda_1, \ldots, \lambda_k$, $f_\theta(t)$ is linear in the parameters $\beta, \alpha_1, \ldots, \alpha_k$ and standard formulas in multiple linear regression can be used to find least squares estimates of the linear parameters $\beta, \alpha_1, \ldots, \alpha_k$. This reduces the problem of minimizing $S(\theta)$ to that of minimizing

$$S^*(\lambda_1, \ldots, \lambda_k) = \min_{\beta, \alpha_1, \ldots, \alpha_k} S(\theta).$$

In the case of the Poisson-type or constant coefficient of variation error model, the weights w_j also involve the unknown parameter θ and can be determined at each iteration from the previous iterate. It is shown in Lai[7] that S^* not only provides a relatively stable numerical algorithm for finding the least squares estimates but also sheds light on the range of models that are compatible with the data. Depending on the experimental design, S^* can be very flat over a broad region containing the minimum or can decrease steeply to the minimum. It is also shown in Lai[7] that although the parameter vector θ may be poorly estimated because S^* is relatively flat, the function $f_\theta(\cdot)$ is typically well estimated by weighted least squares. Therefore derived parameters like AUC can still be well estimated from the estimated $f_{\hat{\theta}}$ even though $\hat{\theta}$ does not estimate θ well because of the experimental design.

Parametric modeling also facilitates the evaluation of standard errors and construction of confidence intervals. For the Emax model (2), which can be rewritten as $E/C = aE + b$ with $a = -1/c_{50}$ and $b = e_{\max}/c_{50}$, Scatchard[9] proposed to estimate a and b by linear regression of the observed E/C on C. This simple method is usually adequate for point estimation because of the large signal-to-noise ratio in the measurements. It is, however, unsatisfactory for constructing confidence intervals of the unknown parameters, as has been noted in the ligand-binding literature related to the mathematically equivalent model (3). Lai and Zhang[10] give a review of the literature and propose a new approach using nonlinear least squares and bootstrap methods to construct confidence regions for the parameters. The numerical studies reported in Lai and Zhang[10] show that these confidence regions are markedly different from the elliptical confidence regions based on asymptotic normal approximations.

So far we have considered estimation of the PK/PD parameters of a subject from the data in a study on the subject. In many PK/PD studies, however, data are collected from a number of subjects, some of whom may have intensive blood sampling while others only have sparse data. A primary objective of these studies is to study the PK/PD characteristics of the entire population, such as how they vary with certain covariates. This requires embedding the individual parametric PK/PD models in a population model. For example, the y_j in model (20) are now replaced by y_{ij}, where i denotes the subject number. Since the dose, volume of distribution, absorption and elimination rate constants may vary from subject to subject, we also have to replace D, V, k_a, k_e, n by D_i, V_i, k_{ai}, k_{ei} and n_i in model (20). Let θ_i be the vector consisting of the logarithms of the PK parameters V_i, k_{ai}, k_{ei}. The unknown θ_i may vary with certain covariates, such as the subject's age and body weight. How can the individual subjects' data be used to analyze such relationships for the target population, of which the subjects can be regarded as a sample? We shall show that nonlinear mixed effects modeling provides a valuable tool to address this problem.

Returning to the PD model (2), the variable C refers to concentration at an effector (tissue) site. It is usually impossible to measure C directly, so some surrogate for C has to be used, as in model (5). On the other hand, if one has a kinetic model for C, then it can be used to impute the value of C from the blood/urine measurements. Chapter 9 of Davidian and Giltinan[11] illustrates how population PK/PD models can be synthesized for such tasks.

2.4. *Nonlinear mixed effects models*

The preceding population PK/PD models are special cases of nonlinear mixed effects models (NONMEM) of the form

$$y_{ij} = f_i(t_{ij}, \theta_i) + \varepsilon_{ij}\,, \quad \theta_i = g(x_i, \beta) + b_i \ (1 \le j \le n_i, 1 \le i \le K)\,, \tag{22}$$

in which θ_i is a $1 \times r$ vector of the ith subject's parameters whose regression function on the subject's observed covariate x_i is given by $g(x_i, \beta)$ with $1 \times s$ parameter vector β, which is the "fixed effect" to be estimated. The "random effects" b_i in model (22) are assumed to be independent and identically distributed, having common distribution G with mean 0. The ith subject's response y_{ij} at t_{ij} has mean $f_i(t_{ij}, \theta_i)$, in which f_i is a known function. Given θ_i, the random errors ε_{ij} are assumed to be normal with mean 0 and standard deviation $\sigma w(\theta_i)$, in which w is a given function and σ is an unknown parameter. The regression function g relates θ_i to the ith subject's physiologic characteristics that constitute the covariate vector x_i in model (22). The first equation of (22) is often called the *individual measurement model* and the second equation the *population structure model.* The population distribution G is usually assumed to be normal with mean 0 and covariance matrix Σ so that β, σ, Σ can be estimated by maximum likelihood. However, unlike linear mixed effects models in which the normal assumption on G yields closed-form expressions of the likelihood, the normality of G in nonlinear mixed effects models leads to computationally intensive likelihoods that involve K integrals. A commonly used approach, as adopted in the software package NONMEM[12] or the `nlme` procedure in S-Plus, is to develop iterative schemes based on first-order approximations of $f_i(t_{ij}, g(x_i, \beta) + b_i)$ in model (22) so that the normal assumption on G can be used to reduce the problem to that of a linear Gaussian mixed effects model at each iterative step.

Unless otherwise stated, we shall assume throughout the sequel that the random errors ε_{ij} in model (22) have common variance σ^2 (so $w(\theta) \equiv 1$). The likelihood function $L(\beta, \sigma, \Sigma)$ is proportional to

$$|\Sigma|^{-K/2} \prod_{i=1}^{K} \int_{\mathbb{R}^r} \sigma^{-n_i} \times \exp\left\{ -\frac{1}{2\sigma^2} \sum_{j=1}^{n_i} [y_{ij} - f_i(t_{ij}, g(x_i, \beta) + b_i)]^2 - \frac{1}{2} b_i \Sigma^{-1} b_i^T \right\} db_i\,, \tag{23}$$

where $|\Sigma|$ denotes the determinant of Σ. For the case of more general $w(\theta_i)$, simply replace σ in model (23) by $\sigma w(g(x_i, \beta) + b_i)$. Computing the maximum likelihood estimate of (β, σ, Σ) via numerical integration and nonlinear optimization becomes difficult for large K. Letting $\eta = (\sigma, \Sigma)$, Lindstrom and Bates[13] proposed the following iterative procedure that involves successive linear approximations to $f_i(t_{ij}, g(x_i, \beta) + b)$. At the mth iteration, the Lindstrom–Bates procedure consists of a pseudo-data step and a linear mixed effects (LME) step.

(a) *The pseudo-data step*: Given the current estimate $\hat{\eta}^{(m)}$ of η, compute $\hat{\beta}^{(m)} = \hat{\beta}(\hat{\eta}^{(m)})$ and $\hat{b}_i^{(m)} = \hat{b}_i(\hat{\eta}^{(m)})$, $1 \le i \le K$, that jointly minimize

$$\sum_{i=1}^{K} \{(\hat{\sigma}^{(m)})^{-2} S_i(b, \beta) + b_i(\hat{\Sigma}^{(m)})^{-1} b_i^T/2\}\,, \quad \text{where}$$

$$S_i(\beta, b) = \sum_{j=1}^{n_i} [y_{ij} - f_i(t_{ij}, g(x_i, \beta) + b)]^2 \Big/ 2\,. \tag{24}$$

This can be carried out by modifying a standard nonlinear least squares routine; see Sec. 6.1 of Lindstrom and Bates.[13] Define the $s \times n_i$, $r \times n_i$ and

$1 \times n_i$ matrices

$$X_i^{(m)} = \left(\frac{\partial f_i}{\partial \beta}(t_{ij}, g(x_i, \beta) + \hat{b}_i^{(m)})|_{\beta = \hat{\beta}^{(m)}} \right)_{1 \le j \le n_i},$$

$$Z_i^{(m)} = \left(\frac{\partial f_i}{\partial b_i}(t_{ij}, g(x_i, \hat{\beta}^{(m)}) + b_i)|_{b_i = \hat{b}_i^{(m)}} \right)_{1 \le j \le n_i},$$

$$Y_i^{(m)} = (y_{ij} - f_i(t_{ij}, g(x_i, \hat{\beta}^{(m)}) + \hat{b}_i^{(m)}))_{1 \le j \le n_i} + \hat{\beta}^{(m)} X_i^{(m)} + \hat{b}_i^{(m)} Z_i^{(m)}.$$

(b) *The LME step*: Linear approximation to $f_i(t_{ij}, g(x_i, \beta) + b_i)$ around $(\hat{\beta}^{(m)}, \hat{b}_i^{(m)})$ leads to the linear mixed effects model

$$Y_i^{(m)} = \beta X_i^{(m)} + b_i Z_i^{(m)} + (\varepsilon_{i1}, \ldots, \varepsilon_{in_i}). \tag{25}$$

The integrals in expression (23) for the likelihood function of the linear mixed effects model (25), instead of model (22), have closed-form expressions, yielding maximum likelihood estimates of the form

$$\hat{\beta} = \left(\sum_{i=1}^{K} Y_i^{(m)} V_{i,m}^{-1} X_i^{(m)T} \right) \left(\sum_{i=1}^{K} X_i^{(m)} V_{i,m}^{-1} X_i^{(m)T} \right)^{-1}, \tag{26}$$

where $V_{i,m} = Z_i^{(m)T} \hat{\Sigma} Z_i^{(m)} + \hat{\sigma}^2 I_{n_i}$ and $\hat{\eta} = (\hat{\sigma}, \hat{\Sigma})$ is computed via the Newton–Raphson algorithm to maximize the likelihood; see Sec. 6.2 of Lindstrom and Bates[13] where a restricted maximum likelihood (REML) variant of the procedure is also given.

Several alternatives to the linearization approach have been proposed in the literature. One is Monte Carlo integration, whose accuracy and computational complexity depend critically on how and how many samples are drawn. Importance sampling and periodic updating of the importance weights during iterative maximization of the likelihood have been proposed.[14–16] Another alternative, proposed by Pinheiro and Bates,[17] is to use an adaptive version of Gaussian quadrature based on ideas similar to importance sampling in Monte Carlo integration. A third approach is to use MCEM (Monte Carlo EM) in which the E-step of the usual EM algorithm is replaced by an empirical estimate based on a random sample generated from the conditional distribution.[15]

Instead of applying Monte Carlo methods to compute the integrals in the likelihood function to be maximized in the maximum likelihood approach, it seems more direct to apply Markov Chain Monte Carlo (MCMC) to evaluate the posterior distribution of (β, σ, Σ) when *a prior* distribution on these parameters is assumed. MCMC enables one to generate a sequence of random samples whose limiting distribution is the target distribution (in this case the posterior distribution of (β, σ, Σ)) and thereby avoids the calculation of normalizing constants and the numerical integration associated with any probability statements of interest. The most popular MCMC method used in the mixed effects model framework is the Gibbs sampler. This is because the (hierarchical) Bayes model allows a natural grouping of the vector of all unknown or unobserved parameters into subvectors β, σ, Σ and $(\theta_i,\ i = 1, \ldots, n)$, where drawing samples for each component is much easier than drawing samples for the whole vector. Successful usage of Gibbs sampler for NONMEM in population PK studies has been reported in Refs. 11, 18–22. The relative efficiencies of different MCMC procedures have been investigated by Bennett *et al.*[23] and Shih.[24] In addition to considerations in choosing transition functions, there are other practical issues one has to deal with when implementing MCMC, such as the number of chains to run, the length of burn-in sequences, and how to monitor convergence. These are no general answers to these questions and they often need to be addressed empirically by numerical experiments; see Chapter 26.

The normality assumption on the population distribution G has been weakened by Davidian and Gallant,[25] who assume that G has a density function of the form of a product of a multivariate normal $N(0, \Sigma)$ density function and the square of a polynomial of degree p, which was introduced in another context and called the "smooth nonparametric" (SNP) model by Gallant and Nychka.[26] The coefficients of the polynomial and the components of the matrix Σ can be estimated by maximum likelihood, while the degree p of the polynomial can be chosen via standard model selection criteria like BIC, AIC or the Hannan-Quinn criterion. Magder and Zeger[27] proposed an alternative method that uses mixtures of normals, while Fattinger *et al.*[28] modeled each component of b_i as a data-dependent monotone spline transformation of the corresponding component of a multivariate normal vector. All these methods require considerably more intensive computation to maximize the likelihood function than the case of normal G assumed before.

Since the normality assumption on G only provides numerically tractable maximum likelihood estimates after various approximations and since attempts to relax that assumption have led to even more computationally intensive procedures, a natural alternative is to try estimating G nonparametrically (by a distribution with finite support, with the number of support points depending on the sample size). However, even for the simple case $n_i \equiv n$ and $f_i(t_{ij}, \theta_i) = \theta_i$ with known β and σ, it is difficult to estimate G well since the optimal rate of convergence of the estimate to G is very slow when G has a smooth density function, as pointed out by Carroll and Hall[29] and Fan.[30] When G has fixed support, Chen[31] showed that the optimal convergence rate is $K^{-1/2}$ if the number of support points is known but decreases to $K^{-1/4}$ otherwise as $K \to \infty$. Lindsay[32] showed that the nonparametric maximum likelihood estimate $\hat{G}$ of G is unique and discrete, with no more than K support points, and Mallet[33] made use of this and other properties of $\hat{G}$ to develop an algorithm to compute $\hat{G}$. The situation becomes considerably worse when σ and β are unknown and $f_i(t_{ij}, \theta_i)$ is nonlinear in θ_i, for which little is known about the performance of nonparametric estimates and it is also difficult to compute $\hat{G}$.

One way to ensure that β and σ can be well estimated is to require the dataset to contain a subset from subjects whose θ_i can be well estimated. This idea was introduced in the work of Ibragimov and Has'minskii[34] who consider estimation of (α, G) from independent random variables $y_1, \ldots, y_J$ such that the conditional density function of y_i given θ_i has the parametric form $f_\alpha(\cdot|\theta_i)$, in the presence of another "direct" sample $\theta_1, \ldots, \theta_I$ from G. Let $K = I + J$. They show that under certain regularity conditions, a variant of the nonparametric maximum likelihood estimate that is initialized at a $\sqrt{n}$-consistent estimate of (α, G) is asymptotically efficient. Their model of the data $\{\theta_1, \ldots, \theta_I; y_1, \ldots, y_J\}$ is commonly called the Ibragimov-Has'minskii (IH) model. We shall relax the model assumptions and extend them to our setting, providing what will be called an "Ibragimov-Has'minskii (IH) environment."

In an IH environment, there are I $(\leq K)$ subjects whose θ_i can be well estimated by the nonlinear least squares estimate $\tilde{\theta}_i$ based on (y_{ij}, t_{ij}), $1 \leq j \leq n_i$. Without loss of generality we can assume that these are the first I subjects. We can determine from the data the standard error of each component of $\tilde{\theta}_i$ using the asymptotic formulas in nonlinear regression.[35] The ith study is deemed "good" if all components of $\tilde{\theta}_i$ have reasonably small standard errors relative to their absolute values. A consistent estimate of σ^2 is given by

$$\tilde{\sigma}^2 = \sum_{i=1}^{I} \sum_{j=1}^{n_i} (w(\tilde{\theta}_i))^{-2} (y_{ij} - f_i(t_{ij}, \tilde{\theta}_i))^2 \Big/ \sum_{i=1}^{I} (n_i - r) . \qquad (27)$$

Such IH environments arise in most population PK studies, which use combined data from several Phases I, II and III trials. The subjects in

Phase I trials are usually healthy volunteers or patients with the intent-to-treat disease, from whom intensive blood sampling is conducted, and thus provide natural candidates for good studies.

Lai and Shih[36] developed the following iterative scheme to compute the MLE of (β, σ, G) in an IH environment. First note that in the case $w(\theta) \equiv 1$ the likelihood function is proportional to

$$L(\beta, \sigma, G) = \prod_{i=1}^{K} \sigma^{-n_i} \sum_{m=1}^{M} \alpha_m \times \exp\left\{ -\frac{1}{2\sigma^2} \sum_{j=1}^{n_i} [y_{ij} - f_i(t_{ij}, g(x_i, \beta) + \zeta_m)]^2 \right\} \tag{28}$$

when G has a finite support $\{\zeta_1, \ldots, \zeta_M\}$ and puts mass α_m at ζ_m. For the case of more general $w(\theta_i)$, simply replace σ in model (28) by $\sigma w(g(w_i, \beta) + \zeta_m)$. The initial estimate $(\hat{\beta}^{(0)}, \hat{\sigma}^{(0)}, \hat{G}^{(0)})$ is obtained as follows: Let $\hat{\sigma}^{(0)} = \tilde{\sigma}$ and $\hat{\beta}^{(0)}$ be the least squares estimate $\hat{\beta}^{(0)}$ which minimizes $\sum_{i=1}^{I} (\widetilde{\theta}_i - g(x_i, \beta))^T (\widetilde{\theta}_i - g(x_i, \beta))$. Let $\widetilde{b}_i = \widetilde{\theta}_i - g(x_i, \hat{\beta}^{(0)})$, $1 \le i \le I$, denote the residuals, and let $\widehat{b}_i = \widetilde{b}_i - (\sum_{j=1}^{I} \widetilde{b}_j)/I$ be the centered residuals. Let $\hat{G}^{(0)}$ be the distribution putting weight $1/I$ at each centered residual. $(\hat{\beta}, \hat{\sigma}, \hat{G})$ is computed via an iterative procedure in which the following two steps are used to compute $(\hat{\beta}^{(k)}, \hat{\sigma}^{(k)}, \hat{G}^{(k)})$ from $(\hat{\beta}^{(k-1)}, \hat{\sigma}^{(k-1)}, \hat{G}^{(k-1)})$; see Ref. 36 where a termination criterion and numerical examples are given.

Step 1. Suppose $\hat{G}^{(k-1)}$ puts mass α_j at ζ_j $(j = 1, \ldots, M_{k-1})$. Find the maximizer $(\hat{\beta}^{(k)}, \hat{\sigma}^{(k)})$ of $L(\beta, \sigma, \hat{G}^{(k-1)})$.

Step 2. Use Mallet's algorithm[33] to maximize $L(\hat{\beta}^{(k)}, \hat{\sigma}^{(k)}, G)$ over the set of distributions G with no more than K support points.

2.5. *Empirical Bayes methods for individualization and diagnostics*

We now consider the prediction problem of estimating a function $h(\theta)$ of the unobservable parameter θ for a new subject with covariate x and from whom some data have been collected. For example, in population PK studies, it is believed that efficacy and toxicity of a drug are directly related to the drug concentrations at the target site, which are generally not available but for which blood concentrations are often good surrogates; therefore the criteria for designing the dosing regimen for a specific subject often involve functions of individual concentrations, or equivalently, functions of the individual parameter θ. The subject's data are often too sparse to provide an adequate estimate $\hat{\theta}$ of θ so that $h(\hat{\theta})$ can be used to estimate $h(\theta)$. If β, σ and G are known, then a natural estimate of $h(\theta)$ in the mixed effects model is the posterior mean $E_{\beta,\sigma^2,G}[h(\theta)\,|\,\text{subject's data}]$. Without assuming β, σ^2 and G to be known, the empirical Bayes approach in Ref. 37 replaces them by their estimates $\hat{\beta}$, $\hat{\sigma}^2$, $\hat{G}$ from the K studies so that $h(\theta)$ is estimated by

$$\widehat{h(\theta)} = E_{\hat{\beta},\hat{\sigma}^2,\hat{G}}[h(\theta)\,|\,\text{subject's data}]\,. \tag{29}$$

This idea of borrowing information from other subjects is in fact one of the main motivations for building population structure models. In particular, because of ethical and practical reasons, intensive blood sampling is often not feasible for clinical patients, for whom this individualization of dosing regimen can be obtained by combining the patient's sparse data and characteristics (as measured by x) with the large database for the population model.

Empirical Bayes ideas can also be used to derive diagnostics for the regression model (22). If the individual parameters θ_i were observed, the residuals $r_i = \theta_i - g(x_i, \hat{\beta})$ would provide approximations for the unobservable i.i.d. random variables b_i. Therefore substantial deviation of these residuals from i.i.d. patterns would suggest inadequacies and possible improvements of the assumed regression model. Since the θ_i are not observed, we propose to replace them by the empirical Bayes estimate $E_{\hat{\beta},\hat{\sigma}^2,\hat{G}}(\theta_i\,|\,y_{i1},\ldots,y_{in_i},t_i,x_i)$, leading to:

$$\hat{r}_i = E_{(\hat{\beta},\hat{\sigma}^2,\hat{G})}(\theta_i\,|\,y_{i1},\ldots,y_{in_i},t_i,x_i) - g(x_i,\hat{\beta})\,, \quad i = 1,\ldots,K\,. \tag{30}$$

The $\hat{r}_i$ can be interpreted as estimates of the independent zero-mean random variables $r_i = E_{(\beta,\sigma^2,G)}(\theta_i\,|\,y_{i1},\ldots,y_{in_i},t_i,x_i) - g(x_i,\beta)$.

Instead of using the posterior mean in Eq. (30), it is popular in population PK studies to use the posterior mode

$$\hat{s}_i = \arg\max_{b_i} p_{(\hat{\beta},\hat{\sigma}^2,\hat{G})}(b_i\,|\,y_{i1},\ldots,y_{in_i},t_i,w_i) \tag{31}$$

to form the residuals $\hat{s}_i - g(x_i,\hat{\beta})$. This was first suggested by Maitre *et al.*[38] in connection with linearization methods under the assumption of normality for the population distribution, but is also used as a general strategy in the semiparametric models of Davidian and Gallant[25] and the hierarchical Bayesian models of Wakefield and Racine-Poon.[39] For linear Gaussian mixed effects models, the mean and the mode of the conditional distribution of θ_i given $y_{i1}, \ldots, y_{in_i}$ coincide since the conditional distribution is Gaussian, so the theoretical justification for the r_i via an empirical Bayes point of view applies also to the s_i. In the case of nonlinear mixed effects models, the posterior mean and mode no longer coincide, and $\hat{r}_i$ is usually easier to compute and more robust. In the above empirical Bayes approach, we have replaced (β, σ^2, G) in the posterior mean $E_{\beta,\sigma^2,G}[h(\theta) \mid \text{subject's data}]$ by an estimate $(\hat{\beta}, \hat{\sigma}^2, \hat{G})$. This estimate $(\hat{\beta}, \hat{\sigma}^2, \hat{G})$ can be either parametric, as in Lindstrom and Bates,[13] or nonparametric, as given above.

We next list some examples of using empirical Bayes/hierarchical Bayes/posterior mode estimates in NONMEM to quantify covariate effects on PK parameters in the literature:

(a) Population PK analysis of felbamate in epileptic patients[40]: Apparent clearance of felbamate was found to decrease with age for children (age ≤ 12) and to stay relatively constant beyond 13 years of age. There were 1–17 blood samples per subject. This study, undertaken by Zhu and his collaborators at Schering-Plough Research Institute and Wallace Laboratories, led to the FDA approval of the labeling of felbamate for its prescription to children.

(b) Population PK analysis of quindine in hospitalized patients treated for atrial fibrillation over ventricular arrhythmias[19,25,41]: The effects of dichotomized creatinine clearance, body weight and α_1-acid glucoprotein concentration on clearance were analyzed from a study consisting of 1–11 blood samples per subject.

(c) Population PK analysis of phenobarbital in neonates[11,25,42]: The effects of birth weight and 5-minute Apgar score on clearance and volume were analyzed from a study with sparse PK data in each subject (having only 1–6 concentration measurements).

Model validation methodology for population PK analysis is still in its infancy. One commonly used approach is to use m-fold cross-validation or bootstrap to estimate the prediction errors based on a fitted model. Here the prediction error may be associated with prediction of concentrations or prediction of PK parameters (that can be estimated nonparametrically only from subjects with intensive measurements). Given the computational complexity associated with fitting nonlinear mixed effects models, m-fold cross-validation (with $m \leq 20$) appears to be more feasible than the bootstrap (for which the FDA recommends using at least 200 bootstrap samples).

2.6. *The Lindstrom–Bates algorithm and related statistical methods*

Vonesh[43] proposed an alternative to the Lindstrom–Bates algorithm (consisting of the pseudo-data and LME steps described in Sec. 2.4) by applying, for fixed β and η, Laplace's asymptotic formula

$$\int_{\mathbb{R}^r} e^{l(b)}\, db \sim (2\pi)^{r/2} | -\ddot{l}(\hat{b})|^{-1/2} e^{l(\hat{b})} \tag{32}$$

to each integral in expression (23), where $\ddot{l}$ denotes the Hessian matrix of second partial derivatives of l and $\hat{b}$ maximizes $l(b)$. Earlier, Wolfinger[44] derived the pseudo-data step of the Lindstrom–Bates algorithm by applying for fixed η Laplace's asymptotic formula to the multiple integral

$$\int \cdots \int \exp\left\{ \sum_{i=1}^{K} l_i(b_i;\beta) \right\} d\beta db_1 db_2 \cdots db_K\,, \tag{33}$$

and then used a Gauss–Newton approximation of $-\ddot{l}$ to derive the REML version of the LME step. Laplace's asymptotic formula has also been used by Breslow and Clayton[45] and Lee and Nelder[46] to derive their estimators in *generalized linear mixed models* (GLMM) and *hierarchical generalized linear models* (HGLM), respectively. The HGLM involves independent random vectors (y_i, x_i^T, z_i^T) such that the conditional density function of y_i given a $1 \times K$ vector of random effects b has the GLM (generalized linear model) form

$$f(y|b, z_i, x_i) = c(y, \phi) \exp\{(\theta_i y - \psi(\theta_i))/a(\phi)\}\,, \tag{34}$$

in which ϕ is a dispersion parameter, θ_i is the canonical parameter such that $E(y|b, z_i, x_i) = g(\beta x_i + b z_i)$ and g is the inverse of a monotone link function. Letting f_α be the density function of b with unknown parameter α, Lee and Nelder[46] define the hierarchical likelihood (h-likelihood) by

$$h(b, \beta, \phi, \alpha) = \log f_\alpha(b) + \sum_{i=1}^{n} \log f(y_i|b, z_i, x_i)\,. \tag{35}$$

They propose to estimate β, ϕ, α by an iterative procedure whose mth iteration consists of the following two steps:

(i) Given the current estimate $(\hat{\phi}^{(m)}, \hat{\alpha}^{(m)})$ of (ϕ, α), compute the maximizer $(\hat{b}^{(m)}, \hat{\beta}^{(m)})$ of $h(b, \beta, \hat{\phi}^{(m)}, \hat{\alpha}^{(m)})$ by solving the score equations $\partial h/\partial \beta = 0$ and $\partial h/\partial b = 0$.

(ii) Given the current estimate $(\hat{b}^{(m)}, \hat{\beta}^{(m)})$ of (b, β), maximize the adjusted profile h-likelihood $h_A(\phi, \alpha) = h(\hat{b}^{(m)}, \hat{\beta}^{(m)}, \phi, \alpha) + (\log |2\pi\phi H^{-1}|)/2$ with

$$H = \left. \begin{pmatrix} \partial^2 h/\partial\beta^2 & \partial^2 h/\partial\beta\partial b \\ \partial^2 h/\partial b\partial\beta & \partial^2 h/\partial b^2 \end{pmatrix} \right|_{(b,\beta)=(\hat{b}^{(m)}, \hat{\beta}^{(m)})},$$

by solving the score equations $\partial h_A/\partial\phi = 0$ and $\partial h_A/\partial\alpha = 0$.

For the special case of normal f_α with mean 0 and covariance matrix $\Sigma(\alpha)$, the HGLM reduces to the GLMM considered by Breslow and Clayton[45] who make use of the normality assumption to come up with an explicit expression for Laplace's approximation to the likelihood function $\int e^{h(b,\beta,\phi,\alpha)} db$, yielding an algorithm similar to that of Lindstrom and Bates for NONMEM. The Lee-Nelder procedure above is somewhat different and is motivated by generalizing Henderson's[47] joint likelihood for linear models with normal random effects. It can be derived by applying Lapalce's approximation to $\int\int e^{h(b,\beta,\phi,\alpha)} db d\beta$, analogous to integral (33).

Let β_0 and σ_0 denote the true values of β and σ. A sufficient condition for the validity of Laplace's asymptotic formula (32) is that $l(b) = N\lambda(b)$, where $N \to \infty$ and λ is a fixed smooth function with a unique maximum. The integral for the ith subject in model(23) has the form

$$\int_{\mathbb{R}^r} \exp\{l_i(b|\beta, \sigma, \Sigma)\} db\,, \quad \text{where}$$

$$l_i(b|\beta, \sigma, \Sigma) = -S_i(b, \beta)/\sigma^2 - b\Sigma^{-1}b^T/2 - n_i \log \sigma\,, \qquad (36)$$

in which S_i is computed via Eq. (24) from n_i observations (y_{ij}, t_{ij}), $1 \leq j \leq n_i$. If these observations are sufficiently informative about the ith subject's parameter vector $\theta_i = g(x_i, \beta_0) + b_i$, then for (β, σ) near (β_0, σ_0), $S_i(b, \beta)$ becomes peaked around b_i and can be approximated by a quadratic function in a neighborhood of the maximizer $\hat{b}_i = \hat{b}_i(\beta, \sigma, \Sigma)$ of $l_i(b|\beta, \sigma, \Sigma)$. Laplace's asymptotic formula basically replaces l_i in integral (36) by the approximating quadratic function of b as $\lambda_{\min}(-\ddot{l}_i(\hat{b}_i|\beta, \sigma, \Sigma)) \to \infty$, where $\lambda_{\min}(\cdot)$ denotes the minimum eigenvalue of a symmetric matrix.

When the ith subject has sparse data (y_{ij}, t_{ij}), $S_i(b, \beta)$ is no longer peaked around $\hat{b}_i$ and Laplace's asymptotic formula may be a poor approximation to integral (36). A better way to compute integral (36) in this case is to use Monte Carlo, expressing integral (36) as the expectation

$$E_\Sigma\{\exp(-S_i(b,\beta)/\sigma^2)\}\,, \tag{37}$$

where E_Σ denotes expectation under the probability measure for which b is a normal random vector with mean 0 and covariance matrix Σ. Lai and Shih[48] proposed the following hybrid method for evaluating model (36). Take $c > 10$ and let $V_i = -\ddot{l}(\hat{b}_i|\beta,\sigma,\Sigma)$.

(i) If $\lambda_{\min}(V_i) < c$, evaluate integral (36) by Monte Carlo approximation to expression (37):

$$B^{-1}\sum_{j=1}^{B}\exp\{-S_i(b_{ij},\beta)/\sigma^2\}\,,$$

where b_{ij}, $j = 1,\ldots,B$, are independent samples from the $N(0,\Sigma)$ distribution.

(ii) If $\lambda_{\min}(V_i) \geq c$, evaluate integral (36) by its Laplace approximation

$$(2\pi)^{r/2}|V_i|^{-1/2}\exp\{l_i(\hat{b}_i|\beta,\sigma,\Sigma)\}\,.$$

By performing simple diagnostics on the appropriateness of using Laplace's asymptotic formula to evaluate the integral in expression (23) for the ith subject, the hybrid approach preserves the computational simplicity of Laplace's method when it can be used and switches to the Monte Carlo method when Laplace's method fails. In practice, the actual population distribution G of the random effects b_i may differ substantially from the assumed normal distribution with unknown covariance matrix, which at best can only be regarded as an approximation to G. If the ith subject has only sparse data so that $S_i(b,\beta)$ is relatively flat in b, then applying the Monte Carlo approach to the subject is tantamount to choosing a certain random distribution G_i, which is the empirical distribution of a sample of size B from a normal distribution, to approximate G. Since the assumed normal distribution is itself also an approximation to G, there is no need for a "high resolution" in the random distribution used to approximate the normal distribution, so using $50 \leq B \leq 200$ samples in the Monte Carlo method should be able to provide enough statistical detail so that the resultant estimator of (β,σ,Σ) still has a low computational cost comparable to that of the Lindstrom–Bates estimator. On the other hand, if the ith subject has enough data so that $S_i(b,\beta)$ is peaked around $\hat{b}_i$ for β near β_0, the Monte Carlo approach becomes unreliable unless B is sufficiently large and importance sampling is needed to generate the B samples from a distribution that is peaked around $\hat{b}_i$, so Laplace's method gives a much better approximation to (36) in this case. Thus the Monte Carlo and Laplace's methods complement each other in the hybrid approach, which uses either $N(0, \Sigma)$ or the empirical distribution of a sample of size B from $N(0, \Sigma)$ as the approximation $G_i(\cdot|\Sigma)$ to the unknown (and possibly non-normal) mixing distribution G. Using this hybrid approach to compute expression (23) approximately, Lai and Shih[48] make use of numerical differentiation and iterative optimization schemes such as conjugate gradient and quasi-Newton methods[49] to maximize this approximation to expression (23), providing the estimator $(\hat{\beta}, \hat{\sigma}, \hat{\Sigma})$ of (β, σ, Σ). Good starting values in this iterative scheme to compute $(\hat{\beta}, \hat{\sigma}, \hat{\Sigma})$ can be obtained by running several steps of the Lindstrom–Bates `nlme` procedure.

Lai and Shih[48] also develop an asymptotic theory of the hybrid estimator $(\hat{\beta}, \hat{\sigma})$ as the number K of subjects becomes infinite. This theory does not require all subjects to have sufficient data to estimate their θ_i consistently, nor does it require the actual G to be normal. Under the assumption that a sufficiently large subset of the subjects have good studies in the sense that their $\lambda_{\min}(V_i)$ exceeds the threshold c for applicability of Laplace's approximation to evaluate integral (36) and some additional regularity conditions, $(\hat{\beta}, \hat{\sigma})$ is shown to converge with probability 1 to (β_0, σ_0) as $K \to \infty$. Let $n = n_1 + \cdots + n_K$. It is also shown in Lai and Shih[48] that $\sqrt{n}(\hat{\beta}_n - \beta_0, \hat{\sigma}_n - \sigma_0)$ has a limiting normal distribution as $K \to \infty$ under these and some other conditions. Moreover, this hybrid estimator and its asymptotic theory have been extended in Lai and Shih[48] to the HGLM (34) and the GLMM of Breslow and Clayton.[45] Lai, Shih and Wong subsequently introduced a refinement of the hybrid estimator by using importance sampling instead of direct Monte Carlo.[50, 51]

3. Bioavailability and Bioequivalence

Generic drug products (manufactured by other companies that are not the innovator) have become increasingly popular since the 1960s. For the approval of a generic drug product, the FDA usually does not require a regular new drug application (NDA) submission to demonstrate the efficacy and safety of the product. Instead, it requires the generic drug company to submit bioavailability (BA) information on the generic drug and to provide evidence of its bioequivalence (BE) to the standard (or reference) drug in an "abbreviated new drug application" (ANDA), following certain regulations that became effective in 1977 and are codified in 21 CFR 320, in which BA is defined as "the rate and extent to which the active ingredient or active moiety is absorbed from a drug product and becomes available at the site of action." In Sec. 2.2 we have discussed how the PK data of a drug can be used to measure its BA. This section focuses on BE and the statistical methods in BE studies.

Two drug products are said to be *bioequivalent* if they contain either identical amounts of the same active ingredient (i.e. are "pharmaceutical equivalents") or an identical therapeutic moiety and if their rates and extents of absorption are not significantly different when administered at the same dose under similar experimental conditions. BE studies are conducted not only for ANDAs of generic drugs but also for formulation change of an approved drug. For example, clinical trials for the NDA of a drug usually use the drug produced in a laboratory setting. After approval, commercial batches produced from manufacturing plants have to be demonstrated to be bioequivalent to the clinical trial batches. Moreover, there may also be changes from tablet to capsule formulations so that BE studies are needed.

BE studies typically use healthy normal subjects and do not involve Phases II and III trials. A pilot study using a small number (e.g. 6) of subjects can be carried out in advance to assess inter-subject and intra-subject variabilities, sample size, time intervals to collect blood or urine samples and to provide other information. Instead of the commonly used randomized designs in Phases II and III studies, in which each subject is randomly assigned to one and only one formulation of a drug (parallel designs), BE studies typically use the crossover design, which is a modified randomized block design in which each block (consisting of a subject or a group of subjects) receives more than one formulation of a drug at different time periods. Crossover designs have the following advantages in BE studies:

(a) Each subject serves as his/her own control, allowing a within-subject comparison between formulations.
(b) Inter-subject variability is removed from the comparison between formulations.
(c) With proper randomization of subjects to the sequence of formulation administrations, a crossover design can provide the best unbiased estimates of the differences (or ratios) between formulations. On the other hand, care must be taken to address the "carry-over" effects in crossover designs. In BE studies, the "washout" period, which is defined as the rest period between two treatment periods for the effect of the preceding

treatment period to taper off, must be long enough so that the carry-over effect from one treatment period to the next is negligible. There is an extensive literature on crossover designs for clinical trials,[52–58] and for BE studies.[59]

Although parallel designs are infrequently used in BE studies since crossover designs usually provide much better ways of identifying and removing the inter-subject variability from the comparison between formulations based on a sample of typically 18–24 subjects, there are situations in which a parallel design is preferable to a crossover design, e.g. when (i) the inter-subject variability is relatively small compared to the intra-subject variability, or (ii) the drug has long elimination half-life so that the long washout period in a crossover design prolongs the study and increases the chance of drop-out of the subjects, or (iii) the cost of increasing the number of subjects is smaller than that of adding an additional treatment period, or (iv) extensive blood collection is not feasible from the subjects.

Suppose there are two formulations, one of which is a test formulation (T) and the other a reference (or standard) formulation (R) of a drug. For a standard 2×2 crossover design, each subject is randomly assigned to either the first sequence RT or the second sequence TR at two dosing periods. A subject assigned RT receives R at the first dosing period and T at the second period. The dosing periods are separated by a washout period of sufficient length to rule out carry-over effects. More generally, an $m \times n$ crossover design involves m sequences of formulations that are administered at n time periods. Examples are the 2×4 crossover design consisting of the two sequences TRTR and RTRT, and Balaam's 4×2 crossover design[52] consisting of the four sequences TT, RR, RT and TR.

A widely used statistical model to perform inference in these designs is the linear mixed effects model

$$y_{ijk} = \mu + a_j + \eta_{ik} + b_{jk} + c_{j-1,k} + \epsilon_{ijk}\,, \tag{38}$$

where i refers to the subject number, j the period number and k the sequence number. Here μ is the overall mean, a_j is the fixed effect of the jth period (with $\Sigma a_j = 0$), η_{ik} is the random effect (assumed to be normal with mean 0) of the ith subject in the kth sequence, b_{jk} is the fixed effect of the formulation in the jth period of the kth sequence, and ϵ_{ijk} is the within-subject random error which is assumed to be normal with mean 0. In particular, for a standard 2×2 crossover design, b_{jk} is the fixed effect of R (resp. T) if $j = k$ (resp. $j \neq k$). Note that model (38) assumes first-order (i.e. one-period) carry-over effects: $c_{j-1,k}$ represents the (fixed) residual effect carried over from period $j-1$ to period j in the kth sequence. For two-period designs, carry-over effects can only occur in the second period. It is also assumed that the η_{ik} and ϵ_{ijk} are independent with $\text{var}(\eta_{ik}) = \sigma_\eta^2$ and $\text{var}(\epsilon_{ijk}) = \sigma_\epsilon^2$. Standard ANOVA techniques can be used to construct unbiased estimates and confidence intervals of linear contrasts of the fixed effects, while the variance parameters σ_η^2 and σ_ϵ^2 can be estimated by the method of moments or restricted maximum likelihood.[59, 60] The y_{ijk} in model (38) is typically some transformation of the observed response (e.g. logarithm of the AUC) to make it approximately normal. Note that the logarithmic transformation converts multiplicative effects into additive effects, as assumed in model (38).

Although model (38) leads to standard F-tests of equality between the formulations T and R, it has been recognized since the 1970s that testing the usual hypothesis of equality is inappropriate for BE, whose purpose is to verify that the two formulations have no "biologically significant" differences.[61, 62] One way to address this difficulty is to change the null hypothesis of equality (versus the alternative hypothesis of inequality) into a null hypothesis of the form $H_0 : \theta \leq \theta_1$ or $\theta \geq \theta_2$, with an interval alternative hypothesis $H_1 : \theta_1 < \theta < \theta_2$, where θ is the parameter of interest and the interval (θ_1, θ_2) is a biological indifference zone. Schuirmann[63, 64] and Anderson and Hauck[65] have developed test procedures for what is now called *average bioequivalence.* Instead of relying on hypothesis testing, Westlake[62] proposed the following confidence interval procedure to assess average bioequivalence. Let $\mu_T(\mu_R)$ denote the mean response of a subject receiving treatment T(R) in model (38). If a $(1-2\alpha) \times 100\%$ confidence interval for $\mu_T - \mu_R$ is within the acceptance limits as recommended by the regulatory agency, then accept the test formulation T as bioequivalent to the reference formulation R.

Average bioequivalence only compares the means of the marginal distributions of the PK parameters of interest, such as AUC or $C_{\max}$, associated with the two formulations. Under normality assumptions, the equivalence between distributions is characterized by the equivalence of their means and variances. *Population bioequivalence* therefore also compares the variances of the two formulations. The intra-subject variability, particularly associated with switching from one formulation to another, leads to another criterion in assessing BE, called *individual bioequivalence.* To explain the underlying motivation, suppose a patient switches from R to T that has a much higher intra-subject variability than R. This may push the AUC of the patient outside the established therapeutic window of R. Consequently, population BE does not guarantee that the two formulations are exchangeable and therapeutically equivalent and individual BE is needed.

To see what is involved in assessing these three criteria of BE, assume for simplicity that there are no carry-over effects and no period-sequence interactions so that (38) can be reduced to a form that involves T and R more directly as

$$y_{i\delta\nu} = \mu_\delta + \alpha_{i\delta} + \epsilon_{i\delta\nu}\,, \tag{39}$$

where i is the subject number, $\delta =$ T or R, ν denotes the number of times that δ appears in a sequence and therefore $1 \le \nu \le n_\delta$ (= largest number of times that δ appears in the available sequences). The $\epsilon_{i\delta\nu}$ are independent normal with mean 0, variance σ_ϵ^2 and are independent of the random effects $(\alpha_{iT}, \alpha_{iR})$ that are independent and have a bivariate normal distribution with $\mathrm{var}(\alpha_{iT}) = v_T$, $\mathrm{var}(\alpha_{iR}) = v_R$ and $\mathrm{var}(\alpha_{iT} - \alpha_{iR}) = \sigma_D^2$. According to the 1999 FDA Guidance on Bioequivalence, average BE is established if the 90% confidence limits for e^{μ_T}/e^{μ_R} are 4/5 and 5/4, or equivalently, if $\pm\ell n(1.25)$ are the 90% confidence limits for $\mu_T - \mu_R$. Note that the total variance of the T formulation is $\sigma_T^2 = \sigma_\epsilon^2 + v_T$, while that of the R formulation is $\sigma_R^2 = \sigma_\epsilon^2 + v_R$. Population BE is established if the 95% upper confidence bound for $\{(\mu_T - \mu_R)^2 + (\sigma_T^2 - \sigma_R^2)\}/\sigma_R^2$ falls below the FDA specified limit of $\{(\ell n 1.25)^2 + 0.02\}/(0.2)^2 = 1.745$. Individual BE is established if the 95% upper confidence bound for $\{(\mu_T - \mu_R)^2 + \sigma_D^2\}/\sigma_\epsilon^2$ falls below another FDA specified limit. These upper confidence bounds can be obtained by appealing to the central limit theorem and using the delta method to compute the asymptotic standard errors. Alternatively, bootstrap methods can be used to compute the confidence bounds and confidence intervals; see in particular Chapter 25 of Efron and Tibshirani[66] and Sec. 4.5.3 of Chow and Liu.[59] The inclusion of population BE and individual BE besides average BE by the FDA in its guidelines for the pharmaceutical industry reflects its concerns about prescribability and switchability of generic drug products. Prescribability means that when a physician prescribes a generic drug product to a patient for the first time, they should both be assured that the drug product yields safety and efficacy results comparable to that of the reference product in the patient population. Switchability means that when a physician switches a reference product to a generic product for a patient, they should both be assured that the generic product will yield comparable safety and efficacy results for the same individual.

Nonparametric and Bayesian approaches to BE have also been developed in the literature.[67] There are intriguing theoretical problems concerning BE in statistical decision theory.[59] Crossover designs and average BE for more than two formulations have also been studied.[59]

4. Assay Development and Validation

The availability of reliable assays is central to determining the drug concentrations in blood, urine, etc., in PK studies. When a pharmaceutical compound is discovered, it is necessary to develop an assay method to measure the substance levels in plasma, serum, etc. The substance that is being measured is called an *analyte*, and the objective is to determine the analyte's *potency*, which refers to its content or activity (e.g. number of particles, gravitometric mass, percent of impurity). There are three types of assays that are commonly used in the pharmaceutical industry: (i) chemical assays such as HPLC (high performance liquid chromatographs), (ii) immunoassays (e.g. radioimmunoassays, enzyme-linked immunosorbent assays), (iii) biological assays (measuring the analyte's potency relative to some standard drug in terms of the magnitudes of their effects on responses from living subjects).

For the development of an assay method of a pharmaceutical compound, the FDA requires that the assay method meet the established specifications, for which instrument calibration is essential. A common approach to calibration is to have a number of known standard concentration preparations put through the instrument to obtain the corresponding responses. Fitting an appropriate statistical model to the data yields an estimated calibration curve, called the *standard curve*. Simple linear regression of the response on the standard is perhaps the most widely used statistical model. The standard curve is used to determine the unknown potency.[68]

Validation of an assay method is the process by which it is established, in laboratory studies, that the performance characteristics of the method indeed meets the specified criteria. As specified in Chow and Liu,[68] these criteria include (i) accuracy (no systematic error in the assay method), (ii) precision (measurement error of the method), (iii) limit of detection/quantitation (LOD/LOQ, which is the lowest concentration of analyte in a sample that can be detected/determined with acceptable precision under the specified experimental conditions), (iv) range (reliable range of the method), (v) linearity (whether the assay generates results that are directly proportional to the concentration of analyte within a given range), (vi) specificity (whether the assay measures the analyte and no other substance in the specimen), (vii) ruggedness (degree of reproducibility of assay results under a variety of normal test conditions, such as different laboratories, assay temperatures, days). Commonly used statistical methods for assay validation include:

(a) regression analysis (particularly with respect to accuracy, linearity and LOD/LOQ),
(b) analysis of variance (particularly with respect to ruggedness); see Chapter 3 of Chow and Liu.[68]

Lin[69] introduces a concordance correlation coefficient to evaluate reproducibility and ruggedness, while Chapter 10 of Davidian and Giltinan[11] applies nonlinear mixed effects models to the analysis of assay data.

5. Drug Discovery

As pointed out in the preceding section, assay development is an important facet in the drug discovery process. Another important facet is of a biological nature and involves the identification of a biological target or pathway. In recent years, advances in bioinformatics and genomics have provided new tools and opportunities in this direction. Besides applications to assay development and bioinformatics, statistical methods are also useful in screening compounds for clinically active drugs, and in searching for novel, active compounds.

A pharmaceutical company typically has a large inventory of compounds, of which an unknown small proportion is truly active. Dunnett[70] developed a model that takes into account the costs and benefits of any screening procedure to derive an optimal procedure; see also the subsequent work of Bergman and Gittins[71] in this direction. Colton[72] and King[73] considered multistage screening procedures, while Redman and King[74] proposed group screening that uses balanced and partially balanced incomplete block designs to increase the rate of compound screening without reducing necessary replication.

Numerical topology is the assignment of numerical values to topologically invariant features of molecules. There is an isomorphism between two-dimensional molecular diagrams and connected graphs; the edges and vertices of the graphs correspond to bonds and atoms of molecules, yielding numerical representation of compounds or parts of compounds. With this representation, search for active compounds involves a very large set of graphs. Moreover, there may also be a large number of potential chemical modifications at different sites that one may want to experiment with. Experimental design techniques are particularly useful for such problems.[75,76]

References

1. Katzung, B. G. (1992). *Basic and Clinical Pharmacology.* Prentice Hall, Englewood Cliffs, NJ.
2. Rowland, M. and Tozer, T. N. (1989). *Clinical Pharmacokinetics*, 2nd edn., Lea and Febiger, Philadelphia.
3. Evans, W. E., Schentag, J. J. and Jusko, W. J. (eds). (1986). *Applied Pharmacokinetics*, 2nd edn., Applied Therapeutics Inc., SF.
4. Welling, P. G. (1986). *Pharmacokinetics: Processes and Mathematics*, American Chemical Society, Washington, DC.
5. Goldstein, A., Aronow, L. and Kalman, S. M. (1974). *Principles of Drug Action*, 2nd edn., Wiley, NY.
6. Wagner, J. G. (1976). Linear pharmacokinetic equations allowing direct calculation of many needed pharmacokinetic parameters from the coefficients and exponents of polyexponential equations which have been fitted to data. *Journal of Pharmacokinetics and Biopharmaceutics* **4**: 443.
7. Lai, T. L. (1985). Regression analysis of compartmental models. *Journal of Research of the National Bureau Standard* **90**: 525.
8. Yeh, K. C. and Kwan, K. C. (1978). A comparison of numerical integration algorithms by trapezoidal, Lagrange and spline approximations. *Journal of Pharmacokinetics and Biopharmaceutics* **6**: 79.
9. Scatchard, G. (1949). The attractions of protein for small molecules and ions. *Annals of New York Academy of Science* **51**: 660.
10. Lai, T. L. and Zhang, L. (1994). Statistical analysis of ligand-binding experiments. *Biometrics* **50**: 782.
11. Davidian, M. and Giltinan, D. M. (1995). *Nonlinear Models for Repeated Measurement Data*, Chapman and Hall, NY.
12. Beal, S. M. and Sheiner, L. B. (1992). *NONMEM User's Guide.* NONMEM Project Group, UCSF.
13. Lindstrom, M. J. and Bates, B. M. (1990). Nonlinear mixed effects models for repeated measures data. *Biometrics* **46**: 673.
14. Geyer, C. J. and Thompson, E. A. (1992). Constrained Monte Carlo maximum likelihood for dependent data. *Journal of the Royal Statistical Society Series* **B54**: 657.
15. Quintana, F. A., Liu, J. S. and del Pino, G. E. (1999). Monte Carlo EM with importance reweighting and its applications in random effects models. *Computational Statistics and Data Analysis* **29**: 429.

16. Gelman, A. (1995). Method of moments using Monte Carlo simulation. *Journal of Computational and Graphical Statistics* **4**: 36.
17. Pinhero, J. C. and Bates, D. M. (1995). Approximations to the loglikelihood function in the nonlinear mixed effects model. *Journal of Computational and Graphical Statistics* **4**: 12.
18. Wakefield, J. C., Smith, A. F. M., Racine-Poon, A. and Gelfand, A. E. (1994). Bayesian analysis of linear and nonlinear population models by using the Gibbs sampler. *Applied Statistics* **43**: 201.
19. Wakefield, J. (1996). The Bayesian analysis of population pharmacokinetic models. *Journal of the American Statistics Association* **91**: 62.
20. Wakefield, J. and Benett, J. (1996). The Bayesian modeling of covariates for population pharmacokinetic models. *Journal of the American Statistical Association* **91**: 917.
21. Gelman, A., Bois, F. and Jiang, J. (1996). Physiological pharmacokinetic analysis using population modeling and informative prior distributions. *Journal of the American Statistical Association* **91**: 1400.
22. Müller, P. and Rosner, G. L. (1997). A Bayesian population model with hierarchical mixture priors applied to blood count data. *Journal of the American Statistical Association* **92**: 1279.
23. Bennett, J. E., Racine-Poon, A. and Wakefield, J. C. (1996). MCMC for nonlinear hierarchical models. In *Markov Chain Monte Carlo in Practice*, eds. W. R. Gills, S. Richardson and D. J. Spiegelhalter, Chapman and Hall, NY, 339–357.
24. Shih, M. (1999). Estimation in nonlinear mixed effects models: Parametric and nonparametric approaches. PhD. dissertation, Dept. Statistics, Stanford University.
25. Davidian, M. and Gallant, A. R. (1992). Smooth nonparametric maximum likelihood estimation for population pharmacokinetics, with applications to quinidine. *Journal of Pharmacokinetics and Biopharmaceutics* **20**: 529.
26. Gallant, A. R. and Nychka, D. W. (1987). Semi-nonparametric maximum likelihood estimation. *Econometrica* **55**: 363.
27. Magder, L. S. and Zeger, S. L. (1996). A smooth nonparametric estimate of a mixing distribution using mixture of gaussians. *Journal of the American Statistical Association* **91**: 1141.
28. Fattinger, K. E., Sheiner, L. B. and Verotta, D. (1995). A new method to explore the distribution of interindividual random effects in nonlinear mixed effects models. *Biometrics* **51**: 1236.
29. Carroll, R. and Hall, P. (1988). Optimal rates of convergence for deconvolving a density. *Journal of the American Statistical Association* **83**: 1184.
30. Fan, J. Q. (1991). On the optimal rates of convergence for nonparametric deconvolution problems. *The Annals Statistics* **19**: 1257.
31. Chen, J. (1994). Optimal rate of convergence for finite mixture models. *The Canadian Journal of Statistics* **22**: 387.
32. Lindsay, B. G. (1983). The geometry of mixture likelihoods: A general theory. *Annals of Statistics* **11**: 86.

33. Mallet, A. (1986). A maximum likelihood estimation method for random coefficient regression models. *Biometrika* **73**: 645.
34. Ibragimov, I. A. and Has'minskii, R. Z. (1983). On asymptotic efficiency in the presence of an inifinite-dimensional nuisance parameter. In *Lecture Notes in Mathematics 1021*, Springer-Verlag, NY, 195–220.
35. Bates, D. M. and Watts, D. G. (1988). *Nonlinear Regression Analysis and Its Applications.* Wiley, NY.
36. Lai, T. L. and Shih, M. (2003). Nonparametric estimation in nonlinear mixed effects models. *Biometrika* **90**: 1.
37. Robbins, H. (1964). The empirical Bayes approach to statistical decision problems. *Ann. Math. Statist.* **35**: 1.
38. Maitre, P. O., Buhrer, M., Thomson, D. and Stanski, D. R. (1991). A three-step approach combining Bayes regression and NONMEM population analysis: Application to midazolam. *Journal of Pharmacokinetics and Biopharmaceutics* **19**: 377.
39. Wakefield, J. and Racine-Poon, A. (1995). An application of Bayesian pharmacokinetic/pharmacodynamic models to dose recommendation. *Statistics in Medicine* **14**: 971.
40. Banfield, C. R., Zhu, G. R., Jen, J. F., Jensen, P. K., Schumaker, R. C., Perhach, J. L., Affrima, M. B. and Glue, P. (1996). The effect of age on the apparent clearance of felbamate: A retrospective analysis using nonlinear mixed effects modeling. *Therapeutic Drug Monitoring* **18**: 19.
41. Verme, C. N., Ludden, T. M., Clementi, W. A. and Harris, S. C. (1992). Pharmacokinetics of quinidine in male patients: A population analysis. *Clinical Pharmacokinetics* **22**: 468.
42. Boeckmann, A. J., Sheiner, L. B. and Beal, S. L. (1992). Part V (Introductory Guide) of *NONMEM User's Guide.* NONMEM Project Group, UCSF.
43. Vonesh, E. F. (1996). A note on the use of Laplace's approximation for nonlinear mixed effects models. *Biometrika* **83**: 447.
44. Wolfinger, R. (1993). Laplace's approximation for nonlinear mixed effects models. *Biometrics* **80**: 791.
45. Breslow, N. E. and Clayton, D. G. (1993). Approximate inference in generalized linear mixed models. *Journal of the American Statistical Association* **88**: 9.
46. Lee, Y. and Nelder, J. A. (1996). Hierarchical generalized linear models. *Journal of the Royal Statistical Society Series* **B58**: 619.
47. Henderson, C. R. (1975). Best linear unbiased estimation and prediction under a selection model. *Biometrics* **31**: 423.
48. Lai, T. L. and Shih, M.-C. (2003). A hybrid estimator in nonlinear and generalised linear mixed effects models. *Biometrika* **90**: 859.
49. Press, W. H., Teukolsky, S. A., Vetterling, W. T. and Flannery, B. P. (1992). *Numerical Recipes in C: The Art of Scientific Computing*, Cambridge Univ. Press.
50. Lai, T. L., Shih, M. C., and Wong, S. P. (2006). Flexible modeling via a hybrid estimation scheme in generalized mixed models for longitudinal data. *Biometrics* **62**: 159.

51. Lai, T. L., Shih, M. C. and Wong, S. P. (2006). A new approach to modelling covariate effects and individualization in population pharmacokinetics-pharmacodynamics. *J. Pharmacokin. Pharmacodyn.* **33**: 49.
52. Balaam, L. N. (1968). A two-period design with t^2 experimental units. *Biometrics* **24**: 61.
53. Brown, B. W. (1980). The crossover experiment for clinical trials. *Biometrics* **36**: 69.
54. Cheng, C. S. and Wu, C. F. (1980). Balanced repeated measurements designs. *The Annals of Statistics* **8**: 1272.
55. Laska, E. M., Meisner, M. and Kushner, H. B. (1983). Optimal crossover designs in the presence of carryover effects. *Biometrics* **39**: 1089.
56. Laska, E. M. and Meisner, M. (1985). A variational approach to optimal two-treatment crossover designs: Applications to carryover effect methods. *Journal of the American Statistical Association* **80**: 704.
57. Jones, B. and Kenward, M. G. (1989). *Design and Analysis of Crossover Trials*, Chapman and Hall, NY.
58. Fleiss, J. L. (1989). A critique of recent research on the two-treatment crossover design. *Controlled Clinical Trials* **10**: 237.
59. Chow, S. C. and Liu, J. P. (1992). *Design and Analysis of Bioavailability and Bioequivalence Studies.* Marcel Dekker, NY.
60. Chinchilli, V. M. and Esinhart, J. D. (1996). Design and analysis of intra-subject variability in cross-over experiments. *Statistics in Medicine* **15**: 1619.
61. Metzler, C. M. (1974). Bioavailability: A problem in bioequivalence. *Biometrics* **30**: 309.
62. Westlake, W. J. (1972). Use of confidence intervals in analysis of comparative bioavailability trials. *Journal of Pharmaceutical Sciences* **61**: 1340.
63. Schuirmann, D. J. (1981). On hypothesis testing to determine if the mean of a normal distribution is continued in a known interval. *Biometrics* **37**: 617.
64. Schuirmann, D. J. (1987). A comparison of the two one-sided tests procedure and the power approach for assessing the equivalence of average bioavailability. *Journal of Pharmacokinetics and Biopharmaceutics* **15**: 657.
65. Anderson, S. and Hauck, W. W. (1983). A new procedure for testing equivalence in comparative bioavailability and other clinical trials. *Communications in Statistics Series* **A12**: 2663.
66. Efron, B. and Tibshirani, R. J. (1993). *An Introduction to the Bootstrap.* Chapman and Hall, NY.
67. Brown, L. D., Hwang, J. T. and Munk, A. (1997). An unbiased test for the bioequivalence problem. *The Annals of Statistics* **25**: 2345.
68. Chow, S. C. and Liu, J. P. (1995). *Statistical Design and Analysis in Pharmaceutical Science.* Marcel Dekker, NY.
69. Lin, L. I. (1989). A concordance correlation coefficient to evaluate reproducibility. *Biometrics* **45**: 255.
70. Dunnett, C. W. (1961). Statistical theory of drug screening. In *Quantitative Pharmacology*, ed. H. DeJonge, North Holland, Amsterdam.
71. Bergman, S. W. and Gittins, J. C. (1985). *Statistical Methods for Planning Pharmaceutical Research.* Marcel Dekker, NY.

72. Colton, T. (1963). Optimal drug screening plans. *Biometrika* **50**: 31.
73. King, E. P. (1964). Optimal replication in sequential drug screening. *Biometrika* **51**: 110.
74. Redman, C. E. and King, E. P. (1965). Group screening utilizing balanced and partially balanced incomplete block designs. *Biometrics* **21**: 865.
75. Thornber, C. W. (1979). Isosterism and molecular modification in drug design. *Chemical Society Reviews* **8**: 563.
76. Martin, E. J., Blaney, J. M., Siani, M. A., Spellmeyer, D. C., Wong, A. K. and Moose, W. H. (1995). Measuring diversity: Experimental design of combinatorial libraries for drug discovery. *Journal of Medicinal Chemistry* **38**: 1431.

About the Author

Tze Leung Lai is Professor of Statistics, and by courtesy, of Health Research and Policy and of the Institute of Computational and Mathematical Engineering at Stanford University, where he is the Director of the Financial and Risk Modeling Institute and Co-director of the Biostatistics Core at the Stanford Cancer Institute and of the Center for Innovative Study Design at the School of Medicine. He made seminal contributions to sequential analysis, innovative clinical trial designs, adaptive methods, survival analysis, nonlinear and generalized mixed models, hybrid resampling methods, and received the Committee of Presidents of Statistical Societies (COPSS) Award in 1983.

Mei-Chiung Shih is Assistant Professor of Biostatistics and a member of the Stanford Cancer Institute and of the Center for Innovative Study Design at the School of Medicine at Stanford University. She is also Associate Director for Scientific and Technical Operations at the Department of Veterans Affairs (VA) Cooperative Studies Program Coordinating Center at Palo Alto Health Care System. She is a leading expert on group sequential and adaptive designs and inference of clinical trials, longitudinal and survival data analysis, and has been leading the design, conduct and analysis of several large trials at the VA.

Guangrui Zhu is Vice President of Biostatistics at Allergan. He previously worked at Eisai, Aventis, Pfizer, Schering-Plough, and US FDA. He has made important contributions to design and execution of clinical studies for new drugs. He also applied population pharmacokinetics and pharmacodynamics, and adaptive design to drug evaluations.

CHAPTER 16

STATISTICS IN TOXICOLOGY*

JAMES J. CHEN

Division of Personalized Nutrition Medicine
National Center for Toxicological Research
Food and Drug Administration
Jefferson, Arkansas 72079, USA
JamesJ.chen@fda.hhs.gov

Toxicology is the study of the adverse effects of chemical substances on biological systems. Toxicological research is typically directed toward providing scientific information for the hazard potential of drugs and chemicals used by humans. Human epidemiology and animal toxicology are two major sources of scientific information for evaluation of toxic chemicals or drugs. Epidemiological studies, which attempt to associate disease or other adverse outcomes with an exposure, have the advantage of directly measuring an effect in humans at exposure conditions. Main limitations on the epidemiological studies are the lack of comprehensive data associated with unintentional or complex exposures, such as quantifying the actual dose concentration and no safety data for new drug or chemical products. Safety evaluation of the use of drug and chemicals are primarily based on animal studies in which animals are considered as surrogates for humans. *In Vitro* mutagenicity studies and structure-activity relationships may be used to support the interpretation of the information from the animal or human studies.

Statistical analyses of various endpoints have been of two aspects: qualitative testing and quantitative estimation for risk assessment. The qualitative testing is to determine if the chemical cause an adverse health effect (if there is a statistically significant difference between treated and control groups). The key is to determine the biological relevance of a change that

*The views presented in this paper are those of the authors and do not necessarily represent those of the U.S. Food and Drug Administration.

is statistical significance. The quantitative estimation is used to determine a safe level of human exposure from the assessment of the dose-response relationship. The quantitative risk estimation for adverse effects is typically used for environmental or workplace exposures and does not apply to pharmaceutical drugs. Risk assessment of pharmaceutical drugs would also require an assessment of benefit. In this chapter, we focus on the qualitative testing for the data from two major toxicological studies, long-term carcinogenicity and reproductive experiment, and mixture experme-nts. Dose-response assessment for quantitative risk estimation is given in Chapter 17.

1. Animal Carcinogenicity Experiments

Long-term rodent bioassays have been the government's primary means of screening chemicals to assess carcinogenic potential to human risk. The United States Food and Drug Administration (FDA) and other countries require that new drugs and certain medical devices must be approved for safety and effectiveness for their intended use before being marketed. As a part of the drug approval process, the FDA requires that the sponsor submit the results of a rodent tumorigenicity bioassay to assess the carcinogenic potential of a drug for chronic use of humans. In the last 25 years the National Toxicology Program (NTP) has conducted about 500 long-term animal carcinogenesis bioassays for safety assessment of environmental compounds, and Food and Drug Administration (FDA) has reviewed hundreds of such studies of pharmaceuticals conducted by drug companies. Data from these studies have been a major database for safety assessment of compounds in the environment and industry.

A standard carcinogenic study is conducted in both sexes of two rodent species, typically rats and mice. A carcinogenicity experiment consists of a control and several dose groups. The *maximum tolerated dose* (MTD) has been used as the high-dose level. The MTD is defined as the dose that causes no more than a 10% body weight decrement, as compared to the appropriate control groups. The MTD is often estimated from the results of subchronic studies (generally three months of duration). Typically, dosage is measured in milligrams per kilogram body weight per day. The number of dose groups and allocation of animals among the dose groups depend on the objective of the study. A typical NTP carcinogenicity experiment consists of a control and three dose levels (0, 1/4 NTD, 1/2 MTD, MTD) with 50 animals per group. Animals are assigned randomly to dose groups or cages. As an example, consider a situation of 200 animals to be assigned to four groups of 50 with four animals from the same group caged together. Thus, 52 cages are used for the 200 animals. Each animal, first, is given to a number according to their order of presentation. A random number sequence of 52 cages numbers each with 4 replicates is, then, generated for placing animals in cages. For example, a sequence may be

Animal number	1	2	3	4	5	6	7	8	9	10	..
random cage number	42	7	8	13	9	11	18	7	22	38	..

The animal #1 would be placed in cage #42, and animal #2 in cage #7, and so on. After randomization of the animals to cages (and into experimental dose groups), the cage position may need to be rotated during the course of the experiment in order to balance the environmental effects.

The animals are given the test substance for a major portion of their lifespan. The test substance may be given in the diet or administered by other routes, such as inhalation, skin paints, or oral gavage. The experiment is terminated according to a predetermined stopping time, for example, 78–104 weeks for mice and 104 weeks for rats. Animal body weights and food consumption are measured weekly, the weeks of death of animals are recorded. Animals which die or are sacrificed are necropsied. Tissues taken from different organs and sites are examined microscopically for the presence of tumors for an evidence of carcinogenic effects.

One main objective of a long-term carcinogenicity experiment is to compare control and dose groups of animals with respect to tumor development. Statistical analysis of tumor responses includes the comparisons between dosed and control groups as well as a test for dose-related trend for each tumor site/organ. A typical experiment investigates approximate 20–50 tumor sites routinely. Because a large number of statistical tests are performed, the chance of false positive findings could increase. For example, the false positive rate is about 0.64 ($\approx 1 - (1 - 0.05)^{20}$) for tests of 20 independent tumor types (sites/organs) all at the 0.05 significance level. For a particular tumor type, the primary response variable (endpoint) for comparison is the incidence of *first* tumors. One factor that affects the performance of methods is the animal survival time. A high degree of animal mortality will cause a significant censoring of the tumor response. Comparisons should be adjusted for the survival time because the crude incidence rate can be biased by the differential mortality (across groups). Another complication is that most tumor types are occult and therefore detectable only after the animal has died; that is, the time to the (first) tumor onset is not directly observable. This section will describe the commonly used statistical procedures for the analysis of animal tumor response data.

1.1. *Time-to-tumor model*

Kodell and Nelson [1] presented a tumor-death model which uses survival/sacrifice data to describe the sequence of events comprised by histological appearance of a tumor followed by death from that tumor. Three random variables can be used to describe the model:

X: The potential time to tumor onset, transition time from the normal state (N) to the tumor-bearing state (T).

T: The potential time from tumor onset to death, transition time from tumor state (T) to the death from the tumor (D_T).

Z: The potential time until death from a competing cause, transition time from the normal state (N) to the death from competing risk (D_{NT}).

Sacrificed animals are considered to be dead from a competing risk. The three random variables X, T, Z completely determined the fate of each animal. The two random variables Y and Z are the survival time of an animal, where $Y = X + T$ is the potential time until death from tumor. Note that X is not observable for the occult tumors.

A survival-adjusted method, that has been widely accepted, is to require that pathologists assign a "context of observation" (cause-of-death) to each tumor.[2] Tumors can be classified as "incidental", "fatal", and "mortality-independent (or observable)". Tumors that do not alter an animal's risk of death and are observed only as the result of a death from an unrelated cause are classified as an incidental context. Tumors that affect mortality by either directly causing death or indirectly increasing the risk of death are classified as a fatal context. Tumors, such as skin tumors, whose detection occurs at times other than when the animal dies are classified as a mortality-independent (or observable) context. It should be noted that the validity of context of observation is under the assumption: tumor-bearing and tumor-free animals of the same age have identical hazard functions for death unrelated to tumor.

In the context of observation, one of the four events will be observed on each animal:

A. appearance of a visible tumor (mortality-independent context, X is observable)
B. animal died from the tumor of interest (fatal context, $Y < Z$)
C. animal had a tumor and died from competing cause (incidental context, $X \leq Z < Y$)
D. animal did not have a tumor and died from a competing cause ($Z \leq X$)

Let $t_1, t_2, \ldots, t_m$ be the distinct times at which the above events are observed, and a_k, b_k, c_k, and d_k, $k = 1, \ldots, m$, are the number of events of A, B, C, and D at time t_k, respectively. Define the tumor resistance (survival) functions for X and Y as $S_X(t) = \Pr(X \geq t)$, and $S_Y(t) = \Pr(Y \geq t)$. Let $f_X(t)$ and $f_Y(t)$ be the density function of X and Y, respectively. For the tumors observed in a mortality-independent context, the likelihood function is given as

$$L_a = \prod f_X(t_k)^{a_k} S_X(t_k)^{d_k}.$$

The likelihood function for the tumors observed in a fatal context is

$$L_b = \prod f_Y(t_k)^{b_k} S_Y(t_k)^{d_k}.$$

The likelihood functions L_a and L_b are essentially the same. The likelihood function for the tumors observed in an incidental context is

$$L_c = \prod [1 - S_X(t_k)]^{c_k} S_X(t_k)^{d_k}.$$

In the general case, when a tumor is observed in a fatal case for some animals and is also observed in an incidental context for other animals, the likelihood function is

$$L_d = \prod [f_Y(t_k)]^{b_k} [S_Y(t_k) - S_X(t_k)]^{c_k} [S_X(t_k)]^{d_k}.$$

Kodell *et al.*[3] showed that

$$S_Y(t) - S_X(t) = [1 - Q(t)] S_Y(t),$$

where $Q(t) = S_X(t)/S_Y(t)$ is the conditional probability of tumor onset after time t, given tumor-free survival through time t. It follows that

$$L_d = \prod [f_Y(t_k)]^{b_k} [S_Y(t_k)]^{c_k + d_k} [1 - Q(t_k)]^{c_k} Q(t_k)^{d_k}.$$

That is, L_d can be expressed as the product of the two likelihood functions

$$L_d^b = \prod [f_Y(t_k)]^{b_k} [S_Y(t_k)]^{c_k+d_k},$$

and

$$L_d^c = \prod [1 - Q(t_k)]^{c_k} Q(t_k)^{d_k}.$$

The L_d^b and L_d^c represent the contributions of the fatal and incidental tumors, respectively.

1.2. *Estimation*

An important first step in the evaluation of animal carcinogenicity data is to estimate the animal survival curve for the assessment of any effects of exposure to the test compound on mortality. The survival curve for each dose group is calculated by the Kaplan-Meier method.[4] In this calculation, the weeks of death for animals killed accidentally or sacrificed are considered as censored observations.[5] For a given group, suppose that the death time of the animals are observed at $t_k, k = 1, \ldots, m$. Let n_k denote the number of animals that died at or after t_k (the number of animals at risk), and x_k denote the number of deaths (out of n_k). The Kaplan-Meier estimate of the conditional probability of survival beyond t_k given survival beyond $t_{(k-1)}$ is $(n_k - x_k)/n_k$. The estimated survival function is

$$\hat{S}(t) = \prod_{t_k \le t} \frac{n_k - x_k}{n_k}, \quad t_k \le t < t_{(k+1)}.$$

The variance of the $\hat{S}(t)$ is calculated by Greenwood's formula

$$V[\hat{S}(t)] = \hat{S}^2(t) \sum_{t_k \le t} \frac{x_k}{n_k(n_k - x_k)} \quad t_k \le t \le t_{(k+1)}.$$

The estimation of the tumor survival functions $S_X(t)$ and $S_Y(t)$ depends on the context of observation. When all tumors are observed in a mortality-independent context or fatal context, the Kaplan-Meier method can be used to estimate the tumor survival function. The calculation is the same as estimating animal survival function. But, the n_k represents the number of animals at risk (have not developed a tumor), and x_k is the number of tumor observed (or death caused by the tumor).

For the tumors observed in an incidental context, these tumors are only discovered at necropsy, either after sacrifice or after has died from the cause unrelated to the presence of tumor. Let the experiment period be partitioned into J sub-interval such that $(t_{j-1}, t_j], j = 1, \ldots, J$, where $t_0 = 0$ and t_J denotes the time at which the terminal sacrifice is scheduled. Let c_j and d_j denote the number of animals that died in the j-th time interval for which the tumor is present or absent, respectively. The total number of deaths in the j-th time interval is $(c_j + d_j)$. Hoel and Walburg[6] proposed the tumor prevalence estimate as

$$\hat{R}(t) = \frac{c_j}{c_j + d_j}, \quad t_{(j-1)} < t \leq t_j.$$

The prevalence method requires to partition the experimental period into several time intervals. The following three partitions have been used in practice: (1) (0, 50], (51–80], (81–104], interim sacrifice (if any), and terminal sacrifice; (2) (0, 52], (53, 78], (79, 92], (93, 104], interim sacrifice (if any), and terminal sacrifice; and (3) the Peto *ad hoc* interval determined by the tumor prevalence data based on the assumption of non-decreasing prevalence function.[2] The maximum likelihood estimate of $R(t)$ is estimated by the 'pooling adjacent violators' method.

For the tumors observed in both incidental and fatal contexts, the maximum likelihood estimate of $S_X(t)$ can be obtained by estimating $S_Y(t)$ and $Q(t)$ separately, provided that $Q(t)$ is monotonically nonincreasing. Consequently, the $S_Y(t)$ and $Q(t)$ are estimated by the Kaplan-Meier estimator and Hoel-Walburg estimator described above. The estimate of tumor onset distribution[3] is

$$\hat{S}_X(t) = \left[\prod_{t_k \leq t} \frac{n_k - b_k}{n_k}\right] \left(\frac{c_j}{c_j + d_j}\right), \quad t_{j-1} \leq t < t_j.$$

The variance and the variance of $\hat{S}_X(t)$ is obtained using a first-order Taylor series,

$$\text{var}[\hat{S}_X(t)] \simeq [\hat{S}_X(t)]^2 \left[\sum_{t_k \leq t} \frac{x_k}{n_k(n_k - x_k)} + \frac{c_j}{(c_j + d_j)d_j}\right].$$

1.3. *Testing*

First, consider testing for difference in animal survival functions, or difference in the incidence of tumors observed in a mortality-independent context or fatal context. The logrank test or the death-rate method[2] is the most widely used procedure for testing the age-specific differences among groups.

Consider a carcinogenicity experiment with g groups $(d_1, \ldots, d_g)$. Taking all dose groups together as one, suppose that the death times are observed at t_k, a time point at which tumors are found in any group, $k = 1, \ldots, m$. Let n_{ik} denote the number of animals in the i-th group that died at or after t_{ik} (at risk), and x_{ik} denote the number of deaths (out of n_{ik}). Animal death-tumor data at time t_k can be summarized in a $2 \times g$ table as

Summary of animal tumor-death data at t_k

Dose	d_1	d_2	$\cdots$	d_g	Total
# with Tumors	x_{1k}	x_{2k}	$\cdots$	x_{gk}	$x_{.k}$
# at risk	n_{1k}	n_{2k}	$\cdots$	n_{gk}	$n_{.k}$

The expected number of tumors in the i-th group at time t_k is $e_{ik} = x_{.k} f_{ik}$, where $f_{ik} = n_{ik}/n_{.k}$, $i = 1, \ldots, g$. Thus, the observed and expected numbers of tumors in the i-th group over the entire experiment are $O_i = \sum_{k=1}^{m} x_{ik}$ and $E_i = \sum_{k=1}^{m} e_{ik}$, respectively. Define

$$D_i = O_i - E_i = \sum_{k=1}^{m} (x_{ik} - e_{ik})$$

and

$$V_{rs} = \sum_{k=1}^{m} \frac{x_{.k}(n_{.k} - x_{.k}) f_{rk}(\delta_{rs} - f_{sk})}{n_{.k} - 1}$$

where δ_{rs} is defined as 1 if $r = s$ and 0 otherwise. Let $\boldsymbol{D_a} = (D_1, \ldots, D_g)'$ and $\boldsymbol{V_a}$ be the $g \times g$ matrix with the (r, s) entry V_{rs}. Then

$$X_a = \boldsymbol{D_a}' \boldsymbol{V_a}^- \boldsymbol{D_a}$$

can serve as a test for heterogeneity among the g groups, where $\boldsymbol{V_a}^-$ is a generalized inverse of $\boldsymbol{V_a}$. Under the null hypothesis, X_H is asymptotically distributed as χ^2 distribution with $g - 1$ degrees of freedom. Also, a dose-related trend test can be considered by using

$$Z_a = \boldsymbol{l}' \boldsymbol{D_a} / \sqrt{\boldsymbol{l}' \boldsymbol{V_a} \boldsymbol{l}},$$

where $\boldsymbol{l} = (d_1, \ldots, d_g)'$.

For the tumors observed in an incidental context, the Mantel and Haenszel[7] test or the prevalence method[2] can be used for comparing the prevalence rates among groups. The prevalence method used is very similar to the death-rate method, except that each interval defines the tumor-death time as described in the estimation. The vector of the differences of observed and expected values $\boldsymbol{D_b}$ is calculated the same way as described for the fatal tumors, and the corresponding covariance matrix V_b is computed. The χ^2 test statistics for heterogeneity and trend can be calculated similarly.

For the tumors observed in both fatal and incidental and contexts, the data for the fatal tumors and for the incidental tumors are analyzed separately by the death-rate and prevalence methods, respectively. The test for the difference in the time of tumor onset is based on the pooled vector $\boldsymbol{D} = \boldsymbol{D}_a + \boldsymbol{D}_b$, with covariance matrix $\boldsymbol{V} = \boldsymbol{V}_a + \boldsymbol{V}_b$.[2] The test statistic for heterogeneity is given by

$$X = (\boldsymbol{D_a} + \boldsymbol{D_b})'(\boldsymbol{V_a} + \boldsymbol{V_b})^-(\boldsymbol{D_a} + \boldsymbol{D_b}).$$

The trend test is given by

$$Z = \boldsymbol{l}'(\boldsymbol{D_a} + \boldsymbol{D_b})/\sqrt{\boldsymbol{l}'(\boldsymbol{V_a} + \boldsymbol{V_b})\boldsymbol{l}}.$$

The choice of time intervals for calculating the incidental tumor component of the test of Peto *et al.*[2] is an important consideration. The use of the *ad hoc* time intervals can be problematic.[8] Moreover, the procedures described above for the analysis of occult tumor all require the information of tumor lethality or cause of death. Some argue that the determination whether a tumor causes an animal's death is a rather complicate and subjective process. It is often difficult for a pathologist to classify accurately and objectively a tumor type as straight causing or not causing animal's death. Furthermore, the validity of context of observation relies on the assumption that tumor-bearing and tumor-free animals of the same age have identical hazard functions for death unrelated to tumor. Chen and Moore[9] showed the Peto test performs poorly when there is a large reduction in survival times in the dosed groups.

1.4. *Other methods*

Dinse and Lagakos[10] proposed a logistic regression model as an alternative prevalence test for the incidental tumors,

$$\exp(\mu + \tau t + \theta d_i)/[1 + \exp(\mu + \tau t + \theta d_i)]. \tag{1}$$

They derived the likelihood score test of $\theta = 0$. The logistic regression analysis assumes that tumor prevalence is a smooth function of ages and it does not require the choice of time intervals. In addition, the logistic regression model can easily incorporate other covariates, and the software is ready available. The logistic regression has been adopted by the NTP as a standard analysis for dose-related trend test.

Bailer and Portier[11] proposed an alternative survival-adjusted approach that do not require the cause of death information. The approach modifies the Cochran-Armitage test to account for the survival times of those animals that die prior to study termination without tumor presence. The Bailer and Portier approach, has been referred to as the Poly-κ test, can be used to replace the Peto's procedure when the cause of death information is not available.

Let y_{ij} be a binary response indicating presence or absence of a tumor type of the j-th animal in the i-th group who dies at time t_{ij}, $i = 1, \ldots, g$, $j = 1, \ldots, n_i$. If all animals survive during the whole experiment period, the probability of developing a tumor for a animal in the i-th group, say, μ_i can be modelled by the linear-logistic model

$$\text{logit}(\mu_i) = \alpha + \beta d_i.$$

Let T denote the length of the experiment and t_{ij} denote the death time of the ij-th animal; Bailer and Portier[11] defined a weight equal to 1 if a tumor is present at death, and a weight equal to $\delta_{ij} = (t_{ij}/T)^{\kappa}$ if the animal dies without tumor presence. The parameter δ_{ij} reflects a less-than-whole animal contribution, and κ depends on the tumor type/site. The Poly-κ trend test for the null hypothesis $\text{H}_0 : \beta = 0$ against $H_1 : \beta > 0$, is given as

$$z = \frac{\sum_i y_{i.} d_i - p'_{..} \sum_i n'_{i.} d_i}{p'_{..}(1 - p'_{..})[\sum_i n'_{i.} d_i^2 - (\sum_i n'_{i.} d_i)^2 / \sum_i n'_{i.}]}$$

where $y_{j.} = \sum_j y_{i.}$, $n'_{i.} = \sum_j \delta_{ij}$, and $p'_{..} = \sum_{ij} y_{ij} / \sum_{ij} \delta_{ij}$. Under the null hypothesis, z is asymptotically standard normally distributed. Bieler and Williams[12] proposed a modification to account for the random variation due to δ_{ijk}.

$$z = \frac{\sum_i a_i p'_{i.} d_i - \left(\sum_i a_i d_i\right)\left(\sum_i a_i p'_{i.}\right) / \sum_i a_i}{\left\{C\left[\sum_i a_i d_i^2 - \left(\sum_i a_i d_i\right)^2 / \sum_i a_i\right]\right\}^{1/2}}$$

where $C = \sum_{ij}(r_{ij} - \bar{r}_i)^2/(N - g)$, $a_i = (n'_i)^2/n_i$, $p'_{i.} = y_{i.}/n'_i$, $r_{ij} = y_{ij} - p'_{..}\delta_{ij}$, $\bar{r}_i = \sum_j r_{ij}/n_i$, $n'_i = \sum_j \delta_{ij}$, $p'_{..} = \sum_i y_{i.}/\sum_i n'_i$, $y_{i.} = \sum_j y_{ij}$, and n_i is the total number of animals in the i-th group, and $N_k = \sum_i n_i$. Under the null hypothesis, z_k is asymptotically standard normally distributed. The values for κ are between 1 to 6 from the examination of the NTP historical data [11]. Recently, the NTP has adopted the modified Poly-3 test ($\kappa = 3$) as a standard test for trend and compares the results against the Poly-1.5 and Poly-6 tests.

1.5. *Example*

Stallard and Whitehead[13] presented the results of a carcinogenicity experiment with four dose groups in male mice. The control, low, medium groups contained 60 animals and the high dose group contained 59 animals. The experiment lasted for 105 weeks. The tumor data are shown in Table 1. Since the data contained mixture of fatal and incidental tumors, the Peto cause-of-death test was used. The fatal tumors and incidental tumors were analyzed separately by the logrank test and the prevalence method, respectively. The vector for the difference between the observed and expected numbers of tumors is $D_a = (1.4976, -6.7991, -7.1938, 12.4952)$ for the fatal tumor and is $D_b = (-0.1489, -8.0581, -8.8191, 17.0532)$ for the

Table 1. Tumor data from a carcinogencity experiment presented by Stallard and Whitehead (1999).

Dose	Deaths without tumors (frequency in parentheses)	Deaths with tumors (frequency in parentheses)
Control	15,62,90,92,96,97,101,105(22)	56,65,66,76,77,80,81,86*,87, 89,93,95,97,98(2),103, 104,105*(14)
Low	24,27,53,64,68,47,82,83,94,96,97, 99,102(2),103,104,105(27)	63,75,78,84,85,95,96,97, 98,101,102,105*(6)
Medium	5,7,39,65,70,75,76,80,82,83, 87,91(2),92,96(2),97,98(2), 99,100(2),102,105(23)	47,52,65,69,70,88,91,95,99, 100,104,105*(3)
High	16,18,49,55,59,77,85(2),105	57*,60,66,70(2),74(2),76,78,83(2), 84(3),85, 88,89,92,93(2),94,95*, 95,96,97,98*,98(2),99,100, 101,102*,102,103,104, 105*(15)

incidental tumor with the variance-covariance matrices

$$V_a = \begin{bmatrix} 6.4575 & -2.7921 & -2.2296 & -1.4358 \\ -2.7921 & 6.2768 & -2.1184 & -1.3663 \\ -2.2296 & -2.1184 & 5.4485 & -1.1005 \\ -1.4358 & -1.3663 & -1.1005 & 3.9026 \end{bmatrix}$$

and

$$V_b = \begin{bmatrix} 7.8714 & -2.8425 & -2.9518 & -2.0772 \\ -2.8425 & 8.7858 & -3.4885 & -2.4549 \\ -2.9518 & -3.4885 & 8.9895 & -2.5493 \\ -2.0772 & -2.4549 & -2.5493 & 7.0813 \end{bmatrix},$$

respectively. Hence, the pooled vector for the fatal and incidental tumors combined is $D = (1.3487, -14.8842, -16.0130, 29.5484)$ with the variance-covariance matrix

$$V = \begin{bmatrix} 14.3289 & -5.6346 & -5.1814 & -3.5130 \\ -5.6346 & 15.0626 & -5.6069 & -3.8212 \\ -5.1814 & -5.6069 & 14.4380 & -3.6498 \\ -3.5130 & -3.8212 & -3.6498 & 10.9839 \end{bmatrix}$$

The χ_3^2 test statistic for heterogeneity among the 4 groups is $X_H = 88.42$ and the Z statistic for dose-response trend is $Z = 4.599$, where the dose metric is $l = (0, 1, 2, 3)$. Both the heterogeneity test and trend test show statistically significant. The z-score from the Poly-3 test is 4.4328.

1.6. *Exact trend tests for incidental tumors*

In animal carcinogenicity bioassay experiments, the number of animals developing certain tumor types of interest is often small. The methods described previously use the asymptotic normal approximation. In general, the mortality patterns, number of intervals used in the partition, and numbers and patterns of tumor occurrence in each interval can have effects on the accuracy of an asymptotic test. When the total number of tumor occurrences is small, the normal approximation may not be reliable.[14] The exact permutation test is recommended. The following will describe an exact permutation trend test for tumors observed in an incidental context. The test is a generalization of the Fisher's exact test to the $2 \times g$ table. The tumors observed in a mortality-independent or fatal context can be tested in a similar way. However, Fairweather *et al.*[15] discussed limitations of applying exact methods to fatal tumors.

The data for the tumors observed in the j-th interval can be summarized as

Summary of animal prevalence data at interval $(t_{(j-1)}, t_j]$.

Dose	d_1	d_2	$\cdots$	d_g	Total
# with Tumors	r_{1j}	r_{2j}	$\cdots$	r_{gj}	$r_{.j}$
# deaths	n_{1j}	n_{2j}	$\cdots$	n_{gj}	$n_{.j}$

where n_{ij}, here, is the total number of animals from the i-th group that died in the j-th time interval, r_{ij} is the number of animals (out of n_{ij}) found to have the tumor of interest, and $r_{.j}$ and $n_{.j}$ are the row marginal totals which are fixed for all $j = 1, \ldots, J$.

Conditional on $r_{.j}$ and $n_{.j}$, under the null hypothesis of no difference among groups, the conditional distribution of $(r_{1j}, r_{2j}, \ldots, r_{gj})$ is the multivariate hypergeometric distribution

$$P(r_{1j}, r_{2j}, \ldots, r_{gj}) = \frac{\binom{n_{1j}}{r_{1j}}\binom{n_{2j}}{r_{2j}}\cdots\binom{n_{gj}}{r_{gj}}}{\binom{n_{.j}}{r_{.j}}}.$$

Assuming independence among the J tables, the joint probability of $(r_{11}, \ldots, r_{21}, \ldots, r_{gJ})$ for a random permutation outcome is

$$P(r_{11}, \ldots, r_{21}, \ldots, r_{gJ}) = \prod_{j=1}^{J} P(r_{1j}, r_{2j}, \ldots, r_{gj}).$$

The trend score associated with $(r_{1j}, r_{2j}, \ldots, r_{gj})$ in the j-interval is defined by

$$S_j = \sum_{i=1}^{g} d_i r_{ij}.$$

The probability distribution for the trend score statistic S_j is

$$P(S_j = s_j) = \sum_{\Omega_j} P(r_{1j}, r_{2j}, \ldots, r_{gj}),$$

where Ω_j consists of all possible permutations of r_{ij} such that $\sum_{i=1}^{g} r_{ij} = r_{.j}$ and $\sum_{i=1}^{g} d_i r_{ij} = s_j$. The trend score associated with a random permutation $(r_{11}, \ldots, r_{21}, \ldots, r_{gJ})$ is

$$S = \sum_{j=1}^{J} S_j = \sum_{j=1}^{J} \sum_{i=1}^{g} d_i r_{ij}.$$

The probability distribution for the trend score S is

$$P(S = s) = \sum_{\Omega} P(S_1 = s_1) \cdots P(S_2 = s_2) \cdots P(S_J = s_J),$$

where Ω consists of all possible permutations $(r_{11}, \ldots, r_{21}, \ldots, r_{gJ})$ such that $\sum_{j=1}^{J} s_j = s$. Let s^* denote the trend score associated with the observed outcome. The exact one-tailed p-value for a positive trend is

$$p\text{-value} = \sum_{s \geq s^*} P(S = s).$$

Note that when k = 1 and g = 2, this procedure becomes the Fisher exact test.

Traditionally, the definition of the p-value of an exact test is the cumulative sum of the probability of the observed outcome and the probabilities of all more extreme outcomes. The trend p-value described above is the sum of the probabilities of all permutations whose *trend scores* are greater than or equal to the trend score of the observed outcome s^*. Thus, every permutation with a trend score equal to s^* is included in the p-value computation irrespective of the magnitude of its probability of occurrence. Chen *et al.*[16] argued that those permutations whose probabilities are greater (less extreme) than the probability of the observed outcome should not be included. A less conservative exact p-value is

$$p\text{-value} = \sum_{s > s^*} P(S = s) + \sum_{\omega} P(S_1 = s_1) \cdot P(S_2 = s_2) \cdots P(S_J = s_J),$$

where ω consists of all permutations such that $\sum_{j=1}^{k} s_j = s^*$ and $P(r_{11}, \ldots, r_{21}, \ldots, r_{gJ}) \leq P^*$, and P^* denotes the probability of the observed outcome.

The lung adenoma data observed in female mice from a two-year feeding study of phenylephrine hydrochloride conducted by the National Toxicology Program (NTP, 1987) is analyzed for illustration. This experiment contained a control and two dose groups, 1,250 and 2,500 ppm. In the

Table 2. The incidence of lung adenoma in female mice in the two-year feeding study of phenylephrine hydrochloride.

Weeks		0 ppm	1,250 ppm	2,500 ppm	Total
0–52	r_{1j}	0	0	0	0
	n_{1j}	1	0	3	4
53–78	r_{2j}	0	0	0	0
	n_{2j}	1	3	3	7
79–92	r_{3j}	1	0	0	1
	n_{3j}	9	5	2	16
93–104	r_{4j}	0	3	5	8
	n_{4j}	39	42	42	123

Table 3. Computations of p-values for the exact trend test.

79–92			93–104			Combined	
Pattern	S_3	P_3	Pattern	S_4	P_4	$S_3 + S_4$	Prob.
						> 16250	.01987
1, 0, 0	0	.5625	1, 1, 6	16250	.008343	16250	.00469
	0	.5625	0, 3, 5	16250	.009482	16250	.00533
0, 1, 0	1250	.3125	2, 0, 6	15000	.003774	16250	.00118
	1250	.3125	0, 4, 4	15000	.012165	16250	.00380
	1250	.3125	2, 0, 6	15000	.027736	16250	.00867
0, 0, 1	2500	.1250	0, 5, 3	13750	.009482	16250	.00118
	2500	.1250	2, 1, 5	13750	.025707	16250	.00321
	2500	.1250	1, 3, 4	13750	.048660	16250	.00608

analysis of tumor incidence data, NTP generally groups the animals into the following four time intervals to adjust for intercurrent mortality: 0–52, 53–78, 79–92, 93–104 weeks. Table 2 shows the number of lung adenomas and the number of deaths occurring in the four time intervals.

The computations of the p-value for the exact trend test are shown in Table 3. Each row in the table corresponds to a permutation for which the score is 16250 from the sum of Columns S_3 and S_4. The exact p-value ($= 0.0540$) is the sum of the probabilities of the right most column, and the exact p-value ($= 0.0393$) by the Chen *et al.*[16] is obtained by excluding two probability values 0.00867 and 0.00608 as they are greater than 0.00533, the probability of the data observed. The MH asymptotic trend test gives a p-value of 0.0347. For a significance level of 5%, the Chen *et al.*[16] adjustment would indicate a statistically significant result, in agreement with the MH trend test.

1.7. *Discussion*

A typical carcinogenicity experiment examines approximately 20–50 tumor types/sites, statistical tests often perform for 10–30 types/sites routinely. Performing several tests without appropriately accounting for the multiplicity effect can inflate the overall Type I error rate or familywise error rate (FWE). Statistical Methods for the analysis of multiple tumor types/sites have been proposed by several authors.[17–20] Haseman[21] presented a rule rejecting a hypothesis for a rare tumor (spontaneous rate at most 0.01) when $p \leq 0.05$ and for a common tumor (spontaneous rate greater than 0.01) with $p \leq 0.01$. The Center for Drug Evaluation and Research (CDER) of FDA has adopted the "Haseman rule" in comparing tumor incidence rates between the control and dose groups in its evaluation of tumorigenicity studies of new drugs, and has recently recommended a new rejection rule for a positive dose-related *trend* test with $p \leq 0.025$ for rare rumors and $p \leq 0.005$ for common tumors.[22]

Interpreting results of carcinogenicity experiments is a complex process, and there are risks of both false negative and false positive results. The relatively small number of animals used, and the low tumor incidence rates can cause carcinogenicity of a compound not to be detected (i.e., a false negative error is committed). Because of the large number of comparisons involved, there is also a great potential or finding statistically significant positive trends or differences in some tumor types that are due to chance alone (i.e., a false positive error is committed). The inflated false-positive rate can invalidate the use of animal carcinogenicity data. Controlling both false positive and false negative rates should be the central issue in the statistical analysis of animal carcinogenicity experiments from the safety assessment viewpoint.

2. Reproductive Studies

Reproductive studies are conducted to assess reproductive risk to mature adults and to the developing individual from the exposure to drugs and environmental compounds. Adverse reproductive and developmental effects include effects on male and female fecundity, spontaneous abortion, infant and child death, congenital malformations, growth retardation, and mental retardation. Three segments of study are required in preclinical animal testing for each new drug depending on how women might be exposed to the drug.[23] These are referred to as Segment I (fertility and general reproductive performance), Segment II (developmental effects), and Segment III (prenatal and postnatal evaluations).

The Segment I study is aimed at providing an overall evaluation of the effects of drugs on fertility in both sexes, the course of gestation, early and late stages of the development of the embryo and fetus, and postnatal development. The studies may be conducted by treating animals of only one sex and mating with untreated animals of the opposite sex, or by treating both male and female animals. Segment II is primarily aimed at detecting teratogenic effects. The drug is given to the pregnant females during the period of organogenesis, e.g., days 6–15 for rats and mice, and days 6–18 for rabbits. The offspring are removed one or two days before term, and corpora lutea, resorption sites, and live and dead fetuses are examined. Fetuses are weighed and examined for anomalies. Segment III is aimed at the evaluation the effects of drugs on the late stages of gestation and on parturition and lactation. The drug is given to pregnant females in the final one-third of gestation and continued throughout lactation to weaning, e.g., gestation day 15 to postnatal day 21 for rats or mice. The effects on duration of gestation is determined. Pup birth and developmental data including litter size, weight, and postnatal growth and mortality, along with impaired maternal behavior are recorded and measured.

Mice, rats, and rabbits are the most commonly used species for reproductive and developmental studies. The experimental design is very similar to the carcinogenicity experiment consisting an untreated control and three dose groups. The U.S. regulatory guidelines generally recommend about 20 pregnant rodents and 15 nonrodent animals per dosage group. The ICH guideline recommends 16 to 20 pregnant animals per group. All adult animals are necropsied at terminal sacrifice.[24, 25]

Regulatory requirements specify that a wide range of endpoints must be measured, recorded, and analyzed. The endpoints can be divided into two categories: parental and embryonic/fetal endpoints. Since the test compound is administered to the adult animal, the effect of the test compound occurs in the female that receives the compound, or that is mated to a male that receives the compound, the treatment affects the fetuses indirectly via the dam. The fetal responses from the same dam are expected to be more alike than responses from different dams. This phenomenon is referred to as the "litter effect". In the analysis of embryonic/fetal endpoints, the experimental unit should be the entire litter rather than an individual fetus. Failure to account for the intra-litter correlations by using each fetus as the experimental unit will inflate the Type I error and will reduce the validity of the test. The classical approach to the analysis of reproductive data is based on the litter mean. However, this approach does account for differences in litter sizes. An alternative approach is to model the fetal endpoints in a litter as correlated outcomes (clustered data). These two approaches will described in this section. Statistical methods described will be according to three measures, continuous, binary, and count.

2.1. *Per-litter based analysis*

Consider a typical experiment of g groups, a control and $g-1$ dose groups. Assume that the i-th group contains m_i female animals. Let y_{ijk} be the response from a fetus out of n_{ij} examined or tested for a particular developmental outcome, $1 \leq i \leq g$, $1 \leq j \leq m_i$, and $1 \leq k \leq n_{ij}$. Note that y_{ijk} may be an indicator variable representing the presence or absence of a particular malformation type or a continuous variable representing a fetal weight or postnatal performance measurement. Depending on the endpoint of interest, n_{ij} may represent the number of viable fetuses, number of implants, or number of measurements. The litter-based analysis is based on the per-litter response $y_{ij} = \sum_k y_{ijk}/n_{ij}$. For a continuous response, y_{ij} will represent the mean fetus response; for a discrete variable, it will represent the sum of the fetal responses. The y_{ij} can be viewed and analyzed as a maternal endpoint.

2.1.1. *Continuous data*

Continuous data such as body weights, organ weights, or behavioral measurements conducted on offspring following birth are measured on a continuous scale. The continuous endpoints are measured either at the litter level in an adult animal (e.g., maternal body weights) y_{ij}, or at the individual fetus level (fetal body weights) y_{ijk}. Analysis of variance (ANOVA) is the most commonly used procedure for the analysis of continuous data.[25] The ANOVA method assumes that data are independently and normally distributed with homogeneous variance. Transformations such as the logarithmic, square-root and arc-sine are often applied to satisfy the normality assumption and stabilize the variance. A simple one-way ANOVA analysis is the comparison of maternal endpoints among groups. Developmental endpoints are analyzed similarly but in terms of the average within each litter as described.[26] Nonparametric methods are used when the assumption of normality fails. The nonparametric analysis is initiated by ranking all observations of the combined groups. The repeated measures ANOVA is often used for the analysis of postnatal behavioral data.[27]

2.1.2. *Binary data*

Binary endpoints can also be measured either at the parent level, such as success or failure of pregnancy, or at the individual fetal level, such as presence or absence of a particular malformation type. Statistical methods for the analysis of the prenatal and fetal responses are different. Asymptotic chi-square test is often used for the analysis of prenatal binary endpoints for comparing the incidence rates among several groups.[28] The Cochran-Armitage test is used to test for trend.[29,30] The Fisher exact test is the best known permutation test for comparing two groups. General computational algorithms and software to perform all possible permutations are given by Mehta *et al.*[31] The general approach to the analysis of fetal binary endpoints is to consider the proportion per-litter such as the proportion of live fetuses with a certain type of malformation. Typically, the proportions are transformed by an arc-sine transformation, and then the parametric ANOVA methods are used. The litter-based approach does not use the data effectively since it does not account for the litter size. For example, one out of two is treated as the same as five out of ten.

2.1.3. *Count data*

A number of primary reproductive endpoints are measured in counts. In a dominant lethal assay, male mice are treated with a suspect mutagen, and then are mated with females. The numbers of corpora lutea, implantations, lives, and dead conceptuses are counted to assess reproductive effects of the test compound. Count data are often normalized by the square root transformation, the transformed data are then analyzed as continuous data using the parametric ANOVA methods. Count data can also be analyzed by nonparemetric methods.

2.1.4. *Example*

A study of the effects of maternal exposure to diethylhexyl phthalate (DEHP) in rats is presented as an example. Table 4 contains a summary of the analysis for selected endpoints. For the detailed design and analysis

Table 4. Reproductive parameters after exposure of pregnant Fisher 344 rats to diethylhexyl phahalate in the feed on gestational days 0 through 20.

	diethylhexyl phahalate % in feed				
Endpoint	0.0	0.5	1.0	1.5	2.0
No. pregnant dams	24	23	22	24	25
Maternal wgt gd 0	173.60 (3.25)	175.37 (3.37)	172.42 (3.12)	171.77 (2.80)	173.33 (2.95)
Maternal wgt gd 20	248.30 (3.64)[a]	246.00 (2.90)	232.73 (3.25)*	217.76 (3.25)*	184.15 (4.28)*
Maternal wgt gain	74.69 (1.71)[a]	70.63 (2.48)	60.31 (1.44)*	45.99 (1.78)*	10.82 (3.00)*
Gravid uterine wgt	49.79 (1.39)[a]	44.83 (2.49)	46.81 (1.31)	43.86 (0.96)	19.08 (3.71)*
Maternal liver wgt	9.75 (0.12)[a]	11.72 (0.17)*	12.06 (0.17)*	12.21 (0.19)*	11.11 (0.15)*
Corpora lutea	10.91 (0.33)	10.96 (0.22)	11.18 (0.30)	11.17 (0.18)	10.52 (0.61)
Implantation sites	10.92 (0.31)	9.83 (0.54)	10.59 (0.24)	10.58 (0.22)	10.40 (0.41)
% viable	10.46 (0.32)[a]	9.39 (0.53)	10.05 (0.26)	10.08 (0.25)	8.00 (0.70)*
% male	53.56 (3.65)	45.77 (4.51)	46.39 (3.31)	54.44 (3.00)	50.66 (6.10)
% malformation	1.27 (0.71)[a]	0.00 (0.00)	1.92 (1.11)	3.13 (1.06)	2.87 (1.64)
Fetal weight	3.022 (.029)[a]	3.143 (.035)*	2.852 (.053)*	2.557 (.034)*	2.266 (.041)*

[a]Significance in linear trend
*Significantly different from control

the reader is referred to Tyl *et al.*[32] As described the ANOVA was used for the analysis of continuous endpoints and per-litter proportion data. Prior to analysis, the arc-sine square root transformation was performed to all maternal or per-litter proportion data. When a significant ($p < 0.05$) dose effect occurred, Duncan's multiple range test was used for pairwise comparisons between control and each dose group. A test of linear dose-response trend was performed using contrast tests. A one-sided test was used for pairwise comparisons except for the maternal and fetal body weights and percentage of males per litter.

2.2. *Likelihood and quasi-likelihood/generalized-estimating-equations approaches*

As discussed, the fetal responses with a litter are not independent. The proper experimental unit in the analysis should be the litter with the fetal responses representing multiple observations from a single experimental unit. The likelihood-based and generalized estimating equations (or quasi-likelihood) are the two commonly used approaches to modeling the correlated data.

2.2.1. *Modeling continuous data*

A general approach to modeling fetal data can be carried out in terms of a mixed-effects model. Dempster *et al.*[33] proposed a normal mixed-effects model with two levels of variance, in which litter effect is modeled by a nested random factor and dose by a fixed factor. The response y_{ijk} in a litter is expressed as a mixed effects model with two sources of variations: the between litter γ_{ij} and within litter variations e_{ijk},

$$y_{ijk} = \mu_{ij} + \gamma_{ij} + e_{ijk}.$$

The random components γ_{ij} and e_{ijk} are independently normally distributed with $\mathrm{E}(\gamma_{ij}) = 0$, $\mathrm{Var}(\gamma_{ij}) = \sigma_a^2$, and $\mathrm{E}(e_{ijk}) = 0$, $\mathrm{Var}(e_{ijk}) = \sigma^2$. Thus, the mean and variance of y_{ijk} are $\mathrm{E}(y_{ijk}) = \mu_i$ and $\mathrm{Var}(y_{ijk}) = \sigma_a^2 + \sigma^2$. The intra-litter correlation between y_{ijk} and $y_{ijk'}$, for $k \neq k'$ is $\phi = \sigma_a^2/(\sigma^2 + \sigma_a^2)$. The mean parameter μ_{ij} is often modeled as a linear function of dose $\mu_{ij} = \beta_0 + \beta_1 d_i$ for trend test $(H_o : \beta_1 = 0)$.

Computation techniques for the maximum likelihood estimation of the parameters of linear mixed effects models have been proposed by many authors.[34–36] The estimates can be obtained using the PROC MIXED procedure of SAS.[37] Alternatively, the generalized estimating equations (GEE) approach[38] can be used to estimate the fixed effects parameters $\boldsymbol{\beta}$. Under the normal model, the likelihood-based and GEE approaches have the same estimating equations for the mean parameters, but unlike the likelihood approach, the GEE uses the method of moments to estimate the variance component parameters.

2.2.2. *Modeling binary data*

Let y_{ijk} denote the presence or absence of a response. Assume that the mean and variance of y_{ijk} are $\mathrm{E}(y_{ijk}) = \mu_i$, and $\mathrm{Var}(y_{ijk}) = \mu_i(1 - \mu_i)$ and the correlation is $\mathrm{Corr}(y_{ijk}, y_{ijk'}) = \phi_i$, where $k, k' = 1, \ldots, n_{ij}$, and

$k \neq k'$. The parameter μ_i is the probability of a developmental effect of the i-th group, and ϕ_i is the intra-litter correlation coefficient. The binary responses $y_{ij1}, \ldots, y_{ijn_{ij}}$ within each litter are assumed exchangeable, that is, if $\{k_1, \ldots, k_l\}$ is a subset of $\{1, \ldots, n_{ij}\}$, then

$$Pr(y_{ij1} = 1, \ldots, y_{ijl} = 1) = Pr(y_{ijk_1} = 1, \ldots, y_{ijk_l} = 1),$$

for all $l = 1, \ldots, n_{ij}$.

Let $y_{ij} = (y_{ij1} + \ldots + y_{ijn_{ij}})$, then the mean and variance of y_{ij} are $\mathrm{E}(y_{ij}|n_{ij}) = n_{ij}\mu_i$ and $\mathrm{Var}(y_{ij}|n_{ij}) = n_{ij}\mu_i(1-\mu_i)[\phi_i(n_{ij}-1)+1]$. The intra-litter correlation coefficient generally is positive ($\phi_i > 0$). Thus, the variance $n_{ij}\mu_i(1-\mu_i)[\phi_i(n_{ij}-1)+1]$ is greater than the nominal binomial variance $n_{ij}\mu_i(1-\mu_i)$. The distribution of y_{ij} is known as an extra-binomial variate. Note that if $\phi_i = 0$, then all y_{ijk}'s are independent binary random variables and y_{ij} is a binomial,

$$P(y_{ij}) = \binom{n_{ij}}{y_{ij}} \mu_{ij}^{y_{ij}} (1-\mu_{ij})^{n_{ij}-y_{ij}}.$$

In a binomial or extra-binomial model, the mean function is often modeled by a logit function, $\mathrm{logit}(\mu_i|\boldsymbol{z}_{ij}) = \boldsymbol{\beta}'\boldsymbol{z}_{ij}$. The dose response model for trend test is given by

$$\mu_i = \frac{\exp(\beta_0 + \beta_1 d_i)}{1 + \exp(\beta_0 + \beta_1 d_i)}.$$

The beta-binomial model is the commonly known distribution used for modeling the extra-binomial variation data.[39] The beta-binomial model assumes that responses within the same litter occur according to a binomial distribution and the probability of responses is assumed to vary among litters according to a beta distribution:

$$P(y_{ij}) = \binom{n_{ij}}{y_{ij}} \frac{\mathrm{B}(a_i + y_{ij}, b_i + n_{ij} - y_{ij})}{\mathrm{B}(a_i, b_i)}$$

where $\mathrm{B}(a_i, b_i) = \Gamma(a_i)\Gamma(b_i)/\Gamma(a_i + b_i)$, where $\Gamma(\cdot)$ is the gamma function, $a_i > 0$, and $b_i > 0$. Under the reparameterization $\mu_i = a_i/(a_i + b_i)$ and $\phi_i = (a_i + b_i + 1)^{-1}$, the parameters μ_i and ϕ_i are, respectively, the mean and the intra-litter correlation parameters in the i-th group. That is, the mean of y_{ij} is $\mathrm{E}(y_{ij}) = n_{ij}\mu_i$, and the intra-litter correlation is $\mathrm{Corr}(y_{ijk}, y_{ijk'}) = \phi_i$. The variance of y_{ij} is $\mathrm{Var}(y_{ij}) = [\phi_i(n_{ij}-1)+1][n_{ij}\mu_i(1-\mu_i)]$. When $\phi_i = 0$, then y_{ij} becomes a binomial variable. The parameters can be estimated by the maximum likelihood method. The likelihood ratio or Wald test is often used to test for the significance of parameters. An advantage of the use of the likelihood-based beta-binomial model is that parameters $\boldsymbol{\beta}$ as well as the intra-litter correlations ϕ's can be tested directly. One problem with the beta-binomial model is the bias and instability of the MLE's of $\boldsymbol{\beta}$ as discussed by Williams.[40] Williams[41] proposed using the quasi-likelihood method as an alternative approach to the beta-binomial model.

In the quasi-likelihood approach, only assumptions on the mean and variance are required: $\mathrm{E}(y_{ij}|n_{ij}) = n_{ij}\mu_i$ and $\mathrm{Var}(y_{ij}|n_{ij}) = n_{ij}\mu_i(1 - \mu_i)[\phi(n_{ij} - 1) + 1]$. Note that in the quasi-likelihood estimation, the intra-litter correlations typically are modeled as constant across groups. The coefficients of the β's can be obtained by solving the quasi-likelihood estimating (score) equations:

$$S(\beta_l) = \sum_{i=1}^{g}\sum_{j=1}^{m_i} z_{ijl}\frac{y_{ij} - n_{ij}\mu_i}{[1 + (n_{ij} - 1)\phi]} = 0, \quad l = 1, \ldots, 2.$$

The intra-litter correlation coefficient is calculated by equating with the mean of Pearson chi-square statistics, i.e.,

$$\phi = \frac{1}{N-2}\sum_{i=1}^{g}\sum_{j=1}^{m_i}\frac{(y_{ij} - n_{ij}\mu_i)^2}{n_{ij}\mu_i(1 - \mu_i)[\phi^{-1} + (n_{ij} - 1)]},$$

where $N = \sum_i^g \sum_j^{m_i} n_{ij}$. The parameters β's and ϕ are estimated by solving $S(\beta_l) = 0$ and ϕ alternatively until convergence. The Wald test is often used to test for the significance of β's.

2.2.3. *Modeling count data*

Count data are generally modeled by a Poisson distribution. Let n_{ij} be an observed count from the j-th animal in the i-th group $1 < i < g$ and $1 < j < m_i$. If n_{ij} has the Poisson distribution

$$p(n_{ij}) = \frac{\mu_i^{n_{ij}} e^{-\mu_i}}{n_{ij}!}, \quad n_{ij} = 0, 1, 2, \ldots,$$

the mean and variance of n_{ij} are $\mathrm{E}(n_{ij}) = \mathrm{Var}(n_{ij}) = \mu_i$. In the Poisson model, the mean function is often modeled by a log-linear function, $\log(\mu_i|\boldsymbol{z}_{ij}) = \boldsymbol{z}_{ij}\boldsymbol{\beta}$. The dose-response model for trend test is $\mu_i = \exp(\beta_0 + \beta_1 d_i)$.

A common complication in the analysis of count data is that the observed variation often exceeds or falls behind the variation that is predicted from a Poisson model. The classical approach is to assume that the mean of the Poisson has a gamma distribution which leads to a negative binomial (gamma-Poisson) distribution for the observed data,

$$p(n_{ij}) = \frac{\Gamma(n_{ij} + \phi_i^{-1})}{\Gamma(n_{ij}+1)\Gamma(\phi_i^{-1})}\left(\frac{\phi_i\mu_i}{1+\phi_i\mu_i}\right)^{n_{ij}}\left(\frac{1}{1+\phi_i\mu_i}\right)^{\frac{1}{\phi_i}}$$

where $\phi_i > 0$. The maximum likelihood estimation of the negative binomial model was described in details by Lawless.[42] The significance of the parameters can be tested using either the likelihood ratio test or Wald test. Like the beta-binomial model, the negative binomial model can be applied to testing for the extra-Poisson variation.

A limitation of the parametric approach is in its restriction on $\phi \geq 0$. In applications, for example, the number of litter implant or the number of corpora lutea may exhibit a sub-Poisson variation. The quasi-likelihood approach[43] provides a method to model sub-Poisson variation data. The quasi-likelihood approach assumes the mean and variance of count data are of a negative binomial form, $\mathrm{E}(n_{ij}) = \mu_i$ and $\mathrm{Var}(n_{ij}) = \mu_i(1+\phi_i\mu_i)$. The coefficients of the β's can be obtained by solving the score equations

$$S(\beta_l) = \sum_{i=1}^{g}\sum_{j=1}^{m_i} z_{ijl}\frac{n_{ij}-\mu_i}{\mu_i+\phi\mu_i^2} = 0.$$

The parameter ϕ is calculated by equating with the mean of Pearson chi-square statistics,

$$\phi = \frac{1}{N-2}\sum_{i=1}^{g}\sum_{j=1}^{m_i}\frac{(n_{ij}-\mu_i)^2}{\mu_i\phi^{-1}+\mu_i^2},$$

where $N = \sum_i^g \sum_j^{m_i} n_{ij}$. The parameters β's and ϕ are estimated by solving $S(\beta_l) = 0$ and ϕ alternatively until convergence. Quasi-likelihood approaches to estimating and testing the mean of various mixed Poisson models are given by Chen and Ahn.[44]

Examples of analyses of fetal response toxicity data using the likelihood and the quasi-likelihood/GEE approaches are given in Chen.[45]

2.3. *Multiple developmental outcomes*

The standard approach for assessment of developmental risks of a compound has been based on the analysis of each developmental endpoint separately. It has been suggested that the developmental toxicity outcomes (i.e., death/resorption, malformation, growth retardation, etc) may represent different degrees of responses to a toxic insult and occur in a dose-related manner.[45,46] These developmental outcomes are likely to be correlated. Therefore, a joint analysis of multiple developmental outcomes can have some advantages: it can increase the power of detecting effects if the multiple outcomes are manifestations of some common biological effects, and it allows investigations of associations among the multiple outcomes if they are the results of different biological mechanisms. Various multivariate models have been developed for simultaneous analysis of multiple endpoints.[47–50]

3. Mixure Experiment

Human population is continuously exposed to many chemical mixtures simultaneously or in sequence. Interactions may occur among chemicals in the mixture. Asessment of the joint toxic effects from exposure to a mixture has been recognized as an important public health issue. In many toxicological mixture experiments, the primary interest is the effect of relative proportions of the components present in the mixture rather than their absolute amount. For example, individual components of air pollution vary from one area to another, a main objective in the study of air quality is to investigate the effects of changes in proportions of individual components on endpoint responses.

Let x_i $(i = 1, \ldots, p)$ denote the proportion of the ith component in the mixture. The effects of the component proportions x_i on the response y is modelled by a Scheffe [51] canonical polynomial

$$E(y|\boldsymbol{x}) = \sum_{i=1}^{p} a_i x_i + \sum_{i<j}^{p} a_{ij} x_i x_j + \sum_{i<j<k}^{p} a_{ijk} x_i x_j x_k + \cdots .$$

Under the normality assumption on y, the parameters a's are estimated by the method of least squares. A comprehensive reference on the design and analysis of continuous response data from a mixture experiment is given by Cornell.[52]

This section will describe a logistic-Weibull mixture model to the analysis of time-to-tumore data. This model will be applied to analyzing a dietary mixture experimental to assess the effects of dietary component proportions in the mixture on tumorigenesis in rats.

3.1. *A mixture model for survival data*

Consider an animal carcinogenesis experiment. Assume the experimental animals consist of two subpopulations. Let $Y = 1$ represent those animals in the susceptible subpopulation, all of which will develop a tumor, and $Y = 0$ represent those in the remaining subpopulation, none of which will develop a tumor. Assume that the treatment can affect susceptibility and that the probability that an animal from the treatment group $\boldsymbol{x}$ will be susceptible is

$$P(Y = 1|\boldsymbol{x}) = E(Y|\boldsymbol{x}) = \frac{exp(\boldsymbol{\beta}'\boldsymbol{x})}{1 + exp(\boldsymbol{\beta}'\boldsymbol{x})},$$

where $\boldsymbol{\beta}'\boldsymbol{x}$ is the Scheffe polynomial,

$$\boldsymbol{\beta}'\boldsymbol{x} = \sum_{i=1}^{p} \beta_i x_i + \sum_{i<j}^{p} \beta_{ij} x_i x_j + \sum_{i<j<k}^{p} \beta_{ijk} x_i x_j x_k + \dots$$

This model is known as a logistic regression model.

For those animals in the susceptible subpopulation that will develop a tumor, let the probability density for time-to-tumor distribution at $\boldsymbol{x}$ follow a Weibull model

$$f(t|\boldsymbol{x}) = \kappa\lambda^{\kappa} t^{\kappa-1} \exp\{-(\lambda t)^{\kappa}\},$$

where $\lambda = \exp(-\boldsymbol{\gamma}'\boldsymbol{x})$ and

$$\boldsymbol{\gamma}'\boldsymbol{x} = \sum_{i=1}^{p} \gamma_i x_i + \sum_{i<j}^{p} \gamma_{ij} x_i x_j + \sum_{i<j<k}^{p} \gamma_{ijk} x_i x_j x_k + \cdots$$

The cumulative distribution of $f(t|\boldsymbol{x})$ is

$$F(t|\boldsymbol{x}) = 1 - exp\{-(\lambda t)^{\kappa}\}.$$

Note that the inverse of λ, $\exp(\boldsymbol{\gamma}'\boldsymbol{x})$, is the characteristic life of the Weibull model, as it is the $100(1-1/e)$ percentile of the Weibull distribution. Here, the canonical link function, the log transformation $\log(1/\lambda) = \boldsymbol{\gamma}'\boldsymbol{x}$, is utilized to rescale the characteristics life of the Weibull distribution by its natural link function in terms of the covariates $\boldsymbol{x}$.

The probability that an animal from the treatment $\boldsymbol{x}$ will develop a tumor at time t is

$$\mu(\boldsymbol{x}) f(t|\boldsymbol{x}),$$

where $\mu(\boldsymbol{x}) = E(Y|\boldsymbol{x})$. The probability that an animal from the treatment $\boldsymbol{x}$ will not have a tumor by time t is

$$[1 - \mu(\boldsymbol{x})] + \mu(\boldsymbol{x})[1 - F(t|\boldsymbol{x})] = 1 - \mu(\boldsymbol{x})F(t|\boldsymbol{x})$$

where $F(t|\boldsymbol{x})$ is the cumulative distribution of the density function $f(t|\boldsymbol{x})$. This model is a mixture of the classical tolerance model commonly used in toxicology (where $F(t_k|\boldsymbol{x})$ is a degenerate distribution) and the Weibull failure time model (where $\mu(\boldsymbol{x}) = 1$).

Let $t_1, t_2, \ldots, t_K$ be the distinct times at which events of tumor occurring or animal death (with or without tumor) were observed, where t t_K is the time at which the experiment was terminated. Further assume the survival time is independent of tumor onset. Thus, the animals dead at time t_k can be viewed as a random sample via an independent censoring scheme. Let d_k be the number of animals with tumor onset at time t_k and c_k be the number of deaths without tumors at time t_k. The likelihood function is

$$L \propto \prod_{k=1}^{K} [\mu(\boldsymbol{x})f(t_k|\boldsymbol{x})]^{d_k}[1 - \mu(\boldsymbol{x})F(t_k|\boldsymbol{x})]^{c_k}.$$

The maximum likelihood estimates of β's, γ's and κ can be computed by the Gauss-Newton method. Since the estimates among β's and among γ's are not independent, the likelihood ratio test is used to assess the significance of the coefficients. The model selection is based on the sequential model fitting approach beginning with the constant and linear models.

In a three-component mixture, if two of the components, say, x_1 and x_2, blend non-linearly but the third x_3 blends linearly with each of the two components as well as their (two-component) mixture, Scheffe[53] pointed out that such a system cannot be represented by the polynomial form

$$\mathrm{a}'\mathrm{x} = a_1x_1 + a_2x_2 + a_3x_3 + a_{12}x_1x_2,$$

Cornell and Gorman[54] showed that the proper model to represent the complete linear blending of x_3 had an expression of the Becker[55] non-polynomial H2 model,

$$\mathrm{a}'\mathrm{x} = a_1x_1 + a_2x_2 + a_3x_3 + a_{12}\frac{x_1x_2}{x_1 + x_2},$$

where $x_1x_2/(x_1 + x_2) = 0$ if $x_1 + x_2 = 0$. The Becker H2 model under the logistic or Weibull model can be derived analogously by following the same argument given by Cornell and Gorman,[54] and it will be applied to analyzing the dietary mixture experiment data.

Table 5. The dietary mixture design: The proportions of dietary fat, carbohydrate, and fiber in percent of total calories.

Diet	1	2	3	4	5	6	7	8	9
Fat	0.175	0.153	0.133	0.491	0.440	0.390	0.701	0.638	0.576
Carbohydrate	0.775	0.820	0.863	0.470	0.538	0.607	0.267	0.343	0.421
Fiber	0.050	0.027	0.004	0.039	0.022	0.003	0.032	0.019	0.003

3.2. *Example*

A dietary mixture experiment was conducted at the National Center for Toxicological Research to study the effects of calories of dietary fat, carbohydrate, and fiber on the promotion of DMBA-induced mammary gland tumors in female rats under conditions of isocaloric consumption at or near ad libitum levels. The mixture experiment contains three components with nine different dietary groups containing combinations of low, medium, and high levels of dietary fat, carbohydrate, and fiber so that their individual contributions can be determined simultaneously over a wide, but physiological, dietary range. Table 5 contains nine diets with different proportions of fat, carbohydrate, and fiber in terms of per cents of the total calorie consumption. Diets 1–3 are low fat and high carbohydrate, Diets 4–6 are medium fat and medium carbohydrate, and Diets 7–9 are high fat and low carbohydrate; and diets 1, 4, 7 are high fiber, diet 2, 5, 8 are medium fiber, diets 3, 6, 9 are low fiber. Diets 2 and 3 are similar to standard diets. Both diets are low fat and high carbohydrate, but diet 2 has medium fiber and diet 3 has low fiber content. In all diets, fat and carbohydrate are the two major sources of calories. Table 6 contains the frequency of the time of tumor onset observed from the nine groups. The primary objective of the statistical analysis is to investigate the effect of changes in proportions of the fat, carbohydrate, and fiber calories in a diet on the tumor response.

In the experiment, female Sprague-Dawley rats (38–42 days of age) were randomly assigned to the nine groups of 30 animals per group. At Day 52, the animals were administered 7.5 mg DMBA in corn oil by stomach tube. One week after the treatment with DMBA, the animals in each group were fed their corresponding diets at equal total calorie consumption but different levels of fat, carbohydrate, and fiber. Animals were palpated for mammary tumors weekly. Twenty six weeks after DMBA administration, the animals were sacrificed and mammary spreads were examined for the presence of tumors. Each tumor was recorded at the time of palpation and

Table 6. The number of animals with the first DMBA-induced mammary gland tumors observed in rats administered different proportions of dietary fat, carbohydrate, and fiber, with each of the nine diet groups having equal total calorie consumption.

	Diets (See Table 1)								
Week	1	2	3	4	5	6	7	8	9
4							1	2	
5								1	1
6					1		2	1	2
7			2		1	1	1	3	1
8		2	3	8	3	4	1		2
9	3	1	1	1	3	6	1	1	4
10	3	2	3		2	2	1	1	2
11	3		1	1	2	3		1	2
12	1	1			1		2	1	2
13		2		1	1	1	3	2	1
14			1		1	1	1	3	1
15	1	2		4	1		2	2	2
16	1					3		2	
17	1		2	2	1				3
18		1		1	1			3	1
19				3					2
20	1	3	1	1					
21							1		
22	1		2	1		1			
23	1				1				
24			1		1	1	1		
25				1	1				
26	1	1	0				1		
26*	13	15	13	6	9	7	12	7	4
26^a	6	8	5	2	5	2	7	3	0
26^b	7	7	8	4	4	5	5	4	4

*Time of sacrifice and necropsy (censored).
^{a}Number of animal censored in susceptible predicted from the mixture model.
^{b}Number of animal in non-susceptible predicted from the mixture model.

necropsy to allow determination of time-to-tumor for each tumor. Tissue sections were prepared and examined by standard histological procedures. Thus, the animals without tumor at week 26 were censored. A detailed description of the study and the mixture design is given in Jackson *et al.*[56]

Since the proportions of the three dietary components were restricted by the lower bounds, the coordinates of the simplex system were redefined in terms of pseudo-component coordinates. The values of the pseudo-component proportions x_1, x_2 and x_3 of the three dietary components were

Table 7. Maximum likelihood estimates (standard errors) and the maximum value of log-likelihood (LL) for the logistic and Weibull models.

Model	Estimate	Logistic	Weibull
Linear	Fat	1.535 (0.300)	2.796 (0.091)
	Carb.	0.526 (0.278)	3.177 (0.111)
	Fiber	−5.979 (4.754)	6.849 (1.627)
	LL	−164.39	−738.28
Quad	Fat	1.513 (0.760)	2.815 (0.192)
	Carb.	0.132 (0.348)	3.370 (0.133)
	Fiber	−15.89 (25.86)	7.724 (8.078)
	Fat*Carb.	2.008 (2.384)	−0.757 (0.662)
	Fat*Fib.	−5.100 (24.07)	3.986 (7.466)
	Carb*Fib.	17.749 (19.84)	−5.690 (5.578)
	LL	−160.89	−733.83
L+F*C	Fat	0.866 (0.397)	3.016 (0.125)
	Carb.	0.189 (0.309)	3.324 (0.109)
	Fiber	−4.281 (4.896)	5.825 (1.613)
	Fat*Carb.	3.635 (1.503)	−1.176 (0.444)
	LL	−161.42	−734.74

computed using the transformation

$$x_1 = \frac{\%\text{Fat} - 13.3\%}{59.7\%}, \quad x_2 = \frac{\%\text{Carb.} - 26.7\%}{59.7\%}, \quad x_3 = \frac{\%\text{Fiber} - 0.3\%}{59.7\%}.$$

The 59.7% is computed by (100 − 13.3 − 26.7 − 0.3)%.

Initially, the Scheffe first-degree (linear) as well as the second-degree (quadratic) polynomials were fitted using the logistic model and Weibull model separately. Table 7 contains the maximum likelihood estimates (standard errors) of regression coefficients of the fitted models and the maximum values of the log-likelihood. Both the fitted Scheffe linear logistic and linear Weibull model show that dietary fat has the most effect on tumor promotion, and fiber has the least effect. The Weibull model shows that fat has the shortest time of tumor onset, and fiber has the longest time of tumor onset. The coefficient estimate for fiber in the linear logistic model is negative, this does not necessary indicate that fiber applied alone has an effect on the reduction of tumor incidence (a dose-response relationship) since the sum of the proportions of fat, carbohydrate, and fiber is restricted to 1.

Both logistic and Weibull models suggest that the (fiber*carbohydrate) and (fiber*fat) interaction terms are unnecessary. It is noticeable that the

Table 8. Maximum likelihood estimates (standard errors) and the maximum values of log-likelihood (LL) for the logistic-Weibull mixture model.

Model	Estimate	Logistic	Weibull
a	Fat	1.736 (0.446)	2.524 (0.106)
	Carb.	0.789 (0.536)	2.756 (0.110)
	Fiber	−0.806 (7.162)	6.915 (2.012)
	LL	−729.67	
b	Fat	0.830 (0.548)	2.530 (0.142)
	Carb.	0.472 (0.426)	2.818 (0.131)
	Fiber	0.909 (7.784)	6.497 (2.081)
	Fat*Carb.	4.474 (2.286)	−0.179 (0.524)
	LL	−726.00	
c	Fat	0.778 (0.520)	2.496 (0.103)
	Carb.	0.441 (0.403)	2.800 (0.107)
	Fiber	1.023 (7.823)	6.575 (2.045)
	Fat*Carb.	4.831 (2.067)	
	LL	−726.02	

estimates of fiber, and the (fiber*carbohydrate) and (fiber*fat) interactions are extremely large. The first-degree polynomial plus (fat*carbohydrate) interaction was fitted using the Becker H2 non-polynomial form subsequently. This model is referred to as $L + F \times C$ model. Note that the coefficient estimates are more similar in size. In both logistic and Weibull models, the likelihood ratio tests show that $L+F \times C$ model provide an adequate fit to the data (results not shown). In the fitted $L+F\times C$ model, the significantly positive (fat*carbohydrate) interaction in the logistic model implies that fat and carbohydrate combined increases the tumor incidence synergistically, and the significantly negative (fat*carbohydrate) interaction in the Weibull model implied that fat and carbohydrate combined reduces the tumor onset time synergistically.

The first-degree polynomial model with and without the (fat*x carbohydrate) interaction was fitted using the logistic-Weibull mixture. Both results are consistent with the results of fitting the logistic model and Weibull model separately. The likelihood ratio test for the Weibull versus logistic-Weibull mixture is $2(-729.67+738.28) = 17.22(P < 0.01)$ with 3 degrees of freedom for the linear model, and is $2(-726.00+733.83) = 15.66(P < 0.01)$ with 4 degrees of freedom for the $L + F \times C$ model. Both tests show that the logistic-Weibull mixture model fits the data better than the Weibull model.

Since the (fat*carbohydrate) interaction in the Weibull component is not significant, the logistic-Weibull mixture model without the (fat*carbohydrate) interaction in the Weibull component was refitted. The maximum likelihood estimates (standard errors) and the maximum values of the log-likelihood for the three fitted mixture models are given in Table 8. These models are referred to as Models a, b, and c, respectively. The likelihood ratio test for Model a versus Model c is $2(-726.02+729.67)=7.30$ with 1 degree of freedom. The likelihood ratio test for Model c versus Model b is $2(-726.00+726.02)=.004$ with 1 degree of freedom. Hence, Model c appears to describe the data adequately.

References

1. Kodell RL and Nelson CJ. (1980) An illness-death model for the study of the carcinogenic process using survival/sacrifice data. *Biometrics*, **36**: 267.
2. Peto R, Pike MC, Day NE *et al.* (1980) Guidelines for simple sensitive significance tests for carcinogenic effects in long-term animals experiments', in *Long-term and Short-term Screening Assays for Carcinogens: A Critical Appraisal*, Annex to Supplement 2. Lyon, International Agency for Research on Cancer, 311.
3. Kodell RL, Shaw GW, and Johnson AM. (1982) Nonparametric joint estimators for disease resistance and survival functions in survival/sacrifice experiments. *Biometrics*, **38**: 43.
4. Kaplan EL and Meier P. (1958) Nonparametric estimation from incomplete observation. *Journal of the American Statistical Association*, **53**: 457. experiments.
5. Gart JJ, Krewski D, Lee PN *et al.* (1986) Statistical Methods in Cancer Research, Vol. 3, *The Design and Analysis of Long-Term Animal Experiments*. Lyon, International Agency for Research on Cancer.
6. Hoel D and Walburg H. (1972) Statistical analysis of survival experiments. *Journal of National Cancer Institute*, **49**: 361.
7. Mantel N and Haenszel W. (1959) Statistical aspects of the analysis of data from retrospective studies of disease. *Journal of the National Cancer Institute*, **22**: 719.
8. Kodell RL, Chen JJ and Moore GE. (1994) Comparing distributions for time to onset of disease in animal tumorigenicity experiments. *Communications in Statistics — Theory and Methods*, **23**: 959.
9. Chen JJ and Moore GE. (1994) Impact of surviving time on tests for carcinogenicity. *Communications in Statistics — Theory and Methods*, **23**: 1375.
10. Dinse GE and Lagakos SW. (1983) Regression analysis of tumor prevalence data. *Applied Statistics*, **32**: 236.
11. Bailer AJ and Portier CJ. (1988) Effects of treatment-induced mortality and tumor-induced mortality on tests for carcinogenicity in small samples. *Biometrics*, **44**: 417.

12. Bieler GS and Williams RL. (1993) Ratio estimates, the delta methods, and quantal response tests for increased carcinogenicity. *Biometrics*, **49**: 793.
13. Stallard N and Whitehead A. (2000) Modified Weibull multi-state models for the analysis of animal carcinogenicity data. *Environmental and Ecological Statistics*, **7**: 117.
14. Chen JJ and Gaylor DW. (1986) The upper percentiles of the distribution of the logrank statistics for small numbers of tumors. *Communications in Statistics — Theory and Methods*, **15**: 991.
15. Fairweather WR, Bhattacharyya PP, Ceuppens G. *et al.* (1998) Biostatistical methodology in carcinogenicity studies. *Drug Information Journal*, **32**: 401.
16. Chen JJ, Kodell RL and Pearce BA. (1997) Significance Levels of Randomization Trend Tests in the Event of Rare Occurrences. *Biometrical Journal*, **39**: 327.
17. Heyse JF and Rom D. (1980) Adjusting for multiplicity of statistical tests in the analysis of carcinogenicity studies. *Biometrical Journal*, **30**: 883.
18. Westfall PH and Young SS. (1989) *p*-value adjustment for multiple tests in multivariate binomial models. *Journal of American Statistical Association*, **84**: 780.
19. Chen JJ. (1996) Global tests for analysis of multiple tumor data from animal carcinogenicity experiments. *Statistics in Medicine*, **15**: 1217.
20. Chen JJ, Lin KK, Huque M. *et al.* (2000) Weighted *p*-value Adjustments for Animal Carcinogenicity. *Trend Test Biometrics*, **56**: 586.
21. Haseman JK, Huff J. and Boorman. (1984) Use of historical control data in carcinogenicity studies in rodents. *Toxicology and Pathology*, **12**: 126.
22. Lin KK and Rahman MA. (1998) Overall false positive rates in tests for linear trend in tumor incidence in animal carcinogenicity studies in new drugs. *Journal of Biopharmaceutical Statistics*, **8**: 1.
23. U.S. Food and Drug Administration, International Conference on Homonisation. (1966) *Guideline on Detection of Reproduction for Medicinal Products.* Rockvill, MD: Food and Drug Administration.
24. Christian MS, Hoberman AM. (1996) Perspectives on the U.S., EEC, and Japanese developmental toxicity testing guidelines. In: RD Hood ed. *Handbook of Developmental Toxicology.* New York, NY: CRC Press, 551.
25. Tyl RW and Marr MC. (1996) Developmental toxicity testing — methodology. In: RD Hood ed. *Handbook of Developmental Toxicology.* New York, NY: CRC Press, 175–225.
26. Healy MJR. (1972) Animal litters as experimental units. *Applied Statistics*, **21**: 155.
27. Karpinski KF. (1991) In: D Krewski, C Frankin eds. *Statistics in Toxicology.* New York, NY: Gordon and Breach Science, 393.
28. Agresti A. (1990) *Categorical Data Analysis.* New York, NY: John Wiley & Sons.
29. Cochran WG. (1954) Some methods for strengthening the common χ^2 tests. *Biometrics*, **10**: 417.
30. Armitage P. (1955) Tests for linear trends in proportions and frequencies. *Biometrics*, **11**: 375.

31. Mehta CR, Patel NR, and Senchaudhuri P. (1992) *Journal of Computation and Graph Statistics*, **1**: 21.
32. Tyl RW, Price CJ, Marr MC, *et al.* (1983) *Teratologic Evaluation of Diethylhexyl Phthalate in Fisher 344 Rats.* Research Triangle Park, NC: Research Triangle Institute.
33. Dempster AP, Selwyn MR, Patel CM *et al.* (1984) Statistical and computational aspects of mixed model analysis. *Applied Statistics*, **33**: 203.
34. Harville DA. (1977) Maximum likelihood approaches to variance component estimation and to related problems. *Journal of the American Statistical Association*, **72**: 320.
35. Laird NM and Ware JH. (1982) Random-effects models for longitudinal data. *Biometrics*, **38**: 963.
36. Lindstrom MJ and Bates DM. (1988) Newton-Raphson and EM algorithms for linear mixed-effects models for repeated measures data. *Journal of the American Statistical Association*, **83**: 1014.
37. SAS Institute Inc. (1994) *Getting Started with PROC MIXED.* SAS Institute Inc., Cary, NC.
38. Liang KY and Zeger SL. (1986) Longitudinal data analysis using generalized linear models. *Biometrika*, **73**: 13.
39. Williams DA. (1975) The analysis of binary responses from toxicological experiments involving reproduction and teratogenicity. *Biometrics*, **31**: 949.
40. Williams DA. (1988) Estimation bias using beta-binomial distribution in teratology. *Biometrics*, **44**: 305.
41. Williams DA. (1982) Extra-binomial variation in logistic linear models. *Applied Statistics*, **31**: 144.
42. Lawless JF. (1987) Negative binomial and mixed Poisson regression. *The Canadian Journal of Statistics*, **15**: 209.
43. Breslow NE. (1984) Extra-Poisson variation in log-linear model. *Applied Statistics*, **33**: 38.
44. Chen JJ and Ahn H. (1996) Fitting mixed Poisson regression models using quasi-likelihood methods. *Biometrical Journal*, **38**: 81.
45. Chen JJ. (1998) Analysis of reproductive and developmental studies. In: SC Chow, JP Liu eds. *Design and Analysis of Animal Studies in Pharmaceutical Development.* New York, NY: Marcel Dekker, 309.
46. Kimmel CA and Gaylor DW. (1988) Issues in qualitative and quantitative risk analysis for developmental toxicology. *Risk Analysis*, **8**: 15.
47. Chen JJ and Gaylor DW. (1992) Correlations of developmental endpoints observed after 2,4,5-trichlorophenoxyacetic acid exposure in mice. *Teratology*, **45**: 241.
48. Lefkopoulou M, Moore D and Ryan LM. (1989) The analysis of multiple correlated binary outcomes: application to rodent teratology experiments. *Journal of the American Statistical Association*, **84**: 810.
49. Chen JJ, Kodell RL, Howe RB *et al.* (1991) Analysis of trinomial responses from reproductive and developmental toxicity experiments. *Biometrics*, **47**: 1049.

50. Catalano PJ and Ryan LM. (1992) Bivariate latent variable models for clustered discrete and continuous outcomes. *Journal of American Statistical Association*, **87**: 651.
51. Scheffe H. (1958) Experiments with mixture. *Journal of the Royal Statistical Society B*, **20**: 344.
52. Cornell JA. (1990) *Experiments with Mixtures, Designs, Models and the Analysis of Mixture Data*, Second Edition. John Wiley and Sons, Inc. New York.
53. Scheffe, H. (1963) The simplex centroid design for experiment with mixtures (with discussion). *Journal of the Royal Statistical Society B*, **25**: 235.
54. Cornell JA and Gorman JW. (1978) On the detection of an additive blending component in multicomponent mixtures. *Biometrika*, **34**: 251.
55. Becker NG. (1968) Models for the response of a mixture. *Journal of the Royal Statistical Society B*, **30**: 349.
56. Jackson CD, Weis C, Chen JJ, *et al.* (1998) Relative contribution of calories from dietary fat, carbohydrates, and fiber in the promotion of DMBA-induced mammary tumors in Sprague-Dawley rats. *Nutrition and Cancer*, **30**: 194.

About the Author

James J. Chen is Mathematical Statistician (SBRS), at the National Center for Toxicological Research (NCTR), U.S. Food and Drug Administration. He heads the Biostatistics Branch at NCTR. He is an Adjunct Professor at the Graduate Institute of Biostatistics and Biostatistics Center, China Medical University, Taiwan, and Department of Biostatistics, University of Arkansas for Medical Sciences, Little Rock, Arkansas. His current research interests are statistical methods for biomarker identification for personalized medicine and statistical modeling for quantitative risk assessment.

CHAPTER 17

DOSE-RESPONSE MODELING AND BENCHMARK DOSES IN HEALTH RISK ASSESSMENT

YILIANG ZHU

Department of Epidemiology and Biostatistics,
University of South Florida,
13201 Bruce B Downs Blvd.
Tampa, FL 33612, USA
yzhu@health.usf.edu

Human health protection against chemical hazards is of fundamental public health importance. Risk assessment is the scientific basis of any regulatory or policy decision. A broad range of statistical methods and tools are used in risk assessment from exposure assessment, dose-response assessment, to risk quantification. Dose-response modeling plays a central role in quantifying how and the degree to which human exposure increase the risk of adverse health effects. From an established dose-response relation, we can then quantify health risk by determining an exposure level (benchmark dose) corresponding to a small risk increase, and use it to inform a safety level. This paper illustrates dose-response modeling in risk assessment through examples of carcinogenicity, developmental toxicity, and neurotoxicity. The examples involve binary, clustered categorical, and longitudinal measurements, requires careful consideration and selection of statistical methods for effective analyses. The methods we use include generalized linear model for binary data, generalized estimating equations for clustered categorical data, and nonlinear mixed-effects models for repeated measurements. We also illustrate benchmark dose estimation and its associated bootstrap confidence limit. While the examples are directly taken from environmental health studies, the issues and approaches are applicable to problems in medicine and biological sciences as well.

1. Introduction

Exposure to environmental chemicals will elevate the risk of adverse health effects, including carcinogenicity, developmental toxicity, mutangenicity, immunotoxicity and neurotoxicity. According the TSCA inventory of the United States Environmental Protection Agency (EPA), there are more than 65,000 chemical substances in active use in the USA, and this number is increasing. However, only about 10% of these substances have been tested for carcinogenicity, and the number of chemicals that have been tested for non-cancer effects is even smaller. For example, of approximately 200 chemicals to which one million or more workers are exposed in the USA, more than one third, including many of the registered pesticide ingredients, are estimated to have adverse effects on the nervous system if sufficient exposure occurs (Anger,1984;1986). Widespread exposure to phthalates in the environment *in utero*, as infants, during puberty, and in adult life is another example of public health threat (NRC, 2008; CDC, 2009). Phthalates are a class of esters of phthalic acid commonly used as plasticizer to make plastics more transparent, flexible, or durable. Toys, cosmetics, plastics and other common household products are a major source of phthalate exposure (EPA, 2012a). Phthalate Syndrome refers to phthalate-induced insufficiency of androgen in fetal life that leads to abnormal development of male reproductive tract (Swan *et al.*, 2005; NRC 2008). Fetals exposure to phthalates is most critical and sensitive. To characterize the health risk of phthalates is a challenge because of cumulative exposure to a mixture of multiple phthalates as well as other chemicals that have similar health effects. The urgent need for better understanding the health risk associated with environmental exposure calls for more research, including research on improved statistical/biological modeling and their applications in risk assessment.

1.1. *Health risk assessment*

Health risk assessment consists of the following components: hazard identification, dose-response assessment, exposure assessment; and risk characterization (EPA, 2004). Hazard identification involves the detection of exposure-induced adverse health effects with respect to dose, route, timing, and duration of exposure. It can be done through either case report or designed human/animal studies. Dose-response analysis is typically done through designed animal experiments or adequate epidemiological studies when available. Dose-response assessment determines how risk changes within a relevant range of exposure. The dose-response relationship within this relevant exposure range provides a basis for risk quantification or characterization. The exposure assessment component identifies the population with respect to its past, present or future exposure in terms of exposure sources, magnitudes, frequencies, and duration. A final statement of the consequence of exposure then arise as a result of the risk characterization.

Until the 1990s, determination of a no-observed-adverse-effect-level (NOAEL) in conjunction with a lowest-observed-adverse-effect-level (LOAEL) largely drove dose-response assessment of non-cancer effects. A NOAEL is the highest experimental dose at which the increase risk of adverse effects is not significantly greater than that of the control group; a LOAEL, on the other hand, is the lowest experimental dose at which the risk is significantly greater. Dividing into a NOAEL(or LOAEL when a NOAEL is unavailable) select uncertainty factors yields a reference dose (RfD) or reference concentration (RfC). Uncertainty factors of 1-10 are chosen to account for uncertainty or variability arising from various sources and stages of the risk assessment process, including for example, species difference, low dose extrapolation, exposure routes, etc (Barnes and Dourson, 1988). The RfD is an estimate, with uncertainty of an order of magnitude, of a daily exposure to the human population that is likely to be without appreciable risks of deleterious health effects during a lifetime (Barnes and Dourson, 1988). It provides a reference for regulatory policy of human safety protection.

Since a NOAEL/LOAEL is restricted to only the experimental doses, it depends heavily the study design (e.g. number of doses, dose spacing, and sample size), and the associated risk varies substantially between experiments (Crump, 1984; Kimmel and Gaylor, 1988; Leisenring and Ryan, 1992). The U.S. EPA and several other international agencies have now recommended the benchmark dose (Crump, 1984) as an alternative to a NOAEL/LOAEL in risk assessment of non-cancer effects (Barnes *et al.*, 1995; EPA, 1991, 1998, 2012). In the following our discussion is focused on dose-response modeling, and the subsequent benchmark dose estimation.

1.2. *Risk of adverse health effects and dose-response models*

Before we describe the benchmark dose method, it helps to make it clear what constitutes adverse effects and how to measure risk. Suppose Y is a measure of a particular health effect or an up-stream biomarker along the disease pathway. Further suppose Y is the dichotomous outcome of a disease diagnosis, i.e. $Y = 1$ indicates the presence of the disease and $Y = 0$ otherwise. Thus the population fraction, or probability $\Pr(Y = 1)$ of diseased is the risk measure. In comparison, suppose Y is a continuous measure whose value may not always clearly define an adverse effect, but indicates abnormality when it is beyond a clinically accepted threshold. For example, elevated blood pressure, rising cholesterol level, or reduced value in forced expiratory volume (FEV) are used to diagnose abnormal cases. In this case a tail area of $\{Y > C\}$ and/or $\{Y < C\}$ defines a region of abnormal outcomes. This approach effectively converts the outcome into a dichotomous diagnose. The risk measure is the population fraction $\Pr(Y > C)$ and/or $\Pr(Y < C)$. Dose-response in these cases is the relationship between risk and exposure level.

There are cases where the biomarker Y indicates exposure-caused systemic effects, but its connection to adverse health effects is unclear. On the premises that man-made effects are unwanted, we can argue that the systemic effects are changes to the population as a whole as a result of the exposure. Even though we cannot use Y to clinically diagnose abnormality individually, population change is in itself a sign of exposure effects, can be utilized to measure the risk associated with exposure. As an example, suppose systemic changes manifest as a mean shift in the population distribution of Y. Also suppose a positive c-unit shift is significant and of physiological concern. We can use $\Pr(\bar{Y} > \mu + c|d)$ as a measure of risk. The case of negative shift can be similarly constructed. The extent of shift can be in reference to the control mean, standard deviation, or physiological range of Y. Still another example is when the systemic effects manifest as c-unit increase of the control scale. We can choose $\Pr(|S^2|/\sigma^2 > c^2)$ with $S^2 = \sum_i (Y_i - \bar{Y})/(n-1)$ being the sample variance. Thus a generic dose-response modeling in these cases of systemic effects or population change is to characterize how the Y-distribution $\Pr(Y < y|d) = F_d(y)$ of a population exposed at d changes compared with that of the control distribution $\Pr(Y < y|d = 0) = F_0(y)$. Here F is the cumulative distribution function.

Exposure-effects on the outcome distribution can take many forms mathematically, so does the functional form of the distribution F. We choose the location-scale family of distributions as a simple example to demonstrate some common scenarios. A location-scale family of distributions $F_d(y) = F((y - \mu_d)/\sigma_d)$ involves the mean μ_d as the location and standard deviation σ_d as the scale. It includes normal distributions as a member. We can conveniently impose $\mu_0 = 0$ and $\sigma_0 = 1$ for the control distribution $F(y)$. If the exposure effects have altered $F_d(y)$ to the extent that it is no longer in the same family of distribution, non-parametric distributions are useful for quantifying the risk (Bosch *et al.*, 1996).

In the brief discussion above we have suggested the use of probabilistic risk $\Pr(d)$ for dose-response modeling of adverse health effects or population changes shown as systemic effects. The choice of $\Pr(d)$ varies from the problems at hand, but depends on the type of measured effects, and the meaning and interpretability of the risk model.

1.3. *Benchmark doses*

A reasonable dose-response model $\Pr(d)$ helps us answer the question what risk is associated with a give level of exposure aside from inevitable uncertainties. Conversely, we can ask what exposure level corresponds to , say, 1% risk increase from that of the control population. In risk assessment terminology, this exposure level is called benchmark dose (BMD) corresponding to a pre-specified level of risk increase called benchmark response (BMR) level. The BMD at a given BMR level γ can be defined by the following excess (extra) risk formula

$$\frac{\Pr(\text{BMD}_\gamma) - \Pr(0)}{1 - \Pr(0)} = \gamma. \tag{1}$$

The BMR level should be chosen within a range that is supported by available data, but is typically between 1 10% under common toxicity testing guidelines. The excess risk intends to measure the true risk due to exposure alone when it is in fact confounded with the background risk. The formula (1) is actually the result of assuming that exposure-caused risk is independent of the background risk.

Solving the equations above yields an estimate of the BMD. This process involves a few steps. First, we establish the dose-response relationship $\Pr(d)$ which should insofar as possible considers all confounding and mediating factors. $\Pr(0)$ denotes the background risk seen in the control population. Second, based on the fitted dose-response models we estimate BMD using equations (1). Third, we compute a lower (upper, if necessary) confidence limit for the estimated BMD to account for statistical uncertainty. Gaylor *et al.*(1998) give a detailed account of the BMD procedures for different types of data. US EPA's guidelines on Benchmark Dose provides a general framework (EPA 2012b). While the principle for determining a BMD is clear, it is important to use appropriate and effective methods according to the type and structure of the data. In this paper we illustrates dose-response modeling and BMD estimation for binary cancer data (section 2), clustered multinomial, developmental toxicity data (section 3), and longitudinal

Table 1. Incidence of adenoma/carcinoma in the liver of medaka exposed to DEN.

Dose (ppm)	0	.075	.15	.3	.6	1.5	3.0
Cases	5	6	11	12	19	27	41
%	0.36	0.43	0.77	0.86	1.36	4.20	6.48
Sample Size	1387	1385	1427	1400	1393	643	633

continuous data from neurobehavioral toxicity screening (section 4). We conclude and discuss further issues in section 5.

2. Binary Data: Carcinogenicity

Binary data are common seen in disease diagnoses. A binary outcome is used to indicate the presence of tumor in a target organ. Animal experiments can designed insofar as possible such that the carcinogenic effects observed in one subject is independent of another. But one should check this assumption. See exceptions in section 3 with developmental toxicity experiments.

Table 1 is a summary of adenoma/carcinoma incidence in the liver of Japanese Medaka (Oryzias latipes) exposed to N-nitrosodiethylamine (DEN), a known carcinogen. This dataset is the 4th replication in a study reported by Brown-Patterson *et al.*(1999). The study aimed to test for nonlinearity in dose-response at or below the 1% BMR level. Lower dose nonlinearity in dose-response has important implication on risk characterization. EPA's current carcinogenicity risk assessment guidelines (EPA 2005) recommends the inclusion of a lowest dose level near the 1% BMR. Once a BMD is determined, a linear extrapolation from the BMD along the dose-response curve to 0-exposure level is performed to derive the cancer slope factor, and subsequently a unit cancer risk (EPA 2005). [1] This starting point for linear extrapolation is termed a *point of departure* (POD). Existence of a nonlinear dose-response below the BMD level challenges the appropriateness and accuracy of the cancer risk estimate based on linear extrapolation.

We can see from Table 1 that the incidence of adenoma and carcinoma combined was elevated by exposure to DEN and the dose corresponding to 1% BMR is around 0.3 to 0.6 ppm. Since Medaka were group-housed

[1] The control is not considered as an experimental exposure, hence the term of extrapolation.

Table 2. Weibul Model fitted to the adenoma/carcinoma incidence.

Coefficient	Estimate	Std. Err.	95%CI
Pr(0)	0.0036	0.0013	(0.0010, 0.0061)
Slope	0.0208	0.0036	(0.0138, 0.0278)
Power	1.0651	0.1726	(0.7267, 1.4035)

in water tanks during both exposure and growing-out periods, similar living condition shared by Medaka in the same tank may have resulted in clustering effects, i.e. data dependence. We checked the sample variance against the binomial variance using the full dataset, but did not find strong evidence of clustering. While a number of mathematical functions can be used to describe the observed shape of dose-response, we chose to report the Weibull model

$$\Pr(d) = \Pr(0) + (1 - \Pr(0))(1 - \exp(-\beta_1 d_2^{\beta}))$$

for its enhanced flexibility through the power parameter. Krewski and Zhu (1994) showed that the Weibull models can describe for instance reversed L-shape or S-shape dose-response in developmental toxicity experiments. The power parameter further makes it possible to approximate threshold models even if the threshold is not explicitly specified as long as it is interior to a contiguous interval (Stiteler *et al.*, 1993). Our investigation revealed negligible and statistically non-significant sex differences. Thus the current model (Table 2) reports the average dose-response with male and female Medaka pooled. The residual deviance for the model was 1.99 on 4 degrees of freedom (goodness-of-fit p-value=0.739), indicating a reasonable fit to the observed data. However, that the estimated power parameter was closer to 1 $(1.065, 95\%CI = (0.727, 1.403))$ suggests that the model is nearly linear within the experimental dose range.

From this model, we computed BMD $= 0.505$ and 95%BMDL $= 0.374$ at 1% BMR level. The default linear extrapolation from the point of departure $(0.01, \text{BMD})$ to the origin of extra risk $(0, 0)$ dictates the following equation:

$$\text{extra risk} = \frac{0.01}{\text{BMD}} d.$$

In contrast, model-based prediction gives

$$\text{extra risk} = \frac{\Pr(d) - \Pr(0)}{1 - \Pr(0)} = \exp(-0.021 d^{1.065})$$

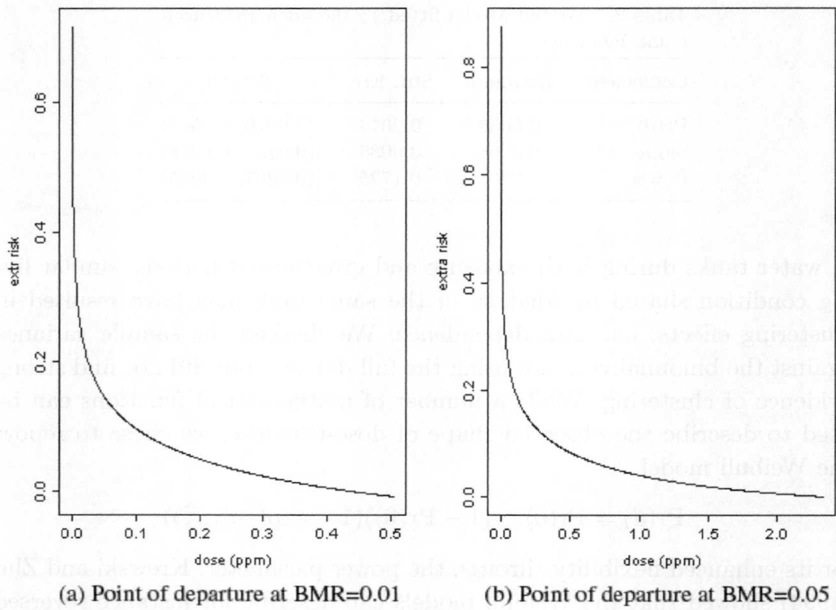

(a) Point of departure at BMR=0.01 (b) Point of departure at BMR=0.05

Fig. 1. Relative difference in excessive risk of linear extrapolation to model-based prediction.

based on the fitted Weibull model. Though minor in magnitude, the impact of nonlinearity can be assessed from the relative difference of the linear extrapolation to the model-based prediction in extra risk. We computed and plotted the relative difference within the dose range (0, BMD) in Figure 1. Liner extrapolation yielded an extra risk estimate what was about 12(the lowest dose level of the experiment) with POD at 0.01 or 0.05, respectively. Mathematically, the overestimation continued to increase as dose decreased, reaching 70% and 86% of the model-predicted risk, in the twoPODcases. Take as a further example, the predicted dose associated with 1/100,000 extra risk is 0.000088 ppm, but would be 0.000050 or 0.000047 ppm by linear extrapolation with PODat BMR = 0.01 or 0.05, respectively. This example has shown the sensitivity of lower dose extrapolation.

3. Clustered Multinomial Data: Developmental Toxicity

One aspect that complicates reproductive and developmental toxicity data is multivariate outcomes of different scales. Because maternal exposure to

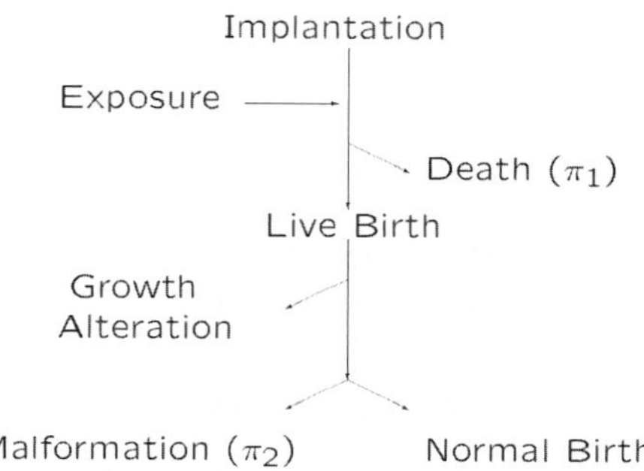

Fig. 2. Multivariate outcomes of developmental toxicity.

a potential developmental toxicant can affect many stages of the reproductive and developmental process, including viability (sperm count, ovulation, etc.), fertilization, and implantation, adverse effects may manifest at each stage. For example, exposure may induce pregnancy loss post implantation, and among live fetus lowered fetal weight, functional deficiency, or malformations. Figure 2 shows the data structure of exposure-induced death rate and growth alterations (e.g. lower fetal weight or malformations). There $\pi_1(d)$ denotes the risk of death including resorption and still birth, and $\pi_2(d)$ the risk of malformations given a live birth under maternal exposure of dose d. Like many previous authors (Ryan, 1992; Zhu *et al.*, 1994; Krewski and Zhu,1994,1995; Chen and Li, 1994), we will illustrate multivariate dose-response modeling using the multinomial outcomes of death and malformations.

Another issue with developmental toxicity data is clustering or *litter* effect, which generally translates into data dependency among offsprings of the same mother. Because exposure often involves dosing pregnant animals during a critical period of organogenesis, the exposure effects on in-utero development is similar on all implants of the same mother. Additionally, the implants share the same genetic traits. As a result, the implants' response to the toxic insult tends to be correlated.

Consider an experiment in which pregnant dams (mothers) are randomized to a control or one of D dose groups at exposure levels $d_0 = 0, d_1, \ldots, d_D$, respectively. Suppose the ith dose group has M_i dams, and of which the $j^{th}, (j = 1, \ldots, M_i)$ dam has n_{ij} implants. Let $y_{ij} = (y_{1ij}, y_{2ij})^T$ denote the number of dead implants and malformed live fetuses in the $(ij)^{th}$ dam, with the true incidence $\pi_1(d)$ and $\pi_2(d)$, respectively. The Weibull models

$$\pi_1(d;\alpha) = 1 - \exp(-(\alpha_0 + \alpha_1 d^{\alpha_2}))$$
$$\pi_2(d;\beta) = 1 - \exp(-(\beta_0 + \beta_1 d^{\beta_2}))$$

have been used to successfully model the incidences of death and malformation (Zhu *et al.*, 1994; Krewski and Zhu, 1995). We will also use them here.

3.1. *Generalized estimating equations*

To fit the Weibull models for the clustered multinomial incidences, we use generalized estimating equations (GEEs) to estimate the parameters $\theta = (\alpha^T, \beta^T)^T$. One mechanism of clustering is mixture of multinomial distributions. Examples include an infinite mixture of Dirichlet-multinomial distributions (Chen *et al.*, 1991; Zhu *et al.*, 1994) and a finite mixture of multinomial (Morel and Neerchal, 1993) which permit extra-multinomial variation. Then maximum likelihood can be applied to fit dose-response models $\pi_1(d)$ and $\pi_2(d)$ simultaneously. When uncertainty arises about the appropriateness of a mixture likelihood, alternative approaches such as generalized estimating equations (GEEs) (Liang and Zeger, 1986) have advantages as demonstrated by several authors within the current context (Ryan, 1992; Zhu *et al.*, 1994; Chen and Li, 1994). The primary advantage is the relaxation of the underlying distribution assumption and subsequent robustness of inference.

To set up the GEEs we only need specification of the mean and variance for the data. For clustered multinomial data we generally the mean and variance function given below:

$$\mu_{ij} = E(Y_{ij}|n_{ij}) = n_{ij}\pi_i$$

where $\pi_i = (\pi_{1i}, \pi_{2i})^T = (\pi_1(d_i), \pi_2(d_i))^T$, and

$$V_{ij} = (1 + (n_{ij} - 1)\rho_i)n_{ij}(\text{diag}(\pi_i) - \pi_i\pi_i^T).$$

In the variance ρ_i is an intra-cluster correlation coefficient, $(n_{ij} - 1)\rho_i$ is the variation component in excess of the multinomial variation, and diag is a diagonal matrix with π_i being the diagonal elements. This variance function appears to cover all exchangeable multinomial data (Zhu and Fung, 1996). GEEs for θ now take the following simple form:

$$\sum_{i,j} \frac{\partial(n_{ij}\pi_i)}{\partial\theta^T} V_{ij}^{-1}(y_{ij} - n_{ij}\pi_i) = 0. \qquad (2)$$

To estimate ρ_i, a separate set of equations is required. The simplest example is the moment estimate given by

$$\sum_{i,j} \frac{\partial E(q(Y_{ij}))}{\partial \rho^T} W_{ij}^{-1} \left(q(y_{ij}) - E(q(Y_{ij}))\right) = 0, \tag{3}$$

where q can be any function beyond a linear function of y_{ij}. For instance it can be a quadratic function of y_{ij} (e.g. y_{ij}^2) as well as θ. In principle, a functional form closer to the score function with respect ρ would be optimal for improved statistical efficiency. Subsequently, W is chosen to approximate the variance of q. The estimates of θ and ρ are obtained iteratively by solving the two sets of equations until convergence. The two sets of equations can be solved simultaneously or alternately. Alternating solution can be more effective computationally because it divides the problem into two of lower dimensions. This is practical especially when the parameters are of higher dimension and the choice of starting value is uncertain.

A validating property of GEEs is that the mean parameters and their variances can be estimated correctly even if the variance (V_{ij}) is incorrect. The correct variance for the estimator of mean parameters is ensured by the inclusion of an empirical variance "fix-up". (See illustration below.) There is still incentive to correctly specifying the variance to improve statistical efficiency (Liang and Zeger, 1986).

Another improvement of the efficiency of estimation is to consider joint GEEs for θ and ρ. This can be done by forming an enlarged "data" vector $(y_{ij}^T, q_{ij}^T)^T$, and use the covariance matrix of the two elements to construct GEEs in the form of (2). Also celled GEE2, this method however requires the specification of the 3rd and 4th moments of Y_{ij}. The computation algorithm is also more complex because the equations for mean parameters θ will most likely also involve ρ and vice versa. Still other variations of GEEs are available. The extended GEEs (Hall and Severini, 1998) rely on the idea of constructing an extended quasi-likelihood by integrating the GEEs (2) and then differentiating the "quasi-likelihood" with respect to ρ to obtain the score-function-like equations for ρ. If the extended quasi-likelihood is somewhat similar to the true likelihood, the second set of equations would be reasonably efficient.

In the illustration below we adopt the first approach, with $q(y_{ij}) = y_{ij}^2 - E(Y_{ij}^2)$ in equation (3). This approach is computationally simple, and numerically equivalent to the GEE2 approach. We further impose a distinct intra-litter correlation ρ_i for each dose group (Krewski and Zhu, 1994).

Still another simple alternative is to transform the data by dividing the so-called *design effects* into the deaths and malformations y_{ij} as well as the number of implants n_{ij}. This transformation effectively removes the over-dispersion component $(n_{ij} - 1)\rho_i$ from the data. As a result, we can use the mean and variance of a multinomial distribution to approximate those of the transformed data. The *design effect* at each dose level is in essence the "ratio" of the true variance to the multinomial variance. Denote the outcomes of malformation, death, and normal birth by an index $k = 1, 2, 3$. The design effect of each dose group can be estimated by

$$\hat{D}_i = \frac{1}{2}\left[\frac{\hat{v}_{i1}}{\hat{\mu}_{i1}} + \frac{\hat{v}_{i2}}{\hat{\mu}_{i2}} + \frac{\hat{v}_{i3}}{\hat{\mu}_{i3}}\right] \tag{4}$$

where $\hat{v}_{ik}$ $(k = 1, 2, 3)$ are the sample variances divided by the average number of implants and $\hat{\mu}_{ik}$ are the mean response rates in each dose group. An added advantage to this transformation procedure is that the usual Chi-squared goodness-of-fit test is applicable. Simulation studies reveals that this transformation procedure is valid even for moderate number of dams per dose group (Fung *et al.*, 1994).

3.2. *Illustration*

Data in Table 3 come from a study (Price *et al.*, 1987) that investigated the developmental effects of diethylene glycol dimenthyl ether(TGDM). The study included a vehicle control group and 3 dose groups, each had some 20 to 30 pregnant rats. Measured outcomes included the number of implantation sites in each dam and the incidence of prenatal death (including resorptions). Live fetuses surviving to sacrifice were weighed and evaluated for the presence of a number of developmental malformations. The data

Table 3. Incidences of death and malformation in pregnant rats exposed to TGDM.

Dose (g/kg)	Dams	Total Impl's	Death[a] No.	Death[a] (%)	Malf's[b] No.	Malf's[b] (%)
0.00	27	340	22	6.5	1	0.3
0.25	26	296	21	7.1	0	0.0
0.50	26	296	34	11.49	2	0.8
1.00	28	327	41	12.54	33	11.5

[a] Including dead or resorbed animals.
[b] Number of live animals exhibiting any malformation.

Table 4. Parameter estimates (S.E.)[a] of joint dose-response models for the incidences of death and malformation in rats exposed to TGDM.

Model	Coefficient	Estimate	Estimates (TR)
Prenatal Death	Intercept(α_0)	0.0617 (0.0180)	0.0642 (0.0154)
	Dose(α_1)	0.0956 (0.0563)	0.0793 (0.0481)
	Power(α_2)	1.2650 (1.0584)	1.2140 (1.0932)
Fetal Malformation	Intercept(β_0)	0.0006 (0.0009)	0.0009 (0.0016)
	Dose(β_1)	0.1209 (0.0346)	0.1222 (0.0356)
	Power (β_2)	4.8157 (2.0224)	2.0224 (1.9803)
Intralitter Correlation	Group 1 (ρ_1)	0.1546 (0.0688)	
	Group 2 (ρ_2)	−0.0369 (0.0315)	
	Group 3 (ρ_3)	0.3288 (0.2829)	
	Group 4 (ρ_4)	0.2846 (0.1021)	

[a] S.E. = standard error.

clearly reveal elevated incidences of death and malformation with increased exposure to TGDM.

The fitted death-malformation models are summarized in Table 4, where the transformation method is labeled by TR. While the incidence of malformation was strongly dose-related, the dose-response relationship of prenatal death was only marginally significant. Litter effects were apparent at the two highest dose levels, as indicated by the estimated intra-litter correlations. The design effects of $1.10, 0.69, 2.78$, and 3.91 were estimated for the four dose groups respectively. The transformation method resulted in a model comparable to that of GEEs; The goodness-of-fit statistic for the model gave $\chi^2 = 2.15$ and p-value $= 0.34$.

We computed benchmark doses based on the extra risks of death (π_1), malformation (π_2), or the overall risk

$$\pi(d) = Pr(\text{death or malformation}|d) = 1 - (1 - \pi_1(d))(1 - \pi_2(d)).$$

Table 5. BMD_{05} (mg/kg/d)(SE)^a based on the joint weibull models for death and malformation.

Prenatal death	Malformation	Multivariate
0.611 (0.333)	0.837 (0.072)	0.548 (0.216)

^{a}S.E. = standard error derived using the delta-method.

The results are given in Table 5 along with their standard error (in parentheses) derived by the delta method. The 95% BMDL can be approximated by BMDL = $BMD_{05} - 1.645 \times$ SE. The results confirm that a BMD estimate based on the joint risk of death and malformation is more sensitive, its corresponding BMD is smaller than the ones based separately on the univariate risk π_1 or π_2 (Gaylor *et al.*, 1998).

4. Longitudinal Data: Neurobehavioral Toxicity Screening

The nervous system controls most human bodily processes in addition to psychological functions. It is sensitive to perturbation from external insults and has limited ability to regenerate. Even anatomical, biochemical, or physiological insults of limited extent to the nervous system can result in adverse effects, either transient or persistent, on human health (EPA, 1998). Hence neurotoxicity is one of the non-cancer endpoints in regulating environmental toxicants (EPA, 1998). Neurotoxicity includes adverse effects in behavior, neurochemistry, neurophysiology, and neuropathology. Neurological development and function outcomes in infants and children can be used to examine neurotoxicity resulting from prenatal and perinatal exposure. The example below is related to neurobehavioral screening.

4.1. *Neurobehavioral screening test*

Jointly developed and endorsed by the International Program on Chemical Safety (IPCS) and the US EPA, the Functional Observational Battery (FOB) was validated and tested for rapid screening of neurobehavioral changes (Moser *et al.*, 1997). The FOB consists of a number of measurements in several domains according to their neurological function: autonomic, neuromuscular, activity, sensorimotor, excitability, and physiology. Except for several in the neuromuscular or physiology domain, most measures are based on behavioral observation. Criteria is not well established to define adversities in individuals. Thus we assess the collective behavioral changes of the exposed group compared to that of a control group. If "rare" behaviors in the control become more common in the exposed group, it is an indication of neurotoxic effects. To define an overall domain-wide score of neurotoxicity, we first converted every single measure, regardless of its binary, continuous, or ordinal scale, to a commonality score of 4 levels, then compute the average score of converted individual measures in the same domain for each subject. For instance, the measure of "ease of removal from cage" in the *excitability* came with six categories: "very easy", "easy", "moderately difficult", "rat flinches", "difficult", and "very difficult". If more than 50% of the control group were either "very easy" or "easy" to remove, then "very easy" and "easy" were converted to "1"; Categories whose frequency is at least one rank away from the mode of the control distribution is assigned a "4". For details on converting a continuous measure see MacDaniel and Moser (1993). Thus after the conversion, level "1" represents the most common observations in the control group, and level "4" the least common. We refer this overall commonality score that is of the average of three measures — handling reactivity, arousal, and ease of removal — in the domain of excitability the *excitability* score. Of course, variations of this conversion can be explored and utilized as well.

Table 6 is a summary of the excitability score. In this EPA study (Moser *et al.*, 1995) 8 rats of the same strain and age from 8 different litters were exposed at one of the four dose levels (150, 500, 1500, 5000 mg/kg) to tetrachloroethylene (PERC), a common chlorinated solvent. In addition, there was a control group. FOB screening was conducted on each subject at just before dosing (time = 0), approximately 4, and 24 hours post exposure. There were four deaths in the 5000 mg/kg dose group by 24 hour so data of the highest dose group was partially missing. This example showcases some common issues that occur simultaneously: small sample size, small number of repeated measurements over time, and missing data likely to occur at higher dose levels or later points in time due to mortality.

Table 6. Mean (S.E.) excitability scores of rats exposed to PERC.

Dose (mg/kg)	0	150	500	1500	5000
0 H	1.7938	2.0413	1.9188	1.7525	1.8350
	(0.0603)	(0.1070)	(0.2442)	(0.0545)	(0.0622)
4 H	1.6238	2.1650	1.9163	2.1650	2.5025
	(0.1414)	(0.1594)	(0.4352)	(0.3168)	(0.1273)
24 H	1.2064	1.5000	1.7088	1.6250	2.3300
	(0.0292)	(0.2876)	(0.6183)	(0.6187)	(0.0000)

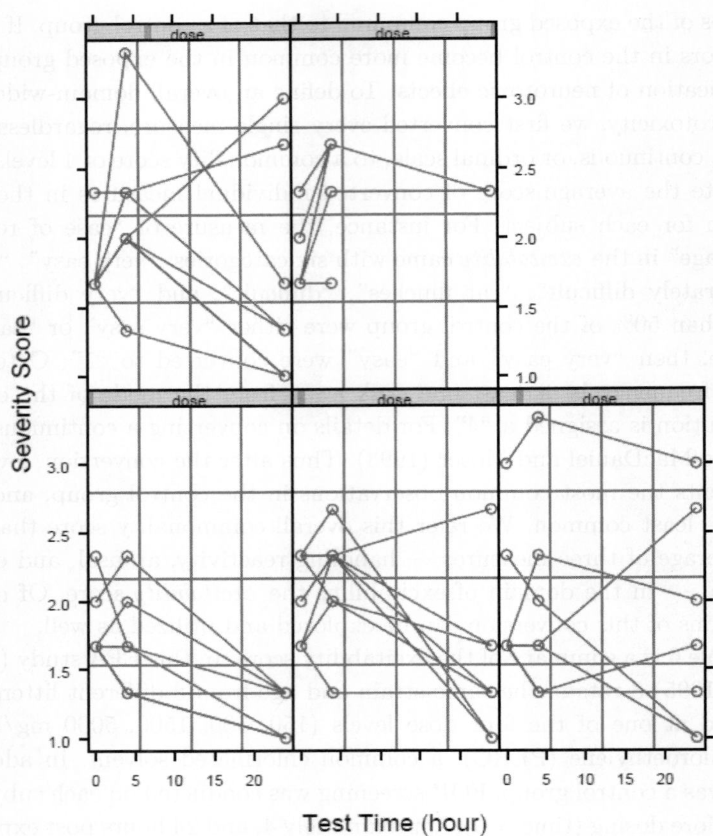

Fig. 3. Individual trajectories of excitability score on rats exposed to PERC.

Figure 3 are the plots of the excitability scores against time for each subject, and the individual trajectories are grouped into separate panels, one for each dose level as indicated by the bar on the panel top, starting from the lower left corner, counter clockwise in increasing dose. Between-subject variation was visible. Figure 4 is 3-dimensional plot with the data smoothed by spline functions to show the average trajectory. The excitability score decreased slightly over time for the control subjects, perhaps because self-adjustment to the caging environment. For exposed subjects, however, there was a dose-dependent tendency of increased excitability near 4H point followed by a drop (150, 500, 1500 mg/kg) towards 24H. At the highest dosing level (5000 mg/kg), the drop was absent, suggesting an extended

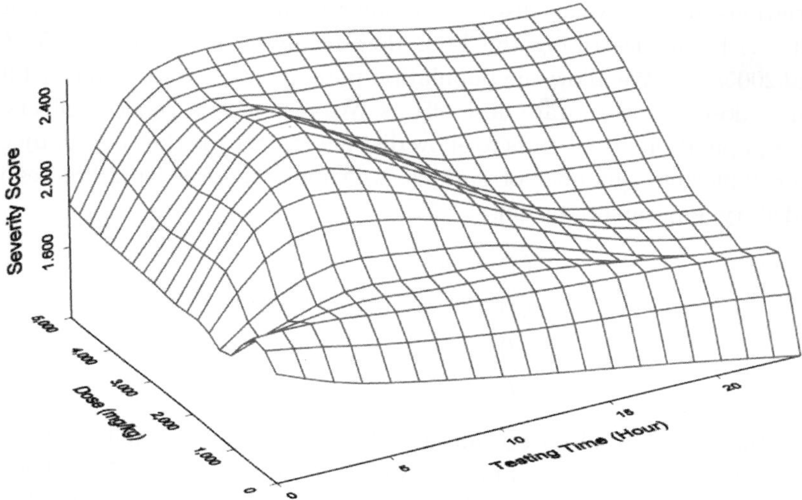

Fig. 4. Averaged changes of excitability score on rats exposed to PERC.

exposure effects over time as compared with somewhat transient effects on subjects in the lower dose groups. In summary, this type of longitudinal data with small number of subjects, potentially non-ignorable between-subject variation, and missing data invites the use of mixed-effects models. To understand the neurotoxicity on behavioral changes, the behavioral trajectory holds the key. Therefore, it is necessary to model not only the dose-response, but also changes in dose-response over with time. Although ANOVA with repeated measures (Moser *et al.*, 1995) if there are differences along time, it falls short to quantify the change along time. Moreover, dose-response modeling is a prerequisite to BMD estimation. Zhu (2005) and Zhu *et al.*(2005a,b) proposed the use of nonlinear kinetic functions, in conjunction with random effects to allow for greater between-subject variation to model this type of *dose-time-response* data.

4.2. *Nonlinear mixed effects models*

To simplify the statistical analysis, the excitability domain score is treated as a continuous variable and modeled using the following hybrid pharmacokinetic function

$$f(\phi(dose), t) = \frac{\phi_1(d) + \phi_2(d)t}{1 + e^{\phi_3(d)}t^{\phi_4(d)}} \tag{5}$$

Variations of the Michaelis-Menton kinetic functions have been found quite useful in describing the FOB dose-response data (Zhu, 2005; Zhu *et al.*2005a, b). We allow the population parameters ϕ_i to be a linear function of dose to incorporate dose effects. We also attach random effects to select population parameters to allow distinct trajectories between subjects. After exploring a number of options, we choose the following "regression model" type parametrization:

$$\begin{aligned}\phi_1(d) &= \beta_{10}\\ \phi_2(d) &= \beta_{20} + (\beta_{21} + b_{21i})d\\ \phi_3(d) &= \beta_{31}d\\ \phi_4(d) &= \beta_{40}.\end{aligned}$$

Note that ϕ_1 determines the initial value (time $= 0$) of excitability that is free of dose because the first test was done before dosing. Therefore we made $\phi_1(d) = \beta_{10}$ a constant. Although we can jitter the intercept β_{10} by random effects to characterize unexplained variation in initial excitability among subjects, the effects seem to be minimal in our actual data analysis. The time-slope ϕ_2 measures how excitability changed over time naturally (β_{20}) as well as under the influence of dosing (β_{21}) with random effects b_{21i} for individual variation. The time-slope β_{31} controls for plausible downturn trajectory within the dose range. A constant term is not essential in β_{31} because it amounts to a scale effect that can be absorbed by reparameterizing ϕ_1 and the 1 on the denominator. Finally, a power parameter β_{40} is employed to increase the flexibility of the dose-time-response shape. Note that although random effects can be mathematically attached to every population parameter, justification should be provided from physiological and data standpoints. Overparameterization should be avoided. Pinheiro and Bates (2000) offers useful guidance for model selection and use of random effects.

A briefly outline is given below for the statistical and computational process for fitting nonlinear mixed-effects models. The notation here follows largely that of Pinheiro and Bates (2000, Chapter 7). One can also find discussion on this topic in Davidian and Glicknan (1995). Consider the following model,

$$Y_{ij} = f(\phi_i, X_{ij}) + \epsilon_{ij}, \quad i = 1, \ldots, M; \quad j = 1, \ldots, n_i \tag{6}$$

where $\epsilon_i = (\epsilon_{i1}, \ldots, \epsilon_{ij}, \ldots, \epsilon_{in_i})^T$ is the error vector for the ith subject in the sample of M; X_{ij} is the covariate vector for the ith subject at the jth

sampling time. The parameter vector $\phi_i = A_i\beta + B_ib_i$ has two components: the first component β is population parameters and the second component b_i ($q \times 1$ vector) represents random effects associated with the ith subject. The matrices A_i and B_i are designed to select population parameters for an individual trajectory as well as for incorporating targeted random effects. In general and the present case in particular, the matrices A_i and B_i would be the same for all individuals. Time-varying coefficients can also be accommodated using extended notation (Pinheiro and Bates, 2000). For convenience we assume that ϵ_i follow the $N_{n_i}(0, \sigma^2\Lambda_i(\theta_1))$ distribution, and are independent between different subjects. Various correlation options may be incorporated into $\Lambda_i(\theta_1)$ through parameterization using θ_1. We also assume the $N_q(0, \sigma^2\Omega(\theta_2))$ distribution for the random effects b_i. In principle non-normal distributions can be considered for both errors and random effects, computational implementation will be more complex, and most computer software is limited to normal distributions.

To fit a non-linear mixed effects model, maximum likelihood estimation is often used via either the EM-algorithm (Dempster *et al.*, 1977) or other numerical algorithms such as Newton-Raphson (Lindstrom and Bates, 1990). Here we use Newton-Raphson algorithm implemented in S-PLUS (Mathsoft, Seattle, Washington). Under the assumption of normality, the marginal distribution of $Y_i = (Y_{i1}, \ldots, Y_{in_i})^T$ is

$$\begin{aligned} p(y_i|\beta, \sigma^2, \theta_1, \theta_2) &= \int p(y_i|b_i; \beta, \sigma^2, \theta_1)p(b_i; \theta_2)db_i \\ &= \frac{1}{(2\pi\sigma^2)^{\frac{n_i+q}{2}}|\Lambda_i|^{\frac{1}{2}}|\Omega|^{\frac{1}{2}}} \int \\ &\quad \times \exp\left\{-\frac{(y_i - f(\phi_i))^T\Lambda_i^{-1}(y_i - f(\phi_i)) + b_i^T\Omega^{-1}b_i}{2\sigma^2}\right\}db_i, \end{aligned}$$

where $f(\phi_i) = (f(\phi_i, X_{i1})), \ldots, f(\phi_i, X_{in_i}))^T$. Using a first order Taylor series expansion about some initial estimates $\hat{\beta}^{(t)}$ and $\hat{b}_i^{(t)}$ to approximate the exponent of the integrand, we can obtain the following approximate marginal log likelihood function

$$\begin{aligned} l(\beta, \sigma^2, \theta_1, \theta_2; y_i) &= -\frac{n_i + q}{2} log(\sigma^2) \\ &\quad - \frac{1}{2}\left\{\log|\Sigma_i| + \frac{1}{\sigma^2}(w_i^{(t)} - Z_{1i}^{(t)}\beta)^T\Sigma_i^{-1}(w_i^{(t)} - Z_{1i}^{(t)}\beta)\right\} \end{aligned}$$

where $w_i^{(t)} = y_i - f(\hat\beta^{(t)}, \hat b_i^{(t)}) + Z_{1i}^{(t)}\hat\beta^{(t)} + Z_{2i}^{(t)}\hat b_i^{(t)}$, and

$$Z_{1i}^{(t)} = \frac{\partial f}{\partial \beta^T} \quad \text{and} \quad Z_{2i}^{(t)} = \frac{\partial f}{\partial b_i^T}$$

are the derivative matrices evaluated at $\hat\beta^{(t)}$ and $\hat b_i^{(t)}$, and

$$\Sigma_i(\theta_1, \theta_2) = \Lambda_i(\theta_1) + Z_{2i}^{(t)}\Omega(\theta_2)(Z_{2i}^{(t)})^T.$$

Maximum likelihood estimates $(\hat\theta_1^{(t)}, \hat\theta_2^{(t)}, \hat\sigma^{2(t)})$ are obtained from maximizing this approximate log-likelihood

$$\max_{\theta_1,\theta_2,\sigma^2} \sum_i^M l(\hat\beta^{(t)}, \sigma^2, \theta_1, \theta_2; y_i). \tag{7}$$

The estimate of the regression parameters β is then updated by a least squares estimator

$$\hat\beta^{(t+1)} = \left\{\sum_1^M (Z_{1i}^{(t)})^T(\Sigma_i^{(t)})^{-1} Z_{1i}^{(t)}\right\}^{-1} \left\{\sum_1^M (Z_{i1}^{(t)})^T(\Sigma_i^{(t)})^{-1} w_i^{(t)}\right\} \tag{8}$$

given the newest estimates of $\hat b_i^{(t)}$ and $(\hat\theta_1^{(t)}, \hat\theta_2^{(t)}, \hat\sigma^{2(t)})$. The estimate of the random effects b_i is updated also by a least squares estimator based on

$$\sum_i^M \left\{(y_i - f(\hat\beta^{(t+1)}, b_i))^T \Lambda_i^{-1}(\hat\theta_1^{(t)})(y_i - f(\hat\beta^{(t+1)}, b_i)) + b_i^T \Omega^{-1}(\hat\theta_2^{(t)}) b_i\right\}.$$

Using a first order Taylor series approximation

$$f(\hat\beta^{(t+1)}, b_i, X_{ij}) = f(\hat\beta^{(t+1)}, \hat b_i^{(t)}, X_{ij}) + Z_{2i}^{(t)}(b_i - \hat b_i^{(t)}),$$

we have the update

$$\hat b_i^{(t+1)} = \left\{\Omega^{-1} + Z_{2i}^T \Lambda_i^{-1} Z_{2i}\right\}^{-1} Z_{2i}^T \Lambda_i^{-1}\left\{y_i - f(\hat\beta^{(t+1)}, \hat b_i^{(t)}) + Z_{2i}\hat b_i^{(t)}\right\}, \tag{9}$$

with all terms evaluated at the most recent parameter estimates. Iteratively solving the three sets of equations (7), (8) and (9) until convergence gives the final MLEs.

The maximization procedure outlined above relies heavily on the normality assumption for both the error terms and random effects. If the random effects follow a non-normal distribution, explicit marginal likelihood

Table 7. Mixed-effects kinetic model fitted to excitability score.

Parameter	Value	S.E.[a]	DF	t-value	p-value
β_{10}	1.8693	0.0763	72	24.51	<.0001
β_{20}	2.2611	0.1723	72	13.12	<.0001
β_{21}	−0.0003	0.0001	72	−4.29	0.0001
β_{31}	−0.0003	0.0001	72	−3.40	0.0011
β_{40}	1.1597	0.0320	72	36.30	<.0001
$\Omega(\theta_2)$	S.E.	7.72e-008			
$\Lambda(\theta_1)$	σ	0.4737			
	corr(i,j)[b]:	(1,2):0.63	(1,3):0.14	(2,3):0.30	

[a]S.E. = standard error.
[b]corr(j,k) = corr(ϵ_{ij},ϵ_{ik}).

is often not available, and the EM-algorithm can be used to numerically approximate the marginal likelihood.

4.3. *Illustration*

Table 7 summarizes the fitted mixed-effects model (5), and Figure 5 presents the predicted dose-time-response surface. A comparison of Figure 5 with Figure 4 reveals that the model captures most of the trends observed in the raw data. The dose effects were highly significant, and altered the group trajectory in a dose-dependent fashion. In particular, the time of peak effects was likely dose-dependent, but cannot be ascertained because of the sparse time points and spacing. Several options were considered for random effects. For example, using random effects for both the intercept β_{10} and the time slope β_{20}, or both β_{10} and the time-dose slope β_{21} led to an almost perfect correlation between the two random effects, suggesting an over-use of random effects. Thus one random effect appeared adequate in the current application. Associating random effects with the time-dose slope β_{21} was more effective under several criteria including likelihood ratio, information criterion and residual plots. Still the standard error for the random effects was $7.72e^{-8}$ (Table 7), a small number compared with the estimate $\hat{\beta}_{21} = -3e^{-4}$, indicating a limited degree of between-subjects variation. We had also considered several correlation structures for the error terms, including that of complete independence, auto-regression with leg 1, compound symmetric, and unrestricted. The unrestricted correlation matrix Λ (Table 7) seemed most flexible.

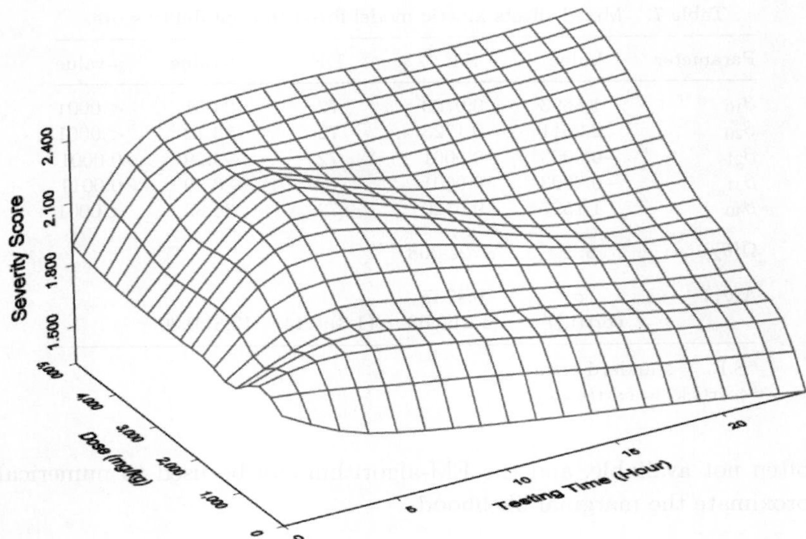

Fig. 5. Model-predicted changes of excitability score on rats exposed to PERC.

4.4. *Benchmark doses*

In the current context of transient neurotoxic effects of PERC, timing of the effects is important and BMD computation must reflect this fact. Common sense suggests that BMD computation can be done at any time-slice of the dose-time-response model at a chosen time point. But it is less clear which time point would correspond to the most sensitive or most conservative BMD value. Intuitively the dose-response slice with the greatest rate of exposure-induced change would be the one to consider. This slice likely to be in the neighborhood of the peak time. Implementation-wise we can compute BMDs over the time-grid. At each grid point the usual BMD approach can be applied. The collection of these individual BMDs form a BMD time-profile to inform the sensitivity of BMD to time as well as a final choice.

Because the excitability score measures the degree to which the observed behaviors are common in the control population, it does not in itself determine abnormality. Instead it measures behavioral change in response to exposure. Thus we measure the proportion of subjects whose excitability score value exceeds a given level that indicates the type of unusual behaviors among the control animals. This threshold c_t is chosen to include the top $\alpha \times 100\%$ of highest excitability scores of the controls. That is $\Pr(0, t) = \Pr(Y > c_t | d = 0, t) = \alpha$. For the exposure group, we use

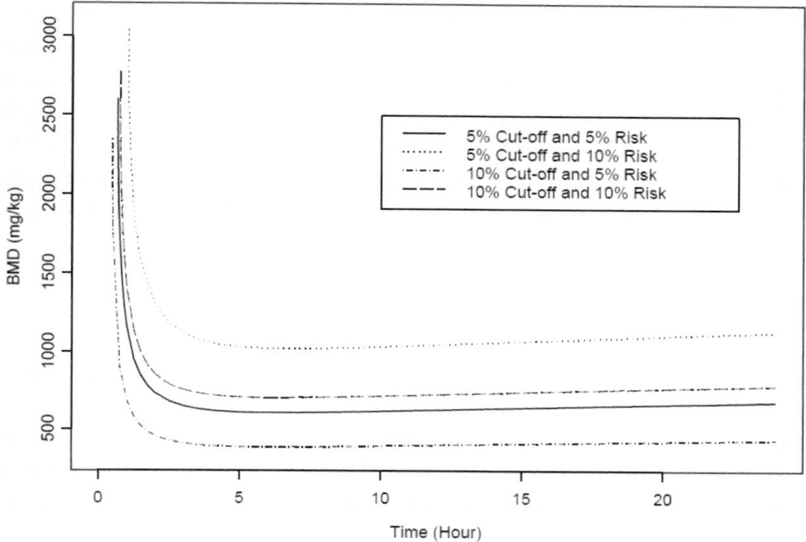

Fig. 6. Time-profile of benchmark dose for excitability score.

$\Pr(d, t) = Pr(Y > c_t | d, t)$ to define risk increase. Note c_t may varies with time as the control behavior could change over time as well. As a result, c_t is determined from the fitted dose-response model. This is necessary because data are available only at the experimental time points (4H and 24H).

Assuming a normal distribution for the excitability score Y,

$$\Pr(d, t) = 1 - \Phi\left(\frac{c_t - f(d, t)}{\sigma_0}\right),$$

where Φ is the cumulative distribution function of the standard normal distribution and with a constant standard deviation $\sigma_0 = 0.4737$ pooled across all dose groups (Table 7). Extra risk (1) simplifies to

$$\Phi\left(\frac{c_t - f(d, t)}{\sigma_0}\right) = \Phi\left(\frac{c_t - f(0, t)}{\sigma_0}\right)(1 - \gamma) = (1 - \alpha)(1 - \gamma),$$

with $c_t = f(0, t) + z_{1-\alpha}\sigma_0$ and $z_{1-\alpha}$ being the $(1 - \alpha)100\%$ percentile of the standard normal distribution. The preceding equation further simplifies to

$$f(\mathrm{BMD}_t, t) = f(0, t) - \sigma_0\left(\Phi^{-1}((1 - \alpha)(1 - \gamma)) - z_{1-\alpha}\right). \quad (10)$$

Solving this equation for BMDwith all parameters replaced with their estimates gives BMD_t estimate at any given time t. In our illustration we computed BMD_t with $\alpha = 0.05, 0.10$ and $\gamma = 0.05, 0.10$. Figure 6 displays

BMD_t over time under the four combinations of α and γ. The plots show that a higher reference "risk" (α) leads to a more conservative or sensitive BMD. A lower level of extra risk (γ) is associated with a more conservative BMD. More importantly, an examination of the time-profile of BMD suggests that the most sensitive or conservative BMD_t is in the neighborhood of 6.25 and 7 hours post exposure. This makes sense because indeed neurotoxicity screening is sensitive to the time window when the test is done.

5. Discussion

We have illustrated in this article several dose-response modes and modeling techniques with examples in health risk assessment, particularly BMD estimation. The examples used include binary, clustered multinomial, and repeated measurement data. Although the basic concepts of modeling and risk assessment are unambiguous, a number of technical issues warrant further discussion.

Defining adversity is not always unequivocal from both clinical and statistical standpoints. We propose to consider population changes in distribution — systemic changes — as a surrogate of adverse effects. Therefore exposure-induced distributional alterations relative to a control population can serve as a basis for risk measure. The nonparametric method of Bosch, Wypij and Ryan (1996) is an interesting example of establishing distributional alterations. Suppose Y_{ij} denotes the observed continuous outcome (e.g. weight or blood pressure) for the jth subject in the ith dose group ($i = 0, \ldots, D$; $j = 1, \ldots, n_i$), with $d_0 = 0$ being the control. If there is no dose effects, $\Pr(d_i) = Pr(Y_{0h} > Y_{ij}) = 1/2$ for all i, including in particular the case $i = 0$, i.e. $\Pr(0) = 1/2$. Thus a "new" response vector of length mn_0 ($m = \sum_{i=1}^{D} n_i$) can be constructed representing the comparisons between each control subject and each exposed subject. That is,

$$\mathbf{W} = (W_{0111}, W_{0112}, \ldots, W_{0hij}, \ldots, W_{0n_0Dn_D})', \quad W_{0hij} = I(Y_{0h} > Y_{ij}),$$

where the indicator function W_{0hij} takes the value 1 if $Y_{0h} > Y_{ij}$ and 0 otherwise. Note that $E(W_{0hij}) = \Pr(d_i)$. Thus inference about $\Pr(d)$ can be done using such methods as logisitc regression for binary data.

Developing generalized linear mixed-effects models for ordinal data (Hedeker and Gibbons, 1994; 1996) would be useful for the analysis of individual measure of FOB data. A major technical issue is how to deal with less common behaviors of zero frequency, a likely situation when sample size is small. Developing multivariate dose-response models is also interesting. Catalano and Ryan (1992) and Regan and Catalano (1998) studied joint dose-response models with both binary (malformation) and continuous outcomes (body weight) in developmental toxicity studies, using a bivariate latent variable model. Attempts have also been made to further include death in the multivariate dose-response model (Catalano *et al.*, 1993; Chen, 1993). Empirical evidences argue that multivariate models should result in improved precision for the purpose of risk assessment, as compared with a univariate approach (Ryan, 1992; Krewski and Zhu, 1994). This improved precision could arise in two ways: (1) a richer class of models and better fit, and (2) more efficient estimators because data of different endpoint contain common information about the toxic mechanism underpinning the adverse effects.

How to deal with uncertainty is a recurring theme in risk assessment. Uncertainty exists in any scientific investigation. In risk assessment uncertainty can arise from all components of the process and from multiple sources. A BMD estimate as a summary characterization of risk is surrounded by uncertainties propagated from many sources. But a full and correct characterization of the overarching uncertainty of a BMD requires an integration of uncertainties across multiple steps of the risk assessment process, a challenge not always practical. Exposure assessment and dose-response assessment are two areas where it is more likely to quantify uncertainties and incorporate them into the final BMD estimate. Reporting the lower confidence limit (BMDL) or even upper confidence limit for the BMD estimate in fact summarizes only a part of the statistical uncertainty. In the BMDL computation, we actually implicitly assume the underlying dose-response model is correct and do not consider other plausible models. Uncertainty can even be introduced when the method used for computing the BMDL is inaccurate. The delta-method (Gaylor *et al.*, 1998) in conjunction with an approximate normal distribution for the BMD has been the most common approach to BMDL computation. Both in essence requires large sample size, a statistical idealistic situation unlikely to be met by toxicity testing guidelines. Better methods can be developed and should be used. Bootstrap method is one such improvement. Zhu *et al.*(2005b) implemented bootstrap method in BMDL computation with longitudinal FOB data.

References

Anger, W.K. (1984) Neurobehavioral testing of chemicals: impact on recommended standards. *Neurobehav. Toxicol. Teratol.* **6**, 147–153.

Anger, W.K. (1986) Workplace exposores. In Neurobehavioral Toxicology Annau, Z.A. Ed. John's Hopkins University Press. 331–347.

Barnes, D.G. and Dourson, M. (1988). Reference dose (RfD): Description and use in health risk assessments. *Regulatory Toxicol. Pharmacol.* **8**: 471–486.

Barnes, D.G. and Daston, G.P., Evans, J.S., Jarabek, A.M., Kavlock, R.J., Kimmel, C.A., Park, C. and Spitzer, W.L. (1995). Benchmark dose workshop: Criteria for use of a benchmark dose to estimate a reference dose. *Regulatory Toxicol. Pharmacol.* **21**, 296–306.

Bosch, R.J., Wypij, D. and Ryan, L.M. (1996). A semiparametric approach to risk assessment for quantitative outcomes. *Risk Analysis* **16**: 657–665.

Brown-Peterson, N., Krol, R., Zhu, Y. and Hawkins, W. (1999). Nitrosodiethylamine Initiation of Carcinogenesis in Japanese Medaka (Oryzias latipes): Hepatocellular Proliferation, Toxicity, and Neoplastic Lesions Resulting from Short Term, Low Level Exposure. *Toxicological Sciences* **50**, 186–194.

Catalano, P.J. and Ryan, L.M. (1992). Bivariate latent variable models for clustered discrete and continuous outcomes. *J. American Statistical Association* **87**: 651–658.

Catalano, P.J., Scharfstein, D.O., Ryan, L., Kimmel, C., and Kimmel, G. (1993). Statistical model for fetal death, fetal weight, and malformation in developmental toxicity studies. *Teratology* **47**, 281–290.

CDC (2009). Centers for Disease Control and Prevention. Fourth National Report on Human Exposure to Environmental Chemicals. http://www.cdc.gov/exposurereport/pdf/FourthReport.pdf (accessed October 2013)

Chen J.J., Kodell, R.L., Howe, R.B., and Gaylor, D.W. (1991) Analysis of trinomial responses from reproductive and developmental toxicity experiments. *Biometrics* **47**, 1049–1058.

Chen, J.J. (1993). A Malformation incidence dose-response model incorporating fetal weight and/or litter size as covariates. *Risk Analysis* **13**, 559–564.

Chen, J.J., and Li, L.A. (1994). Dose-response modeling of trinomial responses from developmental experiments. *Statistica Sinica* **4**, 265–274.

Crump, K.S. (1984). A new method for determining allowable daily intakes. *Fund. Appl. Toxicol.* **4**: 854–871.

Davidian, M and Giltinan, D.M. (1995) Nonlinear models for repeated measurement data, Chapman and Hall: London.

Dempster, A.P., Laird, N.M. and Rubin, D.B. (1977). Maximum likelihood from incomplete data via the EM-algorithm, *J. R. Statist. Soc. B.* **39**, 1–22.

EPA (U.S. Environmental Protection Agency) (1991). Guidelines for developmental toxicity risk assessment. *Federal Register* **56**: 63797–63826.

EPA (U.S. Environmental Protection Agency) (1998) Guidelines for Neurotoxicity Risk Assessment *Federal Register* **63**: 26926–26954.

EPA (U.S. Environmental Protection Agency)(2004) AN EXAMINATION OF EPA RISK ASSESSMENT PRINCIPLES AND PRACTICES. Office of the Science Advisor U.S. Environmental Protection Agency Washington, DC EPA/100/B-04/001.

EPA (U.S. Environmental Protection Agency) (2005) *Guidelines for Carcinogen Risk Assessment.* Risk Assessment Forum U.S. Environmental Protection Agency Washington, DC EPA/630/P-03/001b NCEA-F-0644b

EPA (U.S. Environmental Protection Agency) (2012a). *Phthalates Action Plan.* Available:http://www.epa.gov/oppt/existingchemicals/pubs/actionplans/phthalates_actionplan_revised_2012-03-14.pdf [accessed October 2013].

EPA (U.S. Environmental Protection Agency) (2012b) *Benchmark dose technical guidance.* Risk Assessment Forum U.S. Environmental Protection Agency Washington, DC. EPA/100/R-12/001.

Fung, K.Y., Krewski, D., Rao, J.N.K., Scott, J.A. (1994) Tests for trend in developmental toxicity experiments with correlated binary data. *Risk Analysis* **14**, 639–648.

Gaylor, D.W., Ryan, L., Krewski, D. and Zhu, Y. (1998) Procedures for calculating benchmark doses for health risk assessment. *Regulatory Toxicol. Pharmacol.* **28**, 150–164.

Hall,D.B. and Severini, T.A. (1998) Extended generalized estimating equations for clustered data. *J. American Statistical Association* **93**, 1365–1375.

Hedeker D. and Gibbons, R.D. (1994) A random effects ordinal regression model for multilevel analysis. *Biometrics* **50**, 933–944.

Hedeker, D. and Gibbons, R.D. (1996) MIXOR: a computer program for mixed-effects ordinal regression analysis. *Computer Methods and Programs in Biomedicine* **49**, 157–176.

Kimmel, C.A. and Gaylor, D.W. (1988). Issues in qualitative and quantitative risk analysis for developmental toxicity. *Risk Analysis* **8**, 15–20.

Krewski, D., and Zhu, Y. (1994) Applications of multinomial dose-response models in developmental toxicity risk assessment. *Risk Analysis* **14**: 613–627.

Krewski, D., and Zhu, Y. (1995) A simple data transformation for estimating benchmark dose in developmental toxicity experiments. *Risk Analysis* **15**: 29–39.

Leisenring, W. and Ryan, L. (1992) Statistical properties of the NOAEL. *Regulatory Toxicol. Pharmacol.* **15**: 161–171.

Liang K.Y, Zeger S.L. (1986) Longitudinal Data Analysis Using Generalized Linear Models. *Biometrika* **73**: 13–22.

Lindstrom, M.J. and Bates, D.M. (1990) Nonlinear mixed-effects models for repeated measures data, *Biometrics* **46**, 673–687.

MacDaniel and Moser (1993) Utility of a neurobehavioral screening battery for differ-entiating the effects of two pyrethroids, permethrin and cypermethrin. *Neurotoxicol. Teratol.* **15**, 71–83.

Moser, V.C., Cheek, B.M. and MacPhail, R.C. (1995) A multidisciplinary approach to toxicological screening III: neurobehavioral toxicity. *J. Toxicol. Environ. Health.* **45**,173–210.

Morel, J.G. and Neerchal, N.K. (1993) A finite mixture distribution for modeling multinomial extra variation. *Biometrika* **80**, 363–371.

Moser, V.C., Tilson, H.A., MacPhail, R.C., Becking, G.C., Cuomo, V., Frantik, E., Kulig, B., and Winneke, G. (1997) The IPCS collaborative study on neurobehavioral screening methods: II. protocol design and testing procedures. *NeuroToxicology* **18**, 929–938.

NRC (National Research Council)(2008). *Phthalates and Cumulative Risk Assessment: The Tasks Ahead.* http://dels.nas.edu/dels/rpt_briefs/phthalates_final.pdf (accessed Nov 27, 2013).

Pinheiro, J.C. and Bates, D.M. (2000) Mixed-effects models in S and S-plus. Springer-Verlag: New York.

Price, C.J., Kimmel, C.A., George, J.D. and Marr, M.C. (1987). The developmental toxicity of diethylene glycol dimenthyl ether in mice. *Fund. Appl. Toxicol.* **81**: 113–127.

Regan, M.M. and Catalano, P.J. (1999) Likelihood models for clustered binary and continuous outcomes: applications to developmental toxicology. *Biometrics* **55**, 760–768.

Ryan, L.M. (1992) Quantitative Risk assessment for developmental toxicity. *Biometrics* **48**: 163–174.

Stiteler, W.M., Joly, D.A., and Printup, H.A.T. (1993). Monte carlo investigation of issues relating to the benchmark dose method. Task No. 2-30, Environmental Criteria and Assessment Office. U.S. Environmental Protection Agency, Cincinnati, Ohio.

Swan, S. H.; Main, K. M.; Stewart, S. L.; Kruse, R. L.; Calafat, A. M.; Mao, C. S.; Redmon, J. B.; Ternand, C. L.; Sullivan, S.; Teague. J. L. (2005). Study for Future Families Research Team. Decrease in Anogenital Distance among Male Infants with Prenatal Phthalate Exposure. *Environ. Health Perspect.* **113**(8), 1056–1061.

Zhu Y, Krewski D, and Ross W.H. (1994) Multinomial models for developmental toxicity experiments. *Appl. Statist.* **43**, 583–598.

Zhu, Y., Fung, K.Y. (1996) Statistical methods in developmental toxicity risk assessment. In *Toxicology and Risk Assessment, Principles, Methods and Applications.* Fan and Chang, Eds. 413–446.

Zhu, Y. (2005) Dose-time-response modeling of longitudinal measurements for neurotoxicity risk assessment.*Environmetrics* **16**, 603–617.

Zhu, Y., Wessel, M.R., Liu, T., and Moser, V.C. (2005a). Analyses of Neurobehavioral Screening Data: Dose-Time-Response Modeling of Continuous Outcomes. *Regulatory Toxicology and Pharmacology* **41**, 240–255.

Zhu, Y., Jia, Z., Wang, W., Gift, J., Moser, V.C., and B.J. Pierre-Louis (2005b). Analyses of Neurobehavioral Screening Data: Benchmark Dose Estimation. *Regulatory Toxicology and Pharmacology* **42**, 190–201.

About the Author

Yiliang Zhu is a professor in the Department of Epidemiology and Biostatistics, College of Public Health, University of South Florida. There, he directs the Center for Collaborative Research. He is also joint professor at Morsani College of Medicine's Internal Medicine. His current research involves quantitative methodologies in health risk assessment, including physiologically based pharmacokinetic models, dose-response modeling, benchmark-dose methods, and uncertainty quantification. He also conducts research in health outcome and health system evaluation. Dr. Zhu was a Fulbright Research Fellow (2012–2013) in NW China, where he initiated a 15-year cohort to study rural health and human development in support of evidence-based rural policy especially the new Rural Cooperative Medical Scheme. He was also designated as a 2013–2014 AAAS Science and Policy Fellow. Dr. Zhu has served on a number of advisory boards, including National Research Council committees on Health Risk Assessment of Dioxins, Tetrachloroethylene, Formaldehyde, Sciences at EPA, and EPA's IRIS Process; the Advisory Committee on Organ Transplantation of the Department of Human Health and Services; National Institutes of Health Study Sections, Environmental Protection Agency's external expert panels for IRIS documents, among others. He has advised over 60 master's thesis, PhD dissertations, and various research fellows including post-doctoral fellows. He received a PhD in statistics from the University of Toronto, a master's degree in Statistics from Queen's University in Kingston, and a Bachelor's degree from Shanghai University (of Science and Technology).

CHAPTER 18

SOME FUNDAMENTAL STATISTICAL ISSUES AND METHODOLOGIES IN CONFIRMATORY TRIALS*

GEORGE Y.H. CHI†, HAIYAN XU and QING LIU

Janssen Research and Development L.L.C., USA

†*GChi@its.jnj.com*

1. Introduction

In this section, we will describe the drug development program in general, the importance of confirmatory trials from a regulatory perspective and the two fundamental statistical principles of minimization of bias and maintenance of the overall type I error rate that are of critical importance to the success of such trials.

1.1. *Overview of drug development*

From its initial discovery to final marketing, a new drug in the United States has to go through various stages of development. Typically, preclinical animal studies are needed to determine the toxicity and carcinogenicity potential of a new compound. If these studies offer no suggestion of toxicity and evidence of carcinogenicity, then small studies on human volunteers are conducted in Phase 1 to determine the metabolism and pharmacologic actions of the drug in humans, dose dependent side effects, and if possible evidence of effectiveness. The information collected will permit the design of well-controlled, scientifically valid studies in Phase 2. The clinical studies in Phase 2 are conducted to evaluate the effectiveness of the drug for a

*The reviews expressed in this chapter are those of the authors and not necessarily those of the Janssen R&D, L.L.C.

particular indication or indications in patients with the disease or condition under study and to determine the common short term side effects and risks associated with the drug. In addition, for serious diseases such as cancer, a drug may be approved conditionally based on acceptable surrogate efficacy endpoints in phase 2. The information gathered in these early phases is used to guide the drug sponsor in the planning of phase 3 clinical trials. Phase 3 studies are expanded controlled and uncontrolled studies carried out to obtain confirmatory evidence on the effectiveness of the drug and sufficient safety information to allow a proper benefit-risk assessment prior to regulatory approval. In addition, they should provide sufficient information to form adequate basis for instructions to the physicians on its intended usage to be described in the label [21CFR 312.20 (2001)].

One of the critical requirements for pre-marketing approval of a new drug in the United States is the demonstration of the effectiveness of the drug through phase 3 clinical trials. The United States Code of Federal Regulations [21 CFR 314.126 (a)] requires that to establish the efficacy of a new drug, the sponsor must produce reports of adequate and well-controlled clinical trials that demonstrate its effectiveness. Generally, the evidence of effectiveness is based on at least two adequate and well-controlled studies. Some of the characteristics of an adequate and well-controlled study are described in the regulation [21 CFR 314.126 (b)]. Another critical requirement for pre-marketing approval of a new drug is safety. The safety of the drug is evaluated on the basis of the entire database obtained from all three phases of drug development prior to approval, and continues to be evaluated through phase 4 post-marketing clinical trials, if required as a condition for approval. To be approved, the drug sponsor must demonstrate that there is sufficient information to show that the drug is safe for use under the conditions prescribed, recommended, or suggested in its proposed labeling. Once approved, the safety of the new drug continues to be monitored through post-marketing adverse reaction reports.

A drug that is not yet approved for marketing may be used for treatment in patients with a serious or immediately life-threatening disease condition and for whom no comparable or satisfactory alternative drug or other therapy is available. The regulations allow such treatment to be carried out under a special protocol or treatment IND [21 CFR 312.34, 312.83 (2001)].

For treating serious or life-threatening illnesses, certain new drug products may qualify under accelerated approval [21 CFR 314,500 (2001)]. For treating a serious or life-threatening illness, a new drug that has demonstrated, based on adequate and well-controlled trials, an effect on a surrogate endpoint, or on some clinical benefits other than survival or irreversible morbidity, may be approved for marketing. The drug should provide meaningful therapeutic benefit to patients over existing treatments. For example, it may be effective in treating patients who are unresponsive to available therapy, or it may improve patient response over available therapy. The surrogate endpoint should have been reasonably validated through previous investigations as predictive of clinical benefit.

Accelerated approval is granted under the condition that the drug sponsor will conduct further study to confirm its clinical benefits in relation to the surrogate endpoint, or the ultimate clinical outcome of primary interest.

The following publications provide a good overview and source of reference for the entire drug development process and the United States drug regulatory requirements: Peace (1988), Mathieu (1997), Chow and Liu (1998), the U.S. Code of Federal Regulations [21 CFR 312–314 (2001)], and the U.S. Food and Drug Administration International Conference on Harmonization of Technical Requirements for Registration of Pharmaceuticals for Human Use [(ICH), E1-E10 (1998–1999)]. A corresponding set of regulatory guidance documents issued by the European Union Medicinal Agency also provides a good source of reference (European Medicines Agency).

This chapter focuses primarily some concepts, principles and issues related to establishing the evidence of effectivenessof a drug in a confirmatory trial. The following discussion of selected topics on certain aspects of the design, conduct and analysis of a confirmatory trial focuses on two fundamental statistical principles that are particularly critical from a regulatory perspective, namely, minimization of bias and control of overall type I error.

1.2. *Confirmatory trials*

In drug development, a confirmatory trial is a clinical trial that is prospectively designed to provide the primary source of evidence necessary to support the efficacy claim of the drug under investigation. The evidence from a confirmatory trial must be compelling, especially for mortality or serious morbidity trials where ethical consideration often precludes the possibility of conducting a second trial. This will also be critical for future active control trials where the current drug may be used as the control. The strength of evidence is measured among other things by the overall quality of the trial, internal and external consistency of the trial results. The internal and external consistencies of the trial results are the outcomes of the trial, whereas the overall quality of the trial is to a large extent under the control of the experimenter. The overall quality of a trial should be evaluated with respect to the following aspects of the study. These aspects should include the appropriateness of the design relative to its primary objective, acceptability of the study conduct, quality of the data collected, adequacy of the power, maintenance of the probability of the overall type I error, control of bias and confounding, proper method of analysis, and correct interpretation of trial results.

The accepted standard for the design of a confirmatory trial includes proper randomization, desired level of blinding, absence of confounding and choice of an appropriate control. In addition, other fundamental statistical principles should be closely adhered to in a confirmatory trial. These principles include minimization of the potential for bias and control of the probability of the overall type I error at the desired α-level. These two principles are essential to phase 2 and phase 3 confirmatory trials. A confirmatory trial should have assay sensitivity, that is, the capability of showing a difference when the study treatment is effective, a concept defined in the ICH-E10 (1999) document on the choice of control.

1.3. *Two fundamental statistical principles of clinical trials*

Minimization of the potential for bias and control of the probability of the overall type I error, or the probability of drawing a false positive conclusion, are two fundamental statistical principles that are central to the quality of a trial. Both principles are intimately related to the design, conduct and analysis of the trial, and the final interpretation of the trial results. Deviation from these two principles has the potential of weakening the strength of evidence, rendering the trial results not interpretable, or sometimes, even invalidating the entire trial results. Careful attention to these two principles throughout the trial from design and conduct to the final analysis and interpretation will strengthen the evidence and improve the likelihood of a successful trial.

Minimizing the potential for bias will be discussed first in the next section. In Section 3, the control of the probability of the overall type I error will be discussed through issues and problems related to multiple testing. In Section 4, interim analysis and adaptive design will be discussed. The problems and issues related to the important topic of non-inferiority trial will be discussed in the last section.

2. Minimizing the Potential for Bias

In a clinical trial, bias refers to the consequence of any design deficiency, specific property of the study treatment or control, certain characteristics of the disease, intentional or unintentional trial conduct, and any decision that results in a systematic exaggeration of the treatment difference either in favor or against the study treatment in a show-difference trial. It also refers to the consequence of a systematic dampening of treatment difference in favor of the study treatment in a non-inferiority or equivalence trial. When present, bias affects the estimate of the true treatment effect and may lead to drawing incorrect conclusion regarding the overall effect of the study treatment.

2.1. *Potential sources for bias in a clinical trial*

There are many potential sources for bias in a randomized controlled clinical trial. These sources include confounding, operational bias during trial execution, evaluation bias in outcome measurement, structural bias in the trial design, and statistical bias such as selection bias, in the method of analysis. In any given situation, bias could come from one or more or even a combination of these sources. Some of these sources of bias will be discussed and illustrated by examples below.

2.1.1. *Confounding*

The primary objective of a clinical trial is to demonstrate that the study treatment is effective as expected. Therefore, the trial must allow the experimenter to attribute any observed effect to the study treatment and to the study treatment alone by ruling out all other potential explanations. Confounding occurs when one cannot attribute unequivocally the entire observed treatment difference to the study treatment. The consequence of confounding here is bias, a bias that may be for or against the study treatment. A common source of confounding is an imbalance between the treatment arms in some important baseline covariates or prognostic factors that may have direct influence on the clinical outcomes of interest. A standard technique for avoiding or minimizing confounding is randomization. Randomization may provide some assurance that the treatment arms are relatively balanced with respect to all known or unknown factors that may affect a patient's response to the treatment. Randomization, if carried out properly, can minimize the chances for such imbalances to occur at baseline.

Confounding may occur simply due to failure of the randomization to achieve necessary ***baseline balance*** between the treatment and the control relative to some important and relevant known or unknown demographic or prognostic factors. When there are imbalances in known baseline covariates or prognostic factors, then one will be less assured about absence of imbalances in important but unknown factors. This type of imbalance can often occur when the sample size is modest or when the randomization scheme is flawed. It is important for a confirmatory trial to have sufficient power, proper randomization and stratification relative to some of the most important factors to avoid such potential problems and concerns.

However, even proper randomization may not be able to protect against bias resulting from differential treatment of the experimental and the control arms. Such differential treatment of the two arms may occur through operational bias introduced as a result of unblinding, through inherent structural bias as to be illustrated by the example on duodenal ulcer prevention trial in 2.1.3, or through statistical bias in the method of analysis.

2.1.2. *Operational bias*

If a randomized controlled trial is open label, that is, if there is no blinding, then operational bias can easily be introduced. For instance, in a study of a new treatment for headache, the investigator may consciously or unconsciously allow subjects on study treatment to have concurrent use of aspirins. This type of conduct can introduce bias into the trial favoring the study treatment. *Evaluation bias* can also easily find its way into such trial. For example, if the evaluation involves adjudication of certain event, then the adjudicator may assess the event differently depending upon whether the subject is on study treatment or control.

For certain clinical trials, it is simply impossible to maintain blinding at all. In trials comparing different surgical procedures, it is frequently not possible to have blinding. In some oncology trials, it may not be possible to maintain blinding because the trials may involve comparing treatments with different toxicity profiles and delivery systems, e.g., pill vs. intravenous injection.

In some randomized trials, even though the trials may be blinded, they can still potentially become partially unblinded. For example, it is known that the β blockers, a class of drugs for treating certain heart diseases, can lower heart rate significantly. The mean heart rate of patients treated with

β blockers can be 12 beats per minute lower than that of patients given placebo. Thus, knowing the specific properties of the study treatment, one can correctly guess the patient treatment assignment with a high likelihood of success, resulting in some degree of unblinding.

2.1.2.1. Levels of blinding

Blinding is one of the basic techniques used to control the potential introduction of bias in a randomized controlled trial. It is generally recommended to maintain a level of blinding permissible by the study.

When the individual patients are blinded to their own treatment assignments, the trial is called *single blind.* The blinding is generally achieved by giving patients medications that are identical in appearance but may contain the study treatment, the active comparator, or an inactive ingredient (placebo) depending upon the type of design.

When the investigators, evaluators, raters, or anyone who can influence the course of the trial, are also blinded to the patient treatment assignments during the entire course of the experiment, the trial is called *double-blind.* In a double-blind trial, provisions are made so that the investigators will be able to break the blind in an individual patient during an emergency, or when it is determined that the risk to the patient requires specific cares to be taken by the clinician to protect the patient's safety. In a double-blind trial, all study personnel are blinded to the patient treatment codes and should have no knowledge of or access to the results of any interim treatment comparative analysis.

2.1.2.2. Minimizing the likelihood of unblinding

In a blinded trial, how easy is it for the individual patient to unblind his/her own treatment? Can the study treatment and the control be easily distinguished through appearance, taste, shape, size, route of administration, regimen, frequency of administration, and side effects? Special blinding techniques may be needed in a trial in order to minimize the likelihood that the individual patient will be able to unblind his/her own treatment code. Of course, the investigator and other trial personnel should be instructed not to provide any information to the patient that may help the patient to unblind his/her own treatment code.

How easy is it for the investigator, evaluator, or rater to have access to the patient treatment codes or to unblind the patient treatment assignments? Can the investigator unblind or partially unblind the patient treatment assignments through patient's reported side effects, laboratory, physiological, and clinical parameters? For example, for the congestive heart failure trial involving exercise tolerance test, measures need to be taken to ensure that the administrator who conducts the treadmill test has no access to patient treatment experiences and baseline information so that the likelihood of unblinding patient treatment assignments can be minimized. Or in a trial that requires event adjudication, the adjudicator should not have access to information that may help reveal the patient treatment assignments. However, for the investigator, available blinding techniques may be more limited because the investigator has access to all of the patient data. The attention here should be more on reducing the impact of potential bias in the event of unblinding by the investigator.

How easy is it for the trial personnel to have access to treatment codes, to perform treatment comparative analysis, or to receive treatment comparative analysis results? How easy is it for the trial personnel to make changes to the trial, e.g., patient enrollment criteria, addition or deletion of centers, increasing sample size, changing endpoints, etc. For example, if there is an *Independent Data Monitoring Committee* (IDMC) involved, then how easy is it for the trial personnel to have access to treatment comparative analysis results through members of the IDMC? If the treatment comparative analysis is actually done by the trial personnel, then what safeguard is there to protect the integrity of the trial from changes done to the trial based on knowledge of the interim analysis results? Here, the only available tool to minimize unblinding is to establish a sound clinical trial infrastructure, clear designation of roles and responsibilities, and strict standard operating procedures governing the interaction, communication and dissemination of results among various operating units. These operating units include units within the trial organization such as the safety monitoring group, the data management group, the data analysis group, and the custodian of patient treatment codes. They also include units outside the sponsor's organization such as outside consultants, Contract Research Organization, and IDMC, if there is one. When interim analysis is planned, the standard operating procedures should address some issues including the following. Who is managing the interim data? Who is doing the interim analysis? How is it being carried out? To whom the results should be reported? Who can have access to the results of the interim analysis? How confidentiality of the results can be maintained? For guidance on these issues, one may refer to the Guidance on the Establishment and Operation of Clinical Trial Data Monitoring Committees (2001).

These questions and issues regarding blinding and how to avoid or minimize the potential opportunity for unblinding should be discussed and addressed at the design stage of a confirmatory trial. Appropriate blinding techniques tailored to each trial by taking into consideration the trial design, special properties of the study treatment, and characteristics of the disease should be described in the study protocol. Trial infrastructure and standard operating procedures should be designed in relation to these considerations.

2.1.2.3. Assessing and reducing the impact of unblinding

Of course, the mere occurrence of unblinding will not necessarily result in bias. It is the subsequent conduct on the part of some study personnel intentionally trying to influence or change the outcome either in favor or against the study treatment that results in bias. Thus, in addition to minimize the likelihood of unblinding, one should also consider reducing the severity and impact of potential bias introduced in the event of unblinding.

Generally, the severity and impact of bias introduced subsequent to unblinding depends on the level at which the unblinding occurs, the ease with which the patient response can be altered, the quantifiability of the bias, and the magnitude of the bias relative to the overall study treatment effect size.

When some individual patients are unblinded to their own treatment assignments, then these patients may introduce biases into their own individual responses. These biases introduced by the individual patients may not be consistently in the same direction, nor systematic. So the net effect of all the biases may be much less severe. The impact of the bias depends upon the number of individual patients involved and the magnitude of the net bias relative to the overall study population size and the overall treatment effect size. Occasionally, biases introduced by one or two patients may change the overall conclusion. However, in most cases, these individual biases may not be easily quantified. Various strategies may be taken at the analysis stage to examine the impact of these biases when known. Such strategies may range from excluding some or all of these affected patients from the analysis to imputing conservative values for these patients' responses.

When unblinding occurs at the investigator level, then the potential bias introduced will affect the outcomes from the particular investigator site or center. Such bias tends to be more severe because within each center, the bias introduced tends to be more systematic and consistent, and affects the entire outcome from that particular center. In a trial with only a few centers, or when the centers involved account for a significant proportion of the total patients studied, the result can be devastating. If such biases are known and quantifiable, then appropriate measures may be taken to account for them at the analysis stage. Otherwise, available analysis strategies for examining the impact of such biases may be limited only to dropping the affected centers from the analysis. In such event, randomization stratified within center may become an important issue.

Finally, when unblinding occurs at the study level, treatment comparisons may be made based on the entire available data. Knowledge of such treatment comparative analysis can lead to subtle changes in patient demographics, deletion of sites and sometimes to early trial termination. This type of changes made to the trial may result in bias favoring the study treatment. The impact of this kind of bias may be quite significant because such changes are based on the interim treatment comparative data. The consequences of such bias may include declaring an ineffective study treatment to be effective, prescribing the study treatment for a more general patient population than warranted, and incorrect labeling of the study treatment. It may be difficult to detect this kind of bias as a result of unblinding at the study level, and even when detected, it may be difficult to assess its impact. When unblinding occurs at the study level, the entire study results may be voided.

The potential impact of unblinding may also depend upon the type of efficacy endpoints involved. There are generally two types of endpoints, the objective and the subjective. In general, for subjective endpoints such as scores based on investigator or patient evaluation, concerns for potential unblinding are understandable. In such cases, an investigator or patient can easily assign certain scores, or components of the scores, in a manner that is favoring the study treatment. Subjective endpoints arise frequently in clinical trials. For objective endpoints, the outcomes are less vulnerable to such alterations. However, some forms of operational bias can still be introduced. For example, in many clinical trials, besides the study treatment and the control, concomitant administration of other effective drugs is allowed for all patients. In such cases, differential usage of concomitant medications between the study treatment and the control may potentially lead to bias.

Objective endpoints also may vary in degree of objectivity. For objective endpoints such as mortality or serious morbidity, it is difficult for anyone to alter their outcomes. For some other objective endpoints, operational bias can still be introduced. For example, in congestive heart failure trials, exercise tolerance test is often used to measure a patient's symptomatic improvement. In such trials, patients are asked to walk on treadmill. The administrator of the treadmill test would ask patients to walk until exhaustion. The total walking time will be recorded. Here the exercise tolerance test is an objective endpoint, but it may be affected by how hard the administrator pushes the patient to exhaustion. If the administrator is unblinded or partially unblinded to the patient treatment assignments, then differential handling of patients depending upon their treatment assignments will introduce operational bias. So in such cases, the administrator should not have access to the patient data and the investigator should not communicate to the patient his/her treatment assignment and treatment information.

It is clear that for a confirmatory trial, one should require double blinding. In addition, measures for minimizing the likelihood of unblinding and steps for reducing the impact of bias in the event of unblinding should be described clearly in the protocol. These efforts should include a sound infrastructure for the trial, clear designation of roles and responsibilities, and strict standard operating procedures that are tailored for the trial at hand and that take into account the type of design and specific trial requirements.

2.1.3. *Structural bias*

In a controlled clinical trial, even randomization and blinding may not fully protect against *structural bias* resulting from flaws in the design. Design flaws can occur, and not infrequently. Thus, one should be on guard against such structural bias. When it occurs, it has the potential to invalidate the results of the entire trial. There is usually no satisfactory remedy for structural bias as illustrated in Example 1 and Example 2 below.

Example 1 (Duodenal ulcers): In the late nineteen seventies and early nineteen eighties, it is customary for duodenal ulcer prevention trials to consider a double-blind placebo-controlled design with patients whose duodenal ulcers were recently healed on acute treatment randomized to either the same treatment at half the dose or placebo. Patients were scheduled at regular intervals for endoscopic examination to determine the presence or absence of duodenal ulcers. The intervals are usually of three, four or six month duration, and the entire trial usually lasts twelve months. At the request of the physician, patients could also be endoscoped upon presentation of symptoms such as pain. Patients found to have recurrent duodenal ulcers were discontinued from the study; the remaining patients continued in the trial until symptomatic recurrence, the next scheduled endoscopy, or the end of the trial. So these trials met the basic requirements of being randomized, double-blind and placebo-controlled. What is the problem? For H2-receptor antagonists such as ranitidine and cimetidine, it was generally recognized that they provide symptom relief and promote healing of duodenal ulcers in short term acute treatment trials. In the prevention trial, patients with symptomatic recurrent ulcers are discontinued from the trials. Therefore, if the test drug merely relieves symptoms without actually preventing recurrences, then simply by the present design, more symptomatic recurrences would be observed among patients on placebo. To further compound the problem, regular endoscopies are scheduled three, four or six months apart. It is also known that relatively short time, four to eight weeks, is required for duodenal ulcers to heal either with or without treatment in an acute trial. Thus it is entirely possible that during the intervals between successive endoscopies, symptomatic ulcers may have recurred among patients who remain in the trial, healed before the next scheduled endoscopy, and hence escaped detection. It is clear that there is a bias favoring the H2-receptor antagonist as a result of the properties of the drug and the design flaw. These and related issues were extensively discussed at a FDA Gastrointestinal Advisory Committee meeting [Lewis (1985)]. A renowned gastroenterologist at the time questioned whether duodenal ulcers could recur under maintenance treatment. However, it was demonstrated in a subsequent trial that duodenal ulcers could recur under maintenance treatment [Boyd *et al.*(1988), McManus and Wormsley (1989), and Kurata and Koch (1988)]. A more detailed discussion of this example and the related design issues can be found in Chi (1985), and Elashoff, Koch and Chi (1988). This interesting example illustrates a combination of design flaws, evaluation bias due to the analgesic property of the H2-blockers, and the spontaneous healing of duodenal ulcers over time.

2.1.4. *Statistical bias*

A randomized controlled trial that is blinded and has no design flaw can still have *statistical bias* introduced at the final analysis stage. Statistical bias can arise as a result of the method of analysis, the manner in which patients or data are excluded from the data set, or the manner in which missing data are being handled. This kind of statistical bias can sometimes be fairly subtle.

An important principle in the analysis of clinical trial data is the so-called intent-to-treat principle [See ICH-E9 (1999), Fisher *et al.* (1990), Gillings and Koch (1991), and Lachin (2000)]. The intent-to-treat principle simply espouses the view that the primary analysis should be performed on the outcome measures from all of the randomized patients. When there is no other source of bias, such as design flaw, then the intent-to-treat analysis should provide an unbiased estimate of the treatment effect when there are no patient exclusions and no missing data. When the outcome measures are not available from all of the randomized patients, then efficacy subset analysis is likely to provide biased estimate of the treatment effect. Little and Rubin (1987) and Little (1993) defined three types of missing data mechanisms, missing completely at random (MCAR), missing at random (MAR) and informative missingness. There are various statistical models proposed to handle clinical trial data with these types of missing mechanisms. However, missing data mechanisms in clinical trials are difficult to verify whether they are MCAR, MAR or informative missingness. Generally, clinicians and biostatisticians in the field believe that most missing data mechanisms in clinical trials are likely to be informative missingness for which statistical approaches are less well-developed. One imputation method that has often been used is the so-called Last Observation Carried Forward (LOCF) analysis where the last available observation is substituted for all the subsequent missing observations. The LOCF analysis implicitly assumes that the last observation is an unbiased representation of what the missing observation would have been had the patient been followed, which is also an unverifiable assumption. This assumption would be particularly problematic when the last available observation occurred early on. Various issues related to the LOCF analysis are discussed in Gillings and Koch (1991), Verbeke *et al.* (1997), Lachin (2000), Begg (2000), Myers (2000), and Malinckrodt *et al.* (2001).

The handling of missing data is a difficult problem, and the best strategy is to adhere to the intent-to-treat principle by minimizing the likelihood of missing data. The ICH E-8 Guidance on General Considerations for Clinical Trials (1997) recommends that the study protocol should specify procedures for the follow-up of patients who stop treatment prematurely. Furthermore, the ICH E-9 Guidance on Statistical Principles for Clinical Trials (1998) states that compliance with the intent-to-treat principle requires complete follow-up of all randomized patients for the primary outcome measures. For a confirmatory trial, procedures for such complete follow-up of all randomized patients should be carefully spelled out in the protocol and diligently carried out during the trial. The intent-to-treat principle should be followed with robustness or sensitivity analyses performed if needed. For a recent discussion and recommendation on the problems of missing data, the interested reader can refer to the National Research Council Report (2010).

The following example illustrates an interesting case of structural bias combined with analysis bias in a study for a serious progressive disease.

Example 2: In this example, the investigational new drug is manufactured only in limited quantity; hence only a small percent of the patients can be given the new drug. The study protocol has an unusual design. After a patient satisfies some eligibility criteria, he/she enters a pool and becomes eligible for random selection for the study treatment according to the fixed percentage. If a patient is selected, then the study treatment will be given. On the other hand, if a patient is not selected at a given pool of eligible, then that patient remains unselected until the next selection. If that patient dies before the next selection, then he/she will be counted as an event in the unselected group. Otherwise, at the next selection, this patient enters the pool along with the newly eligible. Again patients in this second pool will have the same probability of being selected for the study treatment. This process continues with selections conducted about every month for over a year. Generally, for the selected patients, there is a delay of about three months between the time of selection and the actual time of administration of the study treatment. There is a one-year follow-up. The primary endpoint of interest is mortality. The length of survival of a patient is measured from the time of first eligibility to subsequent death, lost-to-follow-up, or to the end of the study. The comparison of the survival experience between the selected group and the unselected group from all ten selections is evaluated by the log-rank test statistic.

There are two kinds of bias in this example. The first kind is a structural bias, and the second is an analysis bias. The structural bias can be seen as follows. The definitions of selected and unselected groups are outcome (survival) dependent. This is because a patient who was not selected in any given selection could still be selected in a subsequent selection provided that that patient was able to survive till that selection. A patient who was not selected and died before a selection would automatically remain in the unselected group. This design would enrich the selected group with patients that have better survival experience up to the time of selection, and enrich the unselected group with patients who died before a selection.

There is also a bias in the survival analysis. If a patient who is selected after a given selection, then his/her survival time is measured from the time of first eligibility to death, lost-to-follow-up, or end of the study. But for such patient, the time from first eligibility to the time of selection is actually not under the study treatment. In fact, in general, there is an additional delay of about three months before the study treatment is actually given to a selected patient. Thus a large proportion of his/her survival experience would not be under the study treatment, but would be attributed to the study treatment. Such bias favors the study treatment. However, it is not advisable to consider the survival time as measured from the time of selection or the actual time the selected patient is given the study treatment, because the selected group and the unselected group are outcome dependent and hence there is no valid randomization.

As it turns out, in this example, a majority of the patients were considered for eligibility in the second selection. To maintain randomization and to minimize bias, it was recommended that patients from the second selection be considered for analysis. Thus, the selected patients consist of those who were selected in the second selection, and the unselected patients consist of those who were not selected at the second selection. Now, for these unselected patients, some of them were actually selected at a subsequent selection. So, in the survival analysis, the survival time for the unselected patients are measured from the time of first eligibility to death, lost-to-follow-up, or censored at time of subsequent selection, actual time of study treatment administration, or the end of the study.

Example 3 (Rivaroxaban): In the large ROCKET AF trial, which was randomized double-blind and stratified by country, rivaroxaban is compared to warfarin for the prevention of stroke and systemic embolism in patients with non-valvular atrial fibrillation. Warfarin is known to be effective although it is somewhat difficult to use, since the physicians need to titrate the drug to within a narrow therapeutic range. The overall trial average time in the therapeutic range (TTR) for the ROCKET AF trial is around 55% which is somewhat lower than the average of around 65% or higher in some other recent trials. The reason for this lower average TTR is due to the fact that this was a multiregional trials and the trial protocol did not prescribe a uniform standard procedure for the investigators to adhere to. Thus, due to the varying medical practices across the regions, the average TTR tends to be lower and reflects the actual current practices. An issue was raised in the FDA Clinical Review (U.S. FDA Cardiovascular and Renal Drug Advisory Committee Meeting, September 8, 2011) regarding the potential bias due to the less than optimal use of warfarin in the ROCKET AF trial favoring rivaroxaban. To substantiate this issue, the review describes a sequence of analyses that was performed starting with the analysis of the entire population and then followed by one analysis after another that selectively excluded centers with high average TTR in a decreasing manner. Towards the end of this sequence of analyses, only centers with lower and lower average TTR were left in the analysis set. The overall treatment difference that was favoring rivaroxaban in the beginning gradually gave way to a negative treatment effect in favor of warfarin towards the end of this sequence of analyses. The clinical review suggests that this observation suggests that the treatment effect of rivaroxaban is questionable.

However, there are at least two problems with this sequence of analyses. First, the study was not randomized within center. Therefore, for these analyses, except for the first analysis which is based on the entire population, rivaroxaban and warfarin are not likely to be comparable, especially towards the end, when few centers are left in the analyses. Second, average TTR in a center is a variable derived *only* from the warfarin subjects in the given center and moreover, it is a treatment *outcome dependent* variable. Using average center TTR value to determine the analysis sets in the sequence of analyses is very problematic, not only because these analysis sets are treatment outcome dependent, but also because they involve selection bias. Therefore, the results of this sequence of analyses are not valid and simply cannot be interpreted. A more appropriate analysis would be to compare rivaroxaban to warfarin within certain countries or regions, or some other stratified randomized subgroups, where the average TTR is high and comparable to those observed in the other trials. This was done for the U.S. as a country and North America as a region, and the effect of rivaroxaban was shown in these analyses suggesting that rivaroxaban is effective when warfarin is optimally used. This example points out that selection bias can have serious impact on the proper conclusion of a study if it is inadvertently introduced into the analysis.

2.2. *Some measures to minimize potential bias*

In view of the various potential sources of bias in a clinical trial, it is important for a confirmatory trial to consider adopting appropriate measures at the design stage to minimize the impact of potential biases.

Randomization is the standard technique used in clinical trials to achieve balance in both known important baseline covariates,, prognostic and demographic factors and any unknown important factors between the treatment arm and the control. It is important to use proper randomization scheme that will not lead to unblinding to achieve the necessary balance.

Operational bias is difficult to control. Blinding is the most important technique for controlling operational bias. A confirmatory trial should be blinded at the study level. If necessary, special blinding techniques should be considered at the individual patient level and the investigator level. The aim is to minimize the likelihood of unblinding by the individual patients, the investigators, evaluators or raters, or the study personnel and to minimize its impact in the event of actual unblinding. In order to minimize the impact of bias due to unblinding, randomization should be centralized and stratified within each center, provided that the randomization procedure itself does not lead to potential unblinding. All blinding techniques should be clearly documented, described, standardized and operationalized. At the study level, the only blinding technique that can be implemented is through proper infrastructure, clear delineation of roles and responsibilities, and strict standard operating procedures. For instance, it should be made clear who has custody of the patient treatment codes, circumstances under which the patient treatment codes can be accessed, the parties that may have the authority to access them, and the proper procedure for such accession. These considerations should also include outside consultants, contract research organizations, and IDMC. This is especially critical when the trial involves planned interim analyses and an IDMC. When there is an IDMC, there should be standard operating procedures that define the responsibility and the proper span of authority of this committee, and govern the conduct and communication between the trial sponsor and the committee, whether the committee is independent or not. For example, when an IDMC requests the interim results from the trial sponsor, who in the sponsor's organization is doing the interim analysis, and how can the interim analysis results be kept confidential from the sponsor's study personnel? All of these should be carefully described in an IDMC charter and their executions during the planned interim analyses should be accurately documented.

When the IDMC recommends to the trial sponsor that the study be terminated early, certainly the trial sponsor should be provided with the interim analysis results and the reason for the recommendation. The sponsor's study personnel that receive such recommendation and the interim analysis results would have the interim comparative results. Thus the sponsor's study personnel would now have access to the comparative interim results. If the sponsor decides to continue the trial, then there is a potential opportunity for operational bias to be introduced by the study personnel at this point. How can one prevent such potential opportunity for operational bias to be introduced? The FDA draft document on the Establishment and Operation of Clinical Trial Data Monitoring Committee (2001) provides some relevant guidance on these issues.

To avoid structural bias, properties of the study treatment, type of treatment administration, the nature of the disease, the objective of the trial and other pertinent information should be well understood to insure that the design of the trial is not flawed.

To reduce the problem with missing data, it is recommended that a confirmatory trial should attempt complete follow-up on all missing primary response data from dropouts or others, and better documentation of reasons for dropping out and missing primary response data. This will minimize the impact of bias and may provide the basis for determining the proper method of handling the missing data.

To properly assess the strength of evidence in a trial, one needs to know whether the blind has been broken. If the blind has been broken, what is the extent of unblinding? Whether and how such information was used to bias the trial outcome? Whether the bias can be quantified? What analysis strategies can be applied to examine the impact of the bias, and whether the trial can still provide the strength of evidence sought if at all? These are important issues to be addressed in a confirmatory trial.

3. Control of the Overall Type I Error Rate

The second fundamental statistical principle in clinical trials is to control the overall probability of type I error (sometimes referred to as the false positive error), i.e., the probability of declaring the study treatment to be effective when in truth it is not, at a pre-specified significance level of β. In a test of a simple null hypothesis, the type I error rate may be inflated in various ways. For example, if the distribution of the test statistic involves a nuisance parameter that has to be estimated from the data, then this may lead to inflation of the type I error rate. When one performs multiple testing of the same hypothesis, e.g., the null hypothesis of no treatment effect, through multiple measures of treatment effect, the type I error rate can be substantially inflated as illustrated below.

3.1. *Inflation of the overall Type I error rate under multiple testing*

Consider a clinical trial comparing m doses of a drug to placebo. Let μ_i, $i = 0, 2, \ldots, m$ denote the change from baseline for placebo and m doses of the drug respectively. Let $H_{0,123-m}$: $\Delta\mu_1 = \Delta\mu_2 = \cdots = m\mu_m = 0$ represents the global null hypothesis, and $H_{0,i}$: $\Delta\mu_i = 0$, $i = 1, 2, \ldots, m$ the individual null hypotheses, where $\Delta\mu_i = \mu_i - \mu_0, i = 1, 2, \ldots, m$. Let us suppose that we have a suitable test statistic for testing each of these individual hypotheses and we test each hypothesis at the same significance level of $\alpha_i = \alpha$. Then, the probability of rejecting at least one $H_{0,i}$ is given by

$$\begin{aligned}
&Pr(\text{Reject at least one } H_{0,i}\text{: } \Delta\mu_i = 0,\ i = 1, 2, \ldots, m | H_{0,123-m})\\
&\quad = 1 - \text{Pr}(\text{Fail to reject all } H_{0,i}\text{:}\Delta\mu_i = 0,\ i = 1, 2, \ldots, m | H_{0,123-m}\text{:}\\
&\qquad \Delta\mu_1 = \Delta\mu_2 = \cdots = m\mu_m = 0)\\
&\quad = 1 - \Pi_i\text{Pr}(\text{Fail to reject all } H_{0,i}\text{: } \Delta\mu_i = 0,\ i | H_{0,123-m}\text{:}\\
&\qquad \Delta\mu_1 = \Delta\mu_2 = \cdots = m\mu_m = 0)\\
&\quad = 1 - \Pi_i(1 - \alpha_i), \text{assuming independence}\\
&\quad = 1 - (1 - \alpha)^m,\ \ \text{if } H_{0,i} \text{ is tested at the same significance level of } \alpha.\\
&\quad \geq \alpha. \qquad (1)
\end{aligned}$$

The above inequality (1) shows that when we test m null hypotheses, even when all m null hypotheses are true, the probability of rejecting at least one null hypothesis could be greater than α. This inflation in the type I error increases monotonically as the number of null hypotheses to be tested increases, since the probability of the overall type I error $\geq$0.05. 0.098, 0.143, 0.226, 0.401 as $m = 1, 2, 3, 5$ and 10 comparisons respectively. Thus, it is clear that in order for the probability of the overall type I error to be controlled at a given α level, it is necessary to test the individual null hypothesis $H_{0,i}$ at a significance level $\alpha_i < \alpha$, $i = 1, 2, \ldots, m$, in such a way that the probability of the overall type I error does not exceed α. Various multiple testing procedures have been proposed to accomplish this. We will discuss some of these later in this section.

For this reason and for lack of better concept and methodology, for a long time, confirmatory trials have mostly been designed with a single clinical endpoint in mind, perhaps also encouraged by the recommendation from the regulatory agency [ICH-E9 Guideline (1998)]. The evidence of the effectiveness of a drug/treatment is entirely based on the rejection of the single null hypothesis which was defined in terms of this clinical endpoint. From a statistical and regulatory standpoint, when the primary hypothesis fails to be rejected at the significance level α, then the trial has filed to provide the expected strength of evidence for the efficacy of the drug needed for regulatory approval; additional testing of hypotheses can only result in an inflation of the overall type I error rate. O'Neill (1997) supported the idea that "secondary endpoints cannot be validly analyzed if the primary endpoint does not demonstrate clear statistical significance." D'Agostino (2000) and Moyé (2003) also provide a classification of secondary endpoints. This problem is illustrated by the following carvedilol example.

Example 4: After a trial fails to reject the null hypothesis defined by the designated "primary endpoint" at the specified significance level of α, the sponsor then turns to the "secondary endpoints". When mortality, which is one of several "secondary endpoints", shows "apparent significance", i.e., with a p-value less than α, then can the sponsor claims that the drug is effective based on a mortality benefit? This was the case with carvedilol. For an interesting discussion of the carvedilol study, one may refer to the article by [Fisher (1999a, 1999b) and Moyé(1999, 2000a, 2000b)]. See also Chi (1995) for the SOLVD prevention trial.

However, in many disease areas, the clinical benefit of a treatment may be manifested through multiple ways, such as the disease state, severity, signs and symptoms, survivorship, etc. In certain disease areas, no single clinical endpoint is sufficient to assess the effectiveness of a treatment and would require the joint assessment of several clinical endpoints. Therefore, in these settings, the evaluation of the probability of type I error becomes more complex, and new concepts and methodologies are required. It is the purpose of this section to define these broader concepts and discuss some general methodologies that have been developed to address the multiple test problem.

In this section, we will first make precise the concept of primary family of hypotheses and secondary family of hypotheses from a regulatory perspective. Examples will be given to illustrate some typical families of hypotheses reflecting some of the complex clinical decision rules often encountered in confirmatory trials. After that, we will introduce the general concepts of weak and strong control of familywise error rate. Lastly, general multiple testing procedures will be described and their applications will also be illustrated through some examples.

3.2. *The concept of a family of hypotheses in a confirmatory trial from a regulatory perspective*

3.2.1. *Indication endpoints, clinical decision rules and labeling endpoints in a confirmatory trial*

The indication section of a drug label appears at the very beginning. It succinctly states the patient population that the drug can be prescribed for and the clinical benefits that can be expected. Dosage and safety information appear elsewhere in the label. Despite the brevity of the indication section, it deserves the most serious consideration during the design of confirmatory trials for a drug/treatment therapy, because for a drug/treatment to be approved for its proposed indication, it is necessary for its confirmatory trials to provide sufficient evidence of its effectiveness relative to one or more relevant clinical endpoints at one or more doses of the drug or treatment regimen.

The effectiveness of a treatment is usually assessed by some clinical outcome variables that are deemed relevant and important, and the changes in these variables when compared between treatment groups can provide a reliable and accurate measure of the effectiveness of the treatment. Often these variables may vary in terms of their relative importance, particularly in terms of the approvability of the drug based on evidence they present. Their relative importance would depend on their clinical relevance, reliability, and degree of objectivity. Some clinical outcome variables are very important from these perspectives such as mortality. Some are less important such as signs and symptoms, physician or patient global impression. More specifically, if positive outcome on a clinical variable alone constitutes sufficient evidence for the proposed indication, then we will call such variable an *indication endpoint*. When positive outcome on a clinical variable alone is deemed insufficient evidence for the proposed indication, then such variable will be called a *labeling endpoint*, because they may provide additional useful information for practicing physicians and patients, and may be included in the label somewhere when the drug/treatment has been approved based on positive evidence presented by the indication endpoints. It should be neted however that labeling endpoints together based on some *clinical decision rules* may provide sufficient evidence on the effectiveness of the drug for its proposed indication (see Example 5 & 6). Therefore, clinical decision rules may be viewed as complex indication endpoints.

Example 5: In an epilepsy trial, the decision set consists of three clinical endpoints, $\{A, B, C\}$, where A is a primary endpoint and B and C are secondary endpoints. The clinical decision rule adopted is that either ($\Delta\mu_A > 0$ at ξ_A) or ($\Delta\mu_B > 0$ at ξ_B) and ($\Delta\mu_C > 0$ at ξ_C). Let μ_A, μ_B and μ_C denote the parameters corresponding to the endpoints A, B and C respectively.

This decision rule reflects the following complex null and alternative hypotheses:

$$H_{0,c}\colon \Delta\mu_A = 0 \quad \textit{and} \quad (\Delta\mu_B = 0 \text{ or } \Delta\mu_C = 0)$$
$$H_{a,c}\colon \Delta\mu_A \neq 0 \quad \textit{or} \quad (\Delta\mu_B \neq 0 \text{ and } \Delta\mu_C \neq 0)$$

The sponsor proposes to test instead the restricted null hypothesis:

$$H_{0,r}\colon \Delta\mu_A = 0 \quad \text{and } \Delta\mu_B = 0 \quad \text{and} \quad \Delta\mu_C = 0$$

for no treatment effect. Note that $H_{0,c}$ consists of two axes, ($\Delta\mu_A = 0$ and $\Delta\mu_B = 0$) and ($\Delta\mu_A = 0$ and $\Delta\mu_C = 0$), while $H_{0,r}$ consists of only the origin. It is shown by Jin and Chi (1998) that the probability of the overall type I error for the proposed clinical decision rule under $H_{0,c}$ should be

$$\begin{aligned}\alpha_c &= \sup \Pr(\Delta\mu_A \Delta\mu_B \Delta\mu_C)\{|Z_A| > \xi_A \text{ or } (|Z_B| > \xi_B \text{ and } |Z_C| > \xi_C)\} \\ &\quad [(\Delta\mu_A, \Delta\mu_B, \Delta\mu]_C) \in H_{0,c} \\ &= \max\{\Pr(\Delta\mu_A = 0, \Delta\mu_B = 0)(|Z_A| > \xi_A \text{ or } (|Z_B| > \xi_B), \\ &\quad [Pr]_\downarrow(([\Delta\mu]_\downarrow A = 0[\Delta\mu]_\downarrow C = 0))(|Z_\downarrow A| > \xi_A \text{ or } |Z_\downarrow C| > \xi C)\},\end{aligned}$$

where Z_A, Z_B, and Z_C are the corresponding test statistics and ξ_A, ξ_B and ξ_C are the corresponding critical values.

The probability of the overall type I error corresponding to the restricted null hypothesis is

$$\begin{aligned}\alpha_r = \sup \Pr(\Delta\mu_A \Delta\mu_B \Delta\mu_C)\{|Z_A| > \xi_A \quad \text{or} \\ (|Z_B| > \xi_B \quad \text{and} \quad |Z_C| > \xi_C)\}(\Delta\mu_A, \Delta\mu_B, \Delta\mu_C,) \in H_{0,r}\end{aligned}$$

It is easy to see that $\alpha_C \geq \alpha_r$ with strict inequality holds true in general.

Therefore, if the rejection region, or critical values ξ_A, ξ_B and ξ_C, are defined to preserve α_r at the desired level, say, $\alpha = 0.05$, then the probability of the overall type I error, α_C will be inflated beyond 0.05. Hence, the success of the trial outcomes may be in doubt if it is designed relative to the incorrect null hypothesis.

This example illustrates that it is important to understand clearly a complex clinical decision rule and formulate its corresponding null hypothesis. Otherwise, it can easily weaken the strength of evidence or compromise the validity of the statistical inference.

Conceptually, a clinical decision rule simply defines the alternative region in the multidimensional parameter space that is of interest. More generally, one can extend the concept of a clinical decision rule to include other efficacy assessment schemes involving multiple endpoints, multiple comparisons, repeated testing, multiple indication, etc. The next example illustrates a slightly more complex decision rule that was recently discussed at an FDA Advisory Committee meeting.

Example 6: One of the issues that was presented to the FDA Anti-Infective Advisory Committee in their recent meeting discussing the primary endpoints for assessing effectiveness of a new drug for treating community-acquired bacterial pneumonia (CABP). The FDA had proposed a clinical decision rule defined as (1) improvement in at least two out of four following secondary signs and symptoms endpoints: cough, amount of sputum production, chest pain, and difficulty breathing, and (2) no worsening or new symptoms at day 3 to day 5. Some committee members noted the need to have clinical endpoints that measure how a patient feels, functions and survives. No final decision has been made yet. The interested readers can refer to the materials prepared for this advisory committee meeting (see the November 3, 2011 FDA Anti-Infective Drugs Advisory Committee Meeting Materials).

3.2.2. *Indication and labeling family of hypotheses*

For ease of understanding, consider a confirmatory drug trial intended to provide sufficient evidence of effectiveness for a proposed indication. Suppose that there are only three indication endpoints I_1, I_2 and I_3 and three labeling endpoint primary endpoints L_1, L_2 and L_3, where indication and labeling endpoint have the regulatory implication as defined in the preceding paragraph. Moreover, let $d(L_\downarrow 2,\ L_\downarrow 3) = (\Delta\mu_\downarrow(L_\downarrow 2) > 0$ and $\Delta\mu_\downarrow(L_\downarrow 2) > 0$ be a clinical decision rule defining the criteria for positive evidence in terms of the two labeling endpoints L_2 and L_3 (see Example 5). The set of null hypotheses $F_I = \{H_1^I,\ H_2^I, H_3^I, H^{d(L2,L3)}\}$, where $H^I i$: $\{\Delta\mu_{Ii} \leq 0\}$, $i = 1, 2, 3$ and $H^{d(L2,L3)}$: $\{\Delta\mu_{L2} \leq 0$ or $\Delta\mu_{L3} \leq 0$ is called the indication family of hypotheses, because it consists of the null hypotheses defined by the indication endpoints $\{I_1, I_2, I_3, d(L_2, L_3)\}$

including the complex indication endpoint such that the rejection of nay one of them is considered as sufficient evidence for the effectiveness of the drug/treatment. The family of hypotheses $F_L = \{H_1^L,\ H_2^L,\ H_3^L\}$, where $H^L i$: $\{\Delta\mu_{Li} \leq 0\}$, $i = 1, 2, 3$ is called the labeling family of hypotheses, because it consists of null hypotheses $H^L i$ defined by the labeling endpoints $^L i$ such that the rejection of any one of them is considered insufficient evidence for the effectiveness of the drug/treatment.

Now for confirmatory evidence, we only need to assure the strong control of the familywise error rate, a concept to be defined in the next section, for the indication family $\mathcal{F}_I$. For inclusion in the label, we may need to assure the strong control of the familywise error rate, for the labeling family $\mathcal{F}_L$.

It should be emphasized that it is not necessary to assure strong control of the combined family $\mathcal{F}_I \cup \mathcal{F}_L$, since clearly a positive outcome upon testing the labeling family $\mathcal{F}_L$ cannot possibly inflate the familywise error rate for the indication family $\mathcal{F}_I$, since the positive evidence from the labeling family $\mathcal{F}_L$ alone is not considered sufficient to conclude the effectiveness of the drug/treatment.

3.2.3. *Primary and secondary family of hypotheses*

Now let us consider again the indication family of hypotheses $\mathcal{F}_I$. For a given indication and a given drug/treatment, the effect of the drug/treatment as measured by the various indication endpoints and complex indication endpoint in the indication family $\mathcal{F}_I = \{H_1^I, H_2^I,\ H_3^I,\ H^{d(L2,L3)}\}$ is likely to be different. The various indication endpoints and complex indication endpoint may also have varying probability of success. Therefore, depending upon the given situation, a sponsor may wish to divide the indication family $\mathcal{F}_I$ into disjoint subfamilies called *primary family* $\mathcal{F}_P$ and *secondary family* $\mathcal{F}_S$ (or families) of indication endpoints, where an appropriate multiple testing strategy will be applied to the primary and secondary family of hypotheses to optimize the chances of success while maintaining a strong control of the combined family $\mathcal{F}_P \cup \mathcal{F}_S$ which is just the indication family $\mathcal{F}_I$. For example, we may consider the primary family to be $\mathcal{F}_P = \{I_1, I_2\}$ and the secondary family to be $\mathcal{F}_S = \{I_3, d(L_2, L_3)\}$. Thus, a primary family is a subset of the indication family $\mathcal{F}_I$, and a secondary family is also a disjoint subset of the indication family $\mathcal{F}_I$ and it should not contain any labeling endpoint from $\mathcal{F}_L$. This last point is critical, since we often encounter confirmatory trials where the secondary families often also contain labeling endpoints, which would make it unnecessarily harder for such trials to demonstrate the drug/treatment's effectiveness, since the strong control would then also have to cover the labeling endpoints, which is not necessary as we have just mentioned.

For the rest of this section, the terms primary and secondary family of hypotheses refer to subfamilies of the indication family.

3.3. *Familywise error rate*

When there is more than one hypothesis in a family of m null hypotheses to be tested ($m > 1$), the *Familywise Error Rate* (FWER), which is defined as the probability of rejecting at least one true null hypothesis, is the most commonly used definition of the overall type I error rate in clinical trials.

The FWER can be calculated under the specific assumption (or configuration) that all m null hypotheses are simultaneously true as the probability Pr(Reject at least one $H_\downarrow(0,i)$, $i = 1, 2, \ldots, m-1|H_\downarrow\ (0, 1, 2, 3, \ldots, m)$). The FWER is said to be *controlled in the weak sense at the α level,* if Pr(Reject at least one $H_\downarrow(0,i)$, $i = 1, 2, \ldots, m|H_\downarrow(0, 1, 2, 3, \ldots, m)) \leq \alpha$. Thus, the inequality (1) shows that if we simply test each null hypothesis in the family at the α level, then this multiple testing procedure may not control the FWER in the weak sense. The FWER is said to be *controlled in the strong sense* at α level, if the probability of incorrectly rejecting at least one true null hypotheses is less than or equal to α regardless of which and how many other hypotheses are true. More specifically, suppose we test $H_{0,i}$: $\{\Delta\mu_i \leq 0\}$, $i = 1, 2, \ldots, m$, where $\Delta\mu_i$ is the treatment difference between the ith-dose of the study drug and placebo in the primary efficacy variable, and let T be the index set of true null hypotheses. Then, the FWER is strongly controlled if the following inequality holds:

$$\text{FWER} = \max_{T \sup \Delta\mu_i(T)} Pr\left(\text{Reject at least one } H_{0,i}, i \in T \,\middle|\, \bigcap_{i\in T} H_{0,i}\right) \leq \alpha$$

where the supremum is taken over all $\Delta\mu_i$ satisfying $\Delta\mu_i \leq 0$ for $i \in T$ and $\Delta\mu_i > 0$ for $i \notin T$, and the maximum is taken over all index set T. To illustrate, suppose there is a family of three null hypotheses to be tested in a clinical trial: $[\{H]_{0,1}$, $H_{0,2}$, and $H_{0,3}\}$. In order to control the FWER in the strong sense, we need to make sure that the type I error rate is less than or equal to α for any configuration of true null hypotheses. For example, if all three null hypotheses are true, then we need to make sure that Pr(Reject $H_0, 1, H_0$, 2, or $H_0, 3, |H_0$, 123) $\leq \alpha$; and if only $H_{0,1}$ and $H_{0,2}$ true, then Pr(Reject $H_\downarrow 0$, 1 or $H_\downarrow 0, 2|H_\downarrow 0, 12) needs to be $\leq \alpha$. In particular, if only

$H_{0,1}$ is true, then $Pr(\text{Reject } H_{\downarrow}0,1|H_{\downarrow}0,1)$ needs to be $\leq \alpha$. Thus, it is clear that FWER is controlled in the strong sense at α level implies FWER is controlled in the weak sense at (level and also control of the individual type I error rate at α level. Clearly, FWER controlled in the weak sense at α level does not imply that the control of the individual type I error rates $Pr(\text{Reject } H_{\downarrow}(0,1)|H_{\downarrow}(0,1))$, is necessarily controlled at α level.

The strong control of the FWER for confirmatory trials is usually required by the regulatory agencies. This is for the simple reason that the evidence of effectiveness required for the proposed indication has to be *both endpoint and dose specific.* The strong control of FWER provides both the strength and specificity needed for drug approval — two crucial properties that are missing from the weak control of FWER. Generally, for confirmatory trials, the strong control of the FWER is required for the combined family of $\mathcal{F}_p \cup \mathcal{F}_{S1} \cup \mathcal{F}_{S2} \ldots \cup \mathcal{F}_{Sk}$, where $\mathcal{F}_P$ is a primary family of indication endpoints and $\mathcal{F}_{Si} = 1, 2, \ldots, k$ are secondary families of indication endpoints. If there is a labeling family $\mathcal{F}_L$, then it should be strongly controlled *separately.*

There are other types of overall type I error rates that are not commonly used in clinical trials. For example, the generalized familywise error rate (gFWER) [Lehmann and Romano (2005), Xu and Hsu (2007)], the false discovery rate (FDR) [Benjamini and Hochberg (1995)], and the false discovery proportion (FDP) [Korn *et al* (2004)]. We will not discuss them here.

3.4. *Types of multiple testing settings*

Multiple testing situations surface frequently in clinical trials. Multiple testing may manifest itself in various forms. It often appears in multiple dose-control comparisons, multiple endpoints, multiple patient populations, repeated hypothesis testing, multiple decision rules, or combinations thereof. The basic problem with multiple testing in a clinical trial is that it could inflate the overall type I error rate. This is of particular concern to a regulatory agency because if the effectiveness of a drug can be evaluated arbitrarily through multiple testing, then the probability of falsely concluding that the drug is effective may be inflated. The following are examples of sources of multiplicity commonly encountered in confirmatory clinical trials.

3.4.1. *Multiple dose-control comparisons*

In confirmatory clinical trials, a parallel design that includes multiple doses of the test treatment, placebo, and one or more doses of an active control is often considered and recommended by the regulatory authority. The primary objective of such a trial is to demonstrate that one or more doses of the test drug/treatment is superior to placebo in efficacy, and one or more doses of the test drug/treatment is superior or comparable to the active control in efficacy. In simple dose-response study without a control and placebo, multiplicity is introduced by having multiple dose comparisons.

3.4.2. *Multiple endpoints and clinical decision rules*

In medicine, a disease is often characterized by multiple clinical endpoints which may include signs and symptoms, disease severity, and disease stage that are assessed by various quantitative measures and they may be correlated. Some clinical endpoints provide direct information regarding the state of the disease; Some maybe capable of revealing whether the disease has been modified, such as healing of ulcer as determined by endoscopic examination. Some clinical endpoints provide indirect information regarding the state of the disease; these clinical endpoints include signs and symptoms known to be associated with the disease. In a disease where death is a potential outcome, mortality or survival is considered as a very special and unique clinical endpoint; it is an objective endpoint and due to its seriousness supersedes all other endpoints in importance. On the other end of the spectrum are the so-called surrogate endpoints or surrogate markers, or biomarkers. They are endpoints, usually not clinical in nature, but may be associated or correlated with the clinical endpoints of interests. In a few special instances, surrogate endpoints have been used directly to support drug efficacy claim, as in blood pressure for hypertension trials, CD4 counts in AIDS trials. In some disease areas, due to the lack of good or available treatments, a surrogate endpoint may be used to support drug efficacy claim conditional on subsequent demonstration of meaningful and real clinical benefit under the accelerated approval program [See Mathieu (1997) and 21 CFR 314.500 Subpart H (2001)].

Thus, the effect of a drug may manifest itself in a number of endpoints. From a regulatory perspective (The 1962 Amendment to the 1938 Food, Drug and Cosmetic Act requires drug to show clinical benefit in adequate and well-controlled studies), only endpoints that can provide a measure of relevant clinical benefits for a given proposed indication are of primary interest. This requirement essentially restricts the endpoints to clinical endpoints. But clinical endpoints have varying importance and reliability, and not every clinical endpoint has the potential of leading to an efficacy claim. Only those clinical endpoints that can provide sufficient evidence of effectiveness of the drug/treatment (what we have called the indication endpoints) will be considered as key endpoints. In addition, clinical decision rules that are defined in terms of labeling endpoints may be considered as complex indication endpoints. Therefore, in the design of a confirmatory trial, the investigator should carefully define the primary and secondary family of hypotheses corresponding to a desired strategy and adopt a multiple testing procedure that strongly controls the FWER for the combined family $\mathcal{F}_p \cup \mathcal{F}_{S1} \cup \mathcal{F}_{S2} \ldots \cup \mathcal{F}_{Sk}$.

3.4.3. *Multiple patient populations*

In confirmatory clinical trials, sometimes the trial objectives are to confirm if the general patient population can benefit from the study treatment and/or if some pre-specified sub-population (for example, sub-population defined by some genetic classifiers) can benefit from the study treatment. In this kind of trials, multiplicity is introduced by performing multiple hypotheses testing on different patient populations within a single trial. For a method for testing pre-specified subgroup, the reader may refer to the paper by Yang and Chi (2007).

3.4.4. *Repeated hypothesis testing*

Repeated hypothesis testing occurs in trial designs that have pre-planned interim analyses of accrued data together with formal testing of one or several hypotheses together with the possibility of early rejection or retention of the hypotheses. Such designs are often called a "group sequential" design. Repeated hypothesis testing (without proper adjustment of the significance level) could inflate the overall type I error. Compared to the previously introduced sources of multiplicity, which are focused on a given time point in the trial, the multiplicity issue in repeated hypothesis testing is focused on multiple time points in the trial. There exists a vast literature on technical and operational aspects of such trials: The review paper by Emerson (2007), the books by Jennison and Turnbull (2000), and Proschan, Lan and Wittes (2006). More discussions about controlling the overall type I error rate in repeated hypothesis testing problems can also be found in Section 4.

3.5. *A common method for handling multiple event endpoints*

In this section, we will briefly discuss a general method for handling the multiple event endpoints through a dimension reduction technique.

3.5.1. *Composite endpoint*

In the special situation when there are several types of clinical events of interest, one can define a composite endpoint in one of two ways. Let $\{E_1, E_2, \ldots, E_k\}$ represent k types of events. Then, a composite endpoint T may be defined as a binary outcome variable such that $T = 1$, if one or more of the events E_i had occurred during the study period, $= 0$, if no event was observed. For example, the composite endpoint in a study on sirolimus (Rapamune) on organ transplant patients was defined as the six-month 'failure' rate, where 'failure' = the occurrence of either a biopsy-confirmed acute rejection, a graft loss, or a death [Physicians' Desk Reference (2002)].

On the other hand, a composite endpoint can also be defined as a time-to-event endpoint as follows. Specifically, let us define k time-to-event endpoints, $\{T_1, T_2, \ldots, T_k\}$ with $T_i = t_i$, if an event E_i occurred at t_i, or $= \tau_i$, where τ_i is either the entire duration of the study or censoring time, if no event was observed. The time t_i and τ_i have been adjusted relative to the baseline. The composite endpoint T is defined as $T_i = t$, where $t = t_j$, if the first event observed was at $T = t_j$, where t_j can be an actual event time or censoring time. For example, in cardiovascular trials [Temple (2003)], evaluating therapies for cholesterol and blood pressure control, background mortality rates in the study population are typically not high. To show further improvement in their mortality rates would be difficult and require a sizable study. However, aside from mortality, there may be other outcomes of clinical interest. For example, in acute coronary syndrome (ACS) trials, various studies on low molecular weight heparins, enoxaparin, dalteparin and nadroparin [Kaul & Shih (2000), Gurfinkel *et al.* (1995), Klein *et al.* (1997), Cohen *et al.* (1997), Atman *et al.* (1999)] have used the composite endpoint of death, non-fatal myocardial infarction (MI) and recurrent angina. The CURE study [The CURE Investigators (2001)] of clopidogrel used the composite endpoint of cardiovascular death, non-fatal MI, or non-fatal stroke. The studies EPIC [The EPIC Investigators (1994)], EPILOG [The EPILOG Investigators (1997)] and CAPTURE [The CAPTURE Investigators (1997)] on the platelet GP IIb-IIIa receptor inhibitors, eptifibatide (Integrilin), tirofiban (Aggrastat) and abciximab (ReoPro) used the composite endpoint of death, MI and revascularization.

Composite endpoint is an interesting example of a clinical decision rule. However, there are some attendant issues related to the design and analysis of a trial with a composite endpoint. In particular, the type of censorings, the missing follow-up data after the first event has been observed, and the interpretation of the results are some of the critical issues that need to be addressed at the design stage of such a trial. For a more detailed discussion of these and other related issues, the reader may refer to the review article in Chi (2005).

3.6. *Classical multiple testing problems and testing procedures*

The multiplicity problems in clinical trials can be simply one-dimensional testing problems (i.e., multiplicity comes from a single source, e.g., endpoints or dose comparisons, but not combined sources; also multiple endpoints or multiple dose comparisons are equally important, with no hierarchical ordering). In this case, the null hypotheses of no treatment effect form a single family of hypotheses. This kind of multiplicity problems are referred here as "classical multiplicity problems". There are multiplicity problems that involve more than one dimension of multiplicity (e.g., multiplicity comes from both endpoints and dose comparisons, or multiplicity comes from just endpoints, but endpoints can be ordered and grouped into hierarchical families), which will be discussed in Section 3.7. Some examples of the classical multiplicity problem are as follows.

Example 7 (Two endpoints form a single dimension of multiplicity problem): Osteoporosis/breast cancer trial. The objective of this trial is to evaluate the effects of a study treatment on the risk of new vertebral fractures and incidence of invasive breast cancer in postmenopausal women with osteoporosis. Only placebo and a single dose of the study treatment are included in this trial. The study treatment can be declared to be efficacious if significant improvement is found in at least one of the two endpoints. The multiplicity problem in this trial comes from two endpoints only: incidence of vertebral fractures, and incidence of breast cancer.

Example 8 (Three dose-control comparisons form a single dimension of multiplicity problem): Bipolar I disorder trial. The objective of this trial is to evaluate the anti-manic effect (measured by the change in the Young Mania Rating Scale [YMRS] total score from baseline to end of the trial) of a study treatment in patients with acute manic or mixed episodes associated with Bipolar I Disorder. Placebo and three doses of the study treatment are included in this trial. The multiplicity problem in this trial comes from three dose-placebo comparisons only.

Example 9 (Three patient populations form a single dimension of multiplicity problem): Schizophrenia trial. The objective of this trial is to evaluate the effects of a study treatment in patients diagnosed with schizophrenia. The primary endpoint of this trial is Positive and Negative Symptoms Scale (PANSS) total score. Only placebo and a single dose of the study treatment are included in this trial. There are three patient populations to be studied in this trial: General population, Subpopulation 1 (Females), and Subpopulation 2 (Based on a pre-specified genotypic classifier). The multiplicity problem in this trial comes from these three patient populations only.

In the following, we will introduce some methodologies for controlling the overall type I error rate in classical multiplicity problems.

3.6.1. *P-value based multiple testing procedures*

P-value based multiple testing procedures have been very popular since it is easy to implement compared to other types of testing procedures, and also it is relatively easy to be explained to clinicians. Other than p-value based procedures, there are also resampling-based testing procedures and parametric testing procedures. Resampling-based testing procedures are not widely used in clinical trial applications even though it is more powerful than p-value based procedures. Parametric testing procedures, not like p-value based testing procedures, take into account the joint distribution of test statistics, and therefore, are more powerful than p-value based testing procedures. Parametric testing procedures will be discussed in Section 3.6.2.

There are some commonly used p-value based testing procedures. The Bonferroni procedure and the Simes procedure [Simes (1986)] are the most basic ones. The Bonferroni procedure is a single-step procedure and the Simes procedure is a global procedure. There are stepwise testing procedures which are more powerful than the Bonferroni and Simes procedures: The Holm's step-down [Holm (1979)], the Hochberg step-up [Hochberg (1988)], and the Hommel step-up [Hommel (1988)] procedures; the fixed-sequence [Maurer *et al.* (1995)], the fallback [Wiens (2003) and Wiens and Dmitrienko (2005)], and the chain [Bretz *et al.* (2009) and Millen and Dmitrienko (2011)] procedures. Of these stepwise procedures, the Holm's step-down, the Hochberg step-up, and the Hommel step-up procedures are procedures with data-driven testing sequence; while the fixed-sequence, the fallback, and the chain procedures are procedures with pre-specified testing sequence. The Holm's step-down procedure is a closed testing procedure (the concept of closed testing procedures will be introduced in Section 3.6.3) derived from the Bonferroni procedure and is uniformly more powerful than the Bonferroni procedure. The Hochberg and Hommel step-up procedures are closed testing procedures derived from the Simes procedure and are uniformly more powerful than the Simes procedure.

It is worth mentioning that the Simes procedure may inflate the type I error if test statistics are not independent or positively dependent (more specifically, multivariate totally positive of order two [MTP2]) [Sarkar and Chang (1997) and Sarkar (1998)]. Therefore, the Hochberg and Hommel step-up procedures may inflate type I error as well when the independency or positively dependency condition is not satisfied. If not considering these conditions for ensuring type I error control, the Hochberg and Hommel step-up procedures are more powerful than the Holm's step-down procedure.

As mentioned before, the fixed-sequence, the fallback, and the chain procedures are procedures with pre-specified hypothesis ordering. So when applying these procedures, null hypotheses need to be ordered to reflect clinical importance or probability of success for the associated objectives. For a fixed-sequence procedure, power is maximized under the monotonicity assumption (i.e., null hypotheses are ordered from the largest effect size to the smallest effect size) and power loss is likely when the monotonicity assumption is violated. When the monotonicity assumption is violated, the fallback procedure is a good alternative. Actually, the fixed-sequence procedures derived from the Bonferroni procedure can be viewed as a special case of fallback procedures. Chain procedures are further extension of fallback procedures.

3.6.2. *Parametric multiple testing procedures*

Parametric multiple testing procedures make specific distributional assumptions of test statistics. For example, one may assume that test statistics follow a multivariate t distribution. Since parametric procedures account for correlations among test statistics, they are more powerful than the p-value-based procedures. However, it may not always be feasible to validate certain distribution assumptions in real clinical trials, and also, parametric procedures are usually more difficult to carry out compared to p-value based procedures. Therefore, even though theoretically parametric procedures are more powerful than p-value based procedures, p-value based procedures are still very popular in dealing with multiplicity problems in confirmatory clinical trials.

Some classical parametric testing procedures include the single-step Dunnett procedure [Dunnett (1955)], the step-down Dunnett procedure [Naik (1975); Marcus, Peritz and Gabriel (1976); Dunnett and Tamhane (1991)], and the step-up Dunnett procedure [Dunnett and Tamhane (1992)]. The single-step Dunnett procedure is a parametric version of the Bonferroni procedure and is uniformly more powerful than the Bonferroni procedure. The step-down Dunnett procedure is a parametric version of the Holm's step-down procedure and is uniformly more powerful than the Holm's procedure. The step-up Dunnett procedure is a parametric version of the Hochberg step-up procedure and is uniformly more powerful than the Hochberg procedure. Some more recently developed parametric testing procedures include the parametric fallback procedure [Huque and Alosh (2008)] and the parametric chain procedure [Millen and Dmitrienko (2011)].

3.6.3. *Closure principle and partitioning principle*

It is worth noting that all stepwise procedures discussed above can be constructed using the closure principle (also called the closed testing principle) [Marcus, Peritz and Gabriel (1976)] and the procedures constructed using the closure principle can be referred to as closed testing procedures. The closure principle is a powerful tool for building strongly controlled multiple testing procedures.

We use an example here to illustrate how to build multiple testing procedures using the closure principle. Suppose we have two null hypotheses: $H_{0,1}$: $\{\Delta\mu_1 \le 0\}$, $H_{0,2}$: $\{\Delta\mu_2 \le 0\}$. We then define a closed family of hypotheses which include all intersection of $H_{0,1}$ and $H_{0,2}$: $H_{0,1} \cap H_{0,2}$: $\Delta\mu_1 \le 0 \cap \Delta\mu_2 \le 0$, $H_{0,1}$: $\{\Delta\mu_1 \le 0\}$ and $H_{0,2}$: $\{\Delta\mu_2 \le 0\}$. Note that if we have m null hypotheses then $2^m - 1$ intersection hypotheses can be formed. For example, if there are four null hypotheses in a multiple testing problem, then $2^4 - 1 = 15$ intersection hypotheses can be formed. The closure principle then states that

(1) An original null hypothesis is rejected if all intersection hypotheses H implying this null hypothesis are rejected. For example, the original hypothesis $H_{0,1}$ can be rejected if intersection hypotheses $H_{0,1} \cap H_{0,2}$ and $H_{0,1}$ are both rejected.
(2) If each intersection hypothesis H is tested at the α level, then the closed testing procedure controls the FWER in the strong sense at the α level.

The partitioning principle, introduced by Stefansson, Kim and Hsu (1988) and Finner and Strassburger (2002), is also a powerful tool for building multiple testing procedures. For any family of hypotheses, there is a natural partition of the parameter space. The essential idea behind the partition principle is to partition the parameter space corresponding to a given family of hypotheses under consideration into disjoint sets such that each hypothesis can be written as the union of some of these disjoint sets. One then constructs a level-α test for each of these disjoint sets, and then constructs a multiple level-α test for all hypotheses of interest. It has been shown that procedures constructed using the partitioning principle is at least as powerful as those constructed using the closure principle and can be more powerful under certain situations [Finner and Strassburger (2002)]. For an application of the partition principle to genetic linkage analysis, one may refer to the paper by Rogers, Hsu and Lin (2004).

3.7. *More advanced multiple testing problems and testing procedures*

Multiple testing problems discussed in Section 3.6 deals with one dimension of multiplicity, e.g., two-arm trials with multiple endpoints or single-endpoint trials with multiple dose-control comparisons. However, in more recent clinical trial applications, we have seen more complicated multiplicity problems with more than one dimension of multiplicity where classical multiple testing procedures may not be able to address the complexity of the multiplicity issues (see Examples 5 & 6).

Many recent developments in methodology for dealing with the more complicated multiplicity problems fall into the category of gatekeeping testing strategies. In a gatekeeping testing strategy, null hypotheses are grouped into families. For example, the indication endpoint in a trial can be grouped into two families: A primary family and a secondary family. The effectiveness claims relative to secondary endpoints can only be made subject to successfully passing a test of the primary family of hypotheses, hence the term gatekeeping.

The following are some examples of more complicated multiple testing problems, with corresponding decision trees. These examples are presented with a gatekeeping terminology: "families of hypotheses".

Example 10 (Multiple sets of endpoints): Alzheimer's disease trial. The objective of this trial is to evaluate the effects of a study treatment on cognition and global changes in patients with Alzheimer's disease. Only placebo and a single dose of the study treatment are included in this trial. There are three efficacy endpoints. Two of them are primary endpoints: E_1 = Alzheimer's Disease Assessment Scale-Cognitive Subscale (ADAS-Cog) and E_2 = Clinical Global Impression of Change (CGIC). The third endpoint is a key secondary endpoint: S = an imaging marker. The null hypothesis corresponding to the imaging marker endpoint can be tested only if significant improvement is found in both primary endpoints E_1 and E_2. The null hypotheses H^P_{0,E_1} and H^P_{0,E_2} corresponding to the two primary endpoints E_1 and E_2, say,can be grouped into the primary family of hypotheses $\mathcal{F}_P = \{H^P_{0,E_1}, H^P_{0,E_2}\}$; the null hypothesis H^S_0 corresponding to the key labeling endpoint S forms the labeling family of hypotheses, $\mathcal{F}_L = \{H^S_0\}$. U.S. FDA requires that for the proposed indication, both null hypotheses in the primary family have to be rejected. Rejection of the labeling null hypothesis can provide additional claim in the label other than the indication section *only after* the drug has shown its efficacy based on the rejection of both of the primary null hypotheses (see also Example 5).

Example 10 decision tree

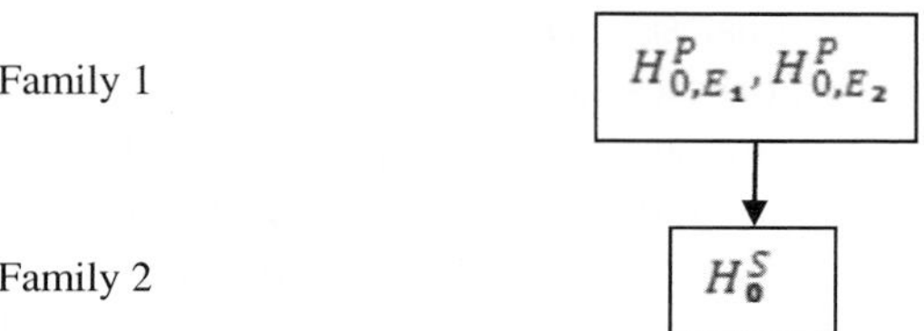

Example 11 (Multiple dose-placebo comparisons and multiple patient populations): Major depressive disorder trial. The objective of this trial is to evaluate of the effect of a study treatment on patients with major depressive disorder. Placebo and two doses of the study treatment are included in the trial. There is only a single primary endpoint in this trial, which is the improvement in depressive symptoms measured by change in the Montgomery-Asberg Depression Scale (MADRS). Two patient populations are to be studied: general population G and a subpopulation S based on a pre-specified genotypic classifier. The null hypotheses corresponding to the general population and the two dose-placebo comparisons, say, H^{G0}, d_1 and H^{G0}, d_2 can be grouped into the primary family of hypotheses, $\mathcal{F}_P = \{H^{G0}, d_1, H^{G0}, d_2\}$ the null hypotheses corresponding to the sub-population and the two dose-placebo comparisons, say, H^{S0}, d_1 and H^{S0}, d_2, can be grouped into the secondary family of hypotheses, $\mathcal{F}_S = \{H^{S0}$,

d_1, H^{S0}, $d_2\}$. Null hypotheses in the secondary family $\mathcal{F}_S$ cannot be tested unless at least one null hypothesis in the primary family $\mathcal{F}_P$ is rejected.

Example 11 decision tree

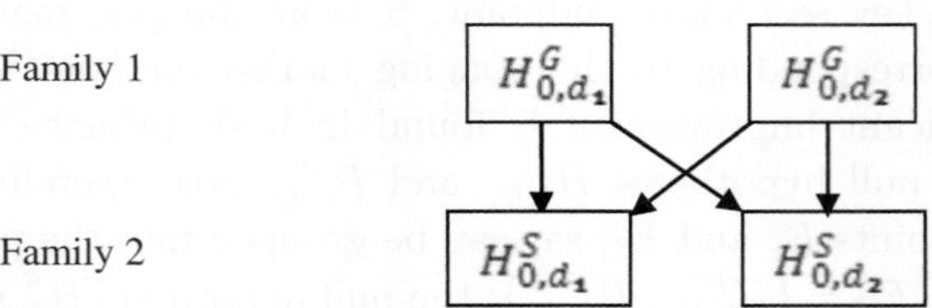

Example 12 (Multiple dose-placebo comparisons and hierarchically ordered endpoints): Osteoarthritis trial. The objective of this trial is to evaluate the effect of a study treatment on patients with osteoarthritis. Placebo and two doses of the study treatment are included in the trial. The primary endpoint of the trial is improvement of pain due to osteoarthritis. The key secondary endpoint is improvement of functioning. The null hypotheses corresponding to the primary endpoint and the two dose-placebo comparisons, say, $H^P_{0,1}$ and $H^P_{0,2}$, can be grouped into the primary family of hypotheses, $\mathcal{F}_P = \{H^P_{0,1}, H^P_{0,2}\}$; the null hypotheses corresponding to the key secondary endpoint and the two dose-placebo comparisons, say, H^S_0, d_1 and H^S_0, d_2, can be grouped into the secondary family of hypotheses, $\mathcal{F}_S = \{H^S_0, d_1, H^S_0, d_2\}$. In addition to the condition that null hypotheses in the secondary family cannot be tested unless at least one null hypothesis in the primary family $\mathcal{F}_P$ is rejected, there is another logical restriction: H^S_0, d_1 cannot be rejected if P^S_0, d_1 is not rejected and H^S_0, d_2 cannot be rejected if H^P_0, d_2 is not rejected.

Example 12 decision tree

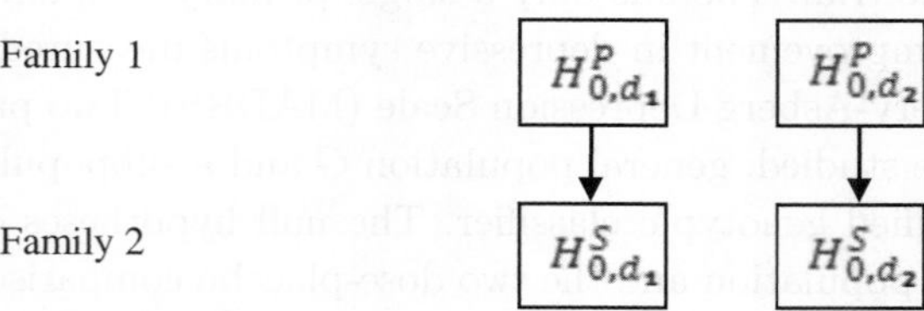

In Sections 3.7.1, 3.7.2, and 3.7.3, we will discuss different types of gatekeeping testing strategies. In Section 3.7.4, partitioning decision paths, a testing strategy different from gatekeeping strategies will be introduced.

3.7.1. *Serial gatekeeping*

Gatekeeping procedures for the case when the primary/gatekeeper family is passed only if all of the hypotheses in the family have been rejected are referred to as "serial" gatekeeping procedures. Example 8 is a case when serial gatekeeping strategy can be applied, since the key secondary endpoint cannot be tested unless both hypotheses corresponding to the two primary endpoints are rejected. Full α level can be used for testing the hypotheses in the primary/gatekeeper family; if all hypotheses in the primary family are rejected, then full α level can be used again for testing the hypotheses in the secondary family.

3.7.2. *Parallel gatekeeping*

There are situations that serial gatekeeping cannot handle. For example, in Example 11 and Example 12, the hypotheses in the gatekeeper family do not need to be all rejected before a hypothesis in the secondary family can be tested. The parallel gatekeeping procedure, first introduced by Dmitrienko *et al.* (2003), requires at least one hypothesis in a gatekeeper family to be declared significant in order to proceed to its subsequent families. This originally proposed parallel gatekeeping procedure was formulated using the closure principle. For each intersection hypothesis in the closed testing framework, a weighted Bonferroni test is applied; therefore, the original parallel gatekeeping procedure can also be called the weighted-Bonferroni-based parallel gatekeeping procedure.

There are extensions on the basis of the weighted-Bonferroni-based procedure. For example, one can replace the weighted Bonferroni test for each intersection hypothesis by a truncated Holm's test or a truncated Hochberg test to improve power (truncation means a convex combination of the Bonferroni test and a more powerful test, e.g., Holm's test, Hochberg test, stepdownDunnett test, etc). There have also been proposals to replace the weighted Bonferroni test by resampling-based tests; however, as we indicated earlier, resampling-based tests are not widely applied in confirmatory clinical trials.

It has been shown that the weighted-Bonferroni-based parallel gatekeeping procedure, which was formulated as a closed testing procedure, admits a shortcut which is a simple stepwise procedure [Dmitrienko *et al.* (2006a)]. Using the stepwise procedure, one can test n null hypotheses in n steps rather than 2^n steps required in the general case.

Dmitrienko *et al.* (2006b) proposed a Dunnett-based parallel gatekeeping method in a clinical study setting with multiple dose-placebo comparisons and hierarchically ordered endpoints, which takes into account distributional assumptions concerning test statistics. However, the Dunnett-based parallel gatekeeping procedure relies on some assumptions that could be difficult to justify in typical clinical trials, namely (a) that the joint distribution of the test statistics from different endpoints can be approximated by a multivariate-t distribution and (b) that the true correlation between multiple endpoints can be well estimated using observed data. The Dunnett-Bonferroni-based parallel gatekeeping procedure [Xu *et al.* (2009)] relaxes the assumptions required for the Dunnett-based parallel gatekeeping procedure, by splitting type I error rate α among families using the Bonferroni inequality. The α-splitting/Bonferronization is applied in testing all intersection hypotheses in a closed testing framework. While it is potentially less powerful than a Dunnett-based parallel gatekeeping procedure when both procedures are applicable, the power loss is very minimal.

Unlike the parallel gatekeeping procedures mentioned above, which are constructed using the closure principle, the multistage parallel gatekeeping procedures are not constructed using the closure principle. The multistage procedures involve two main concepts: the error rate function of a multiple test and the separability condition. For any subset I of the index set $\mathcal{N} = \{1, 2, \ldots, n\}$, the error rate function $e(\Im)$ of a multiple test is the maximum probability of making at least one Type I error when testing $H_{0,i} i \in \Im$. A multiple test meets the separability condition if its error rate function is strictly less than α unless all hypotheses are true, i.e., $e(\Im) < \alpha$ for all $\Im(N)$. The Bonferroni test satisfies this condition, while most other popular multiple tests do not, for example, the Holm's step-down test, the Hochberg step-up test, the Dunnett step-down test, etc. Dmitrienko, Tamhane and Wiens (2008) proposed truncated versions of these popular tests by taking a convex combination of their critical values with the critical values of the Bonferroni test. The multistage procedures start with testing in primary family using a separable multiple test, calculate error rate function of this multiple test, and find out the fraction of α left after testing the primary family; then use the α left for testing next family; and so on and so forth, until the last family.

3.7.3. *Tree-structured gatekeeping*

Tree-structured Gatekeeping procedures are generalization of serial and parallel gatekeeping. Decision-making process no longer exhibits a simple sequential structure but rather relies on a decision tree with multiple branches corresponding to individual objectives. For details, please refer to Dmitrienko, Wiens, Tamhane and Wang (2007), Dmitrienko, Tamhane and Liu (2008), and Kordzakhia *et al.* (2008).

3.7.4. *Partitioning decision paths*

Instead of testing all intersection hypotheses of null hypotheses (as in closed testing procedures), partition testing can form only null hypotheses appropriate for the decision paths of the problem in a way that partitions the parameter space.

Compared to closed testing procedures, the partitioning decision paths method [Liu and Hsu (2009)] significantly reduces the number of hypotheses, for example, just using paths between endpoints within each dose-control comparison reduces the number of hypotheses from $(2^m)^k - 1$ to $(m + 1)^k - 1$. For example, the number of formed hypotheses decreases from 63 to 26 when $m = 2$, $k = 3$.

4. Interim Analysis, Group Sequential and Adaptive Design

In the seventies, clinical trial investigators began to question on ethical grounds whether a trial, with mortality or serious irreversible morbidity as the primary outcomes of interest, should be continued to its intended end when interim analysis based on accumulating data shows that the treatment is effective. In those early days, interim analyses were routinely done by the investigators without any regard to issues of multiple testing and its consequent inflation in the probability of the overall type I error. So in this kind of trials, the decision rule, which is usually defined in terms of one primary endpoint such as mortality, is repeatedly tested at various times in the course of the trial. The problem at that time is that there was no appropriate statistical support structure for the decision process. The desire for stopping the trial early for efficacy has been the driving force behind the development of group sequential procedures in the subsequent decades.

The principal component of a confirmatory trial include the target population, the study design, the decision structure which includes a decision set of key clinical endpoints, a clinical decision rule with its statistical support structure for assessing efficacy, and possibly an interim analysis plan, etc. There is always an interest on the part of the trial sponsor to make changes to the trial based on interim treatment comparative analysis of accumulating data prior to the intended end of the trial. These changes may involve changes in the patient population, in the decision structure including the clinical decision rule, the test statistics, the interim analysis plan, and the sample size. For instance, after an interim analysis, it may be of interest to drop one or more treatment arms, to change or drop one or more endpoints, or in a group sequential trial, to change the interim analysis schedule, to change the stopping boundary, the α-spending function, or to increase the sample size. Since such proposed changes are based on the interim treatment comparative analysis, they may introduce serious bias into the study and inflate the probability of the overall type I error.

4.1. *Group sequential designs*

A *group sequential procedure* is a statistical procedure that provides for a series of test statistics based on the accumulating data. The simple null hypothesis is tested by these statistics. An early termination rule is implemented through a stopping boundary defined by the critical values or in terms of an increasing sequence of nominal significance levels for each test. This boundary is defined so that the probability of the overall type I error will be maintained at a desired α-level for a two-sided test.

Group sequential procedures that allow for interim analyses and early termination had been proposed by many authors. The earlier publications include, Pocock (1977, 1982), O'Brien and Fleming (1979), Tsiatis (1982), Whitehead (1983), Lan and DeMets (1983), DeMets and Lan (1984), and Fleming, Harrington, and O'Brien (1984). These group sequential procedures are used for a type of analysis customarily referred to as *formal interim analysis*, and they are usually implemented for mortality and irreversible morbidity trials.

A group sequential procedure with formal interim analyses is an example of a *sequential clinical decision rule.*

Definition: A *sequential clinical decision rule* is a clinical decision rule, repeatedly applied over some indices, which can be information (i.e., number of subjects or number of events) or information fraction (or information time) expressed as ratio of the information required at an interim analysis and the maximum information.

A *sequential decision structure* is a sequential clinical decision rule with a proper statistical support structure.

The group sequential procedures referred to above that allow for interim analyses and early termination are simple sequential decision structures. They are simple because the clinical decision rule at each time point involves one and the same primary endpoint such as mortality or a composite endpoint consisting of several types of event endpoints.

In a trial with a sequential clinical decision rule, the decision rule itself can be more complex when multiple endpoints and/or multiple doses are involved. This is typical as in clinical trials the totality of accumulating data is made available to the independent data monitoring committee (IDMC) whose decisions can involve clinical judgments that are inherently subjective. The proper statistical support structure involves treating stopping boundaries, which are often developed on the basis of the primary endpoint, with or without considerations of secondary endpoints, as guidance. The IDMC, upon evaluation of the totality of the accumulating data, can overrule these boundaries, when emerging clinical or scientific issues require that the trial needs to be extended. The repeated confidence interval approach proposed by Jenison and Turnbull (1989) provides the framework to carry out group sequential clinical trials. The theoretical foundation for the repeated confidence interval approach was established recently by Liu and Anderson (2008a, 2008b) who provided methods for sequential inference (i.e., sequential p-values, confidence intervals, and point estimates). For example, using sequential p-values at the final analysis, one can perform multiple hypothesis testing involving multiple endpoints or treatment groups using p-value based multiple comparison procedures developed for single stage designs without additional adjustment.

4.2. *Adaptive designs*

Design modification of a clinical trial can also be progressively built into a two- or multi-stage randomized trial. In a two-stage design, modifications may be considered at the end of the first stage. Bauer and Köhne (1995) considered the problem of sample size re-estimation at the end of the first stage. The two-stage combination test is based on Fisher's product test and the assumption that the samples from the two stages are independent. Proschan and Hunsberger (1996) generalized the method of Bauer and Köhne through the concept of conditional error function. Following the conditional error approach, Chi and Liu (1999) and Liu and Chi (2001) proposed a two-stage adaptive design allowing a high probability to stop at the interim for an expected effect size while permitting sample size adjustment that utilizes conditional power at a minimum effect size if the significance boundary is not crossed. The procedure is very efficient as the maximum sample size of the design does not exceed 20% of that of a fixed sample size design at the same minimum effect size. In contrast, other sample size procedures in the literature calculate conditional powers at the current trend (i.e., the observed effect size), resulting in maximum sample sizes that are four times as large. Liu and Chi (2001) also provided methods for statistical inference (i.e., overall p-values, confidence intervals and point estimates).

Cui *et al.* (1999) showed that in a group sequential trial, sample size re-estimation based on observed interim treatment difference can inflate the probability of the overall type I error, essentially because the sample size estimate is interim outcome dependent. They have developed a methodology based on weighted test statistics that would permit sample size re-estimation at any one of the pre-scheduled interim analysis times without inflating the probability of the overall type I error. The methodology retains the original stopping boundary. But the sample size procedure is inefficient as the conditional power calculation is performed at the observed effect size. The Cui *et al.* (1999) design is a special case of a more general adaptive group sequential design by Muller and Schafer (2001) that provides a conditional error rate calculation at any interim analysis of a group sequential design. They then suggested that the remaining trial can be redesigned as long as the conditional error rate is controlled. Thus, the adaptive group sequential design falls into the same conditional error rate framework of Proschan and Hunsberger (1994).

Other than sample size adjustment, adaptive designs can also be used for more innovative clinical development programs, Bauer and Kieser (1999) proposed to use p-value combination test to combine different phases of a clinical development program. Liu and Pledger (2005) proposed a phase 2/3 combination design that incorporates multiple testing with modeling of dose-response relationship. Adaptive designs can also be used to combine phase 2a and phase 2b trials for early clinical development, as well as in clinical development programs of accelerated approval of potentially life-saving drugs in diseases with unmet medical needs (see later discussion).

Liu, Proschan and Pledger (2002) provided a measure-theoretic framework by which the concept of adaptation rule and the validity of adaptive designs are formally established. The theory covers adaptive tests and inference, as well as asymptotic results for adaptive designs with large samples. The measure-theoretic framework relies on the generalization of the conditional error functions to conditional properties with a profound result: Inference of an adaptive design is valid if the conditional inference (e.g., testing) follows the conditional property even if the adaptation rule is not pre-specified. However, for practical applications, one should provide specifics of adaptation in advance so that various operating characteristics of the adaptive design can be evaluated. Providing details of adaptation also helps to facilitate decision making by the IDMC. In addition, it increases transparency to regulatory agencies which translates into confidence on a proposed adaptive design.

Many of the early works assumed independence of the samples form the two stages [Bauer, Brannath and Posch (2001) and Wassmer (1998)]. Following Liu, Proschan and Pledger (2002), Liu and Pledger (2006) provided the theory and methods for two-stage adaptive designs with dependent data. The theory and methods apply to accelerated approval of potentially life-saving drugs in diseases that do not have available treatment [see 4.4 below]. Challenge still remains to develop multi-stage adaptive designs with dependent data.

There are many settings where it is difficult to specify in advance on the type of adaptations needed for clinical trials, and therefore, traditional fixed sample size designs are typically used. Often, there is a need to make certain modifications to an ongoing trial and then followed by study protocol amendments. This often raises concerns on the validity of trial results. Liu and Chi (2010a) has shown that under settings when the underlying statistical inference is based on conditional distributions, such as log-rank or Mantel-Haenszel tests, it is possible to change the fixed sample design to an adaptive design for the ongoing trial. This approach has actually been used in a recent phase 3 confirmative trial.

The past decade has witnessed a tremendous progress in research and applications of adaptive designs. The readers are referred to Liu and Chi (2010b) for a very comprehensive review of the subject.

4.3. *Interim analysis and independent data monitoring committee*

Most mortality or serious irreversible morbidity trials have formal planned interim analysis and stopping rules. There is also an Independent Data Monitoring Committee (IDMC). The primary responsibility of an IDMC is to recommend to the trial sponsor early termination of the trial for either efficacy or safety reason. The requirement of being independent is to maintain the integrity of the trial. It also frequently happens that the IDMC also makes recommendation for changes to the design and conduct of the trial. This kind of recommendations often raises concern. The following are a few important points to consider for an IDMC. For general guidance, one may refer to the FDA's Guidance on the Establishment and Operation of Clinical Trial Data Monitoring Committees (2001).

- The trial protocol should have the prior approval of the IDMC. The IDMC cannot arbitrarily modify the protocol design. Even though IDMC may be independent, its independence refers to the lack of direct interest in the outcome of the trial. It does not imply that the IDMC can recommend design modifications arbitrarily. Any design modification recommended by the IDMC also has the potential for inflation in the probability of the overall type I error. This is because the proposed modification by the IDMC is likely to be based on the interim treatment comparative data. The guideline should clearly define the span of authority of the IDMC.
- The IDMC should have standard operating procedures governing its conduct. It has obligation and responsibility to maintain confidentiality of the interim outcome of the trial. It should not communicate the interim results to anyone outside the IDMC, unless for purpose of early termination according to the pre-specified termination rule or for safety reason.
- There should be clear standard operating procedures governing the communication between the trial sponsor and the IDMC. There should be clear guidelines regarding the documentation of minutes of meetings, decisions reached, and written communications.

The ability to make design modifications is obviously very attractive. However, one should be mindful of the real potential for bias to be introduced as a result of access to the interim unblinded treatment comparative data. As previously noted, if the characteristics of the patients enrolled subsequent to an interim analysis have changed, then this may seriously bias the outcome, unless the drug label can accurately describe the patient population for whom the drug may be prescribed. It is desirable to have an independent third party that is responsible for conducting interim analysis either in a group sequential trial setting or a two- or multi-stage design trial. There should be clear and sound guidelines and standard operating procedures governing the role, responsibility and conduct of the independent third party.

In general, any desired design modification or change should be prespecified at the design stage. Furthermore, one should describe how decisions on modifications are made conditional on the interim outcome data, the distribution of the adapted test statistic, and the overall p-value for assessing the significance of the trial finding. The proposal should also include methods for addressing any adverse impacts such modification or change may introduce, such as, bias, changes in patient population, inflation in the probability of the overall type I error, and proof of the validity of the statistical inference based on the adapted test statistic. Generally, the clinical decision rule should be as complete as possible. The design modification, other than sample size adjustment, should be restricted to deletion of decision branches or paths. The addition of new decision branches or paths should be discouraged.

4.4. *Two-stage design in a randomized trial and accelerated approval*

Accelerated approval of potentially life-saving drugs in diseases that do not have available treatment may be done through an accepted surrogate (or surrogates) whose validity has been established. Validity of the surrogate means it is likely to predict clinical benefit of primary interest. The idea of accelerated approval is to first conditionally approve the use of the drug based on a positive outcome on the surrogate endpoint, and then subsequently confirm its effectiveness through the clinical endpoints of primary interests.

FDA's Oncology Initiatives (1996) recognize that the predictive value of partial responses may still be a matter of discussion for all types of cancer. But for refractory malignant disease or for diseases that have no adequate alternative, clear evidence of anti-tumor activity is a reasonable basis for approving the drug. In these cases, studies confirming a clinical benefit may appropriately be completed after the conditional approval.

So in essence, the Oncology Initiative has gone a step further in permitting a surrogate to be used in certain situations even though the surrogate has not been fully validated. One may refer to the example of gemtuzumabozogamicin in relapsed acute myeloid leukemia as discussed in Bross (2001). It is for this reason that a two-stage design may be well suited for accelerated approval. The drug may be tested at the end of the first stage for conditional approval based on the surrogate, and then confirmed at the end of the second stage by the primary clinical endpoints.

A two-stage design in a randomized trial offers the following advantages. First, it places the evaluation of the surrogate and the clinical outcomes of primary interest in the same trial, and hence would be able to provide some checks on the validity of the surrogate in relation to the clinical benefit of interest.

Secondly, a more appropriate way for conditional approval is to first identify a decision set of clinical endpoints of primary interest that will be used at the end of the second stage to evaluate the efficacy of the drug. Appropriate allocation of α should be considered for multiple endpoints, including the surrogate as well as interim analysis at the end of the first stage, in order to maintain the probability of the overall type I error at α. At the end of the first stage, the efficacy will be evaluated relative to the surrogate endpoint as well as all the clinical endpoints in the decision set. If it fails to demonstrate efficacy relative to the surrogate and all the clinical endpoints, then the trial stops and the drug fails to gain accelerated approval. If any of the clinical endpoints in the decision set demonstrates efficacy, then the trial can be terminated at the end of the first stage. Otherwise, if the test demonstrates efficacy relative to the surrogate only, then one proceeds to calculate the conditional power of showing a positive outcome at the end of the second stage given the current interim outcomes for each of the clinical endpoint in the decision set. If the conditional powers show that the likelihood of such an outcome is very low for all the clinical endpoints, and a sample size increase would be unacceptably large, then the accelerated approval probably should be withheld. Thus, accelerated approval should be granted if at least one such conditional power is sufficiently high, or if sample size can be increased so that at least one clinical endpoint will have sufficient conditional power to suggest a positive outcome at the end of the second stage. If the trial continues to the second stage and the final results show that there is no clinical benefit, then the drug may need to be withdrawn from the market [Sridhara, Yang, Chen and Chi (2001)].

5. Active Control Trials

5.1. *Recent history of the active control trial*

Historically, for trials with mortality or serious morbidity outcome, delaying or withholding available treatments would increase the mortality or irreversible morbidity outcome, the use of a placebo has been considered unethical and active control comparative trials have been proposed [Fleming (1987, 1990)]. An active control superiority trial allows for a direct comparison of a new study treatment against a standard therapy or standard of care. It establishes the efficacy of a new study treatment by demonstrating that the new treatment is superior to the active control [Temple (1983) and Leber (1986, 1989)]. For example, in oncology for cancers that have standard therapies, a new study treatment must be compared to and show superiority to a standard therapy in two randomized controlled clinical trials. In fact, active control superiority trials have often been done not just for trials with serious outcomes, but also for many trials with less serious outcomes. Unless the new treatment represents a new advance in the treatment of the disease, it would be more difficult to show that the new treatment is better than an effective active control. Thus, it is not surprising to find that when a new treatment failed to show superiority to the active control, the sponsor or investigator often would attempt to conclude that the new treatment was either equivalent to, or no worse than the active control. But it is well-known that failing to reject the null hypothesis of equality between the new treatment and the active control does not imply that they are equivalent [Fleming (1990) and Temple (2996)]. As White (1998) aptly puts it, "the lack of evidence of a difference cannot be interpreted as evidence of a lack of difference".

In 2000, the World Medical Association (WMA) made a significant pronouncement at Helsinki that for the first time seriously challenged the ethics of using a placebo control in any clinical trial. This pronouncement led to a series of published debates concerning the merit of an active control trial [Riis (2000), Vastag (2000), Temple and Ellenberg (2000), Ellenberg and Temple (2000)]. The WMA made a subsequent amendment to their Helsinki Declaration in 2004 that ameliorated somewhat the stringency of the original ethical requirements. Nonetheless some debates still ensured. However, today, it has become increasingly difficult to use placebo in trials investigating diseases that involve mortality and/or serious morbidity outcomes, except in situation where there is no available approved treatment for the disease under consideration.

It has been suggested by various authors (e.g., Blackwelder (1982) and Huque, Dubey and Fredd (1989)), that if the intention is to show that the new intervention is equivalent or non-inferior to the active control, then one needs to define the null hypothesis and the corresponding alternative hypothesis appropriately. More specifically, the alternative hypothesis should reflect the hypothesis of interest, namely that of equivalence, or non-inferiority. To do that, these authors suggested that a certain equivalence or non-inferiority margin should be pre-specified in the hypothesis. For example, in bioequivalence studies, an equivalence margin is generally set at $\pm 20\%$ of the control effect. In many active control non-inferiority trials, an arbitrary fixed threshold is pre-specified — for example, a threshold of 1.25 for the hazard ratio of the study treatment relative to the active-control.

If the upper limit of the 95% CI for the study treatment effect relative to the active control lies beneath this threshold, then non-inferiority is inferred.

The major concern with using an arbitrary fixed threshold is that it is unrelated to the active control effect defined as the difference between the control response and the non-existing placebo response. When the active control effect is relatively small, this may lead to a loss of all of the active control effect plus more (or a loss of too great a percent of the active control effect). In other words, if the demonstration of non-inferiority is based on an arbitrary fixed margin, the new treatment may be approved even though it may be less efficacious than a placebo.

Having recognized this problem, it has been proposed that the margin should be set at half the lower limit of the 95% confidence interval for the estimate of the active control effect to ensure that the new drug is better than placebo. A similar approach was used by the FDA Center for Biologics Evaluation and Research in a thrombolytic trial where instead of 95%, they used 90% confidence interval. The null hypothesis of sufficient inferiority will be rejected if the upper limit of the 95% confidence interval for the hazard ratio of the new treatment relative to the active control is below this cutoff. This method has also been called the "two-95% confidence intervals approach". While this fixed margin is not arbitrary and is linked to an estimate of the control effect, it has been criticized as being too conservative because it compares two "statistically worst" cases.

Various authors have proposed not to directly pre-specify a fixed margin, but rather define simply the percent of the control effect one wishes to retain. Non-inferiority is then demonstrated by the new treatment, if it can be shown that the new treatment retains at least the desired percent of the active control effect. The active control effect may be estimated from non-concurrent placebo or standard control studies using mixed effects model. This idea was proposed by Hauck and Anderson (1999), Koch and Tangen (1999), Holmgren (1999), Simon (1999) and Hassalblad and Kong (2001). Rothmann, Li, Chen, and Chi (2001) have further extended this method. This approach is explained in the next section.

5.2. *Non-inferiority trials*

In this section, an *active control* (or *control* for short) refers to a treatment C whose efficacy has previously been demonstrated and approved for marketing, and an *active control trial* refers to a trial with an active control C as the comparator with or without the presence of a placebo control P.

An active control trial with the presence of a placebo is often called a trial with a *gold standard design.* Since the fundamental problems of an active control trial are associated with active control trials without the benefit of the presence of a placebo, we will focus our discussion on active control trials without the presence of a placebo [Chi *et al.* (2010)].

For our subsequent discussion, consider an active control trial involving a new treatment T and an active control C. Event though there is no placebo present in the trial, we'll still let P denotes the putative placebo. Let X denote a primary efficacy endpoint of interest and assume that $X_T \sim N(\mu_T, \sigma_T^2)$, $X_C \sim N(\mu_C, \sigma_C^2)$ and $X_P \sim N(\mu_P, \sigma_P^2)$ represent the variable X under the respective treatment T, C and P with their corresponding normal distributions with their respective means and variances. Furthermore, assume that larger values of X represent better outcomes. The purpose of this article is to discuss the fundamental problems and issues related to active control trials, hence it would suffice to discuss them within the context of normality and differences in means as the efficacy measure. The same issues apply to other types of efficacy measures and distributions.

From a regulatory perspective, the primary objective of an active control trial involving a new treatment T is primarily to provide evidence that T is effective. This can easily be accomplished with a gold standard design, since T can be compared directly to placebo. However, if placebo is not present in a non-inferiority trial, then such comparison is not possible. In the absence of a placebo in an active control trial, how can this objective be met? In this case, the cleanest design would be to do an *active control superiority trial* (superiority to the control) with the following superiority hypothesis:

$$H_o : \mu_T - \mu_C \leq 0 \quad vs. \quad H_a : \mu_T - \mu_C > 0. \tag{2}$$

However, as noted before, unless the new treatment represents a new medical breakthrough, in general, it is less likely for a new treatment to show superiority over a control at comparable doses. Therefore, it is more reasonable to expect that the new treatment, at comparable doses, is no worse than the control by a small quantity δ, called the *non-inferiority margin.* An active control trial without a placebo that is intended to show that a new treatment is no worse than a control by more than a non-inferiority margin δ is called a *non-inferiority trial* with the following non-inferiority hypothesis:

$$H_o : \mu_T - \mu_C \leq -\delta \quad vs. \quad H_a : \mu_T - \mu_C > -\delta \tag{3}$$

Thus, a non-inferiority trial with a non-inferiority margin δ is simply a one-sided therapeutic equivalence trial. To demonstrate that the new treatment T I not worse than the control C by more than δ, we only have to show that the inferiority hypothesis in (3) is rejected based on the non-inferiority trial data. So how is the non-inferiority margin δ determined?

5.2.1. *Fundamental problems of non-inferiority trials*

There are several fundamental problems associated with a non-inferiority trial [Chi *et al.* (2003, 2010), Lawrence (2005) and Koti (2008)]. These problems will be discussed in some details.

Problem 1: In any non-inferiority trial, there is a critical underlying assumption and that is, the active control is an effective treatment, in the sense that it has an effect size that is clinically meaningful as compared to placebo, if a placebo were to be present.

Even though the active control has previously been approved, it does not necessarily mean that the active control will necessarily be shown to be effective in the current non-inferiority trial due to potential changes in the standard clinical practice, to lack of sufficient quality in the current trial, etc. Furthermore, even if the control is effective in the current trial, it may not maintain the same effect size as observed in previous trials. For example, the historical data may show that the control is statistically and clinically significant, but in the current non-inferiority trial, it could be barely clinically significant, or not at all. Worst of all, there is no way to prove it, since there is no placebo in the current trial.

Therefore, it is crucial to have good reasons to belief that in the current non-inferiority trial, the control is not only effective, but maintains a significant clinically meaningful effect size. If one believes that the control in the current trial only has marginal clinical significance, then either one should consider a different control, or perform a superiority trial.

Problem 2: The regulatory requirement for pre-market approval of a new compound only requires that there be substantial evidence from adequate and well-controlled trials to demonstrate its safety and effectiveness. The regulation is silent on how effectiveness is to be demonstrated. However, the FDA paradigm and past practice obviously showed preference for demonstrating effectiveness by comparing the new treatment to a placebo. But this is not possible now in a non-inferiority trial. For a non-inferiority trial, how does one demonstrate that a new treatment is effective relative to a placebo when there is no placebo present in the trial? What should be the requirements for a demonstration of effectiveness of a new treatment in a non-inferiority trial?

Problem 3: In light of Problems 1 and 2 above, how does one determine the non-inferiority margin δ? It is true that non-inferiority trial is used when ethics demands that an active control be used instead of a placebo. Therefore, non-inferiority trials are being considered in trials with mortality and serious morbidity outcomes, such as most cancer trials. For such non-inferiority trials, can the non-inferiority margin δ be so large that the new treatment T is actually substantially worse than the control C, even though T may still be thought to be superior to a putative placebo P? Is it ethical to consider a non-inferiority trial with such a large non-inferiority margin so that patients allocated to the new treatment may be given a substantially inferior treatment than the control?

These are some of the basic problems that the designer of a non-inferiority trial has to contend with. There are currently two approaches to the design and analysis of a non-inferiority trial. Both approaches share some common problems, but in addition each has its own set of individual issues. One approach is called the *fixed margin approach* or *the two-95% confidence interval approach* that we have briefly described and the other is called the *fraction retention approach* or the *synthesis approach.* These two approaches will be described in more detail next. In the recent FDA Guidance on Non-inferiority Trials (March, 2011 FDA Guidance to the Industry on NI Trials), a preference is made for the fixed margin approach.

5.3. *Two current approaches to the design and analysis of non-inferiority trials*

In this section, we will describe these two approaches in some details and will examine the relationship between them which will further elucidate some of the problems inherent in these approaches.

The fraction retention [Holmgren (1999), Rothmann (2003)] or synthesis approach [Hung (2003, 2005, 2007, 2009)] and the fixed margin [Hung (2005, 2007, 2009)] or two-confidence interval approach [Hassalblad (1999)] attempt to address the problem of how to infer the effectiveness of the new treatment in a non-inferiority trial when placebo is not present by formulating the non-inferiority hypothesis (2) in terms of preserving a specified fraction of the control effect relative to placebo that is estimated from historical placebo-controlled studies done on the control. These two approaches and their relationship will be discussed next.

5.3.1. *The fraction retention or synthesis approach*

The fraction retention or synthesis approach starts by considering the following fraction retention ratio hypothesis:

$$H_o \frac{\mu_T - \mu_P}{\mu_C - \mu_P} \leq \delta_o \quad vs. \quad H_a \frac{\mu_T - \mu_P}{\mu_C - \mu_P} > \delta_o. \tag{4}$$

The hypothesis (4) is called the fraction retention hypothesis because the alternative hypothesis states that the fraction $\frac{\mu_T - \mu_P}{\mu_C - \mu_P}$ of the control effect $\mu_C - \mu_P$ that is retained by the new treatment exceeds a fixed desired retention level δ_o, where $0 \leq \delta_o \leq 1$. In order for the fraction retention hypothesis to be meaningful, the control effect $\mu_C - \mu_P$ needs to be positive. Therefore, the *first assumption that the fraction retention approach makes it that the control effect is positive.* Note that this assumption does not say that the control effect has to be clinically meaningful, just that it is greater than zero.

Now it follows that if the control effect $\mu_C - \mu_P > 0$, then the fraction retention hypothesis (4) can be algebraically reformulated into the following equivalent linear hypothesis:

$$\begin{aligned} H_o&: (\mu_T - \mu_C) - (1 - \delta_o)(\mu_C - \mu_P) > 0 \quad vs. \\ H_o&: (\mu_T - \mu_C) - (1 - \delta_o)(\mu_C - \mu_P) \leq 0. \end{aligned} \tag{5}$$

Note that if δ_o represents the retention fraction, then the quantity $(1 - \delta_o)(\mu_C - \mu_P)$ represents the amount of loss of the control effect. Thus, the alternative hypothesis in (5) simply states that the relative difference $(\mu_T - \mu_C)$ between the new treatment T and the control C is less than this amount $(1 - \delta_o)(\mu_C - \mu_P)$.

But in the non-inferiority trial there is no placebo present, hence there is no way one can estimate the control effect $(\mu_C - \mu_P)$ based on data from the current non-inferiority trial. The fraction retention approach [Rothmann *et al.* (2003)] proposes to use the following test statistic to test the null hypothesis in (5):

$$\hat{t} = \frac{(\hat{\mu}_T - \hat{\mu}_C) - (1 - \delta_o)(\hat{\mu}_C - \hat{\mu}_P)}{\sqrt{(\hat{\sigma}_T^2 + \hat{\sigma}_C^2 + (1 - \delta_o)^2(\hat{\sigma}_T^2 + \hat{\sigma}_C^2)}}. \tag{6}$$

Rothmann *et al.* (2003) suggests that $\hat{t}$ is asymptotically standard normal, a claim that was never proven, and the null hypothesis in (5) may be rejected at $\alpha = 0.05$ significance level, if $\hat{t} < -1.96$ and thus claiming retention fraction of at least δ_o. This would seem to suggest that the new treatment is effective in the sense of superior to a placebo that is not present in the current trial. Since, there is actually no placebo in the current trial, therefore the estimate $(\hat{\mu}_C - \hat{\mu}_P)$ for the control effect $(\mu_C - \mu_P)$ is actually based on historical studies external to the current trial. Therefore, the fraction retention approach *assumes that there exist relevant external historical studies that one can use to base the estimate of the control effect on.* Furthermore, it also *assumes that the control effect* $(\mu_C - \mu_P)$ *for the current study is the same as the control effect from the historical study.* This is the so-called constancy assumption. Thus, the test statistic $\hat{t}$ is somewhat meaningful only if these various assumptions are true. However, even when all these assumptions are true, it is still not clear if the test statistic $\hat{t}$ is valid, since it is a statistic derived from data by combining different studies, some of which have already been completed in the past, with the current non-inferiority trial. Thus, the test statistic $\hat{t}$ is not based on data from a prospectively designed studhy.

Let us continue for the moment under the above assumptions and consider the inequality $\hat{t} < -1.96$, that is, when the inferiority hypothesis (4) or (5) is rejected. Upon substituting (6) into this inequality, one obtains the following inequality:

$$(\hat{\mu}_T - \hat{\mu}_C) - (1-\delta_o)(\hat{\mu}_C - \hat{\mu}_P) < -1.96\sqrt{(\hat{\sigma}_T^2 + \hat{\sigma}_C^2) + (1-\delta_o)^2(\hat{\sigma}_T^2 + \hat{\sigma}_C^2)}. \tag{7}$$

After some algebraic operations, one can show that the inequality (7) is equivalent to the following inequality:

$$\begin{aligned}(\hat{\mu}_T - \hat{\mu}_C) + 1.96\sqrt{(\hat{\sigma}_T^2 + \hat{\sigma}_C^2)} &< (1-\delta_o)\left[(\hat{\mu}_C - \hat{\mu}_P) - 1.96\sqrt{(\hat{\sigma}_C^2 + \hat{\sigma}_P^2)}\right] \\ &\quad +1.96\left\{\sqrt{(\hat{\sigma}_T^2 + \hat{\sigma}_C^2)} + (1-\delta_o)\sqrt{(\hat{\sigma}_C^2 + \hat{\sigma}_P^2)}\right. \\ &\quad \left. -\sqrt{(\hat{\sigma}_T^2 + \hat{\sigma}_C^2) + (1-\delta_o)^2(\hat{\sigma}_T^2 + \hat{\sigma}_C^2)}\right\}. \end{aligned} \tag{8}$$

From the property of right triangle, one can see that the quantity inside the parenthesis on the right side of the inequality (8) is always positive. Thus, it follows that if the following inequality

$$(\hat{\mu}_T - \hat{\mu}_C) + 1.96\sqrt{(\hat{\sigma}_T^2 + \hat{\sigma}_C^2)} < (1-\delta_o)\left[(\hat{\mu}_C - \hat{\mu}_P) - 1.96\sqrt{(\hat{\sigma}_C^2 + \hat{\sigma}_P^2)}\right]. \tag{9}$$

holds true, then the inequality (8) will hold true also. We will come back to this inequality (9) in the next section when we compare the two approaches.

The fraction retention approach is also called the synthesis method on account of the test statistic $\hat{t}$ which is defined as a synthesis of two statistics, one for the estimate of the effect of T relative to C obtained from the current non-inferiority trial and the other for the estimate of the effect of the control relative to P obtained from historical study data, and then amalgamated by their combined standard deviations.

The following example illustrates the application of the fraction retention method.

Example 13 (Xeloda): In clinical trials involving colorectal cancer, it is considered unethical to use placebo. In a study of Xeloda for the treatment of colorectal cancer, the objective is to demonstrate that the new treatment is effective in an active control trial [Rothmann *et al.* (2003)]. The clinicians felt that at least 50% retention by Xeloda of the active control effect represents an acceptable level of efficacy in view of its better side effect profile and ease of administration. There are a number of non-concurrent standard control studies involving the active control. These studies demonstrated fairly consistent active control effect. Based on the data from these non-concurrent studies, estimates for the log hazard ratio of the active control effect and its standard error are 0.234 and 0.075 respectively. This is equivalent to a hazard ratio estimate of 1.264 with a 95% confidence interval, (1.091, 1.464). For 50% retention in the active control effect, the largest estimate of the active control effect that is allowed with type I error controlled at 0.025 is 1.228 which corresponds to the lower limit of a 30% confidence interval. Thus, 50% retention of this active control effect produces a cutoff of 1.114. The clinicians believe that the active control effect should not have diminished over time. Thus, in this analysis, the non-inferiority margin $\delta =$ 1.114. The current active control trial produces a hazard ratio estimate of 0.92 with a 97.5% confidence interval upper limit of 1.09 that is below the cutoff of 1.114 (For comparison, the original protocol proposed to consider a fixed cutoff of 1.20). Thus, this trial demonstrates that it rules out a loss of more than 50% of the active control effect. In fact, the new treatment retains at least 61% of the active control effect. The conclusion that one may draw from this trial is that the new treatment is *effective*. It retains at least 61% of the active control effect. However, one cannot claim that this new treatment is non-inferior to the active control.

5.3.2. *The fixed margin or two-confidence interval approach*

The fixed margin or two-95% confidence interval approach simply describes a procedure for testing whether a new treatment is non-inferior to the control based on two confidence intervals. In the two-95% confidence interval approach, a new treatment T is said to be non-inferior to the control if the upper limit of the 95% confidence interval for the relative difference $(\mu_T - \mu_C)$ from the current trial is smaller than the amount of loss of the control effect that can be tolerated. This amount of loos of the control effect that can be tolerated is equal to the fraction $(1 - \delta_o)$ of the control effect, which is defined to be the lower limit of the 95% confidence interval for the control effect $(\mu_C - \mu_P)$, where δ_o is the retention fraction desired, and $(1-\delta_o)$ is the fraction of loss that can be tolerated. This two-95% confidence interval testing procedure is described exactly by the inequality (9). Thus, it follows from our discussion in the preceding section that the two-95% confidence interval approach is a more stringent testing procedure than the fraction retention approach, since whenever the inequality (9) holds true, the fraction retention hypothesis will be true.

Another way of looking at this is by rearranging the inequality in (9) as follows:

$$\hat{t}^* = \frac{(\hat{\mu}_T - \hat{\mu}_C) - (1 - \delta_o)(\hat{\mu}_C - \hat{\mu}_P)}{\sqrt{(\hat{\sigma}_T^2 + \hat{\sigma}_C^2 + (1 - \delta_o)(\hat{\sigma}_T^2 + \hat{\sigma}_C^2)}} < -1.96. \tag{10}$$

The left hand side of the inequality in (10) can be considered as a test statistic $\hat{t}^*$ for testing the fraction retention hypothesis (5). If one assumes that this test statistic $\hat{t}^*$ is asymptotically normal, then one may reject the null hypothesis in (5) at $\alpha = 0.05$, if $\hat{t}^* < -1.96$. Upon comparing the test statistic $\hat{t}$ and $\hat{t}^*$, it is clear that $\hat{t} < \hat{t}^*$ when the numerator of $\hat{t}$ or $\hat{t}^*$ is negative by applying the triangle inequality. Thus, it follows that whenever $\hat{t}^* < -1.96$, then so is $\hat{t}$. Therefore, the two-95% confidence interval testing procedure is more conservative than the fraction retention approach. It is clear from this relationship between the two-95% confidence interval testing procedure and the fraction retention approach that both methods are based on the same set of assumptions. From (10), one can also view the two-95% confidence interval procedure as a fraction retention approach or synthesis method for testing the fraction retention hypothesis (4).

The two-95% confidence interval approach can also be viewed as a fixed margin method. This is because the control effect is estimated based on data from historical studies which are already completed and known. Therefore, the right side of the inequality (9) actually defines the amount of loss of the control effect that one is willing to tolerate. This amount of loss of the control effect that one is willing to tolerate is considered as a fixed non-inferiority margin,

$$\delta - (1-\delta_o)\left[(\hat{\mu}_C - \hat{\mu}_P) - 1.96\sqrt{(\hat{\sigma}_C^2 + \hat{\sigma}_P^2)}\right],$$

and (8) is then simply expressing the inequality

$$(\hat{\mu}_T - \hat{\mu}_C) + 1.96\sqrt{(\hat{\sigma}_T^2 + \hat{\sigma}_C^2)} < \delta. \tag{11}$$

The expression in (11) is simply a test of the following fixed margin non-inferiority hypothesis:

$$H_o\colon \mu_T - \mu_C \geq \delta \quad vs. \quad H_a\colon \mu_T - \mu_C < \delta, \tag{12}$$

where one defines the margin

$$\delta = (1-\delta_o)\left[(\hat{\mu}_C - \hat{\mu}_P) - 1.96\sqrt{(\hat{\sigma}_C^2 + \hat{\sigma}_P^2)}\right].$$

Thus, we see that the two-95% confidence interval approach or the fixed margin approach can be viewed as a fraction retention approach using the test statistic $\hat{t}^*$ given in (10). However, the fraction retention approach cannot be reformulated as a fixed margin hypothesis on account of the denominator of the test statistic, $\hat{t}$, where the two addends under the square root in the denominator are not separable. On the other hand, the fraction retention hypothesis (2) itself is a fixed margin hypothesis, where the fixed margin δ_o is the level of retention desired. There is nothing inappropriate about the fraction retention hypothesis as stated in (2). The difficulty rather lies in the subsequent assumptions required and the make-up of the test statistic which is a composite of statistics from the current trial and from historical studies prior to the actual testing of the non-inferiority hypothesis (5). Rothmann *et al.* (2003) has shown that for time-to-event endpoint, the fraction retention approach actually corresponds approximately to a two-95% confidence interval approach and hence a fixed margin approach, where instead of the 95% confidence interval for the control effect, one is looking at an approximately 41% confidence interval for the control effect.

As discussed above, the two-95% confidence interval approach can be viewed as testing a fixed margin hypothesis with the margin δ defined as

$$\delta = (1-\delta_o)\left[(\hat{\mu}_C - \hat{\mu}_P) - 1.96\sqrt{(\hat{\sigma}_C^2 + \hat{\sigma}_P^2)}\right]. \tag{13}$$

This is simply the right side of the inequality in (8).

As defined in (13), δ is interpreted as the fraction $(1-\delta_o)$ of the control effect $[(\hat{\mu}_C - \hat{\mu}_P) - 1.96\sqrt{(\hat{\sigma}_C^2 + \hat{\sigma}_P^2)}]$ that one can tolerate to lose. Although in past practice, δ_o has often been taken to be 0.5, while the lower limit of the 95% confidence interval has often been used as the estimate of the control effect as shown in (13), these numbers are somewhat arbitrary and can vary depending upon the specific situation at hand.

This fixed margin non-inferiority hypothesis (12) with the non-inferiority margin δ defined by (13) appears to be favored over the fraction retention hypothesis by the regulatory agencies and is the method recommended in the latest FDA Guidance on Non-inferiority Trials (FDA 2010). In the current FDA Guidance, the lower limit of the 95% confidence interval for the control effect is defined to be a margin called M_1. That is,

$$M_1 = \left[(\hat{\mu}_C - \hat{\mu}_P)\ 1.96\sqrt{(\hat{\sigma}_C^2 + \hat{\sigma}_P^2)}\right]. \tag{14}$$

The fraction loss of the control effect estimated by M_1 is called M_2. That is,

$$M_2 = (1-\delta_o)M_1 = (1-\delta_o)\left[(\hat{\mu}_C - \hat{\mu}_P) - 1.96\sqrt{(\hat{\sigma}_C^2 + \hat{\sigma}_P^2)}\right]. \tag{15}$$

M_2 is simply the margin δ of (13) above.

5.3.3. *The fundamental assumptions made in the fraction retention and fixed margin approaches*

Both the fraction retention or synthesis approach and the fixed margin approach have to make three basic assumptions, two of which can never be verified. The first assumption is that there are historical or other concurrent studies available for estimating the control effect. This assumption may not always hold as in some of the anti-infective trials. The second assumption is that this control effect i assumed to exist and maintained in the current non-inferiority trial. This is the so-called constancy assumption. This assumption also may not hold for a variety of reason, such as improving standard of care, drug resistance, etc. The third assumption is that the current non-inferiority trial has assay sensitivity. Assay sensitivity of a trial is the property of a trial to differentiate an active treatment from an inactive treatment. Thus, assay sensitivity of a non-inferiority trial is needed for the second assumption, but is also important for differentiating the new treatment from the control when the control is not effective in the current trial, or if the control is effective but the new treatment is not. The assumption of assay sensitivity may fail for a host of reasons including lack of quality in trial conduct. The fraction retention or synthesis approach has one additional serious problem. This is the question relating to the *validity of the statistical inference of the approach.* Since the test statistic for the fraction retention or synthesis inferiority hypothesis is derived from combined data from the current non-inferiority trial and data from other concurrent or historical studies which have been completed and analyzed, the traditional type I error no longer makes sense, and hence the validity of the inference based on the fraction retention or synthesis approach is questionable. This is perhaps the main reason why the FDA Guidance suggests a preference for the fixed margin approach in addition to its ease of interpretation by the clinicians.

A basic problem with the fixed margin approach is the subjectivity involved in the determination of the margin M_2. Why does one always have to take the lower limit of the 95% confidence interval for the control effect as the estimate of the control effect in the current trial? Why does one usually take half of the control effect estimate as the tolerable loss? To be able to address these questions, we need an objective measure of the degree of closeness between the treatment T and the control C relative to a given metric. This objective measure should be determined theoretically and not dependent on any study data. This is the concept of *inferiority index* introduced in Li and Chi (2011). Inferiority index may be used to measure the tightness of any non-inferiority margin δ no matter how it is derived. In addition, the inferiority index can be used in conjunction with any current approach to arrive at a non-inferiority margin that is more objective. We will not discuss the concept and application of inferiority index to non-inferiority margin specification here further. The interested reader is referred to the recent article by Li and Chi (2011). Research work is currently in progress that relates to non-inferiority margin specification for metrics that are commonly used in binary outcomes.

In summary, if for ethical reason, one has to use an active control, then an active control superiority trial can always be done. The problem is that it may not be easy to demonstrate that the new treatment is superior to the active control, unless the active control happens to be ineffective in the current study. But in the latter case, if one were to claim that the new drug is superior to the active control, then it would be misleading. Thus, even in an active control superiority trial, perhaps one can only conclude that the new treatment is effective, unless one is certain that the active control is effective in the current trial.

On the other hand, due to all the critical assumptions needed in doing an active control non-inferiority trial, most of the times, such trials may not be possible and are not recommended because these assumptions are not verifable. One of the basic concerns is that the active control may not work in the current patient population or trial setting. Another concern is that one may end up demonstrating a drug that is actually inferior to a placebo through such a trial. Therefore, such non-inferiority trials may be contemplated if there are other studies or information that can help to alleviate these concerns which cannot be verified form within the active control trial itself. Even then, the issue regarding bias towards no difference should be properly addressed.

In the actual design of an active control non-inferiority trial, the active control effect, the proportion of control effect to be preserved, the control of the probability of the type I error should be properly determined in light of the objective. One should also pay attention to issues such as multiplicity testing, interim analysis and design modification. These issues may take an already troublesome non-inferiority trial to another level of complexity and risk that should be made fully aware of by the trial sponsor. Proper standard operating procedures should be designed to minimize the introduction of bias towards no difference.

References

Antman EM, McCabe CH, Gurfinkel EP, *et al.* (1999). Enoxaparin prevents death and cardiac ischemic events in unstable angina/non-Q-wave myocardial infarction: results of the Thrombolysis in Myocardial Infarction (TIMI) 121B trial. *Circulation* 100: 1593–1601.

Armitage P, Berry G. (1994). Statistical Methods in Medical Research.

Bauer P (1991). Multiple testings in clinical trials. *Statistics in Medicine* 10: 871–890.

Bauer P, Köhne K (1994). Evaluations of experiments with adaptive interim analyses. *Biometrics* 50: 1029–1041.

Bauer P, Kieser M (1999). Combining different phases in the development of medical treatments within a single trial. *Statistics in Medicine* 18: 1833–1848.

Bauer P, Brannath W, Posch M (2001). Flexible two-stage designs: an overview. *Methods of Information in Medicine* 40: 117–121.

Begg CB (2000). COMMENTARY: Ruminations on the intent-to-treat. *Controlled Clinical Trials* 21: 241–243.

Blackwelder WC (1982). Proving the null hypothesis in clinical trials. *Controlled Clinical Trials* 3: 345–353.

Boyd EJS, Penston JG, Johnston DA, Wormsley KG (1988). Does maintenance therapy keep duodenal ulcer healed? *Lancet* (1988): 1324–1327.

Bretz F, Maurer W, Brannath W, Posch M (2009). A graphical approach to sequentially rejective multiple test procedures. *Statistics in Medicine* 28: 586–604.

Bross PF, Beitz J, Chen G, Chen, XH, Duffy E, Kieffer L, Roy S, Sridhara R, Rahman A, Williams G, Pazdur R (2001). Approval Summary: Gemtuzumabozogamicin in relapsed acute myeloid leukemia. Report from FDA. *Clinical Cancer Research* 7: 1490–1496.

Chi GYH (1985). A design problem in ulcer prevention trials. *Proceedings of the Biopharmaceutical Section of the American Statistical Association*: 100–105.

Chi GYH (1998). Multiple testings: multiple comparisons and multiple endpoints. *Drug Information Journal* 32: Supplement 1347s–1362s.

Chi GYH, Liu Q (1999). The attractiveness of the concept of a prospectively designed two-stage clinical trial. *J. of Biopharmaceutical Statistics* 9: 537–547.

Chi GYH (2000). Clinical decision rules and multiple endpoints: A regulatory perspective. Presented at the Second International Conference on Multiple Comparisons held at the Humboldt University/Charite, Berlin, Germany, June 25–28, 2000.

Chow SC, Liu JP (1998). *Design and Analysis of Clinical Trials: Concept and Methodologies*. John Wiley & Sons, Inc.

Cohen M, Demers D, Gurfinkel EP, *et al.'s*. For the Efficacy and Safety of Subcutaneous Enoxaparin in Non-Q-Wave Coronary Events (ESSENCE) Study Group (1997). A comparison of low molecular weight heparin with unfractionated heparin for unstable coronary artery disease. *New England Journal of Medicine* 337: 447–452.

Committee for Medicinal Producs for Human Use (CHMP) (2005). Guideline on the Choice of the Non-inferiority margin, European Medicines Agency, July 27, 2005.

Cui L, Hung HMJ, Wang SJ (1999). Modification of sample size in group sequential clinical trials. *Biometrics* 55: 853–857.

D'Agostino RB, Sr. (2000). Controlling alpha in a clinical trial: the case for secondary endpoints. *Statistics in Medicine* 19: 763–766.

DerSimonian R, Laird N (1986). Meta-analysis in clinical trials, *Controlled Clinical Trials* 7: 177–188.

Dmitrienko A, Offen W, Westfall PH (2003). Gatekeeping strategies for clinical trials that do not require all primary effects to be significant. *Statistics in Medicine* 22: 2387–2400.

Dmitrienko A, Tamhane AC, Wang X, Chen X (2006a). Stepwise gatekeeping procedures in clinical trial applications. *Biometrical Journal* 48: 984–991.

Dmitrienko A, Offen W, Wang O, Xiao D (2006b). Gatekeeping procedures in dose-response clinical trials based on the Dunnett test. *Pharmaceutical Statistics* 5: 19–28.

Dmitrienko A, Wiens BL, Tamhane AC, Wang X (2007). Tree-structured gatekeeping tests in clinical trials with hierarchically ordered multiple objectives. *Statistics in Medicine* 26: 2465–2478.

Dmitrienko A, Tamhane AC, Wiens BL (2008). General multistage gatekeeping procedures. *Biometrical Journal* 50: 667–677.

Dmitrienko A, Tamhane AC, Liu L (2008). Mixtures of multiple testing procedures with gatekeeping applications. Northwestern University. Department of Industrial Engineering and Management Sciences. Working Paper 08-64.

Dunnett CW (1955). A multiple comparison procedure for comparing several treatments with a control. *J. of the American Statistical Association* 50: 1096–1121.

Dunnett CW, Tamhane AC (1991). Step-down multiple tests for comparing treatments with a control in unbalanced one-way layouts. *Statistics in Medicine* 10: 939–947.

Dunnett CW, Tamhane AC (1992). A step-up multiple test procedure. *J. of the American Statistical Association* 87: 162–170.

Dunnett CW, Tamhane AC (1995). Step-up multiple testing of parameters with unequally correlated estimates. *Biometrics* 51: 217–227.

Elashoff JD, Koch GG and Chi GYH (1988). Designing a clinical trial to demonstrate prevention of ulcer recurrence: modelling simulation approaches. *Statistics in Medicine* 7: 877–888.

Ellenberg SS, Temple R (2000). Placebo-controlled trials and active control trials in the evaluation of new treatments, Part II: practical issues and specific cases. *Annals of Internal Medicine* 133 (6): 464–470.

Emerson S (2007). Frequentist evaluation of group sequential clinical trial designs. *Statistics in Medicine* 26: 5047–5080.

European Medicines Agency. Regulatory Guidance, Guidelines, ICH Documents, Reflection Papers. http://www.emea.europa.eu.

Finner H, Strassburger K (2002). The partitioning principle: a powerful tool in multiple decision theory. *Annals of Statistics* 30: 1194–1213.

Fisher LD, Dixon DO, Herson J, Frankowski RF, Hearron MS, Peace KE (1990). Intention-to-treat in clinical trials. Chapter 7, *Statistical Issues in Drug Research and Development*, edited by Karl E. Peace, Marcel Dekker, Inc.

Fisher LD, Moyé LA (1999a). Carvedilol and the Food and Drug Administration approval process: an introduction. *Controlled Clinical Trials* 20: 1–15.

Fisher LD (1999b). Carvedilol and the Food and Drug Administration (FDA) approval process: the FDA paradigm and reflections on hypothesis testing. *Controlled Clinical Trials* 20: 16–39.

Fleming TR, Harrington DP, O'Brien PC (1984). Designs for group sequential tests. *Controlled Clinical Trials* 5: 348–361.

Fleming TR (1987). Treatment evaluation in active control studies. *Cancer Treatment Reports* 71(11): 1061–1065.

Fleming TR (1990). Evaluation of active control trials in AIDS. *J. of Acquired Immune Deficiency Syndromes* 3: Supplement 2 S82–S87.

Fleming TR (2000). Design and interpretation of equivalence trials. *American Heart Journal* 139: s171–s176.

Follman D (1995). Multivariate tests for multiple endpoints in clinical trials. *Statistics in Medicine* 14: 1163–1175.

Gillings D, Koch G (1991). The application of the principle of intention-to-treat to the analysis of clinical trials. *Drug Information Journal* 25: 411–424.

Goodman S (1999). Toward evidence-based medical statistics. 1: The p-value fallacy. *Ann Intern Med.* 130: 995–1004.

Gurfinkel EP, Manos EJ, Mejail RI *et al.* (1995). Low molecular weight heparin versus regular heparin or aspirin in the treatment of unstable angina and silent ischemia. *J. of American College of Cardiology* 26: 313–318.

Hassalblad V, Kong DF (2001). Statistical methods for comparison to placebo in active-control trials. *Drug Information Journal* 32 2: 435–450.

Hauck WW, Anderson S (1999). Some issues in the design and analysis of equivalence trials. *Drug Information Journal* 33: 109–118.

Hauschke D, Schafer J,Pigeot I (2001). Statistical approaches for the choice of delta. Presented at the 37th Annual Meeting of the Drug Information Association, July 8–12, 2001, Denver, Colorado.

Hochberg Y (1988). A sharper Bonferroni procedure for multiple tests of significance. *Biometrika* 75: 800–802.

Hochberg Y, Tamhane AC (1987). *Multiple Comparison Procedures.* Wiley, New York.

Holm S (1979). A simple sequentially rejective multiple test procedure. *Scandinavian. J. Statistics* 6: 65–70.

Holmgren EB (2001). Establishing equivalence by showing that a specified percentage of the effect of the active control over placebo is maintained. *J. of Biopharmaceutical Statistics* 9(4): 651–659.

Hommel G (1988). A stage wise rejective multiple test procedure based on a modified Bonferroni test. *Biometrika* 75: 383–386.

Hung HMJ, Chi GYH, Lipicky RJ (1993). Testing for the existence of a desirable dose combination. *Biometrics* 49: 85–94.

Hung HMJ, Wang SJ, O'Neill RT (2005). A regulatory perspective on choice of margin and statistical inference issue in non-inferiority trials. *Biometrical Journal* 47: 28–36.

Hung HMJ, Wang SJ, O'Neill RT (2008). Non-inferiority trial. *Wiley Encyclopedia of Clinical Trials*, Wiley, New York.

Hung HMJ, Wang SJ, O'Neill RT (2009). Challenges and regulatory experiences with non-inferiority trial design without placebo arm. *Biometrical Journal* 51(2): 324–334.

Huque M, Dubey S, and Fredd S (1989). Establishing therapeutic equivalence with clinical endpoints. *Proceedings of the Biopharmaceutical Section of the American Statistical Association*: 46–52.

Huque MF and Alosh, M (2008). A flexible fixed-sequence testing method for hierarchically ordered correlated multiple endpoints in clinical trials. *J. Statistical Planning and Inference* 138: 321–335.

Jennison C and Turnbull BW (2000). *Group Sequential Methods with Applications to Clinical Trials.* Chapman and Hall, Boca Raton, FL.

Jin K, Chi GYH (1997). Application of bootstrap in handling multiple endpoints. *Proceedings of the Biopharmaceutical Section of the American Statistical Association*: 150–155.

Jin K, Chi GYH (1998). Clinical decision rules and statistical support structures — a novel approach to handling the multiple endpoints problem. *Proceedings of the Biopharmaceutical Section of the American Statistical Association*: 56–62.

Kaul S, Shah PK (2000). Low molecular weight heparin in acute coronary syndrome: evidence for superior or equivalent efficacy compared with unfractionated heparin? *J. of American College of Cardiology* 35: 1699–1712.

Kieser M, Bauer P, Lehmacher W (1999). Inference on multiple endpoints in clinical trials with adaptive interim analyses. *Biometrical Journal* 41(3): 261–277.

Klein W, Buchwald A, Hillis SE *et al.* for the FRIC Investigators (1997). Comparison of low molecular weight heparin with unfractionated heparin acutely and with placebo for six weeks in the management of unstable coronary artery disease: Frogmin in Unstable Coronary Artery Disease Study (FRIC). *Circulation* 96: 61–68.

Koch GG,Tangen CM (1999). Nonparametric analysis of covariance and its role in noninferiority clinical trials. *Drug Information Journal* 33: 1145–1159.

Koch GG (2000). Discussion for 'Alpha calculus in clinical trials: considerations and commentary for the new millennium'. *Statistics in Medicine* 19: 781–784.

Kordzakhia G, Dinh P, Bai S, Lawrence J, Yang P (2008). Bonferroni-based tree structured gatekeeping testing procedures. Unpublished manuscript.

Korn EL, Troendle JF, McShane LM, Simon RS (2004). Controlling the number of false discoveries: Application to high-dimensional genomic data. *J. of Statistical Planning and Inference* 124: 379–398.

Koti KM (2008). Use and abuse of statistics in design and analysis of active control trials. *Proceedings of the Biopharmaceutical Section of the American Statistical Association.*

Kurata JH, Koch GG (1988). Response to "H2-receptor antagonists and duodenal ulcer recurrence". *The American Journal of Gastroenteroloy* 83(12): 1427–1428.

Lachin JM (2000). Statistical considerations in the intent-to-treat principle. *Controlled Clinical Trials* 21: 167–189.

Lan KKG, DeMets DL (1983). Discrete sequential boundaries for clinical trials. *Biometrika* 70 (3): 659–663.

Lavori PW, Dawson R, Shera D (1995). A multiple imputation strategy for clinical trials with truncation of patient data. *Statistics in Medicine* 14: 1913–1925.

Lawrence J (2005). Some remarks about the analysis of active control studies. *Biometrical Journal* 47: 616–622.

Leber P (1986). The placebo control in clinical trials — A view from the FDA. *Psychopharmacology Bulletin* 22(1):30–32.

Leber P (1989). Hazards of inference: The active control investigation. *Epilepsia*, 30: Supplement 1 s57–s63.

Lehmacher W, Wassmer G, Reitmer P (1991). Procedures for two sample comparisons with multiple endpoints controlling the experimentwise error rate. *Biometrics* 47: 511–521.

Lewis JH (1985). Summary of the Gastrointestical Drug Advisory Committee Meeting — March 21 and 22, 1985. *The American Journal of Gastroenterology* 80: 581–583.

Little RJA, Rubin DB (1987). *Statistical Analysis with Missing Data.* John Wiley and Sons, Inc.

Little RJA (1995). Modeling the drop-out mechanism in repeated-measures studies. *J. of the American Statistical Association* 90 (431): 1112–1121.

Liu A, Hall WJ (1999). Unbiased estimation following a group sequential test. *Biometrika* 86: 71–78.

Liu Q, Chi GYH (2001). On sample size and inference for two-stage adaptive designs. *Biometrics* 57: 172–177.

Liu Q (2001). On general two-stage adaptive designs with dependent data. Personal communication 1–22.

Liu Q, Pledger GW (2005). Phase 2 and 3 combination designs to accelerate drug development. *J. of the American Statistical Association* 100: 493–502.

Liu Q, Pledger GW (2006). On design and inference for two-stage adaptive clinical trials with dependent daa. *J. of Statistical Planning and Inference* 136: 1962–1984.

Liu Q, Anderson KM (2008a). On adaptive extensions of group sequential trials for clinical investigations. *J. of the American Statistical Association* 103: 1621–1630.

Liu Q, Proschan MA, Pledger GW (2002). A unified theory of two-stage adaptive designs. *J. of the American Statistical Association* 97: 1034–1041.

Liu Q, Chi GYH (2010a). Fundamental theory of adaptive designs with unplanned design change in clinical trials with blinded data. *Handbook of Adaptive Designs in Pharmaceutical and Clinical Development* 2-1 to 2-8. Edited by Pong A and Chow SC, Chapman & Hall.

Liu Q, Chi GYH (2010b). Understanding the FDA Guidance on Adaptive Designs: Historical, Legal and Statistical Perspectives. *The 2010 special issue of J. of Biopharmaceutical Statistics* 20: 1178–1219.

Liu Y, Hsu JC (2009). Testing for efficacy in primary and secondary endpoints by partitioning decision paths. *J. of American Statistical Association* 104: 1661–1670.

Malinckrodt C, Clark W, David S (2001). Accounting for dropout bias using mixed-effects models. *J. of Biopharmaceutical Statistics* 11: 9–21.

Marcus R, Peritz E, Gabriel KR (1976). On closed testing procedure with special reference to ordered analysis of variance. *Biometrika* 63: 655–660.

Maurer R, Peritgz E, Gabriel KR (1976). On closed testing procedure with special reference to ordered analysis of variance. *Biometrika* 63: 655–660.

Mathieu M (1997). *New Drug Development: A Regulatory Overview.* Parexel International Corporation, Waltham, Massachusetts.

McManus J, Wormsley KG, (1989). A new perspective on what maintenance therapy of duodenal ulcer achieves — Selected Summaries. *Gastroenterology* 96(4): 1218–1220.

Millen BA, Dmitrienko A (2011). Chain procedures: A class of flexible closed testing procedures with clinical trial applications. *Statistics in Biopharmaceutical Research* 3: 14–30.

Moyé LA (1999). End-point interpretation in clinical trials: the case for discipline. *Controlled Clinical Trials* 20: 40–49.

Moyé LA (2000a). Alpha calculus in clinical trials: considerations and commentary for the new millennium. *Statistics in Medicine* 19: 767–779.

Moyé LA (2000b). Response to commentaries on 'Alpha calculus in clinical trials: considerations and commentary for the new millennium'. *Statistics in Medicine* 19: 795–799.

Moyé LA (2003). *Multiple Analysis in Clinical Trials.* Springer, New York.

Muller H, Schaefer H (2001). Adaptive group sequential designs for clinical trials: Combining the advantages of adaptive and of classical group sequential approaches. *Biometrics* 57: 886–891.

Myers WR (2000). Handling missing data in clinical trials: an overview. *Drug Information Journal* 34: 525–533.

Naik UD (1975). Some selection rules for comparing processes with a standard. *Communication in Statistics, Series A* (4): 519–535.

National Research Council (2010). The Prevention and Treatment of Missing Data in Clinical Trials, Panel on Handling Missing Data in Clinical Trials. http://www.nap.edu/catalog/12955.html.

Neuhäuser M, Steinijans VW, Bretz F (1999). The evaluation of multiple clinical endpoints, with application to asthma. *Drug Information Journal* 33: 471–477.

O'Brien PC, Fleming TR (1979). A multiple testing procedure for clinical trials. *Biometrics* 35: 549–556.

O'Brien PC (1984). Procedures for comparing samples with multiple endpoints. *Biometrics* 40: 1079–1087.

O'Neill RT (1997). Secondary endpoints cannot be validly analyzed if the primary endpoint does not demonstrate clear statistical significance. *Controlled Clinical Trials* 18: 550–556.

O'Neill RT (2000). Commentary on 'Alpha calculus in clinical trials: considerations and commentary for the new millenium'. *Statistics in Medicine* 19: 785–793.

Peace KE (1988). *Biopharmaceutical Statistics for Drug Development.* Marcel Dekker, Inc.

Peace KE (1990). *Statistical Issues in Drug Research and Development.* Marcel Dekker, Inc.

Physicians' Desk Reference (1999). Medical Economics Company, Inc., Montvale, NJ 07645-1742.

Pocock SJ (1977). Group sequential methods in the design and analysis of clinical trials. *Biometrika* 64(2): 191–199.

Pocock SJ (1982). Interim analyses for randomized clinical trials: the group sequential approach. *Biometrics* 38: 153–162.

Pocock SJ, Geller NL, Tsiatis AA (1987). The analysis of multiple endpoints in clinical trials. *Biometrics* 43: 487–498.

Proschan MA, Hunsberger SA (1995). Designed extension of studies based on conditional power. *Biometrics* 51: 1315–1324.

Riis P (2000). Perspectives on the Fifth Revision of the Declaration of Helsinki. *J. of the American Medical Association* 284(23) 3045–3046.

Rogers JA, Hsu JC, Lin S (2004). Using the partititoning principle to construct confidence sets for the location of a disease gene. *J. of Statistical Planning and Inference* 125: 101–118.

Rothmann M, Chen G, Li N, Chi GYH (2001). Design and analysis of non-inferiority mortality trials in oncology. DIA 37th Annual Meeting, July 8–12, 2001, Denver, Colorado.

Rothmann M, Li N, Dhen G, Chi GYH, Temple RO, Tsou HH (2003). Non-inferiority methods for mortality trials. *Statistics in Medicine* 22: 239–264.

Rüger B (1978). Das maximale signifikanzniveau des tests "Lehno Ho ab, wenn k under n gegebenen tests zur Ablehnung fuhren." *Metrika* 25: 171–178.

Samuel-Cahn E (1996). Is the Simes improved Bonferroni procedure conservative? *Biometrika* 83(4): 928–933.

Sankoh AJ, Huque MF, Dubey SD (1997). Some comments on frequently used multiple endpoint adjustment methods in clinical trials. *Statistics in Medicine* 16: 2529–2542.

Sarkar S, Chang CK (1997). Simes' method for multiple hypothesis testing with positively dependent test statistics, *J. of the American Statistical Association* 92: 1601–1608.

Sarkar SK (1998). Some probability inequalities for ordered MTP_2 random variables: A proof of the Simes Conjecture. *Annals of Statistics* 26(2): 494–504.

Shen Y, Fisher L (1999). Statistical inference for self-designing clinical trials with a one-sided hypothesis. *Biometrics* 55: 190–197.

Siegel JP (2000). Equivalence and non-inferiority trials. *American Heart Journal* 139: s166–s170.

Simes RJ (1986). An improved Bonferroni procedure for multiple tests of significance. *Biometrika* 55: 484–487.

Simon R (1999). Bayesian design and analysis of active control clinical trials. *Biometrics* 55: 484–487.

Song Y, Chi GYH (2007). A method for testing a pre-specified subgroup in clinical trials. *Statistics in Medicine* 26: 3535–3549.

Stefansson G, Kim W, Hsu JC (1988). On confidence sets in multiple comparisons. In Gupta SS and Berger JO editors, Statistical Decision Theory and related Topics IV, Volume 2: 89–104. Springer-Verlag, New York.

Tamhane AJ, Hochberg Y, Dunnett CW (1996). Multiple test procedures for dose finding. *Biometrics* 28: 519–531.

Tang DI, Geller, NL, Pocock SJ (1993). On the design and analysis of randomized clinical trials with multiple endpoints. *Biometrics* 49: 23–30.

Tang DI, Gnecco C, Geller NL (1989). An approximate likelihood ratio test for a normal mean vector with non-negative components with application to clinical trials, *Biometrika* 76: 577–583.

Temple R (1983). Difficulties in evaluating positive control trials. *Proceedings of the Biopharmaceutical Section of the American Statistical Association*: 1–7.

Temple R (1996). Problems in interpreting active control equivalence trials. *Accountability in Research*, 4: 267–275.

Temple R, Ellenberg SS (2000). Placebo-controlled trials and active control trials in the evaluation of new treatments, Part I: Ethical and scientific issues. *Annals of Internal Medicine* 133 (6): 455–463.

The Clopidogrel in Unstable Angina to Prevent Recurrent Events (CURE) Trials Investigators (2011). Effects of clopidogrel in addition to asprin in patients with acute coronary syndromes without ST-segment elevation. *New England Journal of Medicine* 345: 494–502.

The EPIC Investigators (1994). Use of a monoclonal antibody directed against the platelet glycoprotein IIb/IIIa receptor in high-risk coronary angioplasty. *New England Journal of Medicine* 330: 956–961.

The EPILOG Investigators (1997). Platelet glycoprotein IIb/IIIa receptor blockade and low = dose heparin during percutaneous coronary revascularization. *New England Journal of Medicine* 336: 1689–1696.

The CAPTURE investigators (1997). Randomized placebo-controlled trial of abciximab before and during coronary intervention in refractory unstable angina. *Lancet* 349: 1429–1435.

Tilley BC, Maler J, Geller NL, Lu M, Legler J, Brott T, Lyden P, Grotta J (1996). Use of a global test for multiple outcomes in stroke trials with application to the National Institute of Neurological Disorders and Stroke t-PA Stroke Trial. *Stroke* 27(11): 2136–2142.

Tsiatis AA (1982). Repeated significance testing for a general class of statistics used in censored survival analysis. *J. of the American Statistical Association* 77 (380): 855–861.

U.S. Code of Federal Regulations 21: Parts 300–499 (2001). U.S. Government Printing Office.

U.S. Food and Drug Administration (1996). Oncology Initiatives. www.fda.gov/opacom/backgrounders/cancerbg/html.

U.S. Food and Drug Administration (1998–2000). International Conference on Harmonization Requirements for Registration of Pharmaceuticals for Human Use (ICH) E-1–E-11. www.FDA.gov/CDER/guidance/index.html.

U.S. Food and Drug Administration (1997). International Conference on Harmonization of Technical Requirements for Registration of Pharmaceuticals for Human Use (ICH). E-8: Guidance on General Considerations for Clinical Trials. Federal Register 62, 242, December 17, 1997/Notices, 66113–66119.

U.S. Food and Drug Administration (1998). International Conference on Harmonization of Technical Requirements for Registration of Pharmaceuticals for Human Use (ICH). E-9: Guidance on Statistical Principles for Clinical Trials. Federal Register 63, 179, September 16, 1998/Notices, 49583–49598.

U.S. Food and Drug Administration (1999). International Conference on Harmonization of Technical Requirements for Registration of Pharmaceuticals for Human Use (ICH). E-10: Guidance on Choice of Control Group in Clinical Trials. Federal Register 64, 185, September 24, 1999/Notices, 51767–51780.

U.S. Food and Drug Administration (2001). On the Establishment and Operation of Clinical Trial Data Monitoring Committees — Draft Guidance. Federal Register: Pending.

U.S. FDA Guidance for Industry (March 1, 2011). Non-inferiority Clinical Trials. The Division of Dockets Management (HFA-305), Food and Drug Administration, White Oaks, Silver Spring, MD.

U.S. FDA http://www.fda.gov/downloads/Drugs/GuidanceComplianceRegulatoryInformation/Guidances/UCM202140.pdf

U.S. FDA Medical-Statisticdal Review for Xeloda (NDA 20-896) dated April 23, 2001. Available at http://www.fda.gov/cder/foi/nda/2001/20896s6Xeloda Medr Statr Pl.pdf.291, 292l.

U.S. FDA Cardivascular and Renal Drugs Advisory Committee Meeting (2011). Meeting materials for the September 8, 2011 Cardiovascular and Renal Advisory Committee Meeting. http://www.fda.gov/AdvisoryCommittees/CommitteesMeetingMaterials/Drugs/Cardiovascularand RenalDrugsAdvisoryCommittee/ucm250287.htnl.

U.S. FDA Anti-Infective Drugs Advisory Committee Meeting (2011). Meeting materials for the November 3, 2011 Anti-Infective Drugs Advisory Committee Meeting. http://www.fda.gov/AdvisoryZCommittees/CommitteesMeetingMaterials/Drugs/Anti-InfectiveDrugsAdvisory Committee/ucm242307.htm.

Vastag B (2000). Helsinki discord? A controversial declaration. *J. of the American Medical Association* 284(23): 2983–2985.

Verbeke G, Molenberghs G, Bijnens L and Shaw D (1997). *Linear Mixed Models in Practice*. New York: Springer.

Wassmer G (1998). A comparison of two methods for adaptive interim analyses in clinical trials. *Biometrics* 54: 696–705.

Wassmer, G, Reitmeir, P, Kieser, M, and Lehmacher, W (1999). Procedures for testing multiple endpoints in clinical trials: An overview. *J. of Statistical Planning and Inference* 82: 69–81.

Westfall PH, Young SS (1992). *Resampling-Based Multiple T esting.* Wiley, New York.

White HD (1998). Thrombolytic therapy and equivalence trials — Editorial Comment. *J. of American College of Cardiology* 31(3): 494–496.

Whitehead J (1983). *The Design and Analysis of Sequential Clinical Trials.* New York: Ellis Horwood.

Whitehead J (1986a). On the bias of maximum likelihood estimation following a sequential test. *Biometrika* 73: 573–581.

Whitehead J (1986b). Supplementary analysis at the conclusion of a sequential clinical trial. *Biometrics* 42: 461–471.

Wiens B (2003). A fixed-sequence Bonferroni procedure for testing multiple endpoints. *Pharmaceutical Statistics* 2: 211–215.

Wiens B, Dmitrienko A (2005). The fallback procedure for evaluating a single family of hypotheses, *J. of Biopharmaceutical Statistics* 15: 929–942.

World Medical Association Declaration of Helsinki — Ethical principles for medical research involving human subjects. *J. of American Medical Association* 284(23): 3043–3045.

Xu H, Hsu JC (2007). Applying the generalized partitioning principle to control the generalized familywise error rate. *Biometrical Journal* 49: 52–67.

Xu H, Nuamah I, Liu J, Lim P, Sampson A (2009). A Dunnett-Bonferroni-based parallel gatekeeping procedure for dose-response clinical trials with multiple endpoints. *Pharmaceutical Statistics* 8: 301–316.

About the Authors

Dr. George Chi is currently a Senior Director, Statistical Science, Biometrics and Reporting, Janssen Research and Development. Prior to that, he was the Director, Division of Biometrics I, Center for Drug Evaluation and Research, Food and Drug Administration (FDA), Rockville, Maryland from 1984–2004. Dr. Chi was elected an ASA Fellow in 2003. Prior to joining FDA, he taught at the University of Pittsburgh, University of Florida, and visited the University of Bucharest as a Senior Fulbright Research Scholar between 1971 and 1976, and was an NIH Research Fellow at the LIPID project at the University of North Carolina and the Highway Safety Research Center at Chapel Hill between 1976 and 1983. Dr. Chi has an active interest in regulatory research. His current research interest includes the design and analysis of active control non-inferiority trials. Recent publications include, "*Inferiority Index and Non-inferiority Trials*" in *Statistics in Biopharmaceutical Research 2011* and "*Inferiority Index and the Behrens-Fisher Problem in NI Trials*" in *2012 Proceeding of the American Statistical Association.*

Dr. Haiyan Xu earned her bachelor degree in international economics and trade from Nankai University (Tianjin, China) in 2001. She then earned her master degree and Ph.D. degree in Statistics from The Ohio State University in 2004 and 2005. Her main research interest is in multiple comparisons. Dr. Xu has been working as a clinical biostatistician at Johnson & Johnson Pharmaceutical Research & Development, L.L.C. (now Janssen Research & Development, L.L.C.) since October 2005. Her job responsibilities mainly include designing late phase clinical trials, planning, conducting, and reporting statistical analyses.

Dr. Qing Liu obtained his Ph.D. degree in statistics from Oregon State University. He is a biostatistician and active researcher in clinical trial designs and statistical methods. Over the years, Dr. Liu has gained broad experience in clinical research and trial experience in oncology, CNS, pain, cardiovascular, anti-infective, anti-virus, and metabolic diseases through employment in academic, regulatory and industry settings. He has leveraged this experience in innovative methodological research in clinical trial designs and statistical inference. His involvement in early methodological research at the U.S. Food and Drug administration (FDA) has helped to pave the way for the current acceptance of the adaptive designs for regulatory applications. Dr. Liu has also published and presented research works extensively. In addition, he has peer-reviewed a substantial number of papers for statistical and medical journals. Dr. Liu is a Fellow of the American Statistical Association.

CHAPTER 19

SURROGATES FOR QUALITATIVE EVALUATION OF TREATMENT EFFECTS

ZHI GENG

School of Mathematical Sciences,
Peking University, Beijing 100871, China
zhigeng@pku.edu.cn

1. Introduction

In a clinical trial, a surrogate may be used for assessing the treatment effect on an endpoint when the measurement of the endpoint may be expensive or infeasible. In recent years, there have been a number of papers questioning the validity of surrogates. Fleming and DeMets (1996), Baker (2006), Manns et al. (2006) and Alonso and Molenberghs (2008) had their papers entitled 'Surrogate end points in clinical trials: are we being misled?', 'Surrogate endpoints: wishful thinking or reality?', 'Surrogate markers in clinical studies: problems solved or created?' and 'Surrogate markers: hopes and perils', respectively. They pointed out that in many real clinical trials, applications of surrogates falsely evaluated treatment effects on endpoints, such as CD4 counts for survival time in clinical trials of AIDS, bone mass for fracture in osteoporosis studies.

Up to now, there have been several criteria of surrogates. The most intuitive one requires that there is a strong correlation between the surrogate and the true endpoint. But Baker and Kramer (2003) and Chen, Geng and Jia (2007) illustrated that for a strongly correlated surrogate, the treatment may have a positive effect on the surrogate but a negative effect on the true endpoint. Prentice (1989) proposed the operational criteria for a statistical surrogate which ensure that the independence of a treatment and the statistical surrogate implies the independence of the treatment and the endpoint, although the inverse of the implication does not always hold (Berger, 2004). Frangakis and Rubin (2002) pointed out that the statistical surrogates based on Prentices criteria do not satisfy the property of causal necessity, and they proposed the criterion for the principal surrogate to satisfy the causal necessity. Lauritzen (2004) used a causal diagram to depict a strong surrogate criterion, and he showed that a strong surrogate requires stronger conditions than a principal surrogate and that they are equivalent for a binary treatment. Chen, Geng and Jia (2007) presented the surrogate paradox for all of these criteria, which means that a treatment has a positive effect on a surrogate and the surrogate has a positive effect or a positive association on the endpoint, but the treatment has a negative effect on the endpoint. To avoid the surrogate paradox, Chen, Geng and Jia (2007), Ju and Geng (2010) and Wu, He and Geng (2011) presented the novel criteria for surrogates based on causation and association among the variables of treatment, surrogate, endpoint and confounder.

Here we discuss the problems on surrogates and introduce the surrogate paradox. We focus only on the qualitative evaluation of treatment effects on the endpoint. Several numerical examples are given to illustrate the phenomena of the surrogate paradox. To avoid the phenomena, we discuss criteria and conditions for surrogates. The goal is that observing a surrogate S instead of the endpoint Y, we use the sign of treatment effect on the observed surrogate S to predict the sign of treatment effect on the unobserved endpoint Y.

We introduce definitions and notation, and then give examples to illustrate that the phenomenon of the surrogate paradox may occur for the statistical, principal and strong surrogates in Section 2. To avoid the surrogate paradox, we discuss the criteria for surrogates based on prior knowledge on causation in Section 3 and the criteria based on prior knowledge on association in Section 4. Finally discussions on the problem of surrogates are given in Section 5.

2. Definitions and Notation

Let T denote a binary treatment, Y an endpoint, and S a surrogate. For a treatment T with more than two levels, we can compare its levels pairwise. Assume that treatment T is randomized. Since the surrogate S may not randomized, there may be a unobserved confounder or a confounder vector U which affects both the surrogate S and the endpoint Y. The relationships among these variables can be depicted by the causal network in Fig. 1.

Let Y_t and S_t denote the potential outcomes of the endpoint and the surrogate under a treatment $T = t$ respectively. Assume that the observed outcomes $Y = Y_t$ and $S = S_t$ for the really treatment $T = t$. Define the

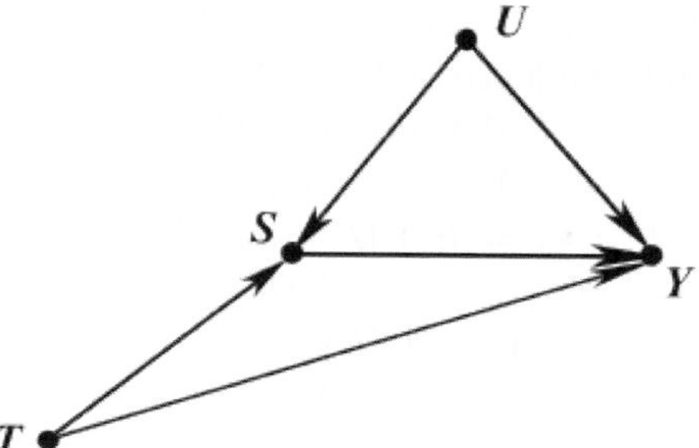

Fig. 1. A causal network with direct and indirect effects on the endpoint.

individual i's causal effect of X on Z as $ICE_{X\to Z}(x, x'; i) = Z_x(i) - Z_{x'}(i)$ for $x > x'$.

Definition 1. For $x > x'$, an average causal effect (ACE) of X on Z is defined as

$$ACE_{X\to Z}(x, x') = E[ICE_{X\to Z}(x, x')] = E(Z_x) - E(Z_{x'}),$$

and the corresponding prima facie average causal effect (FACE) of X on Z is defined as

$$FACE_{X\to Z}(x, x') = E(Z|X = x) - E(Z|X = x').$$

$E(Z_x)$ is the average of the potential outcomes which would be obtained if the treatment $X = x$ were assigned to all individuals including those taking other treatments $x' \neq x$. Without randomization or any untestable assumption, $E(Z_x)$ and $ACE_{X\to Z}(x, x')$ are unidentifiable. Unlike $E(Z_x)$, $E(Z|X = x)$ is the average of outcomes of individuals only in the treatment group of $X = x$, which is identifiable from observed outcomes Z in the treatment group of $X = x$.

In the case where an endpoint or response is a continuous or ordinal discrete variable, a more preferable measure of causal effects than the ACE may be the distributional causal effect.

Definition 2. For $x > x'$, a distributional causal effect (DCE) of X on Z for a specific threshold z is defined as the difference of cumulative distributions of the potential outcomes

$$DCE_{X\to(Z>z)}(x, x') = P(Z_x > z) - P(Z_{x'} > z),$$

and a prima facie distributional causal effect (FDCE) of X on Z is defined as

$$FDCE_{X\to(Z>z)}(x, x') = P(Z > z|X = x) - P(Z > z|X = x').$$

For a binary X, $ACE_{X\to Z}(1,0)$ is simply denoted as $ACE_{X\to Z}$. Let $T \perp\!\!\!\perp Y$ denote the independence of T and Y and $T \perp\!\!\!\perp Y|S$ denote the conditional independence of T and Y given S. Since T is randomized, we have $T \perp\!\!\!\perp (Y_t, \forall t)$ and get that $P(Y_t > y) = P(Y_t > y|T = t) = P(Y > y|T = t)$ and $E(Y_t) = E(Y_t|T = t) = E(Y|T = t)$. Thus we obtain $ACE_{T\to Y} = FACE_{T\to Y}$ and $DCE_{T\to(Y>y)} = FDCE_{T\to(Y>y)}$. Similarly we have $ACE_{T\to S} = FACE_{T\to S}$ and $DCE_{T\to(S>s)} = FDCE_{T\to(S>s)}$. Generally we have neither $ACE_{S\to Y} = FACE_{S\to Y}$ nor $DCE_{S\to(Y>y)}(s,s') = FDCE_{S\to(Y>y)}(s,s')$ since S is not randomized.

We say that X has a non-negative (non-positive or null) DCE on Z if for any two levels $x > x'$, $DCE_{X\to(Z>z)}(x,x') \geq (\leq \text{ or } =)\ 0$ for all z. If, in addition, there exist a threshold z and a pair of levels $x > x'$ such that $DCE_{X\to(Z>z)}(x,x') > (<)0$, then we say that X has a positive (negative) DCE on Z. Similarly we define a non-negative and a positive FDCE. Notice that DCE depends on a specific threshold z but the sign (non-negative, non-positive, negative, positive or null) of DCE does not. A positive DCE and a non-negative DCE imply a positive ACE and a non-negative ACE respectively. However, the converse is not true. Thus DCE describes a stricter causal measurement than ACE.

There are many approaches for using surrogates to quantitatively evaluate the treatment effect on the endpoint, although they require observed data of the endpoint (Burzykowski, Molenberghs and Buyse, 2005). If the endpoint is never observed, we need prior knowledge on the relationship between the endpoint and the surrogate. Based on the prior knowledge, we use the treatment effect on the surrogate to qualitatively evaluate the treatment effect on the endpoint. The qualitative relations between treatment effects on a surrogate and an endpoint means the implication and equivalence relations from the sign of effect on the surrogate to the sign of effect on the endpoint.

There are several criteria for qualifying surrogates. The most intuitive criterion may be that there is a strong association between the endpoint and the surrogate. But only the strong association is not sufficient for using surrogates to evaluate treatment effect on the endpoint. For example, there is a strong association between the shoe size and the number of remembered words for primary school children. It is obvious that a treatment which can increase the shoe size may not increase the number of remembered words for the children.

Prentice's criterion for statistical surrogates further require that the endpoint Y is independent of a treatment T conditionally on an intermediate variable S, denoted as $Y \perp\!\!\!\perp T|S$. Such an intermediate variable S is called a statistical surrogate. The conditional independence means that the intermediate variable S can break the association between the treatment T and the endpoint Y, and thus the association between T and Y can be interpreted by the association between T and S if S and Y have a strong association. Let $T \perp\!\!\!\perp S$ denote the independence of T and S. Under Prentice's criterion, we have that $T \perp\!\!\!\perp S$ implies $T \perp\!\!\!\perp Y$, although the reverse may not be true. For a randomized trial of treatment T, $T \perp\!\!\!\perp S$ and $T \perp\!\!\!\perp Y$ mean $ACE_{T \to S} = DCE_{T \to S} = 0$ and $ACE_{T \to Y} = DCE_{T \to Y} = 0$ respectively. Thus Prentice's criterion can ensure that a null treatment effect on the surrogate S implies a null treatment effect on the endpoint Y in the sense of expectation and distribution.

Frangakis and Rubin (2002) presented that a surrogate should possess the property of causal necessity: an individual effect of treatment on the endpoint Y can occur only if an individual effect of treatment on the surrogate S has occurred. They gave an numerical example to illustrate that the statistical surrogate S does not possess the property of causal necessity. For the individuals in the principal stratum defined by $S_{T=1} = S_{T=0}$, there is no individual treatment effect on the statistical surrogate S, but there may be individual, distributional and average treatment effects on the endpoint Y even if the conditional independence $Y \perp\!\!\!\perp T|S$ required by the statistical surrogate holds. To make a surrogate possess the property of causal necessity, Frangakis and Rubin (2002) defined that S is a principal surrogate if for all fixed s, comparison between the ordered sets

$$\{Y_{T=1}(u)\text{: for every individual } u \text{ of } S_{T=1}(u) = S_{T=0}(u) = s\}$$

and

$$\{Y_{T=0}(u)\text{: for every individual } u \text{ of } S_{T=1}(u) = S_{T=0}(u) = s\}$$

results in equality.

Lauritzen (2004) defined a strong surrogate by the causal network in Figure 2. A strong surrogate S is an intermediate variable which blocks the path from the treatment T to the endpoint Y. Thus a strong surrogate is also a principal surrogate. Lauritzen (2004) showed that if treatment is binary, then a principal surrogate and a strong surrogate are equivalent.

For all of the statistical, principal and strong surrogates, Chen, Geng and Jia (2007) showed that a treatment T has a positive causal effect on a surrogate S, and the surrogate has a positive causal effect on an endpoint Y, but the treatment T may have a negative effect on the endpoint Y.

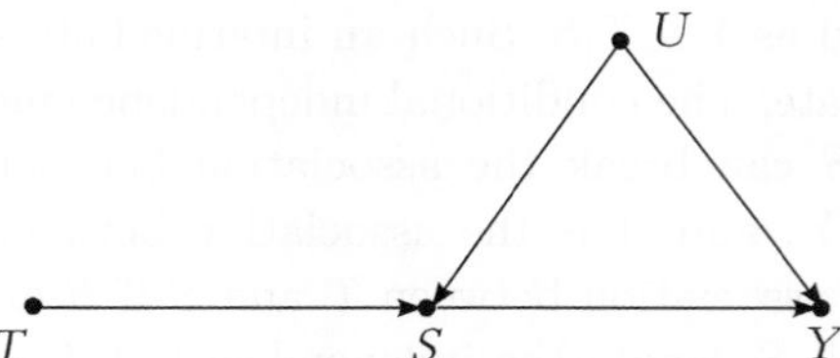

Fig. 2. A strong surrogate without direct effect of treatment on the endpoint.

This phenomenon is called the surrogate paradox or more generally the intermediate variable paradox. The surrogate paradox means that the sign of treatment effect on the endpoint cannot be predicted by the sign of treatment effect on the surrogate and the sign of causal effect of surrogate on the endpoint.

Moore (1995) gave a real example about the surrogate paradox. Doctors have the knowledge on irregular heartbeat that irregular heartbeat is a risk factor for sudden death and that correcting irregular heartbeat would prevent sudden death. Thus 'correction of heartbeat' as a surrogate, several drugs (Enkaid, Tambocor and Ethmozine) were approved by FDA. However a later CAST study showed that the correction of irregular heartbeat by these drugs did not improve survival times but increased mortality.

Below we give several numerical examples to show the surrogate paradox for the statistical, principal and strong surrogates, which also illustrate the difficulty for qualifying a surrogate to avoid the surrogate paradox.

Example 1. Let T denote a binary treatment, 1 for treated and 0 for control. Let S denote the correctness of irregular heartbeat, 1 for corrected and 0 for uncorrected; S_t denote the potential outcome of correctness if assignment of treatment were $T = t$ for $t = 0$ or 1. Let Y denote the survival time and Y_{st} the potential survival time if $T = t$ and $S = s$. Assume that the heartbeat status S is the unique intermediate variable on the path from treatment T to the endpoint Y, which means that the treatment effect on survival time is completely through the intermediate variable S, that is, $Y_{st} = Y_{st'} = Y_s$. Thus we have that $S_1 = S_0 = s$ implies $Y_{s0} = Y_{s1}$, and the heartbeat status is a principal surrogate and also a strong surrogate. Further we assume that correction of irregular heartbeat can increase survival time for every patient i, that is, $Y_{S=0}(i) < Y_{S=1}(i)$. Under these two assumptions, it seems that the correctness of irregular heartbeat can be used as a 'perfect' surrogate. But we give an artificial population with 100 patients of irregular heartbeat in Table 1 to show the phenomenon

Table 1. 100 patients with irregular heartbeat.

Strata	No of patients	$S_{T=0}$	$S_{T=1}$	$Y_{S=0} <$	$Y_{S=1}$	$Y_{T=0}$	$Y_{T=1}$
1	20	0	0	3	5	3	3
2	40	0	1	6	7	6	7
3	20	1	0	5	8	8	5
4	20	1	1	9	10	10	10

of the surrogate paradox. The 100 patients are stratified into four principal strata 1 to 4 defined by $(S_0 = 0, S_1 = 0)$, $(S_0 = 0, S_1 = 1)$, $(S_0 = 1, S_1 = 0)$ and $(S_0 = 1, S_1 = 1)$, as shown in columns 3 and 4. The number of patients in every strata is given in column 2. For simplicity, assume that all patient in the same principal stratum have the same potential survival time. Columns 5 and 6 give the potential survival times for patients in all principal strata, and some of them are prior counterfactual. For example, $Y_{S=1}$ in the strata 1 is prior counterfactual since $S = 1$ cannot be obtained by either treatment $T = 0$ or 1 unless it can be obtained by an intervention. From columns 3 to 6, we can obtain the potential survival times $(Y_{T=0}, Y_{T=1})$. For the population of the 100 patients given in Table 1, we have that the average causal effect of treatment on the correction of irregular heartbeat is positive

$$ACE_{T\to S} = \frac{40+20}{100} - \frac{20+20}{100} = \frac{20}{100} > 0,$$

but we obtain a negative treatment effect on the survival time

$$\begin{aligned} ACE_{T\to Y} = & \frac{3\cdot 20 + 7\cdot 40 + 5\cdot 20 + 10\cdot 20}{100} \\ & - \frac{3\cdot 20 + 6\cdot 40 + 8\cdot 20 + 10\cdot 20}{100} = -\frac{20}{100} < 0. \end{aligned}$$

Thus correction of irregular heartbeat S as a principal and strong surrogate leads to a phenomenon of the surrogate paradox.

In the above example, the surrogate paradox occurs since there is the principal stratum of $(S_{T=0} = 1, S_{T=1} = 0)$, which means that there are some patients for whom the treatment has a reverse effect on correction of irregular heartbeat. Below we give an example without this principal stratum of reverse effect, that is, variable T has a monotonic individual effect on the intermediate variable S.

Example 2. Let T denote the assigned treatment, 1 to the treatment group and 0 to the placebo group. Let S denote the actually accepted

Table 2. A surrogate paradox for $S_{T=1} \geq S_{T=0}$.

No of patients	Principal strata		Effect of S on Y		Effect of T on Y	
	$S_{T=0}$	$S_{T=1}$	$\#\{Y_{S=0}=1\}$	$\#\{Y_{S=1}=1\}$	$\#\{Y_{T=0}=1\}$	$\#\{Y_{T=1}=1\}$
100	0	0	80	80	80	80
100	0	1	60	50	60	50
100	1	1	0	20	20	20

treatment, 1 for treated and 0 for untreated; S_t denote the potentially accepted treatment if a patient were assigned to the treatment group of $T = t$. Let Y denote a binary endpoint, 1 for survival and 0 for death, and Y_{st} the potential survival status if $T = t$ and $S = s$. Also assume that the treatment effect on survival depends only on the actually accepted treatment, that is, $Y_{st} = Y_{st'} = Y_s$. Thus the accepted treatment is a principal and strong surrogate for the survival status. Instead of the monotonicity assumption of accepted treatment on survival status, we assume the monotonicity of treatment assignment on accepted treatment for each patient, that is, $S_{T=0} \leq S_{T=1}$. The artificial population is given in Table 2, where $\#\{Y_s = 1\}$ denotes the number of patients of $Y_s = 1$ in the population. If there is no noncompliance in a clinical trial where accepted treatment S is randomized, then we have

$$ACE_{S\to Y} = \frac{80+50+20}{300} - \frac{80+60+0}{300} = \frac{10}{300} > 0.$$

Thus the treatment is approved and is really applied to clinics. In clinical applications, however, patients may not comply perfectly with doctors' assignment of the treatment. Although the actually accepted treatment $S = 1$ has a positive effect on the endpoint Y and the treatment assignment has a monotonic effect on the actual treatment for every patient, the treatment assignment T may have a negative effect on the endpoint Y

$$ACE_{T\to Y} = \frac{80+50+20}{300} - \frac{80+60+20}{300} = -\frac{10}{300} < 0.$$

A phenomenon of the intermediate variable paradox occurs even for $S_{T=0} \leq S_{T=1}$. A drug S has a positive treatment effect on the endpoint Y, but the assignment T of the effective drug has a negative effect on the endpoint Y even if the assignment T can positively affect every patient to take the drug.

Further for a positive effect of treatment S on the endpoint Y, a higher compliance rate of treatment assignment T may lead to worse effect of

Table 3. Better compliance does not imply a better assignment effect on endpoint.

No of patients	Principal strata		Effect of S on Y		Effect of T on Y	
	$S_{T=0}$	$S_{T=1}$	$\#\{Y_{S=0}=1\}$	$\#\{Y_{S=1}=1\}$	$\#\{Y_{T=0}=1\}$	$\#\{Y_{T=1}=1\}$
50	0	0	30	40	30	30
100+50	0	1	60+50	50+40	110	90
100	1	1	0	20	20	20

treatment assignment T on the endpoint Y. As a numerical example, suppose that 50 of 100 never takers in the stratum of $(S_{T=0}=0, S_{T=1}=0)$ in Table 2 become to be compliance, as shown in Table 3. The compliance in Table 3 is better than that in Table 2, but the assignment effect on the endpoint $ACE_{T\to Y}=-20/300$ becomes worse than that in Table 2.

From columns 2 and 3 in Table 2, we have

$$ACE_{T\to S}=\frac{0+100+100}{300}-\frac{0+0+100}{300}=\frac{100}{300}.$$

Under the monotonicity assumption of treatment assignment on accepted treatment, the instrumental variable (IV) estimate of accepted treatment effect on the endpoint Y for the compliance group presented by Angrist, Imbens and Rubin (1996) is

$$ACE_{S\to Y|S_{T=0}=0,S_{T=1}=1}=\frac{ACE_{T\to Y}}{ACE_{T\to S}}=\frac{-10/300}{100/300}=-\frac{1}{10},$$

which can also be obtained directly from the principal stratum of $(S_{T=0}=0, S_{T=1}=1)$ in Table 2. Similarly, from Table 3, we have $ACE_{S\to Y|S_{T=0}=0,S_{T=1}=1}=-20/150$.

Notice that the IV estimate equation requires the monotonicity assumption of individual effect of T on S, that is, no patients have $(S_{T=0}=1, S_{T=1}=0)$. The monotonicity assumption cannot be assessed from the observed data. In practice, we cannot find such a S as the surrogate, and thus we cannot use the IV estimate equation to evaluate $ACE_{T\to Y}$ even if $ACE_{S\to Y|S_{T=0}=0,S_{T=1}=1}>0$ is known.

We show below two examples to illustrate that a positive treatment effect on a statistical surrogate which satisfies Prentice's criteria is not sufficient to ensure a positive treatment effect on the endpoint, even if the statistical surrogate has a monotonically positive causal effect on the endpoint or there exists a strong positive association between the statistical surrogate and the endpoint.

Table 4. The joint distribution of $(Y_{S=0}, Y_{S=1}, S_{T=0}, S_{T=1})$.

	$(Y_{S=0}, Y_{S=1}) = (0,0)$		$(Y_{S=0}, Y_{S=1}) = (0,1)$		$(Y_{S=0}, Y_{S=1}) = (1,1)$	
	$S_{T=0} = 1$	$S_{T=0} = 0$	$S_{T=0} = 1$	$S_{T=0} = 0$	$S_{T=0} = 1$	$S_{T=0} = 0$
$S_{T=1} = 1$	0.28	0.08	0.02	0.02	0.02	0.06
$S_{T=1} = 0$	0.02	0.10	0.04	0.10	0.02	0.24

Example 3. Also we assume that the sudden death depends only on the correctness of irregular heartbeat, that is, $Y_{st} = Y_{st'} = Y_s$ for $t \neq t'$, and that S has a monotonic effect on Y, that is, $Y_{S=0} \leq Y_{S=1}$. The two assumptions mean that the intermediate variable S has a strong causal mechanism on the endpoint Y. Now we give a distribution of $(Y_{S=0}, Y_{S=1}, S_{T=0}, S_{T=1})$ for an artificial population in Table 4. Assume that treatment T is randomized, that is, $T \perp\!\!\!\perp (Y_{S=0}, Y_{S=1}, S_{T=0}, S_{T=1})$. From this distribution, we can see that

$$p(Y_{S=s} = 1 | S_{T=1} = s) = p(Y_{S=s} = 1 | S_{T=0} = s),$$

which is equal to 0.5 and 0.025 for $s = 0$ and 1 respectively. By

$$\begin{aligned} p(Y_{S=s} = 1 | S_{T=1} = s) &= p(Y_{T=1} = 1 | S_{T=1} = s, T = 1) \\ &= p(Y = 1 | S = s, T = 1) = p(Y = 1 | S = s, T = 0) \\ &= p(Y_{S=s} = 1 | S_{T=0} = s), \end{aligned}$$

Prentice's conditional independence $Y \perp\!\!\!\perp T | S$ holds. From the joint distribution, we have

$$\begin{aligned} ACE_{T\to S} &= E(S_{T=1}) - E(S_{T=0}) \\ &= (0.28 + 0.08 + 0.02 + 0.02 + 0.02 + 0.06) \\ &\quad -(0.28 + 0.02 + 0.02 + 0.04 + 0.02 + 0.02) = 0.08 > 0, \end{aligned}$$

$$\begin{aligned} ACE_{S\to Y} &= E(Y_{S=1}) - E(Y_{S=0}) \\ &\quad [(0.02 + 0.02 + 0.04 + 0.10) + (0.02 + 0.06 + 0.02 + 0.24)] \\ &\quad -(0.02 + 0.06 + 0.02 + 0.24) = 0.18 > 0, \end{aligned}$$

but

$$\begin{aligned} ACE_{T\to Y} &= E(Y_{T=1}) - E(Y_{T=0}) \\ &= \sum_{s=0}^{1} P(Y_{S=s} = 1, S_{T=1} = s) - \sum_{s=0}^{1} P(Y_{S=s} = 1, S_{T=0} = s) \\ &= [(0.02 + 0.24) + (0.02 + 0.02 + 0.02 + 0.06)] \\ &\quad - [(0.06 + 0.24) + (0.02 + 0.04 + 0.02 + 0.02)] \\ &= -0.02 < 0. \end{aligned}$$

Table 5. The joint distribution of T, S and Y satisfying Prentice's criteria.

	$S=0$		$S=1$		$S=2$	
	$T=0$	$T=1$	$T=0$	$T=1$	$T=0$	$T=1$
$Y=0$	0.2565	0.152	0.015	0.002	0.012	0.080
$Y=1$	0.0135	0.008	0.285	0.038	0.018	0.120

Example 4. Consider the joint distribution of T, S and Y given in Table 5. From the joint distribution, we can see that Prentice's criterion $Y \perp\!\!\!\perp T|S$ is satisfied. Although the correlation between S and Y is quite strong ($r(S,Y) = 0.541$), we have a positive treatment effect on S ($DCE_{T\to(S>1)} = 0.45$ and $DCE_{T\to(S>0)} = 0.05$) but a negative treatment effect on Y ($DCE_{T\to(Y>0)} = -0.112$). This example explains that the sign of treatment effect on an endpoint cannot be predicted by the sign of treatment effect on a statistical surrogate.

In the following sections, we shall discuss criteria for surrogates to avoid the phenomenon of the surrogate paradox. The goal is that, instead of observing the endpoint Y, we observe a surrogate S and use the sign of treatment effect on an observed surrogate S to predict the sign of treatment effect on the unobserved endpoint Y.

3. Criteria for Surrogates Based on Prior Knowledge on Causation

Chen, Geng and Jia (2007) and Ju and Geng (2010) presented the criteria for surrogates based on causation. These criteria require the prior knowledge on the causal relationships among the variables of treatment, surrogate, endpoint and confounder.

Assume that a binary treatment T is randomized and that S is a strong surrogate as depicted in Figure 2, and thus the property of causal necessity is satisfied. For a binary treatment, a strong surrogate is equivalent to a principal surrogate. The strong surrogate S blocks the path from treatment T to the endpoint Y. Since the surrogate is an intermediate variable which is not randomized, there may be some confounder U between the surrogate S and the endpoint Y, which may be a confounder vector.

Consider the case that S is a discrete variable with values s_i for $i = 1, \ldots, I$. By the network for the strong surrogate, we have the conditional independence $Y \perp\!\!\!\perp T|(S,U)$, and the conditional DCEs of T on S and S on Y

given U are equal to the corresponding FDCEs. Thus it can be shown that the distributional causal effect of treatment on the endpoint conditionally on $U = u$ can be represented as

$$DCE_{T\to(Y>y)|u} = \sum_{i=1}^{I-1} DCE_{T\to(S>s_i)|u} DCE_{S\to(Y>y)|u}(s_{i+1}, s_i).$$

Similarly for the case of a continuous S, it can be represented as, for any s_0,

$$DCE_{T\to(Y>y)|u} = \int DCE_{T\to(S>s)|u} \frac{\partial DCE_{S\to(Y>y)|u}(s, s_0)}{\partial s} ds.$$

See Chen, Geng and Jia (2007) and Ju and Geng (2010) for details. Thus, given $U = u$, if T has a nonnegative conditional DCE on S and S has a nonnegative conditional DCE on Y, then T has a nonnegative conditional DCE on Y. If there is not any confounder U, a nonnegative (nonpositive) DCE of T on S and a nonnegative DCE of S on Y can predict a nonnegative (nonpositive) DCE of T on Y, and the surrogate paradox cannot occur. If there is a confounder U, then we have $ACE_{T\to Y} = \int ACE_{T\to Y|u} p(u)du$ and $DCE_{T\to(Y>y)} = \int DCE_{T\to(Y>y)|u} p(u)du$. We can predict a nonnegative DCE of treatment T on the endpoint Y by all the nonnegative conditional DCEs of treatment T on the endpoint Y given $U = u$ From the above equations, we can obtain the following result.

Theorem 1. *A nonnegative (nonpositive) DCE of T on S can predict a nonnegative (nonpositive) ACE of T on Y, and a null DCE of T on S can predict a null ACE of T on Y if*

1. *the ACE of S on Y conditional on $U = u$ is non-negative for all u, and*
2. *the DCE of T on S conditional on $U = u$ does not change its sign (nonnegative or nonpositive) with changes in u.*

Further if

3. *conditional on some $U = u$, both the ACE of S on Y is positive and the DCE of T on S has the strict inequality sign ('> 0' or '< 0'),*

then a positive (negative) DCE of T on S can predict a positive (negative) ACE of T on Y.

Also the sign of DCE of T on Y can be predicted by replacing all of the above 'ACE' with 'DCE'.

If the DCE of S on Y conditional on $U = u$ is non-positive for all u, then we can define $S^* = -S$ or $Y^* = -Y$ so that condition 1 holds. According to Theorem 1, we need to know the conditional DCE signs given unobserved confounder U in order to predict the sign of DCE of treatment on the endpoint Y by the sign of DCE of treatment on the surrogate S, and then the phenomenon of the surrogate paradox cannot occur.

Condition 1 means that the surrogate S is a risk (or protective) factor to the endpoint Y conditional on any u. For example, irregular heartbeat is a risk fact to sudden death in every subpopulation of $U = u$. Condition 2 means that conditional DCE of treatment T on the surrogate S given $U = u$ has the same sign for all u, although we may not know whether it is positive or negative. For example, the new drug does not have negative effect to correct irregular heartbeat in every subpopulation of $U = u$ or it does not have positive effect. Condition 3 means the strict sign of inequality (>0 or <0) of conditional causal effects of T on S and S on Y given some $U = u$ simultaneously hold so that the causal effect of T on Y conditional on some u has a strict positive or negative sign, and this probability is not zero.

Let $\alpha_i, \beta_i, \gamma_i$ denote parameters, and let $\alpha_i(), \beta_i(), \gamma_i()$ denote unknown functions in the following models. Chen, Geng and Jia (2007) proved that the equation of ACEs for $s > s'$

$$ACE_{T\to Y} = \frac{ACE_{T\to S}ACE_{S\to Y}(s, s')}{s - s'}$$

holds under the following two models:

- Model I: linear models

$$E(Y|S = s, U = u) = \alpha_1 s + \gamma_1(u),$$

  and
- Model II: semi-parametric models

$$E(Y|S = s, U = u) = s\beta_1(u) + \gamma_1(u),$$
$$\text{and } E(S|T = t, U = u) = \beta_2(t) + \gamma_2(u).$$

On the other hand, this equation gives an IV estimation equation of $ACE_{S\to Y}(s, s')$ for the models more general than linear models when there is a confounder U between S and Y.

Ju and Geng (2010) discussed several commonly-used models including generalized linear models and proportional hazard models, which satisfy the conditions of Theorem 1. Let $g\{\}$ and $h\{\}$ be strictly monotonic link functions in the following models:

- Model A: generalized linear models

$$g\{E(Y|S=s,U=u)\}=\alpha_1 s+\gamma_1(u),$$
$$h\{E(S|T=t,U=u)\}=\alpha_2 t+\gamma_2(u),$$

  where $\alpha_1>0$.

- Model B: extended generalized linear models

$$g\{E(Y|S=s,U=u)\}=\alpha_1(s)\beta_1(u)+\gamma_1(u),$$
$$h\{E(S|T=t,U=u)\}=\alpha_2(t)\beta_2(u)+\gamma_2(u),$$

  where $\alpha_1(s)\geq 0$ and $\alpha_2(t)$ are monotone functions, and both $\beta_1(u)$ and $\beta_2(u)$ do not change their signs with changes in u.

- Model C: proportional hazard models

$$\lambda(y|S=s,U=u)=\lambda_0(y)\exp\{\alpha_1 s+\gamma_1(u)\},$$
$$\lambda^*(s|T=t,U=u)=\lambda_0^*(s)\exp\{\alpha_2 t+\gamma_2(u)\},$$

  where $\lambda()$ and $\lambda^*()$ denote hazard functions, $\lambda_0()$ and $\lambda_0^*()$ are baseline hazards, and $\alpha_1>0$.

- Model D: extended proportional hazard models

$$\lambda(y|S=s,U=u)=\lambda_0(y)\{\alpha_1(s)\beta_1(u)+\gamma_1(u)\},$$
$$\lambda^*(s|T=t,U=u)=\lambda_0^*(s)\{\alpha_2(t)\beta_2(u)+\gamma_2(u)\},$$

  where $\alpha_1(s)\geq 0$ and $\alpha_2(t)$ are monotone functions, and both $\beta_1(u)$ and $\beta_2(u)$ do not change their signs with changes in u.

Models A and B are about the expectations rather than probabilities. Thus the signs of α_1, α_2, $\alpha_1(s)$ and $\alpha_2(t)$ in these models are related to the signs of ACEs, but they are not related to the signs of DCEs. To have them related to the signs of DCEs, we assume that S conditional on T and U is from the exponential family with the density

$$p(s|u,t;\theta_t,\phi)=\exp\{\frac{s\theta_t-b_u(\theta_t)}{a_u(\phi)}+c_u(s,\phi)\}.$$

For example, Poisson, binomial and inverse binomial distributions and the normal distribution belong to the exponential family. In fact, the exponential family makes that $ACE_{T\to S|u}$ and $DCE_{T\to(S>s)|u}$ have the same strict sign (null, positive, or negative).

Under models A and B, the sign of ACE of S on Y is the same as the sign of ACE of S on Y conditional on U (i.e., the sign of α_1 or $\alpha_1(s)$). Thus if the sign of ACE of S on Y is known, condition 1 can always be satisfied (if necessary, define $S^* = -S$ or $Y^* = -Y$). But the sign of DCE of S on Y may not be the same as the sign of DCE of S on Y conditional on U. To make them have the same sign, we further assume that Y conditional on S and U is from the exponential family with the density

$$p(y|u, s; \theta_s, \phi) = \exp\{\frac{y\theta_s - b'_u(\theta_s)}{a'_u(\phi)} + c'_u(y, \phi)\}.$$

Under models A and B, this assumption also makes the signs of ACEs and DCEs conditional on U and not conditional on U have the same sign. Thus to have models A and B satisfy condition 1 and to predict the sign of ACE of T on Y, we need the prior knowledge on the sign of ACE of S on Y; and similarly to predict the sign of DCE of T on Y, we need the prior knowledge on the sign of DCE of S on Y.

For these models A and C, further the conditions 2 and 3 in Theorem 1 hold (i.e., the sign does not change with changes in u and the strict signs hold), and thus the surrogate S can be used to predict the strict sign (positive, negative or null) of distributional causal effect of treatment on the endpoint Y. For these models B and D, only the condition 2 in Theorem 1 hold, but $\alpha_2(t)$ may not be a strictly monotonic function of t, and thus the surrogate S can be used to predict the sign (non-negative, non-positive or null) of distributional causal effect of treatment on the endpoint Y.

Define a model AC as a hybrid model that the first model equation for Y comes from model A, and the second model equation for S comes from model C. Then the hybrid models AC and CA satisfy the conditions 1 to 3 in Theorem 1, and they can be used to predict the strict sign (positive, negative or null) of DCE of treatment effect on the endpoint. The hybrid models BD and DB also satisfy the conditions 1 and 2, and they can be used to predict the sign (non-negative, non-positive or null) of DCE of treatment effect on the endpoint.

Below we give some common parametric models and their combinations in Table 6 where (X, Z) are replaced by (Y, S) and (S, T). If we know $\alpha > 0$ for the model of Y, then all of these models satisfy the conditions 1 to 3, and thus the intermediate variable S for these model can be used to avoid the surrogate paradox and to predict the strict sign of treatment effect on the endpoint.

Table 6. Parametric models which satisfy conditions 1 to 3 of Theorem 1 in Theorem 1.

Model	Form
Linear regression	$E(X\|Z = z, U = u) = \alpha z + \gamma(u)$
Logistic regression	$\text{logit}\{p(X = 1\|Z = z, U = u)\} = \alpha z + \gamma(u)$
Poisson regression	$\log\{E(X\|Z = z, U = u)\} = \alpha z + \gamma(u)$
Cox regression	$\lambda(x\|Z = z, U = u) = \lambda_0(x)\exp\{\alpha z + \gamma(u)\}$

Since U is never observed, these conditions and these models cannot be tested from observed data even if Y is observed in a validation study, and thus we need prior knowledge on causation. On the other hand, the causation-based criteria require that all paths from treatment T to the endpoint Y are blocked by the intermediate variable S, which means no direct effect from T to Y, that is, there is no other paths from T to Y. This requirement can hardly be checked from observed data unless we have a knowledge on the causal mechanism. The advantage of causation-based criteria for surrogates is that the prior knowledge may be obtained by causal mechanisms from experts, but the disadvantages are the empirical untestability and the requirement of no direct treatment effect of on the endpoint.

4. Criteria for Surrogates Based on Prior Knowledge on Association

To remove the disadvantages of the untestability and the requirement of no direct treatment effect for the criteria based on causation, Wu, He and Geng (2011) presented the criteria based on association, which require the prior knowledge on association between the unobserved endpoint and other variables. Unlike the conditions based on causation, these conditions based on association are testable if the endpoint Y is observed in a validation study, and they do not require no direct treatment effect on the endpoint.

Theorem 2. *A non-negative DCE of treatment T on S can predict a non-negative ACE of treatment T on Y if*

1. $FACE_{S\to Y|T=1}(s's'') \geq 0$ *for all* $s' > s''$ *or* $FACE_{S\to Y|T=0}(s's'') \geq 0$ *for all* $s' > s''$, *and*
2. $FACE_{T\to Y|s} \geq 0$ *for all* s.

Notice that a non-negative ACE of T on S is not sufficient to predict a non-negative ACE of T on Y. In addition, a null DCE of T on S cannot ensure a null ACE of T on Y since there may be a direct effect of treatment on the endpoint. If the endpoint Y is observed, the conditions 1 and 2 can be tested by observed data. The condition 1 requires that the monotonicity property of the expectation of Y in s holds for only one of treatment groups not necessary for both groups. Particularly for the control group of $T = 0$, the control treatment (such as a placebo) may be used in the previous trials, and thus a prior knowledge on the condition 1 for $T = 0$ may come from the previous trials. The condition 2 describes the monotonicity property in t that the treatment T non-negatively associates with the endpoint given the surrogate. When Prentice's conditional independence $Y \perp\!\!\!\perp T|S$ holds, the condition 2 holds.

This theorem also shows that to avoid the surrogate paradox, we need to add one more condition to Prentice's criteria: the conditional expectation of the endpoint in the control treatment group is a monotonic function of the surrogate, that is, $FACE_{S \to Y|T=0}(s's'') \geq 0$ for all $s' > s''$. For example, irregular heartbeat is a risk fact to sudden death without treated, while it is not required that irregular heartbeat must also be a risk fact to sudden death in the treatment group.

The condition 2, however, may not hold in some situations. For the stratification defined by the observed intermediate S instead of the principal stratification defined by the potential outcome $(S_{T=1}, S_{T=0})$, the individuals in the treated group of $T = 1$ may not comparable with those in the control group of $T = 0$ (Frangakis and Rubin, 2002). Thus the condition 2 does not means that treatment T has a direct positive effect on the endpoint Y. For example, for two persons who have the regular heartbeat $S = 1$: one from the treated group of $T = 1$ and the other from the control group of $T = 0$, the treated one may have a less probability of survival $Y = 1$ than the control one (i.e., a negative conditional association between T and Y given $S = 1$) since the treated one with worse background got the regular heartbeat by treatment, although, in the causal mechanism, the treatment may have a positive direct effect on the endpoint Y.

Theorem 3. *A non-negative DCE of treatment T on S can predict a non-negative DCE of treatment T on Y if*

1. $FDCE_{S \to (Y>y)|T=1}(s's'') \geq 0$ *for all y and $s' > s''$ or* $FDCE_{S \to (Y>y)|T=0}(s's'') \geq 0$ *for all y and $s' > s''$, and*
2. $FDCE_{T \to (Y>y)|s} \geq 0$ *for all y and s.*

Comparing the conditions for predicting the ACE sign of T on Y, the conditions on the monotonicity of the expectations is replaced by the monotonicity of the distribution function in the above theorem, and the testability and the implication of these conditions are the same. Also a null DCE of T on S cannot ensure a null DCE of T on Y since there may be a direct effect of treatment on the endpoint.

If these conditions for predicting the signs of ACE and DCE do not hold, we may try to redefine $S^* = -S$ or/and $T^* = 1 - T$ and then check these conditions with S^* and T^*. Similarly the prediction of the non-positive ('≤ 0') treatment effect on the endpoint Y can be obtained by defined $Y^* = -Y$. The prediction of the non-negative ('≥ 0') treatment effect on the endpoint can be strengthened to the prediction of strict positive ('> 0') effect if the conditions satisfy stricter inequalities in probability.

The above conditions for the prediction cannot ensure that the reverse prediction is true, and there are the cases that the ACE or DCE sign of treatment on the endpoint cannot be predicted. For example, a null or positive DCE of treatment on the endpoint Y, while $DCE_{T\to(S>s)} < 0$ for some s even if the conditions 1 and 2 hold. Thus the DCE and ACE signs of treatment effect on the endpoint may not be predicted by a negative DCE of treatment on the surrogate S.

Below we discuss the conditions for the equivalence relation between the signs of treatment effects on the surrogate and on the endpoint, under which the prediction and the reverse prediction are simultaneously true.

Assume that the intermediate variable S conditional on $T = t$ is from the exponential family whose density function has the form

$$p(s|t;\theta_t,\phi) = \exp\{\frac{s\theta_t - b(\theta_t)}{a(\phi)} + c(s,\phi)\}.$$

In fact, the exponential family ensures that $ACE_{T\to S}$ and $DCE_{T\to S}$ have the same strict sign (null, positive, or negative).

Theorem 4. *Under the assumptions of S from the exponential family and the conditional independence $Y \perp\!\!\!\perp T|S$, $ACE_{T\to S}$, $DCE_{T\to S}$ and $ACE_{T\to Y}$ have the same sign (null, positive, or negative) if $FACE_{S\to Y}(s', s'') > 0$ for all $s' > s''$. Further $DCE_{T\to Y}$ also has the same strict sign (null, positive, or negative) as them if $FDCE_{S\to(Y>y)}(s', s'') > 0$ for all y and all $s' > s''$.*

The assumption of the conditional independence $Y \perp\!\!\!\perp T|S$ can be relaxed to $Y \perp\!\!\!\perp T|(S, X)$, where X contains all confounders which are simultaneous predictors of S and Y. In this case, we have to assume that X is completely observed, and thus the above results also hold conditionally on $X = x$.

Now we consider the following extension of generalized linear models:

$$h\{E(Y|S = s, T = t)\} = \alpha(s) + \beta t + c,$$

where $\alpha(s)$ is a known function, and $h\{\}$ is a strictly monotonic increasing link function. To make both $FACE_{S\to Y|t}(s', s'')$ and $FDCE_{S\to(Y>y)|t}(s', s'')$ have the same sign and $FACE_{T\to Y|s}$ and $FDCE_{T\to(Y>y)|s}$ have the same sign, assume that Y conditional on $T = t$ and $S = s$ is from the exponential family

$$p(y|s, t; \theta_{st}, \phi) = \exp\left\{\frac{y\theta_{st} - b(\theta_{st})}{a(\phi)} + c(y, \phi)\right\}.$$

Then a positive DCE of T on S predicts a positive DCE of T on Y if

1. $\alpha(s)$ strictly monotonically increases as s increases, and
2. $\beta \geq 0$.

Further if

3. conditional independence $Y \perp\!\!\!\perp T|S$ holds (i.e., $\beta = 0$), and
4. S is from the exponential family conditional on T,

then $DCE_{T\to S}$ and $DCE_{T\to Y}$ have the same strict sign (null, positive, or negative).

Ordinarily, for a generalized linear model, the function $\alpha(s)$ is defined as αs. If $\alpha \neq 0$, then the conditions 1 and 2 always hold for S (or $S^* = -S$) and T (or $T^* = -T$) respectively. Thus for the generalized linear model of Y, the intermediate variable S can always be used as a surrogate to qualitatively assess the DCE on an unobserved endpoint. Furthermore, we have the equivalence relation between the signs of the treatment effects on the surrogate and the endpoint if the intermediate variable S is from the exponential family conditional on T.

Consider the proportional hazard model

$$\lambda(y|S = s, T = t) = \lambda_0(y)\exp\{\alpha(s) + \beta t\},$$

where $\lambda_0()$ is a baseline hazard, and $\alpha(s)$ is a known function. If $\beta \leq 0$ and $\alpha(s)$ strictly monotonically decreases as s increases, then a positive DCE of treatment on S predicts a positive DCE of treatment on Y. Further if $Y \perp\!\!\!\perp T|S$ (i.e., $\beta = 0$) and S is from the exponential family conditional on T, then the DCE of T on S and the DCE of T on Y have the same strict sign (null, positive, or negative).

5. Discussion

We discussed the criteria for surrogates, and we pointed out that many commonly-used criteria cannot avoid the phenomenon of the surrogate paradox, that is, a treatment has a positive effect on a surrogate, and the surrogate has a positive effect on an endpoint, but the treatment has a negative effect on the endpoint. To avoid the surrogate paradox, we described the causation-based criteria and the association-based criteria so that the sign of treatment effect on an unobserved endpoint can be predicted by the sign of treatment effect on an observed surrogate. If the generalized linear models, the proportional hazard models and some of their extended models are assumed for the association and causation relationships among the variables of the treatment, surrogate, endpoint and confounder between surrogate and endpoint, then the nonoccurrence of the surrogate paradox is essentially assumed.

The causation-based criteria for surrogates require the prior knowledge on the causal mechanism which may be derived from experts. But the causal mechanism involves a confounder between the surrogate and the endpoint and require that the surrogate blocks all paths from the treatment to the endpoint. The knowledge on the causal mechanism cannot be checked from the observed data even if the endpoint is observed. The association-based criteria require the prior knowledge on association relationships among the variables of treatment, surrogate and the endpoint, they do not require that the surrogate blocks all paths from treatment to the endpoint and thus the property of causal necessity may not be satisfied. The knowledge on association can be checked from the observed data if the endpoint is observed in a validation study, but it is not always translated directly from knowledge of causal mechanisms.

We only discussed the qualitative evaluation of treatment effects, but the quantitative evaluation may be more important in practice. The quantitative approaches require that the measures of associations in the previous validation studies can be transferred quantitatively to the future studies. For example, the proportion of the treatment effect (PTE) proposed by Freedman and Graubard (1992) assess the surrogate validation based on associations among variables obtained in previous validation studies, and Li, Taylor and Elliott (2010) proposed a Bayesian approach for assessing principal surrogates. Since environments and conditions in future trials may be different from those in previous validation studies, the quantitative results obtained in previous validation studies may not be applicable to future studies. The qualitative evaluation are still applicable as long as the monotonicity of causation or association in the future is the same as that in the previous randomized trials. Both of the qualitative and quantitative approaches have their respective merits and could therefore be used in parallel in real applications.

Acknowledgements

I would like to thank my students, Dr Zhenguo Wu, Dr Ping He, Chuan Ju, Peng Ding, Zhichao Jiang, Peng Luo and Wang Miao, for their discussion on the related topics. The research is supported by Center for Statistical Science, Peking University and NSFC (10931002, 11171365, 10721403, 11021463).

References

1. Alonso, A., Molenbergh, G. (2008). Surrogate end points: hopes and perils. *Expert Review of Pharmacoeconomics and Outcomes Research* **8**: 255–259.
2. Angrist, J., Imbens, G. and Rubin, D. (1996). Identification of causal effects using instrumental variables. *J. Amer. Statist. Assoc.* **91**: 444–472.
3. Baker, S. G. (2006). Surrogate endpoints: wishful thinking or reality? *Journal of the National Cancer Institute* **98**: 502–503.
4. Baker, S. G. and Kramer, B. S. (2003). A perfect correlate does not a surrogate make. *BMC Medical Research Methodology*, **3**: 16.
5. Berger, V. W. (2004). Does the Prentice criterion validate surrogate endpoints? *Statistics in Medicine* **23**: 1571–1578.
6. Burzykowski, T., Molenberghs, G. and Buyse, M. (2005). *The Evaluation of Surrogate Endpoints.* Springer: New York.
7. Chen, H., Geng, Z. and Jia. J. (2007). Criteria for surrogate endpoints. *Journal of the Royal Statistical Society, Series B* **69**: 919–932.
8. Fleming, T. R. and DeMets, D. L. (1996). Surrogate end points in clinical trials: are we being misled? *Annals of Internal Medicine* **125**: 605–613.
9. Frangakis, C. E. and Rubin, D. B. (2002). Principal stratification in causal inference. *Biometrics* **58**: 21–29.
10. Freedman, L. S. and Graubard, B. I. (1992). Statistical validation of intermediate endpoints for chronic diseases. *Statistics in Medicine* **11**: 167–178.
11. Ju, C. and Geng, Z. (2010). Criteria for surrogate endpoints based on causal distributions. *Journal of the Royal Statistical Society, Series B* **72**: 129–142.
12. Lauritzen, S. L. (2004). Discussion on causality. *Scandinavian Journal of Statistics* **31**: 189–192.
13. Li, Y., Taylor, J. M. G. and Elliott, M. R. (2010). A Bayesian approach to surrogacy assessment using principal stratification in clinical trials. *Biometrics* **66**: 523–531.

14. Manns, B., Owen, W. F., Winkelmayer, W. C., Devereaux, P. J. and Tonelli, M. (2006). Surrogate markers in clinical studies: problems solved or created? *American Journal of Kidney Diseases* **48**: 159–166.
15. Moore, T. (1995). *Deadly Medicine: Why Tens of Thousands of Patients Died in America's Worst Drug Disaster*. New York: Simon & Schuster.
16. Prentice, R. L. (1989). Surrogate endpoints in clinical trials: definition and operational criteria. *Statistics in Medicine* **8**: 431–440.
17. Wu, Z. G., He, P. and Geng, Z. (2011). Sufficient conditions for concluding surrogacy based on observed data. *Statistics in Medicine* **30**: 2422–2434.

About the Author

Dr. Zhi Geng is Professor of School of Mathematical Sciences, Peking University. He received the B.S. degree from Shanghai Jiaotong University, Shanghai, China in 1982, and Ph.D. degree from Kyushu University, Fukuoka, Japan in 1989. He has been a faculty member of Peking University since 1989, ISI elected member since 1996, and associated editor of Comp. Statist. & Data Analysis since 1991. His research interests include causal inference, causal networks, and incomplete data analysis.

CHAPTER 20

ADAPTIVE TRIAL DESIGN IN CLINICAL RESEARCH

ANNPEY PONG

Principal Scientist of Biostatistics and
Research Decision Science
Merck Research Laboratories,
126 E. Lincoln Avenue
RY34 A240, Rahway, NJ 07065, USA
annpey.pong@merck.com

SHEIN-CHUNG CHOW

2424 Erwin Road Ste 1102
11068 Hock Plaza Durham,
NC 27705, USA
sheinchung.chow@duke.edu

1. Introduction

In the past several decades, it is recognized that increasing spending of biomedical research does not reflect an increase of the success rate of pharmaceutical (clinical) development. Woodcock (2005) indicated that the low success rate of pharmaceutical development could be due to (i) a diminished margin for improvement that escalates the level of difficulty in proving drug benefits, (ii) genomics and other new science have not yet reached their full potential, (iii) mergers and other business arrangements have decreased candidates, (iv) easy targets are the focus as chronic diseases are harder to study, (v) failure rates have not improved, (vi) rapidly escalating costs and complexity decreases willingness/ability to bring many candidates forward into the clinic.[79] As a result, the United States Food and Drug Administration (FDA) kicked off a *Critical Path Initiative* to assist the sponsors in identifying the scientific challenges underlying the medical product pipeline problems. In 2006, the FDA released a *Critical Path Opportunities List* that calls for advancing innovative trial designs, especially for the use of prior experience or accumulated information in trial design. Many researchers interpret it as the encouragement for the use of innovative adaptive design methods in clinical trials, while some researchers believe it is for the use of Bayesian approach.

The purpose of adaptive design methods in clinical trials is to give the investigator the flexibility for identifying best (optimal) clinical benefit of the test treatment under study without undermining the validity and integrity of the intended study. The concept of adaptive design can be traced back to 1970s when the adaptive randomization and a class of designs for sequential clinical trials were introduced.[77] As a result, most adaptive design methods in clinical research are referred to as adaptive randomization,[1, 24, 33, 44, 67, 68, 77] group sequential designs with the flexibility for stopping a trial early due to safety, futility and/or efficacy,[15, 45, 47, 51, 66, 75] and sample size re-estimation at interim for achieving the desired statistical power.[21, 23, 72] The use of adaptive design methods for modifying the trial and/or statistical procedures of ongoing clinical trials based on accrued data has been practiced for years in clinical research. Adaptive design methods in clinical research are very attractive to clinical scientists due to the following reasons. First, it reflects medical practice in real world. Second, it is ethical with respect to both efficacy and safety (toxicity) of the test treatment under investigation. Third, it is not only flexible, but also efficient in the early phase of clinical development. However, it is a concern whether the p-value or confidence interval regarding the treatment effect obtained after the modification is reliable or correct. In addition, it is also a concern that the use of adaptive design methods in a clinical trial may lead to a totally different trial that is unable to address scientific/medical questions that the trial is intended to answer.[25, 26]

In recent year, the potential use of adaptive design methods in clinical trials have attracted much attention. The Pharmaceutical Research and Manufacturers of America (PhRMA) and Biotechnology Industry Organization (BIO) have established adaptive design working groups and proposed strategies, methodologies, and implementations for regulatory consideration.[30] However, there are no universal agreement in terms of definition, methodologies, and applications. Many journals have published special issues on adaptive design. These journals included, but are not limited to, Biometrics (Vol. 62, No. 3), Statistics in Medicine (Vol. 25, No. 19), Journal of Biopharmaceutical Statistics (Vol. 15, No. 4 and Vol. 17, No. 6), Biometrical Journal (Vol. 48, No. 4), and Pharmaceutical Statistics (Vol. 5, No. 2). For a comprehensive summarization of the issues and recommendations for the use of adaptive design methods, it may look up Chow and Chang (2006), Chang (2007), and Pong and Chow (2010).[8,12,59]

In the next section, commonly employed adaptations and the resultant adaptive designs are briefly described. Also included in this section are regulatory and statistical perspectives regarding the use of adaptive design methods in clinical trials. The impact of protocol amendments, challenges of *by design* adaptations, and obstacles of retrospective adaptations when applying adaptive design methods in clinical trials are discussed in Sections 3–5, respectively. Some concluding remarks are given in the last section.

2. What is Adaptive Design?

In clinical trials, it is not uncommon to modify trial procedures and/or statistical methods during the conduct of clinical trials based on the review of accrued data at interim. The purpose is not only to efficiently identify clinical benefits of the test treatment under investigation, but also to increase the probability of success of the intended clinical trial. Trial procedures are referred to as the eligibility criteria, study dose, treatment duration, study endpoints, laboratory testing procedures, diagnostic procedures, criteria for evaluability, and assessment of clinical responses. Statistical methods include randomization scheme, study design selection, study objectives/hypotheses, sample size calculation, data monitoring and interim analysis, statistical analysis plan, and/or methods for data analysis. In this chapter, we will refer to the adaptations (changes or modifications) made to the trial and/or statistical procedures as the adaptive design methods. Thus, an adaptive design is defined as a design that allows adaptations to trial and/or statistical procedures of the trial after its initiation without undermining the validity and integrity of the trial.[14] With the emphasis of the feature of by design adaptations only (rather than ad hoc adaptations), the PhRMA Working Group on Adaptive Design refers to an adaptive design as a clinical trial design that uses accumulating data to decide on how to modify aspects of the study as it continues, without undermining the validity and integrity of the trial.[30] In February 2010, a draft guidance on *Adaptive Design Clinical Trials for Drugs and Biologics* by the FDA was circulated for comments.[27] The FDA draft guidance defines an adaptive design as a study that includes a *prospectively* planned opportunity for modification of one or more specified aspects of the study design and hypotheses based on analysis of (usually interim) data from subjects in the study. The FDA draft guidance is a document describing the potential use of adaptive designs in clinical trials. It is generally viewed as supportive of the use of adaptive designs if they are employed properly. The FDA draft guidance is not a specific guidance for the implementation of adaptive designs in clinical trials. It, however, noted that adaptive designs have been used at times in confirmatory contexts, for the most part cautiously, limited to changes such as sample size re-estimation and treatment arm consolidation in the early phase of clinical development where there is more uncertainty and regulatory concerns are minimized. In many cases, an adaptive design is also known as a flexible design.[25–26]

2.1. *Adaptations*

An adaptation is referred to as a modification or a change made to trial procedures and/or statistical methods during the conduct of a clinical trial. By definition, adaptations that are commonly employed in clinical trials can be classified into the categories of prospective adaptation, concurrent (or ad hoc) adaptation, and retrospective adaptation. Prospective adaptations include, but are not limited to, adaptive randomization, stopping a trial early due to safety, futility or efficacy at interim analysis, dropping the losers (or inferior treatment groups), sample size re-estimation, and etc. Thus, prospective adaptations are usually referred to as by design adaptations as described in the PhRMA white paper.[30] Concurrent adaptations are usually referred to as any ad hoc modifications or changes made as the trial continues. Concurrent adaptations include, but are not limited to, modifications in inclusion/exclusion criteria, evaluability criteria, dose/regimen and treatment duration, changes in hypotheses and/or study endpoints, and etc. Retrospective adaptations are usually referred to as modifications and/or changes made to statistical analysis plan prior to database lock or unblinding of treatment codes. In practice, prospective, ad hoc, and retrospective adaptations are implemented by study protocol, protocol amendments, and statistical analysis plan with regulatory reviewer's consensus, respectively.

2.2. *Type of adaptive designs*

Based on the adaptations employed, commonly considered adaptive designs in clinical trials include, but are not limited to: (i) an adaptive randomization design, (ii) a group sequential design (iii) an N-adjustable (or sample size re-estimation) design, (iv) a drop-the-losers (or pick-the-winners) design, (v) an adaptive dose finding design, (vi) a biomarker-adaptive design, (vii) an adaptive treatment-switching design, (viii) an adaptive-hypothesis design, (ix) an adaptive seamless (e.g., phase I/II or phase II/III) trial design, and (x) a multiple adaptive design. These adaptive designs are briefly described below.

Adaptive randomization design — An adaptive randomization design is a design that allows modification of randomization schedules based on varied and/or unequal probabilities of treatment assignment in order to increase the probability of success. Commonly applied adaptive randomization procedures include treatment-adaptive randomization,[24,44] covariate-adaptive randomization, and response-adaptive randomization.[33,67,68] For example, a simple randomization may cause an imbalance of prognostic factors among treatment groups (e.g., a greater proportion of "very ill" subjects are assigned to a particular treatment group) for small or moderate clinical trials. The baseline adaptive randomization will improve the chance of having balance among treatment groups with respect to the prognostic factors.

Although an adaptive randomization design could increase the probability of success, it may not be feasible for a large trial or a trial with relatively long treatment duration because the randomization of a given subject depends on the response of the previous subject. A large trial or a trial with a relatively long treatment duration utilizing adaptive randomization design will take a much longer time to complete. Besides, randomization schedule may not be available prior to the conduct of the study. Moreover, statistical inference on treatment effect is often difficult to obtain if it is not impossible due to complicated probability structure as the result of adaptive randomization.

Group sequential design — A group sequential design is a design that allows for prematurely stopping a trial due to safety, futility/efficacy or both with options of additional adaptations based on results of interim analysis. Various stopping boundaries based on different boundary functions for controlling an overall type I error rate are available in the literature.[12,38,39,45,68,76] In recent years, the concept of two-stage adaptive design has led to the development of the adaptive group sequential design.[23,47,51,60]

Unlike a traditional single-stage clinical trial in which the data remain blinded until the conclusion of the study, for example, a two-stage allows adaptive designs that permit increasing the sample size at the end of stage I while still protecting the type I error rate. It should be noted that the standard methods for group sequential design may not be appropriate (i.e., it may not be able to control the overall type I error rate at the desired level of 5%) if there is a shift in target patient population due to additional adaptations or protocol amendments.

Sample size re-estimation design — A sample size re-estimation (or N-adjustable) design is referred to as an adaptive design that allows for sample size adjustment or re-estimation based on the observed data at interim. Sample size adjustment or re-estimation could be done in either a blinding or unblinding fashion based on the criteria of treatment effect-size, conditional power, and/or reproducibility probability.[21,23,29,50,60,64,72] Sample size re-estimation suffers from the same disadvantage as the original power analysis for sample size calculation prior to the conduct of the study because it is performed by treating estimates of the study parameters, which are obtained based on data observed at interim, as true values. It is not a good clinical/statistical practice to start with a small number and then perform sample size re-estimation (adjustment) at interim by ignoring the clinically meaningful difference that one wishes to detect for the intended clinical trial. It should be noted that the observed difference at interim based on a small number of subjects may not be of statistically significant (i.e., it may be observed by chance alone). In addition, there is variation associated with the observed difference which is an estimate of the true difference. Thus, standard methods for sample size re-estimation based on the observed difference with a limited number of subjects may be biased and misleading.

Drop-the-losers design — A drop-the-losers design is a design that allows dropping the inferior treatment groups. A drop-the-losers design also allows adding additional arms. A drop-the-losers design is useful in phase II clinical development especially when there are uncertainties regarding the dose levels.[3,6,61,69] The selection criteria and decision rules play important roles for drop-the-losers designs. Dose groups that are dropped may contain valuable information regarding dose response of the treatment under study. Typically, drop-the-losers design is a two-stage design. At the end of the first stage, the inferior arms will be dropped based on some pre-specified criteria. The winners will then proceed to the next stage. In practice, the study is often powered for achieving a desired power at the end of the second stage (or at the end of the study). In other words, there may not be any statistical power for the analysis at the end of the first stage for dropping the losers (or picking up the winners). In this case, it is a common practice to drop the losers or pick up the winners based on so-called precision analysis, i.e., an approach for determining the confidence level for achieving a statistical significance. Note that some clinical scientists prefer the term pick-the-winners designs.

Adaptive dose finding design — An adaptive dose finding (e.g., escalation) design is often used in early phase clinical development to identify the minimum effective dose (MED) and/or the maximum tolerable dose (MTD), which is used to determine the dose level for the next phase clinical trials.[5,78,80] For adaptive dose finding design, the method of continual re-assessment method (CRM) in conjunction with Bayesian approach is usually considered.[10,56,57] Mugno *et al.* (2004) introduced a nonparametric adaptive urn design approach for estimating a dose-response curve.[53] More details regarding PhRMA's proposed statistical methods, the reader may consult with a special issue recently published at the Journal of Biopharmaceutical Statistics, Vol. 17, No. 6.

Biomarker-adaptive design — A biomarker-adaptive design is a design that allows for adaptations based on the response of biomarkers such as genomic markers. An adaptive-biomarker design involves biomarker qualification and standard, optimal screening design, and model selection and validation. It should be noted that there is a gap between identifying biomarkers that associated with clinical outcomes and establishing a predictive model between relevant biomarkers and clinical outcomes in clinical development. For example, correlation between biomarker and true clinical endpoint makes a prognostic marker. However, correlation between biomarker and true clinical endpoint does not make a predictive biomarker. A *prognostic biomarker* informs the clinical outcomes, independent of treatment. They provide information about the natural course of the disease in individuals who have or have not received the treatment under study. Prognostic markers can be used to separate good- and poor-prognosis patients at the time of diagnosis. A *predictive biomarker* informs the treatment effect on the clinical endpoint.[9]

A biomarker-adaptive design can be used to (i) select right patient population (e.g., enrichment process for selection of a better target patient population), (ii) identify nature course of disease, (iii) early detection of disease, and (iv) help in developing personalized medicine.[9,11,75]

Adaptive treatment-switching design — An adaptive treatment-switching design is a design that allows the investigator to switch a patient's treatment from an initial assignment to an alternative treatment if there is evidence of lack of efficacy or safety of the initial treatment.[7,70] In cancer clinical trials, estimation of survival is a challenge when treatment-switching has occurred in some patients. A high percentage of subjects who switched due to disease progression could lead to change in hypotheses to be tested. In this case, sample size adjustment for achieving a desired power is necessary.

Adaptive-hypotheses design — An adaptive-hypotheses design refers to a design that allows modifications or changes in hypotheses based on interim analysis results.[34] Adaptive-hypotheses designs often considered before database lock and/or prior to data unblinding. Some examples include the switch from a superiority hypothesis to a non-inferiority hypothesis and the switch between the primary study endpoint and the secondary endpoints. For the switch from a superiority hypothesis to a non-inferiority hypothesis, the selection of non-inferiority margin is critical which has an impact on sample size adjustment for achieving the desired power. According to the ICH guideline, the selected non-inferiority margin should be both clinical and statistical justifable.[17,37]

Adaptive seamless trial design — An adaptive seamless trial design is referred to a program that addresses within single trial objectives that are normally achieved through separate trials of clinical development. An adaptive seamless design is an adaptive seamless trial design that would use data from patients enrolled before and after the adaptation in the final analysis.[40,52] Commonly considered adaptive seamless trials in clinical development are an adaptive seamless phase I/II design in early clinical development and an adaptive seamless phase II/III trial design in late phase clinical development. An adaptive seamless phase II/III design is a two-stage design consisting of a learning or exploratory stage (phase IIb) and a confirmatory stage (phase III). A typical approach is to power the study for the phase III confirmatory phase and obtain valuable information with certain assurance using confidence interval approach at the phase II learning stage. Its validity and efficiency, however, has been challenged.[73] Moreover, it is not clear how to perform a combined analysis if the study objectives (or endpoints) are similar but different at different phases.[16] Further research is needed.

Multiple adaptive design — Finally, a multiple adaptive design is any combinations of the above adaptive designs. Commonly considered multiple-adaptation designs include (i) the combination of adaptive group sequential design, drop-the-losers design, and adaptive seamless trial design and (ii) adaptive dose-escalation design with adaptive randomization.[12, 58] In practice, since statistical inference for a multiple-adaptation design is often difficult, it is suggested that a clinical trial simulation be conducted to evaluate the performance of the resultant multiple adaptive design at the planning stage.

Note that as indicated in its draft guidance, the FDA classifies adaptive designs into *well-understood* designs and *less well-understood* designs. Well-understood design refers to the typical group sequential design, which has been employed in clinical research for years. Less well-understood designs include the adaptive dose finding and two-stage phase I/II (or II/III) seamless designs. Many scientific issues surrounding the less well-understood designs are posted in the draft guidance without recommendations for resolution. This raises the question whether the use of adaptive design methods in clinical trials (especially for those less well-understood designs) is ready for implementation in practice.

2.3. *Regulatory/Statistical perspectives*

From regulatory point of view, the use of adaptive design methods based on accrued data in clinical trials may introduce operational bias such as selection bias, method of evaluation, early withdrawal, and modification of treatment. Consequently, it may not be able to preserve the overall type I error rate at the pre-specified level of significance. In addition, p-values may not be correct and the corresponding confidence intervals for the treatment effect may not be reliable. Moreover, it may result in a totally different trial that is unable to address the medical questions that original study intended to answer. Li (2006) also indicated that commonly seen adaptations which have an impact on the type I error rate include, but are not limited to, (i) sample size adjustment at interim, (ii) sample size allocation to treatments, (iii) delete, add, or change treatment arms, (iv) shift in target patient population such as changes in inclusion/exclusion criteria, (v) change in statistical test strategy, (vi) change in study endpoints, and (vii) change in study objectives such as the switch from a superiority trial to a non-inferiority trial.[48] As a result, it is difficult to interpret the clinically meaningful effect size for the treatments under study.[66]

From statistical point of view, major (or significant) adaptations to trial and/or statistical procedures could (i) introduce bias/variation to data collection, (ii) result in a shift in location and scale of the target patient population, and (iii) lead to inconsistency between hypotheses to be tested and the corresponding statistical tests. These concerns will not only have an impact on the accuracy and reliability of statistical inference drawn on the treatment effect, but also present challenges to biostatisticians for development of appropriate statistical methodology for an unbiased and fair assessment of the treatment effect.

Note that although the flexibility of modifying study parameters is very attractive to clinical scientists, several regulatory questions/concerns arise. First, what level of modifications to the trial procedures and/or statistical procedures would be acceptable to the regulatory authorities? Second, what are the regulatory requirements and standards for review and approval process of clinical data obtained from adaptive clinical trials with different levels of modifications to trial procedures and/or statistical procedures of ongoing clinical trials? Third, has the clinical trial become a totally different clinical trial after the modifications to the trial procedures and/or statistical procedures for addressing the study objectives of the originally planned clinical trial? These concerns should be addressed by the regulatory authorities before the adaptive design methods can be widely accepted in clinical research and development.

3. Impact of Protocol Amendments

3.1. *Moving target patient population*

In practice, for a given clinical trial, it is not uncommon to have 3–5 protocol amendments after the initiation of the clinical trial. One of the major impacts of many protocol amendments is that the target patient population may have been shifted during the process, which may have resulted in a totally different target patient population at the end of the trial. A typical example is the case when significant adaptation (modification) is applied to inclusion/exclusion criteria of the study. Denote by the target patient population with the mean μ and standard deviation σ for the primary endpoint. After a given protocol amendment, the resultant (actual) patient population may have been shifted to (μ_1, σ_1), where $\mu_1 = \mu + \varepsilon$ is the population mean of the primary study endpoint and $\sigma_1 = C\sigma$ $(C > 0)$ is the population standard deviation of the primary study endpoint. The shift in target patient population can be characterized by $|\frac{\mu_1}{\sigma_1}| = |\frac{\mu+\varepsilon}{C\sigma}| = \Delta|\frac{\mu}{\sigma}|$, where $\Delta = \frac{1+\varepsilon/\mu}{C}$. Chow and Chang (2006) refer to Δ as a sensitivity index measuring the change in effect size between the actual patient population and the original target patient population.[12]

Denote by, $(\mu_i \ \sigma_i)$ the actual patient population after the ith modification of trial procedure, where $\mu_i = \mu + \varepsilon_i$ and $\sigma_i = C_i\sigma$, $i = 0, 1, \ldots, K$. Note that $i = 0$ reduces to the original target patient population (μ, σ). That is, when $i = 0$, $\varepsilon_0 = 0$ and $C_0 = 1$. After K protocol amendments, the resultant actual patient population becomes (μ_K, σ_K), where $\mu_K = \mu + \sum_{i=1}^{K} \varepsilon_i$ and $\sigma_K = \prod_{i=1}^{K} C_i\sigma$. It should be noted that (ε_i, C_i), $i = 1, \ldots, K$ are in fact random variables. As a result, the resultant actual patient population following certain modifications to the trial procedures is a *moving* target patient population rather than a fixed target patient population.

The impact of protocol amendments on statistical inference due to shift in target patient population (moving target patient population) can be studied through a model that link the moving population means with some covariates.[12, 18, 74] Chow and Shao (2005) derived statistical inference for the original target patient population for simple cases. Their approach and recommendations for improvement are briefly outline below.[17]

3.2. *Statistical inference with covariate adjustment*

Suppose that there are a total of K protocol amendments for a given clinical trial that compares I treatments. Let μ_{i0} be the mean of the study endpoint of the original target patient population under treatment i and μ_{ik} be the mean of the patient population under treatment i after the kth protocol amendment. Suppose that the parameters of interest are μ_{i0}'s (not μ_{ik}) with $k = 1, \ldots, K$. If the differences among $\mu_{i0}, \mu_{i1}, \ldots, \mu_{ik}$ are ignored and statistical inference is made by pooling all data (before and after protocol amendment), then the conclusion drawn on μ_{i0}'s may be biased and misleading. Assuming that there is a relationship between μ_{ik}'s and a covariate vector x. Chow and Shao (2005) considered the following regression model[17]

$$\mu_{ik} = \alpha_i + \beta_i' x_{ik}, \quad k = 0, 1, \ldots, K, \quad i = 1, \ldots, I, \tag{1}$$

where α_i is an unknown parameter, β_i is a vector of unknown parameters, and β_i' is the transpose of β_i. The best example is the change of patient inclusion/exclusion criterion due to the problem of not enough patients. In Model (1), it is assumed x_{ik} is fixed and known so that α_i and β_i can be estimated through a regression between $\bar{y}_{ik}$ and $\bar{x}_{ik}$, where $\bar{y}_{ik}$ and $\bar{x}_{ik}$ are the sample mean of the study endpoint and the sample mean of the fixed known x-covariates, respectively, under treatment i after modification k,

$i = 1, \ldots, I$, $k = 0, 1, \ldots, K$. Once α_i and β_i are estimated, μ_{i0} can be estimated from $\mu_{i0} = \alpha_i + \beta_i' \bar{x}_{i0}$.

In practice, however, x_{ik} is often an observed random covariate vector and model (1) should be replaced by

$$\mu_{ik} = \alpha_i + \beta_i' v_{ik}, \quad k = 0, 1, \ldots, K, \quad i = 1, \ldots, I, \tag{2}$$

where ν_{ik} is the population mean of the covariate under treatment i after modification k. Let y_{ikj} be the observed study endpoint from the jth patient under treatment i after amendment k and x_{ikj} be the associated observed covariate, $j = 1, \ldots, n_{ik}$, $k = 0, 1, \ldots, K$, $i = 1, \ldots, I$. There is room for improvement by the following two directions.

First, under model (2), we estimate μ_{ik} by $\bar{y}_{ik}$ (the sample mean of $\bar{y}_{ik_1}, \ldots, \bar{y}_{ikn_{ik}}$) and ν_{ik} by $\bar{x}_{ik}$ (the sample mean of $\bar{x}_{ik_1}, \ldots, \bar{x}_{ikn_{ik}}$). Then, we estimate α_i and β_i by the weighted least squares estimates $\hat{\alpha}_i$ and $\hat{\beta}_i$ in a "regression" between $\bar{y}_{ik}$ and $\bar{x}_{ik}$ for each fixed i. The parameter μ_{i0} is estimated by $\hat{\mu}_{i0} = \hat{\alpha}_i + \hat{\beta}_i' \bar{x}_{i0}$. Statistical inference (such as hypothesis testing and confidence intervals) can be made using $\hat{\mu}_{i0}$ and its exact or asymptotic distribution can be derived accordingly. Second, a more efficient statistical inference can be made if we replace model (2) by the following stronger model:

$$E(y_{ikj}|x_{ikj}) = \alpha_i + \beta_i' x_{ikj}, \quad j = 1, \ldots, n_{ik}, \quad k = 0, 1, \ldots, K, \quad i = 1, \ldots, I \tag{3}$$

Under this model, we can first fit a regression between y_{ikj} and x_{ikj} for each fixed i to obtain the least squares estimates $\hat{\alpha}_i$ and $\hat{\beta}_i$. Then, μ_{i0} is estimated by $\hat{\mu}_{i0} = \hat{\alpha}_i + \hat{\beta}_i' \bar{x}_{i0}$. Statistical inference can be made using $\hat{\mu}_{i0}$ and its exact or asymptotic distribution can be derived. Note that model (3) is stronger than model (2) so that we need to balance the gain in efficiency over bias due to the violation of model (3).

As an alternative to model (1), we may consider a random-deviation model. Suppose that there exist random variables δ_{ik}, $k = 1, \ldots, K$, $i = 1, \ldots, I$, such that

$$\mu_{ik} = \mu_{i0} + \delta_{ik}, \quad k = 1, \ldots, K, \quad i = 1, \ldots, I. \tag{4}$$

This means that the population mean after the kth protocol amendment deviates from the mean of the target population by a random effect δ_{ik}. Of course, we may consider combining models (1) and (4):

$$\mu_{ik} = \alpha_i + \beta_i' x_{ik} + \delta_{ik}, \quad k = 1, \ldots, K, \quad i = 1, \ldots, I.$$

Under model (4) and the assumptions that, conditional on δ_{ik}'s, y_{ikj}'s are independent with mean μ_{ik} in (4) and variance σ^2, where y_{ikj} is the study endpoint for the jth patient under treatment $i$after modification k. Then, the observed data follow a mixed effects model. Consequently, the existing statistical procedures for mixed effects models can be applied to the estimation or inference. A further assumption can be imposed to model (4).

$$y_{ik} = \mu_{i0} + \lambda_k + \gamma_{ik} + \varepsilon_{ikj}, \quad i = 1, \ldots, I \quad k = 1, \ldots, K, . \tag{5}$$

where λ_k's, γ_{ik}'s (which reflect the "interaction" between treatment and λ_k), ε_{ikj} are independently normal distributed with mean zero and variances $\sigma_\lambda^2, \sigma_\gamma^2$, and σ^2, respectively. Gallo and Khuri (1990) derived an exact test for the unbalanced mixed effects model (5).[31] Although other refinements were developed,[20, 43, 55] these existing tests do not have explicit forms; so the computation is complicated.

Note that model (4) can be modified under the Bayesian frame work. For future methodology development based on statistical inference with covariate adjustment, it is of interest to consider (i) a more complex situations such as unequal sample sizes n_{ik} and/or unequal variances after protocol amendments, (ii) deriving approximations to the integrals involved in the posterior probabilities, (iii) studying robustness of the choices of prior parameters, and (iv) alternative forms of null hypotheses such as $-a \le \theta \le a$ with a given $a > 0$.

3.3. *Inference based on mixture distribution*

The primary assumption of the above approaches is that there is a relationship between μ_{ik}'s and a covariate vector x. In practice, such covariates may not exist or may not be observable. In this case, it is suggested assessing the sensitivity index and consequently deriving a unconditional inference for the original target patient population assuming that the shift parameter (i.e., ϵ) and/or the scale parameter (i.e., C) is random.[12] It should be noted that effect of ϵ_i could be offset by C_i for a given modification i as well as by (ϵ_j, C_j) for another modification j. As a result, estimates of the effects of (ϵ_i, C_i), $i = 1, \ldots, K$ are difficult, if not impossible, to obtain. In practice, it is desirable to limit the combined effects of (ϵ_i, C_i), $i = 0, \ldots, K$ to an acceptable range for a valid and unbiased assessment of treatment effect regarding the target patient population based on clinical data collected from the actual patient population.

4. Challenges in By Design Adaptations

In clinical trials, commonly employed by design (prospective) adaptations include stopping the trial early due to safety, futility, and/or efficacy, sample size re-estimation (adaptive group sequential design), dropping the losers (adaptive dose finding design), and combining two separate trials into a single trial (adaptive seamless design). In this section, major challenges in these by design adaptations will be described. Recommendations for resolution are provided whenever possible.

4.1. *Adaptive group sequential design*

The group sequential design has a long history of application in clinical trials. It is a design in which the accumulating data are analyzed at a series of interim analyses during the course of the trial. The main purpose of the group sequential design is to allow the trail to be stopped for clinical benefit or harm at an interim analysis. The idea of adaptive group sequential design started in early 1990's. It allows a wide range of modifications to the trial design at each interim analysis. For example, the sample size for a future interim analysis may be re-calculated based on the observed treatment differences at the current interim analysis using accumulated data. Results on sample size re-calculation and other modifications can be found in the literature.[23,35,36,39,41,47,49,50,62–65,71]

Consider a group sequential design with K interim analyses without adaptation (i.e., there is no change in the trial design after each interim analysis). Let Z_k be the test statistic at the kth interim analysis such that H_0 is rejected and the trial will be stopped if $|Z_k| > c_{\alpha,k,\kappa}$, where $c_{\alpha,k,\kappa}$ is a constant depending on k, κ, and the significance level α. For $k = 1, \ldots, K-1$, the trial continues if $|Z_k| \leq c_{\alpha,k,\kappa}$. At the last stage $k = K$, the trial stops and H_0 is concluded if $|Z_k| \leq c_{\alpha,k,\kappa}$. Consequently, the overall type I error rate for this procedure is

$$\alpha_K = \sum_{k=1}^{K} P(|Z_k| > c_{\alpha,k,K}, |Z_1| \leq c_{\alpha,1,K}, \ldots, |Z_{k-1}| \leq c_{\alpha,k-1,K} | H_0) \quad (6)$$

If we choose $c_{\alpha,k,\kappa}$'s to satisfy $\alpha_K = \alpha$, then the overall type I error rate is maintained. The selection of $c_{\alpha,k,\kappa}$'s relies on the distributions of Z_k's under H_0. When Z_k is a standard normal random variable based on data accumulated up to the kth interim analysis, the most popular choice of $c_{\alpha,k,\kappa}$'s is Pocock's $c_{\alpha,1,\kappa} = \cdots = c_{\alpha,k,\kappa}$ given in a table by Pocock (1977).[58] Since

$c_{\alpha,k,\kappa}$'s are not uniquely determined, various modifications to Pocock's test have been proposed, for example, O'Brien and Fleming's test, Wang and Tsiatis' test, and the inner wedge test.[38]

The assumption that Z_k's are standard normal, however, does not hold in most practical situations. It holds approximately when the sample size at each interim analysis is large enough, based on the central limit theorem. Consider for example a parallel-group design with two treatments. Let x_{ikj} be the response from patient j under treatment i at the kth interim analysis, $i = 1, 2$, $j = 1, \ldots, n, k = 1, \ldots, K$. Let $\bar{x}_{ik} = \frac{1}{kn}\sum_{j=1}^{n} x_{ikj}$, $i = 1, 2, k = 1, \ldots, K$. Assume x_{ikj}'s are independently normal with mean μ_i and variance σ^2. If H_0: $\mu_1 = \mu_2$ and σ^2 is known, then $Z_k = \sqrt{kn}(\bar{x}_{1k} - \bar{x}_{2k})/\sqrt{2\sigma^2}$ is standard normal under H_0, $k = 1, \ldots, K$, and α_K in (6) is exactly equal to α with Pocock's $c_{\alpha,k,\kappa}$. In practice, σ^2 is usually unknown and has to be estimated. If σ^2 is replaced by the pooled sample variance, then Z_k has a t-distribution instead of the standard normal. As a result, α_K in (6) is not α and the overall type I error rate is not maintained. Of course, $\alpha_K \to \alpha$ as $n \to \infty$, because of the central limit theorem.

One of major challenges for an adaptive group sequential design is that the overall type I error rate may be inflated when there is a shift in target patient population.[28] To overcome this problem, we suggest studying the effect of unknown σ^2 and sample size n in the selection of $c_{\alpha,k,\kappa}$, for various methods and study designs. With Pocock's method, for example, the simulation results in Table 1 show that the overall type I error rate α_K can be much larger than $\alpha(=0.05)$, when σ^2 is replaced by the pooled sample variance (i.e., each Z_k is not normal but t-distributed). The simulation was carried out using two treatments, equal sample size n for any treatment and interim analysis, up to $K = 5$ stages, and simulation size 50,000. For $K = 2, 3, 4, 5$, Pocock's $c_{0.05,k;K}$ values do not depend on k and are 2.178, 2.289, 3.361, 4.413, respectively.

From Table 1, the overall type I error rates are greater than the nominal level 0.05. As the sample size n increases, these error rates are closer to 0.05. But the results for small n are not satisfactory. We also note that the number of stages does not have a large effect, since the overall type I error rates are quite close across the stages when the sample size n is fixed. Thus, developing a new procedure of choosing $c_{\alpha,k,\kappa}$'s is suggested so that the overall type I error rate α_K is exactly equal to α, when σ^2 is replaced by the pooled sample variance in various group sequential tests. The new $c_{\alpha,k,\kappa}$ depends on the sample size n. A statistical table or software for $c_{\alpha,k,\kappa}$ with different n will be constructed.

Table 1. Overall type I error rate for Pocock's test.

	K			
n	2	3	4	5
2	0.197	0.198	0.195	0.198
3	0.129	0.127	0.127	0.124
4	0.100	0.101	0.101	0.100
5	0.089	0.089	0.086	0.086
6	0.081	0.079	0.079	0.079
7	0.076	0.074	0.075	0.075
8	0.071	0.070	0.071	0.071
9	0.069	0.069	0.068	0.069
10	0.067	0.067	0.065	0.067
11	0.066	0.063	0.066	0.066
12	0.063	0.065	0.065	0.064
13	0.061	0.059	0.061	0.061
14	0.063	0.062	0.062	0.061
15	0.062	0.061	0.061	0.060
16	0.061	0.058	0.059	0.059
17	0.058	0.059	0.059	0.058
18	0.060	0.056	0.057	0.060
19	0.058	0.059	0.058	0.058
20	0.058	0.059	0.056	0.058
21	0.059	0.058	0.056	0.056
22	0.057	0.057	0.057	0.057
23	0.058	0.055	0.056	0.057
24	0.057	0.057	0.055	0.058
25	0.056	0.056	0.058	0.054
26	0.057	0.055	0.057	0.056
27	0.056	0.055	0.055	0.053
28	0.056	0.055	0.055	0.055
29	0.054	0.056	0.055	0.055
30	0.054	0.057	0.054	0.055

An adaptive group sequential design is attractive to sponsors in clinical development because it allows adaptations of the trial after each interim to meet specific needs within limited budget or resources and target timelines. However, some adaptations may introduce bias/variation to data collection as the trial continues. To account for these (expected and/or unexpected) biases/variation, statistical tests are necessary adjusted to maintain the overall type I error and the related sample size calculation formulas have to be modified for achieving the desired power. Statistical inference on moving patient population described in the previous section can be applied to the adaptive group sequential design when the adaptations at each interim analysis may alter the patient population. The problem for the adaptive group sequential design is more difficult, since the test procedure is much more complicated. Thus, for future development, it is worthy pursuing the following specific directions that (i) deriving valid statistical test procedures for adaptive group sequential designs assuming model (2) or (3), which relates the data from different interim analyses, (ii) deriving valid statistical test procedures for adaptive group sequential designs assuming the random-deviation model (5), (iii) deriving valid Bayesian methods for adaptive group sequential designs, and (iv) deriving sample size calculation formulas for various situations.

4.2. *Adaptive dose finding design*

Chang and Chow (2005) proposed a hybrid Bayesian adaptive design for dose escalation study, which involves the steps of (i) construction of utility function, (ii) probability model for dose-response, (iii) the selection of a prior, (iv) the re-assessment of model parameters, (v) update of the utility function, (vi) the determination of the next action (i.e., treatment assignment of the next subject near the estimated MTD).[10]

In early clinical development for establishing a dose response relationship, an adaptive multistage design is commonly used.[5] The adaptive multistage design allows various adaptations of the design in one or two prescheduled interim analyses. The idea of an adaptive multistage design for establishing dose response relationship is not only to reassess the sample size by using the observed variability and/or effects, but also to reduce the set of multiple endpoints to suitable subsets. In addition, the adaptive multistage design allows selecting a subset of doses for further experimentation. More specifically, let's consider a two-stage scenario. One would start with two doses from the conjectured therapeutic dose range. If in the pre-scheduled interim analysis there is no sufficient trend, the doses may be changed (e.g., by lowering the low dose and/or increasing the high dose). The second stage of the experiment will be performed and the overall decision relies on a combination test of the test results from the two stages separately. It, however, should be noted that the adaptive multistage design for establishing dose response relationship suffers the disadvantage that only the p-values of the samples are combined but no pooling of the samples itself is performed. This leads to a crucial point of interpretation.

For dose-toxicity studies, the "3 + 3" or more generally, the "m+n" traditional escalation rules (TER) are commonly used in early phase of oncology studies. Recently, many new methods such as the assessment of dose response using multiple-stage designs.[22] and the continued reassessment method (CRM)[2, 56, 57] have been developed. For the method of CRM, the dose-response relationship is continually reassessed based on accumulative data collected from the trial. The next patient who enters the trial is then assigned to the potential MTD level. This approach is more efficient than that of the usual TER with respect to the allocation of the MTD. However, the efficiency of CRM may be at risk due to delayed response and/or a constraint on dose-jump in practice.[2] In recent years, the use of adaptive design methods for characterizing dose response curve has become very popular.[5] An adaptive design is a dynamic system that allows the investigator to optimize the trial (including design, monitoring, operating, and analysis) with cumulative information observed from the trial. For Bayesian adaptive design for dose response trials, some researchers suggest the use of loss/utility function in conjunction with dose assignment based on minimization/maximization of loss/utility function.[32, 78]

Let $X = \{x_1, x_2, \ldots, x_K\}$ be the action space where x_i is the coded value for action of anything that would affect the outcomes or decision-making such as a treatment, a withdrawal of a treatment arm, a protocol amendment, stopping the trial or any combination of the above. In practice, x_i can be either a fixed dose or a variable dose given to a patient. If action x_i is not taken, then $x_i = 0$. Let $y = \{y_1, y_2, \ldots, y_m\}$ be the outcomes of interest, which can be efficacy or toxicity of a test treatment. In each of these outcomes, y_i is a function of action $y_i(x), x. \in X$. The utility is then defined as $U = \sum_{j=1}^{m} w_j \sum_{j=1}^{m} w(y_i)$ where U is normalized such that $0 \leq U \leq 1$ and w_j are pre-specified weights. To allow more patients to be assigned to superior treatment groups, the target randomization probability to x_i group should be proportional to the current estimation of utility or response rate of the group, that is $U(x_i)/\sum_{i=1}^{K} U(x_i)$ where K is the number of groups. As a result, the utility-adaptive randomization can be given. It is to be noted that the hybrid Bayesian adaptive design method for dose response curve is multiple endpoints oriented.[10] Thus, it can be used for various situations. The method can be improved by the following specific directions that (i) studying the relative merits and disadvantage of their method under various adaptive methods, (ii) examining the performance of an alternative method by forming the utility first with different weights to the response levels and then modeling the utility, and (iii) deriving sample size calculation formulas for various situations.

4.3. *Adaptive seamless designs*

As indicated earlier, an adaptive seamless design is a two-stage design that consists of two phases namely a learning (or exploratory) phase and a confirmatory phase. One of the major challenges for designs of this kind is that different study endpoints are often considered at different stages for achieving different study objectives. In this case, the standard statistical methodology for assessment of treatment effect and for sample size calculation cannot be applied.

For a two-stage adaptive design, Bauer and Kohne (1994) proposed a method using Fisher's combination of independent p-values based on subsamples from different stages.[4] Their method provides a great flexibility in the selection of statistical methods for hypothesis testing of subsamples. However, the choices for the stopping boundaries are not flexible to meet practical needs.[54] As an alternative, it was proposed using linear combination of the independent p-values.[8] This method provides great flexibility in the selection of stopping boundaries, which can be calculated manually.[12] Chang's method, however, is valid under the assumption of constancy of the target patient populations, study objectives, and study endpoints at different stages. As pointed out earlier, it is most likely that the study objectives and study endpoints are different at different stages in practice. To have a valid and fair assessment of treatment effect based on combined data from the two stages, appropriate test statistics are necessarily developed.

Assuming that a two-stage adaptive seamless design utilizes two different study endpoints. At the first stage (learning or exploratory phase), the same study endpoint with a much shorter treatment duration or a biomarker is used. At the second stage (confirmatory phase), regular clinical study endpoint is used. Under the assumption that there exists a relationship between the two study endpoints, i.e., the first study endpoint is predictive of the second study endpoint, an appropriate test statistic can be developed. Let x_i be the observation of the study endpoint (e.g., biomarker) at the first stage from the ith subject, $i = 1, \ldots, n$ and y_j be the observation of the study endpoint (the primary clinical endpoint) from the jth subject, $j = 1, \ldots, m$. Assume that x_{i}'s are independently and identically distributed with $E(x_i) = \nu$ and $Var(x_i) = \tau^2$; and $y_j's$ are independently and identically distributed with $E(y_j) = \mu$ and $Var(y_j) = \sigma^2$. Suppose that x and y can be related in a simple relationship as follows:

$$y = \beta_0 + \beta_1 x + \epsilon,$$

where ϵ is an error term with zero mean and variance ξ^2. Furthermore, ϵ is independent of x. Thus μ can be estimated by $\hat{\mu} = w\bar{\hat{y}} + (1-w)\bar{y}$, where $\bar{\hat{y}} = \frac{1}{n}\sum_{i=1}^{n}\hat{y}_i$, $\bar{y} = \frac{1}{m}\sum_{j=1}^{m} y_j$ and $0 \leq w \leq 1$. Note that $\hat{\mu}$ is the minimum variance unbiased estimator among all weighted mean estimators when the weight is given by $w = [n/(\beta_1^2\tau^2)]/[n/(\beta_1^2\tau^2) + m/\sigma^2]$. Based on the result of Khatri and Shah (1974),[42] the variance of $\hat{\mu}$ can be approximated with a given bias order. Thus, under a given set of hypotheses (e.g., hypotheses for non-inferiority or equivalence) for evaluation of treatment effect can be derived accordingly.

In practice, when designing a clinical trial, the first question that the investigator will ask is how many subjects do we need in order to achieve the desired power at the pre-specified significance level. For a two-stage adaptive design with different study endpoints, sample size calculation also involves the allocation of sample sizes n and m at the two different stages. Let $m = \rho n$. Then the total sample size $N = (1+\rho)n$. For simplicity, consider testing the hypotheses for equality, n can be derived accordingly. Note that a two-stage adaptive seamless design can be viewed as a group sequential design with one planned interim analyses.[19]

Remarks — In the previous section for illustration purpose, we only consider the case where the study endpoints are continuous variables. In practice, the study endpoints could be discrete (e.g., binary responses), time-to-event data, or mixed types of data. In these cases, similar idea can be carried out for development of appropriate statistical methods for analysis of the combined data under the assumption that there is a well-established relationship between the two study endpoints.

As indicated earlier, the traditional sample size calculation is often estimated by sample mean and sample variance from a small pilot study. Note that sample size calculation based on $s^2/\hat{\delta}^2$ is rather instable. As an alternative, it is suggested that the median of $s^2/\hat{\delta}^2$ be considered. As it can be seen the bias of the median approach can be substantially smaller than the mean approach for a small sample size and/or small effect size. However, in practice, we do not know the exact value of the median of $s^2/\hat{\delta}^2$. In this case, a bootstrap approach may be useful.[46]

5. Obstacles of Retrospective Adaptations

In practice, retrospective adaptations such as adaptive-hypotheses are commonly encountered prior to database lock (or unblinding) and implemented through the development of statistical analysis plan. To illustrate the impact of retrospective adaptations, for simplicity, we will only consider the common situation for modifying hypotheses is switching a superiority hypothesis to a non-inferiority hypothesis. For a promising test drug, the sponsor would prefer an aggressive approach for planning a superiority study. The study is usually powered to compare the promising test drug with an active control agent. Let μ_T and μ_A be the mean efficacies of the test drug and the active control agent, respectively. Testing for superiority of the test drug over the active control agent amounts to testing the following hypotheses:

$$H_0\colon \mu_T \leq \mu_A + \Delta \quad \text{versus} \quad H_1\colon \mu_T > \mu_A + \Delta, \tag{7}$$

where $\Delta > 0$ is a known mixed superiority margin. If the null hypothesis H_0 in (7) is rejected, then we can conclude that the test drug is superior to the active control agent since μ_T is larger than μ_A by a fixed margin Δ.

However, the collected data may not support superiority. Instead of declaring the failure of the superiority trial, the sponsor may switch from testing superiority to testing the following non-inferiority hypotheses:

$$H_0\colon \mu_T \leq \mu_A - \Delta \quad \text{versus} \quad H_1\colon \mu_T > \mu_A - \Delta. \tag{8}$$

If the null hypothesis H_0 in (8) is rejected, then we can conclude that the test drug is not worse than the active control agent by the margin Δ. Typically, the margin is carefully chosen so that $\mu_A - \Delta$ is larger than the placebo effect and, thus, declaring non-inferiority to the active control agent means that the test drug is superior to the placebo effect. The switch from a superiority hypothesis to a non-inferiority hypothesis will certainly increase the probability of success of the trial because the study objective has been modified to establishing non-inferiority rather than showing superiority. This type of switching hypotheses is accepted to the regulatory agency such as the U.S. FDA, provided that the impact of the switch on statistical issues (e.g., the determination of non-inferiority margin Δ) and inference (e.g., appropriate statistical methods) on the assessment of treatment effect is well justified.

To illustrate the concept of switching a superiority hypothesis to a non-inferiority hypothesis, we consider a parallel-group design with one interim analysis. Both groups for the test drug and active control agent have n patients at the interim analysis, and have additional n patients if the trial continues. For simplicity, assume that data are normally distributed with known variances σ_T^2 and σ_A^2 for the test drug and the active control agent, respectively. At the interim analysis, a superiority test rejects H_0 in (7) if $Z_1 > c_{1,\alpha}$, where $Z_1 = \sqrt{n}(\bar{d}_1 - \Delta)/\sqrt{\sigma_A^2 + \sigma_T^2}$, $\bar{d}_1$ is the difference between the sample mean of the test drug and the sample mean of the active control agent, α is a given significance level, and $c_{1,\alpha}$ is a constant specified according to (9). The trial continues if $Z_1 \leq c_{1,\alpha}$. Let $Z_2 = \sqrt{2n}(\bar{d}_2 - \Delta)/\sqrt{\sigma_A^2 + \sigma_T^2}$, where $\bar{d}_2$ is the difference between the sample mean of the test drug and the sample mean of the active control agent, based on all patients at the end of the trial. The two-stage superiority test rejects H_0 in (7) if $Z_2 > c_{2,\alpha}$, where $c_{1,\alpha}$ and $c_{2,\alpha}$ are chosen so that

$$P(Z_1 > c_{1,\alpha}) + P(Z_2 > c_{2,\alpha}, Z_1 \leq c_{1,\alpha}) = \alpha \quad \text{when } H_0 \text{ in (7) holds.} \tag{9}$$

Now, assume that the hypothesis of interest are switched to (8) when $Z_1 \leq c_{1,\alpha}$ at the interim analysis. Let $\tilde{Z}_2 = \sqrt{2n}(\bar{d}_2 + \Delta)/\sqrt{\sigma_A^2 + \sigma_T^2}$. Consider the following test rule, which is referred to as a two-stage superiority-noninferiority test: If $Z_1 > b_{1,\alpha}$, conclude superiority ($\mu_T > \mu_A + \Delta$) and stop the trial; otherwise, continue the trial and if $\tilde{Z}_2 > b_{2,\alpha}$, conclude non-inferiority, but not superiority ($-\Delta < \mu T - \mu A \leq \Delta$); otherwise, conclude not non-inferiority ($\mu T - \mu A \leq -\Delta$). The constants $b_{1,\alpha}$ and $b_{2,\alpha}$ can be determined according to

$$\begin{aligned} &P(Z_1 > b_{1,\alpha}) = \alpha && \text{when } H_0 \text{ in (7) holds} \\ &P(Z_1 > b_{1,\alpha}) + P(\tilde{Z}_2 > b_{2,\alpha}, Z_1 \leq b_{1,\alpha}) = \alpha && \text{when } H_0 \text{ in (8) holds} \end{aligned} \tag{10}$$

It can be shown that $b_{1,\alpha}$ and $b_{2,\alpha}$ satisfying (10) exist; in fact, $b_{1,\alpha}$ is the $1 - \alpha$ quantile of the standard normal distribution. Note that $c_{1,\alpha}$ satisfying (9) is larger than $b_{1,\alpha}$ satisfying (10). Note that the following pros and cons regarding the two kinds of tests are observed. First, the two-stage superiority-noninferiority test has a better power at the interim stage than the two-stage superiority test. Second, the two-stage superiority-noninferiority test requires smaller sample size since the second stage test is for non-inferiority. Third, at the second stage, the two-stage superiority-noninferiority test can only conclude non-inferiority, whereas the two-stage superiority test may conclude superiority. Thus, in practice, it is worthy of pursuing the following research topics that (i) develop the two-stage superiority-noninferiority tests in more complex situations in terms of the study design and model assumption, (ii) consider a more flexible superiority-noninferiority test by adding a condition at the end of the first stage, i.e., if $Z_1 \leq a_{1,\alpha}$ but $Z_1 > a_{1,\alpha}$, then do not switch hypotheses; otherwise ($Z_1 \leq a_{1,\alpha}$), then switch hypotheses, (iii) derive formulas for sample size calculation. Since the hypotheses in two stages are different, it may not be a good idea to have the same sample size for each stage, and (iv) extend the results to group sequential tests with more than two stages.

Other Adaptive-Hypotheses — For clinical trials comparing several treatments or several doses of the same treatment with a placebo or an active control agent, a parallel-group design is usually considered. After the analysis of interim data, it is desirable to drop some treatment groups or dose groups showing no efficacy. It is also desirable to add some new treatment groups and/or modify the dose regimen for best clinical results. As a result, hypotheses have to be changed in the next stage of analysis.

To illustrate the concept of changing treatment arms, we consider the following simple case. Suppose that a group sequential design with $K = 2$ is adopted. At stage 1, two independent samples of size n are taken from a placebo control and a test drug with dosage x_1. Let $\bar{y}_{01}$ and $\bar{y}_{11}$ be the sample means from the control and test groups, respectively.

Assume $\bar{y}_{01}$ is distributed as $N(\mu_0, \sigma^2/n)$ and $\bar{y}_{11}$ is distributed as $N(\mu_1, \sigma^2/n)$.

Let $Z_1 = \sqrt{n/2}(\bar{y}_{01} - \bar{y}_{11})/s_1$, where s_1^2 is the pooled sample variance. We reject the hypothesis H_{01}: $\mu_0 = \mu_1$ and we stop the trial if $|Z_1| > c_\alpha$. If $|Z_1| \leq c_\alpha$, then the trial continues with two independent samples of size n taken from the placebo control and the test drug with an increased dosage $x_2 > x_1$. At stage 2, the sample mean $\bar{y}_{02}$ from the control group is distributed as $N(\mu_0, \sigma^2/n)$, and the sample mean $\bar{y}_{22}$ from the test group is distributed as $N(\mu_2, \sigma^2/n)$. Hence, the null hypothesis at stage 2 is switched to $H_{02} : \mu_2 = \mu_0$. The test statistic at the second stage depends on what we assume of the relationship between the dosage and mean response. Without any assumption, we can consider the $Z_2 = \sqrt{3n/2}(\bar{y}_0 - \bar{y}_{22})/s_2$, where $\bar{y}_0 = (\bar{y}_{01} + \bar{y}_{02})/2$ and s_2^2 is the pooled sample variance based on 2 stages of data. We reject the null hypothesis H_{02} if $|Z_2| > b_\alpha$, where c_α and b_α are chosen so that

$$P(|Z_1| > c_\alpha) + P(|Z_2| > b_\alpha, |Z_1| \leq c_\alpha) = \alpha \tag{11}$$

when $\mu_0 = \mu_1 = \mu_2$ for a given significance level α. Note that μ_2 is estimated using the second stage data only, although μ_0 and σ^2 are estimated using data from both stages.

Assume now that the mean response and the dose level has the relationship that $\mu_k = \beta x_k$, $k = 1, 2$, where β is an unknown parameter. Then,

μ_2 can be estimated using data from both stages. First, we estimate β by $\hat{\beta} = \frac{x_1\bar{y}_{11}+x_2\bar{y}_{22}}{x_1+x_2}$. Then we estimate μ_2 by $\hat{\mu}_2 = \beta x_2$. The test statistics Z_2 is modified as $Z_2 = (\bar{y}_0 - \hat{\mu}_2)/\sqrt{v}$, where v is an appropriate estimate of the variance of $\bar{y}_0 - \hat{\mu}_2$. We reject H_{02} if $|Z_2| > b_\alpha$, where c_α and b_α are still determined by (11) under $\mu_0 = \mu_1 = \mu_2$. Thus, it is worthy of pursuing the following research topics that (i) deriving valid statistical test procedures for more complex situations, such as designs with multiple dose levels and multiple interim analyses, (ii) employing Bayesian methods to relate dose levels with response means, and (iii) deriving sample size calculation formulas for various situations.

6. Concluding Remarks

As indicated earlier, although the use of adaptive design methods in clinical trials is motivated by its flexibility and efficiency, many researchers are not convinced and still challenge its validity and integrity.[73] As a result, many discussions are around the flexibility, efficiency, validity, and integrity. When implementing an adaptive design in a clinical trial, it is suggested a couple of principles that (i) adaptation should not alter trial conduct and (ii) type I error should be preserved must be followed when implementing the adaptive design methods in clinical trials.[48] Following these principles, some basic considerations such as dose/dose regimen, study endpoints, treatment duration, and logistics should be carefully evaluated for feasibility.[66] To maintain the validity and integrity of an adaptive design with complicated adaptations, it is strongly suggested that an independent data monitoring committee (IDMC) should be established. In practice, IDMC has been widely used in group sequential design with adaptations of stopping a trial early and sample size re-estimation. The role and responsibility of an IDMC for a clinical trial using adaptive design should clearly defined. IDMC usually convey very limited information to investigators or sponsors about treatment effects, procedural conventions, and statistical methods with recommendations in order to maintain the validity and integrity of the study.

When applying adaptive design methods in clinical trials, it is suggested that the feasibility of certain adaptations such as changes in study endpoints/hypotheses be carefully evaluated to prevent from any possible misuse and abuse of the adaptive design methods. For a complicated multiple adaptive design, it is strongly recommended that an independent data monitoring committee be established to ensure the integrity of the study.

It should also be noted that although clinical trial simulation does provide a solution not the solution for a complicated multiple adaptive design. In practice, "how to validate the assumed predictive model for clinical trial simulation?" is a major challenge to both investigators and biostatisticians.

We are moving in the right direction and yet there is still a long way to go until we are able to address all of the scientific issues from clinical, statistical, and regulatory perspectives as described earlier. Detailed design-specific guidances (e.g., guidances regarding sample size calculation/allocation and statistical/clinical considerations for a two-stage phase I/II or phase II/III seamless adaptive trial design) must be developed by the regulatory agencies before implementation of adaptive design methods in pharmaceutical/clinical research and development. In addition, qualification, composition, role/responsibility, and function/activity of an independent data monitoring committee for implantation of adaptive trial design need to be established for an objective and unbiased assessment of the treatment effect of the drug under investigation. Thus, from future perspectives, it is suggested that the escalating momentum for the use of adaptive design methods in clinical trials proceed with caution. At the same time, valid statistical methods for interested adaptive designs with various adaptations should be developed to prevent the possible misuse and/or abuse of the adaptive design methods in clinical trials. More details regarding recent development of statistical methodologies for specific adaptive designs such as adaptive dose finding, genomic-guide target clinical trial design, and two-stage adaptive seamless (phase I/II or phase II/III) designs can be found in Pong and Chow (2010)[59] and Chow and Chang (2012).[13]

References

1. Atkinson, A.C. and Donev, A.N. (1992). *Optimum Experimental Designs*. Oxford University Press, New York, New York.
2. Babb, J. S.. Rogatko, A. (2001). Patient specific dosing in a cancer phase I clinical trial. *Statistics in Medicine* **20**: 2079–2090.
3. Bauer, P. and Kieser, M. (1999). Combining different phases in development of medical treatments within a single trial. *Statistics in Medicine* **18**: 1833–1848.
4. Bauer, P. and Kohne, K. (1994). Evaluation of experiments with adaptive interim analysis. *Biometrics* **50**: 1029–1041.
5. Bauer, P. and Rohmel, J. (1995). An adaptive method for establishing a dose-response relationship, *Statistics in Medicine* **14**: 1595–1607.

6. Brannath, W., Koening, F., and Bauer, P (2003). Improved repeated confidence bounds in trials with a maximal goal. *Biometrical Journal*: 45: 311–324.
7. Branson, M. and Whitehead, W. (2002). Estimating a treatment e ect in survival studies in which patients switch treatment. *Statistics in Medicine* **21**: 2449–2463.
8. Chang, M. (2007). Adaptive design method based on sum of p-values. *Statistics in Medicine* **26**: 2772–2784.
9. Chang, M. (2007). *Adaptive Design Theory and Implementation Using SAS and R.* Chapman and Hall/CRC Press, Taylor and Francis, New York, New York.
10. Chang, M. and Chow, S.C. (2005). A hybrid Bayesian adaptive design for dose response trials. *Journal of Biopharmaceutical Statistics* **15**: 667–691.
11. Charkravarty, A. (2005). Regulatory aspects in using surrogate markers in clinical trials. In The Evaluation of Surrogate Endpoint. Burzykowski, Molenberghs, and Buyse (Eds), Springer.
12. Chow, S.C. and Chang, M. (2006). *Adaptive Design Methods in Clinical Trials.* Chapman and Hall/CRC Press, Taylor and Francis, New York, New York.
13. Chow, S.C. and Chang, M. (2012). *Adaptive Design Methods in Clinical Trials.* 2nd Edition, Chapman and Hall/CRC Press, Taylor & Francis, New York, New York.
14. Chow, S.C., Chang, M., and Pong, A. (2005). Statistical consideration of adaptive methods in clinical development. *Journal of Biopharmaceutical Statistics* **15**: 575–591.
15. Chow, S.C. and Liu, J.P. (2003). *Design and Analysis of Clinical Trials.* 2nd edition, John Wiley & Sons, New York, New York.
16. Chow, S.C., Lu, Q., and Tse, S.K. (2007). Statistical analysis for two-stage adaptive design with different study points. *Journal of Biopharmaceutical Statistics*:17: 1163–1176.
17. Chow, S.C. and Shao, J. (2005). Inference for clinical trials with some protocol amendments. *Journal of Biopharmaceutical Statistics* **15**: 659–666.
18. Chow, S.C. and Shao, J. (2006). On margin and statistical test for noninferiority in active control trials. *Statistics in Medicine* **25**: 1101–1113.
19. Chow, S.C., Shao, J., and Wang, H. (2003). *Sample Size Calculation in Clinical Research.* 2nd edition, Chapman and Hall/CRC Press, Taylor & Francis, New York, New York.
20. Christensen, R. (1996). Exact Tests for Variance Components. *Biometrics* **52**: 309–314.
21. Chung-Stein, C., Anderson, K., Gallo, P., and Collins, S. (2006). Sample size reestimation: A review and recommendations. *Drug Information Journal* **40**: 475–484.
22. Crowley, J. (2001). *Handbook of Statistics in Clinical Oncology*, Marcel Dekker, Inc., New York, New York.
23. Cui. L., Hung, H.M.J., and Wang, S.J. (1999). Modification of sample size in group sequential trials. *Biometrics* **55**: 853–857.

24. Efron, B. (1971). Forcing a sequential experiment to be balanced. *Biometrika* **58**: 403–417.
25. EMEA (2002). Point to Consider on Methodological Issues in Confirmatory Clinical Trials with Flexible Design and Analysis Plan. The European Agency for the Evaluation of Medicinal Products Evaluation of Medicines for Human Use. CPMP/EWP/2459/02, London, UK.
26. EMEA (2006). Reflection paper on Methodological Issues in Confirmatory Clinical Trials with Flexible Design and Analysis Plan. The European Agency for the Evaluation of Medicinal Products Evaluation of Medicines for Human Use. CPMP/EWP/2459/02, London, UK.
27. FDA (2010). *Draft Guidance for Industry — Adaptive Design Clinical Trials for Drugs and Biologics.* The United States Food and Drug Administration, Rockville, Maryland, USA.
28. Feng, H., Shao, J., and Chow, S.C. (2007). Group sequential test for clinical trials with moving patient population. *Journal of Biopharmaceutical Statistics* **17**: 1227–1238.
29. Friede, T. and Kieser, M. (2004). Sample size recalculation for binary data in internal pilot study designs. *Pharmaceutical Statistics* **3**: 269–279.
30. Gallo, P., Chuang-Stein, C., Dragalin, V., Gaydos, B., Krams, M., and Pinheiro, J. (2006). Adaptive design in clinical drug development — an executive summary of the PhRMA Working Group (with discussions). *Journal of Biopharmaceutical Statistics* **16**(3): 275–283.
31. Gallo, J. and Khuri, A. I. (1990). Exact tests for the random and fixed effects in an unbalanced mixed two-way cross-classification model. *Biometrics* **46**: 1087–1095.
32. Gasprini, M. and Eisele, J. (2000). A curve-free method for phase I clinical trials, *Biometrics* **56**: 609–615.
33. Hardwick, J.P. and Stout, Q.F. (2002). Optimal few-stage designs. *Journal of Statistical Planning and Inference* **104**: 121–145.
34. Hommel, G. (2001). Adaptive modifications of hypotheses after an interim analysis. *Biometrical Journal* **43**: 581–589.
35. Hommel, G., Lindig, V., and Faldum, A. (2005). Two stage adaptive designs with correlated test statistics. *Journal of Biopharmaceutical Statistics* **15**: 613–623.
36. Hung, H.M.J., Cui, L, Wang, S.J., and Lawrence, J. (2005). Adaptive statistical analysis following sample size modification based on interim review of effect size. *Journal of Biopharmaceutical Statistics* **15**: 693–706.
37. International Conference on Harmonization Guideline E10: Guidance on Choice of Control Group and Related Design and Conduct Issues in Clinical Trials. The United States Food and Drug Administration, Rockville, Maryland, July 2000.
38. Jennison, C. and Turnbull, B.W. (2000). *Group Sequential Methods with Applications to Clinical Trials.* Chapman and Hall, New York, NY.
39. Jennison, C. and Turnbull, B.W. (2005). Meta-analysis and adaptive group sequential design in the clinical development process. *Journal of Biopharmaceutical Statistics* **15**: 537–558.

40. Kelly, P.J., Sooriyarachchi, M.R., Stallard, N., and Todd, S. (2005). A practical comparison of group-sequential and adaptive designs. *Journal of Biopharmaceutical Statistics* **15**: 719–738.
41. Kelly, P.J., Stallard, N. and Todd, S. (2005). An adaptive group sequential design for phase II/III clinical trials that select a single treatment from several. *Journal of Biopharmaceutical Statistics* **15**: 641–658.
42. Khatri, C. G. and Shah, K. R. (1974). Estimation of location of parameters from two linear models under normality, *Communications in Statistics* **3**: 647–663.
43. Khuri, A. I., Mathew, T., and Sinha, B. K. (1998). *Statistical Tests for Mixed Linear Models*. John Wiley and Sons, New York, NY.
44. Lachin, J.M. (1988). Statistical properties of randomization in clinical trials. *Controlled Clinical Trials* **9**: 289–311.
45. Lan, K.K.G. and DeMets, D.L. (1987). Group sequential procedures: Calendar versus information time. *Statistics in Medicine* **8**: 1191–1198.
46. Lee, Y., Wang, H., and Chow, S.C. A bootstrap-median approach for stable sample size determination based on information from a small pilot study. Unpublished manuscript.
47. Lehmacher, W. and Wassmer, G. (1999). Adaptive sample size calculations in group sequential trials. *Biometrics* **55**: 1286–1290.
48. Li, N. (2006). Adaptive trial design — FDA statistical reviewer's view. Presented at the CRT2006 Workshop with the FDA, Arlington, Virginia, April 4.
49. Li, G., Shih, W.J., Wang, Y. (2005). Two-stage adaptive design for clinical trials with survival data. *Journal of Biopharmaceutical Statistics* **15**: 707–718.
50. Liu, Q. and Chi, G.Y.H. (2001). On sample size and inference for two-stage adaptive designs. *Biometrics* **57**: 172–177.
51. Liu, Q., Proschan, M.A., and Pledger, G.W. (2002). A unified theory of two-stage adaptive designs. *Journal of American Statistical Association* **97**: 1034–1041.
52. Maca, J., Bhattacharya, S., Dragalin, V., Gallo, P., and Krams, M. (2006). Adaptive seamless phase II/III designs — background, operational aspects, and examples. *Drug Information Journal* **40**: 463–474.
53. Mugno, R., Zhus, W., and Rosenberger, W.F. (2004). Adaptive urn designs for estimating several percentiles of a dose response curve. *Statistics in Medicine* **23**: 2137–2150.
54. Muller, H.H., Schafer, H. (2001). Adaptive group sequential designs for clinical trials: Combining the advantages of adaptive and classical group sequential approaches. *Biometrics* **57**: 886–891.
55. Ofversten, J. (1993). Exact Tests for Variance Components in Unbalanced Mixed Linear Models. *Biometrics* **49**: 45–57.
56. O'Quigley, J., Pepe, M., and Fisher, L. (1990). Continual reassessment method: A practical design for phase I clinical trial in cancer, *Biometrics* **46**: 33–48.
57. O'Quigley, J., and Shen, L. (1996). Continual reassessment method: A likelihood approach, *Biometrics* **52**: 673–684.

58. Pocock, S.J. (1977). Group sequential methods in the design and analysis of clinical trials. *Biometrika* **64**: 191–199.
59. Pong, A. and Chow, S.C. (2010). *Handbook of Adaptive Designs in Pharmaceutical and Clinical Development.* Taylor & Francis, New York, New York.
60. Posch, M. and Bauer, P. (1999). Adaptive two stage designs and the conditional error function. *Biometrical Journal* **41**: 689–696.
61. Posch, M., Konig, F., Brannath, W., Dunger-Baldauf, C., and Bauer, P. (2005). Testing and estimation in flexible group sequential designs with adaptive treatment selection. *Statistics in Medicine* **24**: 3697–3714.
62. Posch, M. and Bauer, P. (2000). Interim analysis and sample size reassessment. *Biometrics* **56**: 1170–1176.
63. Proschan, M.A. (2005). Two-stage sample size re-estimation based on a nuisance parameter: A review. *Journal of Biopharmaceutical Statistics* **15**: 539–574.
64. Proschan, M.A. and Hunsberger, S.A. (1995). Designed extension of studies based on conditional power. *Biometrics* **51**: 1315–1324.
65. Proschan, M.A., Leifer, E., and Liu, Q. (2005). Adaptive regression. *Journal of Biopharmaceutical Statistics* **15**: 593–603.
66. Quinlan, J.A., Gallo, P., and Krams, M. (2006). Implementing adaptive designs: Logistical and operational consideration. *Drug Information Journal* **40**: 437–444.
67. Rosenberger, W.F. and Lachin, J. (2002). *Randomization in Clinical Trials.* John Wiley and Sons, New York, New York.
68. Rosenberger, W.F., Stallard, N, Ivanova, A., Harper, C.N., and Ricks, M.L. (2001). Optimal adaptive designs for binary response trials. *Biometrics* **57**: 909–913.
69. Sampson, A.R. and Sill, M.W. (2005). Drop-the-loser design: normal case (with discussions). *Biometrical Journal* **47**: 257–281.
70. Shao, J., Chang, M, and Chow, S.C. (2005). Statistical inference for cancer trials with treatment switching. *Statistics in Medicine* **24**: 1783–1790.
71. Shen, Y. and Fisher, L. (1999). Statistical inference for self-designing clinical trials with a one-sided hypothesis. *Biometrics* **55**: 190–197.
72. Shih, W.J. (2001). Sample size re-estimation — A journey for a decade. *Statistics in Medicine* **20**: 515–518.
73. Tsiatis, A.A. and Mehta, C. (2003). On the inefficiency of the adaptive design for monitoring clinical trials. *Biometrika* **90**: 367–378.
74. Wang, S.J. and Hung, H.M.J. (2005). Adaptive covariate adjustment in clinical trials. *Journal of Biopharmaceutical Statistics* **15**: 605–611.
75. Wang, S.J., O'Neill, R.T., and Hung, H.M.J. (2007). Approaches to evaluation of treatment effect in randomized clinical trials with genomic subset. *Pharmaceutical Statistics* **6**: 227–244.
76. Wang, S.K. and Tsiatis, A.A. (1987). Approximately optimal one-parameter boundaries for a sequential trials. *Biometrics* **43**: 193–200.
77. Wei, L.J. (1978). The adaptive biased-coin design for sequential experiments. *Annal of Statistics* **9**: 92–100.

78. Whitehead, J. (1997). Bayesian decision procedures with application to dose-finding studies. International *Journal of Pharmaceutical Medicine* **11**: 201–208.
79. Woodcock, J. (2005), FDA introduction comments: Clinical studies design and evaluation issues. *Clinical Trials* **2**: 273–275.
80. Zhang, W., Sargent, D.J., and Mandrekar, S. (2006). An adaptive dose-finding design incorporating both toxicity and efficacy. *Statistics in Medicine* **25**: 2365–2383.

About the Author

Shein-Chung Chow, Ph.D. is currently a Professor at the Department of Biostatistics and Bioinformatics, Duke University School of Medicine, Durham, North Carolina and the Founding Director of Global Clinical Trial and Research Center, Tianjin, China. Dr. Chow also held various positions in the pharmaceutical industry. He is the Editor-in-Chief of the *Journal of Biopharmaceutical Statistics*. Dr. Chow is also the Editor-in-Chief of the *Biostatistics Book Series* at Chapman and Hall/CRC Press of Taylor & Francis Group. He was elected Fellow of the American Statistical Association in 1995 and an elected member of the ISI (International Statistical Institute) in 1999. He was the recipient of the DIA Outstanding Service Award (1996), International Chinese Statistical Association (ICSA) Extraordinary Achievement Award (1996), and Chapter Service Recognition Award of the American Statistical Association (1998). Dr. Chow was appointed Scientific Advisor to the Department of Health, Taiwan in 1999–2001 and 2006–2008. Dr. Chow was President of the ICSA in 1997. Dr. Chow is the author or co-author of over 230 methodology papers and over 22 books. Dr. Chow received a B.S. in mathematics from National Taiwan University, Taiwan, and a Ph.D. in statistics from the University of Wisconsin, Madison, Wisconsin.

Annpey Pong is currently a principal scientist at the Department of Biostatistics and Research Decision Sciences, Merck Research Laboratories, Rahway, New Jersey. Dr. Pong has 20 years working experiences in the pharmaceutical industry. Dr. Pong is the Book Review Editor and Associate Editor of the *Journal of Biopharmaceutical Statistics*, co-author of the book "Handbook of Adaptive Designs in Pharmaceutical and Clinical Development", and the author or co-author of over 30 papers in the field of pharmaceutical research. Dr. Pong received a B.S. in mathematics from Providence University, Taiwan, two M.S. in Biostatistics and Mathematics from University of Michigan, Ann Arbor, and Eastern Michigan University, Ypsilanti, respectively, and a Ph.D. in statistics from Temple University, Philadelphia, Pennsylvania.

CHAPTER 21

STATISTICS IN THE RESEARCH OF TRADITIONAL CHINESE MEDICINE

DANHUI YI* and YANG LI

School of Statistics, Renmin University of China, Beijing 100872, People's Republic of China

*xueyi905@yahoo.com.cn

1. Introduction

Traditional Chinese Medicine (TCM) has thousands of years of history. It is a mixture of medicine and traditional Chinese philosophy. The foundation of it is the summarizing of precious experience for the understanding of life, the maintaining of health, and the fighting against diseases. (Hu and Liu, 2012). In China, TCM works well in curing people for many years. However, TCM doctors are facing great challenges nowadays. More and more researchers are suspicious of the objective efficacy of TCM. And some people fail to measure the efficacy in the same way that Western Medicine (WM) does. An article named "Traditional medicine: A culture in the balance" published in the Nature magazine describes the present situation of clinical research in TCM: the treatment itself is a very complex procedure, not to mention the herb (Qiu, 2007). In order to evaluate the objective efficacy of TCM, we should know the basic theory of TCM and how it works. And some corresponding statistical methods should be considered and developed. One of the most important and unique concepts in TCM research is the TCM syndrome. It is one of the foundations of TCM theory. We will introduce statistical methods to discuss the statistics in TCM research related to TCM syndrome in this chapter.

TCM has its own specific viewpoint of physiological functions and pathological changes of the human body. The notation of syndrome is a specific and important term in the theory of TCM. TCM doctors consider the syndrome to be a real factor that causes disease (an imbalance in the patient's body) (Wei, *et al.*, 2005). It means all symptoms and other medical outcomes are manifestations of the underlying syndrome of the patients. In other words, the syndrome is one kind of latent characteristic of the patients which cannot be observed directly. Fundamentally, all the treatments from TCM doctors are based on the evaluation of the specific syndrome of the patients. It is crucial to discuss about the syndrome evaluation as it is one of the most important issues in the clinical efficacy research of TCM. During the past decades, extensive research has been discussed on how to evaluate the syndrome in TCM. In the beginning, most clinical doctors evaluate the syndrome mostly by their subjective judgments (Liu, *et al.*, 2004). An obvious drawback of this traditional method is the influence from the clinical doctors themselves. There would be significant heterogeneity because each doctor made conclusions based on his/her own experience. Recently, mo researchers evaluate syndrome using statistical methods (Lin, 1997; Wang *et al.*, 1999). They build scaling by quantitative questionnaires to measure symptoms or other indicators, and try to evaluate syndromes by the information collected from clinical surveys. Thus, how to determine the scaling weights for each indicator became the most important problem in quantitative syndrome evaluation research. According to the calculation methods of weights for indicators, the syndrome evaluation could be divided into the subjective evaluation and the objective evaluation. Some consulting methods are used in the subjective evaluations, such as the Delphi Method and Analytic Hierarchy Process. However, these methods could also be affected significantly by the experts who determined the weights. The role of a specific indicator could also be exaggerated or reduced significantly by the subjective weights. Objective calculation methods are adopted and developed against this problem, such as Maximizing Deviation Method (Ma, 2007), Factor Analysis Method (Lu *et al*, 2009), and Partial Least Squares (PLS) Path Modeling (Guinot *et al*, 2001; Wang and Fu, 2004; Ruan and Ji, 2006; Liu, 2008; Li *et al*, 2012). All the objective methods involve objective weights determination procedures, which means all the weights were derived based on the relations among indicators. In this chapter, we introduce a second-order latent variable model with the PLS path modeling estimation and illustrate the application in a real analysis of the premenstrual disorder syndrome of TCM liver-qi invasion (PMSNI) syndrome.

With the stimulus for developing TCM from the Chinese government, TCM prevention is also proposed. There are three main advantages in taking TCM prevention to the community health clinic. Firstly, most people usually go to the community health clinic before going to the hospital. So the community health clinic is the best place to popularize the TCM prevention. Secondly, many community health clinics in major cities in China (such as Beijing, Shanghai, and so on) have built up the health files system for the residents in their neighborhoods. It is helpful for healthcare management. The data stored in the health files system make the efficacy evaluation of the TCM prevention relatively easy. Thirdly, TCM treatment not only cures one specific disease but also helps to adjust the inner balance of the patients, which is why most elderly Chinese people prefer it over other treatments. In addition, the treatment cost of TCM is on average cheaper than that of WM. All these reasons make the TCM prevention in the community health clinic very promising nowadays. Compared to WM doctors, the TCM doctors have more information about the patients in the clinic. They have not only the chemistry and biological indicator but also many symptom information from their own four traditional diagnostic methods (inspection; listening and smelling; inquiry; palpation and pulse taking). The symptom information are special in TCM and useful for identification of high risk people for a specific disease or TCM syndrome. But it is not wise to build a complex model with many symptoms and indicator as covariates in clinical research because it requires lots of work to collect the selected independent information and increases the cost of the high risk population identification. Therefore, a suitable symptom selection methodology should be considered. In this chapter, we introduce a group lasso method to select appropriate risk factors for diagnostic prediction in TCM and illustrate the application in a real analysis of the osteoporosis risk prediction model for elderly women.

2. TCM Syndrome Evaluation

As opposed to the definition in WM, TCM explains a disease in terms of symptoms and syndromes together (Guo *et al*, 2002). Under the theoretical assumption, the TCM syndrome is one kind of imbalance of patients, which is represented by specific interrelated symptoms for a fixed phase (Li 1985). Many statistical methods have been applied to syndrome evaluation research. Ren and Guo (1996) analyze the correlations among symptoms and TCM syndromes to build a subjective index for stroke. Yuan *et al.* (1999) make a TCM syndrome index by defining conditional probability in his research. Wu *et al.* (1999) set up an index with the ratios from the result of a logistic regression. However, among all the aforementioned methodologies, two important problems remain: (1) All the symptoms are affected by the underlying TCM syndrome and may be highly inter-correlated.

The researcher could not only consider the relation between each two variables separately, such as correlation between two indicators or correlation between one indicator and one syndrome. We should derive weights for indicators from the relationship among all variables (both symptoms and TCM syndrome) in a specific identified theoretical construct; (2) The distribution of the symptoms from clinic may be skewed and may not be assumed as a classical distribution with close form. We should try to avoid the popular likelihood estimation method because this estimation involves an overly strong joint-distribution assumption for most clinical data, especially in the TCM clinical research. And estimation method without the joint-distribution should be developed in the syndrome evaluation research. To overcome the problems above, we adopt a second-order latent variable model to construct the syndrome-symptoms relationship, and a PLS path modeling algorithm is discussed for parameter estimation.

2.1. *Background of the PMSNI evaluation*

The premenstrual disorder is a common disease for women all over the world. By the indication of several epidemiology investigations, the premenstrual disorder syndrome (PMS) is constructed by a group of typical clinical manifest symptoms such as dysphoria, depression, and others (Table 1). Such symptoms could be identified as the manifestations of a syndrome named liver-qi invasion in TCM, which is abbreviated as PMSNI (Qiao *et al.*, 1997; Wang 2007). The syndrome, PMSNI, is one kind of latent disease-influencing factors that are defined in TCM theory. It indeed influences patient's symptoms but cannot be observed directly. Our goal of analysis is to evaluate the level of the PMSNI syndrome with observed symptom variables. In this study, symptoms are collected by a PMS scale (Table 1) recommended by the American College of Obstetrics and Gynecology. According to the clinical functions, all the symptoms are divided into three groups (dimensions): the body symptom dimension (BSD), the functional condition dimension (FCD), and the mood dimension (MD) (Wang 2007).

2.2. *Methodologies*

The second-order latent variable model we discussed in this section is an evaluation model based on the second-order factor structural equation model. The structural equation model estimates the relations among latent variables by the information from blocks of manifest variables (Yi, 2008).

Table 1. Premenstrual disorder syndrome scale. A research group in Shandong University of Traditional Chinese Medicine translated the premenstrual disorder syndrome scale.

Construct	Indicator
Mood Dimension (MD)	Dysphoria (Dy)
	Depression (De)
Body Symptom Dimension (BSD)	Abdominal Bloating (AB)
	Breast Tenderness (BT)
	Headache (He)
	Nausea (Na)
	Vomiting (Vo)
	Stomachache (St)
Functional Condition Dimension (FCD)	Wakeful & Dreamful (WD)
	Reduced Sex Drive (RSD)
	Tiredness (Ti)
	Increased Appetite (IA)
	Swelling of Extremities (SE)
	Declined Performance (DP)
	Inattention (In)

The latent variable is a characteristic of the subjects in the study without direct observation and should be measured by manifest variables. In the second-order factor structural equation model, the *hth* manifest variable Y_{jh} $(j = 1, \ldots, J;\ h = 1, \ldots, H_j)$ is affected by a unique corresponding first-order latent variable $\xi_j (j = 1, \ldots, J)$, and each first-order latent variable ξ_j is affected by the second-order latent variable η. In other views, the first-order latent variables are the direct factors of the manifest variables, whereas the second-order latent variable is the direct factor of the first-order latent variables. In practice, the second-order latent variable is the TCM syndrome, which we want to evaluate, whereas the first-order latent variables are different dimensions, and the manifest variables are specific indicators (symptoms) for each characteristic (dimension). Although the second-order latent variable affects all the manifestations, it is better to model in the second-order factor structural equation model rather than connecting the second-order factor with all the manifest variables together because manifest variables may not be unidimensional. For example, all the symptoms can be divided into three groups by TCM theory in the PMSNI syndrome evaluation research. Each group of symptoms reflects one specific clinical function, which can be modeled by a corresponding first-order latent variable, and all the three first-order latent variables are affected by the second-order latent variable (syndrome). It is much easier to model all the manifestations by a single latent variable instead of the second-order construct. However, some information that are shared by manifestations in the same group (dimension) may be missed if we model multidimensional manifest variables by a single factor, and we may lose clinical interpretation under such TCM theory assumption.

The second-order factor structural equation model is constructed by the measurement model (2.1) and the structure model (2.2). The measurement model illustrates the relationship among manifest variables Y_{jh}s and the first-order latent variable ξ_j, and the measurement error ε_{jh}s. ε_{jh} is a random measurement error variable with mean 0 and fixed variance for the hth manifest variable Y_{jh} under the jth first-order latent variable ξ_j. The structure model illustrates the relationship among the first-order latent variable ξ_js and the second-order latent variable η and the measurement errors δ_js. And δ_j is a random measurement error variable with mean 0 and fixed variance for the jth first-order latent variable ξ_j.

$$Y_{jh} = \lambda_{jh}\xi_j + \varepsilon_{jh} \tag{2.1}$$

$$\xi_j = \beta_j\eta + \delta_j \tag{2.2}$$

To avoid the joint-distribution assumption, parameters in the second-order latent variable model are estimated by the PLS path modeling method. This is an iterative algorithm proposed by Herman Wold in the 1970s. It was used to be named nonlinear iterative partial least squares (Herman, 1975), for the estimation procedure is divided into several partial linear iterative estimations. It means that we should only assume that each symptom is explained by the first-order latent variable with random measurement errors, and each first-order latent variable is explained by the second-order latent variable with random measurement errors too. These assumptions about random measurement errors are reasonable in practical research and can be validated by residuals. Moreover, the estimation by the PLS path modeling has been proved as a consistent (Herman, 1975) and robust estimator for even skewed manifest variables (Cassel, *et al.*, 1999). Compared with the linear structural relationship method (LISREL), the PLS path modeling estimation does not have strict (hard) requirements for the joint-distribution assumption and the sample size (Fornell and Bookstein, 1982). In the evaluation research, we want to evaluate the latent variable as syndrome by assuming that the indicators are manifest variables. The latent variable cannot be observed directly, and each latent variable should be reflected by some specific manifest variables. The PLS path modeling algorithm constructs an evaluation system by the relationship among the latent variables and the manifest variables. One advantage of this method is that we estimate the weights by the information from the original data (Wang and Fu, 2004). Another advantage is that PLS can estimate the objective weights for each indicator, which cannot be reached by other methods (such as the linear structural relationship). These nice features make the PLS path modeling more suitable for the evaluation research.

The estimation for the weights iterates between the outer estimation procedure and the inner estimation procedure. U_js are defined as outer estimations for the first-order latent variables, whereas U_0 is defined as the outer estimation for the second-order latent variable. In the outer estimation procedure, U_js are estimated by weighted corresponding manifest variables Y_j in Equation (2.3), whereas U_0 is estimated by the first-order latent variables in Equation (2.4).

$$U_{ij} = \varpi_j Y_{ij}, \quad i = 1, \ldots, N; \quad j = 1, \ldots, J; \quad h = 1, \ldots, H_j \tag{2.3}$$

$$U_{i0} = w_j U_{ij}, \quad i = 1, \ldots, N; \quad j = 1, \ldots, J \tag{2.4}$$

where ϖ_js are outer estimations for weights among first-order latent variables and manifest variables, whereas w_js are outer estimations for weights among the second-order latent variable and the first-order latent variables (Bentler and Bonett, 1980).

The inner estimation procedure models the relationship among the second-order latent variable η and the first-order latent variables ξ_j. We assume that V_js are inner estimations for the first-order latent variables and V_0 is the inner estimation for the second-order latent variable, and they can be estimated by Equations (2.5) and (2.6), where e_js are inner estimations for weights among the second-order latent variable and the first-order latent variables by Equation (2.7).

$$V_{ij} = e_j U_{i0}, \quad i = 1, \ldots, N; \quad j = 1, \ldots, J \tag{2.5}$$

$$V_{i0} = \sum e_j U_{ij}, \quad i = 1, \ldots, N; \quad j = 1, \ldots, J \tag{2.6}$$

$$e_j = sign(cor(U_j, U_0)) \tag{2.7}$$

For the reflexive relationship such as Fig. 1, ϖ_js are the covariance coefficients of the manifest variables Y_j and the inner estimations of the first-order latent variables V_j, whereas w_js are the covariance coefficients of the outer estimations of the first-order latent variables U_j and the inner

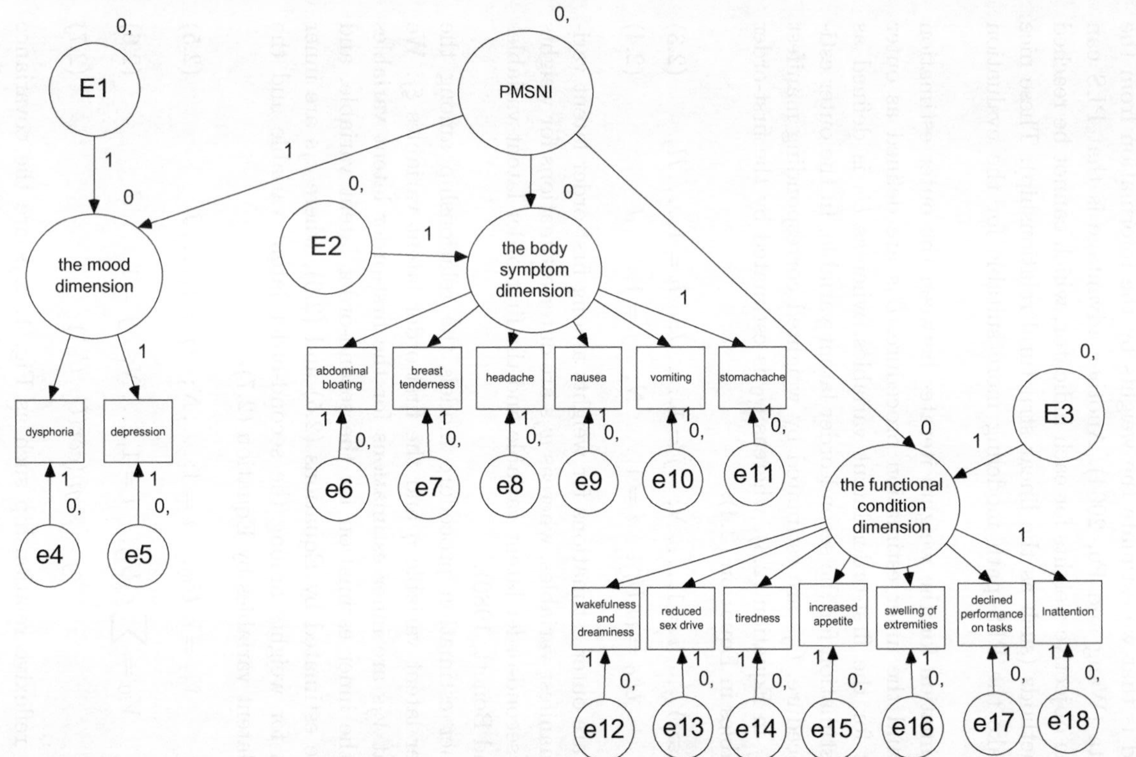

Fig. 1. Premenstrual disorder syndrome of liver-qi invasion (PMSNI) syndrome evaluation model: The ellipse of PMSNI is the second-order latent variable (syndrome) in the model, which affects three first-order latent variables named the mood dimension, the body symptom dimension, and the functional condition dimension. Symptoms are defined as manifest variables in rectangles, and the circles stand for random error terms (with means 0) for the first-order latent variables and manifest variables.

Table 2. Partial least squares path modeling algorithm in second-order factor structural equation model.

(1)	Given initial ϖ_{jh}^1, w_j^1.
(2)	For sth iteration (s = 1, 2, ...), compute U_j^s, U_0^s using ϖ_{jh}^s, w_j^s by (2.3) and (2.4).
(3)	Compute V_j^s, V_0^s using U_j^s, U_0^s by (2.5)–(2.7).
(4)	Compute $\varpi_{jh}^{s+1}, w_j^{s+1}$ using V_j^s, V_0^s by (2.8) and (2.9).
(5)	Repeats step (2)–(4) until convergence, obtain $\hat{\xi}_j = U_j^{\text{last iternation}}$, $\hat{\eta} = U_0^{\text{last iternation}}$.
(6)	Obtain $\hat{\lambda}_{jh}, \hat{\beta}_j$ by OLS in (2.1) and (2.2).

estimation of second-order latent variable V_0.

$$\varpi_j = \frac{1}{n} Y_j' V_j \tag{2.8}$$

$$w_j = \frac{1}{n} U_j' V_0 \tag{2.9}$$

Table 2 shows an iterative algorithm of the PLS path modeling for the second-order factor structural equation model.

After the discussion of the introduced model and the parameter estimation method, we propose a standard procedure for the TCM syndrome evaluation research.

Step 1. Data processing: checking the reliability of data.

Step 2. Model constructing: defining the manifest variables, the first-order latent variables, and the second-order latent variable by TCM prior knowledge.

Step 3. Parameter estimating: estimating the weights (parameters) using the PLS path modeling algorithm under the defined model construct.

Step 4. Syndrome evaluating: calculating the objective score of the syndrome by manifest variables and weights.

2.3. *Application and discussion*

We evaluate the level of the PMSNI syndrome by the data collected under a cluster sampling (we divided the population into different clusters by occupations). It is a self-report investigation at the time points of the first, the third, and the fifth days before and after the individual's normal catamenia.

We measure each symptom by using the interval scale from 0 to 6, and the total sample size is 947.

To simplify the complex relationships among factors, we examine each symptom and find that they can be divided into three groups based on the clinical meaning to patients in TCM theory, and we define that each group of symptoms are affected by a specific first-order factor. Under this TCM theory, we divide all the symptoms into three dimensions, the Mood Dimension (MD), the Body Symptom Dimension (BSD), and the Functional Condition Dimension (FCD). These three dimensions are first-order latent variables (factors) in the model, which affect symptoms directly, and the PMSNI syndrome is the second-order latent variable (factor), which affects the first-order latent factors. The construct of the second-order latent variable, the first-order latent variables, and the manifest variables is shown in Fig. 1.

Firstly, we want to know if the data has good reliability. Table 3 shows that in each dimension, we can obtain a good consistency with Cronbach's alphas being over 0.7, which implies that the data have good reliability. Then, we apply the PLS modeling algorithm to the second-order factor structural equation model in Equations (2.1) and (2.2). Table 4 shows the parameter estimations.

Although the estimated parameters in Table 4 are similar in magnitude under each dimension, they are the objective weights for the indicators (symptoms) under the given model structure. With the measurement of each indicator, we can calculate the factor score of the PMSNI syndrome. In other words, the level of the PMSNI syndrome in TCM can be evaluated by an objective score. It is easy to calculate the score for each patient in Equations (2.10)–(2.13). Therefore, a TCM doctor can evaluate the syndrome level of each patient in his clinical work. According to the different levels of the syndrome, doctors may divide the patients into different groups

Table 3. Reliability. We calculated the Cronbach's alphas for each dimension of manifest variables in SPSS 13.0 (SPSS Inc., Chicago, IL, USA). The symptoms in each dimension have good consistency.

Construct	Cronbach Alpha
the Mood Dimension (MD)	0.72
the Body Symptom Dimension (BSD)	0.77
the Functional Condition Dimension (FCD)	0.86

Table 4. Parameter estimations by partial least squares path modeling. The parameters are estimated by Visual-PLS 1.04.

Construct	Indicator	Weight
MD	Dysphoria	0.55
	Depression	0.55
BSD	Abdominal Bloating	0.31
	Breast Tenderness	0.29
	Headache	0.26
	Nausea	0.22
	Vomiting	0.23
	Stomachache	0.24
FCD	Wakeful & Dreamful	0.23
	Reduced Sex Drive	0.16
	Tiredness	0.24
	Increased Appetite	0.17
	Swelling of Extremities	0.17
	Declined Performance	0.27
	Inattention	0.26
PMSNI	MD	0.37
	BSD	0.38
	FCD	0.38

with different doses of formula or different therapies.

$$PMSNI_i = 0.37 \times MD_i + 0.38 \times BSD_i + 0.38 \times FCD_i \tag{2.10}$$

$$MD_i = 0.55 \times Dy_i + 0.55 \times De_i \tag{2.11}$$

$$\begin{aligned} BSD_i &= 0.31 \times AB_i + 0.29 \times BT_i + 0.26 \times He_i + 0.22 \times Na_i \\ &\quad + 0.23 \times Vo_i + 0.24 \times St_i \end{aligned} \tag{2.12}$$

$$\begin{aligned} FCD_i &= 0.23 \times WD_i + 0.16 \times RSD_i + 0.24 \times Ti_i + 0.17 \times IA_i \\ &\quad + 0.17 \times SE_i + 0.27 \times DP_i + 0.26 \times In_i \end{aligned} \tag{2.13}$$

Further, we can derive the average score of the syndrome from Equation (2.14). It is an averaged level of the PMSNI syndrome for the study sample, and different averaged levels can be compared between different subgroups in the clinical research. In our study, the average level of the patients' syndrome is 17.1 (score ranges from 0 to 100), which implies a mild status.

$$PMSNI_{average} = \frac{E(PMSNI_i) - \min(PMSNI_i)}{\max(PMSNI_i) - \min(PMSNI_i)} \times 100, \quad i = 1, 2, \ldots, N \tag{2.14}$$

As discussed above, we introduce an objective method for the syndrome evaluation in TCM by the second-order latent variable model, which is estimated by the PLS path modeling. We use the second-order latent variable model to construct the relationship between symptoms and the syndrome, which could not be carried out by former syndrome evaluation methods in TCM. This model considers all variables together and their interrelated correlations. The use of the PLS path modeling algorithm for the parameter estimation is another noble feature of the proposed procedure. This 'soft' estimation method releases the joint-distribution for responses and only desires random measurement errors with mean 0 and fixed variance for manifest variables or first-order latent variables, and it is a quick robust estimation even for the skewed manifest data. Through the example in the clinical TCM research, we can conclude that the introduced methodology is meaningful in application with the following advantages: (1) the idea of the evaluation procedure on the basis of the latent and manifest variables coincides the TCM theory of the syndrome; (2) the second-order factor structural equation model, which has simple construct, can evaluate all indicators by a common second-order factor; (3) the PLS path modeling algorithm, which estimates the weights by the relationship among the data, is a good objective evaluation method; and (4) this algorithm only requires for random measurement errors and does not require any joint-distribution assumption for the data.

3. TCM Symptom Selection

Building a disease (or TCM syndrome) risk prediction model is a common topic in the research of TCM. For example, osteoporosis is a systemic skeletal disease of bones, which leads to an increased risk of fractures (Christodoulou and Cooper, 2003; Koda-Kimble *et al.*, 2009). Although the standard procedure for the diagnoses of osteoporosis is the bone mineral density (BMD) measured by the dual energy X-ray absorptiometry (DEXA) (Blake and Fogelman, 2009; 2010), it is too expensive to do the examination for every person. In such case, our research purpose is to identify the people with the high risk of osteoporosis. It will be extremely helpful for the future prevention of osteoporosis if we can establish a risk prediction model based on the epidemiological data. Many risk factors of the osteoporosis have been found by the WM research (Johnell *et al.*, 1995; Turner *et al.*, 1998; Kanis, 1996; Akdeniz *et al.*, 2009; Lane, 2011). On the other hand, according to the TCM theory, every disease is caused by a specific unbalanced status in a person's body (TCM syndrome). All the symptoms and other medical outcomes are manifestation of the underlying TCM syndrome (Liu *et al.*, 2004; Wei *et al.*, 2005). Based on such assumption, the TCM doctors think that the osteoporosis is a result of the TCM syndrome named kidney deficiency (Sheng *et al.*, 2006; Xie *et al.*, 2007; Dai and Yue, 2010; Wang *et al.*, 2010). All these TCM symptoms associated with kidney deficiency are easy to be observed and identified by the doctors even in the community health clinic. Therefore, it will make the prediction model much more accurate and exercisable if we introduce both the WM factors and the TCM symptoms as potential covariates in our study. However, it is not wise to build a complex model with all the symptoms and indicator as covariates in clinical research because it requires lots of work to collect the selected independent information and increases the cost of the high risk population identification. Therefore, a suitable symptom selection methodology should be considered.

In the past few years, many variable selection methods have been widely discussed, such as Lasso (Tibshirani, 1996, 2011; Meinshausen and Buhlmann, 2006; Bickel *et al.*, 2009), Bridge (Frank and Friedman, 1993; Fu, 1998; Huang *et al.*, 2009), SCAD (Wang *et al.*, 2007; Wang *et al.*, 2007) and so on. Among the variable selection methodologies, the Lasso method is one of the best tools to the applied research for its noble features. Three advantages make the lasso method distinguish well for this applied study. Firstly, the lasso method outperforms in simple application by selecting the independent variables and estimating the corresponding parameters simultaneously. Although the lasso method may mislead into the selection inconsistency when irrepresentable conditions fail (Zhao and Yu, 2006; Ma and Huang, 2008), it makes the analysis procedure of the variable selection much simpler than other methods. The second advantage of the lasso method is its computational feasibility. The L_1 and L_2 type estimators in the lasso method are easy to compute which decrease the computation significantly. Most importantly, the lasso method has been proved to have a series of good asymptotic properties (Knight and Fu, 2000; Huang *et al.*, 2009), such as the consistency, which strongly ensures the result of the variable selection meaningful in both the views of statistics and clinical research. However, one important problem comes out in our study is that most symptoms in the TCM are measured in ordinal scale (i.e. none, moderate, sever). Different from the continuous or binary covariates, one categorical covariate involves two or more dummy variables in the prediction model. For example, one of the most important TCM symptoms related to the TCM syndrome kidney deficiency is the muscular spasm of lower limbs, which has five categories in the questionnaire: none, seldom, sometimes, usually and always. Therefore four dummy variables (V1-V4) are introduced in the prediction model representing the last four categories referenced on the first category. If we directly apply the Lasso or other traditional variable selection methods, it is possible that V2 and V4 are selected but V1 and V3 are not. It is not reasonable to select one dummy variable but abandon another one which is generated by the same potential categorical covariate. All the dummy variables generated by the same factor should be either selected or not selected at the same time for the convenience of interpretation. Moreover, the variable selection solution depends on how the dummy variables are encoded. This means the covariate may be selected if we take the first level as the reference, but it may not be selected if we take the last level as reference. This unstable result is not satisfactory. In such a situation, the TCM doctors cannot conclude whether the covariate of the muscular spasm of lower limbs is significantly associated with the response or not. So the variable selection method which only selects individual dummy variables instead of whole factors should be modified. The group lasso (Yuan and Lin, 2006; Wang *et al.*, 2007; Meier *et al.*, 2008; Huang *et al.*, 2009; Duarte *et al.*, 2011; Zhou *et al.*, 2011) is one method which can overcome the above problem by introducing an extension of the lasso penalty. It selects variable by groups instead of individually. And the estimation of the group lasso has been proved to be consistent under specific condition (Bach, 2008).

3.1. *Background of osteoporosis research*

Recent years, the osteoporosis prevention in elderly women in the community health clinic is widely discussed in China. Although the prevalence of the osteoporosis is similar for men and women, epidemiological researches show that the vast majority of the osteoporotic patients occur in the elderly women, especially from the age of 40 to 65 (Kanis and Pitt, 1992; Holroyd *et al.*, 2008; Compston, 2010; Curran *et al.*, 2010). This study has been motivated by the interest of building osteoporosis risk prediction model. The data are from a cohort study of the osteoporosis risk in elderly women, which is conducted by the research team from the Institute of Basic Research in the Clinical Medicine at the China Academy of Chinese Medicine Science. This study is an experimental research which is limited by time and cost. Although the data collection is carried out in only one district of Shanghai, the research of osteoporosis risk of elderly women by the group lasso model can be extended and popularized to entire China if meaningful results are achieved in this study.

In this study, an epidemiology investigation questionnaire with 70 questions is used to record the WM risk factors (demography, lifestyle, and so on) and TCM symptoms. The questionnaire is approved by an independent medical ethics committee at the China Academy of Chinese Medicine Science to comply the requirement of the Declaration of Helsinki (Rid and Schmidt, 2010). The survey is conducted with a standard operating procedure in three communities (the Changqiao community, the Huajingzhen community, and the Lingyun community; the population of women aged between 40 and 65 is 57,996) which are randomly selected out of thirteen communities of Xuhui District (the population of women aged between 40 and 65 is 175,000) in Shanghai. Between April and May in 2009, 1101 women in these three communities who met the inclusion criteria were offered the questionnaire and a free bone density test in Dahua hospital which is also located in Xuhui District. 1087 questionnaires are collected and 983 of them are selected to build the osteoporosis risk prediction model after the data validity checking.

All the elderly women in this study test their BMD in Shanghai Dahua hospital and are divided in two groups (normal and abnormal) by their BMD results. A variable in the dataset, which records this information, is coded as 0 for normal BMD and 1 for abnormal BMD. The number of people with normal BMD is 463 (47.1%) while the number of people with abnormal BMD is 520 (52.9%). After a descriptive statistical analysis, we abandon the covariates with sparse observations (e.g., We abandon the covariate "smoking or not" because only 1.5% women smoke in this study). Finally 52 covariates are selected into the rough osteoporosis risk prediction model. There are 3 continuous covariates (Age, Weight, and Time of Menopause), 16 binary covariates (such as Menopause, Physical Exercise, and so on) and 33 ordinal covariates (such as Times of Fracture, Degree of Feeling fatigue, and so on). As a result of epidemiology research, menopause is one important covariate to the state of osteoporosis (Kanis, 1996; Akdeniz *et al.*, 2009; Lane, 2011). 76.8% women in this study have menopause and the time of menopause ranges from 0 to 34 years. The age difference between women with menopause and women without menopause is considerable (Table 5). The body conditions of these two groups of women are different because the weight does not vary in groups but the height is diverse. This descriptive statistic result implies that the menopause may be a significant covariate to the response of BMD status. As a result of the combination of continuous

Table 5. Descriptive statistics of the elderly women population.

		Non-Menopause N=228 (23.2%)	Menopause N=755 (76.8%)	P-value
Age (year)		49.1 (41, 61)	57.6 (44, 66)	<0.001
Weight (kg)		61.6 (43, 108)	61.1 (35, 135)	0.528
Time of Menopause (year)		—	6.8 (0, 34)	—
Range of Height (cm)	<150	1 (0.4%)	18 (2.4%)	0.206
	150–155	40 (17.5%)	141 (18.7%)	
	156–160	93 (40.8%)	300 (39.7%)	
	161–165	61 (26.8%)	217 (28.7%)	
	166–170	26 (11.4%)	67 (8.9%)	
	>170	7 (3.1%)	12 (1.6%)	
Time of Exercise (hr)	<0.5	76 (33.3%)	208 (27.5%)	0.011
	0.5–1.0	34 (14.9%)	89 (11.8%)	
	1.0–2.0	75 (32.9%)	256 (33.9%)	
	>2.0	43 (18.8%)	202 (26.8%)	
Times of Fracture (times)	0	180 (78.9%)	581 (77.0%)	0.472
	1	41 (18.0%)	137 (18.1%)	
	2	4 (1.8%)	30 (4.0%)	
	3	3 (1.3%)	4 (0.5%)	
	>3	—	3 (0.4%)	

and categorical covariates, the total number of predictors (including dummy variables) is 152. And the significant covariates should be selected by the group lasso from all these predictors.

3.2. *Methodologies*

Suppose that we can observe an independent and identically distributed p-dimensional covariate vector X_i and a $n \times 1$ binary response vector Y_i. Because the p covariates contain both continuous and categorical predictors, we define the degrees of freedom of the gth ($g = 1, \ldots, G$) covariate by df_g and then rewrite X_i as $(X_{i,1}^T, \ldots, X_{i,G}^T)^T$ for the gth group of dummy variables. For example, the degrees of freedom of the muscular spasm of lower limbs are 4 and the degrees of freedom of a continuous (or binary) covariate is 1. Denote β_g as the parameter vector corresponding to the gth group of dummy variables and β as the parameter vector of all β_g's and intercept β_0. The risk prediction model is formulated as the following.

$$\begin{aligned} \text{logit}(p_\beta(X_i)) &= X_i^T \beta \\ &= \beta_0 + \sum_{g=1}^{G} X_{i,g}^T \beta_g \end{aligned} \tag{3.1}$$

The parameter $\hat{\beta}$ is estimated by the minimization of the convex function of (3.2), where λ is the penalty parameter (Meier *et al.*, 2008).

$$S_\lambda(\beta) = -l(\beta) + \lambda \sum_{g=1}^{G} s(df_g)\|\beta_g\|_2 \tag{3.2}$$

where $l(\cdot)$ is the log-likelihood function of the logistic linear regression model (eg. $\sum_{i=1}^{n} y_i(\beta_0 + \sum_{g=1}^{G} x_{i,g}^T \beta_g) - \log[1 + \exp\{\beta_0 + \sum_{g=1}^{G} x_{i,g}^T \beta_g\}]$). The function $s(\cdot)$ is used to rescale the penalty with the degrees of freedom of the parameter vector β_g. Unless stated otherwise, we use $s(df_g) = df_g^{1/2}$ to ensure the penalty term is of the same order of the number of parameter df_g. The same rescaling is used in Yuan and Lin (2006). In addition, the amount of penalization is controlled by the tuning parameter λ. Usually, with the increase of λ, less covariates are selected. For example, Fig. 2 shows

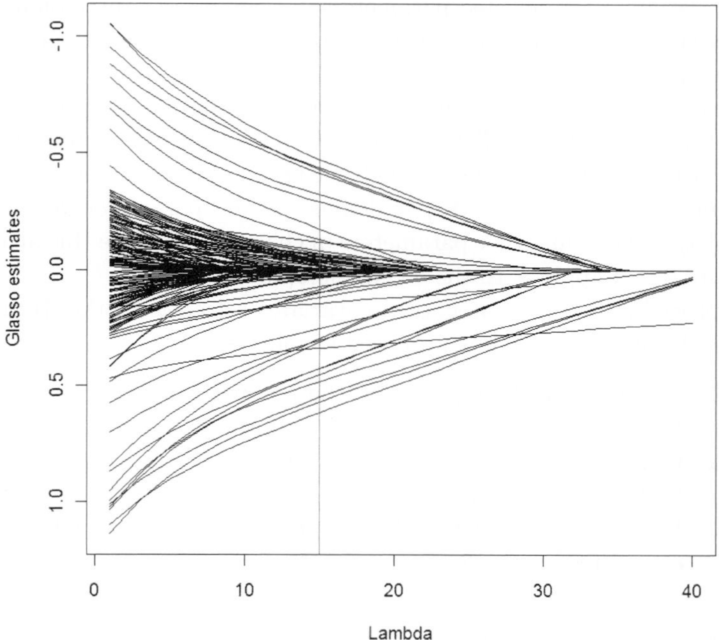

Fig. 2. The parameter estimation in the group lasso model for the simulation data.

The parameters of the potential covariates are estimated in a group lasso logistic model. The estimates decrease or increase significantly with the change of the tuning parameter λ. This figure is illustrated by a simulation results, and the optimal tuning parameter λ is 15.

Table 6. The block coordinate descent algorithm for the group lasso.

Steps	Algorithm
(1)	Give the initial parameter β;
(2)	$\beta_0 = \arg\min_{\beta_0}\{S_\lambda(\beta)\}$;
(3)	For $g = 1, \ldots, G$ if $\|X_g^T(Y - p_{\beta_{-g}})\|_2 \le \lambda s(df_g)$, $\beta_g = 0$;
	else, $\beta_g = \arg\min_{\beta_g}\{S_\lambda(\beta)\}$;
(4)	Repeat step (2) and step (3) until the convergence criterion is reached.

that the change of the penalized parameter estimations in the group lasso logistic model with the change of the tuning parameter λ. The variables can be selected and the corresponding parameters can be estimated simultaneously by the determination of λ. The value of λ can be suggested by the accuracy of the prediction model in a quantitative view, or suggested by the interpretation of the selected parameters in a qualitative discussion. In the real research, it is better to consider from both sides of the quantitative and the qualitative analysis.

We adopt the block coordinate descent algorithm (Tseng, 2001) for the estimation of the risk prediction model. Fixing other parameter estimates, the algorithm (Table 6) cycles through each group by minimizing the convex function (3.2). The vector β_{-g} is defined as the parameter vector when setting $\beta_g = 0$ and all other parameters unchanged. We code this algorithm in R 2.13.0 and apply it to the TCM osteoporosis data.

A procedure for the categorical covariates selection in the Traditional Chinese Medicine research is proposed as follows:

Step 1. Covariates Defining: Denote the potential covariates of both the WM risk factors and the TCM symptoms;

Step 2. Covariates Selection: Select the significant covariates group-wise by the group lasso method;

Step 3. Prediction: Conduct the logistic regression model with the selected covariates in step 2.

3.3. *Application and Discussion*

We establish the osteoporosis risk prediction model using the binary response variable and 52 potential covariates. To compare the prediction accuracy, we establish three models: (1) the logistic model with all potential covariates, and (2) the group lasso logistic model, and (3) the logistic

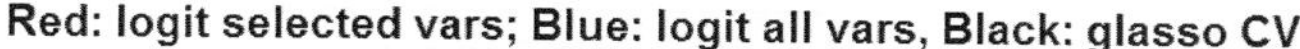

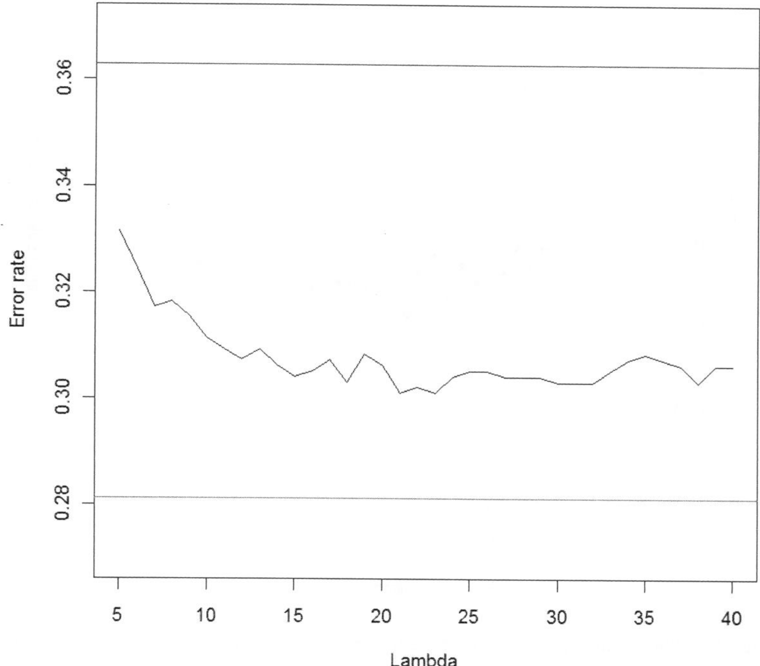

Fig. 3. The error rate of three logistic models.

The upper blue line is the error rate of the logistic regression model with all the potential covariates. The lower red line is the error rate of the logistic regression model with the selected covariates by the group lasso. The black curve is the error rate of the group lasso logistic model using 10 folds cross-validation.

model with the covariates selected by the group lasso method. We conduct the 10 fold cross-validation to estimate the error rate of each model. The error rate of the logistic model with all the potential covariates is 36.3% while the error rate of the logistic model with the covariates selected by the group lasso method is 28.1%. It is reasonable to find out the error rate of the group lasso logistic model varies between these two error rates mentioned above (Fig. 3). It is also reasonable to take variables selected by the group lasso logistic model from all the potential covariates because the error rate is decreased. It is appropriate to see that the error rate for the group lasso logistic model is higher than the error rate of the logistic model with the selected covariates because the likelihood estimator always

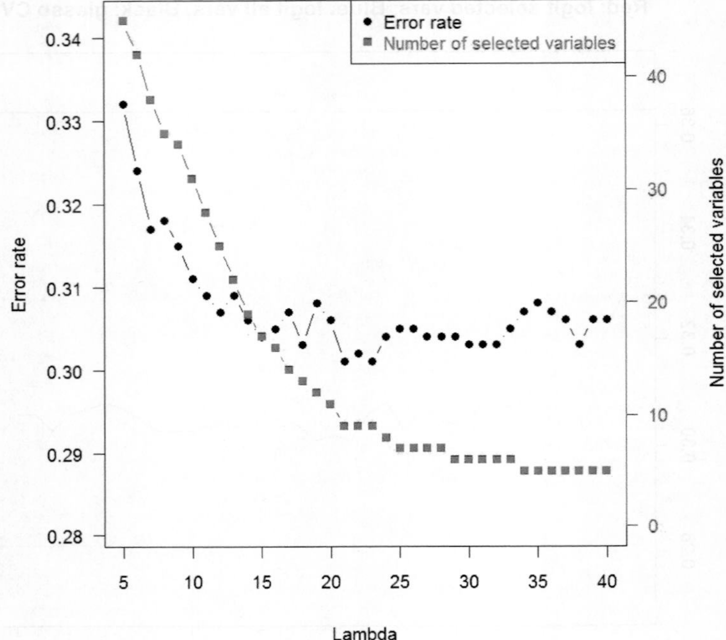

Fig. 4. The tuning parameter and error rate in the group lasso logistic model. The total number of covariates is 52 and the corresponding number of dummy variables is 152. When increasing the value of the tuning parameter λ, the number of selected variables decreases as showed by the red line. The black line is the error rate at different λ.

performs better than the optimal approximation with the finite sample in the Lasso regressions.

Figure 4 shows the corresponding error rates and the numbers of selected covariates at different values of λ. The optimal error rate for the group lasso logistic model is 30.1% with the tuning parameter $\lambda = 21$. Nine groups of covariates (three continuous covariates, three binary covariates, and three ordinal covariates) are selected (Fig. 4). The details of the selected covariates and their estimates are listed in Table 7. As a shrinkage method, the estimates of the group lasso logistic model do not have exact meaning as odds ratios in the logistic regression. But it can reflect the relationship between the covariates and the response. Among the selected covariates, Age and Weight are demographical risk factors for the osteoporosis. The estimate concludes that the risk of being abnormal in BMD increases when the age increases and decreases when the weight increases. After

Table 7. The comparison of the estimates of the group lasso logistic model and the logistics model with the significant selected covariates.

Variable Name	Type	Group Lasso	Logistic
Age	Continuous	0.0406	0.0360
Physical exercise (Yes)	Binary	−0.1639	−0.3788
Weight	Continuous	−0.0352	−0.0518
Menopause (Yes)	Binary	0.7802	1.0638
Time of menopause	Continuous	0.0606	0.0831
Operation	Binary	−0.1452	−0.6375
Times of Fracture	None	—	—
	Once	0.0309	0.2104
	Twice	0.1134	0.9292
	Three times	0.2268	2.2991
	More than three times	0.1051	0.8787
Feeling fatigue	None	—	—
	Seldom	−0.0398	−0.1968
	Sometimes	0.0073	0.0437
	Usually	−0.0266	−0.2835
	Always	0.2537	1.7262
Muscular spasm of lower limbs	None	—	—
	Seldom	0.0055	0.3197
	Sometimes	0.0017	0.1369
	Usually	0.0124	0.7028
	Always	0.0148	0.2091

reviewing the related literature, we find that whether an elderly woman is in menopause is an important risk factor for the osteoporosis: the women after menopause have high risk of the osteoporosis (Kanis, 1996; Akdeniz *et al.*, 2009; Lane, 2011). The estimates of the parameters for the "Menopause" and the "Time of menopause" coincide the above conclusion. The longer the time after menopause is, the higher risk the elderly women are exposed. The "Operation" and the "Times of Fracture" are two other risk factors. The result shows an elderly woman who has taken operations has a higher risk and the risk increases as the number of fractures increases. The "Feeling fatigue" and the "Muscular spasm of lower limbs" are two TCM symptoms associated with the risk. It is interesting to find that the "Muscular spasm of lower limbs" is positively correlated with the risk. In the TCM theory, this symptom reflects the TCM syndrome, Kidney deficiency, which may cause the osteoporosis. According to this result, the TCM doctors can diagnose the person in Kidney deficiency syndrome with the selected symptoms using the "main symptom theory". The intervention or treatment can be suggested against such a TCM syndrome. The estimates of the logistic model with covariates selected by the group lasso method are also shown in Table 7. It is appropriate to find that all the signs of the two sets of estimates from both the group lasso logistic model and the logistic model are the same. It means the similar parameter effects are found by these two models. The difference is due to the shrunk magnitude of parameter estimation. This result, from another perspective, proves appropriateness of using the group lasso for the variable selection.

As discussed above, we use the group lasso to establish the osteoporosis risk prediction model for elderly women in the community health clinic. We conduct model diagnosis and find no obvious model misspecification. The selected covariates and the corresponding parameters of the optimal TCM osteoporosis risk prediction model are shown in the Table 7. We have explored different tuning parameters and found no better results. Finally nine meaningful predictors are selected following the above procedure. Although it is not a comprehensive comparison study, the introduced group lasso method is suitable for the research of the TCM osteoporosis risk prediction model for its asymptotic properties and affordable computational requirement. It simplifies the risk prediction model and makes the future clinic work easier because fewer covariates need to be collected. The prediction error rate is 28.1% for the logistic regression model with the significant covariates. The researcher can identify the elderly women of the high risk of osteoporosis in community health clinic firstly, and take the TCM intervention to the identified population.

Acknowledgement

This research is partly supported by the Special Fund for Chinese Medicine Research in the Public Interest **201207665**, and the Key Research Institute of Humanities and Social Sciences Program **2009JJD910002**.

References

Akdeniz, N., Akpolat, V., Kale, A., Erdemoglu, M., Kuyumcuoglu, U. and Celik, Y. (2009). Risk factor for postmenopausal: anthropometric measurements, age, age at menopause and the time elapsed after menopause onset. *Gynecological Endocrinology* **25**: 125–129.

Bach, F. R. (2008). Consistency of the group lasso and multiple kernel learning. *Journal of Machine Learning Research* **9**: 1179–1225.

Bentler, P.M., Bonett, D.G. (1980). Significance tests and goodness of fit in the analysis of covariance structures. *Psychological Bulletin* **88**(3): 588–606.

Bickel, P. J., Ritov, Y. and Tsybakov, A. B. (2009). Simultaneous analysis of Lasso and Dantzig selector. *Annals of Statistics* **37**: 1705–1732.

Blake, G. M. and Fogelman, I. (2009). The clinical role of dual energy X-ray absorptiometry. *European Journal of Radiology* **71**: 406–414.

Blake, G. M. and Fogelman, I. (2010). An update on dual energy X-ray absorptiometry. *Seminars in Nuclear Medicine* **40**: 62–73.

Cassel, C., Hackl, P., Westlund, H.A. (1999). Robustness of partial least squares method for estimating latent variable quality structures. *Journal of Applied Statistics* **26**(4): 435–446.

Christodoulou, C. and Cooper, C. (2003). What is osteoporosis? *Postgraduate Medical Journal* **79**: 133–138.

Compston, J. (2010). Osteoporosis: social and economic impact. *Radiologic Clinics of North America* **48**: 477–482.

Curran, D., Maravic, M., kiefer, P., Tochon, V. and Fardellone, P. (2010). Epidemiology of osteoporosis-related fractures in France: a literature review. *Joint Bone Spine* **77**: 546–551.

Dai, F. and Yue, L. (2010). The advanced research of the relationship between kidney deficiency and osteoporosis. *Chinese Journal of Osteoporosis* **16**: 67–70.

Duarte, M. F., Bajwa, W. U. and Calderbank, R. (2011). The performance of group lasso for linear regression of grouped variables. Technical Report in Department of Computer Science at Duke University.

Frank, I. E. and Friedman, J. H. (1993). A statistical view of some chemometrics regression tools (with discussion). *Technometrics* **35**: 109–148.

Fu W. J. (1998). Penalized regressions: the Bridge versus the Lasso. *Journal of Computational and Graphical Statistics* **7**: 397–416.

Fornell, C., Bookstein, F.L. (1982). Two structural equation models: LISREL and PLS applied to consumer exit voice theory. *Journal of Marketing Research* **19**(4): 440–452.

Guinot, C., Latreille, J., Tenenhaus, M. (2001). PLS path modeling and multiple table analysis. *Chemometrics and Intelligent Laboratory Systems* **58**(2): 247–259.

Guo, X., Lai, S., Liang, W. (2002). Choice and application of the outcome indexes for clinical effectiveness assessment of traditional Chinese medicine. *Journal of Guangzhou University of Traditional Chinese Medicine* **19**(4): 251–255.

Herman, W. (1975). Path models with latent variable: the NIPALS approach. In *Quantitative Sociology: International Perspectives on Mathematical and Statistical Models Building*, Blalock, H.M., *et al.*, (eds). Academic Press: New York.

Herman, W. (1975). Causal flows with latent variables: partings of the ways in light of NIPALS modeling. *European Economic Review* **5**(1): 67–86.

Holroyd, C., Cooper, C. and Dennison E. (2008). Epidemiology of osteoporosis. *Clinical Endorcrinology and Metabolism* **22**: 671–685.

Hu, J., and Liu, B. (2012). The basic theory, diagnostic, and therapeutic system of traditional Chinese medicine and the challenges they bring to statistics. *Statistics in Medicine* **31**: 602–605.

Huang, J., Ma, S, Xie, H. and Zhang, C-H. (2009). A group bridge approach for variable selection. *Biometrika* **96**: 339–355.

Johnell, O., Gullberg, B., kanis, J. A., Allander, E., Elffors, L., Dequeker, J., Dilsen, G., Gennari, C., Vaz, L. A., Lyritis, G., Mazzuoli, G., Miravet, L., Passeri, M., Cano, P. R., Rapado, A. and Ribot, C. (1995). Risk factors for hip fracture in european women: the MEDOS study. *Journal of Bone and Mineral Research* **10**: 1802–1815.

Kanis, J. A. and Pitt F. A. (1992). The epidemiology of osteoporosis. *Bone* **13**: 7–15.

Kanis, J. A. (1996). Estrogens, the menopause, and osteoporosis. *Bone* **19**: 185–190.

Knight, K. and Fu, W. (2000). Asymptotics for Lasso type estimators. *Annals of Statistics* **28**: 1356–1378.

Koda-Kimble, M. A., Young, L. Y., kradjan, W. A., Guglielmo, B. J., Alldredge, B. K., and Corelli, R. L. (2009). Applied therapeutics: the clinical use of drugs. Lippincott Williams and Wilkins, Philadelphia.

Lane, N. E. (2011). Osteoporosis: yesterday, today and tomorrow. *Rheumatology* **50**: 1181–1183.

Li, Y., Yi, D., Zhang, H., Qin, Y. (2012). Syndrome evaluation in traditional Chinese medicine using second-order latent variable model. *Statistics in Medicine* **31**: 672–680.

Li, D. (1985). Discussion of syndrome identification. *Journal of Liaoning Traditional Chinese Medicine* **8**: 1–3.

Lin, L. (1997). Cooperation of ginseng injection in middle- and late-stage of chemotherapy for malignant tumor. *New Journal of Traditional Chinese Medicine* **29**(2): 19–21.

Liu, F., Fang, J., Wang, J. (2004). Research of clinical efficacy evaluation in TCM. *Traditional Chinese Drug Research and Clinical Pharmacology* **15**(4): 190–192.

Lu, F., Weng, W., Li, R., Tian, Y. (2009). Mid-term evaluation of TCM clinical research with factor analysis. *World Science and Technology: Modernization of Traditional Chinese Medicine and Materia Medica* **11**(6): 800–805.

Liu, X. (2008). The synthesis evaluation of listed company's financial indicators based on partial least square path modeling. *Application of Statistics on Management* **27**(4): 695–700.

Ma, S. and Huang, J. (2008). Penalized feature selection and classification in bioinformatics. *Briefings of Bioinformatics* **9**: 392–403.

Ma, Y. (2007). The method of determining the weights of decision-makers based on the maximizing deviation. *Journal of Beijing University of Chemical Technology* **34**(2): 177–180.

Meier, L., Geer, S. V. D. and Buhlmann, P. (2008). The group lasso for logistic regression. *Journal of Royal Statistical Society: Series B* **70**: 53–71.

Meinshausen, N. and Buhlmann, P. (2006). High dimensional graphs and variable selection with the Lasso. *Annals of Statistics* **34**: 1436–1462.

Qiao, M., Zhang, Z., Xu, X., Han, X., Ci, Y., Ye, Q. (1997). Epidemiological survey on syndromes distribution in PMS. *Chinese Journal of Basic Medicine in Traditional Chinese Medicine* **3**(3): 31–33.

Qiu, J. (2007). Traditional medicine: A culture in the balance. *Nature* **448**: 126–128.

Ren, Z., Guo, R. (1996). Research of syndrome identification for wind stroke disease. *Journal of Beijing University of Traditional Chinese Medicine* **19**(4): 49–50.

Rid, A. and Schmidt, H. (2010). The 2008 declaration of Helsinki-First among equals in research ethics? *The Journal of Law, Medicine and Ethics* **38**: 143–148.

Ruan, J., Ji, H. (2006). Economic development evaluation based on the PLS structural equation model for west of China. *Statistical Education* **8**: 4–7.

Sheng, T., Yang, H., Tian, J. and Han, L. (2006). Symptom characteristics of osteoporosis and related risk factors. *Journal of Beijing University of Traditional Chinese Medicine (Clinical Medicine)* **13**: 15–18.

Tibshirani, R. (1996). Regression shrinkage and selection via the lasso. *Journal of Royal Statistical Society: Series B* **58**: 267–288.

Tibshirani, R. (2011). Regression shrinkage and selection via the lasso: a retrospective. *Journal of Royal Statistical Society: Series B* **73**: 273–282.

Tseng, P. (2001). Convergence of a block coordinate descent method for non-differentiable minimization. *Journal of Optimization Theory and Applications* **109**: 475–494.

Turner, L. W., Leaver-Dunn, D., DiBrezzo, R. and Fort, I. (1998). Physical activity and osteoporotic fracture among older women. *Journal of Athletic Training* **33**: 207–210.

Wang, H. (2007). Differentiation of symptoms and signs standard and curative effect evaluation scale research for liver-qi invasion of PMS. *Doctoral Dissertation of Shandong University of Traditional Chinese Medicine.*

Wang, H., Fu, L. (2004). The application research of PLS path modeling on establishing synthesis evaluation index. *System Engineering: Theory and Practice* **10**: 80–85.

Wang, H., Li, R. and Tsai, C-L. (2007). Tuning parameter selectors for the smoothly clipped absolute deviation method. *Biometrika* **94**: 1005–1011.

Wang, L., Chen, G. and Li, H. (2007). Group SCAD regression analysis for microarray time course gene expression data. *Bioinformatics* **23**: 1486–1494.

Wang, T., Liu, Y., Yang, W., *et al.* (1999). Clinical study on treating chronic fatigue syndrome with Xiao Pi Yi Shen oral fluid. *Journal of Beijing University of Traditional Chinese Medicine* **22**(4): 56–58.

Wang, X., Zhang, Y. and Huang, Q. (2010). Discussion on the main pathogenesis in Traditional Chinese Medicine and etiology about primary osteoporosis. *Journal of Chinese Integrative Medicine* **8**: 1119–1123.

Wei, H., Zheng, P. and Ji, G. (2005). General methods for clinical effect assessment of Traditional Chinese Medicine. *Journal of Chinese Integrative Medicine* **3**: 184–190.

Wu, D., Liang, W., Wen, Z., *et al.* (1999). Establishing standards of measuring blood-stasis syndrome in the patients with acute stroke. *Journal of Guangzhou University of Traditional Chinese Medicine* **16**(4): 249–258.

Xie, Y., Zhu, Y., Ge, J., Piao, H., Yu, J., Wang, H., Chen, W. and Xing, M. (2007). Study on the TCM general syndrome of osteoporosis based on the clinical epidemiological investigation. *World Science and Technology: Modernization of Traditional Chinese Medicine and Materia Medica* **19**: 38–44.

Yang, H., Xu, Z., Wang, X., Yin, S., Tang, G., Liu, D. and Chen, W. (2009). Study on TCM syndrome patterns and distribution of postmenopausal osteoporosis in South Sichuan. *Journal of Sichuan of Traditional Chinese Medicine* **27**: 23–25.

Yi, D. (2008). Structural equation model: theory and application. Renmin University of China Press: Beijing.

Yuan, M. and Lin, Y. (2006). Model selection and estimation in regression with grouped variables. *Journal of Royal Statistical Society: Series B* **68**: 49–67.

Yuan, Z., Zhou, X., Fan, F., *et al.* (1999). Investigation on quantitative diagnosis of clinical manifestations of TCM heart disease diagnosed on the basis of differentiation of blood and qi. *Journal of Traditional Chinese Medicine* **40**(5): 302–304.

Zhao, P. and Yu, B. (2006). On model selection consistency of Lasso. *Journal of Machine Learning Research* **7**: 2541–2563.

Zhou, H., Alexander, D. H., Sehl, M. E., Sinsheimer, J. S., Sobel, E. M. and Lange, K. (2011). Penalized regression for genome-wide association screening of sequence data. *Proceeding of the Pacific Symposium on Biocomputing*, 106–117.

About the Authors

Danhui Yi is currently a professor in the School of Statistics at Renmin University of China (RUC). She is the director of statistical consulting center of RUC. Her main research interests include statistical forecasting, risk management, and other applied statistical methodologies. Recently she is focusing on the study of applied statistical methods in traditional Chinese medicine (TCM).

Dr. Yang Li is an assistant professor in the School of Statistics at Renmin University of China. His main research interests are correlated data analysis, latent variable modeling, joint modeling, and variable selection methodologies in biometrical studies.

Section 3

Statistical Genetics

CHAPTER 22

SPARSE SEGMENT IDENTIFICATIONS WITH APPLICATIONS TO DNA COPY NUMBER VARIATION ANALYSIS

X. JESSIE JENG

North Carolina State University Statistics Department,
2311 Stinson Drive Campus Box 8203,
Raleigh, NC 27695-8203, USA

T. TONY CAI

3730 Walnut St./Jon M. Huntsman Hall,
Department of Statistics, The Wharton School,
University of Pennsylvania,
Philadelphia, PA 19104, USA
tcai@wharton.upenn.edu

HONGZHE LI

Department of Biostatistics and Epidemiology,
215 Blockly Hall University of Pennsylvania,
Perelman School of Medicine, 423 Guardian Drive,
Philadelphia, PA 19014, USA

Copy number variations (CNVs) are alterations of the DNA of a genome that results in the cell having an abnormal number of copies of one or more sections of the DNA. Germline CNVs have been shown to be associated with many complex diseases. Detecting and identifying all the CNVs in a given sample or in multiple population-based samples is an important first step in many CNV analyses. In this chapter, we review statistical methods for CNV identification, focusing on latest developed methods for sparse segment identifications in various settings. We review methods for optimal CNV identification for a single sample based on SNP allele intensity data, methods for robust CNV identification based on the next generation sequence (NGS) data. and methods for detection of recurrent CNVs in a population when a large set of samples are available. Our review focuses on problem formulations and optimal statistical properties of the procedures. We illustrate these methods using data from the 1000 Genomes Project and data from a large genome-wide association study of neuroblastoma. Areas that need further research are also presented.

1. Introduction

Structural variants in the human genome (Sebat *et al.*, 2004; Feuk *et al.*, 2006), including the copy number variants (CNVs) and balanced rearrangements such as inversions and translocations, play an important role in the genetics of complex diseases. Copy number variation refers to duplication or deletion of a segment of DNA sequences compared to a reference genome assembly. In normal genomic regions, there are two copies of DNAs, one from father, one from mother. CNVs are alternations of DNA of a genome that results in the cell having a less or more than two copies of segments of the DNA. CNVs correspond to relatively large regions of the genome, ranging from about one kilobase to several megabases, that are deleted or duplicated. A high proportion of the genome, currently estimated at up to 12%, is subject to copy number variation (Hastings *et al.*, 2009). Hastings *et al.* (2009) further provides possible molecular mechanisms of change in the gene copy number. Analysis of CNV in developmental and neuropsychiatric disorders (Feuk *et al.*, 2006; Stefansson *et al.*, 2008; Stone *et al.*, 2008; Walsh *et al.*, 2008) and in cancer (Diskin *et al.*, 2009), has led to the identification of novel disease-causing copy number variant mutations, thus contributing important new insights into the genetics of these complex diseases.

This chapter reviews a few related statistical problems that arise from the CNV analysis for germline constitutional genomes, focusing on methods for sparse segment identifications. Current high-throughput genotyping technology is able to generate genome-wide observations in very high resolutions. In this type of ultrahigh dimensional data, the number of CNVs is relatively very small and the CNV segments are usually very short. These impose major difficulties in CNV identification (Zhang *et al.*, 2009b). The emerging technologies of DNA sequencing have further enabled the identification of CNVs by the next-generation sequencing (NGS) in high resolution. NGS can generate millions of short sequence reads along the whole human genome. When these short reads are mapped to the reference genome, both distances of paired-end data and read-depth (RD) data can reveal the possible structural variations of the target genome (for reviews, see Medvedev *et al.* (2009) and Alkan *et al.* (2011)). The general statistical problem is to identify sparse and subtle signal segments hidden in a long sequence of noisy data. Let $\mathbb{I}$ be the collection of all signal segments. The goal is two-fold: (1) to detect the existence of segments; and (2) to identify the locations of the segments if they exist. Precisely, we want to test

$$H_0 : \mathbb{I} = \emptyset \qquad \text{against} \qquad H_1 : \mathbb{I} \neq \emptyset, \tag{1.1}$$

and if H_1 is rejected, identify each $I_k \in \mathbb{I}$.

Although many methods have been developed for the CNV analysis, including methods based on hidden Markov models (Wang *et al.*, 2007) and methods based on fused penalized regression (Zhang *et al.*, 2010), these methods do not provide any theoretical results in term of optimality of the procedures. We review three approaches for testing the above null hypothesis and for identifying the CNVs at both individual sample and multiple-sample levels:

(1) optimal CNV identification for a single sample based on single nucleotide polymorphism (SNPs) allele intensity data.
(2) robust CNV identification based on the next generation sequence (NGS) data.
(3) detection of recurrent CNVs in a population when a large set of samples are available.

These three problems can be formulated as general sparse segment identification problems in the high dimensional settings. Our review focuses on the problem formulations and some key steps of the procedure and some theoretical results. We also illustrate these methods with real data analyses. In addition, we discuss a few other interesting problems that require new statistical methodology, including methods for testing CNV associations and methods for CNV analysis based on mapping distances from the pair-end sequencing.

2. Optimal CNV Identification for a Single Sample Based on Log R Ratio Data From the SNP Arrays

2.1. *Statistical formulation and summary of theoretical results*

The SNP data generated from SNP genotyping array platforms, such as the HumanHap550 array can be informative for CNV analysis. At a given SNP location, the observation is the Log R ratio (LRR) calculated as $\log_2(R_{obs}/R_{exp})$, where R_{obs} is the observed total intensity of both major

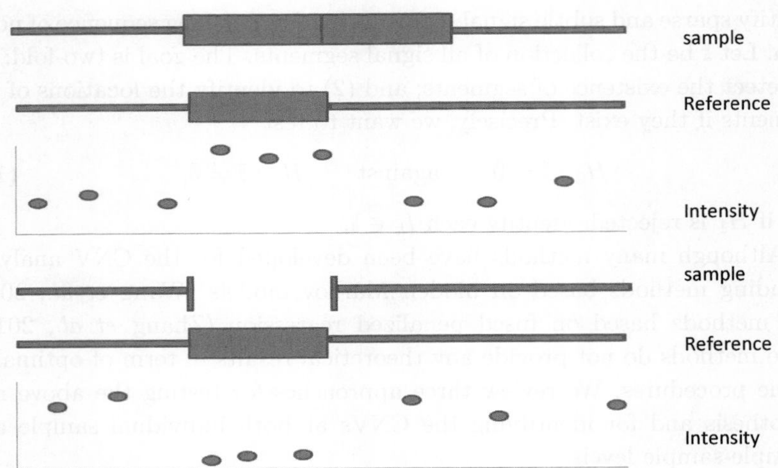

Fig. 1. Illustration of detecting insertions and deletions based on the LRR values. Top panel: duplication; bottom panel: deletion.

and minor alleles for a given SNP, and R_{exp} is computed from linear interpolation of canonical genotype clusters (Peiffer *et al.*, 2006). When there is no copy number change at a SNP location for the observed sample, R_{obs} should be the same as R_{exp}, and the LRR has a baseline level of zero. If there is a copy number deletion/duplication at a SNP location, R_{obs} can be smaller/larger than R_{exp}, therefore the LRR the deviates from zero to the negative/positive side, which implies deletion or duplication. See Figure 1 for an illustration on how different intensities can be used to infer the CNVs.

The problem of CNV identification using LRR data can be generalized as a problem of identifying sparse and short signal segments in a long sequence of noisy data. specifically, we observe $\{X_i, i = 1, ..., n\}$ with

$$X_i = \mu_1 1_{\{i \in I_1\}} + \cdots + \mu_q 1_{\{i \in I_q\}} + \sigma Z_i, \qquad 1 \le i \le n. \tag{2.2}$$

Here $q = q_n$ is the unknown number of the signal segments, possibly increasing with n, $I_1, \ldots I_q$ are disjoint intervals representing signal segments with unknown locations, $\mu_1, \ldots \mu_q$ are unknown positive means, σ is an unknown noise level, and $Z_i \overset{iid}{\sim} N(0, 1)$.

The problem formulated in Section 1 for data described by model (2.2) pertains to statistical research in several areas. Without segment structure, it is closely related to large-scale multiple testing, which has motivated many novel procedures such as false discovery rate (FDR) (Benjamini and Hochberg, 1995) and higher criticism thresholding (HCT) (Donoho and

Jin, 2008). Arias-Castro *et al.* (2005) considered the problem of detecting the existence of signals when there is only one signal segment. This is a special case of the testing part of our problem with $q = 1$. They showed that the detection boundary in this case is $\sqrt{2 \log n}/\sqrt{|I|}$, i.e., the signal mean should be at least $\sqrt{2 \log n}/\sqrt{|I|}$ in order for a signal with length $|I|$ to be reliably detected and that the generalized likelihood ratio test (GLRT) can be used for detecting the segment. A closely related result in Section 6 of Hall and Jin (2010) demonstrates the detection boundary under a wide range of signal sparsity when signals appear in several clusters. Further, Arias-Castro *et al.* (2005) and Walther (2010) studied detection of geometric objects and spatial clusters in 2-dimensional space, respectively, and Arias-Castro *et al.* (2008) provides detection threshold for the existence of an unknown path in a 2-dimensional regular lattice or a binary tree.

The problem considered here is also related to the problem of change-point detection, since it involves shifts in the characteristics of a sequence of data. Change-point detection in a single sequence has been extensively studied. See Zack (1983) and Bhattacharya (1994) for a review of the literature. Olshen *et al.* (2004) used the likelihood ratio based statistics for analysis of DNA copy number data, and Zhang and Siegmund (2007) proposed a BIC-based model selection criterion for estimating the number of change-points. Olshen *et al.* (2004) further developed an iterative circular binary segmentation procedure for segmentation of a single sequence and showed promising results in analysis of DNA copy number data, whereas Zhang *et al.* (2008) extended the problem of change-point detection from single sequence to multiple sequences in order to increase the power of detecting changes.

The problem is studied from another perspective in Jeng *et al.* (2010), which focuses on the recovery of sparse and subtle signals. For any signal segment, a statistical characterization of identifiable region is derived. When a signal segment is in the identifiable region, it is possible to reliably separate the segment from the noise; otherwise, it is impossible to do so. A likelihood ratio selection (LRS) procedure was proposed to identify the signal segments. The LRS involves scanning the linear data sequence of length (n) with all the segment of length less than a pre-specified interval length L and then calculate the likelihood ratio statistics for all these intervals. A threshold of $t_n = \sqrt{2 \log(Ln)}$ is used to control for the genome-wide error rate. Specifically, the LRS has the following steps:

Step 1: Let $\mathbb{J}_n(L)$ be the collection of all possible subintervals in $\{1, \ldots, n\}$ with interval length less than or equal to L. Let $j = 1$. Define $\mathbb{I}^{(j)} = \{\tilde{I} \in \mathbb{J}_n(L) : X(\tilde{I}) > t_n\}$.

Step 2: Let $\hat{I}_j = \arg\max_{\tilde{I} \in \mathbb{I}^{(j)}} X(\tilde{I})$.

Step 3: Update $\mathbb{I}^{(j+1)} = \mathbb{I}^{(j)} \backslash \{\tilde{I} \in \mathbb{I}^{(j)} : \tilde{I} \cap \hat{I}_j \neq \emptyset\}$.

Step 4: Repeat Step 2-4 with $j = j+1$ until $\mathbb{I}^{(j)}$ is empty.

Define the collection of selected intervals as $\hat{\mathbb{I}} = \{\hat{I}_1, \hat{I}_2, \ldots\}$. If $\hat{\mathbb{I}} \neq \emptyset$, we reject the null hypothesis and identify the signal segments by all the elements in $\hat{\mathbb{I}}$.

Jeng *et al.* (2010) showed that the LRS provides consistent estimates for any signal segments in the identifiable region. In other words, the LRS procedure is an optimal procedure, which can reliably separate signal segments from noise as long as the signal segments can be identified. To elucidate the exact meaning of optimality, Jeng *et al.* (2010) introduced a quantity to measure the accuracy of an estimate of a signal segment. Recall that $\mathbb{I}$ is the collection of signal segments. Denote $\hat{\mathbb{I}}$ to be the collection of interval estimates. For any $\hat{I} \in \hat{\mathbb{I}}$ and $I \in \mathbb{I}$, define the dissimilarity between $\hat{I}$ and I as

$$D(\hat{I}, I) = 1 - |\hat{I} \cap I| / \sqrt{|\hat{I}||I|}, \tag{2.3}$$

where $|\cdot|$ represents the cardinality of a set. Note that $0 \leq D(\hat{I}, I) \leq 1$ with $D(\hat{I}, I) = 1$ indicating disjointness and $D(\hat{I}, I) = 0$ indicating complete identity. Similar quantity has been used in Arias-Castro *et al.* (2005) to measure the dissimilarity between intervals.

Definition 1 An identification procedure is *consistent* for a subset $\Omega \subseteq \mathbb{I}$ if its set of estimates $\hat{\mathbb{I}}$ satisfies

$$P_{H_0}(|\hat{\mathbb{I}}| > 0) + P_{H_1}(\max_{I_j \in \Omega} \min_{\hat{I}_j \in \hat{\mathbb{I}}} D(\hat{I}_j, I_j) > \delta_n) \to 0, \tag{2.4}$$

for some $\delta_n = o(1)$. Obviously, the first term on the left measures the type I error. The second term, which is the probability that some signal segments in Ω are not 'substantially matched' by any of the estimates, essentially measures the type II error.

2.2. *Application to CNV analysis of LRR data from a trio*

As an example, Jeng *et al.* (2010) presented an application of using the genotyping data for a father-mother-child trio from the Autism Genetics Resource Exchange (AGRC) collection (Bucan *et al.*, 2009), genotyped on the Illumina HumanHap550 array. For each individual, the LRR data are

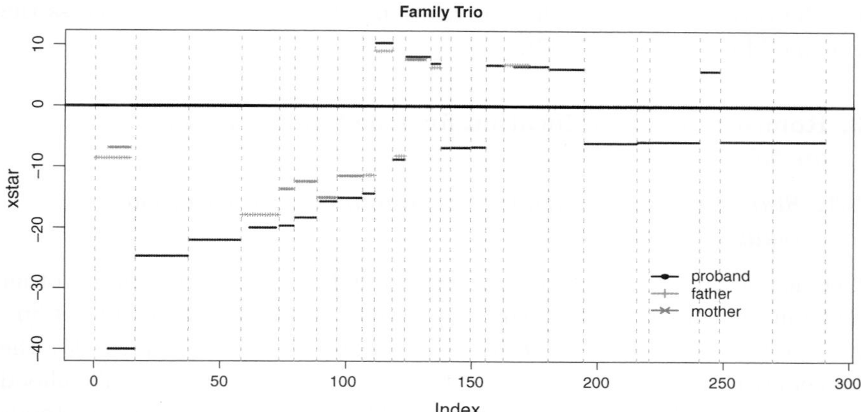

Fig. 2. Summary of results of LRS for CNV detection for a trio: the LR test statistics for the CNV segments identified by the proposed LRS procedure for the child, sorted by the absolute values of the likelihood ratio statistics. One segment with large statistics (−116.70 for the child) is truncated as −40 for better view.

observed at a total of 547,458 SNPs over 22 autosomes, and the numbers of SNPs on each chromosome range from 8,251 on chromosome 21 to 45,432 on chromosome 2. For each individual, the goal is to identify the CNVs by LRS. The purpose of using data from a trio is to partially validate the results since some CNVs are inherited from parents to child. Figure 2 shows the CNV segments with the likelihood ratio test scores (xstar) for the segments that the LRS algorithm selected for the child. The CNV segments identified in the parents are also plotted if they overlap with the CNV segments of the child. It is interesting to note that many of the CNV segments identified in the child were also observed in one of the parents, further indicating that some CNVs are inheritable and the LRS algorithm can effectively identify these CNVs. More details about the selected CNV segments and a comparison with the hidden Markov model (HMM)-based method implemented in PennCNV package (Wang *et al.*, 2007) can be found in Jeng *et al.* (2010).

One of the key assumption made in Jeng *et al.* (2010) is that the noise follows a normal distribution throughout the genomes and the baseline mean values of the data are zero. In real data application, the LRR data can also be affected by genomic features such as GC contents and SNP densities. It is important to pre-process the data to ensure that they roughly follow normal distributions. Loess fitting provides method of normalization for the correction of wave like correlations in signal intensities across the genome Marioni *et al.* (2007).

3. Robust CNV Identification for One Sample Based on NGS Data

3.1. *Statistical formulation and summary of theoretical results*

Classical approaches for signal detection rely heavily on normality or other distributional assumptions on data observed. Examples include but not limited to the false discovery rate (FDR) (Benjamini and Hochberg, 1995), the higher criticism (HC) (Donoho and Jin, 2004) and the generalized likelihood ratio test (GLRT) (Arias-Castro *et al.*, 2005). It is crucial for these methods to specify the tail distribution of the test statistics under null hypothesis, so that false positive errors can be controlled at a desired level. However, the tail behavior critically depends on the noise distribution, which is usually unknown and hard to estimate in real applications. Although the FDR or the HC can be applied to p-values obtained from nonparametric methods, popular nonparametric methods such as permutation are often computationally expensive and not feasible for ultra-high dimensional data.

The emerging technologies of next generation sequencing enable CNV analysis at even higher resolutions. NGS can generate millions of short sequence reads along the whole human genome. When these short reads are mapped to the reference genome, read-depth data are generated to count the number of reads that cover a genomic location or a small bin along the genome. The read counts or read depth (RD) data provide important information about the CNVs (Shendure and Ji, 2008; Medvedev *et al.*, 2009; Yoon *et al.*, 2009; Mills *et al.*, 2011; Sudmant *et al.*, 2010) that a given individual carries. CNVs include large-scale deletions, duplications and insertions and form one type of genetic variation. When the genomic location or bin is within a deletion, one expects to observe a smaller number of read counts or lower mapping density than the background read depth. In contrast, when the genomic location or bin is within an insertion or duplication, one expects to observe a larger number of read counts or higher mapping density. Therefore, these RDs can be used to detect and identify the CNVs. Yoon *et al.* (2009) developed an algorithm for read depth data to detect CNVs, where they convert the read count of a window into a Z-score by subtracting the mean of all windows and dividing by the standard deviation and identify the CNVs by examining the maximum p-value in a given interval. The p-values are obtained by a normality assumption on the RD data. Abyzov *et al.* (2011) developed an approach to first partition the genome into a set of regions with different underlying copy numbers using mean-shift technique and then merge signal and call CNVs by performing t-tests. Xie and Tammi (2009) and Chiang *et al.* (2009) developed methods for CNV detection based on read depth data when pairs of samples are available. The basic idea underlying these two methods is to convert the counts data into ratios and then apply existing copy number analysis methods developed for array CGH data such as the circular binary segmentation (CBS) (Olshen *et al.*, 2004) for CNV detection.

However, the distribution of the RD data is in general unknown due to the complex process of sequencing. Some recent literature assumes a constant read sampling rate across the genome and Poisson distribution or negative-binomial distribution for the read counts data (Xie and Tammi, 2009; Cheung *et al.*, 2011). However, due to GC content, mappability of sequencing reads and regional biases, genomic sequences obtained through high throughput sequencing are not uniformly distributed across the genome and therefore the counts data are likely not to follow a Poisson distribution (Li *et al.*, 2010; Miller *et al.*, 2011; Cheung *et al.*, 2011). The feature of the NGS data also changes with the advances of sequencing technologies. To analyze such data, robust methods that are adaptive to unknown noise distribution and computationally efficient at the same time are greatly needed in order to minimize both false positive and false negative identification of CNVs and to estimate CNV break points more precisely.

The NGS data $\{Y_1, \ldots, Y_n\}$ is modeled as

$$Y_i = \mu_1 1_{\{i \in I_1\}} + \cdots + \mu_q 1_{\{i \in I_q\}} + \xi_i, \qquad 1 \le i \le n, \tag{3.5}$$

where Y_i is the guanine-cytosine (GC) content-adjusted RD counts at genomic location or bin i, which can be regarded as continuous when coverage of the genome is sufficiently high, for example greater than 20 (Yoon *et al.*, 2009; Abyzov *et al.*, 2011). The above model is more general than (2.2) with the distribution of the noise ξ_i unspecified. This model describes the phenomenon that some signal segments are hidden in the n noisy observations. The number, locations, mean values of the segments, and the distribution of the random errors are unknown. Under this more general model, parametric methods designed for Gaussian noise or any other tractable noise may fail completely and provide a large number of misidentifications.

To tackle this difficulty, a computationally efficient method called robust segment identifier (RSI) was proposed in Cai *et al.* (2011), which provides

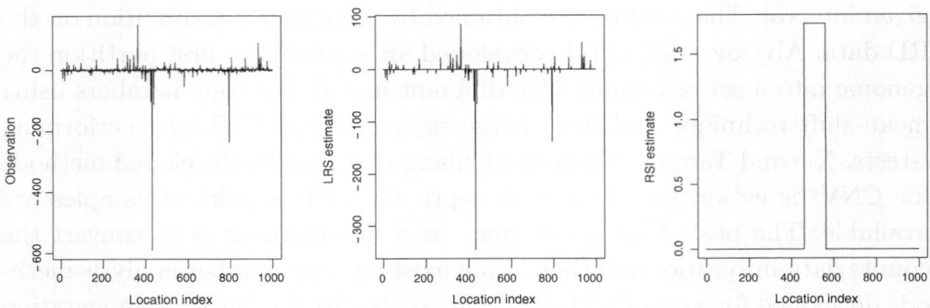

Fig. 3. Effects of long-tailed error distribution on segment identification. Left plot: Data with Cauchy noise and a signal segment at [457 : 556]. Middle plot: Intervals identified and estimated interval means by LRS. Right plot: Interval identified and estimated means by RSI.

a robust and near-optimal solution for segment identification over a wide range of noise distributions. As an illustration, 1000 observations are generated based on Cauchy $(0, 1)$, and the signal segment is set at [457 : 556] with a positive mean. Figure 3 compares the RSI with the LRS, which is an optimal procedure for Gaussian noise. In this example, the LRS fails to work at all by identifying too many false segments, while the RSI, on the other hand, provides a good estimate of the signal segment even when the noise distribution is unknown and heavy-tailed.

A key step of the RSI is a local median transformation, which was first introduced in Brown *et al.* (2008) and Cai and Zhou (2009) in the context of nonparametric regression. The original observations are first divided into T small bins with m observations in each bin and then the median values of the data in these bins are taken as a new data set. The central idea is that the new data set can be well approximated by Gaussian random variables for a wide collection of error distributions. After the local median transformation, existing detection and identification methods that are designed for Gaussian noise, such as LRS, can then be applied to the new data set. Specifically, we first equally divide the n observations into $T = T_n$ groups with $m = m_n$ observations in each group. Define the set of indices in the k-th group as $J_k = \{i : (k-1)m + 1 \le i \le km\}$, and generate the transformed dataset as

$$X_k = \text{median}\{Y_i : i \in J_k\}, \qquad 1 \le k \le T. \tag{3.6}$$

Set

$$\eta_k = \text{median}\{\xi_i : i \in J_k\}, \qquad 1 \le k \le T, \tag{3.7}$$

then the medians X_k can be written as

$$X_k = \theta_k + \eta_k, \qquad 1 \le k \le T, \tag{3.8}$$

where

$$\theta_k = \begin{cases} \mu_j, & J_k \subseteq I_j \text{ for some } I_j, \\ \mu_k^* \in [0, \mu_j], & J_k \cap I_j \neq \emptyset \text{ for some } I_j \text{ and } J_k \not\subseteq I_j, \\ 0, & \text{otherwise.} \end{cases}$$

After the local median transformation, the errors ξ_i in the original observations are re-represented by η_k. The main idea is that η_k can be well approximated by Gaussian random variable for a wide range of noise distributions. Specifically, we assume that the distribution of ξ_i is symmetric about 0 with the density function h satisfying $h(0) > 0$ and

$$|h(y) - h(0)| \leq Cy^2 \tag{3.9}$$

in an open neighborhood of 0. This assumption is satisfied, for example, by the Cauchy distribution, the Laplace distribution, the t distributions, as well as the Gaussian distribution. A similar assumption is introduced in Cai and Zhou (2009) in the context of nonparametric function estimation. The distributions of η_k are approximately normal. This can be precisely stated in the following lemma.

Lemma 3.1. *Assume (4.14), (3.13), and transformation (3.8), then η_k can be written as*

$$\eta_k = \frac{1}{2h(0)\sqrt{m}} Z_k + \frac{1}{\sqrt{m}} \zeta_k, \tag{3.10}$$

where $Z_k \overset{iid}{\sim} N(0,1)$ and ζ_k are independent and stochastically small random variables satisfying $E\zeta_k = 0$, and can be written as

$$\zeta_k = \zeta_{k1} + \zeta_{k2}$$

with

$$E\zeta_{k1} = 0 \text{ and } E|\zeta_{k1}|^l \leq C_l m^{-l}, \tag{3.11}$$

$$P(\zeta_{k2} = 0) \geq 1 - C\exp(-am) \tag{3.12}$$

for some $a > 0$ and $C > 0$, and all $l > 0$.

The proof of this lemma is similar to that of Proposition 1 in Brown *et al.* (2008) and that of Proposition 2 in Cai and Zhou (2009), and is thus omitted. The key fact is that η_k can be well approximated by $Z_k/(2h(0)\sqrt{m})$, which follows $N(0, 1/(4h^2(0)m))$, so that after the data transformation in (3.8), existing methods for Gaussian noise can be applied to $X_k, 1 \leq k \leq T$. It will be shown that by properly choosing the bin size m, a robust procedure can be constructed to reliably detect the signal segments. We note that the noise variance for the transformed data, $1/(4h^2(0)m)$, can be easily estimated and the estimation error does not affect the theoretical results.

It is shown in Cai *et al.* (2011) that the RSI provides robust and near-optimal results as long as the distribution of ξ_i is symmetric about 0 with the density function h satisfying $h(0) > 0$ and

$$|h(y) - h(0)| \leq Cy^2 \tag{3.13}$$

in an open neighborhood of 0. This assumption is satisfied, for example, by the Cauchy distribution, the Laplace distribution, the t distributions, as well as the Gaussian distribution.

Like the LRR data that are subject to local genomic wave effects, the read depth data also depend on the local genomic features such as the GC contents of the genome. GC-content bias describes the dependence between fragment count (read coverage) and GC content found in high-throughput sequencing assays, particularly the Illumina Genome Analyzer technology. This bias can dominate the signal of interest for analyses that focus on measuring fragment abundance within a genome, such as copy number estimation. Benjamini and Speed (2011) proposed a new method to calculate predicted coverage and correct for the bias. This parsimonious model produces single bp prediction which suffices to predict the GC effect on fragment coverage at all scales, all chromosomes and for both strands. This model should be applied to estimate the GC-corrected read depths before our RSI procedure is used in order to reduce the effects of local feature on CNV identifications.

3.2. *Application to CNV analysis of a trio sequencing data from the 1000 Genome Project*

We applied this RSI procedure to a HapMap Yoruban trio and identified the CNVs independently for the parents and the child. After the short reads are mapping to the reference human DNA sequences, we obtain the RD data at $n = 54,361,060$ genomic locations. The statistical challenges for CNV detection based on NGS data include both ultra-high dimensionality of the data that requires fast computation and unknown distribution of the read depths data. A close examination of our data shows that the variance of the data is much larger than its mean, indicating that the standard Poisson distribution cannot be used for modeling these read depth data.

We apply the RSI with $m = 400$ and $L = 150$ to each of the three individuals separately, which assumes that the maximum CNV based on

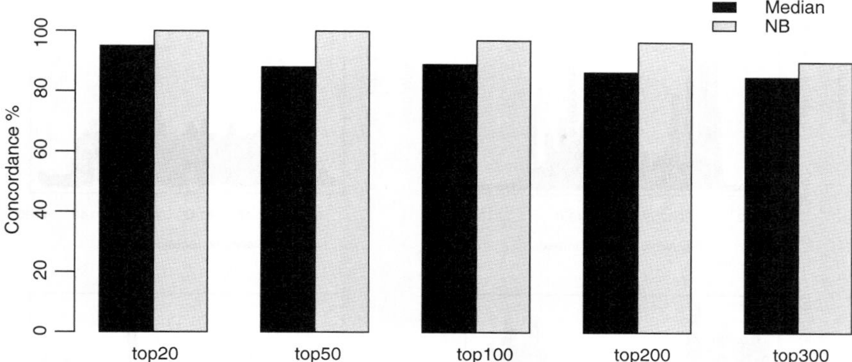

Fig. 4. Parents-child concordant rate of the CNV identified based on median (RSI) and negative binomial (NB) transformation of the RD data for the Yoruban trio.

our pre-processed data is $400 \times 150 = 60,000$ base pairs (bps). This is sensible since typical CNVs include multi-kilobase deletions and duplications. Figure 4 shows the concordant rates of the CNVs identified using the RSI when top 20, 50, 100, 200 and 300 CNVs identified for each of the three individuals on chromosome 19 are compared. We observe a very high concordant rates, which further validates the RSI for CNV detection based on the NGS data. On the same plot, we also present the CNV calling results assuming that the read depth data follow a negative binomial (NB) distribution. The concordant rates based on the NB distribution are slightly higher than the RSI procedure. As an example, Figure 5 shows plots of the read depth data for six different CNVs identified for the child, including two duplications, two deletions, and two regions with the shortest CNVs. It is clear that these identified regions indeed represent the regions with different RDs than their neighboring regions. Examinations of the other CNV regions identified also show that these regions contain more or fewer reads than their neighboring regions, further indicating the effectiveness of the RSI procedure in identifying the CNVs.

4. Detection of Recurrent CNVs Based on a Population-Based Samples

4.1. *Statistical formulation and summary of theoretical results*

Germline CNVs, as a population level genetic variants, often occur recurrently in individuals from a population. Recurrent CNVs are important

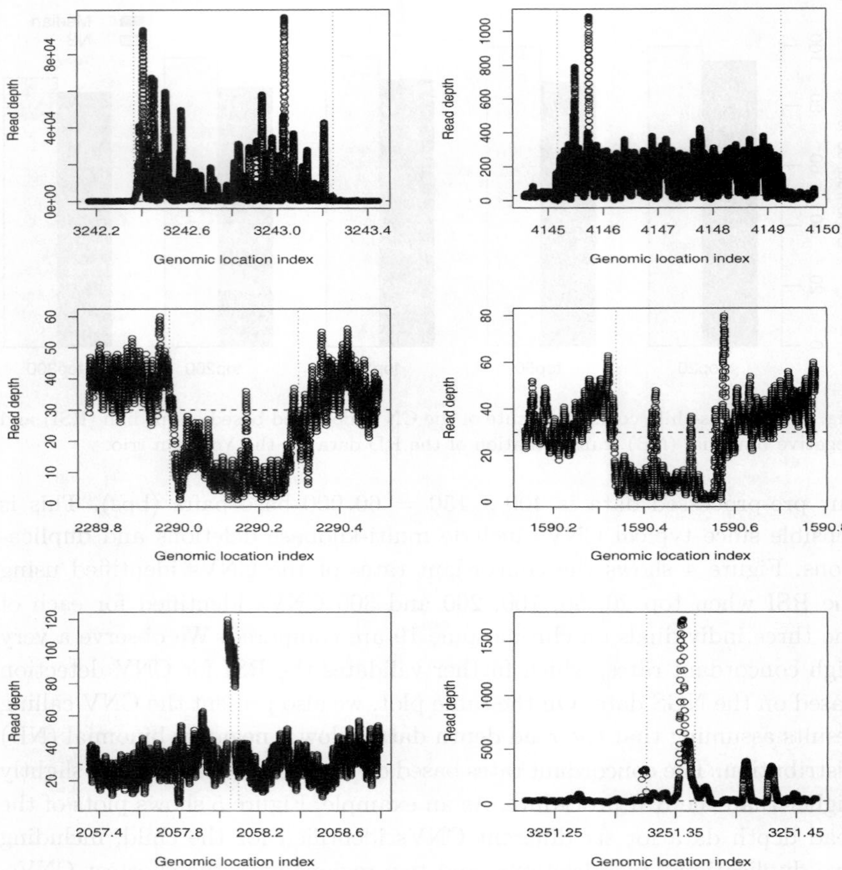

Fig. 5. Examples of CNV identified by the RSI on chromosome 19 of NA19240 from the 1000 Genomes Project. Top two plots: duplications, regions with the highest scores; middle two plots: deletions, regions with the smallest scores; bottom two plots: the two shortest CNVs identified. For each plot, the horizontal line presents the median count of 30 and the vertical dashed lines represent the estimated CNV boundaries. For each plot, x-axis is the genomic location in base pairs/10,000.

targets for association study and other down-stream population genetic analysis. When a large set of samples from a population are available, it is of great interest to pool information from multiple samples to identity recurrent CNVs in the population. This is especially relevant when the CNV signals from one single sample are not strong enough to be detect, however, pooling information across multiple samples can greatly increase the power of detecting such CNVs.

While efficient procedures have been developed for identifying CNVs in a long sequence of genome-wide observations, some type of post-processing is often used to select regions with highly recurrent CNVs. One problem with such an approach is that the power for identifying the recurrent CNVs does not improve with the increase of sample size. An important fact is that the locations of a recurrent CNV are mostly overlapping across samples, so the improvement of identification power is possible if information from multiples samples can be efficiently pooled during the CNV identification step. In addition, most CNVs from the germline constitutional genome are very short and range mostly less than 20 single nucleotide polymorphism (SNPs) (Zhang *et al.* 2009) in typical Illumina 660K chip. Many of these short CNVs cannot be identified even by the optimal method based on data from a single sample (Jeng *et al.* 2010). Efficiently pooling information from multiple samples can greatly benefit the discovery of short CNVs that are missed in single-sample analysis. This has been nicely demonstrated by two recent publications. Zhang *et al.* (2010) introduced a method for detecting simultaneous change-points in multiple sequences that is only effective for detecting common CNVs. Siegmund *et al.* (2010) further extended the method in Zhang *et al.* (2010) for identifying both the rare and common variants by introducing a prior probability of CNV frequencies that needs to be specified. No rigorous power studies were given in these two papers.

The model and the data for multiple sample CNV identification can be summarized as follows. Suppose there are N linear sequences (or samples) of noisy data and each sequence has T observations. Let X_{it} be the observed data for the ith sample at the tth location. If there are no signal variations, X_{it} scatters around 0 for any i and t. Suppose that at certain nonoverlapping segments (subintervals) $I_1, \ldots, I_q$ some samples have elevated or dropped means from the baseline (i.e., carriers) and others do not. Denote the collection of the segments as $\mathbb{I} = \{I_1, \ldots, I_q\}$, the carrier proportion at segment I_k in the population as π_k, and the magnitude of the segment for sample i as A_{ik}. Then an observation for sample $i \in \{1, \ldots, N\}$ at location $t \in \{1, \ldots, T\}$ can be modeled as

$$X_{it} = A_{ik} 1_{\{t \in I_k\}} + Z_{it} \quad \text{for some } I_k \in \mathbb{I}, \tag{4.14}$$

where

$$A_{ik} \sim (1 - \pi_k)\delta_0 + \pi_k N(\mu_k, \tau_k^2), \qquad \mu_k \neq 0, \quad \tau_k^2 \geq 0, \tag{4.15}$$

δ_0 is a point mass at 0, and $Z_{it} \sim N(0, \sigma_i^2)$. The noise variance σ_i^2 for sample i can be easily estimated when T is large and the signal segments are sparse in the linear sequence of data for sample i. For example, the robust median absolute deviation (MAD) estimator can be applied. We assume $\sigma_i^2 = 1$ in theoretical analysis. All of the other parameters $I_k, \pi_k, \mu_k, \tau_k$, $1 \leq k \leq q$ are unknown. From this model, if t is not in any signal segment, X_{it} is Gaussian noise following $N(0, \sigma_i^2)$. If t is in a signal segment I_k, then

$$X_{it} \sim (1 - \pi_k)N(0, \sigma_i^2) + \pi_k N(\mu_k, \sigma_i^2 + \tau_k^2). \tag{4.16}$$

This Gaussian mixture is both heterogenous and heteroscedastic. The τ_k of the second component represents the additional variability introduced by the different magnitudes of signal segments in the population.

Our goal is two-fold: (1) to detect the existence of recurrent segment variants across samples; and (2) to identify the locations of the segments. Precisely, we wish to first test

$$H_0 : \mathbb{I} = \emptyset \qquad \text{agains} \qquad H_1 : \mathbb{I} \neq \emptyset, \tag{4.17}$$

and if H_0 is rejected, detect each $I_k \in \mathbb{I}$.

A major challenge of pooling information from multiple samples to discover recurrent CNVs is that the CNV carrier's proportions vary a lot for different CNVs. Jeng *et al.* (2011) studied the problem from the perspective of sparse signal detection and proposed a proportion adaptive segment selection (PASS) procedure. Denote the set of the intervals with length less than or equal to L by $\mathbb{J}_{T,N}(L)$. For any interval $\tilde{I} \in \mathbb{J}_{T,N}(L)$, we calculate the standardized sum of observations in $\tilde{I}$ for each sample as

$$X_{\tilde{I},i} = \sum_{t \in \tilde{I}} X_{it} / \sqrt{|\tilde{I}|}, \qquad 1 \leq i \leq N. \tag{4.18}$$

By (4.14) and the assumption $\sigma_i^2 = 1$, $X_{\tilde{I},i}$ follows $N(0, 1)$ under H_0. When $\tilde{I}$ overlaps with some signal segment, $X_{\tilde{I},i}$ follows a heterogeneous and heteroscedastic Gaussian mixtures according to (4.16). Specifically, when $\tilde{I} = I_k$ for some $I_k \in \mathbb{I}$,

$$X_{I_k,i} \sim (1 - \pi_k)N(0, \sigma_i^2) + \pi_k N(\mu_k \sqrt{|I_k|}, \sigma_i^2 + \tau_k^2). \tag{4.19}$$

Note that the mean value of the second component includes the information of jump size and length of the segment variant at I_k.

The key of the PASS is to use the HC statistics (Donoho and Jin, 2004) to pool information across multiple samples based on the statistics $X_{\tilde{I},i}$ in order the identify the CNV regions. The PASS procedure can automatically adjusts to the unknown carrier's proportion and optimally detect both the rare and common CNVs. Jeng *et al.* (2011) showed that PASS has desirable theoretical and numerical properties. They further characterized the detection boundary that separates the region where a segment variant is detectable by some method from the region where it cannot be detected by any methods. Despite the fact that the detection boundaries are very different for the rare and common segment variants, Jeng *et al.* (2011) showed that PASS can reliably identify both the rare and common segment variants whenever they are detectable. Compared with methods for single sample analysis, PASS significantly gains power by pooling information from multiple samples.

Similar to the LRS procedure, PASS assumes that the noises of the LRR data follow a normal distribution. Great care must be taken to ensure that the data are approximately normal. An interesting problem for future research is the CNV identification by population-scale genome sequencing (Mills *et al.*, 2011). The next generation sequencing technology can generate billions of counts data along the whole human genome and genotype much more DNA regions with rare variants. Due to complexity of the sequencing process, error distribution of the counts data is unknown and is difficult to characterize parametrically. An promising approach is to apply the median transformation to the read depths data and then to apply the PASS to the transformed data.

4.2. *Application to analysis of neuroblastoma cases*

We applied the PASS procedure to a sample of 674 neuroblamstoma cases that were collected as part of a large-scale genome-wide association study of neuroblastoma (Diskin *et al.*, 2009). For each sample, about 600,000 SNPs were genotyped using the Illumina genotype platform and the log R-ratios data were obtained. In order to account for possible wave-effect or local effects, we performed similar processing as in Zhang *et al.* (2008) to obtain the normalized data, including subtracting the sample median, local adjustment by regressing on the first principal component. In our analysis, we considered only data from the chromosome 1, which includes $T = 40,929$ SNP log R-ratios.

PASS $L = 20$ resulted in selection of 335 CNVs with length of three or more SNPs, including 171 CNVs with three SNPs and 100 CNVs with 4 SNPs, and 11 CNVs with 10 or more SNPs. The median size of the CNVs identified is 4,165 bps with a range of 462 bps and 1,038,000 bps.

Since the identification of the short CNVs are more susceptible to local wave effects or other artifacts of the data, we should interpret the CNVs of three or four SNPs with caution and focus the following comparison on the identified CNVs of 5 or more SNPs. Among the CNVs identified, 64 have five or more SNPs. Among these 64 CNVs, 30 overlap with the CNVs in the database of genomic variants (http://projects.tcag.ca/variation/project.html). Note that this database only includes the CNVs identified in healthy human cases and are relatively common. To further demonstrate the power of PASS, we also performed single-sample CNV identification using the optimal CNV identification procedure LRS. Among the 64 CNVs with 5 or more SNPs identified by PASS, 20 of them did not reach the theoretical threshold of $\sqrt{2\log(TL)} = 5.22$ in any of the 674 samples, indicating a great loss of power of detecting the CNVs based on the single-sample analysis. Of these 20 CNVs missed by single sample analysis, 10 of them overlap with the CNVs in the genomic variants database.

5. Conclusion and Further Discussion

Our review focuses only on the germline CNV detection problems, where the CNVs are short and sparse. There are a few other problems that require further methods development.

5.1. *Statistical tests for CNV associations*

One problem is to identify the CNVs that are associated with a clinical phenotype. This is often performed in a two-step approach. First all the CNVs are identified for all the samples by some CNV identification methods. These identified CNVs are then tested through some simple regression models. One limitation of this approach is the information of shared CNVs across multiple samples are not effectively utilized. In addition, the CNVs identified based on each sample separately often do not have exactly the same staring/ending boundaries. This makes the summaries of CNVs across multiple samples difficult. Finally, since the number of the tests is unknown prior to the CNV calls, it is not clear how one should adjust for multiple comparisons. An alternative to the two-stage procedure is to test for CNV association only for those known CNVs. Barnes *et al.* (2008) developed a robust statistical method for case-control association testing with CNVs using the EM algorithm treating the observed CNVs as latent variables.

Besides testing for association between relatively common CNVs and the clinical phenotypes, statistical methods for testing rare CNV (found in $< 1\%$ of the total sample) association are also needed. Global rare CNV burden are often compared between cases and controls regardless of where the rare CNVs are (Girirajan *et al.*, 2011). Zhang *et al.* (2009a) presented a genome wide copy number variant (CNV) survey of 1001 Bipolar disorder cases and 1034 controls using the Affymetrix SNP 6.0 SNP and CNV platform. Singleton deletions (deletions that appear only once in the dataset) more than 100 kilobases in length are present in 16.2% of BD cases in contrast to 12.3% of controls (permutation $p = 0.007$), indicating potential importance of considering the cumulative effects of rare CNVs on disease risk. Methods that have been developed for testing rare genetic variants associations can also been applied for testing rare CNV association with the difficulty that the carriers of the rare variants have to be inferred from data, which can be challenging unless the signals are very strong.

5.2. *CNV analysis based on mapping distances of pair-end sequencing*

Another area that needs further statistical research is the CNV detection problem based on pair-end sequencing data, where the mapping distances between the mate pairs also provide important information about the structural changes of the genomes. Figure 6 gives an illustration of how mapping

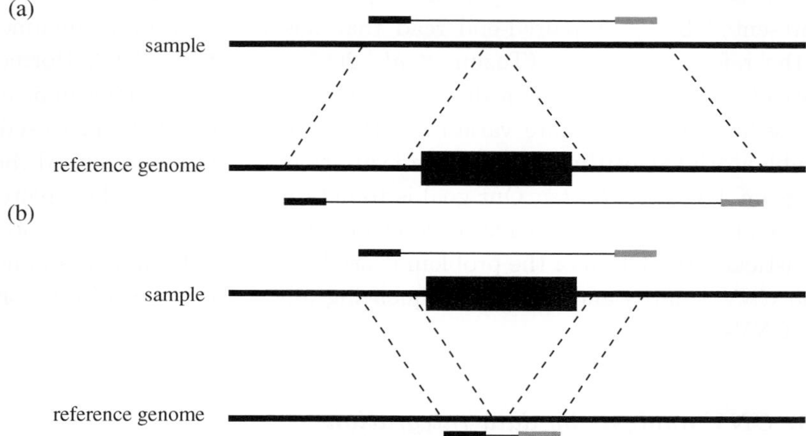

Fig. 6. Illustration of detecting insertions and deletions based on the mapping distances from the paired-end mapping data. The ends of a DNA fragment from a sample individual are mapped to a reference genome (Schrider and Hahn, 2010). (a) If the portion of the reference genome spanned by the fragment ends is larger than expected, then the sample genome probably contains a deletion relative to the reference. (b) If the length of the region spanned by the locations of the end sequences in the reference genome is smaller than expected, then an insertion is inferred to be present in the sample genome.

distances can be used for inferring the deletion and duplication base on the pari-end data. Beside the CNVs, the mapping distances or mapping orientations also provide information on translocations and inversions. Rigorous statistical formulations of both single-sample and multiple-sample CNV detection based on the mapping distances are required. Besides statistical formulation of the problems, efficient computational methods are also necessary since typical data sets often include several billions of end sequences of matepairs.

Methods of CNV analysis based on the matepair mapping distances relies on the computation of the expected distance between matepairs in the donor genome, which is referred to as insert size, d_i for the ith matepair. The distribution of the insert sizes d_i can be determined (Tuzun *et al.*, 2005). An alignment of a paired-end read to reference genome is called concordant (Tuzun *et al.*, 2005), if the distance between aligned ends of a pair in the reference genome is thought to come from the baseline insert size distribution, and both the orientation and the chromosome the paired-end read is aligned to are correct. For instance, in the Illumina platform, a paired-end read is considered to be aligned in the correct orientation if the left matepair is mapped to the "+" strand (which is represented by +), and the right mate pair is mapped to the "-" strand (which is represented by -). A paired-end read that has no concordant alignment in the reference genome (Tuzun *et al.*, 2005; Lee *et al.*, 2008; Hormozdiari *et al.*, 2009) is called a discordant paired-end read, which indicates a possibility of a structure variant. Hormozdiari *et al.* (2009) proposed a combinatorial algorithms for structure variation detection and named their program *VariationHunter*. Our goal is to determine the discordant paired-end reads and use these reads to determine the CNV regions. A rigorous statistical formulation of the problem is needed in order to understand how true CNV lengths and depth of sequencing affect the power of detecting the CNVs.

5.3. *CNV analysis by data integration*

Finally, for the SNP chip data, B-allele frequencies also provide useful information for CNV detection and identifications. How to extend the LRS and PASS procedure to incorporate the B-allele frequencies data is an important topic in CNV research. For NGS data, an interesting research topic is to combine both read depth data and the mapping distances data in a unified framework for CNV detection.

Acknowledgments

This research is supported in part by NIH grant CA127334 and NSF FRG Grant DMS-0854973.

References

Abyzov, A., Urban, A., Snyder, M., and Gerstein, M. (2011). "CNVnator: An approach to discover, genotype and characterize typical and atypical CNVs from family and population genome sequencing," *Genome Research*, **21**, 974–984.

Alkan, C., Coe, B., and Eichler, E. (2011). "Genome structural variation discovery and genotyping," *Nat Rev Genet.*, **12**, 363–375.

Arias-Castro, E., Candes, E. J., Helgason, H., and Zeitouni, O. (2008). "Searching for a trail of evidence in a maze," *Ann. Statist.*, **36**, 1726–1757.

Arias-Castro, E., Donoho, D., and Huo, X. (2005). "Near-optimal detection of geometric objects by fast multiscale methods," *IEEE Transactions on Information Theory*, **51**, 2402–2425.

Barnes, C., Plagnal, V., Fitzgerald, T., Redon, R., Marchini, J., Clayton, D., and Hurles, M. (2008). "A robust statistical method for case-control association testing with Copy Number Variation," *Nature Genetics*, **40**, 1245–1252.

Benjamini, Y. and Hochberg, T. (1995). "Controlling the false discovery rate: a practical and powerful approach to multiple testing," *J. Royal Stat. Soc. B*, **85**, 289–300.

Benjamini, Y. and Speed, T. P. (2011). "Estimation & correction for GC-content bias in high throughput sequencing," *Technical report, UC Berkeley.*

Bhattacharya, P. (1994). "Some aspects of change-point analysis," *In Change-point Problems, IMS Monograph 23, E. Carlstein, H. Muller and D. Siegmund, eds. Institute of Mathematical Statistics, Beachwood, OH*, 28–56.

Brown, L. D., Cai, T. T., and Zhou, H. H. (2008). "Robust nonparametric estimation via wavelet median regression," *Ann. Statist.*, **36**, 2055–2084.

Bucan, M., Abrahams, B., Wang, K., Glessner, J., Herman, E., Sonnenblick, L., Retuerto, A. A., Imielinski, M., Hadley, D., Bradfield, J., Kim, C., Gidaya, N., Lindquist, I., Hutman, T., , Sigman, M., Kustanovich, V., Lajonchere, C., Singleton, A., Kim, J., , Wassink, T., McMahon, W., Owley, T., Sweeney, J., Coon, H., Nurnberger, J., Li, M., Cantor, R., Minshew, N., Sutcliffe, J., Cook, E., Dawson, G., Buxbaum, J., Grant, S., Schellenberg, G., Geschwind, D., and Hakonarson, H. (2009). "Genome-wide analyses of exonic copy number variants in a family-based study point to novel autism susceptibility genes," *PLoS Genetics*, **5**, e1000536.

Cai, T. T., Jeng, J. J., and Li, H. (2011). "Robust Detection and Identification of Sparse Segments in Ultra-High Dimensional Data Analysis," *JRSS-B, in press.*

Cai, T. T. and Zhou, H. H. (2009). "Asymptotic equivalence and adaptive estimation for robust nonparametric regression," *Ann. Statist.*, **37**, 3204–3235.

Cheung, M., Down, T., Latorre, I., and Ahringer, J. (2011). "Systematic bias in high-throughput sequencing data and its correction by BEADS," *Nucleic Acids Research*, **39**(15), e103.

Chiang, D., Getz, G., Jaffe, D., O'Kelly, M., Zhao, X., Carter, S., Russ, C., Nusbaum, C., Meyerson, M., and Lander, E. (2009). "High-resolution mapping of copy-number alterations with massively parallel sequencing," *Nature Methods*, **6**, 99–103.

Diskin, S. J., Hou, C., Glessner, J. T., Attiyeh, E. F., Laudenslager, M., Bossel, K., Colel, K., Moss, Y., Wood, A., Lynch, J. E., Pecor, K., Diamond, M., Winter, C., Wang, K., Kim, C., Geiger, E. A., McGrady, P. W., Blakemore, A. I. F., London, W. B., Shaikh, T. H., Bradfield, J., Grant, S. F. A., Li, H., Devoto, M., Rappaport, E. R., Hakonarson, H., and Maris, J. M. (2009). "Copy number variation at 1q21.1 associated with neuroblastoma," *Nature*, **459**, 987–991.

Donoho, D. and Jin, J. (2004). "Higher criticism for detecting sparse heterogeneous mixtures," *Ann. Statist.*, **32**, 962–994.

Donoho, D. and Jin, J. (2008). "Higher Criticism thresholding: optimal feature selection when useful features are rare and week," *Proc. Natl. Acad. Sci.*, **105**, 14790–14795.

Feuk, L., Carson, A., and Scherer, S. (2006). "Structural variation in the human genome," *Nature Review Genetics*, **7**, 85–97.

Girirajan, S., Brkanac, Z., Coe, B., Baker, C., L, L. V., and *et al.* (2011). "Relative Burden of Large CNVs on a Range of Neurodevelopmental Phenotypes," *PLoS Genetics*, **7**(11), pages.

Hall, P. and Jin, J. (2010). "Innovated Higher Criticism for detecting sparse signals in correlated noise," *Ann. Statist.*, **38**(3), 1686–1732.

Hastings, P. J., Lupski, J. R., Rosenberg, S. M., and Ira, G. (2009). "Mechanisms of change in gene copy number," *Nature Review Genetics*, **10**, 551–564.

Hormozdiari, F., Alkan, C., Eichler, E., and *et al.* (2009). "Combinatorial algorithms for structural variation detection in high-throughput sequenced genomes," *Genome Research*, 19.

Jeng, X. J., Cai, T. T., and Li, H. (2010). "Optimal sparse segment identification with application in copy number variation analysis," *J. Am. Statist. Ass.*, **105**, 1156–1166.

Jeng, X. J., Cai, T. T., and Li, H. (2011). "Simultaneous discovery of rare and common segment variants," *Biometrika*, **100**, 157–172.

Lee, S., Cheran, E., and Brudno, M. (2008). "A robust framework for detecting structural variations in a genome," *Bioinformatics*, **24**, i59–i67.

Li, J., Jiang, H., and Wong, W. (2010). "Modeling non-uniformity in short-read rates in RNA-Seq data," *Genome Biology*, 11, R50.

Marioni, J., Thorne, N., Valsesia, A., Fitzgerald, T., Redon, R., Fiegler, H., Andrews, T., Stranger, B., Lynch, A., Dermitzakis, E., Carter, N., Tavare, S., and Hurles, M. (2007). "Breaking the waves: improved detection of copy number variation from microarray-based comparative genomic hybridization," *Genome Biology*, **8**(1), R228.

Medvedev, P., Stanciu, M., and Brudno, M. (2009). "Computational methods for discovering structural variation with next-generation sequencing," *Nature Methods*, **6**, S13–S20.

Miller, C. A., Hampton, O., Coarfa, C., and Milosavljevic, A. (2011). "ReadDepth: A Parallel R Package for Detecting Copy Number Alterations from Short Sequencing Reads," *PLos ONE*, **6**(1), e16327.

Mills, R. R., Walter, K., Stewart, C., ..., and Korbel, J. O. (2011). "Mapping copy number variation by population-scale genome sequencing," *Nature*, **470**, 59–65.

Olshen, A. B., Venkatraman, E. S., Lucito, R., and Wigler, M. (2004). "Circular binary segmentation for the analysis of array-based DNA copy number data," *Biostatistics*, **5**(4), 557–572.

Peiffer, D. A., Le, J. M., Steemers, F. J., Chang, W., Jenniges, T., Garcia, F., Haden, K., Li, J., Shaw, C. A., Belmont, J., Cheung, S. W., Shen, R. M., Barker, D. L., and Gunderson, K. L. (2006). "High-resolution genomic profiling of chromosomal aberrations using Infinium whole-genome genotyping," *Genome Res*, **16**, 1136–1148.

Schrider, D. R. and Hahn, M. (2010). "Gene copy-number polymorphism in nature," *Proceedings of The Royal Society (B)*, **277**, 3213–3221.

Sebat, J., Lakshmi, B., Troge, J., Alexander, J., Young, J., Lundin, P., Maner, S., Massa, H., Walker, M., Chi, M., and et al. (2004). "Large-scale copy number polymorphism in the human genome," *Science*, **305**, 525–528–97.

Shendure, J. and Ji, H. (2008). "Next-generation DNA sequencing," *Nature Biotechnology*, **26**, 1135–1145.

Stefansson, H., Rujescu, D., Cichon, S., Pietilainen, O., Ingason, A., Steinberg, A., Fossdal, R., Sigurdsson, E., Sigmundsson, T., Buizer-Voskamp, J., and et al. (2008). "Large recurrent microdeletions associated with schizophrenia," *Nature*, **455**, 178–179.

Stone, J., O'Donovan, M., Gurling, H., Kirov, G., Blackwood, D., Corvin, A., Craddock, N., Gill, M., Hultman, C., Lichtenstein, P., and *et al.* (2008). "Rare chromosomal deletions and duplications increase risk of schizophrenia," *Nature*, **455**, 237–241.

Sudmant, P., Kitzman, J., Antonacci, F., Alkan, C., Malig, M., Tsalenko, A., Sampas, N., Bruhn, L., Shendure, J., Project, . G., and Eichler, E. (2010). "Diversity of human copy number variation and multicopy genes," *Science*, **330**, 641–646.

Tuzun, E., Sharp, A. J., Bailey, J., Kaul, R., Morrison, V., Pertz, L., Haugen, E., Hayden, H., Albertson, D., and et al., D. P. (2005). "Fine-scale structural variation of the human genome," *Nature Genetics*, **37**, 727-732.

Walsh, T., McClellan, J., McCarthy, S., Addington, A., Pierce, S., Cooper, G., Nord, A., Kusenda, M., Malhotra, D., Bhandari, A., and *et al.* (2008). "Rare structural variants disrupt multiple genes in neurodevelopmental pathways in schizophrenia," *Science*, **320**, 539–543.

Walther, G. (2010). "Optimal and fast detection of spacial clusters with scan statistics," *Ann. of Stat.*, **38**(2), 1010–1033.

Wang, K., Li, M., Hadley, D., Liu, R., Glessner, J., Grant, S., Hakonarson, H., and Bucan, M. (2007). "PennCNV: an integrated hidden Markov model designed for high-resolution copy number variation detection in whole-genome SNP genotyping data," *Genome Research*, **17**, 1665–1674.

Xie, C. and Tammi, M. (2009). "CNV-seq, a new method to detect copy number variation using high-throughput sequencing," *BMC Bioinformatics*, **10**, 80.

Yoon, S., Xuan, Z., Makarov, V., Ye, K., and Sebat, J. (2009). "Sensitive and accurate detection of copy number variants using read depth of coverage," *Genome Research*, **19**, 1568–1592.

Zack, S. (1983). "Survey of classical and bayesian approaches to the change-point problem: Fixed sample and sequential procedures in testing and estimation," *In Recent Advances in Statistics, Academic Press, San Diego, CA*, 245–269.

Zhang, D., Cheng, L., Qian, Y., Alliey-Rodriguez, N., Kelsoe, J., Greenwood, T., Nievergelt, C., Barrett, T., McKinney, R., and et al (2009a). "Singleton deletions throughout the genome increase risk of bipolar disorder," *Molecular Psychiatry*, **14**, 376–380.

Zhang, F., Gu, W., Hurles, M., and Lupski, J. (2009b). "Copy number variation in human health, disease and evolutions," *Annual Review of Genomics and Human Genetics*, **10**, 451–481.

Zhang, N. R. and Siegmund, D. O. (2007). "A Modified Bayes Information Criterion with Applications to the Analysis of Comparative Genomics Hybridization Data," *Biometrics*, **63**, 22–32.

Zhang, N. R., Siegmund, D. O., Ji, H., and Li, J. (2010). "Detecting Simultaneous Change-points in Multiple Sequences," *Biometrika*, **97**(3), 631–645.

Zhang, Z., Lange, K., Ophoff, R., and Sabatti, C. (2010). "Reconstructing DNA copy number by penalized estimation and imputation," *The Annals of Applied Statistics*, **4**, 1749–1773.

About the Authors

T. Tony Cai received his Ph.D. degree from Cornell University, Ithaca, NY, in 1996. His research interests include high-dimensional inference, large- scale multiple testing, nonparametric function estimation, functional data analysis and statistical decision theory. He is the Dorothy Silberberg Professor of Statistics at the Wharton School of the University of Pennsylvania, Philadelphia. Dr. Cai is the recipient of the 2008 COPSS Presidents Award and a fellow of the Institute of Mathematical Statistics. He was also a past editor of the Annals of Statistics.

Dr. Jeng has been an Assistant Professor of Statistics at North Carolina State University since 2012. Prior to joining NCSU, Dr. Jeng was a post-doctoral researcher in the Department of Biostatistics and Epidemiology at University of Pennsylvania (2009–2012). She received a Ph.D. in Statistics from Purdue University in 2009. Dr. Jeng's research interests include high-dimensional inference, multiple testing, variable selection, mixture model detection, statistical genomics, and bioinformatics.

Dr. Hongzhe Li is a Professor of Biostatistics at the University of Pennsylvania Perelman School of Medicine. His research focuses on developing statistical and computational methods for analysis of high dimensional genomic data, including network-based analysis of genomic, methods for analysis of next generation sequencing data and methods for analysis of metagenomics data. He has published over 130 papers and served as an Associate Editor of Journal of American Statistical Association. He is an Associate Editor of Biometrics and Statistics in Biosciences. His research has been continuously supported by NIH R01 grants since 2007. He is a member of Board of Scientific Counselor for Clinical Sciences and Epidemiology, National Cancer Institute of the US National Institutes of Health. He is an elected Fellow of the American Statistical Association and Institute of Mathematical Statistics.

CHAPTER 23

STATISTICAL METHODS FOR DESIGN AND ANALYSIS OF LINKAGE STUDIES

QIZHAI LI

Academy of Mathematics and Systems Science,
Chinese Academy of Sciences, Beijing 100190, China

HONG QIN

Central China Normal University,
Wuhan 430079, China

ZHAOHAI LI

Department of Statistics, George Washington University,
Washington, DC 20052, USA
zli@gwn.edu

GANG ZHENG

Office of Biostatistics Research,
Division of Prevention and Population Sciences,
National Heart, Lung and Blood Institute,
Bethesda, MD 20892, USA

1. Introduction

With the advance of biological technology, more and more experiments have shown that many human complex diseases, such as type 2 diabetes mellitus, coronary artery disease, schizophrenia, and rheumatoid arthritis, etc, are associated with genetic components. Locating these genetic loci might help understand the etiology of human disorders, and it might result in producing some better treatments for the disease. Since the associated genes with certain diseases are often unknown, the exact orientation of a disease locus is very difficult to find. A feasible way is to find a known marker, which is linked to the unknown disease locus. Since the alleles at two loci are likely to segregate together to the next generation when they are close enough on the same chromosome, the main problem in genetic linkage analysis is to test whether the known marker locus is linked with a disease locus on the same chromosome. This chapter begins with some basic genetic terminology. Then we introduce some common methods for testing linkage. Considering the uncertainty of genetic mode of inheritance, we finally discuss some robust procedures.

1.1. *Basic genetic terminology*

There are totally 23 pairs of chromosomes for each individual, where 22 pairs are autosomal chromosomes, which are focused on here, and one pair is sex chromosome, which determines the sex of an individual (females with XX chromosomes and males with XY chromosomes). The human genome is made up of large units of deoxyribonucleic acid (DNA). Genes are DNA sequences in the genome. A given location in the genome is called a locus, which often indicates single nucleotide polymorphism (SNP)(a DNA sequence variation of single nucleotide between members of a biological species) or a gene (a molecular unit of heredity). At a given locus, there are alleles (the genetic variants), which are often denoted by the letters, for example, A, a, B, or b etc. The proportion of a certain allele in the population is called the allele probability or the allele frequency. Since the concerned allele frequency is often less than 0.5, the allele is called the minor allele and the corresponding allele frequency is called the minor allele frequency (MAF). For example, $\Pr(A) = 0.2$ means the frequency of allele A is 0.2. If we use A and a to denote two alleles at a given locus, then there are three genotypes, AA, Aa and aa, where Aa and aA are not differentiated and taken as the same genotype, which means the order of A and a is not relevant. Usually, AA and aa are called homozygous and Aa is heterozygous. An observable trait of an individual is called phenotype. The genotype and phenotype might not be one-to-one. If both genotype AA and Aa have the same phenotype and it is different from that of aa, allele A is said to be dominant to allele a, or allele a is recessive to allele A. Then phenotype corresponding to AA or Aa is called dominant, and that of aa is recessive. If the phenotype of Aa is different from those of AA and aa, allele A and a are said to be codominant.

1.2. *Hardy-weinberg equilibrium*

Given two alleles A and a at a given locus, we assume that the allele frequency of A is p, that is $\Pr(A) = p$, and $\Pr(a) = 1 - p \mathrel{\widehat{=}} q$. If the genotype frequencies of AA, Aa and aa in the population satisfy to

$$\Pr(AA) = p^2, \quad \Pr(Aa) = 2pq, \quad \text{and} \quad \Pr(aa) = (1-p)^2,$$

this population is said to be in Hardy-Weinberg equilibrium (HWE) (Hardy, 1908; Weinberg, 1908).

In genetic association analysis, HWE in the population is usually assumed. In practice, after getting the observations, we test HWE using Pearson χ^2 test. For a given locus with alleles A and a, a random sample with n individuals are genotyped at this locus, the observed counts of three genotypes, aa, Aa and AA are n_{aa}, n_{Aa}, and n_{AA}, respectively. Then, the maximal likelihood estimators of the allele frequencies of A and a, p_A and p_a, are, respectively,

$$\hat{p}_A = \frac{2n_{AA} + n_{Aa}}{2n}, \quad \text{and} \quad \hat{p}_a = \frac{2n_{aa} + n_{Aa}}{2n}.$$

So, under the null hypothesis H_0 that HWE holds in the population, the expected counts of three genotypes corresponding to AA, Aa, aa, are subsequently, $n\hat{p}_A^2$, $2n\hat{p}_A\hat{p}_a$, and $n\hat{p}_a^2$. The one degree of freedom χ^2 test statistic is

$$T_{\text{HWE}} = \frac{(n_{aa} - n\hat{p}_a^2)^2}{n\hat{p}_a^2} + \frac{(n_{Aa} - 2n\hat{p}_A\hat{p}_a)^2}{2n\hat{p}_A\hat{p}_a} + \frac{(n_{AA} - n\hat{p}_A^2)^2}{n\hat{p}_A^2}.$$

For a given significance level α, if $T_{\text{HWE}} > \chi_1^2(1-\alpha)$, the $1-\alpha$ upper quantile of one degree of freedom χ^2 distribution, we reject H_0.

Consider an example of type II diabetes mellitus. It has been shown that it is correlated with genetic variants and environmental factors and their interactions. Sladek *et al.* (2007) conducted a genome-wide association study using 392,935 SNPs. They reported a SNP rs1005316 that is associated with type II diabetes. The numbers of genotypes of AA, Aa and aa in controls are 44, 211, and 399, respectively. So

$$\hat{p}_A = \frac{44 \times 2 + 211}{2 \times (44 + 211 + 399)} = 0.228.$$

Hence

$$\begin{aligned} T_{\text{HWE}} &= \frac{(44 - 654 \times 0.228^2)^2}{654 \times 0.228^2} + \frac{[211 - 2 \times 0.228 \times (1 - 0.228) \times 654]^2}{2 \times 0.228 \times (1 - 0.228) \times 654} \\ &\quad + \frac{[399 - (1 - 0.228)^2 \times 654]^2}{654 \times (1 - 0.228)^2} \\ &= 4.77. \end{aligned}$$

p-value is 0.029, which is not significance at the significance level 0.0001, which is often used at genome-wide level for testing deviation from HWE. So, we conclude there is no significant deviation from HWE in controls for SNP rs1005316.

1.3. *Linkage*

Each person has a pair of chromosomes, one copy is inherited from his/her father and another copy is inherited from his/her mother. Since 50% genes of a person are from each parent, there is certain correlation between the related individuals for their phenotypes. During human meiosis, these two chromosomes of the parents are generated separately. The two copies of each chromosome line up next to each other and undergo a random progress, which is called recombination. In other words, the alleles at the different loci one person has might be different from his/her parents. This phenomenon is referred to as crossover. When an odd number of crossover events occurs between two loci, the combination of the alleles at the two locus is a new combination that is different from the chromosomes of his/her parent. The probability of an odd number of crossover between two loci is called the recombination fraction, denoted by θ. For example, consider a family with two parents and two sons (squares in Figure 1) and two daughters (circles in Figure 1). Suppose that there are two loci with two alleles A and a at one locus and B and b at another locus. Figure 1 gives the haplotypes each person has in this family. We use "/" to denote the phase-known haplotype. Ab/aB refers to alleles A and b located in the same chromosome and a and B in the the same chromosome. From Figure 1, the recombinations occur

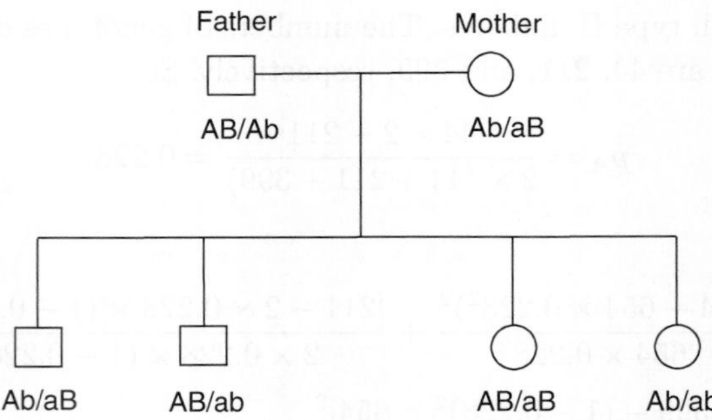

Fig. 1. A pedigree of two parents and 4 offsprings (two sons (squares) and two daughters (circles)).

as for the second son with genotype AB/ab and the second daughter with genotype Ab/ab.

Mendel's first law or the principal of independent segregation states that the probability that an individual receives one of the two alleles from each parent is 1/2. Suppose that the genotype of a parent is Aa, then

$$\Pr(\rightarrow A|Aa) = \Pr(\rightarrow a|Aa) = 1/2,$$

where $\rightarrow A|Aa$ refers to an event that a parent transmits allele A to the offspring given that his/her genotype is Aa, and $\rightarrow a|Aa$ has the similar meaning. If two loci are on different chromosomes, the transmission of alleles at one locus is independent to that at the other locus, which is called Mendel's second law. If two loci locate in the same chromosome and are close together, they tend to transmit together to an offspring, and this phenomenon is referred to as linkage. The recombination fraction for the linked loci is smaller than 0.5. So $\theta \in [0, 0.5]$.

For details on linkage, please refer to the books by Li (1988) and Hartl and Clark (1997).

1.4. *Linkage disequilibrium*

Consider two loci with alleles A and a at the first locus and B and b at the second. Denote the allele frequencies by

$$\Pr(A) = p_A, \quad \Pr(a) = p_a = 1 - p_A, \quad \Pr(B) = p_B, \quad \Pr(b) = p_b = 1 - p_B.$$

There are nine two-locus joint genotypes. If there is no linkage ($\theta = 0.5$) and that the joint genotype probabilities of these two loci for the current generation are given as in Table 1:

Table 1. Joint genotype frequencies of two loci.

$AABB$	$AABb$	$AAbb$	$AaBB$	$AaBb$	$Aabb$	$aaBB$	$aaBb$	$aabb$
$p_A^2p_B^2$	$2p_A^2p_Bp_b$	$p_A^2p_b^2$	$2p_Ap_ap_B^2$	$4p_Ap_ap_Bp_b$	$2p_Ap_ap_b^2$	$p_a^2p_B^2$	$2p_a^2p_Bp_b$	$p_a^2p_b^2$

Then, under the assumption of random mating, the joint genotype frequencies of the next generation is the same as the current one. We say the two loci are in linkage equilibrium. In this case, the two loci are in linkage equilibrium and the haplotype frequencies are given by:

$$\Pr(AB) = p_Ap_B, \quad \Pr(Ab) = p_Ap_b, \quad \Pr(aB) = p_ap_B, \quad \Pr(ab) = p_ap_b.$$

That is, the haplotype frequencies are equal to the product of the corresponding allele frequency of single-locus. $\Pr(AB)$ is the probability that allele A at the first locus and allele B at the second locus are on the same gamete.

On the other hand, the two loci are said in linkage disequilibrium (LD) if the following conditions hold:

$$\Pr(AB) \neq p_A p_B, \quad \Pr(Ab) \neq p_A p_b, \quad \Pr(aB) \neq p_a p_B, \quad \Pr(ab) \neq p_a p_b.$$

Define $\delta = \Pr(AB) - p_A p_B$, which is called the linkage disequilibrium parameter and used to indicate the departure from linkage equilibrium. Then we have

$$\Pr(AB) = p_A p_B + \delta, \quad \Pr(Ab) = p_A p_b - \delta, \quad \Pr(aB) = p_a p_B - \delta,$$
$$\Pr(ab) = p_a p_b + \delta.$$

Under linkage equilibrium, $\delta = 0$.

Now, let δ_0 be the initial LD parameter, which can also be expressed as

$$\delta_0 = \Pr(AB)\Pr(ab) - \Pr(Ab)\Pr(aB).$$

Denote the joint genotype probability matrix of the initial generation by Z_0, which is given by

$$Z_0 = \begin{pmatrix} \Pr(AABB) & \Pr(AABb) & \Pr(AAbb) \\ \Pr(AaBB) & \Pr(AaBb) & \Pr(Aabb) \\ \Pr(aaBB) & \Pr(aaBb) & \Pr(aabb) \end{pmatrix} = \begin{pmatrix} z_{11} & z_{12} & z_{13} \\ z_{21} & z_{22} & z_{23} \\ z_{31} & z_{32} & z_{33} \end{pmatrix}.$$

Then the corresponding gametic probability matrix is

$$g_0 = \begin{pmatrix} \Pr(AB) & \Pr(Ab) \\ \Pr(aB) & \Pr(ab) \end{pmatrix} = \begin{pmatrix} g_{11} & g_{13} \\ g_{31} & g_{33} \end{pmatrix},$$

where

$$\begin{cases} g_{11} = z_{11} + (z_{12} + z_{21})/2 + z_{22}/4, \\ g_{13} = z_{13} + (z_{12} + z_{23})/2 + z_{22}/4, \\ g_{31} = z_{31} + (z_{21} + z_{32})/2 + z_{22}/4, \\ g_{33} = z_{33} + (z_{23} + z_{32})/2 + z_{22}/4. \end{cases}$$

Under the random mating, the joint genotype probability matrix of the first offspring generation is

$$Z_1 = \begin{pmatrix} \Pr(AABB) & \Pr(AABb) & \Pr(AAbb) \\ \Pr(AaBB) & \Pr(AaBb) & \Pr(Aabb) \\ \Pr(aaBB) & \Pr(aaBb) & \Pr(aabb) \end{pmatrix}$$

$$= \begin{pmatrix} g_{11}^2 & 2g_{11}g_{13} & g_{13}^2 \\ 2g_{11}g_{31} & 2(g_{11}g_{33} + g_{13}g_{31}) & 2g_{13}g_{33} \\ g_{31}^2 & 2g_{31}g_{33} & g_{33}^2 \end{pmatrix},$$

and the gametic probability matrix of the first generation is

$$g_1 = \begin{pmatrix} g_{11} - \theta\delta_0 & g_{13} + \theta\delta_0 \\ g_{31} + \theta\delta_0 & g_{33} - \theta\delta_0 \end{pmatrix}.$$

So, the LD parameter of the first generation is

$$\delta_1 = (g_{11} - \theta\delta_0)(g_{33} - \theta\delta_0) - (g_{13} + \theta\delta_0)(g_{31} + \theta\delta_0) = (1 - \theta)\delta_0.$$

Repeat the above step, the LD parameter of the nth generation is

$$\delta_n = (1 - \theta)^n \delta_0.$$

It means that the LD parameter will approach 0 as the number of generations goes to infinity. And also the LD parameter will decrease quickly over generations when the linkage is weak, i.e, the recombination fraction is close to 0.5.

Note that for one locus, if the genotype probabilities of the current generation do not satisfy HWE, the linkage equilibrium will be reached after one generation of random mating (Wentworth and Remick, 1916). For two loci, this equilibrium will be approximately reached after several generations.

2. Linkage Analysis

Linkage analysis is a typical method used to localize disease traits in human genome. It localizes a gene solely on the basis of its location without considering its biochemical functions. Usually, family data or data from biologically related individuals are needed for detecting linkage. Considering the mode of inheritance, linkage analysis can be model-based or model-free. The measurement for linkage between two loci is the recombination fraction θ. The null hypothesis for linkage analysis is $\theta = 0.5$ (no linkage), and the alternative hypothesis is $\theta < 0.5$ (linked).

2.1. *Model-based method for linkage analysis: LOD score*

The maximum likelihood method is commonly employed in linkage analysis. By considering the likelihoods under the null and alternative hypotheses, one can construct a test statistic. The LOD score method was first proposed by Morton (Morton, 1955) for sequential tests for the detection of linkage using the maximum likelihood method. The LOD score method has been considered as a model-based procedure because it depends on the mode of inheritance, and the number of alleles and the penetrance of each genotype are assumed to be known. This method has been considered to be very successful in identifying genes for Mendelian diseases. Ott (1999), and Li, Qin, and Zhang (2006) described the LOD score method in details. Denote the two alleles at a diallelic trait locus by D and d with the allele frequencies being $\Pr(D) = p_D$ and $\Pr(d) = p_d = 1 - p_D$. Let the penetrance of three genotypes be

$$f_{DD} = \Pr(\text{Affected}|DD), \; f_{Dd} = \Pr(\text{Affected}|Dd), \quad \text{and} \\ f_{dd} = \Pr(\text{Affected}|dd).$$

Then the likelihood of θ for the observed data is

$$\Pr(\text{data}|\theta, p_D, p_d, f_{DD}, f_{Dd}, f_{dd}) \\ = \sum_{\text{marker}} \Pr(\text{data, marker}|p_D, p_d, f_{DD}, f_{Dd}, f_{dd})$$

The test statistic is the logarithm to base 10 of the likelihood ratio

$$T(\theta) = \log_{10} \frac{\Pr(\text{data}|\theta, p_D, p_d, f_{DD}, f_{Dd}, f_{dd})}{\Pr(\text{data}|\theta = 0.5, p_D, p_d, f_{DD}, f_{Dd}, f_{dd})},$$

which is termed as the LOD score. Denote the maximum likelihood estimate of θ by $\hat{\theta}$. Asymptotically, under H_0, $4.605 \times T(\hat{\theta})$ follows χ_1^2, a chi-square distribution with one degree of freedom. When $T(\hat{\theta})$ is larger than 3, there is linkage, otherwise no linkage exists. Actually, LOD score > 3 implies that a p-value is less than 0.0001.

2.1.1. *Phase-unknown LOD score*

Consider a rare autosomal dominant disease segregated in a family including two parents and four childrens. We assume that all the individuals have been genotyped at the marker locus, which is depicted in the first panel of Figure 2. In Figure 2, the dark symbols indicate that an individual is affected and the light symbols indicate that an individual is unaffected. A square stands for a male and a circle stands for a female. Let the two alleles at the disease locus be D and d. We assume that an individual is always affected if he/she carries the allele D, that is

$$\Pr(\text{Affected}|DD) = \Pr(\text{Affected}|Dd) = 1, \quad \Pr(\text{Affected}|dd) = 0.$$

We now infer the haplotype of the marker and trait loci. We first infer the father's haplotype. Since the father is unaffected, he is a homozygous dd at the disease locus. We next infer the haplotypes of the four offspring

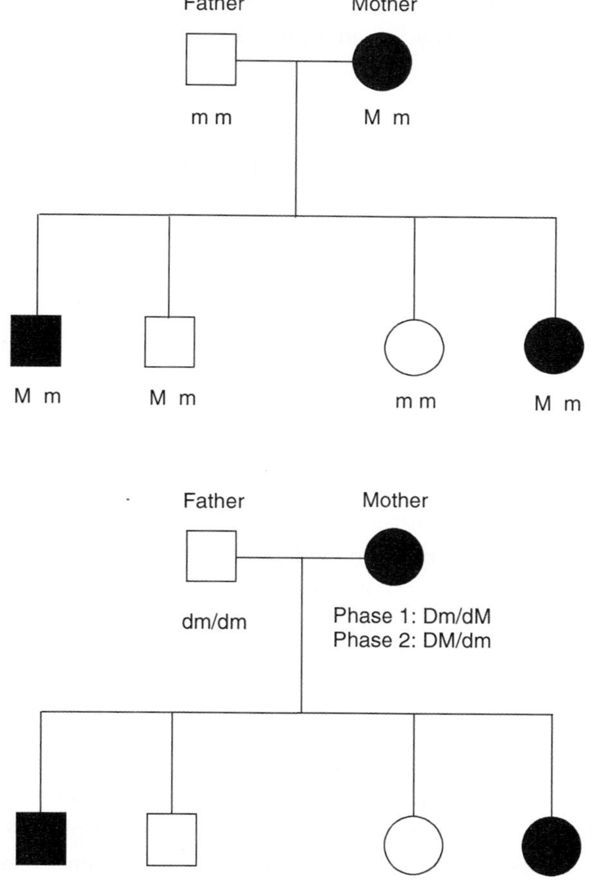

Fig. 2. A pedigree of two parents with one informative parent and 4 offspring with a rare dominant disease.

according to the status that he/she is affected or unaffected, which is shown at the second panel of Figure 2. The phase of the mother cannot be determined with certainty. She has two possible genotype phases, Dm/dM (Phase 1) and DM/dm (Phase 2). There are three recombinants and one non-recombinant for Phase 1 and one recombinant and three non-recombinants for Phase 2. So, under Phase 1, the likelihood for the pedigree in Figure 2 can be written to be

$$\Pr(\text{data}|\theta, p_D, p_d, f_{DD}, f_{Dd}, f_{dd}) = \eta(p_D, p_d, f_{DD}, f_{Dd}, f_{dd}) \times \theta^3(1-\theta),$$

where $\eta(\cdot)$ is a function that integrates the information of the marker and trait loci. In the same way, given Phase 2 of the mother's genotype, the likelihood is

$$\eta(p_D, p_d, f_{DD}, f_{Dd}, f_{dd}) \times \theta(1-\theta)^3.$$

Since we do not know the exact phase of the mother's genotypes, we assume equal probability for each phase, then the likelihood is

$$\begin{aligned}\Pr(\text{data}|\theta, p_D, p_d, f_{DD}, f_{Dd}, f_{dd}) \\ &= 0.5 \times \eta(p_D, p_d, f_{DD}, f_{Dd}, f_{dd}) \times \theta^3(1-\theta) \\ &\quad + 0.5 \times \eta(p_D, p_d, f_{DD}, f_{Dd}, f_{dd}) \times \theta(1-\theta)^3.\end{aligned}$$

The LOD score is

$$T(\theta) = \log_{10} \frac{\Pr(\text{data}|\theta, p_D, p_d, f_{DD}, f_{Dd}, f_{dd})}{\Pr(\text{data}|\theta = 0.5, p_D, p_d, f_{DD}, f_{Dd}, f_{dd})}.$$

The maximum likelihood estimate of θ is $\hat{\theta} = 0.5$. The LOD score is 1, which does not show significance evidence to support the linkage.

When the data is made up of more than one family, the likelihood is the product of the likelihood for each family if the families are independent of each other. The LOD score test is calculated similarly.

2.1.2. *Phase-known LOD score*

The previous section considers phase-unknown LOD score method, however, in practice, additional information might be available for helping us determine the phase of the mother's genotype. For example, we might know the genotype of the unaffected grandmother with the genotype mm on the marker locus. The grandmother's genotype must be dm/dm because of the rare dominant disease with full penetrance. Since the mother is affected, she must have at least one allele D. Given the disease is rare, we assume that her genotype is Dd at the trait locus. Hence, the phase of the mother's genotype is DM/dm, which uses the fact that the mother receives a haplotype dm from the grandmother. We can also infer the genotypes of the four children. The two locus genotypes and their phases for the whole family are given in Figure 3. The father is not informative for the recombination. There are one recombination and three non-recombinations from the mother. The likelihood function is

$$\Pr(\text{data}|\theta, p_D, p_d, f_{DD}, f_{Dd}, f_{dd}) = \eta(p_D, p_d, f_{DD}, f_{Dd}, f_{dd}) \times \theta(1-\theta)^3.$$

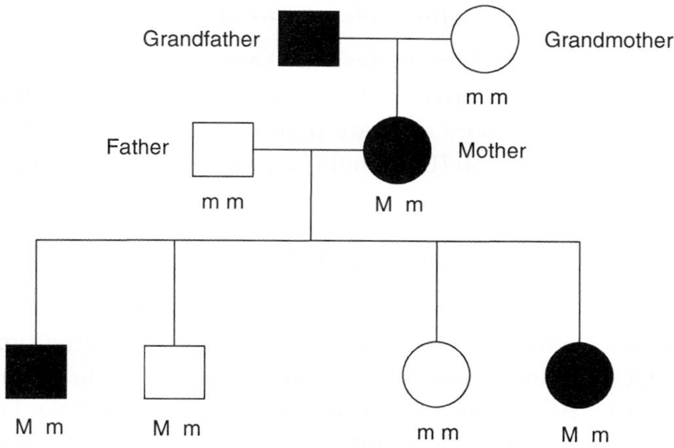

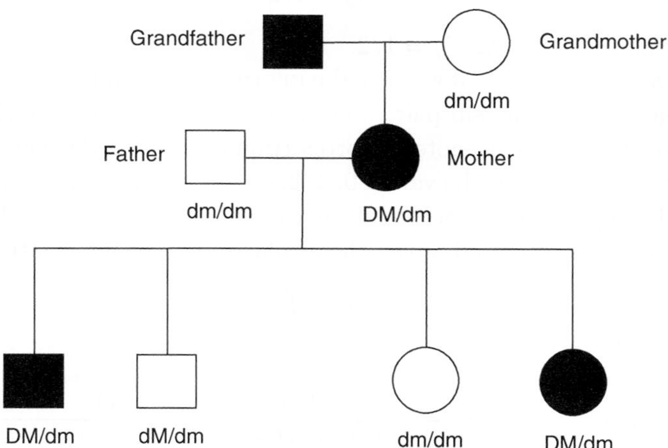

Fig. 3. A pedigree of two grand parents, two parents with one informative parent and 4 offspring with a rare dominant disease.

The LOD score is

$$T(\theta) = \log_{10} \frac{\eta(p_D, p_d, f_{DD}, f_{Dd}, f_{dd}) \times \theta(1-\theta)^3}{\eta(p_D, p_d, f_{DD}, f_{Dd}, f_{dd}) \times \frac{1}{16}}.$$

The maximum likelihood estimate of θ is $\hat{\theta} = 0.25$. Therefore, the LOD score is 1.69, not strong enough to support the linkage.

2.2. Model-free methods for linkage analysis

Model-free methods for linkage analysis are based on the marker IBD (identity by descent) or IBS (identity by status). IBD or IBS measures the marker similarity. Since IBD is more accurate than IBS for measuring the marker similarity, methods based on IBD should be more powerful than those based on IBS.

2.2.1. *Estimating proportion of alleles IBD*

IBD is defined as that two alleles from two related individuals are inherited from the same ancestor. For example, suppose that the mating type of two parents is $AA \times Aa$ and the sib pair's genotypes are both Aa. Then allele a of the sib pair is IBD, allele A of the sib pair might not be IBD. Let I be a random variable indicating the number of alleles IBD by a sib pair. So the distribution of I for a sib pair is

$$\Pr(I = 0) = 1/4, \quad \Pr(I = 1) = 1/2, \quad \text{and} \quad \Pr(I = 2) = 1/4.$$

Hence, $E(I) = 1$ and $\text{Var}(I) = 1/2$.

For any given marker, if we have the information including the genotypes of two parents and the sib pair, we can deduce the number of alleles IBD shared in the sib pair. Denote the proportion of alleles IBD shared in a sib pair by π. Then π takes the values 0, 1/2, or 1. Haseman and Elston (1972) proposed using all the genotype information at the marker locus for the sib pair and parents. In detail, given the available marker information I_m,

$$\hat{\pi} = \hat{f}_2 + \hat{f}_1/2,$$

where

$$\hat{f}_1 = \Pr(I = 1|I_m) = \frac{0.5 \times \Pr(I_m|I = 1)}{\begin{array}{c}0.25 \times \Pr(I_m|I = 0) + 0.5 \times \Pr(I_m|I = 1)\\ +0.25 \times \Pr(I_m|I = 2)\end{array}},$$

and

$$\hat{f}_2 = \Pr(I = 2|I_m) = \frac{0.25 \times \Pr(I_m|I = 2)}{\begin{array}{c}0.25 \times \Pr(I_m|I = 0) + 0.5 \times \Pr(I_m|I = 1)\\ +0.25 \times \Pr(I_m|I = 2)\end{array}}.$$

The Lander-Green algorithm (Lander and Green, 1987) can be used to estimate IBD sharing probabilities for various family structure for multilocus.

2.2.2. *The affected sib pair (ASP) Method*

Because the sib pair has many similarities including an excess of allele sharing for the individuals with similar phenotypes and few allele sharing for the subjects with dissimilar phenotypes, the affected sib pair has been commonly used to detect the linkage for human diseases (Penrose, 1935, 1953). The ASP method used the affected sib pair on the basis of an excess number of allele sharing.

Without loss of generality, we assume that there are two alleles D and d at the trait locus. Denote $p_D = \Pr(D)$ and $p_d = \Pr(d) = 1 - p_D$. Consider a binary trait with $Y = 1$ for a subject being affected and 0 otherwise. The penetrances of the three genotypes are

$$f_{DD} = \Pr(\text{Affected}|DD), \quad f_{Dd} = \Pr(\text{Affected}|Dd), \quad f_{dd} = \Pr(\text{Affected}|dd).$$

Let the disease prevalence be K. Then under HWE, we have

$$\begin{aligned} K &= \Pr(\text{Affected}|DD)\Pr(DD) + \Pr(\text{Affected}|Dd)\Pr(Dd) \\ &\quad + \Pr(\text{Affected}|dd)\Pr(dd) \\ &= p_D^2 f_{DD} + 2p_D p_d f_{Dd} + p_d^2 f_{dd}. \end{aligned}$$

The genetic variance for the binary trait is

$$\begin{aligned} V_G &= \text{var}(E(Y|\text{Genotypes})) \\ &= 2p_D p_d [p_D(f_{Dd} - f_{DD}) + p_d(f_{dd} - f_{Dd})]^2) \\ &\quad + p_D^2 p_d^2 [f_{DD} - 2f_{Dd} + f_{dd}]^2 \\ &\widehat{=} V_A + V_D, \end{aligned}$$

where

$$V_A = 2p_D p_d [p_A(f_{Dd} - f_{DD}) + p_d(f_{dd} - f_{Dd})]^2)$$

is the additive variance, and

$$V_D = p_D^2 p_d^2 [f_{DD} - 2f_{Dd} + f_{dd}]^2$$

is the dominance variance.

Given the parameters (K, V_A, V_D, θ), where θ is the recombination fraction, the affected sib pair provides the most information among the three situations including the both affected sib pair, one affected and another unaffected, and both unaffected. Thus, the ASP method is preferred for detecting linkage. Denote the number of affected sib pairs by n in an experiment, where there are n_2 affected sib pairs with the number of alleles IBD at the marker locus being 2 and n_1 subjects being 1. Based on the above data, many test statistics have been put forward, where the most popular one is the "mean test", which is defined as

$$T_{\mathrm{ASP}} = \frac{2\sqrt{2} \times (n_2 + 0.5 \times n_1 - 0.5 \times n)}{\sqrt{n}}.$$

Under the null hypothesis that there is no linkage, T_{ASP} asymptotically follows a standard normal distribution. So, given the observed value of T_{ASP}, t_{ASP}, p-value is $2 \times (1 - \Phi(|t_{\mathrm{ASP}}|)$, where $\Phi(\cdot)$ is the cumulative distribution function of a standard normal distribution. The parameters (K, V_A, V_D, θ) are often used to calculate the sample size for a given power for ASP design (Knapp *et al.*, 1995; Suarez and Eerdewegh, 1984; Blackwelder and Elston, 1982).

Now, let us consider the ASP method based on the recurrence risk ratio (Risch, 1990). Let Y_1 and Y_2 be the indicator random variables with $Y_1 = 1$ for the first sib being affected and 0 otherwise and Y_2 has the similar meanings for the second sib in a sib pair. Then the recurrence risk of a sib pair is

$$K_R = \Pr(Y_2 = 1|Y_1 = 1).$$

So, K_R is the conditional probability that one sib is affected given the other affected sib. The recurrence risk ratio is

$$\lambda_S = \frac{K_R}{K},$$

the ratio of the sibling recurrence risk over the disease prevalence. Similarly, we can define λ_O, the recurrence ratio between parent and offspring. Denote the number of alleles IBD at the marker locus by I_M and let $\xi = \theta^2 + (1-\theta)^2$. Then we have three conditional probabilities:

$$\Pr(I_M = 0|\text{Two affected sibs}) = \frac{1}{4} - \frac{1}{4\lambda_S}(2\xi - 1) \times [\lambda_S - 1 + 2(1-\xi)(\lambda_S - \lambda_O)],$$

$$\Pr(I_M = 1|\text{Two affected sibs}) = \frac{1}{2} - \frac{1}{2\lambda_S}(2\xi - 1)^2(\lambda_S - \lambda_O),$$

and

$$\Pr(I_M = 2|\text{Two affected sibs}) = \frac{1}{4} + \frac{1}{4\lambda_S}(2\xi - 1) \times [\lambda_S - 1 + 2(1-\xi)(\lambda_S - \lambda_O)].$$

Note that Risch's (1990) parameterization is different from the previous although the test statistics for testing the null hypothesis are the same. The main difference is how to calculate power and sample size. Risch (1990) calculated power and sample size based on $(\lambda_S, \lambda_O, \theta)$. The power and sample calculation for the other method was based on (K, V_A, V_D, θ) .

2.2.3. *The Haseman-Elston approach*

The LOD score method and ASP procedure are often used to test the linkage for qualitative traits, however, there are also many diseases with quantitative traits, such as hypertension and obesity etc. Haseman-Elston (1972) proposed a sib pair procedure for detecting linkage for quantitative trait locus. Suppose that n sib pairs are ascertained. Let y_{1j} and y_{2j} be the trait values for the jth sib pair. We assume that the trait values follow the model:

$$y_{1j} = \mu + g_{1j} + e_{1j},$$

and

$$y_{2j} = \mu + g_{1j} + e_{1j},$$

where μ is the overall mean, g_{1j} and g_{2j} represent genetic effects to the trait values, and e_{1j} and e_{2j} are environmental effects or other effects, $j = 1, 2, \ldots, n$.

Let $z_j = (y_{1j} - y_{2j})^2$, and $\sigma_e^2 = E(e_{1j} - e_{2j})^2$ be the residual variance, $j = 1, 2, \ldots, n$. Denote the genetic variances (variance of g_{ij}) by σ_g^2. Under the assumption of no dominant effect, Haseman-Elston showed

$$E(z_j|\pi_j) = (\sigma_g^2 + \sigma_e^2) - 2\sigma_g^2\pi_j,$$

where π_j is the proportion of alleles IBD for the jth sib pair at the trait locus.

Denote the proportion of alleles IBD for the jth sib pair at the marker locus by π_{mj}. Let $\hat{\pi}_{mj}$ be the estimate of π_{mj}, which is given in Section 2.2.1. When the marker locus is in LD with the trait locus, Haseman and Elston (1972) obtained the regression equation,

$$E(Z_j|\hat{\pi}_{mj}) = 2\sigma_g^2[\theta^2 + (1-\theta)^2] + \sigma_e^2 - 2(1-2\theta)^2\sigma_g^2\hat{\pi}_{mj}.$$

Let $\beta_0 = 2\sigma_g^2[\theta^2 + (1-\theta)^2] + \sigma_e^2$ and $\beta_1 = -2(1-2\theta)^2\sigma_g^2$. The above regression becomes

$$E(Z_j|\hat{\pi}_{mj}) = \beta_0 + \beta_1\hat{\pi}_{mj}.$$

So, the hypothesis testing for linkage is transformed to be $\beta_1 = 0 \longleftrightarrow \beta_1 < 0$. Based on the data $(z_1, \hat{\pi}_{m1}), (z_2, \hat{\pi}_{m2}), \ldots, (z_n, \hat{\pi}_{mn})$, one can conduct a test easily. This method has been extended to a multiple loci and multiple alleles at a locus (Stoesz *et al.*, 1997).

Wright (1997) found that a full likelihood of sib pair data could be expressed in terms of both a sum and a difference of trait values. Both the sum and difference variables of the trait values are dependent (Drigalenko, 1998). So, Elston *et al.* (2000) applied this idea and modified the Haseman-Elston procedure. Later, Xu *et al.* (2000), Forrest (2001), Visscher and Hopper (2001), and Shete *et al.* (2003) considered how to balance the squared sum and squared difference of trait values. Wang and Elston (2005) developed a two-level Haseman-Elston approach for linkage based on quantitative trait. Besides the above regression-based linkage analysis, Amos (1994) used the variance-components to evaluate the LD; Kruglyak and Lander (1998) used the Fourier transforms to do linkage analysis; and Chen *et al.* (2004) considered using generalized estimating equations to model the data.

2.2.4. *The ED and EC sib pair procedure*

The key for the Haseman-Elston method is the regression, which needs the random sample of sib pairs. If we adopted some special sample schemes for choosing sib pairs based on the trait values, it should improve the power intuitively (Blackwelder and Elston, 1982; Carey and Williamson, 1991; Eaves and Meyer, 1994; Risch and Zhang, 1995). Risch and Zhang (1995) concluded that three types of sampling schemes based on the trait values for sib pairs have the most power to detect linkage, which are:

(1) Extremely discordant (ED) (high and low trait values) sib pairs;
(2) Extremely concordant (EC) for high trait values;
(3) Extremely concordant for low trait values.

Denote the number of ED sib pairs in a linkage study by n, where there are n_0, n_1, and n_2 sib pairs with IBD equalling to 0, 1, and 2, respectively. Under the alternative hypothesis that the marker locus and the trait locus are linked, more ED sib pairs should have shared 0 alleles IBD. So, linkage exists when n_0 is significantly larger than n_2. When there is no linkage between the marker locus and the trait locus, (n_0, n_1, n_2) follows a trinomial distribution with the parameter n and $(1/4, 1/2, 1/4)$. Since

$$E_{H_0}(n_0 - n_2) = 0, \quad \text{and} \quad \mathrm{Var}_{H_0}(n_0 - n_2) = n/2,$$

a test statistic is constructed as

$$T_{\mathrm{ED}} = \frac{\sqrt{2}(n_0 - n_2)}{\sqrt{n}},$$

which follows a standard normal distribution asymptotically.

Similarly, the EC sib pair test statistic is

$$T_{\mathrm{EC}} = \frac{\sqrt{2}(n_2 - n_0)}{\sqrt{n}}.$$

Some investigators (Risch and Zhang, 1995, 1996; Zhang and Risch, 1996; Zhao, Zhang and Rotter, 1997) explored the power of the above three designs under different situations, and other investigators (Gu, Todorov and Rao, 1996; Rao, 1998; Li and Zhang, 2000; Li and Gastwirth, 2001) considered combining ED and EC designs to improve the power by using different weights. However, how to choose the weight is a problem.

2.2.5. *The Transmission/Disequilibrium test (TDT)*

It is evident that a given marker allele correlated with the disease trait locus will have higher frequency among the affected ones relative to the unaffected subjects if the marker locus is in the neighborhood of the disease locus and the disease allele is due to a recent mutation. This evidence can help us to detect the linkage between the marker and disease loci.

Consider n parent-offspring trios and a diallelic marker with two alleles M and m. There are six different mating types. The number of six mating types and offspring genotypes with two transmitted/nontransmitted alleles is given in Table 2.

The data in Table 2 can be further summarized in Table 3 according to the transmitted and nontransmitted alleles.

Denote the alleles at the trait locus by D and d, where D is the disease allele. Let $p_M = \Pr(M)$ and $p_D = \mathrm{D}$, where D is the disease allele. Denote the recombination fraction between the marker and trait loci, and LD parameter by θ and δ, respectively. Then $\delta = \Pr(MD) - \Pr(M)\Pr(D)$. Let

$$U = \frac{p_D[p_D(f_{DD} - f_{Dd}) + (1 - p_D)(f_{Dd} - f_{dd})]}{p_D^2 f_{DD} + 2p_D(1 - p_D)f_{Dd} + (1 - p_D)^2 f_{dd}},$$

where $f_{DD} = \Pr(\text{Affected}|DD), f_{Dd} = \Pr(\text{Affected}|Dd), f_{dd} = \Pr(\text{Aff-}$ $\text{ected}|\ dd)$.

Table 2. Transmitted/nontransmitted alleles for six mating types.

Parental		Offspring		Transmitted	
Mating type	Count	Genotype	Count	Yes	No
$MM \times MM$	n_1	MM	n_1	M, M	M, M
$MM \times Mm$	n_2	MM	n_{22}	M, M	M, m
		Mm	n_{21}	M, m	M, M
$MM \times mm$	n_3	Mm	n_3	M, m	M, m
$Mm \times Mm$	n_4	MM	n_{42}	M, M	m, m
		Mm	n_{41}	M, m	M, m
		mm	n_{40}	m, m	M, M
$Mm \times mm$	n_5	Mm	n_{51}	M, m	m, m
		mm	n_{50}	m, m	M, m
$mm \times mm$	n_6	mm	n_6	m, m	m, m

Table 3. Transmitted/nontransmitted alleles.

	Nontransmitted		
Transmitted	M	m	Total
M	x_1	x_2	$x_1 + x_2$
m	x_3	x_4	$x_3 + x_4$
Total	$x_1 + x_3$	$x_2 + x_4$	$2n$

$x_1 = 2n_1 + n_2 + n_3$, $x_2 = n_{22} + 2n_{42} + n_{41} + n_{51}$
$x_3 = n_{21} + 2n_{40} + n_{41} + n_{50}$,$x_4 = 2n_6 + n_3 + n_5$

Table 4. Transmitted/nontransmitted probabilities.

	Nontransmitted	
Transmitted	M	m
M	$p_M^2 + \frac{Up_M\delta}{p_D}$	$p_M(1-p_M) + \frac{U(1-\theta-p_M)\delta}{p_D}$
m	$p_M(1-p_M) + \frac{U(\theta-p_M)\delta}{p_D}$	$(1-p_M)^2 - \frac{U(1-p_M)\delta}{p_D}$

According to Curnow *et al.* (1998), we can get the theoretical transmitted/nontransmitted probabilities corresponding to Table 3, which is given in Table 4.

From Table 4, if $\theta = 1/2$, then

$$p_M(1-p_M) + \frac{U(\theta - p_M)\delta}{p_D} = p_M(1-p_M) + \frac{U(1-\theta-p_M)\delta}{p_D},$$

which means the diagonal in Table 4 are independent of the recombination fraction θ. So, the TDT (Spielman *et al.*, 1993) is

$$T_{TDT} = \frac{(x_2 - x_3)^2}{x_2 + x_3}.$$

Under the null hypothesis with $\theta = 1/2$, T_{TDT} follows a one degree of freedom chi-square test.

Because of the simplicity, the TDT has been extended to handle multi-allelic markers (Sham and Curtis, 1995; Spielman and Ewens, 1996), family data without parental genotype information (Monks *et al.*, 1998; Spielman and Ewens, 1998), and quantitative traits (Allison, 1997; Rabinowitz, 1997; Schaid and Rowland, 1999).

2.3. *Robust tests*

In this section, we will discuss some robust tests (Zheng *et al.*, 2011) for linkage analysis. We mainly focus on the score test based on the data of affected sib pairs.

Let (p_0, p_1, p_2) be the probabilities that an affected sib pair shares $(0, 1, 2)$ alleles IBD, where $p_0 + p_1 + p_2 = 1$. If there is no linkages, $(p_0, p_1, p_2) = (1/4, 1/2, 1/4)$. Suppose that we have n affected sib pairs where n_0, n_1, and n_2 sib pairs share 0, 1, and 2 alleles IBD, respectively. So $n = n_0 + n_1 + n_2$. The likelihood function is

$$L(p_0, p_1) = \frac{n!}{n_0!n_1!n_2!} p_0^{n_0} p_1^{n_1} (1 - p_0 - p_1)^{n_2}.$$

Faraway (1993), and Whittemore and Tu (1998) condiered the triangle constraints for IBD sharing probability, and Whittemore and Tu (1998) provided a "minmax" test that has the minimum of the worst power under the model uncertainty. Here we consider the other robust tests which are often used in current genetic association studies.

Let $p_0 = \frac{1-\lambda}{4}$, $p_1 = \frac{1-\lambda}{2} + \varrho\lambda$. The null hypothesis is transformed to $\lambda = 0$, however $\varrho \in [0, 1/2]$ is a nuisance parameter. Then, we have

$$\begin{aligned} L(\lambda, \varrho) &= \frac{n!}{n_0!n_1!n_2!} \left(\frac{1-\lambda}{4}\right)^{n_0} \left(\frac{1-\lambda}{2} + \varrho\lambda\right)^{n_1} \\ &\quad \times \left(1 - \frac{1-\lambda}{4} - \frac{1-\lambda}{2} - \varrho\lambda\right)^{n_2} \\ &= \frac{n!}{n_0!n_1!n_2!4^{n_0+n_2}2^{n_1}} (1-\lambda)^{n_0} [\lambda(2\varrho - 1) + 1]^{n_1} [1 + \lambda(3 - 4\varrho)]^{n_2}. \end{aligned}$$

The log-likelihood function is

$$l(\lambda, \varrho) = \ln\left(\frac{n!}{n_0!n_1!n_2!4^{n_0+n_2}2^{n_1}}\right) + n_0\ln(1-\lambda) + n_1\ln[\lambda(2\varrho-1)+1] + n_2\ln[1+\lambda(3-4\varrho)]$$

For any given $\varrho \in [0, 1/2]$, the score test is

$$T_{\text{Score}}(\varrho) = \frac{\sqrt{n}\left[4(\varrho-1)\frac{n_0}{n} + (6\varrho-4)\frac{n_1}{n} + (3-4\varrho)\right]}{\sqrt{3-8\varrho+6\varrho^2}}.$$

Under the null hypothesis, $T_{\text{Score}}(\varrho)$ follows the standard normal distribution asymptotically. For any given $\varrho_1 \in [0, 0.5]$ and $\varrho_2 \in [0, 0.5]$, the correlation coefficient between two score tests, $T_{\text{Score}}(\varrho_1)$ and $T_{\text{Score}}(\varrho_2)$ is

$$\rho_{\varrho_1,\varrho_2} = \frac{3-4(\varrho_1+\varrho_2)+6\varrho_1\varrho_2}{\sqrt{(3-8\varrho_1+6\varrho_1^2)(3-8\varrho_2+6\varrho_2^2)}}.$$

Since ϱ is unknown and ϱ vanishes under the null hypothesis, we can apply the robust tests. One robust test is maximin efficiency robust test (MERT) (Gastwirth and Feidlin, 2000; Zheng, Freidlin, and Gaswirth, 2002; Zheng *et al.*, 2011) is given by

$$T_{\text{MERT}} = \frac{T_{Score}(0) + T_{Score}(1/2)}{\sqrt{2(1+\rho_{0,1/2})}} \sim N(0,1) \text{ under } H_0.$$

Another robust test is MAX3 $= \max\{T_{\text{Score}}(0), T_{\text{Score}}(0.25), T_{\text{Score}}(0.5)\}$. Since there is no closed form for the cumulative distribution function, one can use bootstrap method or Rhombus formula (Li *et al.*, 2008, 2010) to obtain its p-value after the observation, t_{MAX3}.

The third robust test is MAX $= \max_{\varrho\in[0,0.5]} |T_{\text{Score}}(\varrho)|$. To calculate the statistical evidence of MAX, one can use the bootstrap method or Davis's formula (Davis, 1977, 1987).

3. Discussion

The main goal in human genetics is to detect the genetic variants that are responsible for human disorders. Since it is difficult to locate the trait locus exactly in genetic studies, finding the marker locus that is linked with the trait locus is very helpful. In this chapter, we discussed the model-based and model-free methods for linkage analysis according to whether the allele frequency, penetrances, and prevalence are assumed. Besides the present methods, there are also many other approaches developed to detect LD. We also provided some robust tests under genetic model uncertainty.

4. Software

(1) LINKAGE (ftp:linkage.rockefeller.edu/software/linkage/)
(2) FASTLINK (http:www.ncbi.nlm.nih.gov/CB-Bresearch/Schaffer/fast-link.html)
(3) S.A.G.E (http:darwin.cwru.edu/sage)
(4) MAPMAKER/SIBS (http:ftp-genome.wi.mit.edu/distribution/softwa-re/sibs/)
(5) ASPEX (http:aspex.sourceforge.net/)
(6) ERPA (http:www.smd.qmul.ac.uk/statgen/dcurtis/software.html)
(7) ···

Acknowledgements

Research of Qizhai Li is partially supported by NSFC, No. 10901155, 61134013.

References

Amos, C.I. (1994). Robust variance-components approach for assessing genetic linkage in pedigrees. *American Journal of Human Genetics* **54**: 535–543.

Allison, D.B. (1997). Transmission-disequilibrium tests for quantitative traits. *American Journal of Human Genetics* **60**: 676–690.

Blackwelder, W.C. and Elston, R.C. (1982). Power and robustness of sib-pair linkage test and extension to larger sibships. *Communication Statistical Theory Methods* **11**: 449–484.

Carey, G. and Williamson, J. (1991). Linkage analysis of quantitative traits: increased power by using selected sample. *American Journal of Human Genetics* **49**: 786–796.

Chen, W.M., Broman, K.W. and Liang, K.Y. (2004). Quantitative trait linkage analysis by generalized estimating equations: unification of variance components and Haseman-Elston regression. *Genetic Epidemiology* **26**: 265–272.

Curnow, R.N., Morris, A.P. and Whittaker, J.C. (1998). Locating genes involved in human disease. *Applied Statistics* **47**: 63–76.

Davies, R.B. (1977). Hypothesis testing when a nuisance parameter is present only under the alternative. *Biometrika* **64**: 247–254.

Davies, R.B. (1987). Hypothesis testing when a nuisance parameter is present only under the alternative. *Biometrika* **74**: 33–43.

Drigalenko, E. (1998). How sib pairs reveal linkage. *American Journal of Human Genetics* **63**: 1242–1245.

Eaves, L. and Meyer, J. (1994). Locating human quantitative trait loci: guidelines for the selection of sibling pairs for genotypes. *Behaviour Genetics* **24**: 443–455.

Elston, R.C., Buxbaum, S., Jacobs, K.B. and Olson, J.M. (2000). Haseman and Elston revisited. *Genetic Epidemiology* **19**: 1–17.

Faraway, J.J. (1993). Improved sib-pair linkage test for disease susceptibility loci. *Genetic Epidemiology* **10**: 225–233.

Forrest, W.F. (2001). Weighting improves the "new Haseman-Elston" method. *Human Heredity* **52**: 47–54.

Gastwirth, J.L. and Freidlin, B. (2000). On power and efficiency robust linkage tests for affected sibs. *Annals of Human Genetics* **64**: 443–453.

Gu, C., Todorov, A. and Rao, D.C. (1996). Combing extremely concordant sib-pairs with extremely discordant sibpairs provides a cost effective way to linkage analysis of QTLs. *Genetic Epidemiology* **13**: 513–533.

Hardy, G. (1908) Mendelian proportions in a mixed population. *Science* **28**: 49–50.

Hartl, D.L. and Clark, A.G. (1997). *Principles of Population Genetics*, Sinauer Associates, Inc. Sunderland, Massachusetts.

Haseman, J.K. and Elston, R.C. (1972). The investigation of linkage between a quantitative trait and a marker locus. *Behaviour Genetics* **2**: 3–19.

Knapp, M., Wassmer, G. and Baur, M.P. (1995). Linkage analysis in nuclear families, I. optimality criteria for affected sib-pair tests. *Human Heredity* **44**: 37–43.

Kruglyak, L. and Lander, E.S. (1998). Faster multipoint linkage analysis using Fourier transforms. *Journal of Computational Biology* **5**: 1–7.

Lander, E.S. and Green, P. (1987). Construction of multilocus genetic linkage maps in humans. *Proceedings of the National Academy of Sciences, USA* **84**: 2363–2367.

Li, C.C. (1988). *First Course in Population Genetics*, The Boxwood Press, Pacific Grove, California.

Li, Q., Zheng, G., Liu, A., Li, Z. and Yu, K. (2010). Approximating probabilities of correlated events. *Science China Mathematics* **53**: 2937–2948.

Li, Q., Zheng, G., Li, Z. and Yu, K., 2008. Efficient approximation of p-value of the maximum of correlated tests, with applications to genome-wide association studies. *Annals of Human Genetics* **72**: 397–406.

Li, Z. and Gastwirth, J.L. (2001). A weighted test using both extreme discordant and concordant sibpairs for detecting linkage. *Genetic Epidemiology* **20**: 34–43.

Li, Z., Qin, H. and Zhang, H. (2006). *Statistics in Genetics*, Science Press, Beijing.

Li, Z. and Zhang, H. (2000). Mapping quantitative trait loci in humans using both extreme discordant and concordant sib pairs: a unified approach for meta-analysis. *Communication Statistical Theory Methods* **29**: 1115–1127.

Monks, S.A., Kaplan, N.L. and Weir, B.S. (1998). A comparative study of sibship tests of linkage and/or association. *American Journal of Human Genetics* **63**: 1507–1516.

Morton, N.E. (1955). Sequential tests for the detection of linkage. *American Journal of Human Genetics* **11**: 1–16.

Ott, J. (1999). *Analysis of Human Genetic Linkage*, The Johns Hopkins University Press, Baltimore and London.

Penrose, L.S. (1935). The detection of autosomal linkage in data which consist of pairs brothers and sisters of unspecified parentage. *Annals of Eugenics* **6**: 133–138.

Penrose, L.S. (1953). The general purpose sib-pair linkage test. *Annals of Eugenics* **18**: 120–124.

Rabinowitz, D. (1997). A transmission disequilibrium test for quantitative trait loci. *Human Heredity* **47**: 342–350.

Rao, D.C. (1998). CAT scans, PET scans, and genomic scans. *Genetic Epidemiology* **15**: 1–18.

Risch, N. (1990). Linkage strategies for genetically complex trait II: the power of affected relative pairs. *American Journal of Human Genetics* **46**: 229–241.

Risch, N. and Zhang H. (1995). Extreme discordant sib pairs for mapping quantitative trait loci in humans. *Science* **268**: 1584–1589.

Risch, N. and Zhang, H. (1996). Mapping quantitative trait with extreme discordant sib pairs: sample size considerations. *American Journal of Human Genetics* **58**: 836–843.

Sham, P.C. and Curtis, D. (1995). An extended transimission/disequilibrium test (TDT) for multi-allele marker loci. *Annals of Human Genetics* **59**: 323–336.

Schaid, D.J. and Rowland, C.M. (1999). Quantitative trait transmission disequilibrium test: allowance for missing parents. *Genetic Epidemiology* **17**: S307–S312.

Shete, S., Jacobs, K.B. and Elston, R.C. (2003). Adding further power to the Haseman and Elston method for detecting linkage in larger sibships: weighting sums and differences. *Human Heredity* **55**: 79–85.

Sladek, R., Rocheleau, G., Rung, J., Dina, C., Shen, L., Serre, D., Boutin, P., Vincent, D., Belisle, A., Hadjadj, S., Balkau, B., Heude, B., Charpentier, G., Hudson, T.J., Montpetit, A., Pshezhetsky, A.V., Prentki, M., Posner, B.I., Balding, D.J., Meyre, D., Polychronakos, C., Froguel, P. (2007). A genome-wide association study identifies novel risk loci for type 2 diabetes. *Nature* **445**: 881–885.

Spielman, R.S. and Ewens, W.J. (1996). The TDT and other family-based tests for linkage disequilibrium and association. *American Journal of Human Genetics* **59**: 983–989.

Spielman, R.S. and Ewens, W.J. (1998). A sibship test for linkage in the presence of association: the sib transmission/disequilibrium test. *American Journal of Human Genetics* **62**: 450–458.

Spielman, R.S., McGinnis, R.E. and Ewens, W.J. (1993). Transmission test for linkage disequilibrium: the insulin gene region and insulin-dependent diabetes mellitus (IDDM). *American Journal of Human Genetics* **52**: 506–516.

Stoesz, M.R., Cohen, J.C., Mooser, V., Marcovina, S. and Guerra, R. (1997). Extension of the Haseman-Elston method to multiple alleles and multiple loci: theory and practice for candidate genes. *Annals of Human Genetics* **61**: 263–274.

Suarez, B.K., Rice, J. and Reich, T. (1978). The generalized sib pair IBD distribution: its use in the detection of linkage. *Annals of Human Genetics* **42**: 87–94.

Suarez, B.K. and van Eerdewegh, P. (1984). A comparison of three affected sib-pair scoring methods to detect HLA-linked disease susceptibility genes. *American Journal of Medical Genetics* **18**: 135–146.

Visscher, P.M. and Hopper, J.L. (2001). Power of regression and maximum likelihood methods to map QTL from sib-pair and DZ twin data. *American Journal of Human Genetics* **65**: 583–601.

Wang, T. and Elston, R.C. (2005). Two-level Haseman-Elston regression for general pedigree data analysis. *Genetic Epidemiology* **29**: 12–22.

Weinberg, W. (1908) Über den nachweis der vererbung beim Menschen. *Jahreshefte des Vereins für vaterländische Naturkunde in Württemberg* **64**: 368–382.

Wentworth, E.N. and Remick, B.L. (1916). Some breeding properties of the generalized Mendelian population. *Genetics* **1**: 608–616.

Whittemore, A.S. and Tu, I.P. (1998). Simple, robust linkage tests for affected sibs. *American Journal of Human Genetics* **62**: 1228–1242.

Wright, F.A. (1997). The phenotypic difference discards sib-pair QTL linkage information. *American Journal of Human Genetics* **60**: 740–742.

Xu, X., Weiss, S., Xu, X. and Wei, L.J. (2000). A unified Haseman-Elston method for testing linkage with quantitative traits. *American Journal of Human Genetics* **67**: 1025–1028.

Zhang, H. and Risch, N. (1996). Mapping quantitative trait loci in humans using extreme concordant sib pair: selected sampling by parental phenotypes. *American Journal of Human Genetics* **59**: 951–957.

Zhao, H., Zhang, H. and Rotter, J.I. (1997). Cost-effective sib-pair designs in the mapping of quantitative-trait loci. *American Journal of Human Genetics* **60**: 1211–1221.

Zheng, G., Freidlin, B. and Gaswirth, J.L. (2002). Robust TDT-type candidate-gene association test. *Annals of Human Genetics* **66**: 145–455.

Zheng, G., Yang, Y.N., Zhu, X.F. and Elston, R. (2012). *Analysis of Genetic Association Studies*, Springer.

About the Authors

Qizhai Li got his Ph.D. in Statistics from Academy of Mathematics and Systems Science, Chinese Academy of Sciences in 2006. Since then he has been an assistant professor and associate professor of the Academy of Mathematics and Systems Science, Chinese Academy of Sciences. His research interests include statistical methods for genetic epidemiology and clinical trials. He has published over 50 works on statistical methodology and their applications in genetic epidemiology and clinical trials.

Hong Qin got his Ph.D. in statistics from Hong Kong Baptist University in 2002. Since then he has been a professor the Department of Statistics,

Central China Normal University. Since 2002, he has published over 60 publications in experiment design and linkage analysis, and a book "Statistical Methods for Genetic Analysis" with Zhaohai Li and Hong Zhang in Science Press in 2006.

Zhaohai Li is a Professor of Statistics and Biostatistics in Department of Statistics at the George Washington University, Washington, DC. He obtained his M.S. degree in Mathematical Statistics from Central China Normal University and Ph.D. in Statistics from Columbia University. He is a Fellow of American Statistical Association. His research interests include statistical methods for genetic epidemiology and empirical Bayes methods for meta-analysis.

Gang Zheng obtained his Ph.D. in statistics from George Washington University in 2000. Since then he has been a mathematical statistician of the Office of Biostatistics, National Heart, Lung and Blood Institute, National Institutes of Health. Since 2000, he has published over 100 publications in statistical methods and their applications to genetic studies, robust statistics, and ordered data, and a Springer book "Analysis of Genetics Association Studies" in 2012.

CHAPTER 24

TRANSCRIPTOME ANALYSIS USING NEXT-GENERATION SEQUENCING

JINGYI JESSICA LI* and HAIYAN HUANG†

Department of Statistics, University of California, Berkeley, CA 94720, USA
**jli@stat.berkeley.edu*
†hhuang@stat.berkeley.edu

MINPING QIAN

School of Mathematical Sciences and Center for Theoretical Biology, Peking University, Beijing 100871, China
qianmp@math.pku.edu.cn

XUEGONG ZHANG

MOE Key Laboratory of Bioinformatics, Department of Automation, Tsinghua University, Beijing 100084, China
zhangxg@tsinghua.edu.cn

1. Introduction

For many years, molecular biology can only study one or a small number of objects such as genes, mRNAs or proteins at a time. This picture has been changed during the last two decades with the development of a series of high throughput technologies, such as SAGE (Velculescu *et al.*, 1995) and DNA microarray (Schena *et al.*, 1995), which can measure thousands of objects in one experiment in a short time. More recently, the emergence of next-generation sequencing (NGS) technologies further opens up the possibility of a wide variety of large-scale genomic research and is transforming genomic science (Schuster, 2008). These new platforms are capable of sequencing billions of bases of DNA in each automated run, offering rapid ways for various genome-wide studies such as RNA profiling (Wang *et al.*, 2009), detection of single nucleotide polymorphisms (SNPs) (Frazer *et al.*, 2007), and identification of transcription factor binding sites (Park, 2009).

A transcriptome analysis utilizing next-generation RNA sequencing (RNA-Seq) has been one of the most attractive topics among recent research activities. The core technique of RNA-Seq is to use NGS technologies to sequence cDNAs to get information about a sample's RNA content (Wang *et al.*, 2009). The RNA-Seq assay, with deep coverage and base level resolution, has provided a view of eukaryotic transcriptomes of unprecedented detail and clarity. Since developed, RNA-Seq has been widely used to reveal the complex landscape and dynamics of transcriptomes for many different species (Nagalakshmi *et al.*, 2008; Wilhelm *et al.*, 2008; Mortazavi *et al.*, 2008; Lister *et al.*, 2008). Compared to previous high-throughput technologies, such as microarray, RNA-Seq does not require probes or primers, and thus in principle is possible to carry out applications that are not possible using traditional microarray-based methods. For instance, RNA-Seq can be used to identify novel genes/isoforms/exons, alternative splice sites, allele-specific expression, and rare transcripts in a single experiment.

This chapter is organized as follows. The detailed procedures for generating RNA-Seq data are introduced in Section 2, following a brief summary of traditional and next-generation sequencing technologies. Basic computational and statistical methods for analyzing RNA-Seq data are introduced in Section 3. Some challenges in transcript assembly and abundance estimation along with some issues in downstream transcriptome analyses are discussed in Section 4. Several other genomic applications facilitated by NGS are described in Appendix.

2. Review on Sequencing Data Generation

Systematic protocols for DNA sequencing, genome mapping and sequence analyses were first established in 1970's (Sanger *et al.*, 1977). In the last two decades, sequencing technology has advanced rapidly and significantly enhanced many genomic studies. The completion of the Human Genome Project, involving contributions from over 100 laboratories worldwide, represents a big accomplishment for the development of sequencing technology and is considered the first scientific milestone of the twenty-first century

(Lander *et al.*, 2001; Venter *et al.*, 2001). In Section 2.1, we overview traditional and next-generation sequencers, and in Section 2.2, we describe their utilization in transcriptomics.

2.1. *Traditional and next-generation DNA sequencing*

Traditional DNA sequencing is based on Sanger sequencing technique, utilizing the complementary basepairing property of DNA. A new DNA strand will be synthesized complementary to an existing single-stranded DNA fragment, when the fragment is isolated and placed with primers, DNA polymerase and the four types of deoxyribonucleoside triphosphate (dNTP). In a DNA sequencing reaction, four types of dideoxyribonucleoside triphosphate (ddNTP) bounded with four different fluorescent dyes are added besides the above components. The synthesis of a new strand will stop when a ddNTP instead of a dNTP is added to the strand. Therefore, with abundant single-stranded DNA templates, a set of complementary DNA segments of all different lengths would be synthesized, with each segment stopped by a colored ddNTP. Under the electrophoresis, these segments will have different migration speeds, with longer segments traveling more slowly than shorter ones. By scanning the colored ddNTPs of all ordered segments, we will be able to read the nucleotide at each position. This technique has been implemented in the first generation of sequencing machines.

The sequencing reaction can only measure DNA sequences up to ~800 base pairs (bp), because current capillary electrophoresis has decreased sensitivity/accuracy in ordering larger DNA molecules by length. Correspondingly, *shotgun strategy* has been used in whole genome sequencing. For instance, in sequencing human genome (Lander *et al.*, 2001; Venter *et al.*, 2001), the first step is fragmentation, in which the genome is first chopped into fragments (~ million bp). In some methods, the chopping positions are marked. These fragments are still too long for sequencing machines; hence they are further randomly broken into shorter segments of 500–800 bp to be sequenced. Multiple overlapping sequencing segments are gathered by several rounds of fragmentation followed by sequencing. These overlapping segments can be aligned and merged into original fragments (e.g. contigs), which will next be assembled.

In 2005, a new generation of sequencing technologies emerged (Margulies *et al.*, 2005; Shendure *et al.*, 2005). They are called next-generation sequencing (NGS), second-generation sequencing or deep sequencing. These new technologies can read huge amount of shorter DNA sequences at much higher efficiency. They constitute various strategies that rely on a combination of template preparation, sequencing and imaging, and genome alignment and assembly. Major platforms of next-generation sequencing technologies include but are not limited to Illumina/Solexa Genome Analyzer, AB SOLiD system (Life Technologies) and 454 Life Sciences (Roche). Among all the platforms, Illuminia/Solexa sequencing is the most popular one nowadays. In its technology, DNA fragments are first cut into short fragments and attached to primers on a slide. Next, in vitro amplification (i.e. bridge PCR) is performed to generate an array of millions of colonies, each of which contains many copies of a single DNA fragment. The colonies will then be sequenced, after four types of reversible dye-terminators are added. During the sequencing, florescence emitted from dye terminators will be captured by a high-resolution image-based detection system. In the end, image data will be processed into nucleotide sequences. Other NGS technologies use similar ideas, but mainly differ in the in vitro amplification step (e.g. emulsion PCR). Compared with the Sanger sequencing technology, the NGS method are highly parallel and can produce gigas of sequence data in a single day.

2.2. *RNA sequencing (RNA-Seq)*

Applying the NGS technology to transcriptomes produces RNA sequencing (RNA-Seq) data. In an RNA-Seq experiment, single-end and/or paired-end reads can be generated. A single-end read is a sequenced end of a cDNA fragment from an mRNA transcript, and a paired-end read is a mate pair corresponding to both ends of a cDNA fragment. The sketch of a typical experiment generating RNA-Seq reads is shown in Figure 1, which is derived from a review article on next-generation transcriptome assembly (Martin and Wang, 2011). To generate RNA-Seq data, the first step is the extraction of RNA transcripts (light blue) that are to be sequenced, followed by the fragmentation of extracted RNAs into short pieces. At the third step, the short fragments are then reversely transcribed into cDNAs (yellow). Sequencing adaptors (purple) are ligated at the following step. Next, PCR amplification is applied to ensure enough concentration of fragments. After undertaking fragment size selection, finally the ends of the cDNAs are sequenced using NGS technologies to produce many short reads. If single-end sequencing protocol is used, reads are sequenced from only the 5'-ends of cDNA fragments; if paired-end sequencing protocol is used, reads are obtained from both ends. One RNA-Seq experiment can generate billions

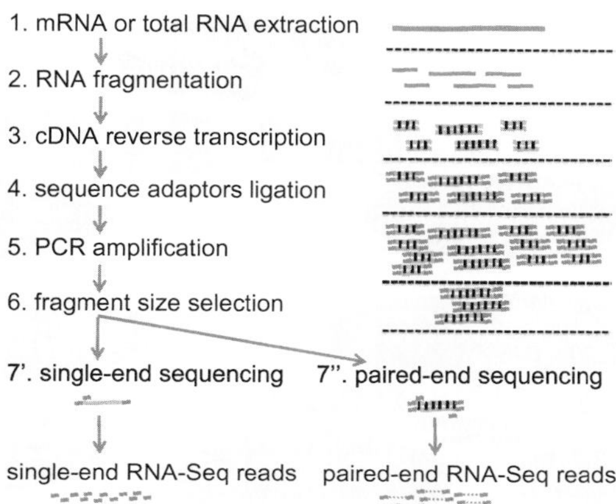

Fig. 1. Data generation steps of a typical RNA-Seq experiment.

of short (25–400 bp) reads. RNA-Seq data generated by different platforms/protocols can have different read-length distributions and sequencing error rates. A detailed discussion of the technical and methodological aspects of these next-generation sequencers can be found in literature (Shendure and Ji, 2008). Despite their technological differences, these major platforms rely on similar work flows for the data production (Figure 1).

3. Methods for Analyzing RNA-Seq Data

Since the year of 2008, enormous methods and software packages have been developed for analyzing RNA-Seq data to discover, profile, and quantify RNA transcripts. The first and most fundamental task is to arrange the RNA-Seq reads by genome positions. One strategy is to map reads to a reference genome, generating the read count data at base level (i.e., counts of reads covering each genome base). This strategy is known as *reference-based*, and the generated read count data can be further analyzed for isoform discovery and quantification. The other strategy is to *de novo* assemble RNA-Seq reads into contigs and transcripts by merging and aligning the overlapping reads. This is known as *de novo strategy*. For species with a reference genome, both strategies can be taken: mRNA isoforms can be either built upon mapped read positions or assembled de novo from reads. For species without a reference genome, RNA-Seq data has to be analyzed by the *de novo* strategy. Figure 2 summarizes the two strategies, which we introduce in details below.

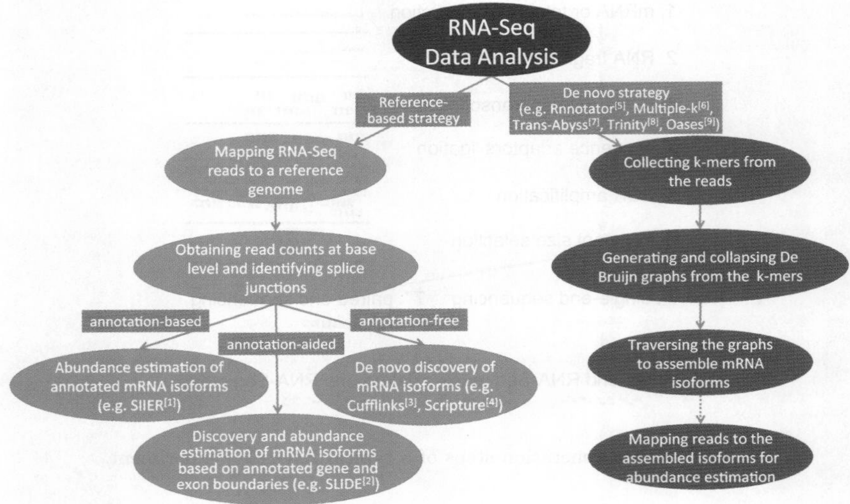

[1] Jiang and Wong, 2009; [2] Li et al., 2011; [3] Trapnell et al., 2010; [4] Guttman et al., 2010; [5] Martin et al., 2010; [6] Surget-Groba and Montoya- Burgos, 2010; [7] Robertson et al., 2010; [8] Grabherr et al., 2011; [9] Schulz et al., 2012

Fig. 2. A sketch of two strategies for RNA-Seq data analysis.

3.1. *Reference-based strategy*

The transcriptome assembly task with RNA-Seq data first involves arranging the RNA-Seq reads by their genome positions and then discovering and quantifying RNA isoforms from the mapped reads. When a reference genome for the target transcriptome is available, the complexity of the task can be reduced tremendously by building the assembly upon the reference genome.

3.1.1. *Reads mapping*

Mapping/aligning RNA-Seq reads to a reference genome with splicing considered is the key first step of transcriptome assembly in a reference-based strategy. This task is usually achieved by a splice-aware aligner such as Blat (Kent, 2002), TopHat (Trapnell *et al.*, 2009), SpliceMap (Au *et al.*, 2010), MapSplice (Wang *et al.*, 2010a), or GSNAP (Wu and Nacu, 2010). Splice-aware aligners can be summarized into two classes: seed-and-extend aligners and Burrows-Wheeler transform (BWT) aligners. Among the above mentioned aligner list, Blat and GSNAP belong to the former class, and TopHat, SpliceMap and MapSplice fall into the latter. Each aligner has clear trade-offs. BWT aligners are generally fast, but better work with shorter reads and few alignment errors.

After the reads are aligned to the genome, base-level read counts can be obtained by counting the number of reads covering each genomic position.

3.1.2. *Isoform discovery*

Given RNA-Seq reads mapped to a reference genome, various attempts have been made to utilize the mapped reads in assembling full length mRNA transcripts/isoforms and subsequently estimating their abundance.

Methods in the field of transcript/isoform discovery can be divided into three categories based on their usage of annotaions: "annotation-based", "annotation-free" and "annotation-aided" methods (see Figure 2). Annotation-based methods take existing annotations to define genes and isoforms. Annotation-free methods, in contrast, assemble mRNA isoforms directly from mapped reads, without using any annotation information. Annotation-aided methods lie somehow in the middle of this annotation usage spectrum from completely ignoring to utilizing as much as possible, combining benefits from both ends.

Cufflinks (Trapnell *et al.*, 2010) and Scripture (Guttman *et al.*, 2010) are two most widely used annotation-free software packages. They use similar deterministic graphical model ideas in isoform discovery, but differ mainly in ways of enumerating candidate isoforms. Cufflinks first defines an "overlap graph" from reads and then uses a parsimony strategy to decompose the graph into a minimum number of paths (i.e. candidate isoforms) covering all the reads. Unlike Cufflinks, Scripture first constructs a "connectivity graph" from exons (i.e, expressed segments assembled from reads), and then enumerates all possible longest paths as candidate isoforms. Cufflinks requires a strict partial order of reads in building the overlap graph, forcing the removal of some reads that could arise from complicated splicing events. These reads are called "uncertain reads" in Trapnell *et al.* (2010). This may lead to an insufficient isoform candidate space. Scripture's candidate space is in contrast bigger but may contain many spurious isoforms that have obvious conflicting splicing events.

IsoLasso (Li *et al.*, 2011b) is another annotation-free method. It starts from the same connectivity graph in Scripture, but introduces two additional steps to remove some spurious isoforms in the candidate set. In general, IsoLasso considers more isoforms than Cufflinks and fewer isoforms than Scripture in the isoform discovery process. At a later stage, IsoLasso quantifies the expression levels of isoform candidates using a simple linear model (see Section 3.1.3). This makes it possible to further reduce the chance of discovering false positive isoforms when LASSO (Least Absolute Shrinkage and Selection Operator) (Tibshirani, 1996) is applied.

These annotation-free methods have been widely applied and helped to (re)construct transcriptomes of various species. However, the discovered isoforms can be easily biased by various RNA-Seq data noises from sequencing errors and mappability issues. The modENCODE consortium (Celniker *et al.*, 2009) recently raised such concerns and suggested using manual annotations to scrutinize the results (Roy *et al.*, 2010; Gerstein *et al.*, 2010). Realizing the same issue, Cufflinks later adds a new assembly feature, known as reference annotation based transcript (RABT), to simulate reads from annotated isoforms and combine them with the mapped reads for isoform discovery (Roberts *et al.*, 2011). This feature to some extent helps Cufflinks to remediate the discovery of isoforms involving exons lowly expressed or missed during the overlap graph building process. However, one obvious drawback of such a method is that annotations in literature can contain exons or isoforms that are possibly non-existing in the target RNA-Seq sample, thus misleading the isoform discovery.

Annotation-aided methods aim to partially use existing annotations to help resolve some of the RNA-Seq data noise issues mentioned above. SLIDE (Sparse Linear model for Isoform discovery and abundance Estimation) (Li *et al.*, 2011a) is such a method. It combines existing annotated gene and exon boundaries with de novo splicing events to construct isoform candidates, and uses a linear model with a probabilistic design matrix to achieve sparse isoform discovery and abundance estimation (see Section 3.1.3). Compared to annotation-based and annotation-free methods, the combination of literature and data information gives the advantage of finding potential novel isoforms without being biased by boundary errors in de novo assembled genes/exons, but this combination also raises the risk of missing isoforms involving novel genes/exons.

3.1.3. *Isoform abundance estimation*

The next challenge faced is to estimate the abundance of isoforms, or equivalently, to quantify the expression levels of the discovered isforms. Available abundance estimation methods include direct computation and model-based approaches. One typical direct computation method is to calculate the number of reads per kilo base of genome per million of reads mapped (RPKM) (Mortazavi *et al.*, 2008). Most model-based methods assume that reads are uniformly sampled from an isoform, leading to a Poisson distribution assumption on the total number of reads mapped to an isoform. Isoform abundance is then a function of the rate parameter in this Poisson model, and can be estimated by maximum likelihood estimation (MLE) methods. RPKM by direct computational methods is equivalent to the MLE estimate if there is no alternative isoforms. The first and most influential model-based method for abundance estimation is Jiang and Wong (2009), which we refer to as SIIER (Statistical Inferences for Isoform Expression in RNA-Seq) for ease of notation. It is an annotation-based method and estimates the abundance of annotated isoforms directly. With the following notations in a given gene,

x_i – number of reads in exon i
l_i – length of exon i
θ_j – abundance of isoform j in RPKM unit
(i.e. $\frac{\text{\# reads from isoform } j}{\text{isoform length} \times (\text{total \# of mapped reads}}$)
a_{ij} – indicator of whether isoform j contains exon i

SIIER assumes that x_i's are independent Poisson variables. The likelihood of θ_j's is

$$L \propto \prod_i \left[\exp\{-l_i \sum_j a_{ij}\theta_j\}(l_i \sum_j a_{ij}\theta_j)^{x_i} \right],$$

where $l_i \sum_j a_{ij}\theta_j$ is the Poisson rate. Then the log-likelihood is

$$\ell = -\sum_i \left(l_i \sum_j a_{ij}\theta_j \right) + \sum_i x_i \log \left(l_i \sum_j a_{ij}\theta_j \right) + C.$$

Since ℓ is a concave function, the isoform abundance parameter θ_j's can be estimated as maximum-likelihood estimates of the above model. SIIER also carries out statistical inference by using importance sampling from the posterior distribution to compute posterior expectation and confidence intervals of θ_j's. More details can be read in the paper (Jiang and Wong, 2009).

There are also efforts on formulating the abundance estimation problem using a linear model. IsoLasso uses the following linear model

$$b_i = \sum_{j=1}^{n} a_{ij} p_j + \epsilon_i, \quad i = 1, \ldots, m,$$

where b_i denotes the number of reads per base pair in the ith exon, a_{ij} denotes the indicator of whether the jth isoform contains the ith exon, p_j denotes the abundance parameter (in RPKM units) of the jth isoform, and ϵ_i is a mean zero error term. Since the number of isoform candidates are often more than the number of exons (i.e. $n > m$ in the model), IsoLasso employs the LASSO method to find sparse estimates of p_j's and subsequently uses them as isoform abundance estimates.

As compared to IsoLasso, SLIDE is based on a similar linear regression framework but has an additional data processing step and employs a more carefully modeled design matrix (a_{ij}) (Li *et al.*, 2011a). The additional data processing step is to retain the exon junction and pairing (for paired-end reads) information, which has not yet been considered in IsoLasso. SLIDE models the design matrix (a_{ij}) compatible with the processed data, taking into account the stochastic nature of the relationships between reads and isoforms. More specifically, SLIDE considers different probabilities of a read coming from the different possible isoforms in deriving (a_{ij}); IsoLasso only considers binary relationships between exons and isoforms. The way of modeling (a_{ij}) makes SLIDE flexible to refine its linear model to incorporate independent transcriptomic data resources (e.g. EST (Adams *et al.*, 1991), CAGE (Shiraki *et al.*, 2003), RACE (Frohman *et al.*, 1988)) in addition to RNA-Seq data.

In general, SLIDE has a larger isoform candidate set than IsoLasso has, thus it is even more critical for SLIDE to apply methods for sparse parameter estimation. Specifically, SLIDE uses modified L_1 sparse estimation for isoform discovery, and then takes a separate step to estimate the abundance of the discovered isoforms by non-negative least squares. Although this two-step approach hinders computational efficiency, it gives more accurate abundance estimates, because non-negative least-squares has smaller bias than L_1 sparse estimation has in parameter estimates.

3.1.4. *Summary of reference-based strategy*

Here we summarize the advantages and disadvantages of the reference-based strategy. Main advantages include:

(1) Mapping reads to a reference genome turns a large scale assembly problem (involving millions of reads) into smaller alignment subproblems,

leading to a much lower computational complexity compared to de novo assembly.

(2) With a reference, it diminishes a concern about contamination or sequencing artifacts, since those reads are not expected to be aligned to the reference genome. Otherwise, a special step would be needed to deal with potential contamination and sequencing errors.
(3) Reference-based mapping can better discern signals from noise, increasing the sensitivity in detecting low abundance transcripts and then reducing the requirement of sequencing depth.
(4) Using a reference genome, small gaps in isoforms caused by low read coverage (i.e., some fragments can be more easily sequenced than others) can be remediated.

There are also a few limitations of the reference-based strategy, including:

(1) Deleting the reads unmappable to the reference genome does diminish a concern on sequencing errors, but also raises the risk of missing interesting genome variations as well as limiting the discovery of novel genes and isoforms.
(2) This strategy heavily relies on high-quality reference genome. Unfortunately, except a few model organisms, most genomes are not available or have a questionable quality.

3.2. *De novo strategy*

In contrast to the reference-based strategy, de novo strategy does not use a reference genome. It takes advantages of vastly improved sequencing depth of next-generation sequencing technology, and directly assembles short reads into full-length transcripts.

Many de novo assembly programs (or assemblers) have been developed. A basic algorithmic technique utilized in most assemblers is De Bruijn graph, which was first applied for de novo assembly in Pevzner *et al.* (2001). Briefly, these algorithms assemble reads by constructing a (directed) De Bruijn graph in which each node represents a k-mer (a sequence of k nucleotides) and connects two nodes if the last $k-1$ nucleotides of one node overlap exactly with the first $k-1$ nucleotides of the other. A longest path of nodes without branches in the graph then corresponds to an assembled sequence, e.g. a full-length transcript. A simple demonstration of constructing a De Bruijn graph is presented in Figure 3. Popular de novo transcriptome assemblers based on De Bruijn graphs include Rnnotator (Martin

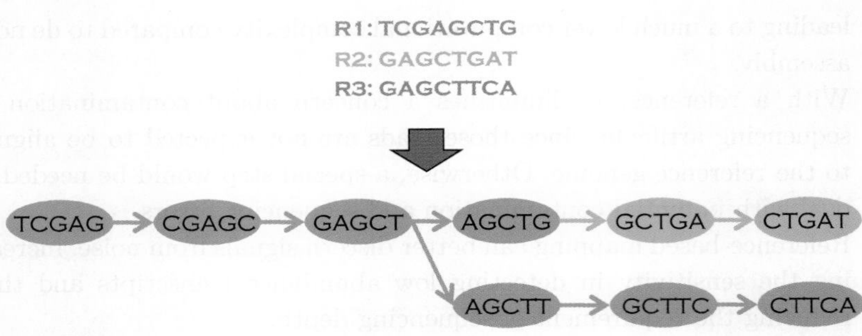

Fig. 3. De Bruijn graph.

et al., 2010), Multiple-k (Surget-Groba and Montoya-Burgos, 2010), Trans-ABySS (Robertson *et al.*, 2010), Trinity (Grabherr *et al.*, 2011) and Oases (Schulz *et al.*, 2012), just naming a few (Figure 2). Another algorithm available for de novo assembly is overlap graph, which is mostly utilized for Sanger sequencing reads and is more computationally intensive compared to De Bruijn graphs (Flicek and Birney, 2009).

As mentioned earlier, the de novo strategy, without depending on a correct alignment of reads to a reference genome, can generate new sequence assemblies for previously uncharacterized genomes. With this advantage, the de novo strategy thus is capable to detect transcripts consisting of unannotated exons or novel splicing events, or to discern transcripts originating from chromosomal rearrangements. This capability is especially important for cancer research, as cancers tend to be genetically diverse. Another important application of the de novo strategy is to recover genetic material (or genes) directly from environmental samples. This broad field of application is known as metagenomics (Handelsman *et al.*, 1998). Metagenomic assembly and whole-metagenome analyses make it possible to view the microbial world and further to achieve a better understanding of the diversity of microscopic life.

Despite its vast popularity, the de novo strategy bears several limitations. One is that it in general requires a much higher sequencing depth (about twice more) than does the reference-based strategy for the same task (Martin and Wang, 2011). This can lead to an overwhelming need for computing resources, especially when assembling large higher eukaryotic transcriptomes. The de novo strategy is also sensitive to sequencing errors. For high-abundance transcripts, sequencing errors can be distinguished from true variation in the reads (e.g. SNPs) by checking nucleotide frequencies

(Brockman *et al.*, 2008; Li *et al.*, 2008). For low-abundance transcripts, it is more difficult for this strategy to recognize sequencing errors. To avoid wrong discoveries, additional steps would be needed to correct/remove those error reads before assembly (Yang *et al.*, 2012). There are also efforts to correct assembly errors through post-assembly steps based on prior biological knowledge (Ronen *et al.*, 2012). Another limitation of the de novo strategy is related to the existence of repetitive sequences. When a De Bruijn graph is used, the sequence repeats can cause branching, and therefore, ambiguity in finding the longest paths during the assembly process (Kingsford *et al.*, 2010).

After de novo assembly, same with the reference-based strategy, the next challenge faced is quantification of assembled transcripts, a necessary step for downstream quantitative analyses (e.g. differential expression analysis). The methods introduced in Sec 3.1.3 for expression quantification are applicable under both strategies.

3.3. *Combined strategy*

As introduced above, both referenced-based and de novo strategies have their own advantages and limitations, and neither is appropriate for every RNA-Seq dataset. It is thus important to properly choose a method or combine the two strategies based on target data and study goal.

Combining the two strategies to take the advantages of both can remediate the limitations of each other. For instance, even with a high-quality reference genome in which situation reference-based strategy seems a natural solution, the removal of unmapped reads in this strategy could be undesirable if the interest is to detect novel genes, splicing isoforms or genome variations. Adding an additional step of de novo assembly of the unmapped reads can be helpful for this problem. This type of combined strategy is known as "align-then-assemble" (Martin and Wang, 2011). Another type of combined strategy practiced in applications is the "assemble-then-align" strategy (Martin and Wang, 2011). In the lack of high-quality reference genomes or when only reference genomes of related species are available, the de novo strategy becomes an obvious choice. But still, aligning the de novo assembled fragments to a related or low-quality reference genome can help close some small assembly gaps or determine ambiguous branches in De Bruijn graphs.

In general, it is wise to consider combining the referenced-based and de novo strategies when possible in order to obtain a more comprehensive transcriptome. Of course, such choices must be properly carried out based on available computation resources and a careful evaluation of target data and study goal.

4. Discussion

We conclude this chapter by further discussing several of the challenges in transcript assembly and abundance estimation using RNA-Seq data, as well as some issues in downstream transcriptomic analyses.

One big challenge to both reference-based and de novo assembly methods is related to the existence of overlapping genes, especially in higher eukaryotic species. Overlapping genes, having partially overlapping expressible nucleotide sequences, can appear on the same strand or opposite strands (i.e., antisense transcripts). For overlapping antisense transcripts, the problem has been resolved by the recent strand-specific RNA-Seq technology, which generates reads with definite strand information (He *et al.*, 2008). For overlapping genes/transcripts on the sand strand, the main difficulty is to identify start/end sites of their open reading frames. Existing annotations and other data resources (e.g. EST (Adams *et al.*, 1991), CAGE (Shiraki *et al.*, 2003), RACE (Frohman *et al.*, 1988)) can aid the identification to some extent. Differences in read coverages can also be helpful to identify overlapped regions; however, unexplained read coverage variations can confound such identification.

Unidentifiability issue in isoform discovery is another challenge faced by both strategies. This issue is attributable to the huge number of potential isoform candidates; that is, the observed read counts can be generated from different sets of isoform candidates. As we present before, this issue can be solved by applying a preselection procedure to reduce the searching space (Trapnell *et al.*, 2010; Guttman *et al.*, 2010; Li *et al.*, 2011b,a) or performing sparse estimation on isoforms (Li *et al.*, 2011b,a; Xia *et al.*, 2011). With further technological development, particularly when high-quality longer reads are available, this issue would be a less concern.

There are more challenges in isoform abundance estimation, caused by various biases introduced during data generation and processing. Some data generation biases are due to technology limitations such as that (1) RNA degradation (Nagalakshmi *et al.*, 2010) and the use of random hexamers introduce bias in library preparation (Hansen *et al.*, 2010); (2) sequencing has positional and base-composition biases (Roberts *et al.*, 2011); and (3) PCR amplification procedure is nonlinear and sensitive to stray impurities (Makrigiorgos *et al.*, 2002). Some other data generation biases are attributable to the complexity of genome structure. For instance, the secondary structure of RNA can cause varied levels of difficulty in sequencing and then a high variation of read coverages across a transcript; presence of transcribed repetitive sequences can give rise to a more desperate situation: a high read coverage of a region in de novo assembly can be a result of repetitive sequences or due to a high expression level of that region. Currently there is no effective method to handle this issue. Data processing biases mainly refer to the read coverage biases introduced by mapping. Particularly, mapping of spliced reads is difficult, inducing low read coverage in proximity of splice junctions compared to exonic regions (Bohnert and Rätsch, 2010). There have been efforts attempting to correct some biases by carefully modeling the data generation process (Roberts *et al.*, 2011; Hansen *et al.*, 2010; Li *et al.*, 2010; Zheng *et al.*, 2011; Gao *et al.*, 2011). However, further improvement of sequencing technology is necessary for more satisfactory solutions.

Since its inception, besides applications in genome annotation, gene expression profiling and alternative splice variants detection, RNA-Seq technology has also been widely used to advance studies in many downstream transcriptomic applications. For example, RNA-Seq data has been used to identify gene fusion events typical in cancer (Maher *et al.*, 2009). RNA-Seq data is also applied to find previously unknown non-coding RNAs (ncRNAs) potentially related to a variety of diseases (Fejes-Toth *et al.*, 2009; Mitchell Guttman *et al.*, 2009). Since RNA-Seq data has advantages in discovering genome-wide SNPs, it is also suitable for studying allele-specific gene expression, an important factor in human phenotypic variability (Skelly *et al.*, 2011). Differential expression analysis using RNA-Seq data also has many biological and medical applications. This analysis can be carried out using similar ideas as for analyzing microarray data, with necessary modifications on statistical models to incorporate the count nature of RNA-Seq data. More discussions on differential expression analysis using RNA-Seq data can be found in Marioni *et al.* (2008), Robinson *et al.* (2010) and Wang *et al.* (2010b).

5. Appendix: Other Applications of *-Seq Data

Since first introduced in 2005, NGS technologies have been applied to a variety of fields in genomic research (Metzker, 2009). Below we briefly introduce a few additional examples of interesting applications, beyond transcriptomes, facilitated by NGS technologies.

NGS technology has promoted research on personalized medicine. For example, the recently launched 1000 Genomes Project (Altshuler *et al.*, 2010) uses NGS to deeply catalog human genetic variants. Gene fusion events and splice variants can also be detected by NGS (e.g. RNA-Seq or genomic DNA sequencing) data. These sequencing variation studies would help understand the association between human genetic variation and health/diseases.

NGS also allows genome-wide mapping of epigenetic events such as DNA methylation (e.g. bisulfite sequencing (Taylor *et al.*, 2007)), histone marks (Bernstein *et al.*, 2007; Goldberg *et al.*, 2007), and open chromatin sites (e.g. DNase sequencing (Boyle *et al.*, 2008)), going beyond previous gene-centric studies. Bisulfite sequencing takes the advantages of NGS to survey DNA methylation status at nucleotide resolution throughout the genome. Genome-wide histone modification sites can be localized by ChIP-Seq (Johnson *et al.*, 2007), in which NGS is used to sequence the immunoprecipitated DNA molecules containing the targeted histone modifications. DNase I hypersensitivity site footprinting coupled with NGS (i.e., DNase-Seq) defines regions of open chromatin structure to indicate potential regulatory sequences. In general, large-scale examination of DNA methylation patterns, histone modification loci and open chromatin sites is useful to characterize cancer genomes.

In functional genomics, NGS technology can be applied to study various interactions between molecules. For example, ChIP-Seq is able to provide genome-wide information on DNA-protein interactions; CLIP-Seq (also known as HITS-CLIP), where NGS is applied to sequence RNA molecules isolated by crosslinking and immunoprecipitation, provides information on RNA-protein and microRNA-mRNA interactions (Licatalosi *et al.*, 2008). In addition, coupling of NGS and chromosome conformation capture (3C) methods can detect long-range genomic interactions (Lieberman-Aiden *et al.*, 2009). Other methods such as circularized chromosome confirmation capture (4C) (Simonis *et al.*, 2006) and carbon-copy chromosome conformation capture (5C) (Dostie *et al.*, 2006) also provide large-scale analyses of genomic interactions but are still limited to selected sites of interrogation. Integration of these interaction study results can provide information on discovering genetic and signaling pathways, such as identifying a number of key genes linked to pathways regulating metastasis, apoptosis and senescence.

In clinical diagnosis of genetic diseases, NGS has also been applied to target the protein-coding parts of a subset of known disease genes for mutation discovery. This type of targeted resequencing is called exome-sequencing (i.e., Exome-Seq) (Ng *et al.*, 2009), which is powerful to capture variants in the coding regions at a reduced cost compared to whole genome sequencing. Followed by linkage or association study on the detected variants, for instance, Exome-Seq can provide a tool for studying disease-associated variants/genes for Mendelian disorders (Bamshad *et al.*, 2011) or complex diseases like cancers (Wang *et al.*, 2012). Of course, Exome-Seq will miss the information in the non-coding regions of the genome, but it is cost-effective for identifying most biologically significant mutations in expressible regions.

There are many other applications of NGS. For instance, combined use of exome and transcriptome sequencing can be used to search for genes with loss of heterozygosity and allele-specific expression (Zhao *et al.*, 2010); non-coding RNA (ncRNA) expression profiling sheds light onto human cancer trancriptomes (Gibb *et al.*, 2011). Overall, NGS brings numerous hope and excitement to genomic research, but challenges regarding data processing and analyses still exist.

References

Adams, M., *et al.*, 1991: Complementary dna sequencing: expressed sequence tags and human genome project. *Science*, **252(5013)**, 1651–1656.

Altshuler, D., *et al.*, 2010: A map of human genome variation from population scale sequencing. *Nature*, **467(7319)**, 1061–1073.

Au, K., H. Jiang, L. Lin, Y. Xing, and W. Wong, 2010: Detection of splice junctions from paired-end rna-seq data by splicemap. *Nucleic Acids Research*, **38(14)**, 4570–4578.

Bamshad, M., S. Ng, A. Bigham, H. Tabor, M. Emond, D. Nickerson, and J. Shendure, 2011: Exome sequencing as a tool for mendelian disease gene discovery. *Nature Reviews Genetics*, **12(11)**, 745–755.

Bernstein, B., A. Meissner, and E. Lander, 2007: The mammalian epigenome. *Cell*, **128(4)**, 669–681.

Bohnert, R. and G. Rätsch, 2010: rquant. web: a tool for rna-seq-based transcript quantitation. *Nucleic acids research*, **38(suppl 2)**, W348–W351.

Boyle, A., S. Davis, H. Shulha, P. Meltzer, E. Margulies, Z. Weng, T. Furey, and G. Crawford, 2008: High-resolution mapping and characterization of open chromatin across the genome. *Cell*, **132(2)**, 311–322.

Brockman, W., *et al.*, 2008: Quality scores and snp detection in sequencing-by-synthesis systems. *Genome Research*, **18(5)**, 763–770.

Celniker, S., *et al.*, 2009: Unlocking the secrets of the genome. *Nature*, **459(7249)**, 927–930.

Dostie, J., *et al.*, 2006: Chromosome conformation capture carbon copy (5c): a massively parallel solution for mapping interactions between genomic elements. *Genome research*, **16(10)**, 1299–1309.

Fejes-Toth, K., *et al.*, 2009: Post-transcriptional processing generates a diversity of 5′-modified long and short rnas. *Nature*, **457(7232)**, 1028–1032.

Flicek, P. and E. Birney, 2009: Sense from sequence reads: methods for alignment and assembly. *Nature Methods*, **6**, S6–S12.

Frazer, K., *et al.*, 2007: A second generation human haplotype map of over 3.1 million snps. *Nature*, **449(7164)**, 851–861.

Frohman, M., M. Dush, and G. Martin, 1988: Rapid production of full-length cdnas from rare transcripts: amplification using a single gene-specific oligonucleotide primer. *Proceedings of the National Academy of Sciences*, **85(23)**, 8998.

Gao, L., Z. Fang, K. Zhang, D. Zhi, and X. Cui, 2011: Length bias correction for rna-seq data in gene set analyses. *Bioinformatics*, **27(5)**, 662–669.

Gerstein, M., *et al.*, 2010: Integrative analysis of the caenorhabditis elegans genome by the modencode project. *Science*, **330(6012)**, 1775.

Gibb, E., *et al.*, 2011: Human cancer long non-coding rna transcriptomes. *PloS one*, **6(10)**, e25 915.

Goldberg, A., C. Allis, and E. Bernstein, 2007: Epigenetics: a landscape takes shape. *Cell*, **128(4)**, 635–638.

Grabherr, M., *et al.*, 2011: Full-length transcriptome assembly from rna-seq data without a reference genome. *Nature biotechnology*, **29(7)**, 644–652.

Guttman, M., *et al.*, 2010: Ab initio reconstruction of cell type-specific transcriptomes in mouse reveals the conserved multi-exonic structure of lincrnas. *Nature biotechnology*, **28(5)**, 503–510.

Handelsman, J., M. Rondon, S. Brady, J. Clardy, and R. Goodman, 1998: Molecular biological access to the chemistry of unknown soil microbes: a new frontier for natural products. *Chemistry & biology*, **5(10)**, R245–R249.

Hansen, K., S. Brenner, and S. Dudoit, 2010: Biases in illumina transcriptome sequencing caused by random hexamer priming. *Nucleic acids research*, **38(12)**, e131–e131.

He, Y., B. Vogelstein, V. Velculescu, N. Papadopoulos, and K. Kinzler, 2008: The antisense transcriptomes of human cells. *Science*, **322(5909)**, 1855–1857.

Jiang, H. and W. Wong, 2009: Statistical inferences for isoform expression in rna-seq. *Bioinformatics*, **25(8)**, 1026–1032.

Johnson, D., A. Mortazavi, R. Myers, and B. Wold, 2007: Genome-wide mapping of in vivo protein-dna interactions. *Science's STKE*, **316(5830)**, 1497.

Kent, W., 2002: Blatthe blast-like alignment tool. *Genome research*, **12(4)**, 656.

Kingsford, C., M. Schatz, and M. Pop, 2010: Assembly complexity of prokaryotic genomes using short reads. *BMC bioinformatics*, **11(1)**, 21.

Lander, E., *et al.*, 2001: Initial sequencing and analysis of the human genome. *Nature*, **409(6822)**, 860–921.

Li, H., J. Ruan, and R. Durbin, 2008: Mapping short dna sequencing reads and calling variants using mapping quality scores. *Genome research*, **18(11)**, 1851–1858.

Li, J., C. Jiang, J. Brown, H. Huang, and P. Bickel, 2011a: Sparse linear modeling of next-generation mrna sequencing (rna-seq) data for isoform discovery and abundance estimation. *Proceedings of the National Academy of Sciences*, **108(50)**, 19 867–19 872.

Li, J., H. Jiang, and W. Wong, 2010: Method modeling non-uniformity in short-read rates in rna-seq data. *Genome Biol*, **11(5)**, R25.

Li, W., J. Feng, and T. Jiang, 2011b: Isolasso: a lasso regression approach to rna-seq based transcriptome assembly. *Research in Computational Molecular Biology*, Springer, 168–188.

Licatalosi, D., *et al.*, 2008: Hits-clip yields genome-wide insights into brain alternative rna processing. *Nature*, **456(7221)**, 464–469.

Lieberman-Aiden, E., *et al.*, 2009: Comprehensive mapping of long-range interactions reveals folding principles of the human genome. *science*, **326(5950)**, 289–293.

Lister, R., R. O'Malley, J. Tonti-Filippini, B. Gregory, C. Berry, A. Millar, and J. Ecker, 2008: Highly integrated single-base resolution maps of the epigenome in arabidopsis. *Cell*, **133(3)**, 523–536.

Maher, C., *et al.*, 2009: Transcriptome sequencing to detect gene fusions in cancer. *Nature*, **458(7234)**, 97–101.

Makrigiorgos, G., S. Chakrabarti, Y. Zhang, M. Kaur, and B. Price, 2002: A pcr-based amplification method retaining the quantitative difference between two complex genomes. *Nature biotechnology*, **20(9)**, 936–939.

Margulies, M., *et al.*, 2005: Genome sequencing in microfabricated high-density picolitre reactors. *Nature*, **437(7057)**, 376–380.

Marioni, J., C. Mason, S. Mane, M. Stephens, and Y. Gilad, 2008: Rna-seq: an assessment of technical reproducibility and comparison with gene expression arrays. *Genome research*, **18(9)**, 1509–1517.

Martin, J. and Z. Wang, 2011: Next-generation transcriptome assembly. *Nature Reviews Genetics*, **12(10)**, 671–682.

Martin, J., *et al.*, 2010: Rnnotator: an automated de novo transcriptome assembly pipeline from stranded rna-seq reads. *BMC genomics*, **11(1)**, 663.

Metzker, M., 2009: Sequencing technologiesthe next generation. *Nature Reviews Genetics*, **11(1)**, 31–46.

Mitchell Guttman, I., *et al.*, 2009: Chromatin signature reveals over a thousand highly conserved large non-coding rnas in mammals. *Nature*, **458(7235)**, 223–227.

Mortazavi, A., B. Williams, K. McCue, L. Schaeffer, and B. Wold, 2008: Mapping and quantifying mammalian transcriptomes by rna-seq. *Nature methods*, **5(7)**, 621–628.

Nagalakshmi, U., K. Waern, and M. Snyder, 2010: Rna-seq: a method for comprehensive transcriptome analysis. *Curr Protoc Mol Biol*, **89(4.11)**, 1–4.

Nagalakshmi, U., Z. Wang, K. Waern, C. Shou, D. Raha, M. Gerstein, and M. Snyder, 2008: The transcriptional landscape of the yeast genome defined by rna sequencing. *Science*, **320(5881)**, 1344.

Ng, S., *et al.*, 2009: Targeted capture and massively parallel sequencing of 12 human exomes. *Nature*, **461(7261)**, 272–276.

Park, P., 2009: Chip–seq: advantages and challenges of a maturing technology. *Nature Reviews Genetics*, **10(10)**, 669–680.

Pevzner, P., H. Tang, and M. Waterman, 2001: An eulerian path approach to dna fragment assembly. *Proceedings of the National Academy of Sciences*, **98(17)**, 9748.

Roberts, A., C. Trapnell, J. Donaghey, J. Rinn, L. Pachter, *et al.*, 2011: Improving rna-seq expression estimates by correcting for fragment bias. *Genome Biol*, **12(3)**, R22.

Robertson, G., *et al.*, 2010: De novo assembly and analysis of rna-seq data. *Nature Methods*, **7(11)**, 909–912.

Robinson, M., A. Oshlack, *et al.*, 2010: A scaling normalization method for differential expression analysis of rna-seq data. *Genome Biol*, **11(3)**, R25.

Ronen, R., C. Boucher, H. Chitsaz, and P. Pevzner, 2012: Sequel: improving the accuracy of genome assemblies. *Bioinformatics*, **28(12)**, i188–i196.

Roy, S., *et al.*, 2010: Identification of functional elements and regulatory circuits by drosophila modencode. *Science*, **330(6012)**, 1787.

Sanger, F., S. Nicklen, and A. Coulson, 1977: Dna sequencing with chain-terminating inhibitors. *Proceedings of the National Academy of Sciences*, **74(12)**, 5463.

Schena, M., D. Shalon, R. Davis, and P. Brown, 1995: Quantitative monitoring of gene expression patterns with a complementary dna microarray. *Science*, **270(5235)**, 467.

Schulz, M., D. Zerbino, M. Vingron, and E. Birney, 2012: Oases: Robust de novo rna-seq assembly across the dynamic range of expression levels. *Bioinformatics*.

Schuster, S., 2008: Next-generation sequencing transforms todays biology. *Nature*, **200(8)**.

Shendure, J. and H. Ji, 2008: Next-generation dna sequencing. *Nature biotechnology*, **26(10)**, 1135–1145.

Shendure, J., *et al.*, 2005: Accurate multiplex polony sequencing of an evolved bacterial genome. *Science*, **309(5741)**, 1728.

Shiraki, T., *et al.*, 2003: Cap analysis gene expression for high-throughput analysis of transcriptional starting point and identification of promoter usage. *Proceedings of the National Academy of Sciences*, **100(26)**, 15 776.

Simonis, M., P. Klous, E. Splinter, Y. Moshkin, R. Willemsen, E. De Wit, B. Van Steensel, and W. De Laat, 2006: Nuclear organization of active and inactive chromatin domains uncovered by chromosome conformation capture–on-chip (4c). *Nature genetics*, **38(11)**, 1348–1354.

Skelly, D., M. Johansson, J. Madeoy, J. Wakefield, and J. Akey, 2011: A powerful and flexible statistical framework for testing hypotheses of allele-specific gene expression from rna-seq data. *Genome Research*, **21(10)**, 1728–1737.

Surget-Groba, Y. and J. Montoya-Burgos, 2010: Optimization of de novo transcriptome assembly from next-generation sequencing data. *Genome research*, **20(10)**, 1432.

Taylor, K., R. Kramer, J. Davis, J. Guo, D. Duff, D. Xu, C. Caldwell, and H. Shi, 2007: Ultradeep bisulfite sequencing analysis of dna methylation patterns in multiple gene promoters by 454 sequencing. *Cancer research*, **67(18)**, 8511.

Tibshirani, R., 1996: Regression shrinkage and selection via the lasso. *Journal of the Royal Statistical Society. Series B (Methodological)*, 267–288.

Trapnell, C., L. Pachter, and S. Salzberg, 2009: Tophat: discovering splice junctions with rna-seq. *Bioinformatics*, **25(9)**, 1105–1111.

Trapnell, C., *et al.*, 2010: Transcript assembly and quantification by rna-seq reveals unannotated transcripts and isoform switching during cell differentiation. *Nature biotechnology*, **28(5)**, 511–515.

Velculescu, V., L. Zhang, B. Vogelstein, and K. Kinzler, 1995: Serial analysis of gene expression. *Science*, **270(5235)**, 484.

Venter, J., *et al.*, 2001: The sequence of the human genome. *Science's STKE*, **291(5507)**, 1304.

Wang, K., *et al.*, 2010a: Mapsplice: accurate mapping of rna-seq reads for splice junction discovery. *Nucleic acids research*, **38(18)**, e178–e178.

Wang, L., Z. Feng, X. Wang, X. Wang, and X. Zhang, 2010b: Degseq: an r package for identifying differentially expressed genes from rna-seq data. *Bioinformatics*, **26(1)**, 136.

Wang, L., *et al.*, 2012: Whole-exome sequencing of human pancreatic cancers and characterization of genomic instability caused by mlh1 haploinsufficiency and complete deficiency. *Genome Research*, **22(2)**, 208–219.

Wang, Z., M. Gerstein, and M. Snyder, 2009: Rna-seq: a revolutionary tool for transcriptomics. *Nature Reviews Genetics*, **10(1)**, 57–63.

Wilhelm, B., *et al.*, 2008: Dynamic repertoire of a eukaryotic transcriptome surveyed at single-nucleotide resolution. *Nature*, **453(7199)**, 1239–1243.

Wu, T. and S. Nacu, 2010: Fast and snp-tolerant detection of complex variants and splicing in short reads. *Bioinformatics*, **26(7)**, 873–881.

Xia, Z., J. Wen, C. Chang, and X. Zhou, 2011: Nsmap: A method for spliced isoforms identification and quantification from rna-seq. *BMC bioinformatics*, **12(1)**, 162.

Yang, X., S. Chockalingam, and S. Aluru, 2012: A survey of error-correction methods for next-generation sequencing. *Briefings in Bioinformatics*.

Zhao, Q., *et al.*, 2010: Systematic detection of putative tumor suppressor genes through the combined use of exome and transcriptome sequencing. *Genome biology*, **11(11)**, R114.

Zheng, W., L. Chung, and H. Zhao, 2011: Bias detection and correction in rna-sequencing data. *BMC bioinformatics*, **12(1)**, 290.

About the Authors

Jingyi Jessica Li, Ph.D. has been an Assistant Professor in Statistics at the Department of Statistics, University of California, Los Angeles from July 1, 2013. She received her Ph.D. in Biostatistics from UC Berkeley in May, 2013, under the supervision of Prof. Peter J. Bickel and Prof. Haiyan Huang. Prior to that, she earned her B.S. (summa cum laude) from the

Department of Biological Sciences and Technology (now School of Life Sciences) at Tsinghua University, China in 2007.

Haiyan Huang, Ph.D. is currently an Associate Professor of Statistics and Biostatistics at the Department of Statistics, University of California, Berkeley. She earned her BS degree in Mathematics in 1997 from Peking University, China. After that, she did her graduate study in the Department of Mathematics at University of Southern California and obtained her PhD degree in 2001. Prior to joining UC Berkeley as a faculty member, she worked as a postdoc in the Departments of Statistics and Biostatistics in Harvard University from 2001 to 2003. Her research interests are in statistical genomics and in general problems at the interface between statistics and data-rich scientific disciplines.

Minping Qian is an Emeritus Professor at the School of Mathematics, Peking University. She started her career as a probabilist, in 1960s. Since late 1990s, she also has been involved in the computational molecular biology. She and her colleagues have been devoted to building mathematical framework and models presenting living systems. She had been a faculty at the School of Mathematics, Peking University since 1962, and retired in 2004.

Xuegong Zhang, Ph.D. earned his BS degree in Industrial Automation in 1989 and Ph.D. degree in Pattern Recognition and Intelligent Systems in 1994, both from Tsinghua University. He joined the faculty of Tsinghua University in 1994, where he is a Professor of Pattern Recognition and Bioinformatics in the Department of Automation since 2002. Dr. Zhang worked at Harvard School of Public Health as a visiting scientist on computational biology in 2001–2002 and in 2006 both in the Biostatistics Department. Currently he is the Director of the Bioinformatics Division, Tsinghua National Laboratory for Information Science and Technology (TNLIST) and the Deputy Director of the Center for Synthetic and Systems Biology (CSSB). His research interests include biological data mining especially for microarray and RNA-Seq data, gene expression and regulation, alternative splicing, RNA regulations and metagenomics methods and applications, etc.

CHAPTER 25

GENETIC STRUCTURE OF HUMAN POPULATION

HUA TANG

Department of Genetics, Alway M335,
300 Pasteur Drive, Stanford University
School of Medicine, Stanford, CA 94305, USA
huatang@stanford.edu

KUN TANG

CAS-MPG Partner Institute for Computational Biology,
Shanghai Institute of Biological Sciences,
Chinese Academy of Science, 320 Yue Yang Road,
Shanghai, 200031 People's Republic of China
tangkun@picb.ac.cn

1. Introduction

The completion of the draft sequence of the human genome (Lander *et al.* 2001; Venter *et al.* 2001) and the rapid advancement in high-throughput technologies have thrust genomics into the center stage of biomedical research. Genomic studies hold tremendous promise to elucidate the biology of diseases and to advance medical science. However, in order to identify and characterize the function of genetic variants that influence disease, it is necessary to appreciate the pattern of genetic variation that is not related to the specific disease. This is because population-based genomic approaches, such as genome-wide association studies (GWAS), are often observational studies in nature, for which randomization of genes is not possible; therefore the design and analysis of genomic studies need to account for the intrinsic genetic structure, arising from the complex human evolutionary history.

The purpose of this chapter is to provide a survey of methods for investigating, and current understanding of, human population genetic structure. We begin by presenting several commonly used statistical methods in

Section 2. Empirical studies characterizing population structure worldwide and within a continent are reviewed in Section 3. Section 4 focuses on studies of genetically admixed populations. Finally, Section 5 discusses the implication of population structure in genetic association studies. To set the stage for the discussion, we first briefly review the four evolutionary forces that shape the genome of natural populations: mutation, genetic drift, gene flow and natural selection.

1.1. *Evolutionary forces shaping patterns of genetic variation*

Mutation, or change in DNA, provides the ultimate source of variation. Mutation occurs through a great number of mechanisms and gives rise to changes ranging from a single base pair alterations to large segments of chromosomal re-arrangements and even the loss or gain of entire chromosomes. For practicality, the discussion in this chapter will focus on variations from small scale mutations: single nucleotide polymorphism (SNP) and short tandem repeat (STR), as these are the two types of variation that can be easily assayed using high-throughput platforms and have been used in a majority of recent surveys of genetic structure. With the accumulation of whole genome sequencing data, we expect that the rare variants and micro-scale insertion/deletion variation will also be cataloged and incorporated in the studies of population structure.

Genetic drift refers to the stochastic variation in allele frequency that occurs as a result of the random sampling of alleles from one generation to the next. Consider a population, whose size remains constant as N diploid individuals (and therefore $2N$ alleles). Suppose in the current generation, the frequency of allele A at a selectively-neutral, bi-allelic, locus, such as a SNP, is p_0, then the distribution of the number of allele A in the next generation follows a binomial distribution, Binom(2N, p_0). If N and p_0 are small, the A allele may not appear in the next generation at all; in other words, genetic drift may completely remove an allele from a population, and the effect of genetic drift is particularly strong in small populations. Furthermore, in the absence of gene flow, reproductively isolated sub-populations undergo independent genetic drift, which leads to divergent allele frequencies across sub-populations. This discrepancy in allele frequencies is the source of information in characterizing genetic structure.

The diversifying effect of genetic drift is countered by gene flow, which occurs when migrants enter a new sub-population and contribute to its gene pool in the next generation. Continuous gene flow is a homogenizing process that reduces genetic distance between sub-populations; in general, the rate of gene flow diminishes with the geographic distance between populations. However, multiple waves of massive trans-continental migration have occurred during the past centuries, giving rise to admixed populations, in which the genome of a single individual consists of mixture of alleles derived from multiple ancestral populations. Fine-scale characterization of genetic structure in admixed populations is discussed in Section 2.4.

The fourth major force that influences the pattern of human genomic variation is natural selection, which can decrease the frequency of a deleterious allele, increase the frequency of an advantageous allele or maintain the intermediate frequency of a variant subject to balancing selection. Recent positive selection, which leads to a rapid increase in the frequency of the adaptive allele, tends to be confined within a specific geographic region. As a result, this type of positive selection often leads to large frequency differences across populations at the selected loci. A great number of methods have been proposed for detecting genomic signature of selection (Nielsen *et al.* 2007). However, theoretical analysis and empirical data suggest that, at the genome level and with a few exceptions, genetic drift and gene flow are much stronger forces than selection in shaping the genome-wide pattern of variation (Kimura 1989; Pickrell *et al.* 2009). Therefore, we will not discuss natural selection further in this chapter.

2. Quantifying Population Structure

In this section, we introduce several commonly used approaches for detecting and quantifying population structure. We begin by describing the classic F-statistics, which measures the degree of genetic differentiation among pre-defined sub-populations. We then focus on methods, which aim to characterize latent and possibly non-discrete population structure. Finally, we touch upon recent developments in finer-scale characterization of structure in genetically admixed populations.

2.1. F_{ST} *and genetic distance*

For the large part of human history, individuals from different continents, separated by expanses of water, do not mate. Within each continent, for a variety of reasons (including geography, language and culture), humans have not and do not currently mate randomly. The intricate mating pattern gives rise to population subdivisions at different levels, which may or may not be hierarchical. Non-random mating has two consequences: first, preferential mating between individuals from the same subpopulation is a form of **inbreeding**, and produces the "Wahlund effect," or a reduction in the observed heterozygotes (Wahlund 1928); second, as the subpopulations experience independent genetic drift, allele frequencies at genetic markers tend to diverge. Originally introduced by Sewall Wright to quantify the effect of population structure on the amount of inbreeding, $\mathrm{F_{ST}}$ has become one of the most widely used measures of population subdivision (Wright 1921).

In explaining the concept of Fst, we will consider a simplified model, in which the entire human population consists of a number of pamictic, or randomly mating, subpopulations. $\mathrm{F_{ST}}$ is defined as the reduction in heterozygosity among subpopulations ($\mathrm{H_S}$) due to genetic drift, relative to the heterozygosity in the total population ($\mathrm{H_T}$):

$$F_{ST} = \frac{H_T - H_S}{H_T}, \tag{1}$$

where $\mathrm{H_S}$ is the average, across sub-populations, of the *expected* heterozygosity across subpopulations, computed under the assumption that mating is random within each subpopulation but not necessarily random with respect to the entire population. Likewise, $\mathrm{H_T}$ is computed assuming random mating in the entire population without population structure.

There is an alternative formula for computing $\mathrm{F_{ST}}$, which is based on the apportioning of variation in allele frequencies at a locus to the subdivision. At a SNP, $\mathrm{F_{ST}}$ can be computed based on the allele frequencies:

$$F_{ST} = \frac{\sigma_p^2}{\bar{p}(1-\bar{p})}, \tag{2}$$

where σ_p^2 is the variance of allele frequencies among subpopulations and $\bar{p}$ denotes the average allele frequency in the total population. For example, suppose the frequency of an allele is 0 and 1 in two subpopulations, respectively, then $\mathrm{F_{ST}} = 1$, meaning the variance in allele frequency is completely explained by the population division. For a pair of subpopulations, $\mathrm{F_{ST}}$ is often taken as a genetic distance measure, with higher values of $\mathrm{F_{ST}}$ reflecting a greater level of genetic divergence. It can be shown that (1) and (2) are mathematically equivalent for biallelic markers, but (2) is often computationally more convenient. Extensions of Fst have been developed to accommodate for multiple alleles (such as STR) and to account for unequal sample sizes among subpopulations (Nei 1977; Weir and Cockerham 1984). It should also be noted that both (1) and (2) define F_{ST} for a specific locus, which can vary considerably from locus to locus due to genetic drift or selection. Therefore, when F_{ST} is reported as a genome-level summary index among subpopulations, it is often calculated by averaging both the numerator and the denominator in (1) or (2) across loci.

While Fst offers a flexible and intuitive measure of genetic differentiation with respect to a pre-defined population subdivision, in many cases we are interested in using the genetic data to define the subpopulations; in other words, the goal is to detect unknown subdivision. In the next two sections, we present two popular and complementary approaches that are used for characterizing hidden population structure.

2.2. *Model-based clustering algorithms*

In the context of inferring genetic structure, the data usually consists of individuals genotyped at multiple genetic markers (e.g., RFLPs, microsatellites, or SNPs). A natural model represents subpopulations as clusters, and an individual's genome is sampled from one of the clusters. The goal of clustering analysis is to simultaneously define clusters (subpopulations) and to assign observational units into these clusters, so that members in the same cluster are similar by some criteria. A rich literature exists for clustering analysis; for a comprehensive survey, readers are referred to (Hastie *et al.* 2009; Mardia *et al.* 1980).

In the discrete population model, all alleles in an individual are assumed to have been drawn randomly from one of the subpopulations, according to a set of allele frequencies that are specific to that subpopulation. The goal of the analysis is to simultaneously estimate subpopulation allele frequencies and group membership. As mentioned earlier, recent migration gives rise to genetically admixed individuals, whose genomes represent a mixture of alleles from multiple clusters [see Section 4]. Mathematically, this means an individual may have partial membership in multiple clusters, which are biologically interpreted as ancestral populations of the admixed individuals. For example, African Americans in the United States are a recently admixed group; most African American individuals deriving ancestry from European and West African ancestral populations (Glass and Li 1953).

A useful concept for characterizing genetic ancestry is the **individual ancestry** (IA) proportion, which will be denoted as a vector, $Q_i =$

$\{q_i^1, \ldots, q_i^K\}$ in what follows. Here q_i^k represents the probability that a randomly selected allele from the individual originates from ancestral population k. Under a discrete subpopulation model, exactly one element in the vector, Q, is set to one and all others are zero, implying all alleles in the individual are traced to one cluster; in contrast, in an admixed individual, alleles are drawn from multiple clusters according to a multinomial distribution with probability vector, Q, which satisfies $\sum_k q_i^k = 1$.

Various frequentist and Bayesian approaches have been developed to jointly infer IA and the allele frequencies in each subpopulation (denoted by P). We begin by explaining the maximum likelihood approach for the admixture model, as this model illustrates the principles that underlie most of the model-based approaches (Satten *et al.* 2001; Tang *et al.* 2005a; Zhu *et al.* 2006). For simplicity, we assume data consists of bi-allelic SNP genotype, although the model can also be used to analyze multiallelic marker data. Let $G_i^m = (g_i^{m,1}, g_i^{m,2})$ denotes the genotype of individual i at marker m, with $g_i^{m,1}$ and $g_i^{m,2}$ being the unordered pair of alleles, and $P = \{p_m^k\}$ be the frequency of (an arbitrarily designated) allele A at marker m in population k. For computational convenience, we augment the data with $Z_i^{m,j} \in (1, \ldots, K)$ (j = 1, 2), which indicate the unobservable subpopulation membership of the corresponding allele, and are considered as independent draws from the multinomial probability vectors, Q_i. Under this conditional independence assumption, the augmented log likelihood function, treating Q and P as parameters and G and Z as data, is simply the product of the probability of observing each allele:

$$l(G, Z|P, Q) = \sum_i \sum_m \sum_{j=1}^{2} u_{imj}, \tag{3}$$

where

$$u_{imj} = \begin{cases} \sum_k \log(p_m^k q_i^k) & \text{if } g_i^{m,j} = 1 \\ \sum_k \log((1 - p_m^k) q_i^k) & \text{otherwise} \end{cases}$$

An Expectation-Maximization (EM) algorithm can be used to find the maximum likelihood estimates for the parameter values, (P, Q), treating Z as missing data. Specifically, in the Expectation step, the expectation of Z is computed based on the current parameter estimates, and in the Maximization step, maximum likelihood estimates of P and Q are updated according to the likelihood function in (3). This EM-algorithm is implemented in program, *frappe* (Tang *et al.* 2005a).

In parallel, Bayesian approaches have been developed based on similar latent cluster models, and use Markov Chain Monte Carlo (MCMC) methods to sample from the posterior distribution of the model parameters. The Bayesian methods offer a flexible framework for incorporating more complex population history models. For example, one of the widely used Bayesian programs, STRUCTURE, includes useful features such as modeling linkage among loci, as well as correlated allele frequencies between evolutionarily related ancestral populations (Pritchard *et al.* 2000; Falush *et al.* 2003).

2.3. *Principal component analysis*

Complementing the model-based approaches, Principal Component Analysis (PCA) is a classic technique for multivariate data analysis, which aims to project high-dimensional data to a much lower dimension while capturing the greatest level of variation (Pearson 1901). Cavalli-Sforza and colleagues were among the first to apply PCA to population-level allele frequency data, and made connection between the principal components (PC) and direction of human migration and expansion throughout the world (Cavalli-Sforza *et al.* 1994).

Applying PCA directly on the matrix of individual-level genotypes, instead of population-level allele frequencies, was proposed in the context of a method for correcting for population stratification [Section 5] (Zhu *et al.* 2002). This approach has been widely adopted for characterizing genetic structure, owing to the availability of software, EIGENSTRAT (Price *et al.* 2006). In this algorithm, the genotype data is represented by an N by M matrix, G^0, where each row represents an individual and each column a SNP; the genotypes are denoted as 0, 1, or 2, corresponding to aa, Aa or AA. Each column, or SNP, in G^0 is centered and scaled by $G_{im} = \frac{(G^0_{im} - 2p_m)}{\sqrt{2p_m(1-p_m)}}$, where G^0_{im} is the genotype of individual i at marker m, and p_m is the sample allele frequency of the marker. Let $\Sigma = GG^t$ be the covariance matrix, where the superscript t denote matrix transpose. PCA seeks the linear transformation $Y = U^tG$, such that U^t is orthogonal, $D = U^t\Sigma U$ is diagonal, with elements $d_1 \geq d_2 \geq \cdots \geq d_N \geq 0$. The i-th column of Y are the scores with respect to the i-th PC. The transformation reduces the high-dimension genotype data to a lower dimension, in the sense that the first k columns of Y span the k-dimensional subspace that captures maximal variance in G. Matrices U^t and D can be computed through singular value decomposition (SVD) on the covariance matrix, Σ, which has the dimension of sample size, $N \times N$. Since N is often much smaller than the number of markers, M, EIGENSTRAT is computationally efficient and have been applied to analyze large data sets generated from high-density SNP arrays (Wellcome Trust Case Control Consortium 2007). Using PCA to characterize genetic structure has gained popularity in genetic analyses due to both computational efficiency and interpretability: as we will see in Sections 3 and 4, when the underlying population structure is driven mainly by reproductive isolation and subsequent genetic differentiation, PCs reveal a close relationship between geographic proximity and genetic similarity; when admixture represents major population structure, PCs often correlate with individual ancestry proportions. A related approach, multidimensional scaling (MDS) has also been using to analyze high-dimensional genotype data. The distinction is that MDS applies eigen-decomposition to a dissimilarity matrix instead of the covariance matrix (Hastie *et al.* 2009; Mardia *et al.* 1980).

Although the underlying model for clustering analysis and PCA differ, both can be considered as a form of decomposing the gentoype matrix, G^0, into two low-rank matrices (Engelhardt and Stephens 2010). Under this unified framework, other matrix decomposition approaches are possible, and some may be more accurate in recapitulate the isolation-by-distance migration model.

2.4. *Fine-scale characterization of genetic structure in admixed populations*

For admixed populations, methods described in the preceding section can be used to infer individual ancestry, which describes the genome-wide average ancestry proportions in an individual. Because chromosomes are transmitted from one generation to the next in large segments, interrupted only through occasional recombination events, the genome of a recently admixed individual resembles a mosaic of long chromosomal blocks derived from one of the ancestral populations. With high-density genotype data, it is now feasible to infer locus-specific ancestry, or ancestry at each location along a chromosome, and thus reconstruct the ancestry blocks. Underlying most methods for inferring locus-specific ancestry is a Hidden Markov Model (HMM), in which the hidden state represents the locus-specific ancestry origin, while the observed state is the genotype or haplotype. A basic HMM algorithm is implemented in the linkage model of STRUCTURE 2.0.

In this model, the initial state, corresponding to the hidden ancestry state at marker 1, is assumed to follow a multinomial distribution, with probability Q_i. Transition in hidden state occurs as a Poisson process, at a rate r per unit of genetic distance, where r can be regarded as the time (in generation) since admixing. For haploid data, let Z_i^m be the ancestry at marker m, $Q_i = \{q_i^1, \ldots, q_i^K\}$ denote IA, and d_m denote genetic distance (in Morgan) between markers m and $m+1$, then,

$$P(Z_i^m = k|r, Q) = q_i^k,$$

and

$$\begin{aligned} &P(Z_i^{m+1} = k'|Z_i^m = k, r, Q) \\ &\quad = \begin{cases} \exp(-d_m r) + (1 - \exp(-d_m r))q_i^{k'} & \text{if } k = k' \\ (1-\exp(-d_m r))q_i^k & \text{otherwise} \end{cases}. \end{aligned}$$

Conditioning on the hidden state, Z = k, the probability of the observed allele at a marker is the allele frequency in population, p_m^k. The HMM is attractive because computationally efficient algorithms have been developed to compute the hidden states and model parameters (Rabiner 1989). However, the HMM makes an important assumption: conditioning on the hidden state, Z, the alleles at neighboring markers are modeled as independently emitted. This is a reasonable assumption when data consists of sparse markers that are in approximate linkage equilibrium (i.e. uncorrelated) within the ancestral populations. As the marker data becomes denser, however, alleles at tightly linked markers form haplotypes, such that the haplotype frequency often deviates substantially from what is expected under linkage equilibrium. (Tang *et al.* 2006a) proposed a Markov-Hidden Markov model, implemented in program SABER, which incorporates the dependency between pairs of neighboring markers. These authors subsequently extended the model to account for higher-order dependency [Johnson, in preparation]. More recently, two similar methods implemented a nest HMM, which features the transition between haplotypes within an ancestral populations using a model originally developed for haplotype phasing (Li and Stephens 2003; Price *et al.* 2009; Sundquist *et al.* 2008). Regardless of the difference between these methods, it is important to realize that the source of information underlying all methods is the different allele and haplotype frequencies among the ancestral populations. As such, the accuracy with which one can infer locus-specific ancestry depends on the genetic divergence between the ancestral populations. The distribution of the ancestry blocks also depends on the admixing history: ancient admixing events result in smaller ancestry fragments, while recent admixing events give rise to extended blocks. With any method, the ability to identify a switch in ancestral state deteriorates when the blocks are very small. Therefore, the accuracy of locus-specific ancestry inference depends on (at least) two aspects of the population history: the divergence time between the ancestral populations, and the time of the admixing events. Simulation studies using HapMap data suggest that current high-density genotype data harbors sufficient information for accurate ancestry inference for admixed groups such as African Americans or Hispanics (Tang *et al.* 2006a). Furthermore, accurate inference of locus-specific ancestry allows the partitioning of an admixed genome into partial genomes, each derived from a specific ancestral population. As we illustrate in Section 3.2, these virtual genomes allow finer-scale characterization of the genetic structure within each ancestral population.

3. Empirical Data on Human Population Structure

One of the earliest efforts to quantify the genetic structure of human population can be traced to a seminal paper by Richard Lewontin, in which he examined variation at 17 polymorphic human loci (including classical blood groups proteins as well as enzymes which exhibit electrophoretic variation) in individuals across classically defined races: Caucasian, African, Mongoloid, S. Asian Aborigines, Amerinds, Oceanians, Australian Aborigines (Lewontin 1972). The key finding of the paper is that 85.4% of the total genetic variation observed occurred between individuals within each group, 8.3% of genetic differences were found between populations within a race, and only 6.3% was attributed to the racial categories. This study concluded that the vast majority of genetic differences are found within populations rather than between them, thus providing no genetic basis for human racial classification. Remarkably, the apportionment of genetic variation has been reproduced in study after study using a variety of genetic data.

Another important source of knowledge in the subject can be found in the canonical book of Luigi Luca Cavalli-Sforza and colleagues, *The History and Geography of Human Genes* (Cavalli-Sforza *et al.* 1994). In addition to documenting and interpreting empirical patterns of genetic variation across 1800 indigenous populations, Cavalli-Sforza and colleagues introduced various statistical techniques to the analysis of genetic data, including the use of maximum likelihood approach for estimating the evolutionary tree and the use of PCA to elucidate major demographic events in human history. This work represents the first full-scale account of human evolution as it occurred across continents, and demonstrated, theoretically and with empirical evidence, that the genome diversity is affected both by the tree-like pattern of historical separation of populations and by spread of genes among population through migration and admixture.

Much of early studies of human population genetic structure focus on two uniparentally-transmitted loci: maternally inherited mitochondrial DNA (mtDNA) and paternally inherited Y chromosome. The lack of recombination at these loci permits haplotype-based analysis; gene trees, or genealogies, have been constructed both at a population level and at an individual level (Underhill *et al.* 2000; van Oven and Kayser 2009). In the remainder of this section, however, we will focus on recent work that analyzes autosomal variation.

3.1. *Global structure of human populations*

It is important to recognize that Lewontin's analyses (and later work that supports his finding) are based on the average F-statistics at *single* genetic loci. While it is an undeniable mathematical fact that the majority of genetic variation observed in the human population is attributed within ethnic groups, this does not mean that genetic ancestry cannot be inferred from genetic data. As we discuss in the next section, numerous studies have now demonstrated that, accumulating minute allele frequency differences across a large number of markers, the joint distribution of alleles in the genome harbors rich information regarding population structure and individual ancestry. With dense SNPs markers that are now routinely generated in GWAS, it is feasible to accurately identify individuals from populations that differ by as little as 1% in F_{ST} on average. It is also important to note that when one looks at correlations in allelic variation across loci, self-identified populations and populations inferred for human subjects using genetic data correspond closely (Edwards 2003; Rosenberg *et al.* 2002; Tang *et al.* 2005b). An epidemiologic perspective on using self-reported race and ethnicity in biomedical and genetic research is provided in (Risch *et al.* 2002).

An important resource for studying human genetic variation is the Human Genome Diversity Panel (HGDP), which consists of immortalized lymphoblastoid cell lines of over 1,000 individuals from 51 populations worldwide (Cann *et al.* 2002). Using genotype data of 377 autosomal microsatellite loci in HGDP and program STRUCTURE, (Rosenberg *et al.* 2002) demonstrated that these individuals could be assigned, with near perfect accuracy, to their continents of origin. Subsequently, high-density genotype data, consisting more than 600,000 SNPs, have also been generated for the complete HGDP cell lines (Li *et al.* 2008). Applying the EM-algorithm implemented in program, *frappe*, the SNP genotype data allows the most comprehensive characterization to date of human genetic variation at a global scale; seven clusters were detected that corresponds to major geographic divisions: Africa, Middle East, Europe, South/Central Asia, East Asia, Oceania and the America. Importantly, under an admixture model, the SNP data not only detected recently admixed populations, such as mixed European and East Asian ancestry in the Uygurs, but also provided clues for ancient relatedness between populations, such as the low level of European and Native American ancestry in the Yakuts, who clustered predominantly with the East Asians.

3.2. *The genetic structure of human populations within continents*

HGDP was established to characterize the genetic diversity at a global level. Recent studies have generated large-scale genomic data, focusing on a specific continent or geographic region within a continent. These datasets reveal aspects of demographic history, such as migration and population bottleneck, in finer detail than geneticists and anthropologists have once envisioned. A recurring theme from these analyses is that geography act as the leading driving force in shaping the pattern of genetic variation that we observe today. This section provides a brief summary of some of these studies.

Africa. Africa and African population represent the origin of all anatomically modern human, and thus play a special role in human evolutionary history. The recent out-of-Africa hypothesis, supported by genetic diversity data and fossil evidence, stipulates that modern humans arose ~200,000 years ago in sub-Saharan Africa, and dispersed throughout the globe within the past 100,000 years (Stringer 2003; White *et al.* 2003). (Tishkoff *et al.* 2009) generate a panel of 121 geographically dispersed African populations, totally over 2400 individuals; each of these individuals was typed at over 1000 STR and insertion-deletion (indels). A model-based clustering algorithm reveals fourteen subpopulation clusters, approximately corresponding to self-identified ethnicity, shared linguistic lineage and cultural practices such as hunting-and-gathering. Likewise, the leading PC separates eastern and Saharan African populations from those representing western, central and Southern Africa. Individuals with mixed ancestry are prevalent, suggesting migration between populations across the continent. The correlation between genetic diversity and geographic location of was used to locate the origin of modern human migration, based on the rationale that, as individuals migrate away from a source population, heterozygosity decays during the serial founding events (Ramachandran *et al.* 2005). This analysis maps the origin to current San homeland near the border of Namibia and Angola in southwestern Africa. The caveat of this analysis, as pointed out by the authors, is that the geographic location of a population today may not accurately reflect its location in early human history.

Asia. The world's largest and most populace continent, the patchwork-quilt linguistic and cultural diversity of Asia has long fascinated anthropologists, linguists and ethnographers. A massive effort by the Hugo Pan-Asian SNP consortium generated the most comprehensive dataset, consisting more than 1900 individuals representing 73 populations and ethnic groups genotyped for more than 50,000 autosomal SNPs (Abdulla *et al.* 2009). Genetic structure, inferred using STRUCTURE and *frappe*, tracks closely with geographic and linguistic barriers; PCA portrays a strong cline that correlates with the latitude of the population. Individuals from the same ethnic group often share similar genetic ancestry despite known gene flow between populations. Significantly, these data provide strong evidence in addressing a long-standing debate regarding the initial peopleing of Asia. Haplotype-based analyses reveal decreasing haplotype diversity along a south-north cline; 90% of haplotypes observed in East Asia are also present in either Southeast Asia or Central-South Asia. Together, these patterns of genetic variation strongly support the hypothesis that a single major wave of migration along a southern coastal route peopled the entire continent, and that Southeast Asia represents a major source of ancestors for East Asian populations.

Europe. To date, the most extensive genetic studies have focused on European populations. Population-level allele frequency data at classic genetic markers enabled Cavalli-Sforza to produce three leading PCs, which correspond to three prominent clines throughout Europe (Northwest-Southeast; East-West; Northeast-Southwest), patterns that have been reproduced in more recent studies (Menozzi *et al.* 1978). For example, analyses of the POPRES collection, consisting over half a million SNPs genotyped in more than 3000 European individuals, found that the first two PCs can be transformed such that the coordinates of these individuals mirror the geography of Europe. (Heath *et al.* 2008; Novembre *et al.* 2008).

Indigenous people of the Americas. The term Indigenous American refers to the pre-Columbian inhabitans of North and South America; in the United States, the terms "Native Americans" or "Amerindians" are also used. Current theory stipulates that the first inhabitants of the New World migrated from Siberia to the Americas via the Bering Land Bridge sometimes after 16,500 years ago (Goebel *et al.* 2008). This theory is partially supported by the HGDP analysis, which identified shared ancestry between the Indigenous American groups and Yakuts, Turkic people from Siberia (Li *et al.* 2008). Population structure in the America has been characterized using STR genotype in a panel of 422 individuals representing 24 indigenous groups sampled from North, Central and South America (Wang *et al.* 2007). Considerable population structure is detected using the model-based clustering algorithm, STRUCTURE. Furthermore, populations further away from the Bering Strait exhibits decreased level of genetic diversity and are genetically more distinct to Siberians. These observations depict a scenario, in which a single wave of migration, originated in Siberia, populated the America landmass from the northwestern tip and dispersed southward mainly along the coastal routes. As a result of multiple population bottlenecks during the expansion through the America, the Indigenous Americans have lower genetic diversity and stronger linkage disequilibrium at the genome-level compared to other populations, a phenomenon termed "serial founder effect" (Ramachandran *et al.* 2005).

Oceania. It is thought that Australia, New Guinea and Melanesia islands were settled by 40,000 years ago, soon after modern humans left Africa (Groube *et al.* 1986). Aboriginal Australian and New Guinean populations have been subject of relatively few genetic studies. Combining a sample of Aboriginal Australian and two Oceanic groups in HGDP (Papuans from New Guinea and Melanesians), (McEvoy *et al.* 2010) argue for a common ancestral population to all the three populations.

The increasingly affordable genomic technologies and the intense effort of GWAS have generated data that permit population genetic analyses focusing a specific geographic region within a continent, including Finland, India, Japan and China (Chen *et al.* 2009; Jakkula *et al.* 2008; Reich *et al.* 2009; Yamaguchi-Kabata *et al.* 2008). A common theme has emerged from these studies that demographic history gives rise to highly complex pattern of genetic structure even within a contiguous geographic region. This observation has significant implication in the design and analysis of genetic association studies, as we discuss in Section 5.

4. Recent Genetic Admixture

While geographic, linguistic and cultural barriers lead to genetic divergence between populations, migration facilitates gene flow. Recent global exploration and colonization have brought into contact individuals from different parts of the world, and tremendously increased gene flow between continents. Their offspring are admixed, whose chromosomes can be thought of as mosaics of segments derived from different ancestral (continental) populations. According to 2010 U.S. census, 28% of the US population consider themselves as having mixed ancestry. This section provides a few examples of studies that focus on characterizing genetic structure in admixed populations.

In the United States, the two largest minority groups, African Americans and Hispanics, have both experienced recent genetic admixture. The African American is largely an African group, with recent European admixture. Numerous studies, using a variety of genetic markers, have estimated an average of 10–20% of European ancestral proportions in African Americans, with some regional variation but also substantial variation among individuals (Parra *et al.* 1998; Tang *et al.* 2006b). As discussed in Section 2.4, high-density genotype data allow inference of locus-specific ancestry and thereby reconstructing ancestry blocks; furthermore, the time since admixing can be estimated based on the transition rate between ancestral states. Assuming a hybrid-isolation model, or one time mixing of ancestral populations followed by random mating, (Falush *et al.* 2003) timed the admixing events at 7–13 generations ago. Considering a more sophisticated demographical model, in which admixture occurs at a constant rate at each generation, (Zhu *et al.* 2006) estimated that admixing has occurred within the past 14 generations. These estimates are consistent with the historical records of transatlantic slave trade, which began in the 16th century.

The terms, "Hispanic" or "Latino," refers to the ethnically diverse groups of Latin America, who typically derive ancestry from Indigenous American, Caucasian and African/African American populations, with the relative proportions varying geographically and among ethnic groups. For example, the Dominican and Puerto Richans, on average, have much higher African ancestry compared to the Mexicans and Ecuadorians (Bryc *et al.* 2010b). Even within Mexico, the Native American ancestry proportions vary among States, ranging from 35% in Sonora in the North to 65% in Guerrero in center-Pacific (Silva-Zolezzi *et al.* 2009). In both African Americans and Hispanics, comparison of the ancestry proportions at the autosomal, X chromosome and uniparentally-transmitted loci (mitochondrial DNA and Y chromosome) have revealed strong evidence of sex-biased admixture (Lind *et al.* 2007; Wang *et al.* 2008).

Genetic admixture is a worldwide phenomenon. The Uyghur population living in the Xinjiang province in western China represents an admixed population in the Eurasian continent. Because of its proximity to the Silk Road, the Uyghur population derives ancestry from East Asian, European and the Middle East ancestral populations (Li *et al.* 2008). Using high-density SNP markers, a recent genetic study estimated approximately equal ancestral contributions from the European and East Asian populations to the Uyghur population (Xu *et al.* 2008).

A few recent studies have aimed to characterize the genetic structure in admixed populations at a sub-continental scale using high-density SNP genotype data. In other words, these studies seek to determine whether the Indigenous American ancestry in a Mexican individual was derived from North, Central or South America. (Johnson *et al.* 2011) developed a hierarchical approach for this purpose: an admixed genome is first partitioned into major components that reflect recent, inter-continental, migration; each of these continental components is then further investigated separately to depict intra-continental structure. In a Mexican cohort from Mexico City, the European ancestry is mapped to Southern Europe (Spaniard and Portuguese); the Indigenous American ancestry is largely attributed to the indigenous groups residing in the southwestern region of Mexico, but some individuals may have varying degrees of ancestry from Mayans of the Yucatan Peninsula, and one individual is likely to have ancestors from South America (Johnson *et al.* 2011). In contrast, analyses of high-density SNP genotype data reveal that African Americans derive their African ancestry to multiple populations from West and West-Central Africa, and it is not possible to trace the African root of an individual to a single African population (Bryc *et al.* 2010a; Zakharia *et al.* 2009). The qualitatively distinct findings in the Mexicans and African Americans are likely due to the different population histories.

5. Population Structure and Confounding in Genetic Association Studies

An accurate depiction of population structure does not only offer clues for reconstructing human evolutionary history, but also has important implications in biomedical research. In population-based genetic association studies, where the frequency of a candidate risk allele is compared between cases and controls, population structure can act as a confounder and give rise to spurious association results. This problem, referred to as population stratification, has been demonstrated in theory and with empirical data; correction for population stratification is now an indispensible element in genome-wide association analyses.

5.1. *Empirical evidence of population stratification*

Population stratification arises because population-based genetic association studies often violate a fundamental epidemiologic principle that underlies all case-control studies: the case and control groups are matched with respect to all factors except the exposures to be evaluated. However, as we explain in preceding sections, population structure leads to difference in allele distribution across the genome. Thus, if the case and control groups represent unmatched population origins, alleles that have different allele frequencies between the subpopulations will appear associated with the disease; this type of association findings do not allow identification of disease risk loci and therefore are referred to as spurious association.

An early empirical demonstration of confounding due to population stratification can be seen in a study of type 2 diabetes in the Pima and Papago tribes (Knowler *et al.* 1988). On the surface, a haplotype Gm3;5,13,14 appears to decrease diabetes risk; it turns out that this haplotype is simply a marker for European admixture: it occurs in Europeans at a frequency of 0.665 while is essentially absent in the Indigenous Americans. Hence, individuals with this Gm haplotype tend to have higher European admixture. On the other hand, the prevalence of type 2 diabetes is lower in the European populations compared to in the Indigenous American populations, and in Hispanics, disease risk is inversely associated with European ancestry proportions. This correlation may or may not be due to genetic factor. Nonetheless, in a population-based genetic association study, in which cases and controls were recruited without matching on ancestry, it is likely that the control group on average has a higher level of European admixture than the case group, and any alleles that occurs more frequently in the Europeans, such as the Gm3;5,13,14, will be over represented among the controls and appear as a protective allele. In this study, the association between the Gm haplotype and disease risk disappeared upon adjusting for the number of European-grandparents, a surrogate of genome-wide ancestry proportion.

In the past few years, genome-wide association studies (GWAS) have become a popular approach for probing the genetic architecture of complex traits. As the sample size used in GWAS increases, even subtle allele frequency difference due to population stratification may give raise to spurious association. As an example, (Price *et al.* 2006) show that adult height is associated with an allele at the LCT locus, which confers lactose persistence trait, but this association is spurious and arose because, on average, the Northern European populations are both taller and have higher frequency of lactose persistence allele compared to Southern Europeans. We next briefly discuss two approaches for correcting population stratification, which have been widely used in GWAS.

5.2. *Correction*

In epidemiology, the most straightforward way for accounting for a confounding variable is to directly model its effect. In the context of genetic association, this approach is termed "structure association test", (SAT). Under this framework, individual ancestry proportions or PCs, are incorporated in the regression model as a covariate. This approach is appealing in GWAS because IA and PC can be accurately constructed using high-density genotype data, and the computation only needs to be done once for each dataset. Based on the large number of GWAS published to date, SAT has proven effective (Redden *et al.* 2006) show, analytically, that adjusting for IA is or PC is not sufficient, and a rigorous adjustment strategy should incorporate the ancestry of the parents. This proposal has not been widely adopted, in part due to the difficulty in obtaining parental genotype data in large-scale case-control studies.

Another popular method for correcting population stratification is the genomic control (GC) approach (Devlin *et al.* 2001). For simplicity, consider the test statistic, Y, of the Armitage's trend test, which test for the association between genotype at a marker and the trait under an additive model [see GWAS chapter for details]. In the absence of population structure, the null distribution of Y has an asymptotic standard χ^2 distribution with one degree of freedom. The rationale behind GC is that, population stratification causes a inflation of the test statistics across the genome, and therefore can be modeled by $Y/\lambda \sim \chi^2$. The inflation, λ, can be estimated based on the overall empirical distribution of Y, assuming most markers do not affect the trait and are sampled from the null distribution. Specifically, GC proposes to estimate $\hat{\lambda} = \text{median}(Y_i)/0.456$, where Y_i are the observed test statistics at marker i, and 0.456 is the median of the standard χ^2 distribution with one degree of freedom. In addition to providing an adjustment procedure, GC is also used as a diagnostic criterion for detecting potential confounding. Many GWAS correct for population stratification by adjusting, as covariate, PC or ancestry proportions, and compute the inflation factors on the adjusted test statistics.

6. Concluding Remarks

For most of the world, human genome structure is shaped by the interplay between ancient geographic isolation and more recent demographic shifts, factors that are captured by the concepts of biogeographic ancestry and admixture, respectively. With the rapidly accumulating genotype and sequencing data, population genetic structure can be characterized at a finer geographic scale, and individual ancestry can be inferred at a greater genomic resolution. As we enter the era of personalized medicine, we envision knowledge of genetic structure will not only shed light on the evolutionary history of our species, but also guide us in designing effective disease prevention and intervention strategies.

References

Abdulla, M. A., I. Ahmed, A. Assawamakin, J. Bhak, S. K. Brahmachari *et al.*, 2009. Mapping human genetic diversity in Asia. *Science* **326:** 1541–1545.

Bryc, K., A. Auton, M. R. Nelson, J. R. Oksenberg, S. L. Hauser *et al.*, 2010a. Genome-wide patterns of population structure and admixture in West Africans and African Americans. *Proc Natl Acad Sci USA* **107:** 786–791.

Bryc, K., C. Velez, T. Karafet, A. Moreno-Estrada, A. Reynolds *et al.*, 2010b. Colloquium paper: genome-wide patterns of population structure and admixture among Hispanic/Latino populations. *Proc Natl Acad Sci USA* **107 Suppl 2:** 8954–8961.

Cann, H. M., C. de Toma, L. Cazes, M. F. Legrand, V. Morel *et al.*, 2002. A human genome diversity cell line panel. *Science* **296:** 261–262.

Cavalli-Sforza, L. L., P. Menozzi and A. Piazza, 1994. *The history and geography of human genes.* . Princeton University Press, Princeton, NJ.

Chen, J., H. Zheng, J. X. Bei, L. Sun, W. H. Jia *et al.*, 2009. Genetic structure of the Han Chinese population revealed by genome-wide SNP variation. *Am J Hum Genet* **85:** 775–785.

Devlin, B., K. Roeder and L. Wasserman, 2001. Genomic control, a new approach to genetic-based association studies. *Theor Popul Biol* **60:** 155–166.

Edwards, A. W., 2003. Human genetic diversity: Lewontin's fallacy. *Bioessays* **25:** 798–801.

Engelhardt, B. E., and M. Stephens, 2010. Analysis of population structure: a unifying framework and novel methods based on sparse factor analysis. *PLoS Genet* **6**.

Falush, D., M. Stephens and J. K. Pritchard, 2003. Inference of population structure using multilocus genotype data: linked loci and correlated allele frequencies. *Genetics* **164:** 1567–1587.

Glass, B., and C. C. Li, 1953. The dynamics of racial intermixture; an analysis based on the American Negro. *Am J Hum Genet* **5:** 1–20.

Goebel, T., M. R. Waters and D. H. O'Rourke, 2008. The late Pleistocene dispersal of modern humans in the Americas. *Science* **319:** 1497–1502.

Groube, L., J. Chappell, J. Muke and D. Price, 1986. A 40,000 year-old human occupation site at Huon Peninsula, Papua New Guinea. *Nature* **324:** 453–455.

Hastie, T., R. Tibshirani and J. Friedman, 2009. *The Elements of Statistical Learning: Data Mining, Inference, and Prediction.* Springer.

Heath, S. C., I. G. Gut, P. Brennan, J. D. McKay, V. Bencko *et al.*, 2008. Investigation of the fine structure of European populations with applications to disease association studies. *Eur J Hum Genet* **16:** 1413–1429.

Jakkula, E., K. Rehnstrom, T. Varilo, O. P. Pietilainen, T. Paunio *et al.*, 2008. The genome-wide patterns of variation expose significant substructure in a founder population. *Am J Hum Genet* **83:** 787–794.

Johnson, A. J., M. A. Coram, M. D. Shriver, I. Romieu, G. S. Barsh *et al.*, 2011. Ancestral Components of Admixed Genomes in a Mexican Cohort. *PLoS Genet* **7:** e1002410.

Kimura, M., 1989. The neutral theory of molecular evolution and the world view of the neutralists. *Genome* **31:** 24–31.

Knowler, W. C., R. C. Williams, D. J. Pettitt and A. G. Steinberg, 1988. Gm3;5,13,14 and type 2 diabetes mellitus: an association in American Indians with genetic admixture. *Am J Hum Genet* **43:** 520–526.

Lander, E. S., L. M. Linton, B. Birren, C. Nusbaum, M. C. Zody *et al.*, 2001. Initial sequencing and analysis of the human genome. *Nature* **409:** 860–921.

Lewontin, R. C., 1972. The apportionment of human diversity. *Evolutionary Biology* **6:** 391–398.

Li, J. Z., D. M. Absher, H. Tang, A. M. Southwick, A. M. Casto *et al.*, 2008. Worldwide human relationships inferred from genome-wide patterns of variation. *Science* **319:** 1100–1104.

Li, N., and M. Stephens, 2003. Modeling linkage disequilibrium and identifying recombination hotspots using single-nucleotide polymorphism data. *Genetics* **165:** 2213–2233.

Lind, J. M., H. B. Hutcheson-Dilks, S. M. Williams, J. H. Moore, M. Essex *et al.*, 2007. Elevated male European and female African contributions to the genomes of African American individuals. *Hum Genet* **120:** 713–722.

Mardia, K. V., J. T. Kent and J. M. Bibby, 1980. *Multivariate Analysis.* Academic Press.

McEvoy, B. P., J. M. Lind, E. T. Wang, R. K. Moyzis, P. M. Visscher *et al.*, 2010. Whole-genome genetic diversity in a sample of Australians with deep Aboriginal ancestry. *Am J Hum Genet* **87:** 297–305.

Menozzi, P., A. Piazza and L. Cavalli-Sforza, 1978. Synthetic maps of human gene frequencies in Europeans. *Science* **201:** 786–792.

Nei, M., 1977. F-statistics and analysis of gene diversity in subdivided populations. *Ann Hum Genet* **41:** 225–233.

Nielsen, R., I. Hellmann, M. Hubisz, C. Bustamante and A. G. Clark, 2007. Recent and ongoing selection in the human genome. *Nat Rev Genet* **8:** 857–868.

Novembre, J., T. Johnson, K. Bryc, Z. Kutalik, A. R. Boyko *et al.*, 2008. Genes mirror geography within Europe. *Nature* **456:** 98–101.

Parra, E. J., A. Marcini, J. Akey, J. Martinson, M. A. Batzer *et al.*, 1998. Estimating African American admixture proportions by use of population-specific alleles. *Am J Hum Genet* **63:** 1839–1851.

Pearson, K., 1901. On lines and planes of closest fit to systems of points in space. *Philosophical Magazine* **2:** 559–572.

Pickrell, J. K., G. Coop, J. Novembre, S. Kudaravalli, J. Z. Li *et al.*, 2009. Signals of recent positive selection in a worldwide sample of human populations. *Genome Res* **19:** 826–837.

Price, A. L., N. J. Patterson, R. M. Plenge, M. E. Weinblatt, N. A. Shadick *et al.*, 2006. Principal components analysis corrects for stratification in genome-wide association studies. *Nat Genet* **38:** 904–909.

Price, A. L., A. Tandon, N. Patterson, K. C. Barnes, N. Rafaels *et al.*, 2009. Sensitive detection of chromosomal segments of distinct ancestry in admixed populations. *PLoS Genet* **5:** e1000519.

Rabiner, L. R., 1989. A tutorial on hidden Markov models and selected applications in speech recognition. *Proc. IEEE* **77:** 257–286.

Ramachandran, S., O. Deshpande, C. C. Roseman, N. A. Rosenberg, M. W. Feldman *et al.*, 2005. Support from the relationship of genetic and geographic distance in human populations for a serial founder effect originating in Africa. *Proc Natl Acad Sci USA* **102:** 15942–15947.

Redden, D. T., J. Divers, L. K. Vaughan, H. K. Tiwari, T. M. Beasley *et al.*, 2006. Regional admixture mapping and structured association testing: conceptual unification and an extensible general linear model. *PLoS Genet* **2:** e137.

Reich, D., K. Thangaraj, N. Patterson, A. L. Price and L. Singh, 2009. Reconstructing Indian population history. *Nature* **461:** 489–494.

Risch, N., E. Burchard, E. Ziv and H. Tang, 2002. Categorization of humans in biomedical research: genes, race and disease. *Genome Biol* **3:** comment2007.

Rosenberg, N. A., J. K. Pritchard, J. L. Weber, H. M. Cann, K. K. Kidd *et al.*, 2002. Genetic structure of human populations. *Science* **298:** 2381–2385.

Satten, G. A., W. D. Flanders and Q. Yang, 2001. Accounting for unmeasured population substructure in case-control studies of genetic association using a novel latent-class model. *Am J Hum Genet* **68:** 466–477.

Silva-Zolezzi, I., A. Hidalgo-Miranda, J. Estrada-Gil, J. C. Fernandez-Lopez, L. Uribe-Figueroa *et al.*, 2009. Analysis of genomic diversity in Mexican Mestizo populations to develop genomic medicine in Mexico. *Proc Natl Acad Sci USA* **106:** 8611–8616.

Stringer, C., 2003. Human evolution: Out of Ethiopia. *Nature* **423:** 692-693, 695.

Sundquist, A., E. Fratkin, C. B. Do and S. Batzoglou, 2008. Effect of genetic divergence in identifying ancestral origin using HAPAA. *Genome Res* **18:** 676–682.

Tang, H., M. Coram, P. Wang, X. Zhu and N. Risch, 2006a. Reconstructing genetic ancestry blocks in admixed individuals. *Am J Hum Genet* **79:** 1–12.

Tang, H., E. Jorgenson, M. Gadde, S. L. Kardia, D. C. Rao *et al.*, 2006b. Racial admixture and its impact on BMI and blood pressure in African and Mexican Americans. *Hum Genet* **119:** 624–633.

Tang, H., J. Peng, P. Wang and N. J. Risch, 2005a. Estimation of individual admixture: analytical and study design considerations. *Genet Epidemiol* **28:** 289–301.

Tang, H., T. Quertermous, B. Rodriguez, S. L. Kardia, X. Zhu *et al.*, 2005b. Genetic structure, self-identified race/ethnicity, and confounding in case-control association studies. *Am J Hum Genet* **76:** 268–275.

Tishkoff, S. A., F. A. Reed, F. R. Friedlaender, C. Ehret, A. Ranciaro *et al.*, 2009. The genetic structure and history of Africans and African Americans. *Science* **324:** 1035–1044.

Underhill, P. A., P. Shen, A. A. Lin, L. Jin, G. Passarino *et al.*, 2000. Y chromosome sequence variation and the history of human populations. *Nat Genet* **26:** 358–361.

van Oven, M., and M. Kayser, 2009. Updated comprehensive phylogenetic tree of global human mitochondrial DNA variation. *Hum Mutat* **30:** E386–394.

Venter, J. C., M. D. Adams, E. W. Myers, P. W. Li, R. J. Mural *et al.*, 2001. The sequence of the human genome. *Science* **291:** 1304–1351.

Wahlund, S., 1928. Zusammensetzung von Population und Korrelationserscheinung vom Standpunkt der Vererbungslehre aus betrachtet. *Hereditas* **11:** 65–106.

Wang, S., C. M. Lewis, M. Jakobsson, S. Ramachandran, N. Ray *et al.*, 2007. Genetic variation and population structure in native Americans. *PLoS Genet* **3:** e185.

Wang, S., N. Ray, W. Rojas, M. V. Parra, G. Bedoya *et al.*, 2008. Geographic patterns of genome admixture in Latin American Mestizos. *PLoS Genet* **4:** e1000037.

Weir, B. S., and C. C. Cockerham, 1984. Estimating F-statistics for the analysis of population structure. *Evolution* **38:** 1358–1370.

Wellcome Trust Case Control Consortium, 2007. Genome-wide association study of 14,000 cases of seven common diseases and 3,000 shared controls. *Nature* **447:** 661–678.

White, T. D., B. Asfaw, D. DeGusta, H. Gilbert, G. D. Richards *et al.*, 2003. Pleistocene Homo sapiens from Middle Awash, Ethiopia. *Nature* **423:** 742–747.

Wright, S., 1921. Systems of mating. *Genetics* **6:** 111–178.

Xu, S., W. Huang, J. Qian and L. Jin, 2008. Analysis of genomic admixture in Uyghur and its implication in mapping strategy. *Am J Hum Genet* **82:** 883–894.

Yamaguchi-Kabata, Y., K. Nakazono, A. Takahashi, S. Saito, N. Hosono *et al.*, 2008. Japanese population structure, based on SNP genotypes from 7003 individuals compared to other ethnic groups: effects on population-based association studies. *Am J Hum Genet* **83:** 445–456.

Zakharia, F., A. Basu, D. Absher, T. L. Assimes, A. S. Go *et al.*, 2009. Characterizing the admixed African ancestry of African Americans. *Genome Biol* **10:** R141.

Zhu, X., S. Zhang, H. Tang and R. Cooper, 2006. A classical likelihood based approach for admixture mapping using EM algorithm. *Hum Genet* **120:** 431–445.

Zhu, X., S. Zhang, H. Zhao and R. S. Cooper, 2002. Association mapping, using a mixture model for complex traits. *Genet Epidemiol* **23:** 181–196.

About the Authors

Hua Tang, Ph.D., is Associate Professor in the Department of Genetics at Stanford University School of Medicine. She is also an Associate Professor, by courtesy, of the Statistics Department at Stanford, a member of the Stanford Cancer Center and the Bio-X program. Previously she was a faculty at the Public Health Sciences Division at the Fred Hutchinson Cancer Research Center in Seattle. Dr. Tang received her PhD in Statistics (with a minor in Genetics) from Stanford University. Research in her laboratory develops and applies statistical methods for analyzing patterns of human genetic variation, which underlie the phenotypic diversity in humans. Her group has collaborated on various genome-wide studies focusing on stratified or recently admixed populations. These studies offer unique opportunities to elucidate the evolutionary forces that have shaped the patterns of genetic variation in humans, to uncover the genetic basis of complex traits, and to shed light on the mechanisms that lead to diverse phenotypes and disparate disease risks among populations.

Kun Tang, PhD is Principle Investigator, Department of Computational Genomics, CAS-MPG Partner Institute of Computational Biology, Shanghai Institute of Biological Sciences, Chinese Academy of Science. He earned his PhD in Biochemistry from National University of Singapore in 2004. Then he did his postdoc work (2004–2007) in Max Planck Institute for Evolutionary Anthropology in Leipzig, Germany, where he mainly focused on the Population Genetic studies of Natural Selection. Currently his research interests include fine characterization of natural selection in human genome and the quantitative study of morphological variation in human face and the underlying evolution and genetic basis.

CHAPTER 26

DATA INTEGRATION METHODS IN GENOME WIDE ASSOCIATION STUDIES

NING SUN and HONGYU ZHAO*

Department of Biostatistics,
Yale School of Public Health, PO Box 208034
60 College Street, New Haven, CT 06520-8034, USA
*hongyu.zhao@yale.edu

Hundreds of genes have been implicated in various human diseases through genome wide association studies (GWAS). A typical GWAS collects genotype information at up to millions of genetic markers in thousands of individuals. Because of the large number of markers being studied, a very stringent threshold, e.g. p-value less than 5×10^{-8}, is commonly adopted to control the overall false positive results. As a result, there is adequate statistical power only to detect genetic variants with relatively large effects or in studies with very large sample sizes. Many methods have been proposed to improve statistical power to detect association signals through the incorporation of prior biological knowledge and/or other data sets. In this chapter, we discuss the types of data and/or prior knowledge that have been considered in GWAS analysis and review statistical methods that have been proposed for integrated analysis.

1. Introduction

Since the landmark paper by Hoh and colleagues (Klein et al. 2005) on the identification of Complement Factor H gene for age-related macular degeneration, genome wide association studies (GWAS) have identified hundreds of genomic loci associated with many human traits and diseases. The results have been annotated and accessible at various web sites, e.g. the catalogue maintained by the National Human Genome Research Institute (http://www.genome.gov/gwastudies/) and GWASdb (Li *et al.* 2012). Many more will likely be discovered in the near future with studies of tens of thousands of subjects through collaborations among research groups, the adoptions of more advanced platforms (e.g. next generation sequencing), and improved statistical and computational methods.

Because up to millions of markers, mostly single nucleotide polymorphisms (SNPs), are analyzed in GWAS, a stringent threshold for statistical significance is needed to control false positive results in a genome scan. For example, when 100,000 SNPs are analyzed, only markers attaining a statistical significance level of 5×10^{-7} would be considered significant using Bonferonni correction if the goal is to control the family-wise false positive rate at 0.05. If we use a normal approximation for the test statistic, this level of statistical significance for a two-sided test corresponds to an observed statistic with an absolute value of 5.03 or higher. Now consider a case-control study with N cases and N controls. For a SNP associated with disease, let A denote the risk allele, a denote the normal allele, and p and q denote the allele frequency of the risk allele A in the cases and controls, respectively. Assuming that the two chromosomes in an individual are independent, i.e. each chromosome has a chance of p or q carrying allele A for a case or control individual, respectively. Note that this assumption holds under a multiplicative disease model, where the two alleles have independent effects on the disease outcome. Under this assumption, the problem of inferring whether there is an association between this SNP and disease is equivalent to a binomial testing problem where the sample size is 2N for both cases and controls, and the p and q represent the success probabilities in these two populations. For example, when the allele frequencies in the cases and controls are 0.55 and 0.5, respectively, N has to be around 3500. This scenario corresponds to a relative risk of about 1.1. When the respective allele frequencies are 0.525 and 0.5, which corresponds to about a relative risk of 1.05, N has to be around 13800. Note that many of the SNPs identified from GWAS have an estimated odds ratio of between 1.05 and 1.1. Realizing the need for very large sample sizes to detect SNPs, many large international consortia have been formed for common diseases to increase the sample size to meet the rigorous demand for statistical significance.

Although only those markers with highly statistically significant SNPs are typically reported in published papers, there is in general an enrichment of markers with small p-values for some studies. It is possible that some of the SNPs with marginal statistical significance, although do not meet the genome wide statistical significance criterion, may represent true signals. In a GWAS for schizophrenia and bipolar disorder, Purcell and colleagues could not identify any marker passing genome wide statistical significance level (Purcell *et al.* 2009). However, when a risk score was derived from one subset of the data, it was indeed correlated with the disease status in an independent cohort, although the correlation was very low. The authors explored various genetics models that could explain the lack of significant findings for single markers yet global overall enrichment for signals, and argued for the presence of hundreds of disease associated SNPs, each with weak effect on disease risk. Given the potential signals in the data, a pressing question is that whether there is any approach to separating them from the noises when up to millions of markers are analyzed.

One area that has received considerable attention to address this challenge is the incorporation of prior knowledge and/or other data in the analysis of GWAS. Our focus in this chapter is on the integration of data types of different nature, instead of meta-analysis of multiple data sets, although it may be considered one type of data integration (Cantor *et al.* 2010). In addition, we focus on the analysis of common SNPs as they are the focus of array-based GWAS analysis. The rest of the chapter is organized as follow. We first review different types of information that has been considered in the literature to facilitate GWAS analysis. We then discuss the basic ideas of various methods introduced in the literature for data integration. The chapter is concluded with discussion on the possible directions for future developments.

2. Different Data Types that can be Incorporated in GWAS Analysis

2.1. *SNP annotations*

With concerted efforts from the community, substantial annotation information has been collected on SNPs, including general genomic features (e.g. physical location in the genome, whether a SNP is in a coding region, splice junction region), population genetics features (e.g. minor allele frequencies in different populations, linkage disequilibrium patterns with other markers, any evidence for natural selection), evolution information (e.g. sequence conservation across different species), and other functional genomics information (e.g. eQTL results). (Cline and Karchin 2011) offered a comprehensive review of the principles and limitations of SNV annotations in the literature. Many computational tools are commonly used. For example, PolyPhen (Adzhubei *et al.* 2010) is often used to predict whether a missense mutation is damaging. More recent efforts for coding variant annotations include those for the loss of function variants, e.g. (MacArthur *et al.* 2012). As for non-coding variants, RegulomeDB (Boyle *et al.* 2012) includes annotations of variants in non-coding regions that includes high-throughput data from ENCODE (Dunham *et al.* 2012) and other data. The regulations information for the regulation of microRNAs and their targets has also been considered in the literature, e.g. (Bulik-Sullivan *et al.* 2013). (Ward and Kellis 2012) reviewed various mechanisms that noncoding variants can influence human diseases. In the context of GWAS and next generation sequencing data analysis, ANNOVAR (Wang *et al.* 2010b), which compiles annotation information from many sources, is often used to infer the functional relevance of candidate SNPs. A comprehensive list of protein-sequence-based and nucleotide-sequence-based annotation tools can be found in the review article by (Cooper and Shendure 2011).

It is conceivable that a coding variant in a gene can disrupt the function of the protein that this gene encodes, therefore affecting relevant biological processes and disease risk. As for the relevance of non-coding variants in GWAS, (Maurano *et al.* 2012) demonstrated that the GWAS hits in non-coding regions are enriched for deoxyribonuclease I (DNase I) hypersensitive sites. (Kindt *et al.* 2013) carried out a comprehensive analysis of enrichment for three annotation categories from GWAS, including genic and regulatory features, conservation and evolutionary signatures, and chromatin states. They found that SNPs annotated with all of the enriched annotations were eight times more likely to be trait associated than those SNPs with none of the annotations. In a similar study by (Knight *et al.* 2011), the authors suggested using a Bayes Factor of 4 for cis eQTL SNPs within regions of open chromatin, 3 for non-synonymous SNPs and 2 for promoter SNPs to improve statistical power to identify disease related SNPs. All these results suggest the potential benefit of incorporating SNP annotations in GWAS analysis. For example, for SNPs with marginal evidence of trait associations that are annotated as "damaging" or "regulatory" regions, they should be given higher priority in follow-up studies those without any functional annotations.

2.2. *Gene and pathway annotations*

In addition to the annotations at the individual levels, SNPs can be organized into genes, which can then be organized into pathways. There are many pathway databases available, e.g. KEGG (http://www.genome.jp/kegg/), BioCarta (http://www.biocarta.com/), and Reactome (www.reactome.org/). Multiple SNPs in a gene may be functionally relevant to a disease outcome. Therefore, joint analysis of all the SNPs in a gene region may prove more powerful than separate analysis of these SNPs. We note that a major focus of rare variant analysis is joint analysis of all the variants identified in a candidate region. Beyond single gene analysis, it is also likely that multiple genes in the same pathway are involved in disease etiology. In the case that each gene only carries small to moderate effects, cumulative evidence from multiple genes in a pathway may be more easily identified as pathway-based analysis involves many fewer analysis units and the penalty for multiple comparisons is less versus SNP or gene based analysis. In addition to treating pathways as a collection of genes, the topological information may also offer additional information in GWAS analysis.

2.3. *Protein interaction*

Protein interactions play key roles in biological functions, especially signaling networks. Various high-throughput technologies and integrated methods have been developed to generate interacting proteins and protein complexes. We can consider each protein complex as a gene set in GWAS analysis. In addition, a protein interaction network may be built from interacting proteins and it is possible that some subnets may be enriched for signals for disease associations due to their related biological roles. Many databases on protein interactions are available, e.g. BIND (Bader *et al.* 2003), BioGRID (Chatr-Aryamontri *et al.* 2013), and HPRD (Peri *et al.* 2004).

2.4. *Functional genomics data*

Genome wide expression data in a sample offer a snapshot of the molecular state of the sample, and such data can also reveal heterogeneity among the samples. In addition, co-expression networks can be constructed through the profiles of many individuals. Genes close to each other in this network have similar expression patterns, and possibly similar biological functions. Therefore, some subnets may be enriched for GWAS signals. (Voineagu *et al.* 2011) found that gene expression modules, i.e. a set of genes with highly coordinated expression profiles, associated with autism are enriched for GWAS signals. In addition to considering a static network across all the samples, separate networks may be constructed from normal and disease individuals and the perturbed section of the overall network may be enriched for GWAS signals (Lin, Cho, and Zhao, unpublished results).

When both expression and SNP data are available from the same set of subjects, it is possible to identify SNPs associated with expression traits. These SNPs, called eQTLs, mark the genomic locations (loci) that are associated with expression levels. Now consider two SNPs with similar statistical evidence of association from a GWAS study. If a SNP is associated with one or more transcripts, whereas the other SNP is not associated with any transcript, and the transcripts examined are from the relevant tissue associated with disease, the first SNP may be more likely associated the disease given the eQTL information. (Mehta *et al.* 2013) showed that the eQTLs identified from whole blood are highly robust and reproducible across studies. Using a GWAS of bone mineral density, (Grundberg *et al.* 2009) showed that the top GWAS signals were more enriched for cis-eQTLs identified from primary human osteoblasts than those from lymphoblastoid cell lines, suggesting the tissue relevance in eQTL data. Examining GWAS hits across different diseases, (Nicolae *et al.* 2010) found that they are enriched for about 1.5 folds among eQTLs from lymphoblastoid cell lines. Many data sets have been collected for eQTL studies and public resources are available for the annotations of eQTLs, e.g. (Gamazon *et al.* 2010).

2.5. *Other information*

Integrating data of distinct nature, many functional networks have been built by researchers, e.g. the HumanNet (Lee *et al.* 2011), functional linkage network (Linghu *et al.* 2009). These networks have proven useful for gene prioritizations. For many diseases, some genes are known to affect disease risk. In this setting, the knowledge of known disease genes may help better prioritize a new set of candidate genes that emerge from a GWAS, e.g. those with the most statistical significant evidence of associations. Endeavour was developed by (Aerts *et al.* 2006) to rank the candidate genes based on their similarities with known genes using multiple heterogeneous data sources, including literature, functional annotation, microarray expression, EST expression, protein domains, protein-protein interactions, pathway membership, cis-regulatory modules, transcriptional motifs, sequence similarity, and other data sources. The authors called their method "genomic data fusion". In the same spirit, (De Bie *et al.* 2007) introduced kernel-based methods for data fusion to prioritize candidate genes.

3. Statistical Methods to Incorporate Different Data Types

3.1. *SNP annotations*

In the simplest set-up, the SNPs can be annotated into two classes, those likely to be involved in disease etiology and those not based prior knowledge. For example, we can group SNPs into those falling into published linkage regions and those not in these regions. In this context, (Roeder *et al.* 2006) proposed to assign higher weights to the observed statistical significance levels for markers within prior linkage peak regions and showed that this approach may improve statistical power to identify SNPs associated with disease where the overall false positive rates can be appropriately controlled. Although recent results suggest that there is a lack of agreement between results from linkage studies and association studies (Kitsios and Zintzaras 2009), the general approach can be adopted with other annotations of the SNPs, e.g. coding versus non-coding regions. In addition to this weighted method, (Lin and Lee 2012) considered another strategy, called prioritized subset analysis. For a list of candidate SNPs, a simple scoring scheme was proposed in (Saccone *et al.* 2008) to rank them based on a weighted linear score from the SNP annotations where each annotation category was assigned a corresponding weight.

In a regression setting, (Chen and Witte 2007) proposed a hierarchical model to analyze GWAS data where the first stage model is a regular regression model $y = \mu_m + x_m\beta_m$, where y is a vector of size N of the phenotypes for the study subjects, x_m is a vector of their coded genotypes for the mth marker, β_m is the regression coefficient, and μ_m is the intercept. The second stage model regresses the β_m for all the M markers against a set of K different types of annotations that characterize the properties of the m markers (e.g. whether the marker is in the coding region, synonymous coding variation), $\beta = Z\pi + U$, where Z is an $M \times K$ matrix and U is the error term. A similar model was studied by (Heron *et al.* 2011) for binary traits. In the same spirit, (Lewinger *et al.* 2007) proposed an empirical Bayes approach to incorporating prior information, where the test statistics across all the markers are assumed to follow a mixture distribution, where one mixture component corresponds to the markers not associated with disease, and the other component corresponds to those associated with the disease. The parameter that defines the likelihood of association is a function of the annotations of each marker, and the parameter that quantifies the degree of association may also be modeled as a function of the annotations for a marker. A full Bayesian version of this modeling approach was proposed in (Fridley *et al.* 2010) and (Fridley *et al.* 2011).

3.2. *Gene-based analysis*

Because genes are the natural units for analysis, we can collect all the SNPs in or around a gene and investigate whether there is any statistical evidence for association between the trait of interest and this gene. The intuition is that when more than one SNP is associated with disease, which is likely the case, joint analysis of all the SNPs in a gene can improve statistical power through information borrowing across the SNPs. In (Wang *et al.* 2007), all SNPs in a genic region are analyzed individually and the one showing the most significant evidence of association is used as representing the gene-level association. However, this approach may be biased in favor of genes with many SNPs on the arrays because, just by chance, a gene with many SNPs is more likely to have one SNP with some significant p-values than a gene represented by fewer SNPs. In (Ballard *et al.* 2010b), the authors compared a number of methods that jointly analyze multiple markers within a gene and disease outcome. It was found that the principal component analysis (PCA) based analysis had an overall good performance in assessing associations between disease and a candidate region. The PCA proceeds by first deriving the principal components of the genotype matrix where each entry in the matrix is the coded genotype of one marker for one individual. One simple way to code is the number of minor alleles (i.e. the allele with its frequency less than 0.5), so the possible values in this matrix are 0, 1, or 2. After the principal components for all the individuals are derived, a (logistic) regression analysis is performed between disease outcome and the first several principal components, where the null hypothesis to be tested is that there is no association between disease and any one of the principal components. As for the number of principal components to be used, the paper considered selecting those that in combination accounting for 85% or more of the total genetic variation. Both simulations and real data analyses suggested the relatively good performance of this approach. One potential limitation of the PCA-based analysis is that only marker information is used and phenotype-genotype correlations are only considered after the PCAs are constructed. It may be more statistically efficient to consider joint marker information in their associations with phenotypes. (Chun *et al.* 2011) proposed to use sparse partial least squares to investigate whether there is association between disease status and all the markers from a gene.

When there are many, e.g. hundreds of, markers in a gene, the methods considered in (Ballard *et al.* 2010b) may not be optimal. (Huang *et al.* 2011) proposed a Bayesian method for model selection and association analysis that is computationally efficient and statistically powerful. (Bacanu 2012) compared the performance of a number of recently developed methods that can more effectively analyze dozens or hundreds of markers in a gene, including VEGAS (Liu *et al.* 2010) and GATES (Li *et al.* 2011), that only require marginal p-values without access to individual genotype data. For example, with m SNPs in a gene region and ranked p-values denoted by $p_{(1)}, p_{(2)}, \ldots, p_{(m)}$, the GATES approach calculates the p-value as $p_G = \min(m_e p_{(j)}/m_{(ej)})$, where m_e is the effective number of independent p-values among the m SNPS, and $m_{(ej)}$ is the effective number of independent p-values among the top j SNPs. Based on the evaluations, (Bacanu 2012) advocated a two-stage procedure where a computationally fast procedure is used to identify interesting regions followed with more refined methods for gene-based analysis.

3.3. *Pathways*

In (Dinu *et al.* 2007), the authors conducted a pathway-based analysis for age-related macular degeneration (AMD) that focused on the complement pathway because the initial GWAS result (Klein *et al.* 2005) suggested the involvement of this pathway in AMD. It was found that there were multiple genes in this pathway showing marginal evidence of association and the whole pathway was enriched for marginal hits. Furthermore, these marginally significant genes corresponded well with the linkage peaks reported in a previous linkage study. For Crohn's disease, dozens of genes have been found to be associated and they belong to a number of pathways. As shown in (Ballard *et al.* 2010a), many pathways are enriched for genes having marginal evidence of association from GWAS. As for height, hundreds of genes have been found related to height from the analysis of hundreds of thousands of individuals. The identified genes fall into a number of plausible pathways (Lango Allen *et al.* 2010). (Wang *et al.* 2007) adapted the gene set enrichment analysis method for gene expression data to GWAS data (Shahbaba *et al.* 2012) proposed a hierarchical Bayesian model to aggregate information from multiple genes in a pathway and rank the pathways based on the posterior distributions of the variance term that is used to characterize the range of the gene-level evidence of association (Wang *et al.* 2011) developed a similar approach to aggregating information from multiple genes in a pathway (Zhang *et al.* 2011) studied how domains are associated with different diseases (Gui *et al.* 2011) compared the performance of seven pathway-based association tests and concluded that those based on raw data-based methods (Wang *et al.* 2010a) reviewed key data sources and approaches for pathway-based GWAS analysis. Another comprehensive review was offered by (Cantor *et al.* 2010). In a more recent review, (Fridley and Patch 2011) discussed the strengths and limitations of different gene set analysis of GWAS data.

3.4. *Topology-based analysis*

One limitation of the methods discussed in the last section is that they treat pathway genes as a collection of entities although much information is available on the relationships among them. It is no surprise that many methods have been proposed to capitalize on the pathway structure, also commonly called topology, information in inference. When a set of seed genes (i.e. genes known to be associated with disease) are available, three types of information can be used to prioritize candidate genes: network connectivity, information flow, and topological similarity (Erten *et al.* 2011). The network connectivity principle is to prioritize genes that have more connections with known genes. Because network connectivity is not able to fully utilize the network information as indirect connections may also be relevant, methods based on information flow consider pathways connecting candidate genes to seed genes. Methods based on topological similarity are motivated by the observation that genes that interact with other genes with similar functions also tend to have similar functions.

Protein-protein interaction (PPI) networks have been extensively explored for gene prioritizations. A PPI network can be represented as an unweighted, undirected graph where the nodes correspond to genes and edges represent interacting proteins. When some genes/proteins are known to be associated with a disease, the relative importance of a set of candidate genes can be evaluated based on their topographical relationships with known genes in this network. (Chen *et al.* 2009a) adopted three algorithms in (White and Smyth 2003) that were designed to rank web pages. One of these three algorithms, the K-step Markov method, was also included in the ToppGene Suite for using protein interaction data to prioritize candidate genes (Chen *et al.* 2009b). Seven methods using PPI information for gene prioritization were compared in (Navlakha and Kingsford 2010) and the authors suggested that the combination of these methods could achieve better performance overall. More recently, (Guney and Oliva 2012) proposed to include the node properties in the constructions of the scores so that nodes known to be associated with disease are given higher scores. When no genes are known to be associated with disease, (Jia *et al.* 2010) proposed to identify dense modules in a PPI network that is enriched for GWAS signals. In this case, randomizations can be used to derive an appropriate statistical significance level.

As for pathway-based analysis utilizing topology information, (Chen *et al.* 2011) found that genes with marginal evidence of association were likely to be neighbors. Based on this observation, (Chen *et al.* 2011) proposed a Markov random field (MRF) model to incorporate topological information in a pathway to increase statistical power to identify disease associated genes from GWAS data. This MRF approach takes GWAS results as input and does not rely on a set of genes known to be associated with disease in the inference.

3.5. *eQTL*

With the idea that genes differentially expressed between cases and controls are likely to be involved in disease, (Xiong *et al.* 2012) proposed to use a combined score from differential expression and gene-based association to rank genes in their relevance for a trait. Nicolae and colleagues observed the eQTLs are enriched for small p-values (Zhong *et al.* 2010) investigated the use of eQTL information to identify pathways relevant to a disease. In their analyses for each gene in a candidate pathway, the GWAS signals for the eQTL SNPs are aggregated and they found 16 (out of 110) pathways were enriched for signals.

3.6. *Combining multiple diseases*

It is likely that the same set of genes may underlie the diseases sharing common characteristics. Even before GWAS era, phenotype similarities were used to cluster diseases and identify genes for a query disease (Freudenberg and Propping 2002). For example, many genes have been found to be associated with multiple autoimmune disorders (Lettre and Rioux 2008), (Frazer *et al.* 2009). Shared genetic basis and heterogeneity across diseases were studied by (Arnold *et al.* 2012). CIPHER developed in (Wu *et al.* 2008) was based on a phenotype network, a gene interaction network, and connections between the two networks.

4. Discussion

As clearly illustrated above, the idea of incorporating prior biological knowledge and different data types has led to developments of many statistical methods in recent years. The primary goal of these approaches has been to better identify genes associated with a phenotype. With an ever increasing sample size, better phenotyping, and refined statistical methods, dozens and, more likely, hundreds of genes will be found to be associated with any specific common disease. With many signals at hands, the focus of data integration methods will be shifting from gene prioritization to a better understanding disease mechanism and heterogeneity. For example, for the dozens of genes associated with Crohn's disease, they fall into a number of distinct pathways. Joint analysis of gene expression data, pathway data, and SNP data from patients may reveal the specific pathways perturbed in a given patient through transcriptome analysis. It is critical to establish a comprehensive statistical framework to facilitate such analysis.

Acknowledgments

Supported in part by NIH grant R01 GM59507.

References

Adzhubei, I. A., S. Schmidt, L. Peshkin, V. E. Ramensky, A. Gerasimova *et al.*, 2010. A method and server for predicting damaging missense mutations. *Nat Methods* **7:** 248–249.

Aerts, S., D. Lambrechts, S. Maity, P. Van Loo, B. Coessens *et al.*, 2006. Gene prioritization through genomic data fusion. *Nat Biotechnol* **24:** 537–544.

Arnold, M., M. L. Hartsperger, H. Baurecht, E. Rodriguez, B. Wachinger *et al.*, 2012. Network-based SNP meta-analysis identifies joint and disjoint genetic features across common human diseases. *BMC Genomics* **13:** 490.

Bacanu, S. A., 2012. On optimal gene-based analysis of genome scans. *Genet Epidemiol* **36:** 333–339.

Bader, G. D., D. Betel and C. W. Hogue, 2003. BIND: the Biomolecular Interaction Network Database. *Nucleic Acids Research* **31:** 248–250.

Ballard, D., C. Abraham, J. Cho and H. Zhao, 2010a. Pathway analysis comparison using Crohn's disease genome wide association studies. *BMC Med Genomics* **3:** 25.

Ballard, D. H., J. Cho and H. Zhao, 2010b. Comparisons of multi-marker association methods to detect association between a candidate region and disease. *Genet Epidemiol* **34:** 201–212.

Boyle, A. P., E. L. Hong, M. Hariharan, Y. Cheng, M. A. Schaub *et al.*, 2012. Annotation of functional variation in personal genomes using RegulomeDB. *Genome Res* **22:** 1790–1797.

Bulik-Sullivan, B., S. Selitsky and P. Sethupathy, 2013. Prioritization of genetic variants in the microRNA regulome as functional candidates in genome wide association studies. *Hum Mutat.* **34:** 1049–1056.

Cantor, R. M., K. Lange and J. S. Sinsheimer, 2010. Prioritizing GWAS Results: A Review of Statistical Methods and Recommendations for Their Application. *The American Journal of Human Genetics* **86:** 6–22.

Chatr-Aryamontri, A., B. J. Breitkreutz, S. Heinicke, L. Boucher, A. Winter *et al.*, 2013. The BioGRID interaction database: 2013 update. *Nucleic Acids Research* **41:** D816–823.

Chen, G. K., and J. S. Witte, 2007. Enriching the Analysis of Genomewide Association Studies with Hierarchical Modeling. *The American Journal of Human Genetics* **81:** 397–404.

Chen, J., B. J. Aronow and A. G. Jegga, 2009a. Disease candidate gene identification and prioritization using protein interaction networks. *BMC Bioinformatics* **10:** 73.

Chen, J., E. E. Bardes, B. J. Aronow and A. G. Jegga, 2009b. ToppGene Suite for gene list enrichment analysis and candidate gene prioritization. *Nucleic Acids Res* **37:** W305–311.

Chen, M., J. Cho and H. Zhao, 2011. Incorporating biological pathways via a Markov random field model in genome-wide association studies. *PLoS Genet* **7:** e1001353.

Chun, H., D. H. Ballard, J. Cho and H. Zhao, 2011. Identification of association between disease and multiple markers via sparse partial least-squares regression. *Genetic Epidemiology* **35:** 479–486.

Cline, M. S., and R. Karchin, 2011. Using bioinformatics to predict the functional impact of SNVs. *Bioinformatics* **27:** 441–448.

Cooper, G. M., and J. Shendure, 2011. Needles in stacks of needles: finding disease-causal variants in a wealth of genomic data. *Nat Rev Genet* **12:** 628–640.

De Bie, T., L. C. Tranchevent, L. M. van Oeffelen and Y. Moreau, 2007. Kernel-based data fusion for gene prioritization. *Bioinformatics* **23:** i125–132.

Dinu, V., P. L. Miller and H. Zhao, 2007. Evidence for association between multiple complement pathway genes and AMD. *Genetic Epidemiology* **31:** 224–237.

Dunham, I., A. Kundaje, S. F. Aldred, P. J. Collins, C. A. Davis *et al.*, 2012. An integrated encyclopedia of DNA elements in the human genome. *Nature* **489:** 57–74.

Erten, S., G. Bebek and M. Koyutürk, 2011. Vavien: An Algorithm for Prioritizing Candidate Disease Genes Based on Topological Similarity of Proteins in Interaction Networks. *Journal of Computational Biology* **18:** 1561–1574.

Frazer, K. A., S. S. Murray, N. J. Schork and E. J. Topol, 2009. Human genetic variation and its contribution to complex traits. *Nature reviews. Genetics* **10:** 241–251.

Freudenberg, J., and P. Propping, 2002. A similarity-based method for genome-wide prediction of disease-relevant human genes. *Bioinformatics* **18 Suppl 2:** S110–115.

Fridley, B. L., E. Iversen, Y. Y. Tsai, G. D. Jenkins, E. L. Goode *et al.*, 2011. A latent model for prioritization of SNPs for functional studies. *PLoS ONE* **6:** e20764.

Fridley, B. L., and C. Patch, 2011. Gene set analysis of SNP data: benefits, challenges, and future directions. *European Journal of Human Genetics* **19:** 837–843.

Fridley, B. L., D. Serie, G. Jenkins, K. White, W. Bamlet *et al.*, 2010. Bayesian Mixture Models for the Incorporation of Prior Knowledge to Inform Genetic Association Studies. *Genetic Epidemiology* **34:** 418–426.

Gamazon, E. R., W. Zhang, A. Konkashbaev, S. Duan, E. O. Kistner *et al.*, 2010. SCAN: SNP and copy number annotation. *Bioinformatics* **26:** 259–262.

Grundberg, E., T. Kwan, B. Ge, K. C. Lam, V. Koka *et al.*, 2009. Population genomics in a disease targeted primary cell model. *Genome Res* **19:** 1942–1952.

Gui, H., M. Li, P. C. Sham and S. S. Cherny, 2011. Comparisons of seven algorithms for pathway analysis using the WTCCC Crohn's Disease dataset. *BMC Res Notes* **4:** 386.

Guney, E., and B. Oliva, 2012. Exploiting protein-protein interaction networks for genome-wide disease-gene prioritization. *PLoS ONE* **7:** e43557.

Heron, E. A., C. O'Dushlaine, R. Segurado, L. Gallagher and M. Gill, 2011. Exploration of empirical Bayes hierarchical modeling for the analysis of genome-wide association study data. *Biostatistics* **12:** 445–461.

Huang, H., P. Chanda, A. Alonso, J. S. Bader and D. E. Arking, 2011. Gene-based tests of association. *PLoS Genet* **7:** e1002177.

Jia, P., S. Zheng, J. Long, W. Zheng and Z. Zhao, 2010. dmGWAS: dense module searching for genome-wide association studies in protein-protein interaction networks. *Bioinformatics* **27:** 95–102.

Kindt, A. S., P. Navarro, C. A. Semple and C. S. Haley, 2013. The genomic signature of trait-associated variants. *BMC Genomics* **14:** 108.

Kitsios, G. D., and E. Zintzaras, 2009. Genomic convergence of genome-wide investigations for complex traits. *Ann Hum Genet* **73:** 514–519.

Klein, R. J., C. Zeiss, E. Y. Chew, J. Y. Tsai, R. S. Sackler *et al.*, 2005. Complement factor H polymorphism in age-related macular degeneration. *Science* **308:** 385–389.

Knight, J., M. R. Barnes, G. Breen and M. E. Weale, 2011. Using Functional Annotation for the Empirical Determination of Bayes Factors for Genome-Wide Association Study Analysis. *PLoS ONE* **6:** e14808.

Lango Allen, H., K. Estrada, G. Lettre, S. I. Berndt, M. N. Weedon *et al.*, 2010. Hundreds of variants clustered in genomic loci and biological pathways affect human height. *Nature* **467:** 832–838.

Lee, I., U. M. Blom, P. I. Wang, J. E. Shim and E. M. Marcotte, 2011. Prioritizing candidate disease genes by network-based boosting of genome-wide association data. *Genome Research* **21:** 1109–1121.

Lettre, G., and J. D. Rioux, 2008. Autoimmune diseases: insights from genome-wide association studies. *Hum Mol Genet* **17:** R116–121.

Lewinger, J. P., D. V. Conti, J. W. Baurley, T. J. Triche and D. C. Thomas, 2007. Hierarchical Bayes prioritization of marker associations from a genome-wide association scan for further investigation. *Genetic Epidemiology* **31:** 871–882.

Li, M.-X., H.-S. Gui, J. S. H. Kwan and P. C. Sham, 2011. GATES: A Rapid and Powerful Gene-Based Association Test Using Extended Simes Procedure. *American Journal of Human Genetics* **88:** 283–293.

Li, M. J., P. Wang, X. Liu, E. L. Lim, Z. Wang *et al.*, 2012. GWASdb: a database for human genetic variants identified by genome-wide association studies. *Nucleic Acids Research* **40:** D1047-D1054.

Lin, W. Y., and W. C. Lee, 2012. Improving power of genome-wide association studies with weighted false discovery rate control and prioritized subset analysis. *PLoS ONE* **7:** e33716.

Linghu, B., E. S. Snitkin, Z. Hu, Y. Xia and C. Delisi, 2009. Genome-wide prioritization of disease genes and identification of disease-disease associations from an integrated human functional linkage network. *Genome Biol* **10:** R91.

Liu, J. Z., A. F. McRae, D. R. Nyholt, S. E. Medland, N. R. Wray *et al.*, 2010. A versatile gene-based test for genome-wide association studies. *American Journal of Human Genetics* **87:** 139–145.

MacArthur, D. G., S. Balasubramanian, A. Frankish, N. Huang, J. Morris *et al.*, 2012. A systematic survey of loss-of-function variants in human protein-coding genes. *Science* **335:** 823–828.

Maurano, M. T., R. Humbert, E. Rynes, R. E. Thurman, E. Haugen *et al.*, 2012. Systematic localization of common disease-associated variation in regulatory DNA. *Science* **337:** 1190–1195.

Mehta, D., K. Heim, C. Herder, M. Carstensen, G. Eckstein *et al.*, 2013. Impact of common regulatory single-nucleotide variants on gene expression profiles in whole blood. *Eur J Hum Genet* **21:** 48–54.

Navlakha, S., and C. Kingsford, 2010. The power of protein interaction networks for associating genes with diseases. *Bioinformatics* **26:** 1057–1063.

Nicolae, D. L., E. Gamazon, W. Zhang, S. Duan, M. E. Dolan *et al.*, 2010. Trait-associated SNPs are more likely to be eQTLs: annotation to enhance discovery from GWAS. *PLoS Genet* **6:** e1000888.

Peri, S., J. D. Navarro, T. Z. Kristiansen, R. Amanchy, V. Surendranath *et al.*, 2004. Human protein reference database as a discovery resource for proteomics. *Nucleic Acids Research* **32:** D497–501.

Purcell, S. M., N. R. Wray, J. L. Stone, P. M. Visscher, M. C. O'Donovan *et al.*, 2009. Common polygenic variation contributes to risk of schizophrenia and bipolar disorder. *Nature* **460:** 748–752.

Roeder, K., S. A. Bacanu, L. Wasserman and B. Devlin, 2006. Using linkage genome scans to improve power of association in genome scans. *American Journal of Human Genetics* **78:** 243–252.

Saccone, S. F., N. L. Saccone, G. E. Swan, P. A. Madden, A. M. Goate *et al.*, 2008. Systematic biological prioritization after a genome-wide association study: an application to nicotine dependence. *Bioinformatics* **24:** 1805–1811.

Shahbaba, B., C. M. Shachaf and Z. Yu, 2012. A pathway analysis method for genome-wide association studies. *Statistics in Medicine* **31:** 988–1000.

Voineagu, I., X. Wang, P. Johnston, J. K. Lowe, Y. Tian *et al.*, 2011. Transcriptomic analysis of autistic brain reveals convergent molecular pathology. *Nature* **474:** 380–384.

Wang, K., M. Li and M. Bucan, 2007. Pathway-based approaches for analysis of genomewide association studies. *American Journal of Human Genetics* **81:** 1278–1283.

Wang, K., M. Li and H. Hakonarson, 2010a. Analysing biological pathways in genome-wide association studies. *Nat Rev Genet* **11:** 843–854.

Wang, K., M. Li and H. Hakonarson, 2010b. ANNOVAR: functional annotation of genetic variants from high-throughput sequencing data. *Nucleic Acids Res* **38:** e164.

Wang, L., P. Jia, R. D. Wolfinger, X. Chen, B. L. Grayson *et al.*, 2011. An efficient hierarchical generalized linear mixed model for pathway analysis of genome-wide association studies. *Bioinformatics* **27:** 686–692.

Ward, L. D., and M. Kellis, 2012. Interpreting noncoding genetic variation in complex traits and human disease. *Nat Biotechnol* **30:** 1095–1106.

White, S., and P. Smyth, 2003. Algorithms for estimating relative importance in networks. *Proceedings of the ninth ACM SIGKDD international conference on Knowledge discovery and data mining*: 266–275.

Wu, X., R. Jiang, M. Q. Zhang and S. Li, 2008. Network-based global inference of human disease genes. *Mol Syst Biol* **4:** 189.

Xiong, Q., N. Ancona, E. R. Hauser, S. Mukherjee and T. S. Furey, 2012. Integrating genetic and gene expression evidence into genome-wide association analysis of gene sets. *Genome Research* **22:** 386–397.

Zhang, W., Y. Chen, F. Sun and R. Jiang, 2011. DomainRBF: a Bayesian regression approach to the prioritization of candidate domains for complex diseases. *BMC Syst Biol* **5:** 55.

Zhong, H., X. Yang, L. M. Kaplan, C. Molony and E. E. Schadt, 2010. Integrating Pathway Analysis and Genetics of Gene Expression for Genome-wide Association Studies. *The American Journal of Human Genetics* **86:** 581–591.

About the Authors

Ning Sun, Ph.D., is a Research Scientist in the Biostatistics Department at Yale School of Public Health. She obtained her B.Sc. from Tsinghua University and Ph.D. from the University of California at Los Angeles. Her current research interests are the development and applications of statistical methods for genome wide association studies and the inference of gene regulation networks.

Hongyu Zhao, Ph.D., is the Ira V. Hiscock Professor of Biostatistics and Professor of Statistics and Genetics at Yale University. He received his B.S. from Peking University and Ph.D. from the University of California at Berkeley. His research interests are the applications of statistical methods in molecular biology, genetics, drug developments, and personalized medicine. Some of his recent projects include large scale genome wide studies to identify genetic variants underlying complex diseases, biological network modeling and analysis, disease biomarker identification through proteomics, genome annotations for the 1000 Genomes Project, microbiome analysis, and systems biology study of herbal medicine.

CHAPTER 27

CAUSAL INFERENCE

ZHI GENG
Peking University, Beijing 100871, PR China
zhigeng@pku.edu.cn

1. Introduction

Causation and correlation are two important and different concepts. Even if there is not any causation between two factors, there may exist spuriously an associational between them. On the other hand, the presence of a causation may not imply the presence of an association. A lot of examples may explain spurious associations. For example, the time of Mr. A's watch is strongly associated with the time of Mr. B's watch, but changing the watch time of Mr. A cannot affect that of Mr. B. Freedman *et al.* (1991) gave an example that reading ability of primary school students is related to sizes of their shoes, but obviously there is no causation between them. Increasing their shoes sizes cannot increase their reading ability. Does a causation between two variables always imply an association between them? In fact, there are also many examples of spurious no association. Suppose that doing *Taijiquan* can enhance health for everybody, that is, doing *Taijiquan* has causal effects on health. However, people doing *Taijiquan* may have similar or even worse health status than people not doing *Taijiquan*, that is, doing *Taijiquan* is not associated with health. It may be because people doing *Taijiquan* are old and sick persons whose health status are enhanced to a normal level by doing *Taijiquan*. Another example is that the health status of uranium miners may be similar to or even better than that of other workers. This cannot explain that exposure to uranium mines does not affect one's health. Perhaps uranium miners were selected from more healthy persons. If they had not been exposed to uranium mines, their health status would have been better. This is the phenomenon of healthy worker effect.

When association-based statistical models and approaches are applied to explain causation, persons often overlook the required assumptions and conditions for causal inference. The association-based models with only observed variables cannot be used to define causation and causal effects. To define causal effects, Neyman (1923) presented the potential outcome model for experiment studies, and Rubin (1974) extended the potential outcome model for observational studies. The potential outcome model requires an explanation of which variable is the cause and which the effect. It can be used to evaluate causal effects but not to discover causal relationships. Holland (1986) gave a review of causal inference. Pearl (1995) proposed the concepts of causal diagrams and external interventions. The causal relationships among variables are depicted by a causal network. For a causal diagram, two topics are parameter learning and structural learning from observed data.

In Section 2, we first introduce Yule-Simpson's paradox to explain the key problem for causal inference. In Section 3, the potential outcome model or the counterfactual model and the definitions of causal effects are introduced. Confounding and confounder are discussed, and the collapsibility-based and comparability-based criteria for checking confounders are discussed in Section 4. Causal diagrams are introduced, and criteria based on diagrams are discussed in Section 5. An algorithm for checking multiple confounders is described in Section 6. Longitudinal causal inference is introduced in Section 7. Finally some discussions are given in Section 8.

2. Yule-Simpson's Paradox

An association measurement between two variables X and Y may be dramatically changed from positive to negative by omitting a third variable Z, which is called Yule-Simpson's paradox (Yule, 1903; Simpson, 1951). To illustrate Yule-Simpson's paradox, suppose that we have the observed data of smoking and lung cancer in Table 1, which may be regarded as a distribution proportion of population. From the data, we get that the relative risk,

Table 1. A numerical example of smoking and lung cancer.

	Case	Control	Total
Smoking	80	120	200
No smoking	100	100	200

Table 2. Stratification by sex.

	Male		Female	
	Case	Control	Case	Control
Smoking	35	15	45	105
No smoking	90	60	10	40

Table 3. Antibiotic prophylaxis (AB-proph.) and urinary tract infections (UTI).

	Hospitals with low UTI		Hospital with high UTI		All hospitals	
AB-proph.	UTI	no-UTI	UTI	no-UTI	UTI	no-UTI
Yes	20	1093	22	45	42	1237
No	5	715	60	10	104	2136

the risk difference and the odds ratio are $RR = (80/200)/(100/200) = 0.80$, $RD = (80/200) - (100/200) = -0.10$ and $OR = (80 \times 100)/(100 \times 120) = 0.67$ respectively. It can be seen that smoking seems to be a preventive factor.

Suppose that we use sex to stratify the observed data and obtain the $2 \times 2 \times 2$ contingency table in Table 2. For male, the relative risk, the risk difference and the odds ratio are $RR_1 = 1.17$, $RD_1 = 0.10$ and $OR_1 = 1.56$ respectively; and for female, the relative risk, the risk difference and the odds ratio are $RR_2 = 1.50$, $RD_2 = 0.10$ and $OR_2 = 1.71$ respectively. Now smoking appears to be a risk factor of lung cancer for both male and female. This phenomenon is called Yule-Simpson's Paradox. The phenomena of Yule-Simpson's paradox happen in many real examples (Bickel *et al.*, 1975; Wagner, 1986; Neufeld, 1995; Reintjes *et al.*, 2000).

However the conclusion obtained by stratification may not always be correct. Reintjes *et al.* (2000) gave such an example from hospital epidemiology. 3519 gynecology patients from eight hospitals in a nonexperimental study were used to study the association between antibiotic prophylaxis (AB-proph.) and urinary tract infections (UTI). The eight hospitals were stratified into two groups with a low incidence percentage (<2.5%) and a high percentage (>2.5%) of UTI. By Table 3, the relative risk is $(42/1279)/(104/2240) = 0.7$ for the overall eight hospitals, which means that AB-proph. had a protective effect on UTI. But the RRs are 2.6 and 2.0 for the low and the high incidence groups respectively, which means that AB-prophylaxis had a risk effect on UTI for both groups. The real effect of AB-prophylaxis on UTI has been shown to be protective by randomized clinical trials, which is consistent with the marginal analysis rather than the stratified analysis. This result explains that there were more unidentified confounders which canceled their effects each other out in the crude analysis.

To avoid the phenomena of Yule-Simpson's paradox, many investigators discussed collapsibility of association measures and related conditions under which association measures are unchanged by omitting other variables (Whittemore, 1978; Cox and Wermuth, 2003; Ma *et al.* 2006). Yule-Simpson's paradox occurs because there are some confounders which are associated with both exposure and response. Thus there is association between the exposure and the response even if there is no causation between them (Greenland, Pearl and Robins, 1999; Pearl, 2000).

Chen *et al.* (2007) presented the surrogate paradox, or called the intermediate variable paradox, which is a variation of Yule-Simpson's paradox. The surrogate paradox means that a treatment has a positive effect on a surrogate endpoint or an intermediate variable, which in turn has a positive effect on the true endpoint, but the treatment has a negative effect on the true endpoint. Moore (1995) described a real story of antiarrhythmic drug trials. By the medical knowledge, an irregular heartbeat is a risk factor of sudden deaths. Several kinds of drugs can significantly corrected irregular heartbeats, but it was found that these drugs really increased sudden deaths. See Geng (2013) in this book for the details.

3. Counterfactual Models for Causal Inference

Neyman (1923) and Rubin (1974) proposed the counterfactual model for causal inference, in which the key notion is the potential outcomes. If we could observe the potential outcomes for each unit under both exposed and unexposed to a treatment, we would assess the causal effect of the treatment on the unit by the difference between these two potential outcomes. Generally in epidemiological and medical studies, however, every unit can be in only one exposure status, either exposed or unexposed to the treatment, but never both. As mentioned in Heraclitus's motto, you cannot step into the same river twice. So only one value of the potential outcomes can be observed and the other cannot. The unobserved value is counterfactual. Some assumptions are required for causal inference by observational studies, while these assumptions cannot be tested empirically.

3.1. *Causal effects*

Three definitions of causal effects in different levels are introduced in this section. Let E denote treatment (or exposure) status. For a binary treatment, $E = e$ denotes that the unit is treated (or exposed) and $E = \overline{e}$ denotes that the unit is untreated (or unexposed). Let $D_e(u)$ denote the potential outcome of a unit u under the treated status $E = e$, and $D_{\overline{e}}(u)$ denote the potential outcome under the untreated or control status $E = \overline{e}$.

Definition 3.1 The individual causal effect (ICE) of treated e versus control $\overline{e}$ for a unit u is defined by $ICE(u) = D_e(u) - D_{\overline{e}}(u)$.

Since every unit u may not be treated and untreated in the same time, it is impossible to observe both D_e and $D_{\overline{e}}$ for the same unit simultaneously, and thus $ICE(u)$ cannot be identified by observed data.

Definition 3.2 Suppose that there are N units in a population U. The average causal effect (ACE) in the population U is defined as the mean of the individual causal effects

$$ACE = \frac{1}{N}\sum_{u \in U} ICE(u) = E(D_e - D_{\overline{e}}).$$

The average causal effect is the difference between the expectation of the potential outcome if all the units were treated and the expectation if all the units were untreated. A covariate is a variable which is not affected by treatment. For example, a variable that occurs before the treatment is a covariate.

Definition 3.3 Let X be a discrete covariate. The population U is stratified into subpopulations by the covariate $X = k$, $k = 1, \ldots, K$. The average causal effect of the subpopulation of $X = k$ is defined as

$$ACE_k = E(D_e - D_{\overline{e}}|X = k).$$

It is well-known that randomized treatment assignment is the most reliable experiment to assess causal effects. Randomization can balance distributions of both known and unknown covariates in the treated group and the control group, and thus it makes these two groups comparable. In a randomized experiment, the treatment variable E is independent of any other covariates, and particularly E is independent of both D_e and $D_{\overline{e}}$, which are covariates, denoted as $E \perp (D_e, D_{\overline{e}})$. Therefore we have

$$E(D_e) = E(D_e|e) = E(D|e) \quad \text{and} \quad E(D_{\bar{e}}) = E(D_{\bar{e}}|\bar{e}) = E(D|\bar{e})$$

and

$$ACE = E(D_e - D_{\overline{e}}) = E(D|E = e) - E(D|E = \overline{e}).$$

Thus ACE can be estimated by the difference between the outcome means in the treatment and control groups.

3.2. *Ignorability of treatment assignment mechanism*

For observational studies, Rosenbaum & Rubin (1983) presented the following assumption to evaluate causal effects.

Assumption 3.1 Treatment assignment E is strongly ignorable given covariates X if the conditional independence $E \perp (D_e, D_{\overline{e}})|X$ and $0 < P(E = e|X = x) < 1$ hold.

If the strongly ignorable treatment assignment (SITA) assumption holds, then the average causal effect in a subpopulation of $X = x$ can be expressed by the expectations of observed variables

$$\begin{aligned} ACE_x &= E(D_e|X = x) - E(D_{\overline{e}}|X = x) \\ &= E(D|E = e, X = x) - E(D|E = \overline{e}, X = x). \end{aligned}$$

Thus ACE_x is identifiable and can be estimated from observed data. The average causal effect in the whole population equals the expectation of the average causal effects in subpopulations defined by X. When X is discrete, it can be written as

$$ACE = E(ACE_X) = \sum_k ACE_k P(X = k).$$

When X is continuous, the sum is replaced by integral. Under the SITA assumption, the average causal effect in the whole population is identifiable.

For an observational study, if we could determine covariates X to ensure the SITA assumption holds, then we may stratify the population on the value of X, estimate the average causal effects in the subpopulations and then estimate the average causal effect in the whole population from the above weighted average formula. This estimation approach is called standardization. It adjusts the treatment and control groups to have the same distribution $P(x)$.

Another approach is the inverse probability weighting. By the SITA assumption, we have

$$\begin{aligned} P(D_e = d, X = k) &= P(D = d|E = e, X = k)P(X = k) \\ &= \frac{P(D = d, E = e, X = k)}{P(E = e|X = k)}, \end{aligned}$$

and thus we get the expectation of the potential outcome

$$\begin{aligned} E(D_e) &= \sum_d \sum_k [d \times I(E = e)] \frac{P(D = d, E = e, X = k)}{P(E = e|X = k)} \\ &= E\left(\frac{D \times I(E = e)}{P(E = e|X)}\right), \end{aligned}$$

where $I(E = e)$ is the indicator function with value 1 if $E = e$, otherwise 0. According to the above equation, $E(D_e)$ can be estimated by the mean of observed outcomes d_i with the inverse probability weights $w_i = 1/P(e|x_i)$ for individuals in the treated group $E = e$. Similarly, $E(D_{\bar{e}})$ can be estimated by the mean of d_i with the weights $w_i = 1/P(\bar{e}|x_i)$ in the control group $E = \bar{e}$. Then ACE for the whole population is estimated by the difference between the inverse probability weighted estimates of $E(D_e)$ and $E(D_{\bar{e}})$.

3.3. *Marginal structural models*

Robins (1997) and Robins, Hernán and Brumback (2000) proposed and introduced the marginal structural models and used the inverse probability weighting method for the parameter estimation. Suppose that the potential outcome D_e has the marginal structural model, for every treatment status e

$$E(D_e) = \alpha + \beta e.$$

This model does not include any covariate and is a marginal model of each single potential outcome D_e. This model cannot be fitted directly with observed data because the potential outcome is counterfactual and cannot be observed. When treatment E is binary ($E = 0, 1$), the model is a saturated model. Under the SITA assumption, as shown in the previous subsection, we can obtain the inverse probability weighted estimates of $E(D_0) = \alpha$ and $E(D_1) = \alpha + \beta$ for E =0 and 1 respectively.

For a multilevel treatment E, suppose that the marginal structural model is $E(D_e) = g(e; \beta)$ where $g(e; \beta)$ is a function with a parameter vector β. Under the SITA assumption, we can write $E(D_e)$ as

$$E\left(\frac{D \times I(E = e)}{P(E = e|X)}|e\right) = g(e; \beta).$$

Covariate X is balanced in the treatment groups (i.e., $X \perp E$) in the pseudo-population constructed by weighting $w_i = 1/P(e_i|x_i)$ for individuals $i = 1, \ldots, n$, and X is not a confounder in the pseudo-population. There is no a potential outcome in the above model, and we can apply the inverse probability weighting method to estimate the parameter vector β. For a continuous treatment E, the stabilized weights are $sw_i = f(e_i)/f(e_i|x_i)$, where $f(e_i)$ and $f(e_i|x_i)$ are the density functions (Robins, Hernán and Brumback, 2000).

3.4. *Propensity score method*

When X is a high dimensional vector of covariates, even if the ignorability treatment assignment assumption holds, stratification analysis by X makes observed data very sparse in strata so that variances of estimates obtained by the standardization and inverse probability weighting methods are very large. Rosenbaum and Rubin (1983) proposed the propensity score by which a population can be stratified most coarsely.

Let X be a covariate vector with continuous and discrete covariates and E a binary treatment. A function $b(X)$ is a balancing score if $X \perp E | b(X)$. The propensity score is defined as the conditional probability

$$s(X) = \Pr(E = e|X).$$

Rosenbaum and Rubin (1983) proved that the propensity score $s(X)$ is the coarsest balancing score in the sense that the propensity score can be expressed by a function of any balancing score, i.e., $s(X) = f(b(X))$. If treatment assignment E is strongly ignorable given covariates X (i.e., $E \perp (D_e, D_{\bar{e}})|X$ and $0 < P(E = e|X = x) < 1$), then treatment assignment E is also strongly ignorable given the propensity score $s(X)$ (i.e., $E \perp (D_e, D_{\bar{e}})|s(X)$ and $0 < P(E = e|s(x)) < 1$). Thus causal effects can be obtained by stratifying the population most coarsely by the propensity score $s(X)$ among all balancing scores. When X is a continuous variable, we may consider a logistic regression model for the propensity score. The standardization and match pair analysis can be performed by using the discretized propensity scores, and the propensity scores may be used for models (Rosenbaum and Rubin, 1983).

4. Confounding Biases and Confounders

Confounding bias and confounders are important concepts in observational studies. The difference between comparison groups is called confounding, and the covariates leading to confounding are called confounders. Greenland, Robins & Pearl (1999) and Greenland and Pearl (2011) gave the overview of confounding, confounders and collapsibility. In epidemiological studies, researchers are often interested in the causal effects of exposure on the exposed population. To eliminate confounding bias, the choice of a control or unexposed group should ensure comparability of the exposure group with the control group. When there exist differences between comparison groups, adjustment of confounders which are unbalanced in the exposed and control groups is necessary to eliminate confounding biases. Criteria for confounders may be classified into two big categories

(1) Collapsibility-based criterion: A factor is not a confounder if the conditional association measures given the factor equal the marginal association measure obtained by omitting the factor;
(2) Comparability-based criterion: A factor is not a confounder if the factor is identically distributed between the exposed and unexposed groups.

Greenland, Robins & Pearl (1999), Geng, Guo, Lau & Fung (2001) and Geng, Guo & Fung (2002) discussed the relation between these two criteria.

4.1. *Collapsibility-based criterion*

Collapsibility of an association measure between two variables over a third variable means that the association remains unchanged conditional on every level of the third variable and after marginalizing over the third variable. Thus the collapsibility may be used to select the variables for the stratification analysis. Kleinbaum *et al.* (1982), Whittemore (1978), Geng (1992), Cox & Wermuth (2003), Ma, Xie & Geng (2006) and Xie, Ma & Geng (2008) discussed the collapsibility of various association measures.

We give the definitions of several commonly-used association measures. Let $f(x, y)$ denote a probability or density function, $F(y|x) = P(Y \leq y|X = x)$ a conditional distribution and $K(x, y)$ an association measure between X and Y. For a general distribution, Cox & Wermuth (2003) presented a distribution association measure $\partial F(y|x)/\partial x$; When X is categorical, the distribution association measure is defined as

$$F(y|x+1) - F(y|x) = P(Y \leq y|x+1) - P(Y \leq y|x).$$

When the measure is negative, the conditional distribution of Y monotonically increases with x increasing. Whittaker (1990) presented a mixture derivative $\partial^2 \log f(x, y)/\partial x \partial y$, called a density association measure. When X is categorical, it is defined as

$$\begin{aligned}&[\log P(y+1|x+1) - \log P(y+1|x)] - [\log P(y|x+1) - \log P(y|x)]\\&\quad = \log OR(x, y),\end{aligned}$$

i.e., the log odds ratio. The expectation association measure is defined as $\partial E(Y|x)/\partial x$. The correlation coefficient is denoted as ρ_{xy}. Xie, Ma & Geng (2008) showed that these measures have the following implication relationships

$$\frac{\partial^2 \log f(x,y)}{\partial x \partial y} \geq 0, \quad \forall x,y \Rightarrow \frac{\partial F(y|x)}{\partial x} \leq 0,$$

$$\forall x,y \Rightarrow \frac{\partial E(Y|x)}{\partial x} \geq 0, \quad \forall x \Rightarrow \rho_{xy} \geq 0.$$

When X and Y have a joint normal distribution or both are binary, the above implications become equivalence relationships.

Let Z denote a covariate. The conditional association measure between X and Y given Z=z is denoted as $K(x,y|z)$. No phenomenon of Yule-Simpson's paradox means that the conditional and marginal association measures have the same direction or sign, called sign-consistent. Xie, Ma & Geng (2008) showed the conditions for the sign-consistence of these measures:

(1) If X and Z are independent (i.e., X⊥Z), then the distribution and expectation association measures and the correlation coefficient are sign-consistent, but the density association measure is not;
(2) If Y and Z are conditionally independent given X (i.e., Y⊥Z | X), then the density, distribution and expectation association measures are sign-consistent, but the correlation coefficient is not.

Below we consider the collapsibility of these association measures. If $K(x,y|z) = K(x,y|z')$ for all $z \neq z'$, we say that $K(x,y|z)$ is consistent over Z. If $K(x,y|z) = K(x,y)$ for all x, y, z, then we say that $K(x,y|z)$ is simply collapsible over Z. Further let I denote a value interval of Z; I is a value set for a nominal Z, and I is an ordinal set $\{i, i+1, \ldots, i+j\}$ for an ordinal categorical Z. If $K(x,y|z \in I) = K(x,y)$ for all x, y, I, then we say that $K(x,y|z)$ is uniformly collapsible over Z.

Ma, Xie & Geng (2006) and Xie, Ma & Geng (2008) presented the conditions for collapsibility of the association measures:

1. the distribution association measure is uniformly collapsible over Z, i.e., for all x, y, I

$$\frac{\partial F(y|x)}{\partial x} = \frac{\partial F(y|x,I)}{\partial x},$$

   if and only if at least one of the following conditions holds

   (1) Y⊥Z | X, or
   (2) X⊥Z, and the conditional distribution measure is consistent over Z, i.e., $\frac{\partial F(y|x,z)}{\partial x} = \frac{\partial F(y|x,z')}{\partial x}$ for all $z \neq z'$.

2. the expectation association measure is uniformly collapsible over Z, i.e., for all x, I

$$\frac{\partial E(Y|x)}{\partial x} = \frac{\partial E(Y|x, I)}{\partial x},$$

if and only if at least one of the following conditions holds

(1) $E(Y|x, z) = E(Y|x, z')$ for all $x, z \neq z'$, or

(2) X⊥Z, and the conditional expectation measure is consistent over Z, i.e., $\frac{\partial E(Y|x,z)}{\partial x} = \frac{\partial E(Y|x,z')}{\partial x}$ for all $x, z \neq z'$.

3. the density association measure is uniformly collapsible over Z, i.e., for all x, y, I

$$\frac{\partial^2 \log f(x, y)}{\partial x \partial y} = \frac{\partial^2 \log f(x, y|I)}{\partial x \partial y},$$

if and only if at least one of the following conditions holds

(1) Y⊥Z | X, or

(2) X⊥Z | Y.

The collapsibility-based criteria for judging confounders depend on the chosen measure of association. It is possible that some measures are collapsible while others are not. The collapsibility-based criteria can be tested by observed data. The collapsibility means only that the confounding bias remains unchanged by collapsing over non-confounders, and thus we still require the SITA assumption to evaluate causal effects.

4.2. *Collapsibility of parameters in models*

In this subsection, we discuss the collapsibility of parameters in models (Wermuth, 1989; Geng and Asano, 1993; Guo & Geng, 1995; Xie, Ma & Geng, 2008). First consider the linear regression model of Y on X. When the background variable Z is categorical, suppose the linear model for $i = 1, \ldots, I$,

$$E(Y|X = x, Z = i) = \alpha(i) + \beta(i)x.$$

If $\beta(i) = \beta$, then the model describes the parallel lines. For a continuous Z, suppose the linear model

$$E(Y|X = x, Z = z) = \alpha + \beta x + \gamma z.$$

If the partial marginal model conditional on any interval I of Z's values has the equation

$$E(Y|X = x, z \in I) = \alpha(I) + \beta(I)x$$

and $\beta(I) = \beta$, then we say that β is uniformly collapsible over Z. Specially, I may be the whole domain of Z. β is uniformly collapsible over Z if and only if

(1) for a categorical Z, $\alpha(i) = \alpha(j), \forall i \neq j$; for a continuous Z, $\gamma = 0$; or
(2) X$\perp$Z.

Suppose that X, Y and Z follow a joint normal distribution or that X and Y follow a conditional normal distribution given a categorical Z, called a conditional Gaussian distribution. Then β is uniformly collapsible over Z if and only if

(1) Y$\perp$Z | X , or
(2) X$\perp$Z.

For a binary response Y, consider a logistic regression model. For a categorical Z, suppose the model

$$\log \frac{P(Y = 1|x, Z = i)}{P(Y = 0|x, Z = i)} = \alpha(i) + \beta(i)x;$$

for a continuous Z, suppose the model

$$\log \frac{P(Y = 1|x, z)}{P(Y = 0|x, z)} = \alpha + \beta x + \gamma z.$$

If the partial marginal model conditional on any interval $I$of Z's values has the equation

$$\log \frac{P(Y = 1|x, Z \in I)}{P(Y = 0|x, Z \in I)} = \alpha(I) + \beta(I)x$$

and $\beta(I) = \beta$, then we say that β is uniformly collapsible over Z. Then β is uniformly collapsible over Z if and only if

(1) Y$\perp$Z | X or
(2) X$\perp$Z.

4.3. *Comparability-based criterion*

Suppose that if the exposed population (e.g., the population of smoking) should not be exposed (i.e., nonsmoking), the distributions of responses (e.g., the probability of disease) would be the same as that in the unexposed population (e.g., the population of nonsmoking); and suppose that if the unexposed population should be exposed, the distributions of responses would be the same as that in the exposed population. Then the exposed population is said to be exchangeable with the unexposed population, or there is no confounding. Comparing the response distributions between the exposed and the unexposed populations which are exchangeable can evaluate the causal effect of the exposure on the response. Therefore we can estimate the averaged causal effect by the difference of observed means of responses in the exposed and unexposed populations. If the exposed and unexposed populations are not exchangeable but their subpopulations stratified by a covariate are exchangeable, then the covariate is called a confounder. Stratifying the population by the confounder can eliminate confounding bias. The averaged causal effects in these subpopulations can be identified, and then the averaged causal effect for the whole population can be obtained by weighting the subpopulation-average causal effects by the distribution of the confounder. But the comparability of exposed and unexposed populations cannot be tested by observed data. The comparability-based criteria for confounders do not depend on the chosen measures of association. These criteria were discussed in Miettinen & Cook (1981), Greenland & Robins (1986), Wickramaratne & Holford (1987), Geng *et al.* (2001) and Geng, Guo & Fung (2002).

In epidemiology studies, researchers often focus only on causal effects of exposure on the exposed population rather than that on the whole population. The average causal effect of exposure on the exposed population is defined as

$$ACE_e = E[D_e(u) - D_{\overline{e}}(u)|E = e] = P(D_e = 1|E = e) - P(D_{\overline{e}} = 1|E = e),$$

where $P(D_{\overline{e}} = 1|E = e)$ denotes the counterfactual probability of response in the case that the exposed population would be unexposed, which cannot be identified by observed data without any assumption. In epidemiological studies, researchers usually select an unexposed reference population of $E = \overline{e}$ and use an estimate of $P(D_{\overline{e}} = 1|E = \overline{e})$ in the reference population to evaluate $P(D_{\overline{e}} = 1|E = e)$.

Miettinen & Cook (1981) (Simply denoted as M & C) used many examples to show the following comparability-based criterion for confounders. A confounder C must satisfy two conditions

(1) C is an independent risk factors, and
(2) C has different distributions in the exposed and unexposed populations.

Now we use counterfactual models to describe the comparability-based criterion. Wickramaratne & Holford (1987) showed under the assumption

$D_{\overline{e}} \perp E|C$ that the exposed population is comparable with the unexposed population, that is, $P(D_{\overline{e}} = 1|E = e) = P(D_{\overline{e}} = 1|E = \overline{e})$ if one of the following conditions holds

(1) $D_{\overline{e}} \perp C|E = \overline{e}$, or
(2) $E \perp C$.

The comparability means no confounding, and then the sufficient conditions (1) and (2) for comparability can be used to interpret M & C's criterion which is the necessary conditions for a confounder.

Further Geng *et al.* (2001) proposed a concept of uniform non-confounding of the coarse subpopulations. If for any set $\omega \subseteq \{1, \ldots, K\}$,

$$P(D_{\overline{e}} = 1|E = e, C \in \omega) = P(D_{\overline{e}} = 1|E = \overline{e}, C \in \omega),$$

then the coarse subpopulations are said to be uniform non-confounding. That is, there is no confounding no matter how to pooling subpopulations defined by C together. For example, when C denotes age, the uniform non-confounding means that there is no confounding no matter how to stratify the age groups, every 5 years, every 10 years or any other interval. Under the assumption $D_{\overline{e}} \perp E|C$, Geng *et al.* (2001) showed that the necessary and sufficient condition for the uniform non-confounding is

(1) $D_{\overline{e}} \perp C|E = \overline{e}$, or
(2) $E \perp C$.

4.4. *Formal definitions and criteria for confounders*

M & C (1981) derived inductively the criterion for confounders without requiring the assumption $D_{\overline{e}} \perp E|C$. Greenland & Robins (1986) illustrated that the comparability-based criterion of M & C is not a sufficient condition, but only a necessary condition. The collapsibility-based criterion depends on the measure of association and the categorization of covariate. In this section, we discuss formal definitions of confounders without the ignorability assumptions, see Geng, Guo & Fung (2002).

Kleinbaum (1982) and Greenland & Robins (1986) gave a qualitative definition for confounders: if controlling for a factor may reduce confounding bias, then the factor is a confounder. Let C be a discrete covariate which is unaffected by the exposure. We use the distribution of the covariate C in the exposed population as the standard distribution and adopt the following standardization to approximate the counterfactual $P(D_{\overline{e}} = 1|E = e)$

$$P_{\Delta}(D_{\overline{e}} = 1|E = e) = \sum_{k=1}^{K} P(D_{\overline{e}} = 1|E = \overline{e}, C = k)P(C = k|E = e).$$

Geng, Guo & Fung (2002) presented the following formal definition of confounder.

Definition 4.1 C is a confounder if

$$\begin{aligned} &|P(D_{\overline{e}} = 1|E = e) - P_{\Delta}(D_{\overline{e}} = 1|E = e)| \\ &\quad < |P(D_{\overline{e}} = 1|E = e) - P(D_{\overline{e}} = 1|E = \overline{e})|. \end{aligned}$$

The definition means that the probability $P_{\Delta}(D_{\overline{e}} = 1|E = e)$ standardized with a confounder C is closer to the counterfactual probability than the conditional probability $P(D_{\overline{e}} = 1|E = \overline{e})$.

Definition 4.2 C is an irrelevant factor if

$$P_{\Delta}(D_{\overline{e}} = 1|E = e) = P(D_{\overline{e}} = 1|E = \overline{e}).$$

An irrelevant factor is not a confounder. Adjustment by an irrelevant factor cannot reduce confounding bias. However, this definition of a confounder depends on the categorization of covariate C. Below we give a definition of an occasional confounder which does not depend on the categorization.

Definition 4.3 If there exists a partition p of C's categories (i.e., $p = \{\omega_1, \ldots, \omega_M\}$, where $\omega_k \neq \phi$, $\omega_i \cap \omega_j = \phi$, $\cup_k \omega_k = \{1, \ldots, K\}$, $M \leq K$) such that

$$\begin{aligned} &|P(D_{\overline{e}} = 1|E = e) - P_p(D_{\overline{e}} = 1|E = e)| \\ &\quad < |P(D_{\overline{e}} = 1|E = e) - P(D_{\overline{e}} = 1|E = \overline{e})|, \end{aligned}$$

then C is an occasional confounder, where $P_p(D_{\overline{e}} = 1|E = e)$ is the standardized probability obtained by the partition p

$$P_p(D_{\overline{e}} = 1|E = e) = \sum_{m=1}^{M} P(D_{\overline{e}} = 1|E = \overline{e}, C \in \omega_m)P(C \in \omega_m|E = e).$$

Definition 4.4 C is a uniformly irrelevant factor if for any possible partition p of C's categories,

$$P_p(D_{\overline{e}} = 1|E = e) = P(D_{\overline{e}} = 1|E = \overline{e}).$$

Definition 4.3 means that C is an occasional confounder if there exists a partition p such that adjustment by p can reduce the confounding bias.

Definition 4.4 means that C is a uniformly irrelevant factor if there does not exist any partition p such that adjustment by p can reduce the confounding bias.

It can be shown from the formal definitions of confounders that the collapsibility-based and comparability-based criteria are not contradictory, but mutually complementary. Combination of these two criteria can eliminate more non-confounders from the set of confounder candidates.

Three necessary conditions for a covariate C to be a confounder are

(A1) $C \perp E$ and $D_{\overline{e}} \perp C | E = \overline{e}$,
(A2) the risk difference is not collapsible over C, and
(A3) the relative risk is not collapsible over C.

The condition (A1) is the comparability-based criterion of M & C, and (A2) and (A3) are the collapsibility-based criteria. If C is a confounder by Definition 4.1, then it must satisfy all of three conditions in (A1), (A2) and (A3). In the next subsection, we illustrate that the three necessary conditions are complementary.

Three necessary conditions for a covariate C to be an occasional confounder are

(B1) $C \perp E$ and $D_{\overline{e}} \perp C | E = \overline{e}$,
(B2) the risk difference is not strongly collapsible over C, and
(B3) the relative risk is not strongly collapsible over C.

If C is an occasional confounder by Definition 4.3, then it must satisfy all of three conditions in (B1), (B2) and (B3). Condition (B1) is just the comparability-based criterion of M & C. It can be shown that condition (B1) implies conditions (B2) and (B3), and thus (B2) and (B3) can be removed.

4.5. *Numerical examples of confounders*

The comparability-based criterion of M & C is only a necessary condition of a confounder and it cannot be used as a definition of confounder. Greenland & Robins (1986) gave an example that the criterion of M & C is not a sufficient condition. The collapsibility-based criterion is not sufficient either, which depends on association measures and categorization of covariate. In the section we use the notion of individual effects proposed by Greenland & Robins (1986) to give some examples to illustrate these criteria for confounders.

Table 4. Artificial data: a non-confounder C, but not collapsible.

	$C=1$		$C=2$		Crude ($C \in \{1,2\}$)	
Type	$E=e$	$E=\overline{e}$	$E=e$	$E=\overline{e}$	$E=e$	$E=\overline{e}$
1("doomed")	15	5	40	50	55	55
4("immune")	85	95	60	50	145	145
Total	100	100	100	100	200	200
RD	0.10		−0.10		0.00	
RR	3.00		0.80		1.00	

Suppose that the response of every individual is determinate under a given exposure. Then all individuals in the population may be divided into the four types

Type 1. No causal effect (individual "doomed"): $D_e = D_{\overline{e}} = 1$;

Type 2. Exposure causative (individual susceptible): $D_e = 1$, $D_{\overline{e}} = 0$;

Type 3. Exposure preventive (individual susceptible): $D_e = 0$, $D_{\overline{e}} = 1$;

Type 4. No causal effect (individual immune to disease): $D_e = D_{\overline{e}} = 0$.

In the following examples, suppose that exposure has no causal effect, i.e., there are only Types 1 and 4 of individuals in the population. But by observed data, we do not know whether this supposition holds or not. We can observe only the disease status of every individual, but we cannot determine which type any individual belongs to.

Example 4.1 For the artificial data shown in Table 4, neither the risk difference (RD) nor the relative risk (RR) are collapsible, and thus we cannot decide from the collapsibility-based criterion whether C is a confounder. But the joint distribution has the independence $C \perp E$, and thus we can judge by the comparability-based criterion that C is not a confounder. Without adjustment for C, we obtain from the marginal table that $RD = 0$ and $RR = 1$, which correctly assess that exposure has no causal effect.

Example 4.2 Consider the artificial data shown in Table 5. Both RD and RR are collapsible, and thus we can judge from the collapsibility-based criterion that C is not a confounder. By Table 5, we have $C \perp E$ and $D_{\overline{e}} \perp C | E = \overline{e}$, and thus we cannot decide from the comparability-based criterion that C is not a confounder. Without stratifying and adjustment on C, we can obtain directly from the marginal table that $RD = 0$ and $RR = 1$, which correctly assess that exposure has no causal effect.

Table 5. Artificial data: a non-confounder C and collapsible.

	$C=1$		$C=2$		$C=3$		Crude ($C \in \{1,2,3\}$)	
Type	$E=e$	$E=\overline{e}$	$E=e$	$E=\overline{e}$	$E=e$	$E=\overline{e}$	$E=e$	$E=\overline{e}$
1("doomed")	95	95	5	5	75	25	175	125
4("immune")	5	5	95	95	75	25	175	125
Total	100	100	100	100	150	50	350	250
RD	0.00		0.00		0.00		0.00	
RR	1.00		1.00		1.00		1.00	

Table 6. Artificial data: non-confounder C, simply collapsible.

	$C=1$		$C=2$		$C=3$		$C=4$		Crude ($C \in \Delta$)	
Type	$E=e$	$E=\overline{e}$	$E=e$	$E=\overline{e}$	$E=e$	$E=\overline{e}$	$E=e$	$E=\overline{e}$	$E=e$	$E=\overline{e}$
1("doomed")	60	66	40	184	160	46	20	26	280	322
4("immune")	40	34	60	216	240	54	80	74	420	378
Total	100	100	100	400	400	100	100	100	700	700
RD	−0.06		−0.06		−0.06		−0.06		−0.06	
RR	0.91		0.87		0.87		0.77		0.87	

Example 4.3 For the artificial data shown in Table 6, RD is simply collapsible, but RR is not. Therefore, we can judge from the collapsibility-based criterion that C is not a confounder. But by Table 6, we have $C \perp E$ and $D_{\overline{e}} \perp C|E=\overline{e}$, and so we cannot decide from the comparability-based criterion that C is not a confounder. Using the standardization by the distribution of C, we obtain

$$P_{\Delta}(D_{\overline{e}}=1|E=e)=\frac{66}{100}\cdot\frac{100}{700}+\frac{184}{400}\cdot\frac{100}{700}+\frac{46}{100}\cdot\frac{400}{700}+\frac{26}{100}\cdot\frac{100}{700}=0.46,$$

which is the same as the crude $P(D_{\overline{e}}=1|E=\overline{e})=\frac{322}{700}=0.46$. It shows that C is an irrelevant factor.

Further we consider whether C is an occasional confounder. Let $p=\{\{1,2\},\{3,4\}\}$. Table 7 shows the distribution for the partially pooled subpopulations obtained by combining levels 1 and 2 and combining levels 3 and 4 based on the partition p of C's categories. It can be seen that the risk differences RD in Table 7 do not equal those in Table 6, and thus RD is not strongly collapsible. Under the assumption that exposure has no causal

Table 7. $p = \{[1,2],[3,4]\}$, an accidental confounder C.

	$C \in [1,2]$		$C \in [3,4]$	
Type	$E = e$	$E = \overline{e}$	$E = e$	$E = \overline{e}$
1("doomed")	100	250	180	72
4("immune")	100	250	320	128
Total	200	500	500	200
RD	0.00		0.00	
RR	1.00		1.00	

effect, we have

$$P(D_{\overline{e}} = 1|E = e) = P(D_e = 1|E = e) = \frac{280}{700} = 0.40.$$

We can compute the standardized probability $P_p(D_{\overline{e}} = 1|E = e)$ based on the partition p

$$P_p(D_{\overline{e}} = 1|E = e) = \frac{250}{500} \cdot \frac{200}{700} + \frac{72}{200} \cdot \frac{500}{700} = \frac{280}{700} = 0.40.$$

From $|P(D_{\overline{e}} = 1|E = e) - P_p(D_{\overline{e}} = 1|E = e)| = 0$, we have that confounding bias is completely eliminated by standardization with the partition p. Since this zero bias is less than $|P(D_{\overline{e}} = 1|E = e) - P(D_{\overline{e}} = 1|E = \overline{e})| = 0.06$, we could find that C is an occasional confounder. The adjusted risk difference $P(D_e = 1|E = e) - P_p(D_{\overline{e}} = 1|E = e) = 0$ and the adjusted relative risk $P(D_e = 1|E = e)/P_p(D_{\overline{e}} = 1|E = e) = 1$ correctly assess that exposure has no causal effect. Since the counterfactual probability $P(D_{\overline{e}} = 1|E = e)$ is unknown, we cannot decide only by observed data whether C is an occasional confounder.

5. Criteria for Confounders Based on Causal Diagrams

Robins (1986), Sprites, Glymour & Scheines (1993) and Pearl (1993, 1995, 2000) proposed causal diagrams to derive causal inferences from nonexperimental data. They supposed first a completely constructed causal diagram. Pearl (1995) presented the sufficient conditions for no confounding and established a set of inference rules to identify causal effects based on the causal diagram. Greenland, Pearl & Robins (1999) applied causal diagrams to epidemiological studies and provided a criterion for confounders, which can determine confounders and non-confounders more exactly than the traditional criteria, although the criterion requires a known causal diagram.

In many practical cases, however, it is difficult to know a whole causal diagram. Geng & Li (2002) presented conditions of non-confounding without the requirement of a whole causal diagram.

5.1. *Definitions and notation of causal diagrams*

A directed graph has a set of nodes $X = \{X_1, \ldots, X_n\}$ and a set of directed edges. X_i is called a parent node of X_j, or X_j is a son of X_i, if there is a directed edge $X_i \to X_j$. Let pa_i denote the parent set of X_i. A path between X_i and X_j is a succession of edges from X_i to X_j regardless of their directions. If all directions of edges on the path between X_i and X_j point to X_j, then this path is a directed path from X_i to X_j and X_j is a descendant of X_i. A directed path from X_i to itself is a cycle. A directed graph without any cycle is a directed acyclic graph (DAG), also called a diagram.

Definition 5.1 Let C is a set of nodes in a DAG Γ. A path between X_i and X_j is not blocked by C if every node X_k on the path satisfies the following two conditions:

(1) if the node X_k is a collider ($\to X_k \leftarrow$), then either the node X_k or one of its descendants is in C; and
(2) if the node X_k is not a collider, then it is not in C.

Otherwise the path is blocked by C.

Definition 5.2 (*d-separation*) Let A, B and C be three disjoint subsets of nodes in a DAG Γ. C is said to d-separate A from B, denoted $d(A, B, C)$, if and only if C blocks every path from a node in A to a node in B.

Example 5.1. The directed graph in Figure 1 is a DAG. Let $C = \{X_1\}$. C blocks the path $X_2 \leftarrow X_1 \to X_3$. Since neither X_4 nor X_5 is in C, C blocks the path $X_2 \to X_4 \leftarrow X_3$. Therefore C d-separates $A = \{X_2\}$ from $B = \{X_3\}$. Let $C' = \{X_1, X_4\}$. Then X_4 is a collider on the path $X_2 \to X_4 \leftarrow X_3$ and it is in C'. So C' does not d-separate $A = \{X_2\}$ from $B = \{X_3\}$.

For the graphical model depicted by a DAG Γ, variables $X_1, \ldots, X_n$ have a joint probability distribution

$$P(x_1, \ldots, x_n) = \prod_{i=1}^{n} P(x_i \,|pa_i),$$

where $P(x_i \,|pa_i)$ is the conditional probability of $X_i = x_i$ given $Pa_i = pa_i$. We assume that $P(x_1, \ldots, x_n) > 0$ for every $x_1, \ldots, x_n$.

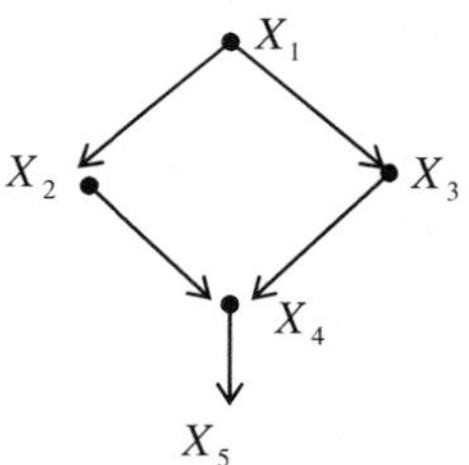

Fig. 1. A directed acyclic graph.

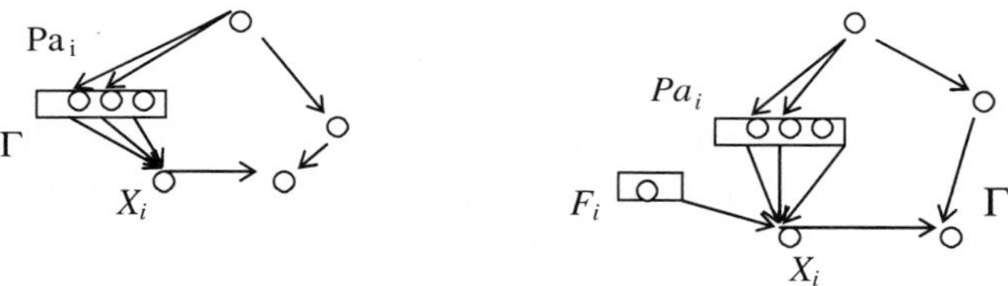

Fig. 2. A external intervention F_iX_i.

Example 5.2. For the DAG in Figure 1, the joint probability distribution is

$$P(x_1, x_2, x_3, x_4, x_5) = P(x_1)P(x_2|x_1)P(x_3|x_1)P(x_4|x_2, x_3)P(x_5|x_4).$$

Assume that a causal system can be represented by a DAG, where a directed edge $X_i \to X_j$ presents that X_i is a cause of X_j. The causal effect of variable X_i is described by an external intervention on X_i. In Figure 2, Γ is a DAG and Γ' represents the DAG under a possible external intervention on X_i, where the directed edge $F_i \to X_i$ in Γ' represents the external intervention on X_i. F_i is a new parent node of X_i with value $set(x_i)$ and *idle*, where $set(x_i)$ denotes that F_i externally forces X_i to a fixed value x_i, and *idle* denotes that there is no external intervention on X_i.

In the DAG Γ', the set of X_i's parent nodes is extended to $Pa_i' = Pa_i \cup \{F_i\}$. The conditional distribution of X_i given Pa_i' is defined by

$$P'(x_i|pa_i) = \begin{cases} p(x_i|pa_i), & \text{if } F_i = idle; \\ 0, & \text{if } F_i = set(x_i') \ \& \ x_i \neq x_i'; \\ 1, & \text{if } F_i = set(x_i') \ \& \ x_i = x_i'. \end{cases}$$

The joint distribution after the intervention $set(x_i')$ is given by

$$P_{x_i'}(x_1, \ldots, x_n) = P'(x_1, \ldots, x_n|F_i = set(x_i')),$$

where $P_{x'_i}(x_1, \ldots, x_n)$ represents the joint distribution of $X_1, \ldots, X_n$ when all X_i of the units in the population are externally forced to x'_i.

The transformation formula between the pre-intervention and the post-intervention distributions is given by

$$P_{x'_i}(x_1, \ldots, x_n) = \begin{cases} \dfrac{P(x_1, \ldots, x_n)}{P(x_i|pa_i)}, & \text{if } x_i = x'_i; \\ 0, & \text{if } x_i \neq x'_i. \end{cases} \tag{5.1}$$

Let X_j and X_i denote the response and treatment variables respectively, and Ω_j and Ω_i their domains. The causal effect of X_i on X_j is defined as $P_{x'_i}(x_j)$, which means the post-intervention distribution of X_j under the intervention on $X_i = x_i$.

Given a causal diagram, we say that there is no confounding for the causal effect of X_i on X_j if $P_{x'_i}(x_j)$, the post-intervention distribution of X_j under the external intervention on $X_i = x_i$ in the whole target population, is equal to $P(x_j|x'_i)$, the conditional distribution of X_j in the subpopulation of $X_i = x'_i$ without the external intervention.

Definition 5.3 (*no confounding*) There is no confounding for the causal effect of X_i on X_j if for every $x_j \in \Omega_j$ and $x'_i \in \Omega_i$,

$$P_{x'_i}(x_j) = P(x_j|x'_i).$$

No confounding means that the conditional distribution $P(x_j|x'_i)$ has the same interpretation as the causal distribution $P_{x'_i}(x_j)$. The confounding bias is defined as the difference between $P_{x'_i}(x_j)$ and $P(x_j|x'_i)$. If there is confounding for the population, but there is no confounding for all the subpopulations stratified by some other variables, we call these variables confounders. Let $C = \{X_{t_1}, \ldots, X_{t_k}\}$ be a set of variables, Ω_{t_k} be the domain of X_{t_k}, and $P_{x'_i}(x_j|x_{t_1}, \ldots, x_{t_k}) = \frac{P_{x'_i}(x_j, x_{t_1}, \ldots, x_{t_k})}{P_{x'_i}(x_{t_1}, \ldots, x_{t_k})}$ denote the conditional distribution under the external intervention $set(X_i = x_i)$. This conditional distribution means that the condition is taken after the external intervention $set(X_i = x_i)$.

Given a causal diagram together with the corresponding joint distribution, we can infer the post-intervention distribution from the transformation formula (5.1). Thus we can evaluate the causal effects of interventions using the diagram and the distribution. The joint distribution, usually is unknown and cannot be estimated since some variables may be unobservable. Let $X = X_O \cup X_U$, where X_O denotes the set of observed variables and X_U

denotes the unobserved. The goal is to identify the causal effect $P_{x'_i}(x_j)$ of X_i on X_j by the distribution of observed variables $P(X_O)$. The causal effect of X_i on X_j is identifiable if there is a unique $P_{x'_i}(x_j)$ which can be interpreted by $P(X_O)$. No confounding is equivalent to the identifiability of the causal effect $P_{x'_i}(x_j)$ when only X_i and X_j are observed.

Pearl (1995a) gave the following properties which can be shown from the transformation (5.1)

(1) an intervention $set(x_i)$ affects only the descendants of X_i;
(2) $P_{x'_i}(S|pa_i) = P(S|x'_i, pa_i)$ holds for any set S of variables;
(3) $X_j \perp Pa_i | X_i$ is a sufficient condition for no confounding.

Property (1) implies that $P_{x'_i}(S) = P(S)$ if S is not the descendants of X_i. Property (2) implies no confounding, which means that the causal effect of X_i on any set S is equal to the distribution conditional on the parent set of X_i. Spiegelhatter *et al.* (1993) gave some examples to show that the conditional independence in property (3) is not necessary for no confounding. Geng & Li (2002) proved that the conditional independence in property (3) is a necessary and sufficient condition for uniform non-confounding.

5.2. *Criteria for confounders*

To check whether there are other confounders outside a set S, we delete all directed edges emanating from exposure E in a given causal diagram, that is, remove all effects of exposure. If there still exists a path between E and response D which is not blocked by S, then there may exist some association between E and D conditional on S. The association cannot be interpreted by the causal effect of E on D, and thus there are some confounders outside S. Greenland, Pearl & Robins (1999) presented the following algorithm. Given a set of variables $S = \{S_1, \ldots, S_n\}$ which does not include descendants of E and D,

(1) Delete the arrows emanating from E (i.e., remove all exposure effects).
(2) In the new DAG without exposure effects, check whether there is any path between E and D which is not blocked by S.
(3) If yes, then there are some other confounders outside S; otherwise S is a sufficient set of confounders, but there may be some redundant non-confounders in S.

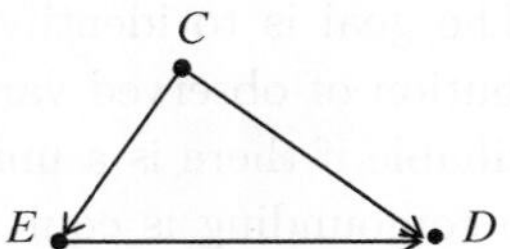

Fig. 3. C is a confounder.

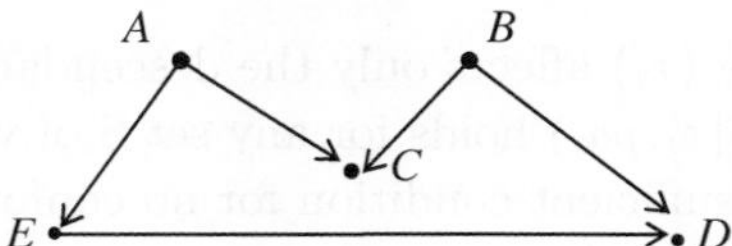

Fig. 4. None of A, B and C is not a confounder.

Example 5.3 Consider the causal diagram in Fig. 3. After deleting $E \to D$, there is still some association between E and D. Thus there exists some confounder. Let $S = \{C\}$ be a confounder set. The path between E to D is blocked by S and $S = \{C\}$ is a sufficient set of confounders.

Example 5.4 Consider the causal diagram in Fig. 4. After deleting $E \to D$, E is independent of D. Thus the association between E and D in the original graph is due to the causal effect of E on D. None of A, B and C is a confounder. However, if controlling for C, then the path $E \leftarrow A \to C \leftarrow B \to D$ is unblocked by C. Thus deleting $E \to D$, E is not independent of D conditional on C. That is, controlling for C introduces confounding bias.

6. Multiple Confounders

The criteria for checking confounders introduced in Section 4 are discussed only for a single confounder. The criteria based on causal diagrams introduced in Section 5 require a whole diagram, although usually such a diagram is unknown. Below we introduce the algorithm for deleting non-confounders from a sufficient set of confounders presented by Wang *et al.* (2009). This algorithm does not require a known diagram, and it removes non-confounders from the sufficient confounder set.

Let D_e denote the potential outcome, E the treatment, and $S = \{S_1, \ldots, S_n\}$ a sufficient confounder set such that the treatment assignment assumption $D_e \perp E | S$ holds. In many cases, we may be interested not only in the causal effect of a treatment in the population, but also those in some subpopulations stratified by a covariate set of interest. For example, even in a randomized clinical trial, we may be interested in treatment effects at different age and sex. Let C be the covariate set of interest which is a subset of the sufficient confounder set S, and the goal is to assess the treatment effects in the subpopulations defined by C, such as the average effect $E(D_e - D_{\bar{e}}|C = c)$ for the subpopulation of $C = c$. For the assessment, the key issue is to identify the counterfactual distribution $p(D_e = d|c)$. Below we describe the algorithm of Wang *et al.* (2009):

Input: a sufficient set of confounders $S = \{S_1, \ldots, S_n\}$ and the covariate set C of interest,

where $C \subseteq S$ and C may be an empty set.

Step 1: Set $F = S \backslash C$ as the initial set from which non-confounders will be deleted.

Step 2: Delete the non-confounders which are not risk factors to the outcome. Define

$$U^a = \{S_i : S_i \in F, D \perp S_i | (E, C, F \backslash S_i)\},$$

and then set $F = F \backslash U^a$.

Step 3: Delete the non-confounders which are balanced in the treatment groups. Define

$$U^b = \{S_i : S_i \in F, E \perp S_i | (C, F \backslash S_i)\},$$

and then set $F = F \backslash U^b$.

Step 4: Repeat Steps 2 and 3 until F is empty or both U^a and U^b are empty.

Output: the reduced confounder set F.

Using the reduced confounder set F, we can identify the counterfactual distribution $p(D_e = d|f, c)$ by

$$p(D_e = d|f, c) = p(D = d|e, f, c),$$

where the right hand side is the distribution of observed variables. The target counterfactual distribution $p(D_e = d|c)$ can be obtained by

$$p(D_e = d|c) = \sum_f p(D = d|e, f, c)p(f|c).$$

When F contains some continuous variables, the corresponding sums in the above equation are replaced by integrals.

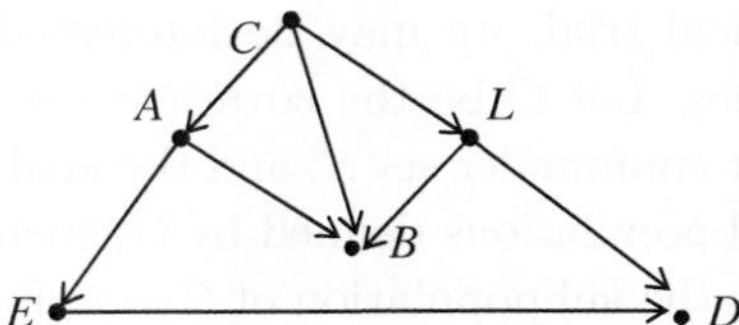

Fig. 5. A sufficient confounder set $\{A, B, C\}$ and a latent L.

Example 6.1. Suppose that the diagram as shown in Fig. 5 is unknown, where C denotes education of patient, L salary, B type of car owned by patient, A profession, E exposure and D disease. Further suppose that we know that the observed covariate set $S = \{A, B, C\}$ is a sufficient confounder set. L is an unobservable latent variable. We are interested in the causal distributions $p(D_e = d|c)$ in the subpopulations of different education levels. In the first iteration, the initial set $F = \{A, B\}$; at step 2, we have $U^a = \phi$ an empty set, and thus no covariates in Z can be deleted; at step 3, we have $U^b = \{B\}$ and thus delete B from F. In the second iteration, at step 2, we have $U^a = \{A\}$ and then further delete A from F. Finally we obtain an empty F. Thus we obtain the causal distribution$p(D_e = d|c) = p(D = d|e, c)$.

7. Causal Inference in Longitudinal Studies

Robins (1989, 1997) and Robins, Greenland & Hu (1999) explored causal inference and confounders in longitudinal studies. In a longitudinal study, the same unit is repeatedly observed in multiple time points. Let $m = 1, \ldots, M$ denote the time points of longitudinal observation; $Y_{m,i}$ and $A_{m,i}$ denote the response and the exposure status for unit i at time m respectively; X_i denote a set of background covariates for unit i which does not depend on time; and let $L_{m,i}$ denote a set of covariates of unit i which depends on time. Suppose that $Y_{m,i}$ and $L_{m,i}$ occur before $A_{m,i}$ at the same time m.

Based on the counterfactual model, let $Y^{(0)}_{m,i}$ denote the response of unit i at m if the unit i were not exposed at any time from the beginning of follow-up to m (i.e. continuous unexposed). Similarly, $Y^{(1)}_{m,i}$ denote the response of the same unit i at m if the unit i were exposed at any time from the beginning of follow-up to m (i.e. continuous exposed). If the unit i changes its exposure status during follow-up, its response at m is neither $Y^{(0)}_{m,i}$ nor $Y^{(1)}_{m,i}$. Therefore neither $Y^{(0)}_{m,i}$ nor $Y^{(1)}_{m,i}$ can be observed for such a unit. For an arbitrary process Z, let $\overline{Z}_m = (Z_1, \ldots, Z_m)$ if $m \geq 1$ and $\overline{Z}_m = 0$ if $m \leq 0$. Assume that N series of data, $(\overline{Y}^{(0)}_{M,i}, \overline{Y}^{(1)}_{M,i}, \overline{Y}_{M,i}, \overline{A}_{M,i}, \overline{L}_{M,i}, X_i)$for $i = 1, \ldots, N$, are independently identical distributed random variables. Define

$$\theta^{(0)}_m(x) = E[Y^{(0)}_m | X = x], \quad \theta^{(1)}_m(x) = E[Y^{(1)}_m | X = x].$$

In the subpopulation of $X = x$ at the time m, the average causal effect of continuous exposed versus continuous unexposed is defined as

$$\delta_m(x) = \theta^{(1)}_m(x) - \theta^{(0)}_m(x).$$

The average causal effect cannot be identified without any assumptions. Robins, Greenland & Hu (1999) proposed the following assumption similar to the strongly ignorable treatment assignment assumption

$$\{(Y^{(0)}_m, Y^{(1)}_m); m = k+1, k+2, \ldots, M\} \perp A_k | (\overline{A}_{k-1}, \overline{Y}_k, \overline{L}_k, X) \tag{7.1}$$

for every $k \geq 1$. This assumption means that the SITA assumption holds for every k, and it cannot be tested by observed data.

If there are no time-dependent confounders, that is, the set $\overline{L}_k$ in (7.1) is empty, then the counterfactual conditional probabilities of the potential responses can be expressed by the probabilities of observed variables

$$\begin{aligned} P(Y^{(j)}_m = 1 | \overline{Y}^{(j)}_{m=1} = \overline{y}_{m-1}, X = x) = P(Y_m = 1 | \overline{Y}_{m-1} \\ = \overline{y}_{m-1}, \overline{A}_{m-1} = j^{[m-1]}, X = x), \end{aligned}$$

where $j^{[m-1]}$ is a vector with $m-1$ elements that are all equal to j. Substituting the expression into the following g-algorithm formula given by Robins (1986, 1987), we can identify the causal parameter $\theta^{(j)}_m(x)$

$$\begin{aligned} \theta^{(j)}_m(x) &= P(Y^{(j)}_m = 1 | X = x) \\ &= \sum_{\forall \overline{y}_{m-1}} P(Y^{(j)}_m = 1 | \overline{Y}^{(j)}_{m-1} = \overline{y}_{m-1}, X = x) \\ &\quad \times \prod_{k=1}^{m-1} P(Y^{(j)}_k = y_k | \overline{Y}^{(j)}_{k-1} = \overline{y}_{k-1}, X = x). \end{aligned}$$

If there are time-dependent confounders, that is, the set $\overline{L}_k$ in (7.1) is not empty, then the causal parameter $\theta_m^{(j)}(x)$ can be identified by the following expression:

$$\begin{aligned}
\theta_m^{(j)}(x) &= P(Y_m^{(j)} = 1|X = x) \\
&= \sum_{\forall \overline{y}_{m-1}, \overline{l}_{m-1}} P(Y_m = 1|\overline{Y}_{m-1} = \overline{y}_{m-1}, \\
&\qquad \overline{L}_{m-1} = \overline{l}_{m-1}, \overline{A}_{m-1} = j^{[m-1]}, X = x) \\
&\qquad \times \prod_{k=1}^{m-1} P(Y_k = y_k|\overline{Y}_{k-1} = \overline{y}_{k-1}, \\
&\qquad \overline{L}_{k-1} = \overline{l}_{k-1}, \overline{A}_{k-1} = j^{[k-1]}, X = x) \\
&\qquad \times P(L_k = l_k|\overline{Y}_k = \overline{y}_k, \overline{L}_{k-1} = \overline{l}_{k-1}, \overline{A}_{k-1} = j^{[k-1]}, X = x),
\end{aligned}$$

where l_k and $\overline{l}_{k-1}$ consist of part elements of $\overline{l}_{m-1}$. Therefore, from the causal parameter $\theta_m^{(j)}(x)$, we can identify the average causal effect $\delta_m(x)$ of continuous exposed versus continuous unexposed in the subpopulation of $X = x$ at the time m.

8. Conclusions

We introduced Yule-Simpson's paradox and then discussed the confounding and confounders. Comparability-based and collapsibility-based criteria can be used to determine non-confounders. Given a sufficient confounder set, these criteria can be used to remove non-confounders from the set. A causal diagram can depicts the confounders more clearly. For a given sufficient confounder set, the standardization, the inverse probability weighting and the propensity score approaches can be used to evaluate the causal effects. The SITA assumption is the key assumption for causal inference, and the sequentially ignorable treatment assignment assumption is required for longitudinal studies. The topic on the surrogate endpoints is introduced in another chapter of this book (Geng, 2013).

Acknowledgements

I would like to thank Professor Jiqian Fang and Professor Hua Jin for their valuable comments and suggestions on the article. The research is supported by Center for Statistical Science, Peking University and NSFC (10931002, 11171365, 10721403, 11021463).

References

1. Bickel, P. J., Hammel, E. A. and O'Connell, J. W. (1975). Sex bias in graduate admissions: data from Berkeley. *Science* **187**, 398–404.
2. Chen, H., Geng, Z. and Jia, J. (2007). Criteria for surrogate end points. *J. Royal Statist. Soc.*, **B 69**, 919–932.
3. Cox, D. R. and Wermuth, N. (2003). A general condition for avoiding effect reversal after marginalization. *J. Royal. Statist. Soc.*, **B 65**, 937–941.
4. Freedman, D., Pisani, R., Purves, R. and Adhikari, A. (1991). *Statistics.* (the second Edition). New York: W. W. Norton & Company, Inc.
5. Geng, Z. (1992). Collapsibility of relative risks in contingency tables with a response variable. *J. Roy. Statist. Soc.* **B 54**, 585–593.
6. Geng, Z. (2013). Surrogates for qualitative evaluation of treatment effects. In Ying, L *et al.* eds., *Advanced Medical Statistics*, 2nd Edn., World Scientific., Singapore.
7. Geng, Z. and Asano, Ch.(1993). Strong collapsibility of association measures in linear models. *J. Royal Statist. Soc.* **B 55**, 741–747.
8. Geng, Z., Guo, J. and Fung, W. (2002). Criteria for confounders in epidemiological studies. *J. Roy. Statist. Soc.* **B 64**, 3–15.
9. Geng, Z., Guo, J., Lau, T. and Fung, W. (2001). Confounding, homogeneity and collapsibility for causal effects in epidemiologic studies. *Statistica Sinica*, **11**, 63–75.
10. Geng, Z. and Li, G. W. (2002). Conditions for non-confounding and collapsibility without knowledge of completely constructed causal diagrams. *Scand. J. Statist.*, **29**, 169–181.
11. Greenland, S., Pearl, J. and Robins, J. M. (1999). Causal diagrams for epidemiologic research. *Epidemiology*, **10**, 37–48.
12. Greenland, S. and Pearl, J. (2011). Adjustments and their consequences — collapsibility analysis using graphical models. *Inter. Statist. Rev.*, **79**, 401–426.
13. Greenland, S. and Robins, J. M. (1986). Identifiability, exchangeability, and epidemiologic confounding. *Int. J. of Epid.*, **15**, 413–419.
14. Greenland, S., Robins, J. and Pearl, J. (1999). Confounding and collapsibility in causal inference. *Statist. Sci.*, **14**, 29–46.
15. Guo, J.H. and Geng, Zhi (1995). Collapsibility of logistic regression coefficients. *J. Royal Statist. Soc.*, **B 57**, 263–267.
16. Holland, P. W. (1986). Statistics and causal inference. *J. Am. Statist. Asso.*, **81**, 945–970.
17. Kleinbaum, D. G., Kupper, L. L. and Morgenstern, H. (1982). *Epidemiologic Research: Principles and Quantitative Methods.* Van Nostr and Reinhold, New York.
18. Ma, Z. M., Xie, X. C. and Geng, Z. (2006). Collapsibility of distribution dependence. *J. Royal Statist. Soc.*, **B 68**, 127–133.
19. Miettinen, O. S. and Cook, E. F. (1981). Confounding: essence and detection. *Am. J. Epid.*, **114**, 593–603.

20. Moore, T. J. (1995). *Deadly Medicine: Why Tens of Thousands of Patients Died in America's Worst Drug Disaster*. Simon & Schuster.
21. Neufeld, E. (1995). Simpson's paradox in artificial intelligence and in real life. *Computational Intelligence*, **11**, 1–10.
22. Neyman, J. (1923). On the application of probability theory to agricultural experiments: Essay on principles, Section 9. Ann. Agric. Sci. Translated in *Statist. Sci.*, 1990, **5**, 465–480.
23. Pearl, J. (1993). Comments: graphical models, causality, and intervention. *Statist. Sci.*, **8**, 266–269.
24. Pearl, J. (1995). Causal diagrams for empirical research (with discussion). *Biometrika*, **83**, 669–710.
25. Pearl, J. (2000). *Causality: Models, Reasoning, and Inference*. Cambridge University Press, Cambridge, England.
26. Reintjes, R., de Boer, A., van Pelt, W., Mintjes-de Groot, J. (2000). Simpson's paradox: an example from hospital epidemiology. *Epidemiology* **11**, 81–83.
27. Robins, J. M. (1986). A new approach to causal inference in mortality studies with sustained exposure periods–application to control of the healthy worker survivor effects. *Math. Modelling*, **7**, 1393–1512.
28. Robins, J. M. (1987). A graphical approach to the identification and estimation of causal parameters in mortality studies with sustained exposure periods. *J. Chronic Disease*, **40 supp.**, 139s–161s.
29. Robins, J. M. (1989). The control of confounding by intermediate variables. *Statist. Medicine*, **8**, 679–701.
30. Robins, J. M. (1997). Causal inference from complex longitudinal data. In Berkane, M. ed., *Latent Variable Modeling and Applications to Causality.* Springer-Verlag, New York. 69–117.
31. Robins, J. M., Greenland, S. and Hu, F. C. (1999). Estimation of the causal effect of a time-varying exposure on the marginal mean of a repeated binary outcome (with discussion). *J. Am. Statist. Asso.*, **94**, 687–712.
32. Robins, J. M., Hernán, R. M. and Brumback, B. (2000). Marginal structural models and causal inference in epidemiology. *Epidemiology*, **11**, 550–560.
33. Rosenbaum, P. R. and Rubin, D. B. (1983). The central role of the propensity score in observational studies for causal effects. *Biometrika*, **70**, 41–55.
34. Rubin, D. B. (1974). Estimating causal effects of treatments in randomized and nonrandomized studies. *J. Educ. Psychology*, **66**, 688–701.
35. Simpson, E. H. (1951). The interpretation of interaction in contingency tables. *J. Roy. Statist. Soc.* **B 13**, 238–241.
36. Spiegelhalter, D. J., Dawid, A. P., Lauritzen, S. L. and Cowell, R. C. (1993). Bayesian analysis in expert systems (with discussion). *Statist. Sci.*, **8**, 219–283.
37. Spirtes, P., Glymour, C. and Scheines, R. (1993). *Causation, Prediction and Search*. Springer, New York.
38. Wagner, C. H. (1982). Simpson's paradox in real life. *The Am. Statist.*, **36**, 46–48.

39. Wang, X., Geng, Z., Chen, H. and Xie, X. (2009). Detecting multiple confounders. *J. Statist Plan. & Inf.*, **139**, 1073–1081.
40. Wermuth, N. (1989). Moderating effects of subgroups in linear models. *Biometrika*, **76**, 81–93.
41. Whittaker, J. (1990). *Graphical Models in Applied Multivariate Statistics.* Wiley, Chichester.
42. Whittemore, A. S. (1978). Collapsibility of multidimensional contingency tables. *J. Roy. Statist. Soc.* **B 40**, 328–340.
43. Wickramaratne, P. J. and Holford, T. R. (1987). Confounding in epidemiologic studies: the adequacy of the control groups as a measure of confounding. *Biometrics* **43**, 751–765.
44. Xie, X., Ma, Z. and Geng, Z. (2008). Some association measurements and their collapsibility. *Statistica Sinica*, **18**, 1165–1183.
45. Yule, G. U. (1903). Notes on the theory of association of attributes in statistics. *Biometrika* **2**, 121–134.

About the Author

Dr. Zhi Geng is Professor of School of Mathematical Sciences, Peking University. He received his B.Sc. degree from Shanghai Jiaotong University, Shanghai, China in 1982, and Ph.D. degree from Kyushu University, Fukuoka, Japan in 1989. He has been a faculty member of Peking University since 1989, ISI elected member since 1996, and associated editor of Comp. Statist. & Data Analysis since 1991. His research interests include causal inference, causal networks and incomplete data analysis.

Section 4

General Methods

CHAPTER 28

SURVIVAL ANALYSIS

D. Y. LIN

Department of Biostatistics, University of North Carolina,
3101E McGavran-Greenberg Hall, CB#7420,
Chapel Hill, NC 27599-7420, USA
Tel: 919-843-5134; lin@bios.unc.edu

1. Introduction

The primary response variables in many medical studies pertain to the time to occurrence of a clinically important event, such as death, development or progression of a disease, or occurrence of a clinically significant morbid event such as a serious infection, stroke or major organ failure. A complexity that frequently arises in studies having time-to-event outcome measures is that a substantial fraction of the study subjects have not experienced the event of interest at the time of data analysis. These subjects who provide this incomplete information are referred to as being censored, or more precisely right-censored, since it is only known that the true time-to-event for that subject exceeds the duration of follow-up.

The complexities created by the presence of censored observations have led to the development of a special field of statistical methodology. Because the analysis of clinical trials data with time-to-death outcomes provided the original motivation for this development, the field has become known as survival analysis. This article provides an overview of the key ideas and methods in survival analysis. After introducing some basic terminology, we will discuss the estimation of the survival distribution, the comparison of two survival distributions as well as regression models. We will focus on non- and semi-parametric methods, which do not impose parametric assumptions on the survival distribution.

2. Basic Concepts

Let T denote the true time-to-event or failure time for a study subject in a medical study. Primary interest usually lies in estimation and testing regarding the distribution of T. This distribution can be characterized by the survival function $S(t) \equiv \Pr(T > t)$. Because of censoring, it is more convenient to deal with the hazard function, which is the instantaneous probability of dying at time t given that the subject is alive just prior to t. If T is continuous with density function f, then the hazard function is defined by

$$\lambda(t) = \lim_{\Delta t \downarrow 0} \Pr(t \leq T < t + \Delta t | T \geq t)/\Delta t = f(t)/S(t) .$$

The function $\Lambda(t) \equiv \int_0^t \lambda(u)du$ is called the cumulative hazard function for T, and it is easily shown that $S(t) = e^{-\Lambda(t)}$ for a continuous survival time T.

Let U denote the censoring time, that is, the time beyond which the study subject cannot be observed. Then (T, U) are referred to as latent data, while the observed data are denoted by (X, δ), where $X = \min(T, U)$, $\delta = I(T \leq U)$, and $I(\cdot)$ is the indicator function. The study subjects having $\delta = 0$ are referred to as having censored observations.

While the distribution function $S(t)$ can be consistently estimated when data are uncensored, neither $\lambda(t)$ nor $S(t)$ is identifiable or consistently estimable if one only observes (X, δ).[18,78] Observing (X, δ) rather than T for all subjects only allows one to consistently estimate $S^{\#}(t) \equiv \exp\{-\int_0^t \lambda^{\#}(u)du\}$ for all t such that $\Pr(X > t) > 0$, where

$$\lambda^{\#}(t) = \lim_{\Delta t \downarrow 0} \Pr(t \leq T < t + \Delta t | T \geq t, U \geq t)/\Delta t . \tag{1}$$

We refer to $\lambda^{\#}(t)$ as the *crude* hazard and $\lambda(t)$ as the *net* hazard.[14] In most survival analysis applications, a key assumption is made regarding the equality of the crude hazard (that is estimable) and the net hazard (that is of interest), i.e.

$$\lambda^{\#}(t) = \lambda(t) \text{ for all } t \text{ such that } \Pr(X > t) > 0 . \tag{2}$$

A sufficient condition for the validity of assumption (2) is the independence of T and U.

3. Estimation of the Survival Distribution

A fundamental problem in survival analysis is the estimation of the hazard function $\lambda(t)$ and the survival function $S(t)$. Several parametric models are available, and the maximum likelihood approach can be used for estimation of the parameters under the assumption of independent censoring. For example, assuming a constant hazard function, i.e. $\lambda(t) = \lambda$ for all $t > 0$, one obtains the exponential distribution, where the maximum likelihood estimator for λ is the number of observed events divided by the summation of duration of follow-up over all subjects. Kalbfleisch and Prentice[37] and Lawless[42] provided detailed discussion of parametric methods.

It is more desirable to estimate the failure time distribution without parametric modelling. Nelson[60] introduced a nonparametric estimator of the cumulative hazard function $\Lambda(t)$. This estimator is given by a step function, with steps occurring at times of observed events and having size D/Y, where D events occur among Y subjects at risk. Recognizing the relationship between $S(t)$ and $\Lambda(t)$ through the differential equation, $-\{dS(t)/dt\}/S(t-) = \lambda(t)$, one motivates the relationship,

$$-\{\Delta\hat{S}(t)\}/\hat{S}(t-) = \Delta\hat{\Lambda}(t)\,,$$

where one estimates $\Lambda(t)$ using Nelson's estimator and then recursively solves for the estimator of $S(t)$. The resulting estimator is that proposed by Kaplan and Meier.[38] It is a step function, with value reduced by the multiplicative factor $\{1 - (D/Y)\}$ at times of observed events. The asymptotic properties of the Kaplan–Meier estimator have been studied by Breslow and Crowley,[9] Gill[30] and Ying[84] among others.

Figure 1 displays the Kaplan–Meier estimates for the survival probabilities in a randomized clinial trial, which was designed to assess whether a new therapy, levamisole plus fluorouracil, prolongs the survival time for patients with Duke's Stage C colon cancer.[47] There are 315 and 304 patients in the observation and therapy groups. By the end of the study, 155 patients in the observation group and 108 patients in the therapy group had died. The Kaplan–Meier estimates given in Fig. 1 show the average survival experiences of the patients in the two groups over the entire follow-up period. Clearly, the patients on the therapy tend to have higher survival probabilities than the patients in the observation group.

4. Counting Process Theory

It is difficult to study the properties of the statistics used in survival analysis, such as the Nelson and Kaplan–Meier estimators, by using standard statistical techniques because they are not sums of independent random variables. Aalen[1] introduced an elegant martingale-based approach

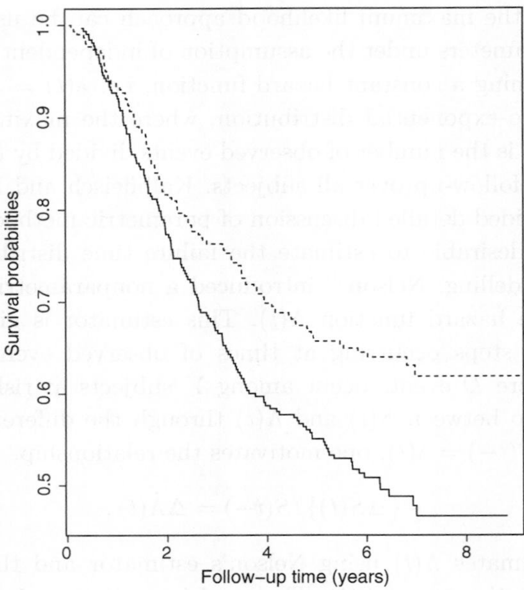

Fig. 1. Kaplan–Meier estimates for the survival probabilities in the colon cancer study: ———: observation groups, - - - - - - - - -: therapy groups.

to survival analysis, where statistical methods can be cast within a unifying counting process framework. This approach uses an integral representation for censored data statistics that provides a simple unified form for estimators, test statistics and regression methods. These martingale methods allow one to obtain simple expressions for moments of complicated statistics and asymptotic distributions for test statistics and estimators, and to examine the operating characteristics of censored data regression methods. Detailed presentation of this approach has been provided in textbooks by Fleming and Harrington[27] and Andersen *et al.*[4]

In the counting process approach for analyzing data on time-to-a-single-event, the data for the ith subject, (X_i, δ_i), is represented as $\{N_i(t), Y_i(t)\}$ $(t > 0)$, where

$$N_i(t) = I(X_i \leq t, \delta_i = 1)\,, \quad \text{and} \quad Y_i(t) = I(X_i \geq t)\,. \tag{3}$$

The right-continuous process $N(t)$ is referred to as the counting process, since it essentially counts the number of events observed up to and including time t, while the left-continuous process $Y(t)$ is referred to as the at-risk process, indicating whether the subject is at risk at time t.

A simple yet important illustration of the counting process approach is provided by examining the properties of the Nelson estimator $\hat{\Lambda}(t)$ of $\Lambda(t)$. The hazard integrated over the region in which one has data is

$$\Lambda^*(t) \equiv \int_0^t I\{\bar{Y}(u) > 0\}\lambda(u)du\,,$$

where $\bar{Y}(t) = \sum_{i=1}^n Y_i(t)$, and n is the sample size. One can write

$$\hat{\Lambda}(t) - \Lambda^*(t) = \sum_{i=1}^n \int_0^t H_i(u)dM_i(u)\,, \tag{4}$$

where $H_i(t) \equiv I\{\bar{Y}(t) > 0\}/\bar{Y}(t)$ is a left-continuous process, and

$$M_i(t) \equiv N_i(t) - \int_0^t Y_i(u)\lambda(u)du \tag{5}$$

is the subject-specific martingale. The martingale M_i in Eq. (5) represents the difference over the interval $(0, t]$ between the observed number and the model-predicted number of events for the ith subject. The left-continuity of the process H_i and the martingale property for M_i render the entire expression in Eq. (4) to be a martingale transform. This structure directly yields moments and large-sample properties. For example, since the martingale M_i has expectation zero, it follows that the Nelson estimator $\hat{\Lambda}(t)$ has expectation $\int_0^t \Pr\{\bar{Y}(u) > 0\}\lambda(u)du$. This martingale-based approach enables an elegant development of the small- and large-sample properties of the Nelson and Kaplan–Meier estimators, as shown by Gill.[29]

5. Two-Sample Statistics

The primary objective of many clinical trials is to provide a reliable comparison of the efficacy and safety of two treatments, where efficacy often is assessed in terms of a time-to-event outcome measure. Similarly, many epidemiologic studies are concerned with the comparisons of exposed and unexposed groups in the time to disease occurrence. A variety of parametric and nonparametric two-sample statistics have been proposed to compare two survival distributions based on censored data. Parametric methods are described by Kalbfleisch and Prentice[37] and Lawless.[42]

The most popular nonparametric two-sample statistic is the so-called logrank statistic, which was originally proposed by Mantel.[55] The subjects at risk at the time of an event are classified into a 2×2 table, according to event status (yes versus no) and group membership. The numerator of the logrank statistic is obtained by computing the observed and the expected (conditioning on the margins of the 2×2 table) events in the first group, and by summing the differences of these over all distinct event times. Within each 2×2 table, the variance of the number of events in the first group is obtained using the hypergeometric distribution. These are then summed over all distinct event times to provide the variance estimator for the logrank statistic. For the colon cancer study mentioned in Sec. 3, the observed chi-squared value of the logrank statistic is 11.2, providing strong evidence for the benefit of the therapy.

The logrank statistic has been extended to a broad class of weighted logrank statistics. Any member of this class can be written as a weighted sum of the "observed minus expected" events in Mantel's 2×2 tables. These statistics can be formulated as in Eq. (4). Using this structure, Gill[29] derived small- and large-sample properties for statistics of this wide class. He developed criteria for consistency of these tests against ordered hazards and stochastic ordering alternatives. He also provided asymptotic distribution results, not only under the null hypothesis of equality of survival distributions, but also under contiguous alternatives, allowing him to provide a characterization of the alternatives against which the tests are efficient. Among these results was a proof that the logrank statistic provides an efficient test under proportional hazards alternatives.

6. Regression Models

In medical studies designed to assess the effect of a treatment or exposure on a time-to-event outcome, it is important to be able to explore or adjust for the effect of an array of other covariates that may be associated with that outcome. Hence, the information collected on each study subject (X, δ) is expanded to be $(X, \delta, \mathbf{Z})$, where $\mathbf{Z}$ represents a p-vector of covariates. The covariates can be treatment indicators or exposure levels; demographic variables, such as age, gender or race; laboratory measurements, such as levels of bilirubin, blood pressure or viral load; histologic assessments based on biopsy; or other descriptive measurements such as time from diagnosis of disease, type of disease, prior therapeutic exposures, or functional status of the subject. In regression models, these covariates can take a variety of functional forms, being dichotomous, ordered or continuous. The continuous variables may be transformations of original measures, such as the logarithm of bilirubin.

The linear regression model for survival time data takes the form

$$\log T = \boldsymbol{\beta}'\mathbf{Z} + \epsilon\,, \tag{6}$$

where $\boldsymbol{\beta}$ is a set of unknown regression parameters, and ϵ is an error variable independent of $\mathbf{Z}$. The logarithmic transformation is employed because T is positive; other appropriate transformations of T may also be selected. Exponentiation of Eq. (6) yields $T = e^{\boldsymbol{\beta}'\mathbf{Z}}T_0$, where $T_0 = e^{\epsilon}$. This expression shows that the role of $\mathbf{Z}$ is to accelerate (or decelerate) the time to failure. Thus, Eq. (6) is referred to as the accelerated failure time model.

Because of censoring, it is more convenient to model the survival data through the hazard function. Let $\lambda(t|\mathbf{Z})$ denote the hazard function associated with $\mathbf{Z}$, i.e.

$$\lambda(t|\mathbf{Z}) = \lim_{\Delta t \downarrow 0} \Pr(t \le T < t + \Delta t | T \ge t, \mathbf{Z})/\Delta t\,.$$

The proportional hazards model specifies that

$$\lambda(t|\mathbf{Z}) = \lambda_0(t)e^{\boldsymbol{\beta}'\mathbf{Z}}\,, \tag{7}$$

where $\lambda_0(t)$ is the so-called baseline hazard function, i.e. the hazard function under $\mathbf{Z} = \mathbf{0}$, and $\boldsymbol{\beta}$ is a set of unknown regression parameters. Under this model, the covariates have multiplicative effects on the hazard function, and the regression parameters are interpreted as the logarithms of the hazard ratios or relative risks.

Equation (6) can be rewritten as

$$\lambda(t|\mathbf{Z}) = \lambda_0(te^{-\boldsymbol{\beta}'\mathbf{Z}})e^{-\boldsymbol{\beta}'\mathbf{Z}}\,, \tag{8}$$

where $\lambda_0(t)$ is the hazard function of T_0. A comparison of Eq. (8) with Eq. (7) reveals that the only overlap in the accelerated failure time and proportional hazards models arises when $\lambda_0(t)$ is Weibull.[37]

In the regression setting, the independent censoring assumption given by Eq. (2) is extended so that, conditional on $\mathbf{Z}$, the crude and net hazard functions are equal. Survival models, such as Eqs. (6) and (6.2), are referred to as parametric models if the distributional form of the failure time, i.e. $\lambda_0(t)$, is specified, and as semiparametric models otherwise. Analysis of parametric survival models has been discussed by Kalbfleisch and Prentice,[37] Lawless,[42] Cox and Oakes,[21] and Andersen *et al.*[4] Due to the complex nature of human diseases, it is difficult to specify the parametric form. Thus, semiparametric models are preferable to parametric models in most medical applications.

7. Cox Proportional Hazards Model

Cox[19,20] introduced an ingenious semiparametric approach to inference based on the proportional hazards model. These methodologic results are among the developments in the field of survival analysis that have had the most profound impact on medical research.

By fitting the proportional hazards model in Eq. (7) with an unspecified baseline hazard function $\lambda_0(t)$, Cox obtained a robust approach for studying the influence of covariates on outcome. However, with an infinite-dimensional nuisance function $\lambda_0(t)$, modifications to the classical likelihood approach would be needed. Thus, Cox[20] introduced the partial likelihood, which is based on the data that does not carry information about $\lambda_0(t)$. Specifically, one discards the times of observed events, and the number of events at those times. Assuming that censoring is independent and is uninformative for $\boldsymbol{\beta}$ (see Definition 4.3.1 of Fleming and Harrington[27]), one also discards the censoring times and the identity of subjects associated with the censored times. The partial likelihood is then based on, for all event times, the identity of the subject(s) failing at each event time, given the number failing and the identity of the subjects at risk at that time. It takes the form

$$L(\boldsymbol{\beta}) = \prod_{i \in \mathcal{D}} \frac{e^{\boldsymbol{\beta}' \mathbf{Z}_{(i)}}}{\sum_{j \in \mathcal{R}_i} e^{\boldsymbol{\beta}' \mathbf{Z}_j}}, \tag{9}$$

where $\mathcal{D}$ is the set of indices of observed event times, $\mathbf{Z}_{(i)}$ is the covariate vector for the subject failing at the ith observed event time T_i^0, and $\mathcal{R}_i$ is the set of subjects at risk at T_i^0. The maximum partial likelihood estimator $\hat{\boldsymbol{\beta}}$ is the value of $\boldsymbol{\beta}$ that maximizes $L(\boldsymbol{\beta})$. Given $\hat{\boldsymbol{\beta}}$, the cumulative baseline hazard function $\Lambda_0(t) \equiv \int_0^t \lambda_0(u)du$ is estimated by the Breslow estimator:[8]

$$\hat{\Lambda}_0(t) \equiv \sum_{i \in \mathcal{D}; T_i^0 \le t} \frac{1}{\sum_{j \in \mathcal{R}_i} e^{\hat{\boldsymbol{\beta}}' \mathbf{Z}_j}}. \tag{10}$$

Cox[19,20] conjectured that $L(\boldsymbol{\beta})$ shares the asymptotic properties of a full likelihood. This conjecture was confirmed by a number of authors. The first published proof was provided by Tsiatis.[78] Andersen and Gill[5] provided an elegant asymptotic theory for $\hat{\boldsymbol{\beta}}$ and $\hat{\Lambda}_0(t)$ by observing that the partial likelihood score function can be formulated as a martingale transform, of the form given in Eq. (4).

The left panel of Table 1 summarizes the results of the Cox regression analysis for the Mayo primary biliary cirrhosis data.[27] The database

Table 1. Regression analysis of the Mayo primary biliary cirrhosis data.

	Proportional Hazards			Accelerated Failure Time		
Parameter	Est	SE	95% conf int	Est	SE	95% conf int
Age	0.039	0.008	(0.024, 0.054)	−0.026	0.004	(−0.035, −0.018)
log(Albumin)	−2.533	0.648	(−3.803, −1.263)	1.656	0.368	(0.934, 2.378)
log(Bilirubin)	0.871	0.083	(0.709, 1.033)	−0.585	0.046	(−0.674, −0.496)
Oedema	0.859	0.271	(0.328, 1.391)	−0.734	0.178	(−1.083, −0.385)
log(Protime)	2.380	0.767	(0.877, 3.883)	−1.944	0.462	(−2.850, −1.038)

contains 418 patients who were referred to the Mayo Clinic. As of the date of data listings, 161 patients had died. The Cox regression analysis not only quantifies the effects of the five covariates on the risk of death but also allows one to estimate the survival probabilities for patients associated with specific covariate values.[48]

8. Multiplicative Intensity Model

In many medical studies, the outcome of primary interest extends beyond the time of the first event to exploration of the rate of recurrent events over time. These recurrent events, for example, may be repeated otitis media infections in an infant, or repeated hospitalizations in an adult with a serious disease. To analyze such data, Aalen[2] introduced the multiplicative intensity model as a generalization of the proportional hazards model. In this model, the subject-specific martingale is

$$M(t) = N(t) - \int_0^t Y(u)\lambda_0(u)e^{\boldsymbol{\beta}'\mathbf{Z}(u)}du\,, \tag{11}$$

where N and Y are of more general forms than given in Eq. (3). Specifically, the counting process $N(t)$ still reflects the number of events that have occurred by time t, but now has range over all non-negative integers. The at-risk process $Y(t)$ can be any left-continuous process indicating, by 1 versus 0, whether or not the subject is at risk at time t. In addition, the covariate vector is allowed to be a stochastic process.

In the semiparametric setting where $\lambda_0(t)$ in Eq. (11) is unspecified, one can use the partial likelihood principle to make inference about $\boldsymbol{\beta}$ and the Breslow estimator to estimate $\Lambda_0(t)$, although now the set $\mathcal{D}$ in Eqs. (9) and (10) may involve multiple event times from the same subject. The corresponding large-sample theory was again provided by Andersen and Gill.[5]

9. Regression Model Diagnostics

Extensive development of residuals has provided a wide variety of model diagnostics that are useful for the Cox proportional hazards model as well as for the broader multiplicative intensity model. For simplicity, we consider the subject-specific martingale in Eq. (5) for the special case of the Cox model given by Eq. (7). The corresponding martingale residual is

$$\hat{M}_i(t) \equiv N_i(t) - \hat{\Lambda}_0(t \wedge X_i)e^{\hat{\boldsymbol{\beta}}'\mathbf{Z}_i},$$

where $a \wedge b = \min(a, b)$. This residual, introduced by Barlow and Prentice[6] and explored by Therneau *et al.*[76] can be interpreted as the "observed" minus "estimated model predicted" events for subject i over the interval $(0, t]$. As $t \to \infty$, the martingale residual reduces to

$$\hat{M}_i \equiv \delta_i - \hat{\Lambda}_0(X_i)e^{\hat{\boldsymbol{\beta}}'\mathbf{Z}_i}.$$

These residuals, symmetrized using the deviance transformation[56] can be used to detect outliers. The partial residuals, defined by

$$\hat{M}_i/\{\hat{\Lambda}_0(X_i)e^{\hat{\boldsymbol{\beta}}'\mathbf{Z}_i}\} + \hat{\beta}_j Z_{ij}, \quad i = 1, \ldots, n; \ j = 1, \ldots, p,$$

where Z_{ij} and $\hat{\beta}_j$ are the jth components of $\mathbf{Z}_i$ and $\hat{\boldsymbol{\beta}}$, can be used to suggest the proper functional form for covariates in the model.

A class of martingale-transform residuals can be obtained by replacing $M_i(u)$ with $\hat{M}_i(u)$ for each i in Eq. (4). Important members of this class are the p "score residuals" for each subject. These residuals are defined by

$$L_{ij} \equiv \int_0^\infty H_{ij}(t)d\hat{M}_i(t), \quad i = 1, \ldots, n; \ j = 1, \ldots, p,$$

where $H_{ij}(t)$ is chosen such that $\sum_i L_{ij}$ reduces to the jth component of the partial likelihood score statistic. These p score residuals can be used to assess the influence of each subject on the parameter estimates $\hat{\beta}_j$ $(j = 1, \ldots, p)$. They are also related to a class of residuals, proposed by Schoenfeld,[74] that are useful for detecting departures from the proportional hazards assumption.

Lin *et al.*[52] studied the cumulative sums of martingale-based residuals over covariates or event times. The distributions of these stochastic processes under the assumed model can be approximated by zero-mean Gaussian processes. Each observed process can then be compared, both graphically and numerically, with a number of realizations from the approximate null distribution by computer simulation. These comparisons enable one to determine objectively whether a seemingly abnormal residual pattern reflects model misspecification or natural random variation. This methodology can be used to assess the functional forms of covariates, the proportional hazards assumption, as well as the overall fit of the model.

10. Alternatives to the Cox Model

Despite the great popularity and versatility of the Cox regression model, there are reasons to explore alternative models. First, the proportional hazards assumption may not be satisfied in some applications. Second, alternative models characterize different aspects of the associations between covariates and survival time. In this section, we describe briefly some alternative semiparametric models.

In contrast to the proportional hazards model, the additive hazards model specifies that covariates have additive rather than multiplicative effects on the hazard function, i.e.

$$\lambda(t|\mathbf{Z}) = \lambda_0(t) + \boldsymbol{\beta}'\mathbf{Z}(t)\,. \tag{12}$$

This model was discussed by Cox and Oakes,[21] Thomas[77] and Breslow and Day.[10] Using the counting-process martingale approach, Lin and Ying[54] obtained closed-form estimators for the regression parameters $\boldsymbol{\beta}$ and the cumulative baseline hazard function $\Lambda_0(t)$.

Semiparametric transformation models take the form

$$h(T) = \boldsymbol{\beta}'\mathbf{Z} + \epsilon\,, \tag{13}$$

where ϵ is a random error with a given distribution function F, and h is a completely unspecified function. If F is the extreme value distribution, then Eq. (13) is the proportional hazards model. If F is the standard logistic function, then Eq. (13) is the proportional odds model, under which the hazard ratio approaches unity as time increases. This class of models was studied by Clayton and Cuzick[17] and Dabrowska and Doksum,[24] and the proportional odds model was studied by Pettitt,[68] Bennet[7] and Murphy *et al.*[59] A significant breakthrough was made by Cheng *et al.*[13] who provided simple and relatively efficient estimators of $\boldsymbol{\beta}$ for all members of Eq. (13).

The semiparametric accelerated failure time model takes the same form as Eq. (13), but with h specified, usually as $h(T) = \log T$, and ϵ unspecified. Various methods of estimation for this model were proposed around 1980. Specifically, Koul *et al.*[39] suggested to include in the least-squares estimator only the uncensored survival times, but to weigh them by the inversed probabilities of being uncensored. The resulting estimator is highly inefficient, especially in the presence of heavy censoring. However, the underlying idea of weighting uncensored observations by their inversed probabilities of being uncensored, to be referred to as the inverse probability of censoring weighting (IPCW) technique, turns out to be extremely useful in many other contexts. In fact, the Cheng *et al.*[13] estimators were based on this idea. A more efficient modification of the least-squares estimator was provided by Buckley and James,[11] which replaces the conditional expectations for the censored survival times by their estimates based on the Kaplan–Meier estimator of the residual lifetime distribution and which involves an iterative estimation scheme analogous to the EM algorithm.[25] Prentice,[69] on the other hand, showed how to adapt the rank estimation method for non-censored data to the censored data setting. The asymptotic properties of the Buckley–James and rank estimators were established in the early 1990's by Tsiatis,[80] Ritov,[72] Wei *et al.*[83] Lai and Ying[40,41] and Ying.[85]

Despite the theoretical advances, semiparametric methods for the accelerated failure time model have not been widely used in medical applications due to the lack of simple and reliable numerical algorithms. Recently, Jin *et al.*[36] provided a practical method for implementing the rank estimators. Using their method, we obtain the results for the accelerated failure time regression of the primary biliary cirrhosis data shown in the right panel of Table 1. These results are based on the log-rank estimating function. Although the conclusions are not qualitatively different, the analysis under the accelerated failure time model provides an alterative and more direct interpretation of the effects of the covariates on the survival time, as compared to the Cox regression analysis.

11. Multivariate Failure Time Data

Under the multiplicative intensity model described in Sec. 8, the risk of a recurrent event for a subject is unaffected by earlier events that occurred to the subject unless time-dependent covariates that capture such dependence are included explicitly in the model. In medical applications, the dependence structures are complex and the forms of time-dependent covariates are unknown. Furthermore, the inclusion of such time-dependent covariates which are part of the response results in biased estimation of the overall treatment effect in a randomized clinical trial. Thus, it would be desirable to model the marginal distribution of the recurrent event times while leaving the dependence structures unspecified.

It is particularly appealing to consider the cumulative mean function $\mu(t) \equiv E\{N^*(t)\}$, where $N^*(t)$ is the number of events that the subject has actually experienced by time t (in the absence of censoring). This function was first considered by Nelson[61] and further studied by Lawless and Nadeau.[43] A number of authors[44, 51, 65] studied the following regression models for the cumulative mean function

$$E\{N^*(t)|\mathbf{Z}\} = \mu_0(t)e^{\boldsymbol{\beta}'\mathbf{Z}}, \tag{14}$$

where $\mu_0(t)$ is an arbitrary baseline mean function, and $\boldsymbol{\beta}$ is a set of regression parameters. If $N^*(t)$ is a (non-homogeneous) Poisson process, then Eq. (14) is equivalent to the intensity model determined by Eq. (11). Although in general N^* is not a Poisson process, the maximum partial likelihood estimator for $\boldsymbol{\beta}$ of Eq. (11) remains consistent and asymptotically normal under Eq. (14). The covariance matrix, however, can no longer be estimated by the inversed information matrix. A sandwich variance estimator has to be used instead.

In the one-sample case, $\mu(t)$ can be consistently estimated by the Nelson estimator. Under model (14), the baseline mean function $\mu_0(t)$ can be consistently estimated by the Breslow estimator, and the covariate-specific mean function can be estimated in a similar fashion.[51] It is particularly informative to display the estimated mean functions for different treatment arms and for specific covariate patterns.

In some medical studies, each subject can potentially experience more than one type of event. Examples include the developments of physical symptoms or diseases in several organ systems (e.g. stroke and cancer) or in several members of the same organ system (e.g. eyes or teeth). Models such as Eqs. (11) and (14) are not applicable since the multiple events on the same subject are of different natures and in fact may not even be ordered.

It is convenient to formulate the marginal distributions of the multiple event times through the proportional hazards models while leaving the dependence structures completely unspecified. Let K denote the number of potential events per subject. The hazard function for the kth event of the ith subject is postulated to take the form

$$\lambda(t|\mathbf{Z}_{ki}) = \lambda_{k0}(t)e^{\boldsymbol{\beta}'\mathbf{Z}_{ki}(t)}, \quad k = 1, \ldots, K; \quad i = 1, \ldots, n, \tag{15}$$

where $\mathbf{Z}_{ki}$ is the covariate vector for the ith subject with respect to the kth event, λ_{k0} $(k = 1, \ldots, K)$ are arbitrary baseline hazard functions, and $\boldsymbol{\beta}$ is a set of regression parameters. In some applications (e.g. an ophthalmologic study involving the left and right eyes), it is natural to impose the restriction that $\lambda_{10} = \cdots = \lambda_{K0}$ wheareas in others (e.g. the setting of multiple diseases) it is necessary to allow the λ_{k0}'s to be different.

If the event times were independent, then the partial likelihood could be easily constructed for $\boldsymbol{\beta}$ of model (15). The resulting estimator turns out to be consistent and asymptotically normal even if the event times are correlated. However, a sandwich variance estimator is again needed to account for the intra-class dependence. This approach was pioneered by Wei *et al.*[82] and further developed by Lee *et al.*,[45] Liang *et al.*[46] and Cai and Prentice[12] among others.

The marginal approach discussed above treats the dependence of related event times as a nuisance. An alternative approach is to explicitly formulate the nature of dependence by the so-called frailty. The term frailty was first introduced by Vaupel *et al.*[81] to illustrate the consequences of a lifetime being generated from several sources of variation. The use of frailty in bivariate survival time data was considered by Clayton.[15] Frailty models were studied extensively in the 1980s by Clayton and Cuzick,[16] Hougaard[34] and Oakes[63] among others. The frailty-model analog of Eq. (15) specifies that the hazard function for the kth event of the ith subject, given the frailty ν_i, takes the form

$$\lambda_{ki}(t|\mathbf{Z}_{ki};\nu_i) = \nu_i \lambda_{k0}(t) e^{\boldsymbol{\beta}'\mathbf{Z}_{ki}(t)}, \tag{16}$$

where ν_i $(i = 1, \ldots, n)$ are independent random variables. Conditional on ν_i, the event times on the ith subject are assumed to be independent.

The parameter vector $\boldsymbol{\beta}$ has a population-average interpretation under model (15) and a subject-specific interpretation under model (16). Models (15) and (16) cannot hold simultaneously unless ν is a positive-stable variable. It is very challenging, both theoretically and computationally, to deal with frailty models such as (16). Major progress was made in the 1990s. In the special case of gamma frailty models, maximum likelihood estimation via the EM algorithm was studied by Nielsen *et al.*,[62] Murphy,[57,58] Andersen *et al.*[3] and Parner[64] among others.

Nonparametric estimation for the multivariate survival function is a fundamental problem in the analysis of multivariate failure time data. Using the IPCW technique, Lin and Ying[53] developed a simple estimator for the special case where there is a common censoring time for all event times of the same subject. Estimation in the general setting has been studied by Dabrowska,[23] Prentice and Cai,[70] and van der Laan[81] among others.

The occurrence of one event (e.g. death) may preclude the development of another (e.g. relapse of cancer). In some applications, such as cause-specific mortality studies, the subject can only experience one of several potential events. This type of data is referred to as competing risks. The simplest solution to this problem is to censor the event time of interest at the time of the competing events, and then apply the standard survival analysis methods such as the logrank test and Cox regression. The results pertain to the so-called cause-specific hazard function, which is given by Eq. (1) with U representing the time to the competing events.

An important limitation of the cause-specific hazard function is that the associated $S^{\#}(t)$ is not a survival function unless the cause of interest is independent of other risks and the other risks could be eliminated without altering the distribution of the cause of interest. Thus, in general the Kaplan–Meier estimator does not pertain to the survival function or disease incidence. Special methods have been developed to estimate disease incidence functions.[26,31,66]

12. Concluding Remarks

We have reviewed many areas of survival analysis in the previous sections. All these methods require the assumption of independent censoring. As discussed in Sec. 2, the survival distribution is not identifiable in the presence of dependent censoring. If one is willing to model certain aspects of the dependent censoring mechanism, then it is possible make inference about the survival distribution under dependent censoring.[50,73]

When the event of interest is asymptomatic, as is the case with cancer progression or HIV infection, the event time cannot be measured exactly, but is rather known to lie in an interval determined by two successive examinations. The resulting data are said to be interval censored. Non- and semi-parametric analysis of such data has been studied by Groeneboom and Wellner,[32] Huang,[35] Lin *et al.*[49] and Rabinowitz *et al.*[71] among others.

The applications of survival analysis methods to medical studies have been greatly facilitated by the developments of software packages. Standard methods such as the Kaplan–Meier estimator, weighted logrank tests, Cox regression and parametric regression with (univariate) right-censored data are now available in virtually all software packages. The multiplicative intensity model and the sandwich variance estimators for models (14) and (15) have been implemented in major packages, such as SAS, S-Plus and STATA. However, most of the newer methods, such as those for the semi-parametric analysis of models (6), (12) and (13), and those mentioned in this section, are not available in software packages.

Further developments are anticipated in many areas of survival analysis. For example, the Cheng *et al.*[13] estimators for Eq. (13) require modelling the censoring distribution, and it would be worthwhile to explore estimation procedures which do not involve such modelling. In the area of multivariate failure time data, efficient estimators for model (15) have yet to be identified, and further theoretical and numerical advances are warranted for model (16). Considerable activities are also expected in the areas of dependent censoring, interval censored data, causal inference, and joint modelling of longitudinal and failure time data. Finally, further expansion of software is anticipated.

References

1. Aalen, O. O. (1975). *Statistical Inference for a Family of Counting Processes.* PhD. Dissertation, University of California, Berkeley.
2. Aalen, O. O. (1978). Nonparametric inference for a family of counting processes. *The Annals of Statistics* **6**: 701–726.
3. Andersen, P. K., Klein, J. P., Knudsen, K. M. and Palacios, R. T. (1997). Estimation of variance in Cox's regression model with shared gamma frailties. *Biometrics* **53**: 1475–1484.
4. Andersen, P. K., Borgan, Ø., Gill, R. D. and Keiding, N. (1993). *Statistical Models Based on Counting Processes.* Springer-Verlag, London.
5. Andersen, P. K. and Gill, R. D. (1982). Cox's regression model for counting processes: A large sample study. *The Annals of Statistics* **10**: 1100–1120.
6. Barlow, W. E. and Prentice, R. L. (1988). Residuals for relative risk regression. *Biometrika* **75**: 65–74.
7. Bennett, S. (1983). Analysis of survival data by the proportional odds model. *Statistics in Medicine* **2**: 273–277.
8. Breslow, N. E. (1972). Contribution to the discussion on the paper by D. R. Cox cited below. *Journal of the Royal Statistical Society* **B34**: 216–217.
9. Breslow, N. E. and Crowley, J. J. (1974). A large sample study of the life table and product limit estimates under random censorship. *The Annals of Statistics* **2**: 437–453.
10. Breslow, N. E. and Day, N. E. (1987). *Statistical Methods in Cancer Research. The Design and Analysis of Cohort Studies* **2**, IARC, Lyon.
11. Buckley, J. and James, I. (1979). Linear regression with censored data. *Biometrika* **66**: 429–436.
12. Cai, J. and Prentice, R. L. (1995). Estimating equations for hazard ratio parameters based on correlated failure time data. *Biometrika* **82**: 151–164.
13. Cheng, S. C., Wei, L. J. and Ying, Z. (1995). Analysis of transformation models with censored data. *Biometrika* **82**: 835–845.
14. Chiang, C. L. (1968). *Introduction to Stochastic Processes in Biostatistics.* John Wiley, New York.
15. Clayton, D. G. (1978). A model for association in bivariate life tables and its application in epidemiological studies of familial tendency in chronic disease incidence. *Biometrika* **65**: 141–151.
16. Clayton, D. G. and Cuzick, J. (1985). Multivariate generalizations of the proportional hazards model (with discussion). *Journal of the Royal Statistical Society* **A148**: 82–117.
17. Clayton, D. G. and Cuzick, J. (1986). The semiparametrics Pareto model for regression analysis of survival times. In *Proceedings of the International Statistical Institute*, International Statistical Institute, Amsterdam, 23. 3-1–18.

18. Cox, D. R. (1959). The analysis of exponentially distributed life-times with two types of failure. *Journal of the Royal Statistical Society* **B21**: 411–421.
19. Cox, D. R. (1972). Regression models and life tables (with discussion). *Journal of the Royal Statistical Society* **B34**: 187–220.
20. Cox, D. R. (1975). Partial likelihood. *Biometrika* **62**: 269–276.
21. Cox, D. R. and Oakes, D. (1984). *Analysis of Survival Data.* Chapman and Hall, London.
22. Cuzick, J. (1985). Asymptotic properties of censored linear rank tests. *The Annals of Statistics* **13**: 133–141.
23. Dabrowska, D. M. (1988). Kaplan–Meier estimate on the plane. *The Annals of Statistics* **16**: 1475–1489.
24. Dabrowska, D. M. and Doksum, K. A. (1988). Partial likelihood in transformation models with censored data. *Scandinavian Journal of Statistics* **15**: 1–23.
25. Dempster, A. P., Laird, N. M. and Rubin, D. (1977). Maximum likelihood estimation for incomplete data via the EM algorithms (with discussion). *Journal of the Royal Statistical Society* **B39**: 1–38.
26. Fine, J. P. and Gray, R. J. (1999). A proportional hazards model for the subdistribution of a competing risk. *Journal of the American Statistical Association* **94**: 496–509.
27. Fleming, T. R. and Harrington, D. (1991). *Counting Processes and Survival Analysis.* Wiley, New York.
28. Gehan, E. A. (1965). A generalized Wilcoxon test for comparing arbitrarily single-censored samples. *Biometrika* **52**: 203–223.
29. Gill, R. D. (1980). *Censoring and Stochastic Integrals.* Mathematical Centre Tracts 124, Mathematisch Centrum, Amsterdam.
30. Gill, R. D. (1983). Large sample behavior of the product-limit estimator on the whole line. *The Annals of Statistics* **11**: 49–58.
31. Gray, R. J. (1988). A class of K-sample tests for comparing the cumulative incidence of a competing risk. *The Annals of Statistics* **16**: 1141–1154.
32. Groeneboom, P. and Wellner, J. A. (1992). *Information Bounds and Nonparametric Maximum Likelihood Estimation.* Birkhäuser, Basel.
33. Harrington, D. P. and Fleming, T. R. (1982). A class of rank test procedures for censored survival data. *Biometrika* **69**: 553–566.
34. Hougaard, P. (1987). Modelling multivariate survival. *Scandinavian Journal of Statistics* **14**: 291–304.
35. Huang, J. (1996). Efficient estimation for the proportional hazards model with interval censoring. *The Annals of Statistics* **24**: 540–568.
36. Jin, Z. Lin, D. Y., Wei, L. J. and Ying, Z. (2003). Rank-based inference for the semiparametric accelerated failure time model. *Biometrika*, in press.
37. Kalbfleisch, J. D. and Prentice, R. L. (1980). *The Statistical Analysis of Failure Time Data.* Wiley, New York.
38. Kaplan, E. L. and Meier, P. (1958). Nonparametric estimator from incomplete observations. *Journal of the American Statistical Association* **53**: 457–481.
39. Koul, H., Susarla, V. and Van Ryzin, J. (1981). Regression analysis with randomly right censored data. *The Annals of Statistics* **9**: 1276–1288.

40. Lai, T. L. and Ying, Z. (1991a). Rank regression methods for left-truncated and right-censored data. *The Annals of Statistics* **19**: 531–556.
41. Lai, T. L. and Ying, Z. (1991b). Large sample theory of a modified Buckley–James estimator for regression analysis with censored data. *The Annals of Statistics* **19**: 1370–1402.
42. Lawless, J. F. (1982). *Statistical Models and Methods for Lifetime Data.* Wiley, New York.
43. Lawless, J. F. and Nadeau, C. (1995). Some simple robust methods for the analysis of recurrent events. *Technometrics* **37**: 158–168.
44. Lawless, J. F., Nadeau, C. and Cook, R. J. (1997). Analysis of mean and rate functions for recurrent events. In *Proceedings of the First Seattle Symposium in Biostatistics*: *Survival Analysis*, eds. D. Y. Lin and T. R. Fleming, Springer-Verlag, New York, 37–49.
45. Lee, E. W., Wei, L. J. and Amato, D. A. (1992). Cox-type regression analysis for large numbers of small groups of correlated failure time observations. In *Survival Analysis*: *State of the Art*; eds. J. P. Klein and P. K. Goel, Kluwer Academic Publishers, Dordrecht, 237–247.
46. Liang, K. Y., Self, S. G. and Chang, Y. C. (1993). Modelling marginal hazards in multivariate failure time data. *Journal of the Royal Statistical Society* **B55**: 441–453.
47. Lin, D. Y. (1994). Cox regression analysis of multivariate failure time data: The marginal approach. *Statistics in Medicine* **13**: 2233–2247.
48. Lin, D. Y., Fleming, T. R. and Wei, L. J. (1994). Confidence bands for survival curves under the proportional hazards model. *Biometrika* **81**: 73–81.
49. Lin, D. Y., Oakes, D. and Ying, Z. (1998). Additive hazards regression with current status data. *Biometrika* **85**: 289–298.
50. Lin, D. Y., Robins, J. M. and Wei, L. J. (1996). Comparing two failure time distributions in the presence of dependent censoring. *Biometrika* **83**: 381–393.
51. Lin, D. Y., Wei, L. J., Yang, I. and Ying, Z. (2000). Semiparametric regression for the mean and rate functions of recurrent events. *Journal of the Royal Statistical Society* **B62**: 711–730.
52. Lin, D. Y., Wei, L. J. and Ying, Z. (1993). Checking the Cox model with cumulative sums of martingale-based residuals. *Biometrika* **80**: 557–572.
53. Lin, D. Y. and Ying, Z. (1993). A simple nonparametric estimator of the bivariate survival function under univariate censoring. *Biometrika* **80**: 573–581.
54. Lin, D. Y. and Ying, Z. (1994). Semiparametric analysis of the additive risk model. *Biometrika* **81**: 61–71.
55. Mantel, N. (1966). Evaluation of survival data and two new rank order statistics arising in its consideration. *Cancer Chemotherapy Report* **50**: 163–170.
56. McCullagh, P. and Nelder, J. (1989). *Generalized Linear Models*, 2nd ed. Chapman and Hall, London.
57. Murphy, S. A. (1994). Consistency in a proportional hazards model incorporating a random effect. *The Annals of Statistics* **22**: 712–731.
58. Murphy, S. A. (1995). Asymptotic theory for the frailty model. *The Annals of Statistics* **23**: 182–198.

59. Murphy, S. A., Rossini, A. J. and van der Vaart, A. W. (1997). Maximum likelihood estimation in the proportional odds model. *Journal of the American Statistical Association* **92**: 968–976.
60. Nelson, W. B. (1969). Hazard plotting for incomplete failure data. *Journal of Qual Technology* **1**: 27–52.
61. Nelson, W. B. (1988). Graphical analysis of system repair data. *Journal of Quality Technology* **20**: 24–35.
62. Nielsen, G. G., Gill, R. D., Andersen, P. K. and Sorensen, T. I. A. (1992). A counting process approach to maximum likelihood estimation in frailty models. *Scandinavian Journal of Statistics* **19**: 25–43.
63. Oakes, D. (1989). Bivariate survival models induced by frailties. *Journal of the American Statistical Association* **84**: 487–493.
64. Parner, E. (1998). Asymptotic theory for the correlated gamma-frailty model. *The Annals of Statistics* **26**: 183–214.
65. Pepe, M. S. and Cai, J. (1993). Some graphical displays and marginal regression analyses for recurrent failure times and time dependent covariates. *Journal of the American Statistical Association* **88**: 811–820.
66. Pepe, M. S. and Mori, M. (1993). Kaplan–Meier, marginal or conditional probability curves in summarizing competing risks failure time data? *Statistics in Medicine* **12**: 737–751.
67. Peto, R. and Peto, J. (1972). Asymptotically efficient rank invariant test procedures (with discussion). *Journal of the Royal Statistical Society* **A135**: 185–206.
68. Pettitt, A. N. (1982). Inference for the linear model using a likelihood based on ranks. *Journal of the Royal Statistical Society* **B44**: 234–243.
69. Prentice, R. L. (1978). Linear rank tests with right censored data. *Biometrika* **65**: 167–179.
70. Prentice, R. L. and Cai, J. (1992). Covariance and survival function estimation using censored multivariate failure time data. *Biometrika* **79**: 495–512.
71. Rabinowitz, D., Tsiatis, A. and Aragon, J. (1995). Regression with interval censored data. *Biometrika* **82**: 501–513.
72. Ritov, Y. (1990). Estimation in a linear regression model with censored data. *The Annals of Statistics* **18**: 303–328.
73. Robins, J. M. and Rotnitzky, A. (1992). Recovery of information and adjustment for dependent censoring using surrogate markers. In *AIDS Epidemiology: Methodological Issues*, eds. N. P. Jewell, K. Dietz and V. T. Farewell, Birkhäuser, Boston, 297–331.
74. Schoenfeld, D. (1982). Partial residuals for the proportional hazards regression model. *Biometrika* **69**: 239–241.
75. Tarone, R. E. and Ware, J. (1977). On distribution-free tests for equality of survival distributions. *Biometrika* **64**: 156–160.
76. Therneau, T., Grambsch, P. and Fleming, T. R. (1990). Martingale-based residuals for survival models. *Biometrika* **77**: 147–160.
77. Thomas, D. C. (1986). Use of auxiliary information in fitting nonproportional hazards models. In *Modern Statistical Methods in Chronic Disease Epidemiology*, eds. S. H. Moolgavkar and R. L. Prentice, Wiley, New York, 197–210.

78. Tsiatis, A. A. (1975). A nonidentifiability aspect of the problem of competing risks. *Proceedings of the National Academy of Science USA* **72**: 20–22.
79. Tsiatis, A. A. (1981). A large sample study of Cox's regression model. *The Annals of Statistics* **9**: 93–108.
80. Tsiatis, A. A. (1990). Estimating regression parameters using linear rank tests for censored data. *The Annals of Statistics* **18**: 354–372.
81. van der Laan, M. J. (1996). Efficient estimation in the bivariate censoring model and repairing NPMLE. *the Annals of Statistics* **24**: 596–627.
82. Vaupel, J. W., Manton, K. G. and Stallard, E. (1979). The impact of heterogeneity in individual frailty on the dynamics of mortality. *Demography* **16**: 439–454.
83. Wei, L. J., Lin D. Y. and Weissfeld, L. (1989). Regression analysis of multivariate incomplete failure time data by modeling marginal distributions. *Journal of the American Statistical Association* **84**: 1065–1073.
84. Wei, L. J., Ying, Z. and Lin, D. Y. (1990). Linear regression analysis of censored survival data based on rank tests. *Biometrika* **77**: 845–851.
85. Ying, Z. (1989). A note on the asymptotic properties of the product-limit estimator on the whole line. *Statisitics and Probability Letters* **7**: 311–314.
86. Ying, Z. (1993). A large sample study of rank estimation for censored regression data. *The Annals of Statistics* **21**: 76–99.

About the Author

Dr Danyu Lin received his Bachelor degree from East China Normal University, Shanghai, in 1983, Ph.D degree in Biostatistics at University of Michigan, Ann Arbor, in 1989. He was a professor at the University of Washington before joining the Department of Biostatistics, University of North Carolina at Chapel Hill in 2001. Dr. Lin is the Dennis Gillings Distinguished Professor of Biostatistics. He is primarily interested in developing statistical methods for the designs and analyses of medical and public health studies, including genetic association studies. His current research focuses on two areas: statistical methods and computer programs for genetic association studies. Dr. Lin in particularly interested in genome-wide association studies (GWAS) and next-generation sequencing studies; (2) semiparametric regression models and associated inference procedures for potentially censored survival (failure) times. Dr. Lin is particularly interested in transformation models and accelerated failure time models and seek efficient inference procedures based on nonparametric maximum likelihood and related approaches. For his distinguished contribution, Dr. Lin received numerous awards including the Mortimer Spiegelman Award from the American Public Health Association (APHA).

CHAPTER 29

NONPARAMETRIC REGRESSION MODELS FOR THE ANALYSIS OF LONGITUDINAL DATA

COLIN O. WU* and XIN TIAN†

Office of Biostatistics Research
National Heart Lung and Blood Institute,
Bethesda, MD 20892, U.S.A
**wuc@nhlbi.nih.gov*
†tianx@nhlbi.nih.gov

KAI F. YU

Department of Mathematical Sciences and
Mathematical Sciences Center
Tsinghua University, Beijing 100084, P.R.China
kfyu@math.tsinghua.edu.cn

and

MI-XIA WU

College of Applied Sciences
Beijing University of Technology,
Beijing 100124, P.R.China
wumixia@bjut.edu.cn

1. Introduction

1.1. *Scientific objectives of longitudinal studies*

In biomedical studies interests are often focused on evaluating the effects of treatments, medication dosage, risk factors or other biological or environmental covariates on the outcomes of interest, such as disease progression and change of health status, over time. Because the changes of outcomes and covariates over time within each subject usually provide important information of scientific relevance, longitudinal samples that contain repeated measurements of the subjects over time are often more preferable than the classical cross-sectional samples. By combining the characteristics of random sampling and time series observations, the usefulness of longitudinal samples goes far beyond biomedical studies, and their trace is often found in economics, psychology, sociology and many other fields of natural and social sciences.

In general, there are two main approaches for obtaining longitudinal observations in biomedical studies: (a) clinical trials with repeated measurements, and (b) epidemiological studies, which are often referred as observational cohort studies. The main difference between a clinical trial and an observational cohort study is at their designs. In a clinical trial, the selection of subjects, randomized study treatments, length of the trial period, visiting times and methods of the measurement process are determined by the study investigators, although, in some occasions, non-randomized concomitant treatments or interventions may also be given to some subjects due to ethical and logistical reasons. An observational cohort study, on the other hand, is more complicated, because the risk factors, treatments and the measurement process depend on the participants of the study and are not controlled by the investigators.

In a longitudinal clinical trial, the main scientific objective is to evaluate the efficacy of the experimental treatments versus placebo or standard treatment on the primary outcomes, such as certain health status indicators, over time during the trial period. In many situations, a follow-up period is added at the end of the treatment period, so that time-to-event variables, such as time to hospitalization or death, may be included as a primary outcome in addition to the repeatedly measured health outcomes. In a particular analysis, the trial period may be defined based on the objectives of the analysis. For example, if the objective is to evaluate the treatment effects on the time-trend of a health indicator within the treatment period, it is appropriate to consider the treatment period as the trial period. On the other hand, if it is also of interest to consider certain time-to-event variables beyond the treatment period, it is then appropriate to include both the treatment period and the follow-up period into the trial period. Effects of the study treatments may be evaluated through the conditional means, conditional distributions or conditional quantiles of the outcome variables. Although regression models based on conditional means of the outcome variables are by far the most popular methods used in the analysis of longitudinal clinical trials, regression methods based on conditional distributions or conditional quantiles are often valuable statistical tools in situations when the outcome variables have highly skewed or other distributions that are not easily approximated by normality. In addition to the evaluation of randomized study treatments, an important secondary objective is to evaluate the effects of concomitant interventions or other covariates on the time-varying trends of the outcome variables. Regression analyses involving covariates other than the randomized study treatments are often useful for evaluating treatment-covariate interactions or identifying sub-groups of patient populations to whom the experimental treatments are effective.

In a longitudinal observational cohort study, there are no randomized experimental treatments to be tested, and the main objective is to evaluate the potential associations of various covariates, such as demographic and environmental factors, with the outcome variables of interest and their trends over time. Observational cohort studies are often used for the purpose of data exploration, so that more specific scientific hypotheses may be generated and tested in a future properly designed clinical trial. Because the variables are repeatedly measured over time, long-term longitudinal observational cohort studies are useful for understanding the natural progression of certain diseases both on a population-wide level and for certain subsets of subjects. In practice, an observational cohort study usually involves a large number of subjects with sufficient numbers of repeated measurements over time, so that novel findings with adequate statistical accuracy can be obtained from the study. Similar to longitudinal clinical trials, the choices of statistical approaches for the analysis of data from observational cohort studies depend on the scientific objectives, and may involve regression models for the conditional means and conditional distributions.

1.2. *Structures of longitudinal data*

For a typical framework of longitudinal data, we define t to be a real-valued variable of time, $Y(t)$ a real-valued outcome variable and $\mathbf{X}(t) = \big(X^{(0)}(t), \ldots, X^{(K)}(t)\big)^T$, $K \geq 1$, a R^{K+1}-valued covariate vector at time t. Depending on the choice of origin, the time variable t is not necessarily non-negative. As part of the general methodology, interest of statistical analysis with regression models is often focused on modeling and determining the effects of $\big\{t, \mathbf{X}(t)\big\}$ on the population means, subject-specific deviations from the population means, conditional distributions or conditional quantiles of $Y(t)$. For n randomly selected subjects and each subject repeatedly measured over time, the longitudinal sample of $\big\{Y(t), t, \mathbf{X}(t)\big\}$ is denoted by $\{(Y_{ij}, t_{ij}, \mathbf{X}_{ij}); i = 1, \ldots, n,\ j = 1, \ldots, n_i\}$, where t_{ij} is the jth measurement time of the ith subject, Y_{ij} and $\mathbf{X}_{ij} = \big(X_{ij}^{(0)}, \ldots, X_{ij}^{(D)}\big)^T$ are the observed outcome and covariate vector, respectively, of the ith subject at time t_{ij}, and n_i is the ith subject's number of repeated measurements. The total number of measurements for the study is $N = \sum_{i=1}^{n} n_i$. In contrast to the independent identically distributed (i.i.d.) samples in classical cross-sectional studies, the measurements within each subject are possibly correlated, although the inter-subject measurements are assumed to be independent.

A longitudinal sample is said to have a balanced design if all the subjects have their measurements made at a common set of time points, i.e. $n_i = m$ for some $m \geq 1$ and all $i = 1, \ldots, n$ and $t_{1j} = \cdots = t_{nj}$ for all $j = 1, \ldots, m$. An unbalanced design arises if the design time points $\mathbf{t}_i = \{t_{ij}; 1 \leq j \leq n_i\}$ are different for different subjects. In practice, unbalanced designs may be caused by the presence of missing observations in an otherwise balanced design or by the random variations of the time design points. In long-term clinical trials or epidemiological studies, study subjects are often assigned to a set of prespecified "design visiting times", but their actual visiting times could be different from the "design visiting times" because of missing visits or changing visiting times due to various reasons. It is possible to observe balanced longitudinal data from a well-controlled longitudinal clinical trial, because the randomized study treatments and clinical visiting times are determined by the study investigators. However, for various reasons that are out of the investigators' control, most observational cohort studies have unbalanced longitudinal designs.

1.3. *Examples of longitudinal studies*

These real-life examples, three epidemiological studies and a longitudinal clinical trial, illustrate some typical features and scientific objectives of longitudinal studies. Although these examples share some similarities in study designs, they have different data structures and objectives.

Example 1. Alabama Small-for-Gestational-Age Study (ASGA)

This is a prospective study of risk factors and intrauterine growth retardation involving 1475 women who had their fetal anthropometry measurements made by ultrasound repeatedly during pregnancy. All women were scheduled to have their measurements made at approximately 17, 25, 31 and 36 weeks of gestation. In the dataset, however, their actual clinical visit times do not exactly follow this schedule and are scattered between 12 to 43 weeks of gestation. The numbers of visits range between 1 and 7 during pregnancy. This results in an unbalanced design that not all the subjects have measurements at the same time design points. Associated covariates that may affect fetal development include maternal behavioral factors, such as cigarette smoking, alcohol consumption and drug abuse, and maternal anthropometric measurements, such as pre-pregnancy weight, height and body mass index, and placental development measured by placental thickness at different stages of gestation. Some of these covariates, such as the maternal anthropometric measurements are time-dependent. But, the others, such as maternal behavioral factors, may be either time-dependent or time-invariant, depending on how these variables are defined in an analysis. The outcome variables of fetal development, which, of course, are all time-dependent, include fetal abdominal circumference, biparietal diameter, femur length and other ultrasound measurements.

Figure 1 shows the observed fetal abdominal circumferences (in centimeters) at their corresponding gestational age in weeks. To see the temporal

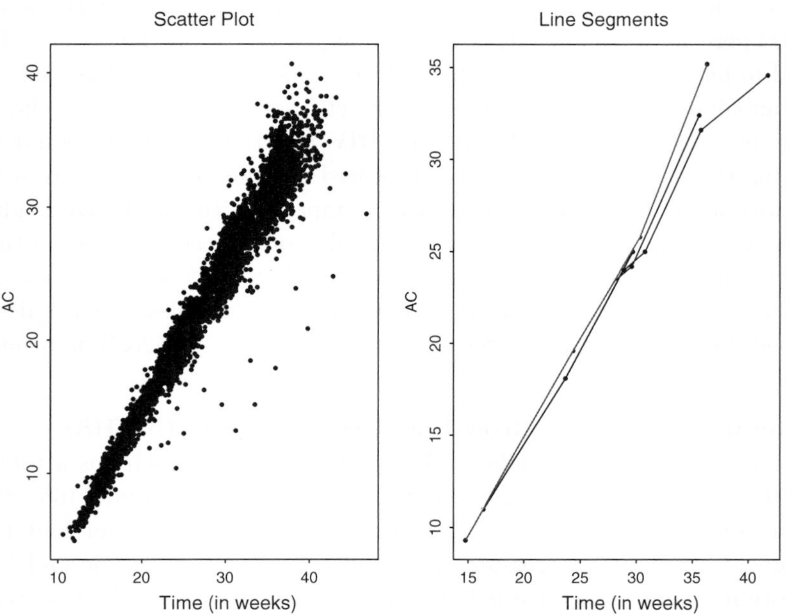

Fig. 1. Relationship between fetal abdominal circumference (in centimeters) and fetal gestation (in weeks). Left Panel: individual measurement; Right Panel: sequences of measurements for some randomly selected subjects.

trend of the individual repeated measurements, the line segments indicate the measurement sequences for three randomly selected subjects. Heuristically, we observe a linear upward trend on the growth of fetal size. But, there has been no prior study which justifies the goodness of a linear growth model for this population or any other statistical model on the covariate effects on fetal growth. A statistical analysis should then focus on two objectives: establishing an appropriate statistical model so that the effects of these covariates on the outcome of interest can be clearly interpreted; developing estimation and inference procedures to adequately quantify the covariate effects based on the chosen statistical models.

Example 2. Baltimore Multicenter AIDS Cohort Study (BMACS)

This dataset is from the Baltimore site of the Multicenter AIDS Cohort Study (MACS), and includes 400 homosexual men who were infected by the human immunodeficiency virus (HIV) between 1984 and 1991. Because CD4 cells (T-helper lymphocytes) are vital for immune function, an important component of the study is to evaluate the effects of risk factors, such as cigarette smoking and drug use, and health status, such as CD4 cell levels before the infection, on the post-infection depletion of CD4 percent (CD4 percent of lymphocyte cells). Although all the individuals were scheduled to have their measurements made at semi-annual visits, the study has an unbalanced design because the subjects' actual visiting times did not exactly follow the schedule and the HIV infections happened randomly during the study. The numbers of repeated measurements range from 1 to 14 with a median of approximately 6. Compared with the ASGA Study of Example 1, this dataset has a smaller number of subjects and a wider range of repeated measurements. The covariates of interest in these data also include both time-dependent and time-invariant variables. Further details of the statistical design and scientific importance of the MACS data can be found in Kaslow *et al.* (1987).

Example 3. National Growth and Health Study (NGHS)

This is a 3-center population-based cohort study, which has a total of 2379 girls, among them 1213 (51%) African-Americans and 1166 (49%) Caucasians, who were 9 or 10 years old at enrollment and had their height, weight, blood pressure (BP) and other anthropometric and laboratory measurements recorded once a year until they reached 19 years old. The main objective of the study is to evaluate the patterns of obesity and cardiovascular risks during childhood and adolescence. The three centers, University of California, Berkeley, University of Cincinnati/Cincinnati

Children's Hospital Medical Center, and Westat, Rockville, Maryland, were selected on the basis of census tract data to include a wide distribution of household income and parental education within each race. Observations were collected at clinical centers or home visits between 1986 and 1997 based on a standard protocol (NGHSRG, 1992), which contained the scientific objectives, justifications, study design and methods of measurements.

Major findings of the study have been reported, for example, in Daniels *et al.* (1998), Kimm *et al.* (2000, 2001, 2002), Thompson *et al.* (2007) and Obarzanek *et al.* (2010). Among these results, Daniels *et al.* (1998) studied the longitudinal mean effects of race, height and body mass index (BMI, measured in kg/m^2) on the levels of systolic blood pressure (SBP) and diastolic blood pressure (DBP). Kimm *et al.* (2000, 2001, 2002) studied the effects of race on obesity, and the relationship between the changes in physical activity and BMI. Thompson *et al.* (2007) investigated the associations between childhood overweight and cardiovascular disease risk factors such as hypertension and unhealthy levels of low-density lipoprotein cholesterol (LDL) and triglyceride (TG), and Obarzanek *et al.* (2010) investigated the effects of race, obesity, and a range of socioeconomical and nutritional variables on the prevalence and incidence rates of hypertension and prehypertension as defined in NHBPEP Working Group (2004). The statistical methods used by these authors depend on summarizing the effects of childhood obesity and other variables on the cardiovascular risk variables through their conditional-means or the probabilities of unhealthy risk levels specified by certain threshold values. Although these results present some useful snapshots of the harmful effects of childhood obesity on cardiovascular risks, a further question is whether similar associations between childhood obesity and cardiovascular risks still hold if other definitions of unhealthy risk levels are used. It is desirable to have a flexible conditional-distribution based regression method so that the covariate effects on the entire distribution of a risk variable are described. This study gives a typical example that motivates the development of longitudinal estimation and inference methods based on conditional distributions and conditional quantiles, instead of the usual regression methods based on conditional means.

Example 4. Enhancing Recovery in Coronary Heart Disease (ENRICHD) Study

This study is a randomized clinical trial that evaluated the efficacy of a cognitive behavior therapy (CBT) versus usual cardiological care (UC) on survival and depression severity in 2481 patients who had depression and/or low perceived social support after acute myocardial infarction. Details of the study design, objectives, and major findings of the trial have been described in ENRICHD (2001, 2003). The primary objective of the study is to determine whether mortality and recurrent myocardial infraction are reduced by treatment of depression and low perceived social support with cognitive behavior therapy, supplemented with the use of selective serotonin reuptake inhibitor (SSRI) or other antidepressants as needed, in patients enrolled within 28 days after myocardial infarction (MI). The intervention of the trial consists of cognitive behavior therapy initiated at a median of 17 days after the index of MI for a median of 11 individual sessions throughout 6 months. Depression severity was measured by Hamilton Rating Scale for Depression (HRSD) and Beck Depression Inventory (BDI) with higher HRSD and BDI scores indicating worsened depression severity. Group therapy was conducted when feasible, with antidepressants, such as SSRIs, as a pharmacotherapy for patients scoring higher than 24 on the HRSD or having a less than 50% reduction in BDI scores after 5 weeks. Antidepressants were also prescribed at the requests of the patients or their primary-care physicians, therefore, could be treated as a concomitant treatment in addition to the randomized CBT psychosocial treatment or usual cardiological care specified in the trial design. The main outcome measures consist of a composite primary end point of death or recurrent MI, and secondary outcomes including change in HRSD and BDI for depression or the ENRICHD Social Support Instrument scores for low perceived social support at 6 months (ENRICHD, 2001 and 2003).

In addition to the primary objective of the trial, an important question of secondary objective is whether the use of antidepressants has added benefits for reducing mortality and recurrent MI and lowering the BDI scores for this patient population. To evaluate the effects of pharmacotherapy with the use of antidepressants, Taylor *et al.* (2005) compared the survival rates for death and cardiovascular morbidity and mortality among 1834 depressed patients in this trial and found that the use of SSRIs seemed to reduce subsequent cardiovascular morbidity and mortality. Bang and Robins (2005) analyzed the same data but only with a cross-sectional component. By treating the patient's starting time of pharmacotherapy as a subject-specific "change-point time" and evaluating the effects of pharmacotherapy on the patient's BDI scores over time using different model patterns before and after the "change-point", Wu, Tian and Bang (2008) and Wu, Tian and Jiang (2011) showed that the use of SSRIs was beneficial for lowering the patient's depression severity measured by the BDI scores.

This study is used throughout Section 5 as a motivating example for the development of appropriate regression models and their estimation and inference procedures for situations when some of the time-dependent covariates are adaptive depending on the outcome trajectories at previous time points. In such situations, where some time-dependent covariates are adaptive to the previous outcome trajectories, the commonly used parametric or nonparametric mixed-effects models may be misspecified and lead to biased and erroneous conclusions.

1.4. *Regression models for longitudinal analysis*

Generally speaking, a proper longitudinal analysis should achieve at least three objectives:

(1) The model under consideration must give an adequate description of the scientific relevance of the data and be sufficiently simple and flexible to be practically implemented. In biomedical studies, an appropriate regression model should give a clear and meaningful biological interpretation and also has a simple mathematical structure.
(2) The methodology must contain proper model diagnostic tools to evaluate the validity of a statistical model for a given data set. Two important diagnostic methods are confidence regions and tests of statistical hypotheses.
(3) The methodology must have appropriate theoretical and practical properties, and can adequately handle the possible intra-subject correlations of the data. In practice, the intra-subject correlations are often completely unknown and difficult to be adequately estimated, so that it is generally preferred to use estimation and inference procedures that do not depend on modeling the specific correlation structures.

1.4.1. *Parametric models*

Naturally, the most commonly used approach in longitudinal analysis is through parametric regression models, such as the generalized linear and nonlinear mixed-effects models. The simplest case of these models is the marginal linear model of the form

$$Y_{ij} = \sum_{l=0}^{K} \beta_l X_{ij}^{(l)} + \epsilon_i(t_{ij}), \tag{1.1}$$

where $\beta_0, \ldots, \beta_K$ are constant linear coefficients describing the effects of the corresponding covariates, $\epsilon_i(t)$ are realizations of a mean zero stochastic process $\epsilon(t)$ at t and $\mathbf{X}_{ij}$ and $\epsilon_i(t_{ij})$ are independent. Similar to all regression models where a constant intercept term is desired, we set $X^{(0)} \equiv 1$, which produces a baseline coefficient β_0, representing the mean value of $Y(t)$ when all the covariates $X^{(l)}(t)$ are set to zero. A popular special case of the error process is to take $\epsilon(t)$ to be a mean zero Gaussian stationary process. Although (1.1) appears to be overly simplified for many practical situations, its generalizations lead to many useful models which form the bulk of longitudinal analysis.

Estimation and inference methods based on parametric models, including the weighted least squares, the quasi-likelihoods and the generalized estimating equations, have been extensively investigated in the literature. The details can be found, for example, in Laird and Ware (1982), Pantula and Pollock (1985), Ware (1985), Liang and Zeger (1986), Diggle (1988), Zeger, Liang and Albert (1988), Jones and Ackerson (1990), Jones and Boadi-Boteng (1991), Davidian and Giltinan (1995), Vonesh and Chinchilli (1997), Verbeke and Molenberghs (2000) and Diggle, Heagerty, Liang and Zeger (2002). The main advantage of parametric models is that they generally have simple and intuitive interpretations. User friendly computer programs are already available in most popular statistical software packages, such as SAS, STATA and R. However, these models suffer the potential shortfall of model misspecification, which may lead to erroneous conclusions. At least in exploratory studies, it is necessary to relax some of the parametric restrictions.

1.4.2. *Semiparametric models*

A useful semiparametric model, investigated by Zeger and Diggle (1994) and Moyeed and Diggle (1994), is the partially linear model of the form

$$Y_{ij} = \beta_0(t_{ij}) + \sum_{l=1}^{K} \beta_l X_{ij}^{(l)} + \epsilon_i(t_{ij}), \tag{1.2}$$

where $\beta_0(t)$ is an unknown smooth function of t, β_l are unknown constants and $\epsilon_i(t)$ and $\mathbf{X}_{ij}$ are defined in (1.1). This model is more general than the marginal linear model (1.1), because $\beta_0(t)$ is allowed to change with t, rather than setting to be a constant over time. On the other hand, by including the linear terms of $X_{ij}^{(l)}$, (1.2) is also more general than the nonparametric regression studied by Hart and Wehrly (1986), Altman (1990), Hart (1991),

Rice and Silverman (1991), among others, which involves only (t_{ij}, Y_{ij}). However, because (1.2) describes the effects of $X_{ij}^{(l)}$ on Y_{ij} through constant linear coefficients, this model is still, to some degree, based on mathematical convenience rather than scientific relevance. For example, there is no reason to expect that the influences of maternal risk factors on fetal development in the ASGA Study or the effects of cigarette smoking and pre-infection CD4 level on the post-infection CD4 cell percent in the HIV/CD4 Depletion Data are linear and constant throughout the study period. Thus, further generalization of (1.2) is needed in many situations.

1.4.3. *Nonparametric models*

Although it is possible in principle to model $\{Y_{ij}, t_{ij}, \mathbf{X}_{ij}\}$ through a completely nonparametric high dimensional function, such approach is often impractical due to the well-known problem of "curse of dimensionality". Moreover, numerical results obtained from high dimensional nonparametric fittings are often difficult to interpret. These problems motivate the consideration of nonparametric models that have certain meaningful structures. An important class of structural nonparametric regression models is the varying-coefficient models of the form

$$Y_{ij} = \mathbf{X}_{ij}^T \beta(t_{ij}) + \epsilon_i(t_{ij}), \tag{1.3}$$

where $\beta(t) = (\beta_0(t), \ldots, \beta_K(t))^T$ is a $(K+1)$-vector of smooth functions of t and $\epsilon_i(t)$ and $\mathbf{X}_{ij}$ are defined as in (1.1). Because (1.3) gives a linear model between $Y(t)$ and $\mathbf{X}(t)$ at each fixed t, the linear coefficients $\beta_l(t)$, $l = 0, \ldots, K$, can be interpreted the same way as in (1.2). Taking $X_{ij}^{(0)} \equiv 1$, $\beta_0(t)$ represents the intercept at time t. On the other hand, because all the linear coefficients may change with t, we may obtain different linear models at different time points. Model (1.3) is a special case of the general varying-coefficient models discussed by Hastie and Tibshirani (1993).

Methods of estimation and inferences based on this class of models have been subjected to intense investigation in the literature. A number of different smoothing methods for the estimation of $\beta(t)$ have been proposed. These include the ordinary least squares local polynomials, the penalized least squares, the two-step and componentwise methods and the basis approximation approaches. Targeted to specific types of longitudinal designs, each of these methods has its own advantages and disadvantages in practice. We will present in Section 3.2 and Section 3.3 an overview of the above estimation and inference methods and demonstrate in Section 3.4 the applications of these methods.

1.4.4. *Regression models for conditional distributions*

In addition to the regression models described above, which are mostly based on modeling the conditional means of the repeatedly measured outcome variables, regression models based on conditional distributions are often used in longitudinal analysis when the response variables are not normally distributed. Well-known approaches with non-Gaussian data, such as the generalized linear models (e.g., Molenberghs and Verbeke, 2005), are often used for discrete outcome variables or the discretized versions of continuous outcome variables defined by some prespecified threshold values. In some situations when the outcome variable has non-Gaussian conditional distributions, a known transformation, such as the Box-Cox transformation, may be applied so that the conditional distribution of the transformed variable is approximately normal. In many situations, however, there are no appropriate threshold values or transformations for the outcome variables being considered, and the scientific objectives are better studied by directly modeling the conditional distributions.

Nonparametric estimation of conditional distribution functions for independent identically distributed data and certain time series samples without incorporating any modeling structures has been studied by Hall, Wolff and Yao (1999) based on two kernel-based smoothing methods, namely the local logistic estimation method and the adjusted Nadaraya-Watson method. Since the estimation methods based on unstructured nonparametric models could be numerically unstable when the number of covariates is large and the corresponding results are often difficult to interpret, Wu, Tian and Yu (2010) proposed a dimension-reduction strategy by extending the linear transformation modeling structures studied by Cheng, Wei and Ying (1995, 1997) to longitudinal data, and studied a time-varying linear transformation model with a two-step local polynomial method for the estimation of covariate effects and conditional distributions. As a result, the time-varying transformation models proposed by Wu, Tian and Yu (2010) give a flexible and convenient structural nonparametric framework for characterizing the conditional distributions of the outcome variables, when the conditional-mean based regression models are insufficient for the scientific objectives of the study. Applying this conditional-distribution based structural nonparametric modeling approach to the NGHS data of Example 3, the statistical estimates, predictions and their inferences presented in Section 4 yield useful insights on the temporal trends of blood pressure for children and adolescents.

2. An Overview of Parametric and Semiparametric Methods

2.1. *Linear mixed-effects models*

As a popular regression approach for modeling the covariate effects on the longitudinal outcome variables, the mixed-effects models generally serve two purposes: (i) describing the effects of the treatments and other factors on the mean response profile; (ii) describing the differences in response profiles between individuals. A regression model serving the first purpose is generally classified as a marginal model or a population average model. A regression model serving the second purpose is a random effects model or a subject specified model (e.g. Zeger, Liang and Albert, 1988). A mixed effects model then combines both the marginal and random effects. In particular, a linear mixed effects model is obtained when the marginal and random effects are additive and follow a linear relationship.

It is convenient to describe the model through a matrix representation. Let $\mathbf{Y}_i = (Y_{i1}, \ldots, Y_{in_i})^T$ be the $[n_i \times 1]$ vector of the response for the ith subject, $t_i = (t_{i1}, \ldots, t_{in_i})^T$ be the subject's time design points and $\mathbf{X}_i$ be the corresponding $[n_i \times (k+1)]$ covariate matrix whose jth row, for $j = 1, \ldots, n_i$, is $\big(1, X_{ij}^{(1)}, \ldots, X_{ij}^{(k)}\big)$. Assuming that the error term $\epsilon_i(t)$ of (1.1) is a mean zero Gaussian process with covariate matrix $\mathbf{V}_i(t_i)$, the responses $\mathbf{Y}_i$ are then independent Gaussian random vectors such that

$$\mathbf{Y}_i \sim \mathbf{N}\left(\mathbf{X}_i \beta, \mathbf{V}_i(t_i)\right), \tag{2.1}$$

where $\beta = (\beta_0, \ldots, \beta_k)^T$ with β_j being defined in (1.1) and $\mathbf{N}(\mathbf{a}, \mathbf{b})$ denotes a multivariate normal distribution with mean vector $\mathbf{a}$ and covariance matrix $\mathbf{b}$. Note that, because (2.1) represents the conditional mean of $\mathbf{Y}_i$ at $\mathbf{X}_i$ through $\mathbf{X}_i\beta$, it is a marginal model.

The covariance structures of (2.1) are usually influenced by three factors: random effect, serial correlation and measurement error. The random effects characterize the stochastic variations between subjects within the population. In particular, we may view that, when the covariates affect the response linearly, some of the linear coefficients may vary from subject to subject. The serial correlations are the results of time-varying associations between different measurements of the same subject. Such correlations are typically positive in biomedical studies, and become weaker as the time interval between the measurements increases. Finally, the measurement errors, which are normally assumed to be independent both between and within the subjects, are induced by the measurement process or random variations within the subjects.

Suppose that, for each subject i, there is a $[r \times 1]$ vector of explanatory variables $\mathbf{U}_{ij}$ measured at time t_{ij}, which may or may not overlap with the original covariate vector $\mathbf{X}_{ij}$. Using the additive decomposition of random effects, serial correlations and measurement errors, $\epsilon_i(t_{ij})$ can be expressed as

$$\epsilon_i(t_{ij}) = \mathbf{U}_{ij}^T b_i + W_i(t_{ij}) + Z_{ij}, \tag{2.2}$$

where b_i is the $[r \times 1]$ random vector with multivariate normal distribution $\mathbf{N}(\mathbf{0}, \mathbf{D})$, $\mathbf{D}$ is a $[r \times r]$ covariate matrix with (p,q)th element $d_{pq} = d_{qp}$, $W_i(t_{ij})$ for $i = 1, \ldots, n$ are independent copies of a mean zero Gaussian process whose covariance at time points t_{ij_1} and t_{ij_2} is $\rho_W(t_{ij_1}, t_{ij_2})$, and Z_{ij} for $i = 1, \ldots, n$ and $j = 1, \ldots, n_i$ are independent identically distributed random variables with $N(0, \tau^2)$ distribution. Writing $\delta_i(t_{ij}) = W_i(t_{ij}) + Z_{ij}$, $\delta_i = \left(\delta_i(t_{i1}), \ldots, \delta_i(t_{in_i})\right)^T$ and $\mathbf{U}_i$ the $[n_i \times r]$ matrix whose jth row is $\mathbf{U}_{ij}^T$, (2.1) and (2.2) reduce to the linear mixed effects model of Laird and Ware (1982)

$$\mathbf{Y}_i = \mathbf{X}_i \beta + \mathbf{U}_i b_i + \delta_i. \tag{2.3}$$

The marginal effect β represents the influence of $\mathbf{X}_i$ on the population average of the response profile, while b_i describes the variation of the ith subject from the population conditioning on the given explanatory variable $\mathbf{U}_i$. Thus, conditioning on $\mathbf{X}_i$ and $\mathbf{U}_i$, (2.3) implies that $\mathbf{Y}_i$ for $i = 1, \ldots, n$ are independent Gaussian vectors such that

$$\mathbf{Y}_i \sim \mathbf{N}\left(\mathbf{X}_i \beta, \mathbf{U}_i \mathbf{D} \mathbf{U}_i^T + \mathbf{P}_i + \tau^2 \mathbf{I}_i\right), \tag{2.4}$$

where $\mathbf{P}_i$ is the $[n_i \times n_i]$ covariance matrix whose (j_1, j_2)th element is $\rho_W(t_{ij_1}, t_{ij_2})$ and $\mathbf{I}_i$ is the $[n_i \times n_i]$ identity matrix.

A number of special cases can be derived for the variance-covariance structure of (2.2). The classical linear models for the independent cross-sectional data (or the independent identically distributed data) is a special case of (2.4) where $\epsilon_i(t_{ij})$ are only affected by the measurement errors Z_{ij}. When neither random effects nor measurement errors are present, the error term is of pure serial correlation $\epsilon_i(t_{ij}) = W_i(t_{ij})$. Moreover, if $W_i(t_{ij})$ are from a mean zero stationary Gaussian process, the covariance of $\epsilon_i(t_{ij_1})$ and $\epsilon_i(t_{ij_2})$, hence, Y_{ij_1} and Y_{ij_2}, can be specified by

$$\mathrm{Cov}\left(\epsilon_i(t_{ij_1}), \epsilon_i(t_{ij_2})\right) = \sigma^2 \rho\left(|t_{ij_1} - t_{ij_2}|\right), \tag{2.5}$$

where σ is a positive constant and $\rho(\cdot)$ is a continuous function. Useful choices of $\rho(\cdot)$ include the exponential correlation $\rho(s) = \exp(-as)$ for some constant $a > 0$ and the Gaussian correlation $\rho(s) = \exp(-as^2)$, among others. When $\epsilon_i(t_{ij})$ are affected by a mean zero stationary Gaussian process and a mean zero Gaussian white noise (measurement error), the variance of Y_{ij} is $\sigma^2\rho(0) + \tau^2$, while the covariance of Y_{ij_1} and Y_{ij_2}, for $j_1 \neq j_2$, is $\sigma^2\rho(|t_{ij_1} - t_{ij_2}|)$, for some $\sigma > 0$, $\tau > 0$ and continuous correlation function $\rho(\cdot)$. When serial correlations are not present, the intra-subject correlations are only induced by the random effects, so that $\mathbf{P}_i$ is not present in (2.4).

2.2. *Likelihood based estimation and inferences*

2.2.1. *Conditional maximum likelihood estimation*

Suppose that the variance-covariance matrix $\mathbf{V}_i(t_i)$ of (2.2) is determined by a R^q-valued parameter vector α. Denote $\mathbf{V}_i(t_i; \alpha)$ to be the variance-covariance matrix parametrized by α. The log-likelihood function for (2.1) is

$$L(\beta, \alpha) = c + \sum_{i=1}^{n} \left\{ -\frac{1}{2} \log |\mathbf{V}_i(t_i; \alpha)| - \frac{1}{2} (\mathbf{Y}_i - \mathbf{X}_i\beta)^T \mathbf{V}_i^{-1}(t_i; \alpha) (\mathbf{Y}_i - \mathbf{X}_i\beta) \right\}, \tag{2.6}$$

where $c = \sum_{i=1}^{n} [(-n_i/2)\log(2\pi)]$. For a given α, (2.6) can be maximized by

$$\widehat{\beta}(\alpha) = \left[\sum_{i=1}^{n} \left(\mathbf{X}_i^T \mathbf{V}_i^{-1}(t_i; \alpha) \mathbf{X}_i \right) \right]^{-1} \left[\sum_{i=1}^{n} \left(\mathbf{X}_i^T \mathbf{V}_i^{-1}(t_i; \alpha) \mathbf{Y}_i \right) \right]. \tag{2.7}$$

It is easy to verify that, under (2.1), $\widehat{\beta}(\alpha)$ is an unbiased estimator of β. Direct calculation also shows that the covariance matrix of $\widehat{\beta}(\alpha)$ is

$$\begin{aligned} \mathrm{Cov}\left[\widehat{\beta}(\alpha)\right] &= \left[\sum_{i=1}^{n} \left(\mathbf{X}_i^T \mathbf{V}_i^{-1}(t_i; \alpha) \mathbf{X}_i \right) \right]^{-1} \\ &\quad \times \left[\sum_{i=1}^{n} \left(\mathbf{X}_i^T \mathbf{V}_i^{-1}(t_i; \alpha) \mathrm{Cov}(\mathbf{Y}_i) \mathbf{V}_i^{-1}(t_i; \alpha) \mathbf{X}_i \right) \right] \\ &\quad \times \left[\sum_{i=1}^{n} \left(\mathbf{X}_i^T \mathbf{V}_i^{-1}(t_i; \alpha) \mathbf{X}_i \right) \right]^{-1} \\ &= \left[\sum_{i=1}^{n} \left(\mathbf{X}_i^T \mathbf{V}_i^{-1}(t_i; \alpha) \mathbf{X}_i \right) \right]^{-1}. \end{aligned} \tag{2.8}$$

It is interesting to note that the second equality sign of (2.8) does not hold when the structure of the variance-covariance matrix is not correctly specified. Further derivation using (2.1), (2.7) and (2.8) shows that $\widehat{\beta}(\alpha)$ has a multivariate Normal distribution,

$$\widehat{\beta}(\alpha) \sim \mathbf{N}\left\{\beta, \left[\sum_{i=1}^{n}\left(\mathbf{X}_i^T \mathbf{V}_i^{-1}(t_i;\alpha)\mathbf{X}_i\right)\right]^{-1}\right\}. \tag{2.9}$$

When α is known, this result can be used to develop inference procedures, such as confidence regions and test statistics, for β.

2.2.2. *Maximum likelihood estimation*

When α is unknown, as in most practical situations, a consistent estimate of α has to be used. An intuitive approach is to estimate β and α by maximizing (2.6) with respect to β and α simultaneously. Maximum likelihood estimators (MLE) of this type can be computed by substituting (2.7) into (2.6) and then maximizing (2.6) with respect to α. Denote the resulting ML estimators by $\widehat{\beta}_{ML}$ and $\widehat{\alpha}_{ML}$. The asymptotic distributions of $(\widehat{\beta}_{ML}, \widehat{\alpha}_{ML})$ can be developed using the standard approaches in large sample theory.

Although $(\widehat{\beta}_{ML}, \widehat{\alpha}_{ML})$ has some justifiable statistical properties, as for most likelihood-based methods, it may not be desirable in practice. To see why an alternative estimation method might be warranted in some situations, we consider the simple linear regression with independent errors and $n_1 = \cdots = n_n = m$,

$$\mathbf{Y}_i \sim \mathbf{N}\left(\mathbf{X}_i\beta, \sigma^2\mathbf{I}_m\right), \tag{2.10}$$

where $\mathbf{I}_m$ is the $[m \times m]$ identity matrix. The parameters involved in the model are β and σ. Let $\widehat{\beta}_{ML}$ and $\widehat{\sigma}_{ML}$ be the MLEs of β and σ, respectively, and RSS be the residual sum of squares defined by

$$\mathrm{RSS} = \sum_{i=1}^{n}\left(\mathbf{Y}_i - \mathbf{X}_i\widehat{\beta}_{ML}\right)^T\left(\mathbf{Y}_i - \mathbf{X}_i\widehat{\beta}_{ML}\right).$$

The MLE of σ^2 is $\widehat{\sigma}^2_{ML} = \mathrm{RSS}/(nm)$. However, it is well-known that, for any finite n and m, $\widehat{\sigma}^2_{ML}$ is a biased estimator of σ^2. On the other hand, a slightly modified estimator $\widehat{\sigma}^2_{REML} = \mathrm{RSS}/[nm - (k+1)]$ is unbiased for σ^2. Here, $\widehat{\sigma}^2_{REML}$ is the restricted maximum likelihood (REML) estimator for the model (2.10).

2.2.3. *Restricted maximum likelihood estimation*

This class of estimators was introduced by Patterson and Thompson (1971) for the purpose of estimating variance components in the linear models. The main idea is to consider a linear transformation of the original response variable so that the distribution of the transformed variable does not depend on β. Let $\mathbf{Y} = \left(\mathbf{Y}_1^T, \ldots, \mathbf{Y}_n^T\right)^T$, $\mathbf{X} = \left(\mathbf{X}_1^T, \ldots, \mathbf{X}_n^T\right)^T$ and $\mathbf{V}$ be the block-diagonal matrix with $\mathbf{V}_i(t_i)$ on the ith main diagonal and zeros elsewhere. Then, with $\mathbf{V}$ parameterized by α, model (2.1) is equivalent to

$$\mathbf{Y} \sim \mathbf{N}\left(\mathbf{X}\beta, \mathbf{V}(\alpha)\right). \tag{2.11}$$

The REML estimator of α, the variance component of (2.11), is obtained by maximizing the likelihood function of $\mathbf{Y}^* = \mathbf{A}^T\mathbf{Y}$, where $\mathbf{A}$ is a $[N \times (N-k-1)]$, $N = \sum_{i=1}^n n_i$, full rank matrix such that $\mathbf{A}^T\mathbf{X} = \mathbf{0}$. A specific construction of $\mathbf{A}$ can be found in Diggle, Heagerty, Liang and Zeger (2002, Section 4.5). It follows from (2.11) that $\mathbf{Y}^*$ has a mean zero multivariate Gaussian distribution with covariance matrix $\mathbf{A}^T\mathbf{V}(\alpha)\mathbf{A}$. Harville (1974) showed that the likelihood function of $\mathbf{Y}^*$ is proportional to

$$\begin{aligned} L^*(\alpha) = & \left|\sum_{i=1}^n \mathbf{X}_i^T\mathbf{X}_i\right|^{1/2} \left|\sum_{i=1}^n \mathbf{X}_i^T\mathbf{V}_i^{-1}(t_i;\alpha)\mathbf{X}_i\right|^{-1/2} \left\{\prod_{i=1}^n \left|\mathbf{V}_i(t_i;\alpha)\right|^{-1/2}\right\} \\ & \times \exp\left\{-\frac{1}{2}\sum_{i=1}^n \left(\mathbf{Y}_i - \mathbf{X}_i\widehat{\beta}(\alpha)\right)^T \mathbf{V}_i^{-1}(t_i;\alpha)\left(\mathbf{Y}_i - \mathbf{X}_i\widehat{\beta}(\alpha)\right)\right\}. \end{aligned} \tag{2.12}$$

The REML estimator $\widehat{\alpha}_{REML}$ of α maximizes (2.12). The REML estimator $\widehat{\beta}_{REML}$ of β is obtained by substituting α of (2.7) with $\widehat{\alpha}_{REML}$. Because (2.12) does not depend on the choice of $\mathbf{A}$, the resulting estimators $\widehat{\beta}_{REML}$ and $\widehat{\alpha}_{REML}$ are free of the specific linear transformations.

The log-likelihood of $\mathbf{Y}^*$, $\log[L^*(\alpha)]$, differs from the log-likelihood $L(\widehat{\beta}, \alpha)$ only through a constant, which does not depend on α, and

$$-\frac{1}{2}\log\left|\sum_{i=1}^n \mathbf{X}_i^T\mathbf{V}_i^{-1}(t_i;\alpha)\mathbf{X}_i\right|,$$

which does not depend on β. Because both REML and ML methods are based on the likelihood principle, they all have important theoretical properties such as consistency, asymptotic normality and asymptotic efficiency. In practice, neither one is uniformly superior to the other for all the situations. Their numerical values are also computed from different algorithms.

For the ML method, the fixed effects and the variance components are estimated simultaneously, while for the REML method, only the variance components are estimated.

2.2.4. *Inferences*

The results established in the previous sections are useful to construct inference procedures for β. For the purpose of illustration, only a few special cases are presented here. A more complete account of inferential and diagnostic tools may be found in Diggle (1988), Zeger, Liang and Albert (1988), Diggle, Heagerty, Liang and Zeger (2002) or Vonesh and Chinchilli (1997), among others.

Suppose that there is a consistent estimator $\widehat{\alpha}$ of α, which may be either the ML estimator $\widehat{\alpha}_{ML}$ or the REML estimator $\widehat{\alpha}_{REML}$. Substituting α of (2.9) with $\widehat{\alpha}$, the distribution of $\widehat{\beta}(\widehat{\alpha})$ can be approximated, at least when n is large, by

$$\widehat{\beta}\left(\widehat{\alpha}\right) \sim \mathbf{N}\left(\beta, \widehat{\mathbf{V}}\right), \tag{2.13}$$

where $\widehat{\mathbf{V}} = \left[\sum_{i=1}^{n} \left(\mathbf{X}_i^T \mathbf{V}_i^{-1}(t_i; \widehat{\alpha})\mathbf{X}_i\right)\right]^{-1}$. Suppose that $\mathbf{C}$ is a known $[r \times (k+1)]$ matrix with full rank. It follows immediately from (2.13) that, when n is sufficiently large, the distribution of $\mathbf{C}\widehat{\beta}(\widehat{\alpha})$ can be approximated by

$$\mathbf{C}\widehat{\beta}\left(\widehat{\alpha}\right) \sim \mathbf{N}\left(\mathbf{C}\beta, \mathbf{C}\widehat{\mathbf{V}}\mathbf{C}^T\right). \tag{2.14}$$

Consequently, when $r = 1$, an approximate $[100 \times (1 - a)]\%$, $0 < a < 1$, confidence interval for $\mathbf{C}\beta$ can be given by

$$\mathbf{C}\widehat{\beta}\left(\widehat{\alpha}\right) \pm Z_{1-a/2}\left(\mathbf{C}\widehat{\mathbf{V}}\mathbf{C}^T\right)^{1/2}.$$

Taking $\mathbf{C}$ to be the $(k + 1)$ row vector with 1 at its lth place and zero elsewhere, an approximate $[100 \times (1 - a)]\%$ confidence interval for β_l can be given by

$$\widehat{\beta}_l\left(\widehat{\alpha}\right) \pm Z_{1-a/2}\sqrt{\widehat{V}_l}, \tag{2.15}$$

where $\widehat{V}_l$ is the lth diagonal element of $\widehat{\mathbf{V}}$.

The approximation in (2.14) can also be used to construct test statistics for linear statistical hypotheses. For example, suppose that we would like to test the null hypothesis of $\mathbf{C}\beta = \theta_0$ for a known vector θ_0 against the general alternative that $\mathbf{C}\beta \neq \theta_0$. A natural test statistic would be

$$\widehat{T} = \left[\mathbf{C}\widehat{\beta}(\widehat{\alpha}) - \theta_0\right]^T \left(\mathbf{C}\widehat{\mathbf{V}}\mathbf{C}^T\right)^{-1} \left[\mathbf{C}\widehat{\beta}(\widehat{\alpha}) - \theta_0\right], \tag{2.16}$$

which has approximately a χ^2-distribution with r degrees of freedom, denoted by χ_r^2, under the null hypothesis. A level $(100 \times a)\%$ test based on $\widehat{T}$ then rejects the null hypothesis when $\widehat{T} > \chi_r^2(a)$ with $\chi_r^2(a)$ being the $[100 \times (1-a)]$th percentile of χ_r^2. For the special case of testing $\beta_l = 0$ versus $\beta_l \neq 0$, a simple procedure equivalent to (2.16) is to reject the null hypothesis when

$$\left|\widehat{\beta}_l(\widehat{\alpha})\right| > Z_{1-a/2}\sqrt{\widehat{V}_l},$$

where $Z_{1-a/2}$ and $\widehat{V}_l$ are defined in (2.15).

2.3. *Partially linear models*

As discussed in Section 1.4, this class of models has been studied by Zeger and Diggle (1994) and Moyeed and Diggle (1994) as a means to generalize the marginal linear models. With further restrictions on the error process, (1.2) is equivalent to

$$Y(t) = \beta_0(t) + \sum_{l=1}^{D} \beta_l X^{(l)}(t) + \epsilon(t), \tag{2.17}$$

where $\epsilon(t)$ is a mean zero stochastic process with variance σ^2 and correlation function $\rho(t)$, and $X^{(l)}(t)$, $l = 1, \ldots, D$, and $\epsilon(t)$ are independent. The errors $\epsilon_i(t_{ij})$ specified in (1.2) are then independent copies of $\epsilon(t)$. A useful way to view $\epsilon_i(t_{ij})$ is through the decomposition

$$\epsilon_i(t_{ij}) = W_i(t_{ij}) + Z_{ij}, \tag{2.18}$$

where $W_i(t)$ are independent copies of a mean zero stationary process $W(t)$ with covariance function $\sigma_W^2\rho(t)$ and Z_{ij} are independent identically distributed measurement errors with mean zero and variance σ_Z^2. The covariance structure of the measurements Y_{ij} for $i = 1, \ldots, n$ and $j = 1, \ldots, n_i$ are

$$\mathrm{Cov}\left(Y_{i_1 j_1}, Y_{i_2 j_2}\right) = \begin{cases} \sigma_Z^2 + \sigma_W^2, & \text{if } i_1 = i_2 \text{ and } j_1 = j_2, \\ \sigma_W^2 \rho(t_{i_1 j_1} - t_{i_2 j_2}), & \text{if } i_1 = i_2 \text{ and } j_1 \neq j_2, \\ 0, & \text{otherwise.} \end{cases} \tag{2.19}$$

Although the above models can be classified as a special case of (1.3), a class of the structural nonparametric models to be discussed in later sections, their estimation methods are quite different, a fact owing to the structural differences between these two classes of models. The rest of this section focuses on an iteration procedure for the estimation of $\beta_0(t), \beta_1, \cdots, \beta_k$. Inferential and alternative estimation methods, which constitute some major research activities in longitudinal analyses, are still not well-understood and warrant considerable effort in further investigation.

2.4. *Unstructured smoothing methods for mean responses*

Suppose for the moment that no covariate other than time is considered in modeling the mean response. The model (2.17) then reduces to

$$Y(t) = \beta_0(t) + \epsilon(t). \tag{2.20}$$

Equivalently, with $\epsilon(t)$ defined in (2.17), $\beta_0(t)$ is the mean response of $Y(t)$ conditioning on time t; that is, $\beta_0(t) = E[Y(t)|t]$.

A natural approach for estimating $\beta_0(t)$ nonparametrically is to borrow smoothing techniques from the classical independent identically distributed (i.i.d.) setting, while evaluating the statistical performances of the resulting estimators by taking the influences of the intra-subject correlations into account. A simple method is to use kernel smoothing, which amounts to estimate $\beta_0(t)$ through a weighted average using the measurements obtained within a neighborhood of t defined by a kernel function. Let $K(u)$ be a continuous kernel function, usually a continuous probability density function, defined on the real line, and h a positive bandwidth sequence which shrinks to zero as n tends to infinity. A kernel estimator similar to the well-known Nadaraya-Watson type kernel estimators in the i.i.d. setting is

$$\widehat{\beta}_0^K(t) = \frac{\sum_{i=1}^{n}\sum_{j=1}^{n_i}\{Y_{ij}K[(t-t_{ij})/h]\}}{\sum_{i=1}^{n}\sum_{j=1}^{n_i}K[(t-t_{ij})/h]}. \tag{2.21}$$

Here, (2.21) uses uniform weight on each measurement, hence, makes no distinction between the subjects that have unequal numbers of repeated measurements. Thus subjects with more repeated measurements are used more often than those with fewer repeated measurements. A general formulation is to assign a specific weight to each subject and estimate $\beta_0(t)$ by

$$\widehat{\beta}_0^K(t;w) = \frac{\sum_{i=1}^{n}\sum_{j=1}^{n_i}\{Y_{ij}w_iK[(t-t_{ij})/h]\}}{\sum_{i=1}^{n}\sum_{j=1}^{n_i}\{w_iK[(t-t_{ij})/h]\}}, \tag{2.22}$$

where the weights, $w = (w_1, \ldots, w_n)$, satisfy $w_i \geq 0$ for all $i = 1, \ldots, n$ with strict inequality for some $1 \leq i \leq n$. Clearly, (2.22) reduces to (2.21) when

$w_i = 1/N$. An intuitive weight choice other than $w_i = 1/N$ is to uniformly weight each subject, rather than each measurement, so that the resulting kernel estimator is (2.22) with $w_i = 1/(nn_i)$.

Other approaches for the estimation of (2.19) have also been studied by Hart and Wehrly (1986), Müller (1988), Altman (1990), Hart (1991), Rice and Silverman (1991), among others. These methods are not discussed here, and their details can be found in these original articles. These methods, including (2.22) and the above alternative approaches, are essentially based on the fundamental spirit of local smoothing, hence, often lead to similar results in practice. This is in contrast to the smoothing methods to be discussed in the next section, where, because of the model complexity, different smoothing methods often produce very different results.

A crucial step in obtaining an adequate kernel estimator for $\beta_0(t)$ is to select an appropriate bandwidth h, while the choices of kernel functions are relatively less important. For estimation methods other than kernel smoothing, such as splines, this amounts to selecting an appropriate smoothing parameter. Rice and Silverman (1991) suggested a simple cross-validation for selecting a data-driven smoothing parameter which does not depend on the intra-subject correlation structures of the data. Applying their cross-validation to the kernel estimator (2.22), we first define $\widehat{\beta}_0^{(-i,K)}(t; w)$ to be the estimator computed using (2.22) and the remaining data after deleting the entire set of repeated measurements of the ith subject. Predicting the ith subject's outcome at time t by $\widehat{\beta}_0^{(-i,K)}(t; w)$, the cross-validation score of (2.22) is

$$\mathrm{CV}(h) = \sum_{i=1}^{n} \sum_{j=1}^{n_i} \left\{ w_i \left[Y_{ij} - \widehat{\beta}_0^{(-i,K)}(t_{ij}; w) \right]^2 \right\}. \tag{2.23}$$

Suppose that (2.23) can be uniquely minimized. The "leave-one-subject-out" cross-validated bandwidth h_{cv} is the minimizer of (2.23). Heuristically, the use of h_{cv} can be justified because, by minimizing (2.23), it approximately minimizes an average prediction error of (2.22). More details for the implementations and generalizations of this cross-validation will be discussed in Section 4.7.

Direct calculation of (2.23) can often be time consuming, as the algorithm repeats itself each time a new subject is deleted. Denote $K_{ij} = K[(t - t_{ij})/h]$,

$$K_{ij}^* = \frac{w_i K[(t - t_{ij})/h]}{\sum_{i=1}^{n} \sum_{j=1}^{n_i} w_i K[(t - t_{ij})/h]} \qquad \text{and} \qquad K_i^* = \sum_{j=1}^{n_i} K_{ij}^*$$

for $i = 1, \ldots, n$. A computationally simpler approach, also suggested by Rice and Silverman (1991), is to compute $[Y_{ij} - \widehat{\beta}_0^{(-i,K)}(t_{ij}; w)]$ using the following expression:

$$\begin{aligned}
Y_{ij} &- \widehat{\beta}_0^{(-i,K)}(t_{ij}; w) \\
&= Y_{ij} - \left[\widehat{\beta}_0^K(t_{ij}; w) - \sum_{j=1}^{n_i} \left(Y_{ij} K_{ij}^*\right)\right]\left(1 + \frac{K_i^*}{1 - K_i^*}\right) \\
&= \left[Y_{ij} - \widehat{\beta}_0^K(t_{ij}; w)\right] + \sum_{j=1}^{n_i} \left(Y_{ij} K_{ij}^*\right) \\
&\quad - \left[\widehat{\beta}_0^K(t_{ij}; w) - \sum_{j=1}^{n_i} \left(Y_{ij} K_{ij}^*\right)\right]\left(\frac{K_i^*}{1 - K_i^*}\right) \\
&= \left[Y_{ij} - \widehat{\beta}_0^K(t_{ij}; w)\right] + \left(\frac{K_i^*}{1 - K_i^*}\right)\left[\frac{\sum_{j=1}^{n_i} \left(Y_{ij} K_{ij}^*\right)}{K_i^*} - \widehat{\beta}_0^K(t_{ij}; w)\right].
\end{aligned} \tag{2.24}$$

The above expression, as currently stated, is specifically targeted to kernel estimators defined in (2.22). When other smoothing methods, such as splines, are used, we may not get an explicit expression as the right side of (2.24), hence, direct calculation of (2.23) has to be carried out by deleting the subjects one at a time.

Large sample inferences of $\widehat{\beta}_0^K(t; w)$ can be derived based on the asymptotic expressions of its means and variances and its asymptotic distributions. Because $\widehat{\beta}_0^K(t; w)$ is a linear statistic of Y_{ij}, its means and variances can be directly computed and, consequently, its asymptotic distributions can be easily established by checking the triangular array central limit theorem after taking the intra-subject correlations into account; see, for example, Wu, Chiang and Hoover (1998) and Wu and Chiang (2000). Because $\widehat{\beta}_0^K(t; w)$ is a special case of the kernel estimators of Section 4, details of pointwise and simultaneous inferences for $\beta_0(t)$ are discussed in Section 5.1.

2.5. *Estimation of covariate effects in partially linear models*

With covariates other than time entered into the model, the estimation of $(\beta_0(t), \beta_1, \ldots, \beta_k)$ can be proceeded by an iteration that combines smoothing with parametric estimation techniques. Suppose that the error terms $\epsilon_i(t)$ of (2.18) have known variance-covariance matrices $\mathbf{V}_i(t_i)$ for

$\mathbf{t}_i = (t_{i1}, \ldots, t_{in_i})$ and all $i = 1, \ldots, n$. The iteration can be proceeded as follows:

(a) Set $\beta_0(t)$ to zero and calculate an initial estimate of $(\beta_1, \ldots, \beta_k)^T$ using (2.7), an expression also for the generalized least squares, with $\mathbf{V}_i(\mathbf{t}_i; \alpha)$ replaced by $\mathbf{V}_i(\mathbf{t}_i)$.

(b) Based on the current estimate $(\widehat{\beta}_1, \ldots, \widehat{\beta}_k)$, calculate the residual $r_{ij} = Y_{ij} - \sum_{l=1}^{k} \widehat{\beta}_l X_{ij}^{(l)}$ and compute the kernel estimator $\widehat{\beta}_0^K(t; w)$ of $\beta_0(t)$ using (2.21) with Y_{ij} replaced by r_{ij}.

(c) Based on the current kernel estimator $\widehat{\beta}_0^K(t; w)$, calculate the residual $r_{ij} = Y_{ij} - \widehat{\beta}_0^K(t_{ij}; w)$ and update the estimate of $(\beta_1, \ldots, \beta_k)$ using (2.7) with $(\mathbf{V}_i(\mathbf{t}_i; \alpha), Y_{ij})$ replaced by $(\mathbf{V}_i(\mathbf{t}_i), r_{ij})$.

(d) Repeat steps (b) and (c) until the estimates converge.

This algorithm is a special case of the more general backfitting algorithm described in Hastie and Tibshirani (1993).

The assumption of having a known correlation structure is unrealistic and can be relaxed. Although an incorrectly specified correlation structure may cost the efficiency of the estimators, it generally does not affect the consistency. When the variance-covariance matrix is parametrized by a parameter α and the error terms are from a mean zero Gaussian stationary process, the above iteration algorithm can be used in conjunction with the likelihood and restricted likelihood methods of the previous section, i.e. the generalized least squares estimators used in Steps (a) and (c) can be replaced by the likelihood based estimators $\widehat{\beta}_{ML}$ or $\widehat{\beta}(\widehat{\alpha}_{REML})$. Further computational details, statistical properties of the resulting estimators and a modified estimation procedure can be found in Zeger and Diggle (1994) and Moyeed and Diggle (1994). Inferences based on the resulting estimators have not been systematically investigated, hence, warrant substantial further development.

3. Nonparametric Time-Varying Coefficient Models

This section presents a series of different smoothing methods for estimating the coefficient curves $\beta(t) = (\beta_0(t), \ldots, \beta_k(t))^T$ of (1.2) and some asymptotic and bootstrap inference procedures based on the smoothing estimators of $\beta(t)$. Applications of the estimation and inference procedures are illustrate through the Alabama Small-for-Gestational-Age Study (ASGA) of Example 1 and the Baltimore Multicenter AIDS Cohort Study (BMACS) of Example 2.

3.1. *Some useful expressions*

In observational studies, the covariates are usually random as the subjects are randomly chosen, although they could in principle be either random or fixed. For generality, it is assumed throughout that $\mathbf{X}(t)$ is random and the matrix $E[\mathbf{X}(t)\mathbf{X}^T(t)] \equiv E_{\mathbf{XX}^T}(t)$ exist. With a proper change of the notation, the methods here can be modified to accommodate the case of nonrandom covariates. An equivalent expression of (1.3) is then

$$Y(t) = \mathbf{X}^T(t)\beta(t) + \epsilon(t), \tag{3.1}$$

where $\epsilon(t)$ is a mean zero stochastic process and $\epsilon(t)$ and $\mathbf{X}(t)$ are independent. Suppose that $E_{\mathbf{XX}^T}(t)$ is invertible and its inverse is $E^{-1}_{\mathbf{XX}^T}(t)$. It directly follows from (3.1) that $\beta(t)$ uniquely minimizes the second moment of $\epsilon(t)$ in the sense that

$$E\left\{\left[Y(t) - \mathbf{X}^T(t)\beta(t)\right]^2\right\} = \inf_{\text{all } b(\cdot)} E\left\{\left[Y(t) - \mathbf{X}^T(t)b(t)\right]^2\right\}, \tag{3.2}$$

and is given by

$$\beta(t) = E^{-1}_{\mathbf{XX}^T}(t)E\left[\mathbf{X}(t)Y(t)\right]. \tag{3.3}$$

When the covariates are time-invariant, we have $\mathbf{X}(t) \equiv \mathbf{X}$ and $E_{\mathbf{XX}^T}(t) \equiv E_{\mathbf{XX}^T}$, so that the equation (3.3) reduces to

$$\beta_r(t) = E\left[\left(\sum_{l=0}^{k} e_{rl}X^{(l)}\right)Y(t)\right], \tag{3.4}$$

where e_{rl} is the element of $E^{-1}_{\mathbf{XX}^T}$ at the rth row and lth column.

3.2. *Smoothing based on least squares*

3.2.1. *General formulation*

Intuitively, (3.2) suggests that $\beta(t)$ can be estimated by a method of local least squares using the measurements observed within a neighborhood of t. Assume that, for each l and some integer $p \geq 0$, $\beta_l(t)$ is p times differentiable and its pth derivative is continuous. Approximating $\beta_l(t_{ij})$ by a pth order polynomial $\sum_{r=0}^{p}\{b_{lr}(t)(t_{ij}-t)^r\}$ for all $l = 0, \ldots, k$, a local pol$\beta(t) = (\beta_0(t), \ldots, \beta_k(t))^T$ based on a kernel neighborhood is $\widehat{b}_0(t) = \left(\widehat{b}_{00}(t), \ldots, \widehat{b}_{k0}(t)\right)^T$, where $\{\widehat{b}_{lr}(t);\ l = 0, \ldots, k,\ r = 0, \ldots, p\}$

minimizes

$$L_p(t) = \sum_{i=1}^{n}\sum_{j=1}^{n_i} w_i \left\{ Y_{ij} - \sum_{l=0}^{k}\left[X_{ij}^{(l)} \left(\sum_{r=0}^{p} b_{lr}(t)(t_{ij}-t)^r \right)\right]\right\}^2 K\left(\frac{t_{ij}-t}{h}\right), \tag{3.5}$$

where w_i are the non-negative weights as in (2.22), $K(\cdot)$ is a kernel function, usually chosen to be a probability density function, and h is a non-negative bandwidth. ynomial estimator of As a by-product of (3.5), $(r!)\widehat{b}_{lr}(t)$ may be used to estimate the rth derivative $\beta_l^{(r)}(t)$ of $\beta_l(t)$, $r = 1, \ldots, p$.

3.2.2. *Least squares kernel estimators*

The simplest case of (3.5) is the ordinary least squares kernel estimator, also known as the local constant fit, obtained by minimizing (3.5) with $p = 0$. Using the matrix representation $\mathbf{Y}_i = (Y_{i1}, \ldots, Y_{in_i})^T$,

$$\mathbf{X}_i = \begin{pmatrix} 1 & X_{i1}^{(1)} & \cdots & X_{i1}^{(k)} \\ \vdots & \vdots & \vdots & \vdots \\ 1 & X_{in_i}^{(1)} & \cdots & X_{in_i}^{(k)} \end{pmatrix} \quad \text{and} \quad \mathbf{K}_i(t) = \begin{pmatrix} K_{i1} & \cdots & 0 \\ \vdots & \vdots & \vdots \\ 0 & \cdots & K_{in_i} \end{pmatrix}$$

with $K_{ij} = K[(t_{ij} - t)/h]$, if $\sum_{i=1}^{n} \mathbf{X}_i^T \mathbf{K}_i(t) \mathbf{X}_i$ is invertible, then (3.5) with $p = 0$ can be uniquely minimized and its minimizer, the kernel estimator of $\beta(t)$, is given by

$$\widehat{\beta}^{LSK}(t) = \left(\sum_{i=1}^{n} w_i \mathbf{X}_i^T \mathbf{K}_i(t) \mathbf{X}_i \right)^{-1} \left(\sum_{i=1}^{n} w_i \mathbf{X}_i^T \mathbf{K}_i(t) \mathbf{Y}_i \right). \tag{3.6}$$

When the model incorporates no covariate other than time, i.e. $k = 0$, (3.6) reduces to a Nadaraya-Watson type kernel estimator of the conditional expectation $E[Y(t)|t]$; see, for example, Härdle (1990).

3.2.3. *Least squares local linear estimators*

Although (3.6) has a simple mathematical expression, it often leads to significant bias when t is at the boundary of its support. An automatic procedure to reduce such boundary bias is to use higher order local polynomial fits. But, a high order local polynomial fit can be impractical in some applications because it usually requires large sample sizes and may be computationally intensive. A practical approach that provides automatic boundary bias adjustment is to use local linear fit that minimizes (3.5) with $p = 1$. Denote

$$\mathcal{N}_{lr} = \begin{pmatrix} \sum_{i,j} \left[w_i X_{ij}^{(l)} X_{ij}^{(r)} K_{ij}\right] & \sum_{i,j} \left[w_i X_{ij}^{(l)} X_{ij}^{(r)} (t_{ij} - t) K_{ij}\right] \\ \sum_{i,j} \left[w_i X_{ij}^{(l)} X_{ij}^{(r)} (t_{ij} - t) K_{ij}\right] & \sum_{i,j} \left[w_i X_{ij}^{(l)} X_{ij}^{(r)} (t_{ij} - t)^2 K_{ij}\right] \end{pmatrix},$$

$\mathcal{N}_r = (\mathcal{N}_{0r}, \ldots, \mathcal{N}_{kr})$, $\mathcal{N} = (\mathcal{N}_0^T, \ldots, \mathcal{N}_k^T)^T$,

$$\mathcal{M}_r = \left(\sum_{i,j} \left[w_i X_{ij}^{(r)} Y_{ij} K_{ij}\right], \sum_{i,j} \left[w_i X_{ij}^{(r)} (t_{ij} - t) Y_{ij} K_{ij}\right] \right)^T,$$

$\mathcal{M} = (\mathcal{M}_0^T, \ldots, \mathcal{M}_k^T)^T$, $b_l(t) = (b_{l0}(t), b_{l1}(t))^T$ and $b(t) = (b_0(t), \ldots, b_k(t)^T$ for $r, l = 0, \ldots, k$. Setting the partial derivatives of $L_1(t)$ with respect to $b_{lr}(t)$ to zero, the normal equation of (3.5) with $p = 1$ is

$$\mathcal{N} b(t) = \mathcal{M}. \tag{3.7}$$

Suppose that the matrix $\mathcal{N}$ is invertible at t. The solution of (3.7) exists and is uniquely given by $\widehat{b}(t) = \mathcal{N}^{-1}\mathcal{M}$. The least squares local linear estimator $\widehat{\beta}_l^{LSL}(t)$ of $\beta_l(t)$ is then

$$\widehat{\beta}_l^{LSL}(t) = e_{2l+1}^T \widehat{b}(t), \tag{3.8}$$

where e_q is the $[2(k+1) \times 1]$ column vector with 1 at its qth place and zero elsewhere. Explicit expressions for the general higher order least squares local polynomial estimators can be similarly derived; see Hoover *et al.* (1998). Details of these general higher order estimators are omitted, since a local linear fitting is sufficiently satisfactory in almost all the biomedical studies that have appeared in the literature.

3.2.4. *Least squares with centered covariates*

In some situations, some of the covariates used in (3.1) can not have values at zero, so that the baseline coefficient curve $\beta_0(t)$ does not have a practical interpretation. Strictly positive covariates appear naturally both in the ASGA Study (Section 1.2.1), such as the mother's placental thickness and pre-pregnancy height, and the HIV/CD4 Depletion Data (Section 1.2.2), such as the subject's pre-infection CD4 level. A useful remedy when such a situation arises is to use a centered version of the covariates in the model, so that the corresponding baseline coefficient can be interpreted as the conditional mean of $Y(t)$ when the centered covariates are set to zero.

Let $X^{(*l)}(t) = X^{(l)}(t) - E[X^{(l)}(t)]$ be the centered version of $X^{(l)}(t)$ and $\mathbf{X}^{(*)}(t)$ be the covariate vector with some or all of its components being centered. An equivalent form of (3.1) is

$$Y(t) = \left(\mathbf{X}^{(*)}(t)\right)^T \beta^*(t) + \epsilon(t), \tag{3.9}$$

where $\beta^*(t) = (\beta_0^*(t), \beta_1(t), \ldots, \beta_k(t))^T$. Note that $\beta_0^*(t)$, the baseline coefficient curve of (3.9), represents the mean of $Y(t)$, when $X^{(*l)}(t)$, rather than $X^{(l)}(t)$, for $l = 1, \ldots, k$ are set to zero. Other coefficient curves of (3.9) can be interpreted the same way as those of (3.1).

The estimation of $\beta^*(t)$ can be obtained by first estimating the centered covariates $X_{ij}^{(*l)}$ of $X_{ij}^{(l)}$ and then minimizing (3.5) with $X_{ij}^{(l)}$ replaced by $X_{ij}^{(*l)}$. If $X^{(l)}(t)$ is a time-dependent covariate, then, using a kernel smoothing, a centered version of $X_{ij}^{(l)}$ can be estimated by $X_{ij}^{(*l)} = X_{ij}^{(l)} - \widehat{\mu}_l(t_{ij})$ with

$$\widehat{\mu}_l(t) = \frac{\sum_{i=1}^n \sum_{j=1}^{n_i} \left\{ w_i X_{ij}^{(l)} \Gamma_l[(t - t_{ij})/\gamma_l] \right\}}{\sum_{i=1}^n \sum_{j=1}^{n_i} \{ w_i \Gamma_l[(t - t_{ij})/\gamma_l] \}}, \tag{3.10}$$

where $(\Gamma_l(\cdot), \gamma_l)$ is a set of kernel and bandwidth. On the other hand, if $X^{(l)}(t) \equiv X^{(l)}$ is time-invariant, then $X_{ij}^{(l)} \equiv X_i^{(l)}$ for all $j = 1, \ldots, n_i$, and $X_i^{(*l)}$ can be taken as $X_i^{(l)} - \bar{X}^{(l)}$, where $\bar{X}^{(l)} = n^{-1} \sum_{i=1}^n X_i^{(l)}$ is the weighted sample mean for $X^{(l)}$. Let $\mathbf{X}_i^{(*)}$ be the $n_i \times (k+1)$ centered covariate vector whose jth row is $(1, X_{ij}^{(*1)}, \ldots, X_{ij}^{(*k)})$. A least squares kernel estimator of $\beta^*(t)$ is

$$\widehat{\beta}^{*LSK}(t) = \left[\sum_{i=1}^n w_i \left(\mathbf{X}_i^{(*)}\right)^T \mathbf{K}_i(t) \left(\mathbf{X}_i^{(*)}\right)^T \right]^{-1} \left[\sum_{i=1}^n w_i \left(\mathbf{X}_i^{(*)}\right)^T \mathbf{K}_i(t) \mathbf{Y}_i \right], \tag{3.11}$$

where $\mathbf{K}_i(t)$ and $\mathbf{Y}_i$ are defined as in (3.6).

Wu, Yu and Chiang (2000) investigated the large sample properties of $\widehat{\beta}^{*LSK}(t)$. Their results suggest that neither $\widehat{\beta}^{LSK}(t)$ nor $\widehat{\beta}^{*LSK}(t)$ is uniformly superior to the other. In particular, when the covariates are time-invariant, $\widehat{\beta}^{LSK}(t)$ and $\widehat{\beta}^{*LSK}(t)$ are asymptotically equivalent. However, when $X^{(l)}(t)$ for $l \geq 1$ changes significantly with t, theoretically and practically superior estimators of $\beta_l(t)$ may be obtained by centering $X^{(l)}(t)$.

Of course, after a covariate is centered, the baseline coefficient curve of the model is changed. The decision on whether a covariate should be centered or not primarily depends on the biological interpretations of the corresponding baseline coefficient curve. Such a decision should be made based on the statistical properties of the estimators only if the effects of the covariates, rather than the baseline coefficient curve, is of primary interest in the investigation. Clearly, methods other than kernel smoothing may also be applied to the estimation with centered covariates. But, because of the complication caused by smoothing the covariates, statistical properties for estimators other than (3.11) have not been investigated in the literature.

3.2.5. *A simple modification*

The estimators mentioned above, both with and without covariate centering, rely on a single bandwidth to estimate all $(k+1)$ coefficient curves. This simple approach may work well when all the curves roughly belong to the same smoothness family. However, such an idealized scenario is often not anticipated in practice. A flexible method which automatically adjusts for the possibly different smoothing needs for different coefficient curves is always preferred.

In the literature, the potential deficiency associated with the use of a single bandwidth has been reported by Hoover *et al.* (1998), Fan and Zhang (2000), Wu, Yu and Chiang (2000), among others. These authors have also proposed a number of alternative approaches (see Sections 4.3–4.6) to overcome this potential drawback. A simple method suggested by Wu, Yu and Chiang (2000) is to use a linear combination of the form

$$\widehat{\beta}(t;\mathbf{K},\mathbf{h}) = \sum_{l=0}^{k} e_{l+1}^T \widehat{\beta}(t;K_l,h_l), \tag{3.12}$$

where $\mathbf{K}(\cdot) = (K_0(\cdot),\ldots,K_k(\cdot))$, $\mathbf{h} = (h_0,\ldots,h_k)$, e_p is the $[(k+1)\times 1]$ vector with 1 at its pth place and zero elsewhere and $\widehat{\beta}(t;K_l,h_l)$ is the kernel estimator of $\beta(t)$ or $\beta^*(t)$ obtained from (3.6) or (3.11), respectively, using kernel $K_l(\cdot)$ and bandwidth h_l. Intuitively, $\widehat{\beta}(t;\mathbf{K},\mathbf{h})$ relies on a specific pair of kernel and bandwidth to estimate the corresponding component of $\beta(t)$ or $\beta^*(t)$. As a general methodology, (3.12) is not limited to kernel estimators and may be applied to other local polynomial estimators as well.

3.2.6. *Choices of w_i*

An important factor that affects the theoretical and practical behaviors of the least squares local polynomial estimators of $\beta(t)$ is the choice of w_i in (3.5). For cross-sectional studies with independent identically distributed data, a uniform weight choice, $w_i \equiv 1/N$, is often desirable. For the current sampling, it is conceivable that a proper choice of w_i may depend on the intra-subject correlation structures and the numbers of repeated measurements n_i. In practice, however, the correlation structures of the data are often completely unknown and may be difficult to estimate, so that subjective choices such as $w_i = 1/N$ and $w_i = 1/(nn_i)$ are often considered. Intuitively, $w_i = 1/N$ assigns equal weight to each observation point, while $w_i = 1/(nn_i)$ assigns equal weight to each subject. Theoretically, the choice of $w_i = 1/N$ may produce inconsistent least squares kernel estimators when some n_i are much larger than the others. On the other hand, the least squares kernel estimators based on $w_i = 1/(nn_i)$ are always consistent regardless the choices of n_i (Hoover *et al.*, 1998, and Wu and Chiang, 2000).

3.3. *Penalized least squares*

Suppose that all the components of $\beta(t)$ are twice continuously differentiable and have bounded and square integrable second derivatives with respect to t. A natural penalized least squares criterion is to minimize

$$J(\beta, \lambda) = \sum_{i=1}^{n} \sum_{j=1}^{n_i} \left\{ Y_{ij} - \sum_{l=0}^{k} X_{ij}^{(l)} \beta_l(t_{ij}) \right\}^2 + \sum_{l=0}^{k} \lambda_l \int \left[\beta_l''(t) \right]^2 dt \quad (3.13)$$

with respect to $\beta_l(t)$, where $\lambda = (\lambda_0, \ldots, \lambda_k)^T$ and λ_l are positive smoothing parameters. The existence and uniqueness of the minimizer of (3.13) depend on t_{ij} and $X_{ij}^{(l)}$. Suppose that (3.13) can be uniquely minimized. The penalized least squares estimator $\widehat{\beta}^{PLS}(t) = (\widehat{\beta}_0^{PLS}(t), \ldots, \widehat{\beta}_k^{PLS}(t))^T$ of $\beta(t)$ is then defined to be the unique minimizer of (3.13). Using similar techniques as in univariate smoothing, it can be shown that $\widehat{\beta}_l^{PLS}(t)$ are natural cubic splines with knots at the distinct values of $\{t_{ij} : i = 1, \ldots, n,\ j = 1, \ldots, n_i\}$ and can be expressed as linear functions of $\{Y_{ij} : i = 1, \ldots, n,\ j = 1, \ldots, n_i\}$.

One feature that distinguishes $\widehat{\beta}^{PLS}(t)$ from the estimators obtained from (3.5) is the use of multiple smoothing parameters λ_l in the penalty term. In (3.13), all $(k+1)$ smoothing parameters λ_l, $l = 0, \ldots, k$, can be adjusted in the penalty term. Numerical results presented in Hoover *et al.* (1998) demonstrated that the extra flexibility created by multiple smoothing parameters could indeed lead to better estimators than the least squares local polynomials that rely on a single smoothing parameter.

However, because $\widehat{\beta}^{PLS}(t)$ has knots at all the distinct time points, it can be extremely computationally intensive when the number of distinct time points is large, a case often happened in unbalanced longitudinal studies.

3.4. *Two-step smoothing method*

In an attempt to provide flexible smoothing estimators that are computationally accessible with large longitudinal data, Fan and Zhang (2000) proposed to estimate $\beta(t)$ by a two-step smoothing method which uses $(k+1)$ smoothing parameters in a different way from (3.12) and (3.13). Their procedure calls for the following two steps:

(i) computing the raw estimates $\widehat{\beta}^{RAW}(s)$ of $\beta(s)$ at a set of distinct time points, say $s_1, \ldots, s_m$, where m may depend on n and n_i, $i = 1, \ldots, n$;
(ii) estimating each coefficient curve $\beta_l(t)$ by smoothing the raw estimates $\widehat{\beta}_l^{RAW}(s_r)$, $r = 1, \ldots, m$.

Although Fan and Zhang (2000) used local polynomials to illustrate the method, other smoothing methods such as splines may in principle be used.

For the special case of balanced longitudinal data where all the subjects are observed at a same set of time points $\{s_j; j = 1, \ldots, m\}$ with $m = n_i$, $i = 1, \ldots, n$, the raw estimates can be computed by fitting linear models between Y_{ij} and X_{ij} at s_j for all $j = 1, \ldots, m$. However, when the design is unbalanced and the numbers of subjects on some time points are sparse, as in most practical situations, it may be necessary to computing the raw estimates by grouping the observations from the adjacent time points. In particular, we can first compute $\widehat{\beta}_l^{RAW}(s_r)$, $l = 0, \ldots, k$, using the local polynomial method (3.5) with a small bandwidth, and then, treating $\widehat{\beta}_l^{RAW}(s_r)$ as the new data, estimate $\beta_l(t)$ by minimizing

$$L_{p,l}^{TS}(t) = \sum_{j=1}^{m} \left\{ \widehat{\beta}_l^{RAW}(s_j) - \sum_{r=0}^{p} b_{lr}(t)(s_j - t)^r \right\}^2 K_l\left(\frac{s_j - t}{h_l}\right) \tag{3.14}$$

with respect to $b_{lr}(t)$, where $(K_l(\cdot), h_l)$ is a set of kernel and bandwidth. Similar to (3.5), if $\widehat{b}_{lr}^{TS}(t)$ for $r = 0, \ldots, k$ uniquely minimize (3.14), $\widehat{b}_{l0}^{TS}(t)$ is the two-step pth order local polynomial estimator of $\beta_l(t)$, while $(r!)\widehat{b}_{lr}^{TS}(t)$ can be used to estimate the rth derivative of $\beta_l(t)$.

In contrast to the estimators obtained from (3.5) where a single bandwidth must be used for all $\beta_l(t)$, the two-step method has in principle the flexibility to adjust for the specific smoothing need of each coefficient curve.

However, a main difficulty in current version of two-step smoothing is that it lacks a specific and practical guideline to construct the raw estimates for unbalanced longitudinal data. Certain data-driven bandwidth procedures would be desirable for computing both the raw and the final estimates. Impacts of different raw estimates on the theoretical and practical properties of the final two-step estimators are still not well-understood and require substantial further development.

3.5. *Component-wise smoothing with time-invariant covariates*

When the covariates of interest are time-invariant, such as in clinical trials when the treatments are kept fixed throughout the study periods, an effective way motivated by (3.3) to provide flexible and computational feasible estimators of $\beta(t)$ is to smooth each component of $\beta(t)$ separately.

Let $Z^{(r)}(t)=[\sum_{l=0}^{k} e_{rl}X^{(l)}]Y(t)$, $\mathbf{X}_i=(1,X_i^{(1)},\ldots,X_i^{(k)})^T$ be the covariate vector of the ith subject and $\widehat{e}_{rl}$ be the (r,l)th element of the matrix $(\widehat{E}_{\mathbf{XX}^T})^{-1}$, the inverse of the sample mean $\widehat{E}_{\mathbf{XX}^T}=(1/n)\sum_{i=0}^{n}\mathbf{X}_i\mathbf{X}_i^T$. A natural estimator of $Z^{(r)}(t)$ is $Z_{ij}^{(r)}=[\sum_{l=0}^{k}\widehat{e}_{rl}X_i^{(l)}]Y_{ij}$. By (3.3), a componentwise smoothing estimator of $\beta_r(t)$ can be obtained by smoothing $Z_{ij}^{(r)}$ for $i=1,\ldots,n$ and $j=1,\ldots,n_i$. Specifically, a local polynomial estimator of $\beta_r(t)$ with order $p\geq 0$ is $\widehat{b}_{r0}^{COM}(t)$, such that $\widehat{b}_{rl}^{COM}(t)$, $l=0,\ldots,p$, uniquely minimize

$$L_{p,r}^{COM}(t)=\sum_{i=1}^{n}\sum_{j=1}^{n_i}w_i\left\{Z_{ij}^{(r)}-\sum_{l=0}^{p}b_{rl}(t)(t_{ij}-t)^l\right\}^2K_r\left(\frac{t_{ij}-t}{h_r}\right), \tag{3.15}$$

with respect to $b_{rl}(t)$. For the local constant fitting with $p=0$, (3.15) leads to the componentwise kernel estimator

$$\widehat{\beta}_r^{COM}(t)=\frac{\sum_{i=1}^{n}\sum_{j=1}^{n_i}\left\{w_iZ_{ij}^{(r)}K_r\left[(t_{ij}-t)/h_r\right]\right\}}{\sum_{i=1}^{n}\sum_{j=1}^{n_i}\left\{w_iK_r\left[(t_{ij}-t)/h_r\right]\right\}}. \tag{3.16}$$

Wu and Chiang (2000) established the large sample mean squared errors of $\widehat{\beta}_r^{COM}(t)$, while Wu, Yu and Yuan (2000) developed a procedure for constructing approximate asymptotic pointwise and simultaneous confidence regions for $\beta_r(t)$. These results shed some light on the asymptotic behaviors of the higher order estimators $\widehat{b}_{r0}^{COM}(t)$, although specific asymptotic risks and asymptotic distributions have not been established for the case with $p \geq 1$. The results of Wu and Chiang (2000) and Wu, Yu and Yuan (2000) indicate some clear advantages of $\widehat{\beta}_r^{COM}(t)$ over the kernel estimator (3.6) both in terms of theoretical convergence rates and practical flexibilities. Similar advantages over the least squares method of (3.5) are also expected for the componentwise local polynomial estimators.

Obviously, minimizing (3.15) is not the only componentwise smoothing approach. Suppose that the support of the design time points is contained in a compact set $[a, b]$ and $\beta_r(t)$ is twice differentiable with respect to t in $[a, b]$. A viable alternative is to estimate $\beta_r(t)$ by penalized least squares estimator $\widetilde{\beta}_r^{COM}(t)$, where $\widetilde{\beta}_r^{COM}(t)$ minimizes

$$J_r^{COM}(\beta_r, \lambda_r) = \sum_{i=1}^{n} \sum_{j=1}^{n_i} \left\{ w_i \left[Z_{ij}^{(r)} - \beta_r(t_{ij}) \right]^2 \right\} + \lambda_r \int_a^b \left[\beta_r^{''}(s) \right]^2 ds, \tag{3.17}$$

with λ_r being a non-negative smoothing parameter. By the same rationale as in Section 2.3, it is easy to verify that $\widetilde{\beta}_r^{COM}(t)$ is a natural cubic spline with knots at the distinct points of $\{t_{ij};\ i = 1, \ldots, n,\ j = 1, \ldots, n_i\}$. Furthermore, using the approach of equivalent kernels, Chiang, Rice and Wu (2001) derived the asymptotic mean squared errors and the asymptotic distributions of $\widetilde{\beta}_r^{COM}(t)$. In contrast to the multiple penalized least squares of (3.13) whose solution is obtained by solving a large linear system involving all $(k + 1)$ components, (3.17) significantly simplifies the computation by solving $(k + 1)$ separate linear systems. This computational advantage ensures the practical implementability of (3.17) in many situations, while the intensive computational needs often make the optimization of (3.13) impracticable.

3.6. *Smoothing via basis approximations*

All the smoothing methods described above depend on local smoothing in the sense that only the measurements obtained within some neighborhood of t are effectively used to estimate $\beta(t)$. Although local smoothing works well when all the coefficient curves $\beta_r(t)$ are nonparametric, it is not adequate when some of the coefficient curves have known parametric forms, as in the partially linear model (1.1).

Compared with local smoothing, estimation using basis approximations has three important advantages. First, it can be used to estimate $\beta(t)$

whether its components are parametric or nonparametric, hence, is suitable for both nonparametric and semiparametric varying-coefficient models. Second, when a random effect is desired, it provides a natural means to incorporate random effects into a nonparametric or semiparametric model. Third, because popular basis estimators, such as truncated polynomials or B-splines, often rely on far fewer knots or approximation terms than smoothing splines, they often enjoy considerable computationally advantage over smoothing splines or even local polynomials. Although estimation with mixed effects is of great interest in various settings, we only discuss here the case of marginal models. Extension to mixed effects models can be found in Rice and Wu (2001).

The main idea is to first approximate $\beta_r(t)$ by a basis function expansion with K_r terms, where K_r may or may not tend to infinity as n tends to infinity, and then estimate $\beta_r(t)$ by estimating the coefficients of this expansion. For each $r = 0, \ldots, k$, let $B_{rs}(t)$, $s = 1, \ldots, K_r$, be a set of basis functions. If $\beta_r(t)$ can be approximated by an expansion based on $B_{rs}(t)$, $s = 1, \ldots, K_r$, there is a set of constants γ_{rs} so that

$$\beta_r(t) \approx \sum_{s=1}^{K_r} \gamma_{rs} B_{rs}(t). \tag{3.18}$$

Substituting (3.18) into (1.2), an approximation of the varying-coefficient model is

$$Y_{ij} \approx \sum_{r=0}^{k} \sum_{s=1}^{K_r} X_{ij}^{(r)} \gamma_{rs} B_{rs}(t) + \epsilon_i(t_{ij}). \tag{3.19}$$

The approximation sign in (3.19) will be replaced by the equality sign if, for all $r = 0, \ldots, k$, $\beta_r(t)$ belongs to a linear space spanned by $\{B_{rs}(t);\ s = 1, \ldots, K_r\}$.

Using (3.19), the least squares estimators $\widehat{\gamma}_{rs}$ of γ_{rs} can be obtained by minimizing

$$\ell(\gamma) = \sum_{i=1}^{n} \sum_{j=1}^{n_i} \left\{ w_i \left[Y_{ij} - \sum_{r=0}^{k} \sum_{s=1}^{K_r} \left(X_{ij}^{(r)} \gamma_{rs} B_{rs}(t_{ij}) \right) \right]^2 \right\}, \tag{3.20}$$

where $\gamma = (\gamma_0^T, \ldots, \gamma_k^T)^T$ and $\gamma_r = (\gamma_{r1}, \ldots, \gamma_{rK_r})^T$. If the minimizer of (3.20) uniquely exists, the basis function estimator of $\beta_r(t)$ is

$$\widehat{\beta}_r^{BAS}(t) = \sum_{s=1}^{K_r} \left[\widehat{\gamma}_{rs} B_{rs}(t) \right], \tag{3.21}$$

where K_r may depend on n and n_i, $i = 1, \ldots, n$. Clearly, if K_r is finite and known and $\beta_r(t)$ belongs to the linear space spanned by $B_{rs}(t)$, $s = 1, \ldots, K_r$, then (3.21) returns a parametric estimator of $\beta_r(t)$. On the other hand, if (3.18) holds with K_r unknown, a consistent nonparametric estimator produced by (3.21) may require K_r to be a function of n and n_i, $i = 1, \ldots, n$, which may tend to infinity as n tends to infinity.

Depending on the underlying scientific nature of the data, many different bases may be used to approximate the components of $\beta(t)$. The most popular basis system in the classical linear models is the polynomial basis $\{1, t, \ldots, t^{K_r - 1}\}$. A general class of bases that have certain numerical advantages over the above polynomial basis is the class of piecewise polynomials. Examples of piecewise polynomial bases include B-spline bases, such as linear, quadratic or cubic splines, or other types of truncated power series; see de Boor (1978) for further details of the explicit expressions of piecewise polynomials and their numerical properties. If $\beta_r(t)$ is believed to exhibit periodicity, Fourier series are often natural basis choices.

Huang, Wu and Zhou (2002) established the consistency of (3.21) and studied the practical performance of (3.21) with B-splines through an intensive simulation. Further asymptotic properties for the B-splines estimators of (3.21) are developed in Huang, Wu and Zhou (2004). In general, a B-spline estimator requires a smoothing parameter consisted of three aspects: degrees of the polynomials and number and location of the knots. Although generally desired, it is difficult, however, to simultaneously determine all three of these aspects from the data. Rice and Wu (2001) showed that the simple approach of using equally spaced knots often works well in practice, a finding also corroborated by the simulation of Huang, Wu and Zhou (2002).

3.7. *A cross-validation procedure*

The most important factor that affects all of the above smoothing methods is the selection of appropriate smoothing parameters, such as the bandwidth, the positive penalty weight λ and the number and location of knots. It is of both theoretical and practical interest to select these values directly from the data.

Selecting data-driven smoothing parameters for nonparametric regression with independent identically distributed data has been a subject of intense investigation in the literature. Under the current context, a widely used method, suggested by Rice and Silverman (1991), is a cross-validation that deletes the entire repeated measurements of a subject, rather than an individual measurement, one at a time. Hart and Wehrly (1993) derived the consistency of this cross-validation for a simple nonparametric regression without the presence of covariates other than time. Without loss of generality, we denote ξ to be a vector of smoothing parameters, $\widehat{\beta}(t;\xi)$ a smoothing estimator based on ξ and $\widehat{\beta}^{(-i)}(t;\xi)$ an estimator computed using the same method as $\widehat{\beta}(t;\xi)$ but with the ith subject's measurements deleted. The cross-validation score for $\widehat{\beta}(t;\xi)$ is

$$\mathrm{CV}(\xi) = \sum_{i=1}^{n}\sum_{j=1}^{n_i}\left\{w_i\left[Y_{ij} - X_{ij}^T\widehat{\beta}^{(-i)}(t;\xi)\right]^2\right\}, \tag{3.22}$$

which measures the predictive error of $\widehat{\beta}(t;\xi)$. The cross-validated smoothing parameter ξ_{cv} is then the minimizer of $\mathrm{CV}(\xi)$, provided that the unique minimizer of $\mathrm{CV}(\xi)$ exists.

The above cross-validation criterion is directly applicable to all the smoothing methods presented above, except the two-step smoothing of Section 2.4. For the estimators of Sections 2.2, 2.3 and 2.5 and B-splines with equally spaced knots, minimizing the corresponding cross-validation scores would either return a univariate bandwidth or a R^{k+1}-valued vector. An automatic search of the global minima usually requires a sophisticated optimization software. In practice, particularly when the smoothing parameter is multivariate, it is often reasonable to use a smoothing parameter whose cross-validation score is close to the global minima.

There are three intuitive reasons to use the cross-validation criterion (3.22). First, by deleting the subjects one at a time, it preserves the correlation structure of the data. Second, in contrast to alternatives such as the AIC, the BIC and the generalized cross-validation (e.g. Akaike, 1970, Schwarz, 1978, Shibata, 1981, and Wahba, 1990), (3.22) does not depend on the structure of the intra-subject correlations, hence, can be implemented in almost all the practical situations. Third, when the number of subjects is sufficiently large, minimizing (3.22) leads to a smoothing parameter that approximately minimizes the average squared error:

$$\mathrm{ASE}\left(\widehat{\beta}(\cdot;\xi)\right) = \sum_{i=1}^{n}\sum_{j=1}^{n_i}\left\{w_i\left[X_{ij}^T\left(\beta(t_{ij}) - \widehat{\beta}(t_{ij};\xi)\right)\right]^2\right\}. \tag{3.23}$$

The last assertion can be heuristically seen by the decomposition:

$$\mathrm{CV}(\xi) = \sum_{i=1}^{n}\sum_{j=1}^{n_i}\left\{w_i\left[Y_{ij} - X_{ij}^T\beta(t_{ij})\right]^2\right\} \tag{3.24}$$

$$+2\sum_{i=1}^{n}\sum_{j=1}^{n_i}\left\{w_i\left[Y_{ij}-X_{ij}^T\beta(t_{ij})\right]\left[X_{ij}^T\left(\beta(t_{ij})-\widehat{\beta}^{(-i)}(t_{ij};\xi)\right)\right]^2\right\}$$

$$+\sum_{i=1}^{n}\sum_{j=1}^{n_i}\left\{w_i\left[X_{ij}^T\left(\beta(t_{ij})-\widehat{\beta}^{(-i)}(t_{ij};\xi)\right)\right]^2\right\}.$$

Here, (3.23) and the definition of $\widehat{\beta}^{(-i)}(t;\xi)$ imply that the third term at the right side of (3.24) is approximately the same as $\mathrm{ASE}(\widehat{\beta}(\cdot;\xi))$. Because the first term at the right side of (3.24) does not depend on the smoothing parameter and the second term is approximately zero, ξ_{cv} approximately minimizes $\mathrm{ASE}(\widehat{\beta}(\cdot;\xi))$.

3.8. *Asymptotic inferences for kernel estimators*

Confidence statements can be made either based on the asymptotic distributions of the estimators or through a bootstrap procedure. Currently, explicit expressions of asymptotic distributions have only been developed for the kernel estimators (3.6) and (3.16).

3.8.1. *Pointwise confidence intervals*

For both (3.6) and (3.16), their asymptotic distributions have been developed based on two important assumptions. First, the numbers of repeated measurements n_i are non-random and may or may not tend to infinity as n tending to infinity. Second, the time design points t_{ij} are random and independent identically distributed according to an unknown density function $f(\cdot)$. These assumptions are made for practical considerations as well as mathematical tractability.

Consider first the confidence procedures based on (3.6). Under the above assumptions and some additional mild regularity conditions, Wu, Chiang and Hoover (1998) showed that, if $w_i = 1/N$, $h = N^{-1/5}h_0$ and

$$\lim_{n\to\infty} N^{-6/5}\sum_{i=1}^{n} n_i^2 = \theta$$

for some constants $h_0 > 0$ and $0 \le \theta < \infty$, $\widehat{\beta}^{LSK}(t)$ has an asymptotically multivariate normal distribution in the sense that

$$(Nh)^{1/2}\left[\widehat{\beta}^{LSK}(t)-\beta(t)\right] \longrightarrow \mathbf{N}\left(B(t), D^*(t)\right), \tag{3.25}$$

in distribution as $n \to \infty$. The bias, $B(t)$, and the variance-covariance matrix, $D^*(t)$, of (3.25) are

$$B(t) = [f(t)]^{-1} E^{-1}_{XX^T}(t)(b_0(t), \ldots, b_k(t))^T \tag{3.26}$$

and

$$D^*(t) = [f(t)]^{-2} E^{-1}_{XX^T}(t) D(t) E^{1}_{XX^T}(t) \tag{3.27}$$

where $D(t)$ is a $(k+1) \times (k+1)$ matrix whose (l,r)th element is

$$D_{lr}(t) = \sigma^2(t) E\left[X^{(l)}(t)X^{(r)}(t)\right] f(t) \left\{\int [K(u)]^2 du\right\}$$
$$+\theta h_0 \rho_\epsilon(t) E\left[X^{(l)}(t)X^{(r)}(t)\right] [f(t)]^2,$$

$\sigma^2(t) = E[\epsilon^2(t)]$, $\rho_\epsilon(t) = \lim_{a\to 0} E[\epsilon(t+a)\epsilon(t)]$ and

$$b_l(t) = h_0^{3/2} \sum_{c=0}^{k} \left\{\left[\int u^2 K(u) du\right] \left\{\beta_c'(t) \left[E\left[X^{(l)}(t)X^{(c)}(t)\right]\right]' f(t)\right.\right.$$
$$+\beta_c'(t) E\left[X^{(l)}(t)X^{(c)}(t)\right] f'(t)$$
$$\left.\left. + (1/2)\beta_c''(t) E\left[X^{(l)}(t)X^{(c)}(t)\right] f(t)\right\}\right\}.$$

Then, there are lower and upper end points $L_\alpha(t)$ and $U_\alpha(t)$ given by

$$\left\{A^T \widehat{\beta}^{LSK}(t) - (Nh)^{-1/2} A^T B(t)\right\} \pm Z_{\alpha/2}(Nh)^{-1/2} \left[A^T D^*(t) A\right]^{1/2}, \tag{3.28}$$

where $Z_{\alpha/2}$ is the $(1-\alpha/2)$ quantile of the standard normal distribution, so that

$$\lim_{n\to\infty} P\left\{L_\alpha(t) \le A^T\beta(t) \le U_\alpha(t)\right\} = 1 - \alpha. \tag{3.29}$$

Because $B(t)$ and $D^*(t)$ depend on unknown quantities, (3.28) is not implementable in practice. If $B(t)$ and $D^*(t)$ can be consistently estimated by $\widehat{B}(t)$ and $\widehat{D}^*(t)$, a pointwise $(1-\alpha)$ confidence interval for $A^T\beta(t)$ can be approximated by $(\widehat{L}_\alpha(t), \widehat{U}_\alpha(t))$ with $\widehat{L}_\alpha(t)$ and $\widehat{U}_\alpha(t)$ being the lower and upper end points given by

$$\left\{A^T \widehat{\beta}^{LSK}(t) - (Nh)^{-1/2} A^T \widehat{B}(t)\right\} \pm Z_{\alpha/2}(Nh)^{-1/2} \left[A^T \widehat{D}^*(t) A\right]^{1/2}. \tag{3.30}$$

Wu, Chiang and Hoover (1998) suggested to compute $\widehat{B}(t)$ and $\widehat{D}^*(t)$ by substituting $f(t)$, $\sigma^2(t)$, $\rho_\epsilon(t)$, $E[X^{(l)}(t)X^{(r)}(t)]$ and the required derivatives in (3.26) and (3.27) with their kernel estimators. Suppose that the kernel function $K(\cdot)$ is at least twice continuously differentiable in the interior of its support. These authors proposed to estimate $f(t)$, $\sigma^2(t)$, $\rho_\epsilon(t)$ and $E[X^{(l)}(t)X^{(r)}(t)]$ by

$$\widehat{f}(t) = (Nh)^{-1}\sum_{i=1}^{n}\sum_{j=1}^{n_i} K\left(\frac{t_{ij}-t}{h}\right),$$

$$\widehat{\sigma}^2(t) = \frac{1}{Nh\widehat{f}(t)}\sum_{i=1}^{n}\sum_{j=1}^{n_i}\left\{\widehat{\epsilon}_i^2(t_{ij})K\left(\frac{t_{ij}-t}{h}\right)\right\},$$

$$\widehat{\rho}_\epsilon(t) = \frac{\sum_{i=1}^{n}\sum_{j_1\neq j_2}\left\{\widehat{\epsilon}_i(t_{ij_1})\widehat{\epsilon}_i(t_{ij_2})K\left(\frac{t_{ij}-t}{h}\right)K\left(\frac{t_{ij}-t}{h}\right)\right\}}{\sum_{i=1}^{n}\sum_{j_1\neq j_2}\left\{K\left(\frac{t_{ij}-t}{h}\right)K\left(\frac{t_{ij}-t}{h}\right)\right\}}$$

and

$$\widehat{E}\left[X^{(l)}(t)X^{(r)}(t)\right] = \frac{1}{Nh\widehat{f}(t)}\sum_{i=1}^{n}\sum_{j=1}^{n_i}\left\{X_i^{(l)}(t_{ij})X_i^{(r)}(t_{ij})K\left(\frac{t_{ij}-t}{h}\right)\right\},$$

where $\widehat{\epsilon}_i(t_{ij}) = Y_{ij} - X_i^T(t_{ij})\widehat{\beta}(t_{ij})$ are the residuals, and to estimate the first and second derivatives of $f(t)$, $\beta_l(t)$ and $E[X^{(l)}(t)X^{(r)}(t)]$ by the corresponding derivatives of $\widehat{f}(t)$, $\widehat{\beta}_l^{LSK}(t)$ and $\widehat{E}[X^{(l)}(t)X^{(r)}(t)]$. Through an intensive simulation, these authors also suggested that the cross-validation bandwidth h_{cv} obtained from (3.22) may be used to compute all of the above estimators, although, in general, different bandwidths may be used for these estimators.

The above plug-in approach can also be extended to $\widehat{\beta}_r^{COM}(t)$ of (3.16) when the covariates are time-invariant. Wu, Yu and Yuan (2000) have derived the explicit expressions of the bias, $\mathrm{B}(\widehat{\beta}_r^{COM};t)$, and the standard deviation, $\mathrm{SD}(\widehat{\beta}_r^{COM};t)$, of $\widehat{\beta}_r^{COM}(t)$, and suggested to use the approximate $(1-\alpha)$ confidence interval for $\beta_r(t)$ with end points

$$\left\{\widehat{\beta}_r^{COM}(t) - \widehat{\mathrm{B}}\left(\widehat{\beta}_r^{COM};t\right)\right\} \pm Z_{1-\alpha/2}\widehat{\mathrm{SD}}\left(\widehat{\beta}_r^{COM};t\right),$$

where $\widehat{\mathrm{B}}(\widehat{\beta}_r^{COM};t)$ and $\widehat{\mathrm{SD}}(\widehat{\beta}_r^{COM};t)$ are plug-in estimators of $\mathrm{B}(\widehat{\beta}_r^{COM};t)$ and $\mathrm{SD}(\widehat{\beta}_r^{COM};t)$. Because of the similarity it shares with $\widehat{\beta}^{LSK}(t)$, we omit the details for this case.

The above asymptotic intervals differ from their counterparts with independent identically distributed data in the inclusion of intra-subject correlations in the variance term. When n_i are not negligible relative to n, θ in

(3.27) may not be negligible, so that the contribution of the correlations may not be ignored. For the HIV/CD4 data (Section 1.2.2), the numbers of repeated measurements range from 1 to 14, while the number of subjects is 400. Asymptotic results that do not take the intra-subject correlations into account may not lead to adequate approximations. In this case, it is appropriate to estimate the correlations directly from the data. When the numbers of repeated measurements are negligible relative to the numbers of subjects, as in the ASGA data (Section 1.2.1), the contribution of the intra-subject correlation structures becomes negligible in the variances of the kernel estimators. The resulting confidence intervals are then similar to that with independent identically distributed samples.

3.8.2. *Simultaneous bands*

In most applications, the main interest of inference lies in the overall confidence regions of $\beta_l(t)$ within a proper range of t values, rather than the confidence intervals at a particular time point. When the data are from independent identically distributed samples, simultaneous confidence regions for regression curves may be constructed using either extreme value theory of Gaussian processes (e.g. Eubank and Speckman, 1993) or variability bands bridged by pointwise intervals over a grid points (e.g. Knafl, Sacks and Ylvisaker, 1985, Hall and Titterington, 1988, and Härdle and Marron, 1991). For longitudinal samples, analogous asymptotic theory of extreme values has not been developed. This leaves the latter approach to be the only practical simultaneous inferential tool in longitudinal analysis.

To construct a simultaneous band for $A^T\beta(t)$ over $t \in [a, b]$ based on the least squares kernel estimator $\widehat{\beta}^{(LSK)}(t)$, we choose a positive integer M and partition $[a, b]$ into M equally spaced intervals with grid points $a = \xi_1 < \cdots < \xi_{M+1} = b$, such that $\xi_{j+1} - \xi_j = (b-a)/M$ for $j = 1, \ldots, M$. A set of approximate $(1-\alpha)$ simultaneous confidence intervals for $A^T\beta(\xi_j)$, $j = 1, \ldots, M+1$, is then the collection of intervals $(\widehat{l}_\alpha(\xi_j), \widehat{u}_\alpha(\xi_j))$, $j = 1, \ldots, M+1$, which satisfies

$$\lim_{n\to\infty} P\Big\{\widehat{l}_\alpha(\xi_j) \le A^T\beta(\xi_j) \le \widehat{u}_\alpha(\xi_j) \\ \text{for all } j = 1, \ldots, M+1\Big\} \ge 1-\alpha. \tag{3.31}$$

The Bonferroni adjustment suggests

$$(\widehat{l}_\alpha(\xi_j), \widehat{u}_\alpha(\xi_j)) = (\widehat{L}_{\alpha/(M+1)}(\xi_j), \widehat{U}_{\alpha/(M+1)}(\xi_j)), \tag{3.32}$$

where $(\widehat{L}_\alpha(\xi_j), \widehat{U}_\alpha(\xi_j))$ are defined in (3.30).

To establish a band that covers all the points between the grid points ξ_j, $j = 1, \ldots, M+1$, we first consider the interpolation of $A^T\beta(\xi_j)$ defined by

$$(A^T\beta)^{(I)}(t) = \left\{\frac{M(\xi_{j+1} - t)}{b-a}\right\}[A^T\beta(\xi_j)] + \left\{\frac{M(t - \xi_j)}{b-a}\right\}[A^T\beta(\xi_{j+1})], \tag{3.33}$$

for $t \in [\xi_j, \xi_{j+1}]$. A simultaneous band for $(A^T\beta)^{(I)}(t)$ over $t \in [a, b]$ is $(\widehat{l}_\alpha^{(I)}(t), \widehat{u}_\alpha^{(I)}(t))$, where $\widehat{l}_\alpha^{(I)}(t)$ and $\widehat{u}_\alpha^{(I)}(t)$ are the linear interpolations of $\widehat{l}_\alpha(\xi_j)$ and $\widehat{u}_\alpha(\xi_j)$, similarly defined as in (3.33). The gaps between the grid points are then bridged by the smoothness conditions of $A^T\beta(t)$. If $A^T\beta(t)$ satisfies

$$\sup_{t\in[a,b]} \left|(A^T\beta)'(t)\right| \le c_1, \quad \text{for a known constant } c_1 > 0, \tag{3.34}$$

then it follows that

$$\left|A^T\beta(t) - (A^T\beta)^{(I)}(t)\right| \le 2c_1\left[\frac{M(\xi_{j+1} - t)(t - \xi_j)}{b-a}\right],$$

for all $t \in [\xi_j, \xi_{j+1}]$, and consequently

$$\left(\widehat{l}_\alpha^{(I)}(t) - 2c_1\left[\frac{M(\xi_{j+1} - t)(t - \xi_j)}{b-a}\right], \widehat{u}_\alpha^{(I)}(t) + 2c_1\left[\frac{M(\xi_{j+1} - t)(t - \xi_j)}{b-a}\right]\right) \tag{3.35}$$

is an approximate $(1-\alpha)$ confidence band for $A^T\beta(t)$. If $A^T\beta(t)$ satisfies

$$\sup_{t\in[a,b]} \left|(A^T\beta)''(t)\right| \le c_2, \quad \text{for a known constant } c_2 > 0, \tag{3.36}$$

then

$$\left|A^T\beta(t) - (A^T\beta)^{(I)}(t)\right| \le \frac{c_2}{2}\left[\frac{M(\xi_{j+1} - t)(t - \xi_j)}{b-a}\right],$$

for all $t \in [\xi_j, \xi_{j+1}]$, and an approximate $(1-\alpha)$ confidence band can be given by

$$\left(\widehat{l}_\alpha^{(I)}(t) - \frac{c_2}{2}\left[\frac{M(\xi_{j+1} - t)(t - \xi_j)}{b-a}\right], \widehat{u}_\alpha^{(I)}(t) + \frac{c_2}{2}\left[\frac{M(\xi_{j+1} - t)(t - \xi_j)}{b-a}\right]\right). \tag{3.37}$$

For smoothness conditions other than the ones considered in (3.34) and (3.36), the corresponding confidence bands may be similarly established. When the covariates are time-invariant, the same approach can be used to establish simultaneous confidence bands based on $\widehat{\beta}^{COM}(t)$; see Wu, Yu and Yuan (2000) for details.

3.9. *Bootstrap variability bands*

The above asymptotic inferences subject to two restrictions which, to some degree, limit their applications in longitudinal analysis. First, because the asymptotic distributions have so far only been developed for the two kernel type estimators, $\widehat{\beta}^{LSK}(t)$ and $\widehat{\beta}^{COM}(t)$, confidence procedures for other estimators are still not available. Given that smoothing methods such as splines and local polynomials have exhibited a number of theoretical and practical advantages over the kernel methods, particularly at the boundary of the support of t, inferential procedures based on these smoothing methods are in demand. Second, because the plug-in estimators require the estimation of the design densities, covariance functions and the other quantities appeared in the bias and variance terms of the estimators, the procedure is usually computationally intensive and may introduce additional errors in its coverage probabilities.

A more appealing inferential procedure that has been suggested in the literature is the "resampling-subject" bootstrap. This approach has broader appeal in longitudinal analysis since it resamples the subjects of the original data, which may preserve the intra-subject correlations. Although its theoretical properties have not been well-understood, practical performances of this "resampling-subject" bootstrap have been investigated by a number of simulation studies. Let $\widehat{\beta}(t) = (\widehat{\beta}_0(t), \ldots, \widehat{\beta}_k(t))^T$ be an estimator of $\beta(t)$ constructed based on any of the previously mentioned smoothing method. An approximate $(1-\alpha)$ pointwise percentile interval for $A^T E[\widehat{\beta}(t)]$ can be constructed by the following steps:

(1) Randomly draw n subjects with replacement from the original dataset and denote the resulting bootstrap sample to be $\{(Y_{ij}^*, t_{ij}^*, X_{ij}^*);\ i = 1, \ldots, n, j = 1, \ldots, n_i\}$.
(2) Compute the bootstrap estimator $\widehat{\beta}^{boot}(t)$, hence $A^T\widehat{\beta}^{boot}(t)$, based on the above bootstrap sample and the smoothing method specified for $\widehat{\beta}(t)$.
(3) Repeating the above two steps B times, so that B bootstrap estimators $A^T\widehat{\beta}^{boot}(t)$ are obtained.

(4) Calculate $L_\alpha^{boot}(t)$ and $U_\alpha^{boot}(t)$, the lower and upper $[100 \times (\alpha/2)]$th percentiles, respectively, of the B bootstrap estimators $A^T \widehat{\beta}^{boot}(t)$. The approximate $(1-\alpha)$ bootstrap interval is then $(L_\alpha^{boot}(t), U_\alpha^{boot}(t))$.

When $A^T E[\widehat{\beta}(t)]$ satisfies the smoothness conditions (3.34) or (3.36), simultaneous confidence bands for $A^T E[\widehat{\beta}(t)]$ can be constructed using (3.35) and (3.37) with (3.32) replaced by $(L_{\alpha/(M+1)}^{boot}(\xi_j), U_{\alpha/(M+1)}^{boot}(\xi_j))$.

The main advantages of this bootstrap are its generality and simplicity. It is not limited to kernel type estimators and does not depend on the correlations and designs of the data. Despite its potential, several related theoretical and practical issues have still yet to be resolved. Because the biases of the estimators have not been adjusted, the resulting intervals or bands may not always have desirable coverage probabilities for $A^T \beta(t)$. If a consistent estimator of the bias is also available, improved confidence regions for $A^T \beta(t)$ may be obtained by adjusting the bias appeared in $(L_{\alpha/(M+1)}^{boot}(\xi_j), U_{\alpha/(M+1)}^{boot}(\xi_j))$. Currently, consistent bias estimators can only be obtained on a case-by-case basis, and no general procedure is available. A natural alternative to the percentile end points used in Step 4 is to consider normal approximated intervals with end points $A^T \widehat{\beta}(t) \pm z_{(1-\alpha/2)} \widehat{se}^{boot}(t)$, where $\widehat{se}^{boot}(t)$ is the sample standard error of the B bootstrap estimators $A^T \widehat{\beta}^{boot}(t)$. Asymptotic properties for both the percentile and the normal approximation bootstrap procedures have not been investigated.

3.10. *Application to alabama fetal growth study*

Normal fetal growth is naturally thought to influence infant survival and proper child development. Our objective is to investigate the effects of maternal risk factors and maternal anthropometric measurements on the patterns of fetal growth. Although the outcomes measured by fetal abdominal circumference, biparietal diameter and femur length are all time-dependent, the covariates of interest may be either time-dependent or time-invariant. A typical time-dependent covariate is the maternal placental thickness measured by ultrasound at each visit. On the other hand, mother's height, weight and body mass index measured at the beginning of pregnancy, are time-invariant. Other variables, such as maternal habits of cigarette smoking and alcohol consumption, may be either time-dependent or time-invariant depending on how these variables are defined. A simple way to define time-invariant maternal smoking and drinking status is to categorize the mothers as smokers (ever smoked cigarettes during the pregnancy) versus non-smokers (never smoked cigarettes during the pregnancy) and non-drinkers/light-drinkers (consumed one beer/one glass of wine or less per day in average during the pregnancy) versus heavy-drinkers (consumed more than one beer or one glass of wine per day in average during the pregnancy). As in most self-reported questionnaires, the data contain the average numbers of cigarettes smoked and the average amount of alcohol consumed per day per subject. These actual cigarette and alcohol consumptions are clearly time-dependent as some of the participating subjects change their behaviors during the study. Depending on the specific scientific questions, both smoking and drinking categories and the actual consumptions could be considered in the analysis.

For the purpose of illustration, the analysis present here focuses on the effects of maternal smoking/drinking categories and placental thickness on the growth of fetal abdominal circumference. Other covariate and outcome measurements can be similarly investigated, provided that the models have clear and meaningful biological interpretations. Although the general trend of Figure 1 shows an upward growth pattern, it hardly provides any clue on the relationship between fetal growth and the covariates of interest. A nonparametric analysis with (1.2) seems a natural start.

Let $Y(t)$ and $X^{(1)}(t)$ be the fetal abdominal circumference and placental thickness, respectively, at t weeks of gestation; $X^{(2)}$ and $X^{(3)}$ be the mother's drinking and smoking categories defined by

$$X^{(2)} = \begin{cases} 1 & \text{if she is a non-drinker/light-drinker,} \\ 0 & \text{if she is a heavy-drinker,} \end{cases}$$

$$X^{(3)} = \begin{cases} 1 & \text{if she is a smoker,} \\ 0 & \text{otherwise;} \end{cases}$$

and $X^{(4)}$ be the mother's height (in centimeters) at the beginning of the pregnancy.

In view that proper placental development may also be affected by drinking and smoking, we first consider the effects of the time-invariant covariate vector $X = (1, X^{(2)}, X^{(3)}, X^{(4)})^T$. Although we can fit (1.2) directly with $(Y(t), t, X)$ and describe the covariate effects by $\beta(t) = (\beta_0(t), \beta_2(t), \beta_3(t), \beta_4(t))^T$, a better biological interpretation can be obtained if $X^{(4)}$ were replaced by its centered version $X^{(*4)} = X^{(4)} - E[X^{(4)}]$, so that the covariate effects are characterized by $\beta^*(t) = (\beta_0^*(t), \beta_2(t), \beta_3(t), \beta_4(t))^T$. For the latter case, the baseline coefficient curve

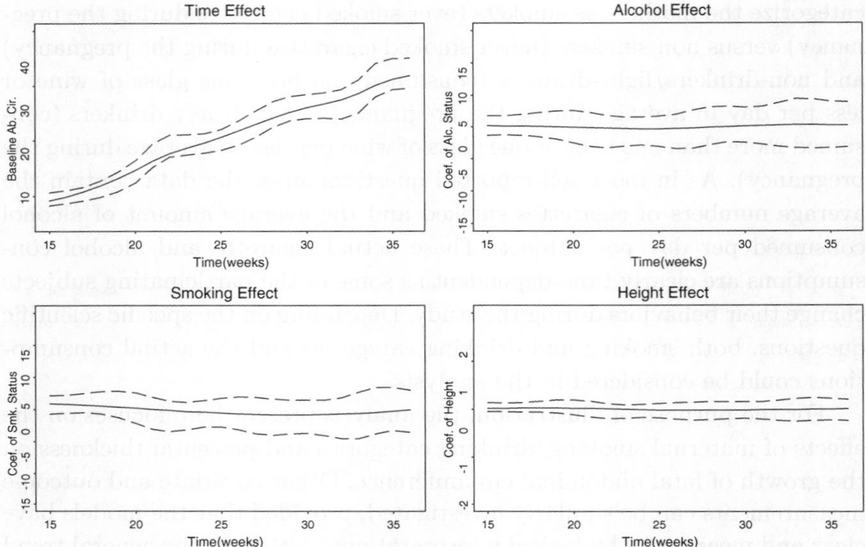

Fig. 2. Solid lines: componentwise kernel estimates of the coefficient curves (covariate effects) computed using the Epanechnikov kernel, the cross-validated bandwidths and $w_i = 1/(nn_i)$. Dashed lines: the 95% Bonferroni-type confidence bands.

$\beta_0^*(t)$ represents the mean abdominal circumference at t weeks of gestation for a non-smoking and non-drinking/light-drinking mother whose height is at average, while, for the former, $\beta_0(t)$ itself does not have a biological interpretation.

To fit model (1.2) with $(Y(t), t, X^{(*)})$, $X^{(*)} = (1, X^{(2)}, X^{(3)}, X^{(*4)})^T$, we computed $X_i^{(*4)}$, $i = 1, \ldots, 1475$, by subtracting the sample average of $\{X_j^{(4)};\ j = 1, \ldots, 1475\}$ from $X_i^{(4)}$. Figure 2 shows the estimated coefficient curves, including the baseline growth curve and the covariate effects characterized by alcohol consumption, cigarette smoking and mother's height, and their corresponding 95% simultaneous confidence bands. These coefficient curves were computed using the componentwise estimators of (3.16) with the Epanechikov kernel, the cross-validated bandwidths described in (3.22) and $w_i = 1/(nn_i)$. It is worthwhile noting that in this data set the numbers of repeated measurements, most of which are around 4, are much smaller compared with the number of subjects $n = 1475$. Thus, asymptotic results obtained by assuming n tending to infinity and n_i remaining finite are expected to give adequate approximations. For kernel smoothing estimators, this means that both $w_i = 1/(nn_i)$ and $w_i = 1/N$ lead to very similar estimates, and the inter-subject correlations can be ignored in the asymptotic variances of the estimators. Thus, no covariance estimators are needed in the construction of asymptotically approximate confidence bands. Based on the same kernel and bandwidths used in the coefficient curve estimates, the simultaneous confidence bands were computed using the asymptotic approximation (3.35) and the Bonferroni adjustment with $M = 40$ and $c_1 = 5$. These graphs suggest an upward linear baseline curve $\beta_0^*(t)$ and undetectable effects from alcohol consumption, cigarette smoking and mother's height. However, because the confidence bands used here tend to be conservative, they may not be sensitive enough to detect small influences of the covariates. The curve estimates and their corresponding confidence bands can also be computed using the least squares kernel method of (3.6). These results are omitted from the presentation, because they are similar to the ones shown in Figure 2.

The above nonparametric results, i.e. graphs shown in Figure 2, suggest that the relationship between fetal abdominal circumference $Y(t)$, gestational age t, alcohol consumption $X^{(2)}$, cigarette smoking $X^{(3)}$ and centered maternal height $X^{(*4)}$ can be reasonably described by the linear model

$$Y(t) = \beta_{00} + \beta_{01}t + \beta_2 X^{(2)} + \beta_3 X^{(3)} + \beta_4 X^{(*4)} + \epsilon(t)$$

with unknown parameters $(\beta_{00}, \beta_{01}, \beta_2, \beta_3, \beta_4)$ and a mean zero error process $\epsilon(t)$. This model can be fitted using the *Mixed-Effects Procedure* in S-plus (Bates and Pinherio, 1999). Table 1 shows the parameter estimates and the corresponding standard errors computed from the above linear model and the S-plus procedure. The results from this linear model suggested clearly non-significant effects for alcohol consumption and maternal height and a very weak, but slightly positive, effect for cigarette smoking. The weak smoking effect shown in this linear analysis is likely caused by the random variations of the data, rather than any substantial association between fetal

Table 1. Parameter estimates and their standard errors computed using the *Mixed-Effects Procedure* in S-plus.

	Parameter Estimate	Standard Error	Z-ratio
β_{00}	−6.5496	0.0614	−106.5880
β_{01}	1.0645	0.0021	496.1262
β_2	0.0026	0.0551	0.0478
β_3	0.1009	0.0516	1.9555
β_4	0.0007	0.0035	0.1996

size and smoking. These results generally agree with the findings obtained from the above nonparametric analysis.

When placental thickness $X^{(1)}(t)$ is added to the model, smoothing has to be carried out with time-dependent covariates. In order to obtain a meaningful biological interpretation for the baseline coefficient curve, we use the centered covariate $X^{(*1)}(t) = X^{(1)}(t) - E[X^{(1)}(t)]$, the difference between a subject's placental thickness at time t and the conditional mean at t. To avoid starting with a model that has too many covariates, we consider first fitting (1.2) with $(t, X^{(*1)}(t), X^{(*4)})$ as the covariate vector. The top panel of Figure 3 shows the estimated coefficient curve

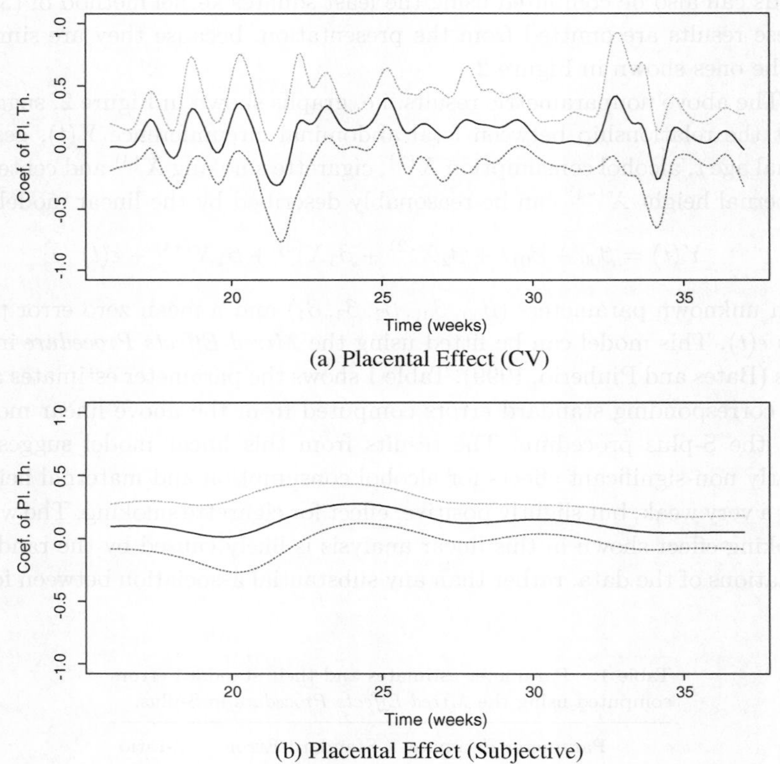

(a) Placental Effect (CV)

(b) Placental Effect (Subjective)

Fig. 3. Solid lines: estimated coefficient curve (covariate effect) for placental thickness, computed using (3.11) with the standard Gaussian kernel, $w_i = 1/N$, cross-validated bandwidths (top panel) and bandwidth vector $(\gamma_1, h_0, h_1, h_4) = (1.5, 1.0, 2.0, 1.0)$ (bottom panel). Dashed lines: the 95% pointwise intervals computed using the "resampling-subject" bootstrap percentiles.

for $X^{(*1)}(t)$ computed using the kernel method of (3.11) with the standard Gaussian kernel, the cross-validated bandwidths and $w_i = 1/N$. This estimate appears to be undersmoothed, as it can not be explained by a clear biological interpretation. An alternative, perhaps biologically more transparent, estimated coefficient curve of $X^{(*1)}(t)$, shown in the bottom panel of Figure 3, is computed using the same method except with bandwidth vector $(\gamma_1, h_0, h_1, h_4) = (1.5, 1.0, 2.0, 1.0)$. This bandwidth vector was chosen because its cross-validation score was very close to that of the cross-validated bandwidths. Bootstrap percentile intervals are used to demonstrate the variability of the estimates, while inferences based on asymptotic approximations are still not yet available for this type of estimators.

Figure 3 suggests, at least qualitatively, some positive association between placental thickness and fetal abdominal circumference. The estimated coefficient curve for the centered maternal height $X^{(*4)}(t)$ stays constantly close to zero, suggesting a non-significant effect for the maternal height. The estimated baseline coefficient curve is also very close to the one presented in Figure 2. Hence, these curves are omitted from the presentation. Also omitted are the analysis with the mother's drinking and smoking status, $X^{(2)}$ and $X^{(3)}$, added to the model, as their effects are very similar to the ones shown in Figure 2.

3.11. *Application to BMACS CD4/HIV study*

Let t_{ij} denote the ith subject's time length (in years) for his jth measurement since HIV infection. Our objective is to evaluate the effects of two factors, the pre-HIV infection CD4 percent $X^{(1)}$ and the smoking status $X^{(2)}(t)$, on the post-HIV infection depletion of CD4 percent $Y(t)$ over time. The first covariate $X^{(1)}$ does not depend on the time since HIV infection. The second covariate $X^{(2)}(t)$ equals 1 if the subject is classified as a smoker at time t and zero otherwise. Because some of the subjects change their smoking habits during the study, $X^{(2)}(t)$ is a time-dependent variable. Owing to the lack of an existing parametric or semiparametric model that is known to describe the scientific relevance between these variables, it is reasonable to consider an initial analysis with the nonparametric model (1.2).

The same rationale used in the analysis of the ASGA study suggests that, in terms of biological interpretability, the center variable $X^{(*1)} = X^{(1)} - E[X^{(1)}]$ is more preferable than its uncentered version $X^{(1)}$ in the model (1.2). However, because $X^{(2)}(t)$ is a time-dependent binary variable, it is unnecessary to be centered. Thus, with $X_i^{(*1)}$ estimated by subtracting the corresponding sample mean from $X_i^{(1)}$, the model (1.2) can be fitted with the data $\{(Y_{ij}, t_{ij}, X_{ij}^*);\ i = 1, \ldots, 400, j = 1, \ldots, n_i\}$. The baseline coefficient curve $\beta_0^*(t)$ represents the mean CD4 percent at t years after the infection for those who are non-smokers at time t and have average level of CD4 percent before the infection. The effects $\beta_1^*(t)$ and $\beta_2(t)$ of $X^{(*1)}$ and $X^{(2)}(t)$, respectively, can be interpreted the usual way.

Besides the difference in covariate centering, there is another important difference in the estimation and inferences between this and the previous example. The numbers of repeated measurements in this data set can not be simply ignored compared with the number of subjects. Thus, at least for the known case of kernel estimation, the asymptotic approximations assuming n tending to infinity and n_i remaining bounded may not lead to adequate estimators of the variances, although both $w_i = 1/(nn_i)$ and $w_i = 1/N$ seem to be reasonable weight choices. Because the correlation structure of the data is completely unknown and difficult to be estimated accurately, Wu, Chiang and Hoover (1998) suggested that it is appropriate in this case to obtain conservative Bonferroni-type bands with the covariance $\rho_\epsilon(t)$ in (3.28) replaced by the variance $\sigma^2(t)$, an upper bound for $|\rho_\epsilon(t)|$. The graphs in Figure 4 show the individuals' depletion of CD4 percent over time, the estimated coefficient curves and their corresponding conservative Bonferroni-type 95% asymptotic confidence bands. The estimated coefficient curves were computed using (3.6) with Epanechnikov kernel, the cross-validated bandwidth and the $w_i = 1/N$ weight. The confidence bands were computed using (3.30) and (3.35) with $M = 138$, $c_1 = 3$ and $\rho_\epsilon(t)$ replaced by $\sigma^2(t)$. The same kernel and bandwidth used in computing (3.6) were also used in computing all the plug-in kernel estimators required in (3.30).

Figure 4(b) shows a declining baseline CD4 percent curve over time since HIV infection, which coincides with the basic trend suggested by the plot shown in Figure 4(a). The simultaneous band for the coefficient curve of the pre-infection CD4 percent stays positive at least for the first four years after HIV infection, suggesting strongly the benefit of high pre-infection CD4 level for the initial period since the infection. However, the positive effect of the pre-infection CD4 percent on the post-infection CD4 percent appears tapering down at the later stage of the infection. Although the estimated curve in Figure 4(c) stays positive throughout the seven-year time range considered in this data set, the confidence band obtained for this curve does not show any significant positive association between

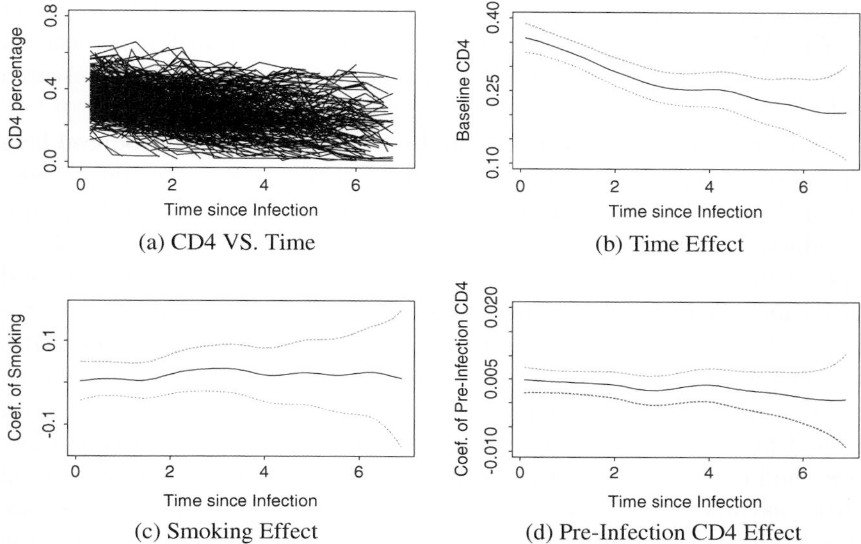

(a) CD4 VS. Time

(b) Time Effect

(c) Smoking Effect

(d) Pre-Infection CD4 Effect

Fig. 4. (a) Individuals' CD4 percent versus time (in years) since HIV infection. (b)–(d) Estimated baseline CD4 percent, coefficient curve for smoking and coefficient curve for pre-HIV infection CD4 percent (solid curves) and their corresponding 95% simultaneous confidence bands (dotted curves).

cigarette smoking and post-infection CD4 level. This may be either caused by the weak association between these two variables or the conservative nature of our confidence bands. Clearly, our findings here only provide some exploratory insights on the data. Biomedical implications and parametric models that provide additional meaningful descriptions of the biological mechanisms have to be further developed and independently confirmed by other studies. Nevertheless, the usefulness of nonparametric regression, particularly the varying-coefficient models, in the initial exploration of longitudinal data is transparent, as was shown in this and the previous examples.

3.12. *Discussion and further remarks*

This section has presented a series of parametric, semiparametric and nonparametric models and their estimation and inferential methods for the analysis of longitudinal data. These methods have a wide range of applications in biomedical studies. Theory and methods for parametric models, particularly the linear models, have been extensively studied in the literature. Estimation and inferences based on parametric models can be easily implemented using existing statistical software packages, such as SAS and S-plus. Methods based on semiparametric and nonparametric models, on the other hand, represent the most current progress in this active research field.

The nonparametric estimation and inferential methods introduced here are all based on the general framework of varying-coefficient models. These methods have the advantage of being flexible while applicable to large longitudinal studies. Smoothing methods for these models have been developed using local polynomials and splines, each has its own advantages and disadvantages in practice. Generally speaking, the componentwise smoothing methods are flexible and computationally feasible when the covariates are time-invariant, while methods based on ordinary and penalized least squares and basis approximations can be applied to models with both time-dependent and time-invariant covariates. Pointwise and simultaneous confidence bands for the coefficient curves can be constructed using either asymptotic approximations or the "resampling-subject" bootstrap. The asymptotic confidence procedures have only been developed for the kernel methods. The "resampling-subject" bootstrap may in principle be used with any smoothing estimators. However, despite the usefulness of this bootstrap shown by a number of simulation studies, its theoretical properties have not been investigated. The approach of two-step smoothing appears to be useful to overcome some of the drawbacks of the ordinary least squares. But, in order for this approach to be useful in an unbalanced longitudinal study, further research is needed to establish specific methods for calculating the raw estimates and the asymptotic properties of the final estimators. Finally, a practical consideration is the use of the uniform weight $w_i = 1/N$ versus the uniform subject weight $w_i = 1/(nn_i)$. Although none of these weight uniformly dominates the other in all the longitudinal designs and an ideal weight may depend on the unknown correlation structure and how fast n_i, $i = 1, \ldots, n$, tending to infinity relative to n, simulation studies that have been reported in the literature so far suggest that both weight choices are appropriate when all the subjects have approximately the same numbers of repeated measurements, while the $w_i = 1/(nn_i)$ weight is usually preferred when the numbers of repeated measurements differ from each other significantly.

There are a number of topics that warrant further investigation. First and foremost, although estimation and confidence tools are important in longitudinal analyses, methods that are enormously useful in biomedical studies are testing procedures that can evaluate the statistical evidence for different hypotheses. Such procedures distinguish a parametric submodel that explains a given scientific hypothesis from the general nonparametric model. The main task of decision making is to determine the distributions of the appropriate test statistics. Another practically important problem is to improve the confidence procedures. The procedures presented in this article are known to be conservative, which often hinders their usefulness in practice. Further work needs to focus on reducing the widths of the bands while maintaining satisfactory coverage probabilities. Finally, in view that the varying-coefficient models are still inadequate for a number of longitudinal settings, there is a need to further extend these models. A useful extension is to consider regression models where the outcome variable depends on the history as well as the current values of the covariates. All the estimation and inference methods will have to be redeveloped for this extension.

4. Nonparametric Models for Distribution Functions

4.1. *Motivation and justification*

The regression methods discussed in Section 2 and Section 3 are generally based on modeling the conditional mean and covariance structures of the response variables given a set of covariates, which could be either time-varying or time-invariant. Since the mean and covariance structures could be either parametric or nonparametric, the conditional-mean based regression models are undoubtedly the primary tools in a longitudinal analysis, and constitute the majority of techniques developed in the literature. Although popular in practice, this class of methods could be inadequate when the conditional means and covariances are ill-suited for answering the scientific questions being investigated. Such scenarios could arise when the scientific objectives are defined by the outcome variables through their conditional distribution functions which can not be adequately approximated by the normal distributions.

The NGHS data of Example 3, Section 1.3, is a typical example where many relevant scientific questions would better answered by evaluating the conditional distribution functions. As described in Section 1.3, an important objective of the NGHS is to evaluate the effects of age, race and obesity on several cardiovascular risk factors and the temporal trends of cardiovascular health status determined by the corresponding risk factors, such as blood pressure (BP) and hypertension, during adolescence. Since the conditional distributions of the cardiovascular risk factors observed in the NGHS are unknown *a priori* and usually non-Gaussian, statistical inferences for the effects of age, race and obesity on the conditional means of these risk factors may not have meaningful clinical interpretations, because statistical effects on the conditional means may not have direct implications on the distributions of cardiovascular health status for the population of interest. A more meaningful approach is to investigate the statistical effects of age, race and obesity on the distributions of the risk factors, so that various options of clinical interventions may be explored to reduce the chance of developing undesired health status.

4.2. *Unstructured conditional-distribution models*

Let $F_t\big[y|\mathbf{X}(t)\big] = P\big[Y(t) \le y|\mathbf{X}(t), t\big]$ be the conditional cumulative distribution function (CDF) of $Y(t)$ given $\{t, \mathbf{X}(t)\}$. If there is no structure imposed on the relationship between $\{t, \mathbf{X}(t)\}$ and $F_t\big[y|\mathbf{X}(t)\big]$, the estimation of $F_t\big[y|\mathbf{X}(t)\big]$ based on the longitudinal sample $\big\{\big(Y_{ij}, t_{ij}, \mathbf{X}_{ij}\big) : i = 1, \ldots, n, j = 1, \ldots, n_i\big\}$ may be carried out by extending the kernel methods of Hall, Wolff and Yao (1999) to the current sampling framework. This extension may be straightforward when the number of covariates involved in $\mathbf{X}(t)$ is small, for example, $K = 0$ or 1. In particular, when $K = 0$, the univariate local logistic method and adjusted Nadaraya-Watson Estimator described in Section 3 of Hall, Wolff and Yao (1999) may be directly applied. When $K \ge 1$, the multivariate estimators described in Section 3.2 of Hall, Wolff and Yao (1999) have to be considered. However, as noted in Hall, Wolff and Yao (1999), when the number of covariates K is large, the multivariate kernel smoothing methods may be computationally unstable due to the well-known problem of "curse of dimensionality" (Fan and Gijbels, 2006, p.264). In addition, statistical results and inferences obtained from a completely unstructured nonparametric estimator for $F_t\big[y|\mathbf{X}(t)\big]$ could be difficult to interpret in practical situations. These potential drawbacks, namely computational instability and difficulty in interpretations, often render the unstructured smoothing estimation of $F_t\big[y|\mathbf{X}(t)\big]$ impractical. The rest of this section describes the estimation and inference based on a class of structural nonparametric models for $F_t\big[y|\mathbf{X}(t)\big]$, the time-varying transformation models.

4.3. *Time-varying transformation models*

Transformation models with time-to-event data have been studied extensively in survival analysis. Methods of estimation and inference with various right-censored time-to-event data may be found in Cheng, Wei and Ying

(1995, 1997), Lu and Ying (2004), Lu and Tsiatis (2006), and Zeng and Lin (2006), among others. In contrast to the conditional-mean based regression models, the transformation models provide a class of functional structures for the conditional CDFs, which has been shown to be an effective dimension-reduction strategy to approximate the conditional distribution functions.

By extending the varying-coefficient approach to the transformation models, Wu, Tian and Yu (2010) suggests that $F_t\big[y|\mathbf{X}(t)\big]$ can be modeled by the time-varying linear transformation models of the form:

$$g\big\{S_t\big[y|\mathbf{X}(t)\big]\big\} = h(y,t) + \mathbf{X}^T(t)\,\beta(t), \tag{4.1}$$

where $g(\cdot)$ is a known decreasing link function, $S_t\big[y|\mathbf{X}(t)\big] = 1 - F_t\big[y|\mathbf{X}(t)\big]$, $h(\cdot,\cdot)$ is a unknown baseline function strictly increasing in y, $\beta(t) = \big(\beta_0(t), \ldots, \beta_K(t)\big)^T$, and $\beta_k(t)$ are smooth functions on the time range $\mathcal{T}$. For each fixed t within the time range, the model (4.1) is a semiparametric linear transformation model with a nonparametric baseline function $h(y,t)$ and the linear coefficients $\big(\beta_0(t), \ldots, \beta_K(t)\big)^T$. The covariate effect $\beta_k(t)$ at any given t represents the change of $g\big\{S_t\big[y|\mathbf{X}(t)\big]\big\}$ for all $y \in R$ associated with a unit increase of $X^{(k)}(t)$. Since the effect of y on $F_t\big[y|\mathbf{X}(t)\big]$ is summarized in $h(y,t)$, the covariate effects of $X^{(k)}(t)$, $k = 0, \ldots, K$, on $F_t\big[y|\mathbf{X}(t)\big]$ are constant for all possible values of y when t is fixed. Thus, by imposing a functional linear structure, the model complexity of (4.1) is greatly reduced compared with that of the unstructured nonparametric conditional-distribution models.

It is assumed throughout this section that the form of the link function $g(\cdot)$ is known and chosen by the investigators depending on the goals of the specific analysis. Well-known special cases include the proportional hazard model $g\big\{S_t\big[y|\mathbf{X}(t)\big]\big\} = \log\big\{-\log\big[S_t\big(y|\mathbf{X}(t)\big)\big]\big\}$ and the proportional odds model $g\big\{S_t\big[y|\mathbf{X}(t)\big]\big\} = -\log\big\{S_t\big[y|\mathbf{X}(t)\big]/F_t\big[y|\mathbf{X}(t)\big]\big\}$. In practice, the fitness of (4.1) may be graphically evaluated by first dividing the time range into small time bins and then examining the linearity of the plots of $g\big\{S_t\big[y|\mathbf{X}(t)\big]\big\}$ versus $X^{(k)}(t)$ for $k = 0, \ldots, K$ and t within all the time bins. Estimation and prediction based on the model (4.1) with unknown link function $g(\cdot)$ deserve substantial investigation, but these results have not been well-established in the present literature. To simplify the notation, each of the n subjects is observed at a randomly selected subset of

$J > 1$ distinct design time points $\mathbf{t} = (t_{(1)}, \ldots, t_{(J)})^T$. Since not all the subjects are observed at every $t_{(j)}$, $\mathcal{S}_j$ denotes the set of subjects whose observations are available at time $t_{(j)}$, $\mathcal{Z} = \{Y_i(t_{(j)}),\ \mathbf{X}_i(t_{(j)}),\ t_{(j)};\ i \in \mathcal{S}_j,\ j = 1, \ldots, J\}$ the longitudinal sample of $\{Y(t), \mathbf{X}(t), t \in \mathcal{T}\}$, and $\mathcal{D} = \{\mathbf{X}_i(t_{(j)}),\ t_{(j)};\ i \in \mathcal{S}_j,\ j = 1, \ldots, J\}$ the set of observed covariates. Here $Y_i(t_{(j)})$ and $\mathbf{X}_i(t_{(j)}) = (X_{i0}(t_{(j)}), \ldots, X_{iK}(t_{(j)}))^T$ are the outcome and covariate vector, respectively, at $t_{(j)}$ for the ith subject when $i \in \mathcal{S}_j$. Let $m_j = \#\{i \in \mathcal{S}_j\}$ be the number of subjects in $\mathcal{S}_j$, and $m_{j_1 j_2} = \#\{i \in \mathcal{S}_{j_1} \bigcap \mathcal{S}_{j_2}\}$ the number of subjects in both $\mathcal{S}_{j_1}$ and $\mathcal{S}_{j_2}$ when $j_1 \neq j_2$. Clearly $m_{j_1 j_2} \leq \min(m_{j_1}, m_{j_2})$.

The main results of this section are focused on the estimation and inference of the time-varying covariate effects $\beta(t)$ in (4.1) and the practical interpretations of the statistical results. In addition to the estimation of $\beta(t)$, nonparametric smoothing estimation and prediction of $h(y, t)$, $F_t\big[y|\mathbf{X}(t)\big]$ and their functions, such as the conditional quantiles, also have important applications in biomedical studies. For example, appropriate nonparametric predictors of $F_t\big[y|\mathbf{x}\big]$ for any given $\mathbf{X}(t) = \mathbf{x}$ may be used to identify subgroups of the population who may have excessive risks at different time periods. But, methods and theory for the nonparametric estimation and prediction of $h(y, t)$, $F_t\big[y|\mathbf{X}(t)\big]$ and their functions based on (4.1) are currently still under development, hence, are not included in the present discussion. In survival analysis with the linear transformation models, most estimation methods are developed for time-to-event data with random censoring, for example, Cheng, Wei and Ying (1995, 1997). In longitudinal studies, however, repeatedly measured outcome variables and covariates are usually not censored, although censoring remains a theoretical possibility. Thus, in the estimation of $\beta(t)$ in (4.1), none of the variables in the dataset are censored.

4.4. *Two-step smoothing methods*

As discussed above, when t is fixed, the model (4.1) reduces to the linear transformation model of Cheng, Wei and Ying (1995), so that $\beta(t)$ may be estimated by the estimating equations developed in their paper. When t changes within $\mathcal{T}$, a useful smoothing method for the estimation of the coefficient curves in (4.1) is to first compute a set of raw estimate the coefficient curves at time design points $\mathbf{t}$, and then compute the smoothing estimates of the coefficient curves at $t \in \mathcal{T}$ based on the raw estimates at $\mathbf{t}$.

4.4.1. *Raw estimates of coefficients*

The coefficients $\beta(t_{(j)})$ of (4.1) can be estimated by adapting the estimating equations of Cheng, Wei and Ying (1995) to the observations at $t_{(j)}$. Denote

$$\epsilon_{i(j)} = g\Big\{S_{t_{(j)}}\Big[Y_i(t_{(j)})\Big|\mathbf{X}_i(t_{(j)})\Big]\Big\}.$$

It can be verified from

$$P\Big[\epsilon_{i(j)} \le u\big|\mathbf{X}_i(t_{(j)}), t_{(j)}\Big] = P\Big\{S_{t_{(j)}}\Big[Y_i(t_{(j)})\Big|\mathbf{X}_i(t_{(j)})\Big] \ge g^{-1}(u)\Big|\mathbf{X}_i(t_{(j)}), t_{(j)}\Big\}$$

and the similar derivation used in the equation (1.4) of Cheng, Ying and Wei (1995), that (4.1) is equivalent to

$$h\left[Y_i(t_{(j)}), t_{(j)}\right] = -\mathbf{X}_i^T(t_{(j)})\beta(t_{(j)}) + \epsilon_{i(j)}, \tag{4.2}$$

where $\epsilon_{i(j)}$ are random errors with distribution function $G(\cdot) = 1 - g^{-1}(\cdot)$. Let

$$Z_{i_1,i_2}(t_{(j)}) = 1_{[Y_{i_1}(t_{(j)}) \ge Y_{i_2}(t_{(j)})]}, \qquad \mathbf{X}_{i_1,i_2}(t_{(j)}) = \mathbf{X}_{i_1}(t_{(j)}) - \mathbf{X}_{i_2}(t_{(j)})$$

and $\xi(s) = \int_{-\infty}^{\infty}\{1 - G(t+s)\}dG(t)$. It follows from (4.2) that

$$\begin{aligned} E\left[Z_{i_1,i_2}(t_{(j)})\big|\,\mathbf{X}_{i_1}, \mathbf{X}_{i_2}, t_{(j)}\right] &= P\Big\{h\Big[Y_{i_1}(t_{(j)}), t_{(j)}\Big] \\ &\qquad \ge h\Big[Y_{i_2}(t_{(j)}), t_{(j)}\Big]\Big|\,\mathbf{X}_{i_1}, \mathbf{X}_{i_2}, t_{(j)}\Big\} \\ &= P\left[\epsilon_{i_1,(j)} - \epsilon_{i_2,(j)} \ge \mathbf{X}_{i_1,i_2}^T(t_{(j)})\beta(t_{(j)})\right] \\ &= \xi\left[\mathbf{X}_{i_1,i_2}^T(t_{(j)})\beta(t_{(j)})\right]. \end{aligned} \tag{4.3}$$

A raw estimator for $\beta(t_{(j)})$ is a solution $\tilde{\beta}(t_{(j)})$ to the estimating equation

$$\sum_{i_1 \ne i_2 \in \mathcal{S}_j} U_{i_1 i_2}\Big[\tilde{\beta}(t_{(j)})\Big] = 0, \tag{4.4}$$

where, with $w(\cdot)$ being a known weight function,

$$\begin{aligned} U_{i_1 i_2}\Big[\beta(t_{(j)})\Big] &= w\Big[\mathbf{X}_{i_1,i_2}^T(t_{(j)})\beta(t_{(j)})\Big]\,\mathbf{X}_{i_1,i_2}(t_{(j)}) \\ &\quad \times\Big\{Z_{i_1,i_2}(t_{(j)}) - \xi\Big[\mathbf{X}_{i_1,i_2}^T(t_{(j)})\beta(t_{(j)})\Big]\Big\}. \end{aligned}$$

It has been shown in Cheng, Wei and Ying (1995, Section 2 and Appendix 1) that, if the weights $w(\cdot)$ are positive, their estimating equation has asymptotically a unique solution, and when $w(\cdot) = 1$ and the matrix $\sum\sum Z_{ij} Z_{ij}^T$ of their equation (2.1) is positive definite, their estimating equation has a unique solution. For each fixed $t_{(j)}$, the estimating equation (4.4) is identical to the estimating equation (2.2) of Cheng, Wei and Ying (1995) without censoring, so that the conclusions of uniqueness and asymptotically uniqueness of the solutions also hold for the estimating equation (4.4). Although the explicit expressions for the finite sample mean and variance of $\tilde{\beta}(t_{(j)})$ are not yet available the asymptotic properties of $\tilde{\beta}(t_{(j)})$ for a fixed time point $t_{(j)}$ are the same as properties developed in Cheng, Wei and Ying (1995). When different time points in $\mathbf{t}$ are involved, the potential intra-subject correlations of the data imply that our raw estimators at different time points are potentially correlated. Large sample approximations of the mean, covariance and variance of $\tilde{\beta}(t_{(j)})$ are presented later in this section.

It is worthwhile to note that the assumption of having J distinct design time points $\mathbf{t} = (t_{(1)}, \ldots, t_{(J)})^T$ is a mathematical simplification for the purpose of simplifying the theoretical discussion. In practical biomedical samples, the design time points are usually not prespecified, and $\mathbf{t}$ may be chosen from a practical round-off of the time points based on biological or clinical justifications. When the number of distinct time points is large and there are very few subjects observed at t_j, the raw estimates $\tilde{\beta}(t_j)$ may not exist at some time points $t_{(j)}$. In such situations, a practical approach is to group the observed time points into small time bins with $t_{(j)}$ being the center of the jth time bin, so that the raw estimates can be computed at each bin. Fan and Zhang (2000) considered this binning approach for a two-step estimation with conditional-mean based varying-coefficient models. When a binning method is used, we require the bin sizes to be small so that the raw estimates are undersmoothed relative to the smoothing parameters computed in the smoothing step. Practical effects of various bin choices deserves have not been systematically investigated. We assume throughout this section that $\mathbf{t}$ already contains the centers of the properly chosen time bins, so that no further binning is necessary. A practical implication of this assumption is that there are sufficient numbers of subjects having observations at all the time points in $\mathbf{t}$.

4.4.2. *Smoothing estimates of coefficient curves*

Based on the raw estimates at time points $\mathbf{t} = \{t_{(1)}, \ldots, t_{(J)}\}$, a smoothing estimator of $\beta(t)$ can be constructed for all $t \in \mathcal{T}$. To see why the smoothing step is necessary in addition to the raw estimates, it is important to note that the raw estimates are only for the coefficients at $\{t_{(1)}, \ldots, t_{(J)}\}$ and the smoothing step computes the curve estimates for all t within $\mathcal{T}$. In addition, the raw estimates often have large variations over different time design points and such "spiky" estimates generally do not have meaningful biological interpretations. Through the smoothing step, the resultant estimators have reduced variations by sharing information from the adjacent time points.

Applying the least squares kernel approach of Section 3.2 to the raw estimates $\tilde{\beta}(t_{(j)})$ for $j = 1, \ldots, J$, a kernel estimator of $\beta_d(t)$ for $0 \le d \le K$ can be obtained by

$$\widehat{\beta}_d(t) = \frac{\sum_{j=1}^{J} \tilde{\beta}_d(t_{(j)}) K_h(t - t_{(j)})}{\sum_{j=1}^{J} K_h(t - t_{(j)})}, \tag{4.5}$$

where $K_h(s) = (1/h)K(s/h)$ and $K(\cdot)$ is a non-negative kernel function. Given the known drawbacks of potentially having large boundary biases for kernel estimators (Fan and Gijbels, 1996), a more preferable smoothing approach for the estimation of $\beta_d(t)$ is through the local polynomial method. More generally, if $\beta_d(t)$ is $(Q+1)$ times continuously differentiable with respect to t, a local polynomial estimator of the qth derivatives of $\beta_d^{(q)}(t)$ is given by

$$\widehat{\beta}_d^{(q)}(t) = \sum_{j=1}^{J} w_{q,Q+1}(t_{(j)}, t) \tilde{\beta}_d(t_{(j)}), \tag{4.6}$$

where $w_{q,Q+1}(t_{(j)}, t)$ is determined by the smoothing method.

When $q = 0$, $\widehat{\beta}_d(t) = \widehat{\beta}_d^{(0)}(t)$ are local polynomial estimators of $\beta_d(t)$, and specific choices of $w_{q,Q+1}(t_{(j)}, t)$ in (4.6) determine the smoothness and statistical properties of the smoothing estimators. Let $C_j = (1, t_{(j)} - t, \ldots, (t_{(j)} - t)^Q)^T$, $C = (C_1, \ldots, C_J)^T$, $W_j = K\{(t_{(j)} - t)/h\}$ with $K(\cdot)$ being a non-negative kernel function, and $W = diag(W_1, \ldots, W_J)$. The weight function for the qth order local polynomial estimator of (4.6) is

$$w_{q,Q+1}(t_{(j)}, t; h) = q! e_{q+1,Q+1}^T (C^T W C)^{-1} C_j W_j, \; j = 1, \ldots, T, \tag{4.7}$$

where $e_{q+1,Q+1} = (0, \ldots, 0, 1, 0, \ldots, 0)^T$ with 1 at its $(q+1)$th place. This expression, (4.7) is the same as Equation (3.5) of Fan and Zhang (2000).

Coefficient curves in the conditional-mean models may also be estimated by a "one-step smoothing method", such as Hoover *et al.* (1998), Lin and

Carroll (2000) and Wu and Chiang (2000). Since the estimation of (4.1) is generally obtained through rank-based methods, similar one-step smoothing methods are not yet available for the current setting, because there currently lacks a rank-based smoothing method which does not depend on the initial raw estimation. The two-step smoothing approach is considered in Wu, Tian and Yu (2010) because it is computationally simple. This two-step approach is also capable of automatically adjusting different smoothing needs for different coefficient curves. A potential drawback, however, is that the two-step smoothing approach often requires that there are sufficient observations available at each time design point $t_{(j)}$.

In practice, it is often important to estimate and predict the conditional quantiles and cumulative distributions of the response variable $Y(t)$ at given covariates $\{\mathbf{X}(t), t\}$. Under this circumstance, this implies that there is a need to construct a nonparametric estimator of $h(y, t)$ that is monotone increasing or "order-preserving" in y for all $t \in \mathcal{T}$. In principle, $h(y, t)$ can be estimated by smoothing some raw estimators obtained at the distinct time points $\{t_{(j)};\ j = 1, \ldots, J\}$, and a set of raw estimators can be constructed using the approach described in Cheng, Wei and Ying (1997). However, as demonstrated in Hall and Müller (2003), the local polynomial method does not automatically lead to "order-preserving" smoothing estimators except for the simple case of kernel estimators with non-negative kernels. The construction of "order-preserving" nonparametric estimators for the conditional quantiles and cumulative distribution functions based on (4.1) require different methods and theory from the ones used in this section.

4.4.3. *Bandwidth choices*

The choices of bandwidth h in (4.5) and (4.7) are crucial for obtaining an appropriate smoothing estimator. In practice, subjective bandwidths may be chosen by examining the fitted curves and evaluating the specific clinical settings. Although subjectively chosen bandwidths may lead to scientifically meaningful estimators, data-driven bandwidths are often required as a useful alternative bandwidth choice in practical studies.

For conditional-mean based regression models, a popular choice for selecting bandwidths with longitudinal data is the "deleting-subject" cross-validation (CV) approach, which deletes the entire observations of a subject one at a time, e.g., Hoover *et al.* (1998) and Wu and Chiang (2000). Extending the CV approach to our setting, we consider here two CV methods for selecting the bandwidths in (4.5) and (4.6) based on the data. The first approach is a direct extension of the "deleting-subject" CV bandwidth, which minimizes the cross-validation score

$$CV_Z(\mathbf{h}) = \sum_{j=1}^{J} \sum_{i_1 \neq i_2 \in \mathcal{S}_j} \left[Z_{i_1,i_2}(t_{(j)}) - \xi \left\{ \mathbf{X}_{i_1,i_2}^T(t_{(j)}) \widehat{\beta}_{-(i_1,i_2)}(t_{(j)}; \mathbf{h}) \right\} \right]^2, \tag{4.8}$$

where $\widehat{\beta}_{-(i_1,i_2)}(t_{(j)}; \mathbf{h})$ is the two-step local polynomial or kernel estimator computed with all the observations from the subject pair (i_1, i_2) deleted and $\mathbf{h} = (h_0, \ldots, h_D)^T$ is the vector of bandwidths for $\left(\widehat{\beta}_0(t), \ldots, \widehat{\beta}_D(t)\right)^T$. In practice, it can be computationally intensive when (4.8) involves a large sample size n. An alternative approach to speed up the computation is to replace (4.8) with a "M-fold" cross-validation score, which is calculated by deleting a block of subjects each time. To do this, we randomly divide the subjects into M blocks, $\{b(m);\ m = 1, \ldots, M\}$, and compute $\mathbf{h}_{CV_Z}$ which minimizes

$$CV_Z^{(M)}(\mathbf{h}) = \sum_{j=1}^{J} \sum_{m=1}^{M} \sum_{i_1 \neq i_2 \in \mathcal{S}_j; (i_1,i_2) \in b(m)} \times \left[Z_{i_1,i_2}(t_{(j)}) - \xi \left\{ \mathbf{X}_{i_1,i_2}^T(t_{(j)}) \widehat{\beta}_{-b(m)}(t_j; \mathbf{h}) \right\} \right]^2, \tag{4.9}$$

where $\widehat{\beta}_{-b(m)}(t_{(j)}; \mathbf{h})$ is the two-step kernel or local polynomial estimator computed with the entire block $b(m)$ deleted.

In both (4.8) and (4.9), $CV_Z(\mathbf{h})$ and $CV_Z^{(M)}(\mathbf{h})$ are minimized over $\mathbf{h} = (h_0, \ldots, h_K)^T$, which could still be computationally intensive when K is large. Another approach, which relies on a component-wise approach, is to find a CV bandwidth, $h_{d,CV}$, which minimizes

$$CV_{\beta_d}(h_d) = \sum_{j=1}^{J} \left\{ \tilde{\beta}_d(t_{(j)}) - \widehat{\beta}_{d,-(j)}(t_{(j)}; h_d) \right\}^2, \tag{4.10}$$

for each d with $0 \leq d \leq K$, where $\widehat{\beta}_{d,-(j)}(t_{(j)}, h_d)$ is the smoothing estimator computed with the raw estimate $\tilde{\beta}_d(t_{(j)})$ at time point $t_{(j)}$ deleted. It is straightforward to see from (4.10) that, by minimizing the CV scores for each d, substantial amount of computation is saved in (4.10) compared with (4.8) or (4.9). A clear implication of (4.10) is that, by deleting raw estimates at each time design point $t_{(j)}$, it ignores the potential intra-subject correlations of the data, and consequently the theoretical properties of (4.10) are potentially different from the CV bandwidths obtained from (4.8) and (4.9). Theoretical properties of these CV procedures have not been systematically investigated.

4.5. *Inferences*

Asymptotic distributions for the smoothing estimators of the conditional-distribution based regression models under the current setting have not been systematically developed. Given the lack of a reliable asymptotic result, asymptotically approximated statistical inferences for the smoothing estimators of this section have not been established. Two difficult issues for establishing adequate statistical inferences are: (a) correcting the potential biases of the smoothing estimators; (b) quantifying the standard errors of the smoothing estimators. In practice, the estimation biases are often difficult to estimate. However, it has been shown in the literature (e.g., Fan and Zhang, 2000; Huang, Wu and Zhou, 2002) that a "$\pm Z_{1-\alpha/2}$ standard error band", which ignores the bias, can often be used to approximate a $[100 \times (1-\alpha)]\%$ pointwise confidence interval for a smoothing estimator. If the variances of $\widehat{\beta}_d^{(q)}(t)$ given $\mathcal{D}$ can be consistently estimated, say, by $\widehat{var}\{\widehat{\beta}_d^{(q)}(t)|\mathcal{D}\}$, a "$\pm Z_{1-\alpha/2}$ standard error band" for $\beta_d^{(q)}(t)$ can be expressed as

$$\widehat{\beta}_d^{(q)}(t) \pm Z_{1-\alpha/2}\Big[\widehat{var}\{\widehat{\beta}_d^{(q)}(t)|\mathcal{D}\}\Big]^{1/2}. \tag{4.11}$$

To obtain an appropriate estimate $\widehat{var}\{\widehat{\beta}_d^{(q)}(t)|\mathcal{D}\}$, a practical approach is to use a "resampling-subject" bootstrap in which a bootstrap sample is generated by randomly resampling n "bootstrap subjects" from the original sample with replacement. Let $\widehat{\beta}_{d,b}^{(q)}(t)$ be the smoothing estimator of $\beta_d^{(q)}(t)$ computed from the bth bootstrap sample. The conditional variance estimator $\widehat{var}\{\widehat{\beta}_d^{(q)}(t)|\mathcal{D}\}$ are then computed by the sample variances of $\{\widehat{\beta}_{d,b}^{(q)}(t);\ b = 1, \ldots, B\}$.

An alternative approach for constructing an $[100 \times (1-\alpha)]\%$ confidence intervals for $\beta_d^{(q)}(t)$ without using the normal approximation as in (4.11) is to use the bootstrap quantile intervals

$$\Big(L_{\alpha/2}, U_{\alpha/2}\Big), \tag{4.12}$$

where $L_{\alpha/2}$ and $U_{\alpha/2}$ are the lower and upper $[100 \times (\alpha/2)]$th percentiles of $\{\widehat{\beta}_{d,b}^{(q)}(t);\ b = 1, \ldots, B\}$. Both (4.11) and (4.12) may be used as approximate inference tools in practice. When the sample size is large, such as the examples of Section 1.3, the approximate confidence intervals constructed by (4.11) and (4.12) are similar and may be used interchangeably.

4.6. *Applications to the NGHS data*

Applying the conditional-distribution based regression approach to the NGHS data, the age-specific covariate effects of race, height and BMI on the distribution functions of systolic blood pressure (SBP) and diastolic blood pressure (DBP) can be evaluated using the time-varying transformation model (4.1). Before fitting the SBP and DBP data with either a conditional-mean based regression model or a conditional-distribution based regression model, Wu, Tian and Yu (2010) reported in a series of preliminary evaluations for normality, including the Shapiro-Wilk tests, the Kolmogorov-Smirnov tests and visual inspections of the quantile-quantile plots, that the conditional distributions of SBP and DBP for this population of girls given age, race, height (in dm) and BMI (in kg/m^2) were clearly not normal. In particular, many of these conditional distributions were skewed and were rejected for normality by the goodness-of-fit tests at 5% significance level.

The preliminary findings reported in Wu, Tian and Yu (2010) suggest that the existing results obtained in Daniels *et al.* (1998) or Thompson *et al.* (2007) may not give an adequate description of the covariate effects on the overall conditional distributions of SBP and DBP. In particular, Daniels *et al.* (1998) used the conditional-mean regression models, which may not be adequate for describing the effects of these covariates on the probabilities of unhealthy levels of cardiovascular risks, and the conclusions of Thompson *et al.* (2007) depend on their specific threshold choices for the outcome variables, which may not hold if other threshold values were used. Thus, there are two major advantages for using (4.1) over the conditional-mean based regression analyses. First, it has a flexible and parsimonious structure to summarize the age-specific effects of these covariates on the overall distributions of the outcome variables. Second, statistical inferences for the age-dependent coefficient curves have the same biological interpretations as in Cheng, Wei and Ying (1995) and do not depend on the normality assumption of the outcome variables or the threshold values for defining unhealthy risk levels.

Because the repeated measurements are obtained for girls between 9 and 19 years of age, the analysis presented here is confined to the age range $\mathcal{T} = [9, 19)$. For a girl at age $t \in \mathcal{T}$, the outcome variable, $Y(t)$, is either the girl's SBP or DBP value at age t, and the covariate vector is $\mathbf{X}(t) = (Race,\ Height(t),\ BMI(t))^T$, where $Race = 0$ or 1 if the girl is Caucasian or African–American, and $Height(t)$ and $BMI(t)$ are the girl's height and body mass index, respectively, at age t. Since the visit time for this study is not regularly spaced, it is clinically meaningful to round up the age to one tenth of a year, so that the age range can be grouped into equally spaced bins $[9.0, 9.1), \ldots, [18.9, 19.0)$ with time design points $\mathbf{t} = \{9.0, 9.1, 9.2, \ldots, 18.9\}$. The ith girl's age, covariates and outcome are denoted by $\{t_j, \mathbf{X}_i(t_j), Y_i(t_j)\}$ if her actual age at the visit falls into the bin $[t_j, t_{j+1})$. This binning scheme is based on the clinical definition of age and the assumption that $Height(t)$, $BMI(t)$ and $Y(t)$ are smooth functions of age t.

In the exploratory analysis reported in Wu, Tian and Yu (2010), the odds-ratios plots of SBP with a range of threshold values under various strata of age, race, height and BMI showed that the proportional odds models gave reasonable approximations to the relationships between the conditional distribution functions of SBP and the covariates $\mathbf{X}(t)$. Thus, for this analysis, the following time-varying proportional odds model is considered:

$$\log\left\{\frac{P\Big[Y(t) > y | t, Race, Height, BMI\Big]}{P\Big[Y(t) \leq y | t, Race, Height, BMI\Big]}\right\}$$
$$= -h(y,t) + \beta_0(t) \times Race + \beta_1(t) \times Height(t) + \beta_2(t) \times BMI(t), \tag{4.13}$$

where a positive (negative) value for $\beta_0(t)$ suggests that African-American girls tend to have higher (lower) SBP or DBP values than Caucasian girls at age t, and $\beta_1(t)$ and $\beta_2(t)$ represent the changes of the log-odds of $Y(t) > y$ associated with a unit increase of $Height(t)$ and $BMI(t)$, respectively, at age t.

Following the estimation procedure of Section 4.4, the raw estimates are first computed at the time design points $\mathbf{t} = \{9.0, 9.1, 9.2, \ldots, 18.9\}$ with the $w(\cdot) = 1$ weight, and then the smoothing estimates $\widehat{\beta}(t) = \left(\widehat{\beta}_0(t), \widehat{\beta}_1(t), \widehat{\beta}_2(t)\right)^T$ are computed using the local linear method with the Epanechnikov kernel and the cross-validated bandwidths chosen from (4.9) and (4.10). For the M-block CV bandwidths, ten subject blocks, $M = 10$, are used to minimize the CV score (4.9). Figure 5 shows the two-step local linear estimators of $\beta(t) = (\beta_0(t), \beta_1(t), \beta_2(t))^T$ computed from the CV

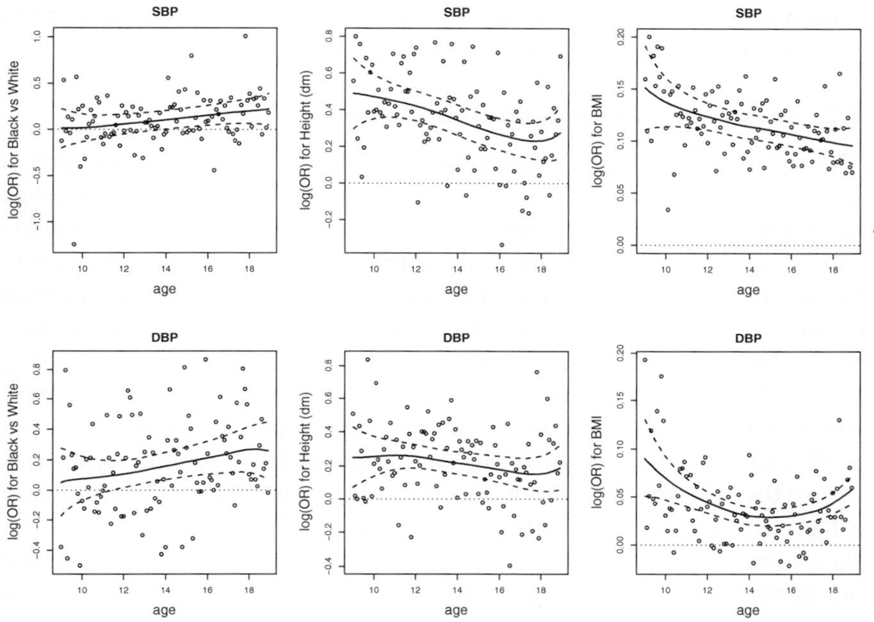

Fig. 5. Top panels: systolic blood pressure (SBP). Bottom panels: diastolic blood pressure (DBP). Each row shows the raw estimates, the two-step local linear estimates (solid lines) computed with the CV bandwidths from (4.10), and their ± 1.96 bootstrap standard error bands (dashed lines) for $\beta_0(t)$, $\beta_1(t)$ and $\beta_2(t)$ of (4.1).

bandwidths based on (4.10) and the "± 1.96 standard error bands" computed from 500 bootstrap repetitions. In order to ease the computational burden, the CV bandwidths obtained from the original sample are used for the bootstrap standard error bands. The covariate effects shown in Figure 5 are similar for both SBP and DBP. The contribution of race $\beta_0(t)$ is close to zero and slightly increases with age, suggesting that African-American girls tend to have slightly higher odds of SBP and DBP than Caucasian girls at later years. The positive estimates of $\beta_1(t)$ and $\beta_2(t)$ suggest that both height and BMI contribute positively to the odds of SBP and DBP. The effects $Height(t)$ and $BMI(t)$ on the conditional distribution of SBP appear to decrease as the girls are getting older. The $BMI(t)$ seems to have different effects on the conditional distribution of SBP and the conditional distribution of DBP. For the conditional distribution of SBP, the effects of $BMI(t)$, $\beta_2(t)$, appears decreasing linearly as t increases. For the conditional distribution of DBP, the effects of $BMI(t)$, $\beta_2(t)$, appears to be a nonlinear function of the girl's age t.

4.7. *Discussion and potential extensions*

The time-varying linear transformation models discussed in this section use a conditional-distribution based regression approach for modeling the entire conditional distribution functions and evaluating the covariate effects on these distributions. This approach is conceptually superior to the conditional-mean based models when the scientific objective depends on the conditional distribution functions. As illustrated in the application to the NGHS blood pressure data, the practical advantages of modeling the conditional distribution functions may be generalized to other typical biomedical studies. Similar to the conditional-mean based varying-coefficient models, the time-varying transformation models effectively reduce the problem of "curse-of-dimensionality" and at the same time retain a high degree of model flexibility. From the computational point of view, the two-step estimation procedure is conceptually simple and can be carried out by combining the existing rank-based estimation procedures in survival analysis and the smoothing procedures in nonparametric curve estimation.

Given the practical implications of conditional-distribution based regression models, further research based on this approach is warranted. First, notice that, in the application to the NGHS blood pressure data, the fitness of the model (4.1) is examined in an *ad hoc* fashion by a series of exploratory plots. More rigorously, appropriate goodness-of-fit tests should be developed to formally test the adequacy of the time-varying models under appropriate statistical hypotheses. Second, the model (4.1) considered in this section involves only a univariate outcome variable. In many situations the scientific objective is better described through the joint distributions of a multivariate outcome variable. Extensions to conditional distributions with multivariate outcome variables warrant further investigation. Third, the two-step procedure discussed in this section is limited to the estimation of the covariate effects over time. Smoothing methods for the estimation and prediction of conditional distributions and conditional quantiles have useful applications in longitudinal studies and should be developed as well.

5. Regression Methods for Outcome-Adaptive Covariates

It is well-known in the literature (for example, Pepe and Anderson, 1994) that when the values of a covariate depend on the outcome values at the previous time points, the wide range of conditional-mean based regression methods of Section 2 and Section 3 may lead to unsatisfactory results. This type of covariates, whose values may depend on the previous outcome values, are referred herein as "outcome-adaptive" covariates. As a special case of longitudinal analysis with "outcome-adaptive" covariates, this section presents the modeling and estimation approaches for longitudinal data with the presence of a concomitant intervention. After a brief introduction of data with a concomitant intervention, the rest of this section summarizes the similarities and differences between the modeling approaches of Wu, Tian and Bang (2008) and Wu, Tian and Jiang (2011) and their corresponding estimation and inference procedures.

5.1. *Outcome-adaptive covariates*

For longitudinal clinical trials with randomly assigned study treatments, longitudinal effects of the study treatments are modeled through a time-invariant categorical covariate vector, while other factors of interest, such as age, gender, ethnicity and disease risk factors, can be modeled through either time-invariant or time-dependent covariates. In many longitudinal studies, some time-dependent covariates are "outcome-adaptive" in the sense that their potential values at a time point may depend on the values or time-trends of the outcome variable prior to that time point.

A typical scenario which involves "outcome-adaptive" covariates is the presence of concomitant interventions in longitudinal clinical trials. Unlike the study treatments of a clinical trial which are randomly assigned to the study subjects, concomitant interventions are not randomly assigned, because they are initiated, usually due to ethical reasons, to study subjects who exhibit less satisfactory trends in their health outcomes. The scenario of concomitant interventions bears some similarities to longitudinal studies with informative missing data. In the case of informative missing data, the study subjects with undesirable outcome time-trends tend to drop out from the study earlier than those with more desirable outcome time-trends. The only difference is that, in studies with concomitant interventions, the outcomes of the study subjects continue to be observed after the start of the concomitant interventions. In a randomized longitudinal clinical trial with randomly assigned study treatments, study subject who have taken a concomitant intervention in addition to their assigned study treatments may generally have different disease pathology from those who do not need the concomitant intervention. Thus, in addition to the primary objective of evaluating the effects of the study treatments, an important secondary objective is to evaluate the effects of the additional concomitant interventions on the outcome variables of the study populations.

The Enhancing Recovery in Coronary Heart Disease (ENRICHD) Study described in Example 4 is a typical example which involves a concomitant intervention in addition to the randomly assigned treatment regimens. In this randomized clinical trial for evaluating the efficacy of a six-month cognitive behavior therapy (CBT) versus usual cardiovascular care (UC), the Beck Depression Inventory (BDI) scores for patients in the CBT arm were repeatedly measured at weekly visits during the treatment and four yearly follow-up visits, while BDI scores for patients in the UC arm were only measured at baseline, the six-month visit and the yearly follow-up visits. By the study design (ENRICHD, 2001), pharmacotherapy with antidepressants was allowed as a concomitant intervention in both the CBT and the UC arms if a patient had high baseline BDI scores or nondecreasing BDI trends five weeks after enrollment or antidepressants were requested by the patient or the primary-care physicians. Although Taylor *et al.* (2005) reported that pharmacotherapy improved survival among 1834 depressed ENRICHD patients, their results, however, did not address the question of whether pharmacotherapy was beneficial for lowering the patients' depression severity.

Using the repeatedly measured BDI scores in a subsample of 91 ENRICHD patients in the CBT arm who received pharmacotherapy within the treatment period, Wu, Tian and Bang (2008) showed that the naïve mixed-effects models gave misleading results for the pharmacotherapy effects on the BDI trends over time, and proposed a varying-coefficient mixed-effects model to reduce the potential bias associated with the estimated pharmacotherapy effects. A main drawback of Wu, Tian and Bang (2008) is the potential loss of information because their regression model can not be applied to patients who have already received pharmacotherapy at baseline or have not received pharmacotherapy during the study.

As a generalization of the varying-coefficient mixed-effects model, Wu, Tian and Jiang (2011) proposed a comprehensive regression method for evaluating the concomitant intervention effects which is capable to incorporate information from all the study subjects in a longitudinal study. Using the framework of shared-parameter models in Follmann and Wu (1995), the approach of Wu, Tian and Jiang (2011) describes the covariate effects on the response variable through a change-point mixed-effects model, and incorporates the random coefficients and the intervention starting time (change-point time) through a series of joint distributions. Patients who have received a concomitant intervention at baseline or have not received any concomitant intervention during the study period are treated as censored. A likelihood-based method is established for statistical estimation and inferences, and its computation is implemented through a two-stage iteration procedure. Applying their procedures to the ENRICHD pharmacotherapy data, the results of Wu, Tian and Jiang (2011) suggest that their proposed method leads to adequate estimates when a concomitant intervention is present, while the naïve mixed-effects model is likely misspecified under such situations.

5.2. *Structure for data with one concomitant intervention*

Following the notation of Section 1.2, let $\mathcal{T}_0$ and $\mathcal{T}_1$ be the beginning and ending times of a study, and n be the total number of randomly selected subjects. The ith subject has n_i visits and observations $(T_{ij}, Y_{ij}, \mathbf{X}_i)$ at the jth visit, where T_{ij}, the study time, is the time elapsed from the beginning of the study to the jth visit, $\mathbf{X}_i$ is a time-invariant covariate vector, and Y_{ij} is the real-valued outcome variable. For simplicity, we assume throughout the section that the study involves only one concomitant intervention, and the ith subject can change from "without concomitant intervention" to "concomitant intervention" only once during the study with S_i being the concomitant intervention starting time or change-point time. Let $\lambda_{ij} = 0$ or 1, if $T_{ij} \leq S_i$ or $T_{ij} > S_i$, respectively, be the concomitant intervention indicator for the ith subject. Since not every subject has a change-point time during the study, the ith subject's change-point time is observed if $T_{i1} \leq S_i \leq T_{in_i}$. If $S_i < T_{i1}$ or $S_i > T_{in_i}$, the subject's change-point time is left or right censored, respectively. The indicator variable for censoring $\delta_i^{(c)}$ is defined by $\delta_i^{(c)} = 0$ if $T_{i1} \leq S_i \leq T_{in_i}$, 1 if $S_i > T_{in_i}$, and 2 if $S_i < T_{i1}$. The observed change-point times are $\{\mathcal{S}_i^{(c)} = (S_i^{(c)}, \delta_i^{(c)});\ i = 1, \ldots, n\}$, where $S_i^{(c)} = S_i$ if $\delta_i^{(c)} = 0$, T_{in_i} if $\delta_i^{(c)} = 1$, and T_{i1} if $\delta_i^{(c)} = 2$.

5.3. *Model formulations and interpretations*

5.3.1. *Näive mixed-effects change-point models*

Since a concomitant intervention is not randomly assigned, it is understood in practice that the effects of a concomitant intervention can not be properly evaluated by directly comparing the outcome values between the subjects who received the intervention and those who did not receive the intervention. This fact has been noted in ENRICHD (2003) and Taylor *et al.* (2005) for the ENRICHD Study. A better approach that has been suggested by Wu, Tian and Bang (2008) and Wu, Tian and Jiang (2011) is to use a change-point model, which assumes that the outcome variable Y_{ij} follows different trajectories before and after the concomitant intervention, so that the effects of the concomitant intervention can be evaluated through the differences of the mean trajectories.

Let $\mu_0(T_{ij}, \mathbf{X}_i; \mathbf{a}_i)$ be the ith subject's trajectory before the concomitant intervention, which is parameterized by the subject-specific parameter $\mathbf{a}_i^T = (a_{i1}, \ldots, a_{id_0})^T$, $d_0 \geq 1$, and let $\mu_1(T_{ij}, \mathbf{X}_i, R_{ij}; \mathbf{b}_i)$ be the change of the trajectory after the concomitant intervention, which is parameterized by the subject-specific parameter $\mathbf{b}_i = (b_{i1}, \ldots, b_{id_1})^T$, $d_1 \geq 1$, and may depend on the "intervention duration time" $R_{ij} = T_{ij} - S_i$ as well as T_{ij} and $\mathbf{X}_i$. The usual mixed-effects model framework (Davadian and Giltinan, 1995; Verbeke and Molenberghs, 2000; Diggle *et al.*, 2002) suggests that a naïve mixed-effects model for evaluating the pre- and post-intervention trajectories can be expressed as

$$\begin{cases} Y_{ij} = \mu_0(T_{ij}, \mathbf{X}_i; \mathbf{a}_i) + \lambda_{ij}\, \mu_1(T_{ij}, \mathbf{X}_i, R_{ij}; \mathbf{b}_i) + \epsilon_{ij}, \\ \left(\mathbf{a}_i^T, \mathbf{b}_i^T\right)^T \sim \text{ joint distribution } G(\cdot), \end{cases} \tag{5.1}$$

where $(\mathbf{a}_i^T, \mathbf{b}_i^T)^T$ has unknown mean $(\alpha^T, \beta^T)^T$ and covariance matrix Σ, ϵ_{ij} are mean zero random errors with $cov(\epsilon_{ij_1}, \epsilon_{ij_2}) = \sigma_{ij_1j_2}$, and $\epsilon_{i_1j_1}$ and $\epsilon_{i_2j_2}$ are independent if $i_1 \neq i_2$. For mathematical convenience, the joint distribution of $\mathbf{a}_i$ and $\mathbf{b}_i$ may be assumed to be multivariate Gaussian $\mathcal{N}\{(\alpha^T, \beta^T)^T, \Sigma\}$. Under (5.1), a positive (or negative) value for $\mu_1(T_{ij}, \mathbf{X}_i, R_{ij}; \mathbf{b}_i)$ would suggest that the intervention tends to increase (or decrease) the mean of Y_{ij} given $(T_{ij}, \mathbf{X}_i, R_{ij})$.

5.3.2. *An example for the biases of Näive mixed-effects models*

Because the "self-selectiveness" of the intervention is ignored, Wu, Tian and Bang (2008) shows that (5.1) can be a misspecified model even if $\mu_0(\cdot; \mathbf{a}_i)$, $\mu_1(\cdot; \mathbf{b}_i)$, ϵ_{ij} and $G(\cdot)$ are correctly specified. Sometimes misleading conclusions may occur even under simple situations where (5.1) appears to have natural interpretations. The following simple synthetic example illustrates the potential erroneous conclusions which may result from the standard estimation procedures of a näive mixed-effects model.

Suppose that a longitudinal study has $n = 24$ independent subjects, and, for $1 \le i \le 24$, $j = 1, \ldots, n_i$, $n_i = 10$ and $T_{ij} = j$. Let S_i be the change-point time for the ith subject changing from "no concomitant intervention" to "with concomitant intervention", and let λ_{ij} be the corresponding "concomitant intervention indicator" such that $\lambda_{ij} = 0$ if $S_i < T_{ij}$, and $\lambda_{ij} = 1$ if $S_i \ge T_{ij}$. For the first 12 subjects, i.e., $1 \le i \le 12$, their change-point time is $S_i = 2$, and their outcomes are generated by $Y_{ij} = 20 + e_{ij}$ for $\lambda_{ij} = 0$ and $1 \le j \le 2$, and $Y_{ij} = 19 + e_{ij}$ for $\lambda_{ij} = 1$ and $3 \le j \le 10$, where e_{ij} are independent identically distributed with the $N(0, 3)$ distribution. For the remaining 12 subjects, i.e., $13 \le i \le 24$, their change-point time is $S_i = 8$, and their outcomes are generated by $Y_{ij} = 19 + e_{ij}$ for $\lambda_{ij} = 0$ and $1 \le j \le 8$, and $Y_{ij} = 17 + e_{ij}$ for $\lambda_{ij} = 1$ and $9 \le j \le 10$, where e_{ij} are independent identically distributed with the $N(0, 3)$ distribution. Suppose that it is known that Y_{ij} does not depend on T_{ij} for all $1 \le i \le 24$ and $1 \le j \le 10$. Then, a special case of the näive mixed-effects change-point model of (5.1) which may be considered for the current situation is

$$\begin{cases} Y_{ij} = a_i + b_i \lambda_{ij} + \epsilon_{ij}, \\ \big(a_i, b_i\big)^T \sim \text{joint distribution } G(\cdot), \end{cases} \tag{5.2}$$

where, for all $1 \le i \le 24$ and $1 \le j \le 10$, ϵ_{ij} are independent identically distributed with the $N(0, 3)$ distribution, $E(a_i) = \alpha$ and $E(b_i) = \beta$ are the fixed-effects, and $G(\cdot)$ is an unknown distribution. Since, for $1 \le i \le 12$, the true effect of the concomitant intervention is $b_i = -1$, and, for $13 \le i \le 24$, the true effect of the concomitant intervention is $b_i = -2$, the true fixed mean effect for the population is $\beta = -1.5$, which is unknown and needs to be estimated from the data.

Given a sample $\{(Y_{ij}, T_{ij}, S_i); i = 1, \ldots, 24, \ j = 1, \ldots, 10\}$ generated from the above specification, the mean and covariance parameters of (5.1) can be estimated using a number of standard statistical analysis software packages, such as SAS and R. Although the exact distribution function $G(\cdot)$ is generally unknown, adequate estimates of the mean parameters $\{\alpha, \beta\}$ may often be obtained in practice by assuming $G(\cdot)$ to be a multivariate normal distribution with a suitable correlation structure. Since the correlation structures of the data are generally unknown, three LME procedures in the R statistical package can be used to estimate $\{\alpha, \beta\}$: LME with working independent correlation structure (LMEWI), LME with random intercept (LMERI), and LME with random intercept and slope (LMERIS). Similarly,

Table 2. Averages of the parameter estimates and their standard errors (SE) and the empirical coverage probabilities of their corresponding 95% confidence intervals (CI) covering the true parameter $\beta = -1.5$ computed from 10,000 simulated samples with the näive mixed-effects change-point model (5.2).

R Procedure with Correlation Structure	Estimate	SE	Empirical Coverage Probability of 95% CI
LME Working Independence	−0.598	0.395	37.8%
LME Random Intercept	−0.731	0.403	51.0%
LME Random Intercept & Slope	−0.788	0.431	60.4%
GEE Working Independence	−0.598	0.385	36.2%
GEE Exchangeable	−0.709	0.385	46.7%
GEE Unstructured	−0.752	0.572	43.9%

parameter estimates can also be obtained using the generalized estimation equation procedure with three correlation structures: GEE with working independent correlation structure (GEEWI), GEE with exchangeable correlation structure (GEEEC), and GEE with unstructured correlation structure (GEEUC). Further details for the parameter estimations with linear mixed-effects models can be in Verbeke and Molenberghs (2000).

To examine whether the näive mixed-effects change-point model (5.2) can lead to appropriate estimates for the mean concomitant intervention effect β, 10,000 independent samples of $\{(Y_{ij}, T_{ij}, S_i); i = 1, \ldots, 24,\ j = 1, \ldots, 10\}$ were generated in a simulation study. The estimators $\widehat{\beta}$ and their standard errors were computed from each of the simulated samples using each of the estimation procedures, namely LMEWI, LMERI, LMERIS, GEEWI, GEEEC and GEEUC, in SAS. Table 2 summarizes the averages of the estimators and their standard errors (SE) and the empirical coverage probabilities of the corresponding 95% confidence intervals covering the true parameter $\beta = -1.5$ computed from the 10,000 simulated samples and the näive mixed-effects model (5.2). These results suggest that all these LME and GEE procedures with different correlation structure assumptions give similar estimates for β, which are around -0.6 and -0.7 and far from the true value of $\beta = -1.5$, with comparable standard errors. Consequently, the 95% confidence intervals shown in Table 2 have low empirical coverage probabilities, which suggests that the model (5.2) leads to excessive biases and inadequate estimates for β.

Are there simple approaches which can lead to better estimates of the mean concomitant intervention effect β? Obviously, for the simple setup considered here, one can consider an "individual fitting" estimator of β

based on (5.2), which is given by

$$\widehat{\beta}_{ind} = (1/n)\sum_{i=1}^{n}\left\{\frac{\sum_{j=1}^{n_i}\left(Y_{ij}1_{[\delta_{ij}=1]}\right)}{\sum_{j=1}^{n_i}1_{[\delta_{ij}=1]}} - \frac{\sum_{j=1}^{n_i}\left(Y_{ij}1_{[\delta_{ij}=0]}\right)}{\sum_{j=1}^{n_i}1_{[\delta_{ij}=0]}}\right\}. \tag{5.3}$$

A simple application of (5.3) to our simulated samples led to estimates of β very close to its true value of -1.5. However, it is known in the literature that "individual fitting" estimation methods based on the repeated measurements separately from each subject, such as (5.3), are generally less efficient than the well-known procedures, such as MLEs, REML estimates and GEEs (e.g., Verbeke and Molenberghs, 2000; Diggle *et al.*, 2002). In addition, it is also difficult to generalize the "individual fitting" approaches to regression models with more complicated terms and patterns than the simple cases exhibited in (5.2).

Comparing the underlying mechanism for generating $\{(Y_{ij}, T_{ij}, S_i); i = 1, \ldots, 24,\ j = 1, \ldots, 10\}$ with the model (5.2), one potential flaw of using (5.2) with its LME and GEE estimation procedures is that the model does not take the potential relationship between the change-point time S_i and the values of Y_{ij} before the change-point time, i.e., the values of Y_{ij} when $\delta_{ij} = 0$. Indeed, under the real data generating mechanism, subjects with subject-specific mean value of Y_{ij} at $j = 1$ to be 20 have change-point time at $S_i = 2$, while subjects with subject-specific mean value of Y_{ij} at $j = 1$ to be 19 have change-point time at $S_i = 8$. Although this fact is unknown at the estimation stage, the possibility of the potential relationship between S_i and Y_{ij} when $\delta_{ij} = 0$ is not allowed in the MLEs, REML estimates and GEEs based on the näive model (5.2). To see whether the potential bias for the estimation of β could be reduced by incorporating the change-point time S_i into the model, we consider here the following simple generation of (5.2):

$$\begin{cases} Y_{ij} = a_{0i} + a_{1i}S_i + b_i\lambda_{ij} + \epsilon_{ij}, \\ \left(a_{0i}, a_{1i}, b_i\right)^T \sim N\Big((\alpha_0, \alpha_1, \beta)^T, \Gamma\Big), \end{cases} \tag{5.4}$$

where $(\alpha_0, \alpha_1, \beta)^T$ is the vector of mean parameters and Γ is the unknown covariance matrix. The structures of Γ generally do not have major influences on the estimation of $(\alpha_0, \alpha_1, \beta)^T$, and many commonly used parametric structures may be used when implementing the estimation procedures (Diggle *et al.*, 2002). It is important to note that the interpretation of β is the same in both (5.2) and (5.4). Strictly speaking, the model (5.4) is not

Table 3. Averages of the parameter estimates and their standard errors (SE) and the empirical coverage probabilities of their corresponding 95% confidence intervals (CI) covering the true parameter $\beta = -1.5$ computed from 10,000 simulated samples with the mixed-effects model (5.4).

R Procedure with Correlation Structure	Estimate	SE	Empirical Coverage Probability of 95% CI
LME Working Independence	−1.498	0.485	94.7%
LME Random Intercept	−1.498	0.483	94.6%
LME Random Intercept & Slopes	−1.498	0.496	95.2%

correct for the underlying data generating mechanism, since Y_{ij} does not depend on S_i through a simple linear model. Although (5.4) is at best a rough approximation of the true underlying data generating mechanism, the main intent here is to evaluate whether the bias for the estimation of the concomitant intervention effect can be reduced by incorporating S_i into the model. Details on the justifications of (5.4) and interpretations of its parameters are given in Section 5.4, where it is described as a special case of the varying-coefficient mixed-effects models of Wu, Tian and Bang (2008).

Table 3 summarizes the averages of the estimators and their standard errors (SE) and the empirical coverage probabilities of the corresponding 95% confidence intervals covering the true parameter $\beta = -1.5$ computed from the 10,000 simulated samples, the mixed-effects model (5.4) and the same LME procedures as the ones used in Table 2. The mean estimates for β in Table 3 are very close to the true value of $\beta = -1.5$, with comparable standard errors in both Table 2 and Table 3. The 95% confidence intervals shown in Table 3 have empirical coverage probabilities which are very close to the nominal level of 95% and much higher than the ones shown in Table 2. Clearly, (5.4) leads to much smaller bias for the estimation of β than (5.2).

5.3.3. *General shared-parameter models*

The data structure of Section 5.2 is a special case of outcome-adaptive covariates, which involves only one concomitant intervention and each study subject has at most one change-point from "without concomitant intervention" to "concomitant intervention". This simple structure of outcome-adaptiveness suggests that a natural extension for the mixed-effects approach of (5.1) is to incorporate the initiation of the concomitant intervention into the regression model. This extension of (5.1) can be achieved by allowing the intervention starting time S_i to be correlated with the pre-intervention random coefficients $\mathbf{a}_i$ or more generally $\{\mathbf{a}_i, \mathbf{b}_i\}$. Let $\mu_0(\cdot; \mathbf{a}_i)$ and $[\mu_0(\cdot; \mathbf{a}_i) + \mu_1(\cdot; \mathbf{b}_i)]$ be the subject-specific response curves before and after the start of the concomitant intervention, respectively. With $\mu_1(\cdot; \mathbf{b}_i)$ being interpreted as the concomitant intervention effect, a shared-parameter change-point model for the given dataset $\{Y_{ij}, T_{ij}, \mathbf{X}_i, S_i\}$ is

$$\begin{cases} Y_{ij} = \mu_0(T_{ij}, \mathbf{X}_i; \mathbf{a}_i) + \delta_{ij}\, \mu_1(T_{ij}, \mathbf{X}_i, R_{ij}; \mathbf{b}_i) + \epsilon_{ij}, \\ \left(\mathbf{a}_i^T, \mathbf{b}_i^T, S_i\right)^T \sim \text{ Joint Distribution}, \end{cases} \tag{5.5}$$

where $R_{ij} = T_{ij} - S_i$, ϵ_{ij} are mean zero errors with $cov(\epsilon_{ij_1}, \epsilon_{ij_2}) = \sigma_{ij_1j_2}$, $\epsilon_{i_1j_1}$ and $\epsilon_{i_2j_2}$ are independent if $i_1 \neq i_2$, and, conditioning on $\{\mathbf{a}_i, \mathbf{b}_i\}$, S_i and $\{T_{ij}, \mathbf{X}_i\}$ are independent. In addition, we assume that $\{\mathbf{a}_i, \mathbf{b}_i\}$ and $\{T_{ij}, \mathbf{X}_i\}$ are independent. Using the matrix representation $\mathbf{Y}_i = (Y_{i1}, \ldots, Y_{in_i})^T$ and $\mathbf{T}_i = (T_{i1}, \ldots, T_{in_i})^T$, the joint likelihood function of $(\mathbf{Y}_i^T, S_i)^T$ given $\{\mathbf{T}_i, \mathbf{X}_i\}$ based on (5.5) is

$$f(\mathbf{Y}_i, S_i|\mathbf{T}_i, \mathbf{X}_i) = \int f(\mathbf{Y}_i|\mathbf{T}_i, \mathbf{X}_i, S_i, \mathbf{a}_i, \mathbf{b}_i) f(S_i|\mathbf{a}_i, \mathbf{b}_i)\, dH(\mathbf{a}_i, \mathbf{b}_i), \tag{5.6}$$

where $f(\cdot|\cdot)$ denotes the conditional density and $H(\cdot, \cdot)$ is the joint distribution function of $\{\mathbf{a}_i, \mathbf{b}_i\}$. The extra $f(S_i|\mathbf{a}_i, \mathbf{b}_i)$ in the integrand distinguishes (5.6) from the usual likelihood functions for the mixed-effects models (Verbeke and Molenberghs, 2000, p. 24).

In (5.5), the parameters $\{\mathbf{a}_i, \mathbf{b}_i\}$ are associated with both the response curves of Y_{ij} and the distribution of S_i. The shared parameters approach was proposed in Follmann and Wu (1995) for the purpose of modeling the behaviors of informative missing data. However, in (5.5), the subjects are still being observed after the change-point time. The correlation between S_i and $\mathbf{a}_i$ suggests that the ith subject's change-point time is affected by the pre-intervention response curve $\mu_0(\cdot)$, and the correlation between S_i and $\mathbf{b}_i$ suggests that S_i may also influence the response curve $\mu_1(\cdot)$, which characterizes the intervention effects.

5.4. *Varying-coefficient mixed-effects models — a special case*

5.4.1. *Formulation of varying-coefficient mixed-effects models*

The joint likelihood function (5.6) requires a known distribution function for $\{\mathbf{a}_i, \mathbf{b}_i, S_i\}$, and maximizing this likelihood can be computationally intensive in practice. When all the subjects have observed change-point times within the study period, that is, $\mathcal{T}_0 < S_i < \mathcal{T}_1$ for all $1 \le i \le n$, a simpler regression method, which does not depend on the distribution function of S_i, may be considered. Since S_i are observed for all $1 \le i \le n$, we can consider the conditional distribution

$$f(\mathbf{Y}_i|S_i, T_i, \mathbf{X}_i) = \int f(\mathbf{Y}_i|T_i, \mathbf{X}_i, S_i, \mathbf{a}_i, \mathbf{b}_i) dG(\mathbf{a}_i, \mathbf{b}_i|S_i) , \tag{5.7}$$

and rewrite (5.5) as a varying-coefficient model using the conditional distribution of $\{\mathbf{a}_i, \mathbf{b}_i\}$ given S_i. Although $\mu_0(\cdot)$ and $\mu_1(\cdot)$ are allowed to take general parametric or nonparametric forms, this approach is illustrated here assuming that $\mu_0(\cdot)$ and $\mu_1(\cdot)$ are linear functions of the form $\mu_0(T_{ij}, \mathbf{X}_i; \mathbf{a}_i) = \mathbf{Z}_{ij}^T \mathbf{a}_i$ and $\mu_1(T_{ij}, \mathbf{X}_i, S_i; \mathbf{b}_i) = \mathbf{W}_{ij}^T \mathbf{b}_i$, where $\mathbf{Z}_{ij} = (Z_{ij0}, \ldots, Z_{ijD_1})^T$ is generated by $\{(T_{ij}, \mathbf{X}_i);\ 1 \le j \le n_i,\ \delta_{ij} = 0\}$, and $\mathbf{W}_{ij} = (W_{ij0}, \ldots, W_{ijD_2})^T$ is generated by $\{(T_{ij}, \mathbf{X}_i, S_i);\ 1 \le j \le n_i, \delta_{ij} = 1\}$.

Let $\alpha(S_i) = E(\mathbf{a}_i|S_i)$, $\beta(S_i) = E(\mathbf{b}_i|S_i)$, $\mathbf{a}_i^* = \mathbf{a}_i - \alpha(S_i)$ and $\mathbf{b}_i^* = \mathbf{b}_i - \beta(S_i)$. A varying-coefficient mixed-effects model for the data $\{Y_{ij}, T_{ij}, S_i; 1 \le i \le n, 1 \le j \le n_i\}$ is

$$\begin{cases} Y_{ij} = \mathbf{Z}_{ij}^T \left[\alpha(S_i) + \mathbf{a}_i^*\right] + \delta_{ij} \mathbf{W}_{ij}^T \left[\beta(S_i) + \mathbf{b}_i^*\right] + \epsilon_{ij}, \\ \left(\mathbf{a}_i^{*T}, \mathbf{b}_i^{*T}\right)^T \Big| \, S_i \sim G(\cdot|S_i) \end{cases} \tag{5.8}$$

where, for $S_i = s$, $G(\cdot|s)$ is a distribution function with mean zero and covariance matrix $cov[(\mathbf{a}_i^{*T}, \mathbf{b}_i^{*T})^T|s] = \mathbf{C}(s)$. The population-mean parameters of interest are $\alpha(s)$ and $\beta(s)$, which, in this case, are both smooth functions of s. When $S_i = s$, the mean concomitant intervention effect is $\beta(s)$. The special choice of $\beta(s) = 0$ for all $s \in (\mathcal{T}_0, \mathcal{T}_1)$ implies that the concomitant intervention has no population-mean effect on the time-trend curve of Y_{ij}.

A number of interesting special cases of (5.8) may be considered in real applications by specifying the forms of $\alpha(\cdot)$, $\beta(\cdot)$ and $G(\cdot|\cdot)$. An obvious choice for $G(\cdot|S_i)$ is the multivariate normal distribution with mean zero and covariance matrix $\mathbf{C} = cov[(\mathbf{a}_i^{*T}, \mathbf{b}_i^{*T})^T|s]$, which is assumed to be time-invariant for simplicity. Extension to time-dependent covariances can be made by modeling $\mathbf{C}(s)$. Since the main objective is to evaluate the population-mean effects of the concomitant intervention and explicit forms of $G(\cdot|S_i)$ are often unknown, using appropriate models for $\alpha(s)$ and $\beta(s)$ is often more important than using a suitable model for $\mathbf{C}(s)$. Linear models for $\alpha(s)$ and $\beta(s)$ can be expressed as $\alpha(s;\gamma) = (\alpha_0(s;\gamma_0),\ldots,\alpha_{D_1}(s;\gamma_{D_1}))^T$ and $\beta(s;\tau) = (\beta_0(s;\tau_0),\ldots,\beta_{D_2}(s;\tau_{D_2}))^T$, where

$$\alpha_d(s;\gamma) = \sum_{l=0}^{L_d} \gamma_{dl}\mathcal{T}_{dl}(s) \qquad \text{and} \qquad \beta_d(s;\tau) = \sum_{m=0}^{M_d} \tau_{dm}\mathcal{T}^*_{dm}(s) \tag{5.9}$$

where $\{L_d, M_d\}$ are fixed, and $\{\mathcal{T}_{dl}(s), \mathcal{T}^*_{dm}(s)\}$ are known transformations of s. The choice of $\mathcal{T}_{dl}(s) = s^l$ and $\mathcal{T}^*_{dm}(s) = s^m$ leads to the global polynomials $\alpha_d(s;\gamma)$ and $\beta_d(s;\tau)$.

When the parametric forms of $\alpha(s)$ and $\beta(s)$ are unknown, nonparametric analysis can be performed by approximating $\alpha(s)$ and $\beta(s)$ with basis expansions. If $\{\mathcal{B}_{d_1}(s) = (\mathcal{B}_{d_10}(s),\ldots,\mathcal{B}_{d_1\mathcal{L}_{d_1}}(s))^T;\ 0 \le d_1 \le D_1\}$ and $\{\mathcal{B}^*_{d_2}(s) = (\mathcal{B}^*_{d_20}(s),\ldots,\mathcal{B}_{d_2\mathcal{M}_{d_2}}(s))^T;\ 0 \le d_2 \le D_2\}$ are two sets of pre-specified basis functions, their basis approximations for $\alpha(s)$ and $\beta(s)$ are given by

$$\alpha_d(s;\gamma) \approx \sum_{l=0}^{\mathcal{L}_d} \gamma_{dl}\mathcal{B}_{dl}(s) \qquad \text{and} \qquad \beta_d(s;\tau) \approx \sum_{m=0}^{\mathcal{M}_d} \tau_{dm}\mathcal{B}^*_{dm}(s), \tag{5.10}$$

where $\mathcal{L}_d$ and $\mathcal{M}_d$ may tend to infinity as $n \to \infty$. Common choices of basis functions include truncated polynomial bases, Fourier bases or B-splines. Currently, only B-splines with fixed knot sequences have been investigated for the model (5.8) in the literature (Wu, Tian and Bang, 2008) because of the superior numerical stability of B-spline approximatoins. An alternative smoothing approach is to approximate $\alpha(s)$ and $\beta(s)$ by smoothing splines (Lin and Zhang, 1999; Chiang, Rice and Wu, 2001). But nonparametric estimation and inference with smoothing splines in (5.8) have not been studied, since the explicit expressions and statistical properties of smoothing spline estimators are very different from B-splines.

5.4.2. *Least-squares estimation*

Likelihood-based estimates of $\alpha(s)$ and $\beta(s)$ for (5.8) can not be computed if the explicit forms of $G(\cdot|S_i)$ and the distribution of ϵ_{ij} are unknown. When $\alpha(s) = \alpha(s;\gamma)$ and $\beta(s) = \beta(s;\tau)$ are parametrized by Euclidean valued parameters γ and τ, respectively, a practical approach, which does not require the explicit distribution functions, is to compute the weighted least-squares estimators $\widehat{\gamma}_{LS}$ and $\widehat{\tau}_{LS}$ which minimize

$$\begin{aligned}\ell(\gamma,\tau) = \sum_{i=1}^{n} \Big\{ \big[\mathbf{Y}_i - \big(\mathbf{Z}_i^T\alpha(S_i;\gamma) + (\delta\mathbf{W})_i^T\beta(S_i;\tau)\big)\big]^T \\ \times \Lambda_i \big[\mathbf{Y}_i - \big(\mathbf{Z}_i^T\alpha(S_i;\gamma) + (\delta\mathbf{W})_i^T\beta(S_i;\tau)\big)\big]\Big\},\end{aligned} \tag{5.11}$$

where $\mathbf{Z}_i = (\mathbf{Z}_{i1}, \ldots, \mathbf{Z}_{in_i})^T$, $(\delta\mathbf{W})_i = (\delta_{i1}\mathbf{W}_{i1}, \ldots, \delta_{in_i}\mathbf{W}_{in_i})^T$, and Λ_i are pre-specified symmetric nonsingular $n_i \times n_i$ weight matrices. Explicit expressions of the weighted least-squares estimators are

$$\begin{pmatrix} \widehat{\gamma}_{LS}(\mathcal{T}) \\ \widehat{\tau}_{LS}(\mathcal{T}) \end{pmatrix} = \left\{ \sum_{i=1}^{n} [\mathcal{W}_i \mathcal{T}_i]^T \Lambda_i [\mathcal{W}_i \mathcal{T}_i] \right\}^{-1} \left\{ \sum_{i=1}^{n} [\mathcal{W}_i \mathcal{T}_i]^T \Lambda_i \mathbf{Y}_i \right\}, \quad (5.12)$$

where $\sum_{i=1}^{n} [\mathcal{W}_i \mathcal{T}_i]^T \Lambda_i [\mathcal{W}_i \mathcal{T}_i]$ is nonsingular, and the jth row of $\mathcal{W}_i$ is $\left(\mathbf{Z}_{ij}^T, \delta_{ij}\mathbf{W}_{ij}^T\right)$.

For nonparametric functions of $\alpha(s)$ and $\beta(s)$ with basis approximations (5.10), the least-squares based nonparametric estimators of $\alpha(s)$ and $\beta(s)$ are computed by substituting the right-hand side terms of (5.10) into (5.11), which lead to

$$\left(\widetilde{\alpha}_{LS}^T(s; \mathcal{B}), \widetilde{\beta}_{LS}^T(s; \mathcal{B})\right)^T = \mathcal{B}(s) \left(\widetilde{\gamma}_{LS}^T(\mathcal{B}), \widetilde{\tau}_{LS}^T(\mathcal{B})\right)^T, \quad (5.13)$$

where $\{\widetilde{\gamma}_{LS}(\mathcal{B}), \widetilde{\tau}_{LS}(\mathcal{B})\}$ are given in (5.12) with $\mathcal{T}(s)$ replaced by $\mathcal{B}(s)$.

When $\Lambda_i = \mathbf{V}_i^{-1}$ and the distribution functions are assumed to be normal, (5.12) and (5.13) are the same as the maximum likelihood estimators or their approximated versions based on B-splines. When $\mathbf{V}_i$ are unknown, as often the case in practice, subjective choices for Λ_i may be used. One potential "plug-in" approach is to estimate $\mathbf{V}_i$ from the data and compute the estimates by substituting Λ_i with the estimates of $\mathbf{V}_i^{-1}$. But, in practice, $\mathbf{V}_i$ is often difficult to estimate, it is unclear whether such "plug-in" estimators have superior statistical properties than the estimators with subjective Λ_i choices.

5.5. *Estimation with shared-parameter models*

5.5.1. *Linear and additive shared-parameter models*

For many situations where concomitant interventions are involved, the change-point time S_i, which depends on the pre-intervention trend of Y_{ij}, may not be observed for all the study subjects, since some subjects may have the concomitant intervention change-points before or after the study period. In such situations, where S_i is referred in Section 5.2 as double censored, a natural strategy is to further simply (5.2) into a sufficiently general model that is practically useful. Suppose that the concomitant intervention effects only depend on the pre-intervention trends $\mathbf{a}_i$ of the outcome variable but not on the change-point time S_i. A useful special case of (5.2) is

$$\begin{cases} Y_{ij} = \mu_0(T_{ij}, \mathbf{X}_i; \mathbf{a}_i) + \lambda_{ij}\, \mu_1(T_{ij}, \mathbf{X}_i, R_{ij}; \mathbf{b}_i) + \epsilon_{ij}, \\ \mathbf{a}_i \sim F_a(\cdot),\ S_i|\mathbf{a}_i \sim F_s(\cdot|\mathbf{a}_i),\ \mathbf{b}_i|\mathbf{a}_i \sim F_b(\cdot|\mathbf{a}_\mathrm{i}), \end{cases} \tag{5.14}$$

where $F_a(\cdot)$ is the cumulative distribution function (CDF) of $\mathbf{a}_i$, $F_s(\cdot|\mathbf{a}_i)$ and $F_b(\cdot|\mathbf{a}_i)$ are the conditional CDF's of S_i and $\mathbf{b}_i$, respectively, given $\mathbf{a}_i$, and $\mathbf{b}_i$ and S_i are independent given $\mathbf{a}_i$. In contrast to the varying-coefficient model (5.8), where the conditional means of $\mathbf{a}_i$ and $\mathbf{b}_i$ given S_i are used, (5.14) incorporates S_i through $F_s(\cdot|\mathbf{a}_i)$. By modeling the conditional distribution of S_i given $\mathbf{a}_i$, (5.14) allows S_i to be left or right censored. For simplicity, (5.14) assumes that $\mathbf{b}_i$ does not depend on S_i, although further generalizations may allow the distribution of $\mathbf{b}_i$ to depend on $(S_i, \mathbf{a}_i)$.

Further specifications of $F_a(\cdot)$, $F_s(\cdot|\mathbf{a}_i)$ and $F_b(\cdot|\mathbf{a}_i)$ may be considered in practice to balance the computational feasibility and flexibility of the model. A useful and mathematically tractable specification for (5.14) is to assume that S_i and $\mathbf{b}_i$ depend on $\mathbf{a}_i$ only through their conditional means, which are linear functions of $\mathbf{a}_i$. A linear shared-parameter model for (5.14) is

$$\begin{cases} Y_{ij} = \mu_0(T_{ij}, \mathbf{X}_i; \mathbf{a}_i) + \lambda_{ij}\, \mu_1(T_{ij}, \mathbf{X}_i, R_{ij}; \mathbf{b}_i) + \epsilon_{ij}, \\ \mathbf{a}_i = \alpha + e_i^{(a)},\ S_i = \gamma^T(1, \mathbf{a}_i^T)^T + e_i^{(s)},\ \mathbf{b}_i = \beta^T(1, \mathbf{a}_i^T)^T + e_i^{(b)}, \end{cases} \tag{5.15}$$

where $\alpha = (\alpha_1, \ldots, \alpha_{d_0})^T$, $\alpha_d \in R$, $\beta = (\beta_1^T, \ldots, \beta_{d_1}^T)^T$, $\beta_l = (\beta_{l0}, \ldots, \beta_{ld_0})^T$, $\beta_{ld} \in R$, $\gamma = (\gamma_0, \ldots, \gamma_{d_0})^T$, and $\{\epsilon_i = (\epsilon_{i1}, \ldots, \epsilon_{in_i})^T, e_i^{(a)}, e_i^{(b)}, e_i^{(s)}\}$ are independent mean zero random errors with covariance matrices $\{\mathbf{V}_y, \mathbf{V}_a, \mathbf{V}_b, \sigma_s^2\}$, respectively. The unknown parameters in (5.15) are the mean components $\theta = (\alpha^T, \beta_1^T, \ldots, \beta_{d_1}^T, \gamma^T)^T$ and the covariance structures $\mathbf{V} = \{\mathbf{V}_y, \mathbf{V}_a, \mathbf{V}_b, \sigma_s^2\}$.

When the relationship between S_i and $\mathbf{a}_i$ in (5.14) are unknown, a nonparametric model for $\{S_i, \mathbf{a}_i\}$ is $S_i = \mu^{(s)}(\mathbf{a}_i) + \epsilon_i^{(s)}$, where $\mu^{(s)}(\mathbf{a}_i) = E(S_i|\mathbf{a}_i)$ is a smooth function of $\mathbf{a}_i$. Since unstructured estimation of $\mu^{(s)}(\mathbf{a}_i)$ could be difficult when $\mathbf{a}_i$ is a high dimensional vector, a simple additive approach is to replace the relationship between S_i and $\mathbf{a}_i$ in (5.15) with

$$S_i = \sum_{d=0}^{d_0} \mu_d^{(s)}(a_{id}) + \epsilon_i^{(s)}, \tag{5.16}$$

where $\mu_d^{(s)}(a_{id})$ are smooth functions of a_{id}, so that an additive shared-parameter model for (5.14) is

$$\begin{cases} Y_{ij} = \mu_0(T_{ij}, \mathbf{X}_i; \mathbf{a}_i) + \lambda_{ij}\, \mu_1(T_{ij}, \mathbf{X}_i, R_{ij}; \mathbf{b}_i) + \epsilon_{ij}, \\ \mathbf{a}_i = \alpha + e_i^{(a)},\ S_i = \sum_{d=0}^{d_0} \mu_d^{(s)}(a_{id}) + \epsilon_i^{(s)},\ \mathbf{b}_i = \beta^T (1, \mathbf{a}_i^T)^T + e_i^{(b)}. \end{cases} \tag{5.17}$$

Further generalizations of (5.17) are theoretically possible but at the expense of computational complexity.

5.5.2. *Maximum likelihood estimation methods*

If the distribution functions are explicitly specified with a known parametric form, the parameters in (5.14) can be estimated by a maximum likelihood (ML). Denote by $\mathbf{Y}_i = (Y_{i1}, \ldots, Y_{in_i})^T$, $\mathbf{T}_i = (T_{i1}, \ldots, T_{in_i})^T$, $\mathcal{D}_i = (\mathbf{T}_i, \mathbf{X}_i)$, and $f_y(\cdot)$, $f_b(\cdot)$, $f_s(\cdot)$ and $f_a(\cdot)$ the densities of Y_{ij}, $\mathbf{b}_i$, S_i and $\mathbf{a}_i$. The joint density of $(\mathbf{b}_i, S_i, \mathbf{a}_i)$ can be expressed as

$$f(\mathbf{b}_i, S_i, \mathbf{a}_i) = f_b(\mathbf{b}_i|\mathbf{a}_i) f_s(S_i|\mathbf{a}_i) f_a(\mathbf{a}_i).$$

Then the conditional density of $(\mathbf{Y}_i, S_i)$ given $\mathcal{D}_i = (\mathbf{T}_i, \mathbf{X}_i)$ can be derived by integrating over $\mathbf{a}_i$ and $\mathbf{b}_i$ and is given by

$$f_{(y,s)}(\mathbf{Y}_i, S_i|\mathcal{D}_i) = \iint f_y(\mathbf{Y}_i|\mathcal{D}_i, S_i, \mathbf{a}_i, \mathbf{b}_i) f_b(\mathbf{b}_i|\mathbf{a}_i) f_s(S_i|\mathbf{a}_i)\, f_a(\mathbf{a}_i)\, d\mathbf{a}_i\, d\mathbf{b}_i. \tag{5.18}$$

Since the observed change-point time is the double censored version $\{S_i^{(c)}, \delta_i^{(c)}\}$, the conditional density function (5.18) may not be directly used in estimation, and one has to consider the following conditional density of $\mathcal{S}_i^{(c)} = (S_i^{(c)}, \delta_i^{(c)})$ given $\mathbf{a}_i$:

$$f_s\Big(S_i^{(c)}, \delta_i^{(c)}|\mathbf{a}_i\Big) = \begin{cases} f_s(S_i|\mathbf{a}_i), & \text{if } \delta_i^{(c)} = 0, \\ 1 - F_s(T_{in_i}|\mathbf{a}_i), & \text{if } \delta_i^{(c)} = 1, \\ F_s(T_{i1}|\mathbf{a}_i), & \text{if } \delta_i^{(c)} = 2. \end{cases} \tag{5.19}$$

By (5.18) and (5.19), the log-likelihood function for $(\mathbf{Y}_i, \mathcal{S}_i^{(c)})$ conditioning on $\mathcal{D}_i$, $i = 1, \ldots, n$, is

$$L_c = \frac{1}{n} \sum_{i:\delta_i^{(c)}=0} \log f_{(y,s)}(\mathbf{Y}_i, S_i|\mathcal{D}_i) + \frac{1}{n} \sum_{l=1,2} \sum_{i:\delta_i^{(c)}=l} \log f_{(y,l)}(\mathbf{Y}_i|\mathcal{D}_i) \tag{5.20}$$

where $f_{(y,s)}(\cdot|\cdot)$ is given above, $f_{(y,1)}(\cdot|\mathcal{D}_i, \mathbf{a}_i)$ and $f_{(y,2)}(\cdot|\mathcal{D}_i, \mathbf{a}_i, \mathbf{b}_i)$ are the densities of $\mathbf{Y}_i$ given $\{\mathcal{D}_i, \mathbf{a}_i, \delta_i^{(c)} = 1\}$ and $\{\mathcal{D}_i, \mathbf{a}_i, \mathbf{b}_i, \delta_i^{(c)} = 2\}$, respectively,

$$f_{(y,1)}(\mathbf{Y}_i|\mathcal{D}_i) = \int f_{(y,1)}(\mathbf{Y}_i|\mathcal{D}_i, \mathbf{a}_i)\{1 - F_s(T_{in_i}|\mathbf{a}_i)\} f_a(\mathbf{a}_i)\, d\mathbf{a}_i$$

and

$$f_{(y,2)}(\mathbf{Y}_i|\mathcal{D}_i) = \iint f_{(y,2)}(\mathbf{Y}_i|\mathcal{D}_i, \mathbf{a}_i, \mathbf{b}_i) F_s(T_{i1}|\mathbf{a}_i) f_b(\mathbf{b}_i|\mathbf{a}_i) f_a(\mathbf{a}_i)\, d\mathbf{a}_i\, d\mathbf{b}_i.$$

If the parametric family for $f_{(y,s)}(\cdot|\cdot)$ is denoted by $\{f_{(y,s)}(\cdot; \phi|\mathcal{D}_i);\ \phi = (\theta, \mathbf{V})\}$, the ML estimators for $\phi = (\theta, \mathbf{V})$ can be obtained by maximizing the log-likelihood function (5.20).

5.5.3. *Approximate maximum likelihood estimation methods*

Estimation for the additive shared-parameter model (5.17) can be achieved by maximizing an approximate likelihood function for (5.17). Under some mild smoothness conditions on $\mu_d^{(s)}(\cdot)$ (e.g., Huang, Wu and Zhou, 2004), $\mu_d^{(s)}(\cdot)$ can be approximated by the B-spline expansion

$$\mu_d^{(s)}(a_{id}) \approx \sum_{p=1}^{P_d} \gamma_p^{(d)} B_p^{(d)}(a_{id}) = \left(\gamma^{(d)}\right)^T \mathbf{B}^{(d)}(a_{id}) \tag{5.21}$$

where, for some P_d, $\{B_p^{(d)}(\cdot);\ 1 \le p \le P_d\}$ is a spline basis,

$$\mathbf{B}^{(d)}(a_{id}) = \left(B_1^{(d)}(a_{id}), \ldots, B_{P_d}^{(d)}(a_{id})\right)^T$$

and $\gamma^{(d)} = (\gamma_1^{(d)}, \ldots, \gamma_{P_d}^{(d)})^T$ is a set of real-valued coefficients. It follows from (5.16) that

$$S_i \approx \sum_{d=0}^{d_0} (\gamma^{(d)})^T \mathbf{B}^{(d)}(a_{id}) + \epsilon_i^{(s)}. \tag{5.22}$$

By substituting $\sum_{d=0}^{d_0} \mu_d^{(s)}(a_{id})$ of (5.16) with $\sum_{d=0}^{d_0} \left(\gamma^{(d)}\right)^T \mathbf{B}^{(d)}(a_{id})$, the parameters are

$$\theta = \left(\alpha^T, \beta_1^T, \ldots, \beta_{d_1}^T, \gamma^T\right)^T,\ \gamma = \left((\gamma^{(0)})^T, \ldots, (\gamma^{(d_0)})^T\right)^T \text{ and}$$
$$\mathbf{V} = \left\{\mathbf{V}_y, \mathbf{V}_a, \mathbf{V}_b, \sigma_s^2\right\}.$$

Let $f_s^*(\cdot; \gamma, \sigma_s|\mathbf{a}_i)$ be the conditional density of $\sum_{d=0}^{d_0}\{(\gamma^{(d)})^T \mathbf{B}^{(d)}(a_{id})\} + \epsilon_i^{(s)}$ given $\mathbf{a}_i$. If the distributions of ϵ_{ij}, $e_i^{(a)}$, $e_i^{(b)}$ and $e_i^{(s)}$, which all have zero means, are parameterized by the vector of variance parameters $\mathbf{V}$, the density $f_s(S_i|\mathbf{a}_i)$ can be approximated by $f_s^*(S_i;\gamma,\sigma_s|\mathbf{a}_i)$, and the parameters of (5.17) can be obtained by maximizing the following approximate log-likelihood function for $(\mathbf{Y}_i,\mathcal{S}_i^{(c)})$ given $\mathcal{D}_i$,

$$L_c^*(\phi)=\frac{1}{n}\sum_{i:\delta_i^{(c)}=0}\log f_{(y,s)}^*(\mathbf{Y}_i,S_i;\phi|\mathcal{D}_i)+\frac{1}{n}\sum_{l=1,2}\sum_{i:\delta_i^{(c)}=l}\log f_{(y,l)}^*(\mathbf{Y}_i;\phi|\mathcal{D}_i) \tag{5.23}$$

where $\phi=(\theta,\mathbf{V})$, $f_{(y,s)}^*(\cdot|\mathcal{D}_i)$, $f_{(y,k)}^*(\cdot|\mathcal{D}_i)$, $k=1,2$, are given in (5.20) with $f_s(S_i|\mathbf{a}_i)$ replaced by $f_s^*(S_i;\gamma,\sigma_s|\mathbf{a}_i)$. If $L_d^*(\phi)$ satisfies the regularity conditions for MLE's, the approximate MLE $\hat{\phi}$ satisfy $L_c^*(\hat{\phi})=\max_\phi L_c^*(\phi)$.

5.5.4. *A two-stage estimation procedure*

The likelihood functions (5.20) and (5.23) involve nonlinear terms of the parameters. A global maximization of (5.20) or (5.23) over θ and $\mathbf{V}$ simultaneously could be computationally unfeasible in practice. In order to alleviate the computational burden, Wu, Tian and Jiang (2011) suggests to use the following two-stage procedure, which combines REMLE with the Newton-Raphson algorithm:

(*S1*) Assume that $\{\epsilon_{ij},\mathbf{a}_i,\mathbf{b}_i,S_i\}$ of (5.15) or (5.17) are independent random variables with covariance matrices $\mathbf{V}=\{\mathbf{V}_y,\mathbf{V}_a,\mathbf{V}_b,\sigma_s^2\}$, that is, the naïve mixed-effects model (5.1) holds. Compute $\widehat{\mathbf{V}}$ of $\mathbf{V}$ using the REMLE procedure.

(*S2*) Substitute $\mathbf{V}$ with $\hat{\mathbf{V}}$, and maximize $L_c(\theta,\hat{\mathbf{V}})$ with respect to θ using the Newton-Raphson procedure. The maximizer $\hat{\theta}=\arg\max_\theta L_c(\theta,\hat{\mathbf{V}})$ is the approximate ML estimator for θ.

From the expressions of $f_{(y,s)}(\mathbf{Y}_i,S_i|\mathcal{D}_i)$ and $f_{(y,k)}(\mathbf{Y}_i|\mathcal{D}_i)$ for $k=1,2$, it is easy to see that the Newton-Raphson algorithm for maximizing $L_c(\theta,\hat{\mathbf{V}})$ at stage (S2) involves multi-dimensional integrations over the functions of $\mathbf{a}_i$, $\mathbf{b}_i$ and S_i with respect to the joint distributions of $\mathbf{a}_i$ and $\mathbf{b}_i$. All the necessary quantities involved in the Newton-Raphson algorithm, including the log-likelihood functions, and their gradients and Hessian matrices, can be computed using Monte Carlo simulations, in which case large Monte-Carlo samples are required to compute the gradient and the Hessian matrix in each iteration, so that a complete Newton-Raphson algorithm can be costly to implement. If a suitable initial estimator is available, computation of the algorithm can be significantly reduced by a "one-step" Newton-Raphson procedure (Bickel, 1975). In Wu, Tian and Jiang (2011), the authors suggest to use the estimators computed from the REMLE procedure as a natural candidate for the initial estimator $\hat{\theta}_0$ and to compute the initial estimators of γ by fitting the regression model $S_i = \gamma^T(1, \tilde{\mathbf{a}}_i^{pred}) + \epsilon_i^{(s)}$ using the subjects with S_i observed (i.e., $\delta_i^{(c)} = 0$), where $\tilde{\mathbf{a}}_i^{pred}$ is the predicted value for $\mathbf{a}_i$.

5.6. *Bootstrap confidence intervals*

In theory, approximate inferences for the parameter vector ϕ can be constructed using the asymptotic distribution of the ML estimator $\hat{\phi}$, when n is large and the model (5.15) follows a known parametric family. Under suitable regularity conditions (Serfling, 1980, Ch. 4), the asymptotic normality of the MLE's implies that $\hat{\phi}$ has approximately the multivariate normal distribution $\mathcal{N}(\phi,\ Var(\phi))$, so that an approximate $[100\times(1-\alpha)]$th confidence interval for $\ell(\phi)$, a linear combination of ϕ, is $\ell(\hat{\phi}) \pm Z_{\alpha/2}\big[\hat{Var}\{\ell(\phi)\}\big]^{1/2}$, where $\hat{Var}\{\ell(\phi)\}$ is the variance estimator and $Z_{\alpha/2}$ is the $[100\times(1-\alpha/2)]$th percentile of the standard normal distribution. For the additive model (5.17), where nonparametric components are present, asymptotic distributions of the approximate MLE in (5.23) have not yet been developed. As a practical alternative, a bootstrap procedure is to generate bootstrap samples by resampling the subjects with replacement and compute the corresponding bootstrap estimators. The estimates obtained from the original sample are natural choices for the initial estimates for the bootstrap samples. A $[100 \times (1-\alpha)]$th confidence interval based on percentiles is given by the corresponding lower and upper $[100 \times (\alpha/2)]$th percentiles $(L_{\alpha/2}, U_{\alpha/2})$ of the bootstrap estimators. This bootstrap approach has been used in Wu, Tian and Bang (2008) and Wu, Tian and Jiang (2011). Alternatively, one can also compute $\hat{Var}\{\ell(\phi)\}$ from the bootstrap samples, and use the approximate confidence interval $\ell(\hat{\phi}) \pm Z_{\alpha/2}\big[\hat{Var}\{\ell(\phi)\}\big]^{1/2}$.

5.7. *Applications to the ENRICHD pharmacotherapy data*

5.7.1. *Application to subjects with observed change-points*

A brief summary of the ENRICHD study has been described in Example 4 of Section 1.3. The objective here is to evaluate the additional effects of pharmacotherapy (antidepressants) on the trends of depression severity measured by BDI scores for patients who received pharmacotherapy during the six-month cognitive behavior therapy (CBT) treatment period. Pharmacotherapy with antidepressants is a concomitant intervention in this trial because the decision of using antidepressants and its starting time was made by the patients or their primary care physicians.

Using the regression framework of Section 5.4, this analysis includes 91 patients with a total of 1,446 observations in the CBT arm who received pharmacotherapy during the treatment period and had clear records of their pharmacotherapy starting time. Data from patients in the usual care (UC) arm are excluded, since the pharmacotherapy starting time and repeated BDI scores were not accurately recorded for these patients. Excluded are also data from patients in the CBT arm who did not have pharmacotherapy starting time accurately recorded during the six month CBT treatment period. Among the 91 patients analyzed here, 43 of them started pharmacotherapy at baseline and 48 started pharmacotherapy between 7 and 172 days. The number of visits for these patients ranges from 5 to 36 and has the median of 16.

Following Section 5.2, Y_{ij}, T_{ij}, S_i, $R_{ij} = T_{ij} - S_i$ and $\delta_{ij} = 1_{[T_{ij} \geq S_i]}$ are the ith subject's BDI score, trial time (in months), starting time of pharmacotherapy, time from initiation of pharmacotherapy, and pharmacotherapy indicator, respectively, at the jth visit. A simple case of the näive mixed-effects models for evaluating the trends of BDI score over T_{ij} is the linear mixed-effects model

$$Y_{ij} = a_{0i} + a_{1i} T_{ij} + b_{0i} \delta_{ij} + b_{1i} \delta_{ij} R_{ij} + \epsilon_{ij}, \tag{5.24}$$

where $E(a_{0i}, a_{1i}, b_{0i}, b_{1i})^T = (\alpha_0, \alpha_1, \beta_0, \beta_1)^T$. When $\delta_{ij} = 1$ and $R_{ij} = r$, $(\beta_0 + \beta_1 r)$ describes the mean pharmacotherapy effect at r months since the start of pharmacotherapy.

Since (5.24) ignores the possible correlation between S_i and the pre-pharmacotherapy depression trends, which may lead to potential bias, its varying-coefficient generalization is

$$Y_{ij} = \alpha_0(S_i) + \alpha_1(S_i) T_{ij} + \beta_0 \delta_{ij} + \beta_1 \delta_{ij} R_{ij} + e_{ij}, \tag{5.25}$$

where $e_{ij} = a^*_{i0} + a^*_{i1} T_{ij} + b^*_{i0} \delta_{ij} + b^*_{i1} \delta_{ij} R_{ij} + \epsilon_{ij}$, $\alpha_0(S_i) = \gamma_{00} + \gamma_{01} S_i$ and $\alpha_1(S_i) = \gamma_{10} + \gamma_{11} S_i$. The mean pre-pharmacotherapy BDI trend in (5.25) is associated with S_i through intercept $\alpha_0(S_i)$ and slope $\alpha_1(S_i)$. The mean pharmacotherapy effect at r months after the start of pharmacotherapy is $\beta_0 + \beta_1 r$. A negative (positive) value for $\beta_0 + \beta_1 r$ corresponds to a beneficial (harmful) effect for reducing depression.

Table 4. Parameter estimates for β_0 and β_1 and their standard errors (SE), 95% confidence intervals (CIs) and p-values were obtained by restricted maximum likelihood with unstructured correlations for the näive linear mixed-effects model (Näive LME) (5.24) and the shared-parameter linear mixed-effects model (SP-LME) (5.25).

Model	Parameter	Estimate	SE	95% CI	p-value
Näive LME	β_0	−3.410	0.994	(−5.399, −1.422)	0.0013
	β_1	−1.584	0.521	(−2.626, −0.542)	0.0039
SP-LME	β_0	−4.302	1.041	(−6.385, −2.220)	0.0001
	β_1	−2.062	0.773	(−3.608, −0.516)	0.0105

For mathematical simplicity, (5.25) assumes that $\beta_0(S_i) \equiv \beta_0$ and $\beta_1(S_i) \equiv \beta_1$, so that the effects of pharmacotherapy only depend on how long the antidepressant has been used. Under this assumption, β_0 and β_1 have the same interpretations in both the näive linear mixed-effects model (Näive LME) (5.24) and the shared-parameter linear mixed-effects model (SP-LME) (5.25), although the mean BDI scores have different pre-pharmacotherapy time trends.

Table 4 summarizes the estimates for β_0 and β_1 and their corresponding standard errors, 95% CIs and p-values obtained by the REML procedure with unstructured correlations. The negative estimates for (β_0, β_1) suggest that the beneficial effect of pharmacotherapy for this patient population is detected under both the Näive LME and SP-LME models, when only the patients who had pharmacotherapy change-point time within the CBT period are included in the analysis.

5.7.2. *Application to subjects with censored change-points*

The previous analysis uses only a sub-sample of 91 depressed patients in the ENRICHD CBT arm who had their change-point time S_i observed during the CBT treatment period. Thus, the conclusion of the beneficial effects of antidepressants for lowering the BDI scores ignores the information from patients who did not start pharmacotherapy during the CBT period. Using the shared-parameter models, the analysis here is based on 557 depressed patients who had their exact dates of antidepressant starting time recorded and attended 5 or more CBT sessions during the six-month treatment period. For practical considerations, patients in the UC arm, patients whose starting dates of antidepressant use were not recorded, and patients who had poor adherence to the required weekly CBT sessions (attended less than 5 sessions) are excluded from the analysis. Because antidepressant use for each patient was individually monitored and recorded as accurate as possibly by study psychiatrists (Taylor *et al.*, 2005, page 794), it is reasonable to assume that the missing records on antidepressant starting dates were missing at random. The longitudinal sample then includes 11 patients who used antidepressants before baseline, 92 patients who started antidepressant during the treatment period, and 454 patients who did not use antidepressants before and during the treatment period. The number of visits for these patients ranges from 5 to 36 and has a median of 12.

With a slight modification of the notation in Section 5.7.1, Y_{ij}, T_{ij}, $S_i^{(c)}$, and $R_{ij} = T_{ij} - S_i^{(c)}$ denote the ith patient's BDI score, trial time (months), starting time (months) of antidepressant use, and antidepressant duration time (months), respectively, at the jth visit. For all $1 \leq i \leq n$, the observed $(S_i^{(c)}, \delta_i^{(c)})$ is $(S_i^{(c)} = S_i, \delta_i^{(c)} = 0)$ if the ith patient used antidepressants within the CBT period, $(S_i^{(c)} = T_{in_i}, \delta_i^{(c)} = 1)$ if the patient did not use antidepressant within the CBT period, and $(S_i = 0, \delta_i^{(c)} = 2)$ if the patient used antidepressants before baseline. When $\lambda_{ij} = 1_{[S_i < T_{ij}]}$ and the linear models $\mu_0(T_{ij}; a_{i0}, a_{i1}) = a_{i0} + a_{i1} T_{ij}$ and $\mu_1(R_{ij}; b_{i0}, b_{i1}) = b_{i0} + b_{i1} R_{ij}$ are used, (a_{i0}, a_{i1}) represents the intercept and slope of the ith subject's BDI trajectory before antidepressant use, and (b_{i0}, b_{i1}) is the intercept and slope of the change of the subject's BDI trajectory after antidepressant use. A series of preliminary analyses described in Wu, Tian and Jiang (2011, Appendix D.1 of the Web-Supplementary Materials) suggest that the above linear models for $\mu_0(T_{ij}; a_{i0}, a_{i1})$ and $\mu_1(R_{ij}; b_{i0}, b_{i1})$ can be used as a parsimonious approximation to the BDI time trends for this study.

Similar to (5.24), the REMLE procedure is applied to the following näive mixed-effects model to estimate the unknown population-mean parameters α_0, α_1, β_{00} and β_{10}:

$$\begin{cases} Y_{ij} = a_{i0} + a_{i1} T_{ij} + \lambda_{ij}(b_{i0} + b_{i1} R_{ij}) + \epsilon_{ij}, \\ (a_{i0}, a_{i1}, b_{i0}, b_{i1})^T \sim \mathcal{N}((\alpha_0, \alpha_1, \beta_0, \beta_1)^T, \Sigma), \end{cases} \tag{5.26}$$

where $(\alpha_0, \alpha_1, \beta_0, \beta_1)^T$ is the unknown mean vector and Σ is the unstructured covariance matrix for the multivariate normal distribution $\mathcal{N}(\cdot, \cdot)$. The population-mean concomitant intervention effects are β_0 and β_1, which are the mean intercept and slope for the "correction term" after antidepressant use, and zero value of $\beta_0 + \beta_1 R_{ij}$ indicates ignorable antidepressant effect on the mean BDI scores.

Table 5. Parameter estimates, standard errors (SE) and 95% confidence intervals (CI) computed for the ENRICHD pharmacotherapy data based on the naïve linear mixed–effects model (Näive-LMEM) (5.26), the linear shared-parameter model (LSPM)(5.27).

Effect	Näive-LMEM			LSPM		
Parameter	Estimate	SE	95% CI	Estimate	SE	95% CI
α_0	14.454	0.312	(13.842, 15.066)	15.867	0.375	(15.216, 16.771)
α_1	−1.887	0.067	(−2.018, −1.756)	−1.816	0.070	(−1.989, −1.714)
β_0	3.579	0.825	(1.962, 5.196)	−6.646	0.915	(−8.239, −4.990)
β_1	0.036	0.227	(-0.409, 0.481)	−0.453	0.284	(−0.962, 0.122)
γ_0	—	—	—	15.162	1.134	(13.497, 17.652)
γ_1	—	—	—	0.480	0.050	(−0.593, −0.392)

To account for the possible link between pharmacotherapy change-point time and the BDI trend before the use of antidepressants, a shared-parameter model that directly generalizes (5.26) is

$$\begin{cases} Y_{ij} = a_{i0} + a_{i1} T_{ij} + \lambda_{ij}(b_{i0} + b_{i1} R_{ij}) + \epsilon_{ij}, \ (a_{i0}, a_{i1})^T = (\alpha_0, \alpha_1)^T + \epsilon_i^{(a)}, \\ b_{i0} = \beta_0 + \epsilon_{i0}^{(b)}, \ b_{i1} = \beta_1 + \epsilon_{i1}^{(b)}, \ S_i = \gamma_0 + \gamma_1 a_{i0} + \epsilon_i^{(s)}, \end{cases} \tag{5.27}$$

where $\epsilon_i^{(a)}$ and $\epsilon_i^{(b)} = (\epsilon_{i0}^{(b)}, \epsilon_{i1}^{(b)})^T$ are mean zero bivariate normal random vectors with unstructured covariance matrices $\Sigma^{(a)}$ and $\Sigma^{(b)}$, respectively, $\epsilon_i^{(s)}$ is a mean zero normal random variable with variance σ_s^2, and $\epsilon_i^{(a)}$, $\epsilon_i^{(b)}$ and $\epsilon_i^{(s)}$ are independent. The interpretations of the population-mean parameters α_0, α_1, β_0 and β_1 in (5.27) are the same as their counterparts specified in (5.26).

Table 5 shows the estimates of α_0, α_1, β_0 and β_1, and their standard errors and 95% confidence intervals (CI) computed using REMLE with unstructured covariance matrix Σ under the näive linear mixed-effects model (Näive-LMEM) (5.26) and the two-stage ML procedure with ten Newton-Raphson iterations under the linear shared-parameter model (LSPM) (5.27). Under Näive-LMEM, the negative estimate $\tilde{\alpha}_1 = -1.887$ suggests that the mean BDI score for these patients tends to decrease over the trial time since the start of the CBT sessions, while the positive estimate $\tilde{\beta}_0 = 3.579$ and its 95% CI seem to suggest that the use of antidepressants increase the patients' mean BDI scores. Since the "self-selectiveness" of the antidepressant use as a concomitant intervention is not considered in (5.26), the positive estimate of β_0 under this model does not reflect the real effect of pharmacotherapy on depression severity. On the other hand, under the

LSPM (5.27), the negative estimates $\hat{\beta}_0 = -6.646$ and $\hat{\beta}_1 = -0.453$ suggest that pharmacotherapy has on average a beneficial effect for lowering a patient's depression severity. The 95% CI's for γ_0 and γ_1 obtained from (5.27) suggest that (5.26) is likely a misspecified model for this dataset.

5.8. *Discussion and further remarks*

The main results of this section show that, in general, outcome-adaptive covariates, such as concomitant interventions, should not be treated as usual time-dependent covariates in näive mixed-effects models. For the simple case of a concomitant intervention, a shared-parameter model may be considered to reduce the estimation bias and correct the "self-selectiveness" of the concomitant intervention. The methods presented here have a narrow focus on a single concomitant intervention in a longitudinal clinical trial. Concomitant interventions may commonly appear in other settings, such as in an epidemiological study where study subjects may take antihypertensive medication during the study when their blood pressure levels either exhibit some undesirable trends or stay in an intolerable range. In the ENRICHD pharmacotherapy data, pharmacotherapy as a concomitant was initiated under a vague guideline and a linear shared-parameter model appears to be a reasonable to choice. However, this model may not be suitable when the intervention selection mechanism is changed, and in some situations the entire shared-parameter approach may have to be re-evaluated.

As a special case of the shared-parameter models, a varying-coefficient mixed-effects model may be considered mainly because it has a simple and clear biological interpretation for the simple situation where there is only one concomitant intervention and the change-point time is observed for all subjects in the study. Compared with the shared-parameter models, the least-squares based estimation method for the varying-coefficient mixed-effects models does not require the known parametric forms of the distribution functions. The shared-parameter models, on the other hand, may be applied to concomitant interventions with double censored change-point time, but their estimation requires computationally intensive ML and approximate ML algorithms.

Future research in this area may be pursued with several potentially worthy extensions. First, subjects in longitudinal studies may have single or multiple concomitant interventions which can be turned on or off at different time points. In such situations, more general shared-parameter models may be needed to accommodate the possibility of multiple interventions and/or multiple change-points. Second, all the shared-parameter models studied in this section rely on linear functions to describe the time-trends before and after the intervention, but it is possible that linear response curves are inadequate for certain disease outcomes. Models with nonlinear response curves can be justified in practice and should be investigated. Third, the estimation approach of this section depends on the classical frequentist's framework for the B-spline methods. In a different context, Fahrmeir and Lang (2000) demonstrated a promising Bayesian inference procedure for generalized additive mixed models based on Markov random field priors. Similar Bayesian estimation and inference approaches for the shared-parameter models of this section may lead to computationally simpler estimation and inference procedures. Fourth, large sample properties, such as convergence rates and asymptotic distributions, of the ML and approximate ML estimators are still not well-understood and should be systematically developed to provide theoretical justifications for these estimators. Finally, since it may not be always clear whether an intervention is a concomitant intervention, a model diagnostic method for evaluating the appropriateness of a shared-parameter model would be a valuable tool to be developed.

References

1. Akaike, H (1970). Statistical predictor identification. *Ann. Inst. Statist. Math.* **22**, 203–217.
2. Altman, N. S (1990). Kernel smoothing of data with correlated errors. *J. Amer. Statist. Assoc.* **85**, 749–759.
3. Bang, H and Robins, J. M (2005). Doubly robust estimation in missing data and causal inference models. *Biometrics* **61**, 962–972.
4. Bates, D. M and Pinheiro, J. C (1999) *Mixed Effects Models in S.* Springer-Verlag, New York.
5. Bickel, P. J (1975). One-step Huber estimates in linear models. *Journal of the American Statistical Association* **34**, 584–653.
6. Cheng, S. C., Wei, L. J and Ying, Z (1995). Analysis of transformation models with censored data. *Biometrika* **82**, 835–845.
7. Cheng, S. C., Wei, L. J and Ying, Z (1997). Predicting survival probabilities with semiparametric transformation models. *Journal of the American Statistical Association* **92**, 227–235.
8. Chiang, C.-T., Rice, J. A and Wu, C. O (2001). Smoothing spline estimation for varying coefficient models with repeatedly measured dependent variable. *J. Amer. Statist. Assoc.* **96**(454):605–619.
9. Daniels, S. R., McMahon, R. P., Obarzanek, E., Waclawiw, M. A., Similo, S. L., Biro, F. M, Schreiber, G. B., Kimm, S. Y. S., Morrison, J. A. and

Barton, B. A (1998). Longitudinal correlates of change in blood pressure in adolescent girls. *Hypertension* **31**, 97–103.

10. Davidian, M and Giltinan, D.M (1995).*Nonlinear Models for Repeated Measurement Data.* London; New York: Chapman Hall.
11. De Boor, C (1978). *A Practical Guide to Splines.* Springer-Verlag, New York.
12. Diggle, P. J (1988). An approach to the analysis of repeated measurements. *Biometrics* **44**, 959–971.
13. Diggle, P. J., Heagerty, P., Liang, K.-Y and Zeger, S. L (2002). *Analysis of Longitudinal Data.*, 2nd ed. Oxford: Oxford University Press, England.
14. Eubank, R. L and Speckman, P. L (1993). Confidence bands in nonparametric regression. *J. Amer. Statist. Assoc.* **88**, 1287–1301.
15. ENRICHD Investigators. (2001). Enhancing recovery in coronary heart disease patients (ENRICHD): study int ervention rationale and design *Psychosomatic Medicine* **63**, 747–755.
16. ENRICHD Investigators. (2003). Enhancing recovery in coronary heart disease patients (ENRICHD): the effects of treating depression and low perceived social support on clinical events after myocardial infarction. *Journal of the American Medical Association* **289**, 3106–3116.
17. Fahrmeir, L and Lang, S (2000). Bayesian inference for generalised additive mixed models based on Markov random field priors. *Applied Statistics*, **50**, 201–220.
18. Fan, J and Gijbels, I (1996). *Local Polynomial Modeling and Its Applications.* London: Chapman and Hall.
19. Fan, J and Marron, J. S (1994). Fast implementations of nonparametric curves estimators. *J. Comput. Graph. Statist.*, **3**, 35–56.
20. Fan, J. Q and Zhang, J.-T. (2000). Functional linear models for longitudinal data. *J. Roy. Statist. Soc. B* **62**, 303–322.
21. Follmann, D and Wu, M. C (1995). An approximate generalized linear model with random effects for informative missing data. *Biometrics* **51**, 151–168.
22. Hall, P., and Müller, H.G (2003). Order-preserving Nonparametric regression, with applications to conditional distributions and quantile function estimation. *J. Amer. Statist. Assoc.* **98**, 598–608.
23. Hall, P and Titterington, D. M (1988). On confidence bands in nonparametric density estimation and regression. *J. Multi. Anal.* **27**, 228–254.
24. Hall, P., Wolff, R. C. L and Yao, Q (1999). Methods for estimating a conditional distribution function. *J. Amer. Statist. Assoc.* **94**, 154-163.
25. Härdle, W (1990). *Applied Nonparametric Regerssion*, Cambridge University Press, Cambridge, U.K.
26. Härdle, W and Marron, J. S (1991). Bootstrap simultaneous error bars for nonparametric regression. *Ann. Statist.* **19**, 778–796.
27. Hart, T. D (1991). Kernel regression estimation with time series errors. *J. Roy. Statist. Soc., Ser. B* **53**, 173–187.
28. Hart, T. D and Wehrly, T. E (1986). Kernel regression estimation using repeated measurements data. *J. Amer. Statist. Assoc.* **81**, 1080–1088.

29. Harville, D. A (1974). Bayesian inference for variance components using only error contrasts. *Biometrika* **61**, 383–385.
30. Hastie, T. J and Tibshirani, R. J (1993). Varying-coefficient models. *J. Roy. Statist. Soc. B* **55**, 757–796.
31. Hoover, D. R., Rice, J. A., Wu, C. O and Yang, L.-P (1998). Nonparametric smoothing estimates of time-varying coefficient models with longitudinal data. *Biometrika* **85**, 809–822.
32. Huang, J., Wu, C. O and Zhou, L (2002). Varying coefficient models and basis function approximations for the analysis of repeated measurements. *Biometrika* **89**, 111–128.
33. Huang, J. Z., Wu, C. O and Zhou, L (2004). Polynomial spline estimation and inference for varying coefficient models with longitudinal data. *Statistica Sinica* **14**, 763–788.
34. Jones, R. H and Ackerson, L. M (1990). Serial correlation in unequally spaced longitudinal data. *Biometrika* **77**, 721–731.
35. Jones, R. H and Boadi-Boteng, F (1991). Unequally spaced longitudinal data with serial correlation. *Biometrics* **47**, 161–175.
36. Kaslow, R. A., Ostrow, D. G., Detels, R., Phair, J. P., Polk, B. F. and Rinaldo, C. R (1987). The Multicenter AIDS Cohort Study: Rationale, Organization and Selected Characteristics of the Participants. *American Journal of Epidemiology* **126**, 310–318.
37. Kimm, S. Y., Barton, B. A., Obarzanek, E., McMahon, R. P., Sabry, Z. I., Waclawiw, M. A., *et al.* (2001). Racial divergence in adiposity during adolescence: the NHLBI Growth and Health Study. *Pediatrics* 2001;107:E34.
38. Kimm, S. Y., Barton, B. A., Obarzanek, E., McMahon, R. P., Kronsberg, S. S., Waclawiw, M. A., *et al.* (2002). Obesity development during adolescence in a biracial cohort: the NHLBI Growth and Health Study. *Pediatrics* 2002;110:E54.
39. Kimm, S. Y., Glynn, N. W., Kriska, A. M., Fitzgerald, S. L., Aaron, D. J., Similo, S. L, *et al.* (2000). Longitudinal changes in physical activity in a biracial cohort during adolescence. *Med. Sci. Sports Exerc.* 2000;**32**: 1445–1454.
40. Knafl, G., Sacks, J and Ylvisaker, D (1985). Confidence bands for regression functions. *J. Amer. Statist. Assoc.* **80**, 683-691.
41. Laird, N. M and Ware, J. H (1982). Random-effects models for longitudinal data. *Biometrics* **38**, 963–974.
42. Liang, K.-Y and Zeger, S. L (1986). Longitudinal data analysis using generalized linear models. *Biometrika* **73**, 13–22.
43. Lin, X and Carroll, R. J (2000). Nonparametric function estimation for clustered data when the predictor is measured without/with error. *J. Am. Statist. Assoc.* **95**, 520–534.
44. Lin, X and Zhang, D (1999). Inference in generalized additive mixed models by using smoothing splines. *Journal of the Royal Statistical Society: Series B*, **61**(2), 381–400.
45. Lu, W and Tsiatis, A. A (2006). Semiparametric transformation models for the case-cohort study. *Biometrika* **93**, 207–214.

46. Lu, W and Ying, Z (2004). On semiparametric transformation cure models. *Biometrika* **91**, 331–343.
47. Molenberghs, G and Verbeke, G (2005). *Models for Discrete Longitudinal Data.* Springer: New York, NY.
48. Moyeed, R. A and Diggle, P. J (1994). Rates of convergence in semiparametric modeling of longitudinal data. *Austral. J. Statist.* **36**, 75–93.
49. Müller, H.-G (1988). Nonparametric Regression Analysis of Longitudinal Data. *Lecture Notes in Statistics,* **46.** Springer-Verlag, Berlin.
50. National High Blood Pressure Education Program Working Group on High Blood Pressure in Children and Adolescents (NHBPEP Working Group) (2004). The fourth report on the diagnosis, evaluation, and treatment of high blood pressure in children and adolescents. *Pediatrics* **114**, 555–576.
51. National Heart, Lung, and Blood Institute Growth and Health Research Group (NGHSRG) (1992). Obesity and cardiovascular disease risk factors in black and white girls: the NHLBI Growth and Health Study. *Am J. Public Health* **82** 1613–1620.
52. Obarzanek, E., Wu, C. O., Cutler, J. A., Kavey, R. W., Pearson, G. D and Daniels, S. R (2010). Prevalence and incidence of hypertension in adolescent girls. *The Journal of Pediatrics* **157**(3), 461–467.
53. Pantula, S. G and Pollock, K. H (1985). Nested analysis of variance with autocorrelated errors. *Biometrics*, **41**, 909–920.
54. Patterson, H. D and Thompson, R (1971). Recovery of inter-block information when block sizes are unequal. *Biometrika* **58**, 545–554.
55. Pepe, M. S and Anderson, G (1994). A cautionary note on inference of rmarginal regression models with longitudinal data and general correlated response data. *Communications in Statistics: Simulation and Computation*, **23**, 939–951.
56. Rice, J. A and Silverman, B. W (1991). Estimating the mean and covariance structure nonparametrically when the data are curves. *J. Roy. Statist. Soc. Ser. B* **53**, 233–243.
57. Rice, J. A and Wu, C. O (2001). Nonparametric mixed effects models for unequally sampled noisy curves. *Biometrics* **57**, 253–259.
58. Schwarz, G (1978). Estimating the dimension of a model. *Ann. Statist.* **6**, 461–464.
59. Serfling, R. J (1980). *Approximation Theorems of Mathematical Statistics.* New York: Wiley & Sons.
60. Shibata, R (1981). An optimal selection of regression variables. *Biometrika* **68**, 45–54.
61. Taylor, C. B., Youngblood, M. E., Catellier, D., Veith, R. C., Carney, R. M., Burg, M. M., Kaufmann, P., Shuster, J., Mellman, T., Blumenthal, J. A., Krishnan, R. and Jaffe, A. S (2005). Effects of antidepressant medication on morbidity and mortality in depressed patients after myocardial infarction. *Archives of General Psychiatry*, **62**, 792–298.
62. Thompson, D. R., Obarzanek, E., Franko, D. L., Barton, B. A., Morrison, J., Biro, F. M., Daniels, S. R. and Striegel-Moore, R. H (2007). Childhood overweight and cardiovscular disease risk factors: The National Heart, Lung,

and Blood Institute Growth and Health Study. *Journal of Pediatrics* **150**, 18–25.
63. Verbeke, G and Molenberghs, G (2000). *Linear Mixed Models for Longitudinal Data.* Springer, New York.
64. Vonesh, E. F and Chinchilli, V. M (1997). *Linear and Nonlinear Models for the Analysis of Repeated Measurements.* Marcel Dekker, New York.
65. Wahba, G (1990). *Spline Models for Observational Data.* SIAM, Philadelphia.
66. Ware, J. H (1985). Linear models for the analysis of longitudinal studies. *The American Statistician*, **39**, 95–101.
67. Wu, C. O and Chiang, C.-T (2000). Kernel smoothing on varying coefficient models with longitudinal dependent variable. *Statistica Sinica* **10**, 433–456.
68. Wu, C. O., Chiang, C.-T and Hoover, D. R (1998). Asymptotic confidence regions for kernel smoothing of a varying-coefficient model with longitudinal data. *J. Amer. Statist. Assoc.* **93**, 1388–1402.
69. Wu, C. O., Tian, X.d and Bang, H (2008). A varying-coefficient model for the evaluation of time-varying concomitant intervention effects in longitudinal studies. *Statistics in Medicine* **27**, 3042–3056.
70. Wu, C. O., Tian, X and Jiang, W (2011). A shared parameter model for the estimation of longitudinal concomitant intervention effects. *Biostatistics* **12**(4):737–749.
71. Wu, C. O., Tian, X and Yu, J (2010). Nonparametric estimation for time-varying transformation models with longitudinal data. *Journal of Nonparametric Statistics* **22**, 133–147.
72. Wu, C. O., Yu, K. F. and Chiang, C.-T (2000). A two-step smoothing method for varying-coefficient models with repeated measurements. *Ann. Inst. Statist. Math.* **52**, 519–543.
73. Wu, C. O., Yu, K. F and Yuan, V. W. S (2000). Large sample properties and confidence bands for component-wise varying-coefficient regression with longitudinal dependent variable. *Commun. Statist.–Theory Meth.* **29**, 1017–1037.
74. Zeger, S. L and Diggle, P. J (1994). Semiparametric models for longitudinal data with application to CD4 cell numbers in HIV seroconverters. *Biometrics* **50**, 689–699.
75. Zeger, S. L., Liang, K.-Y and Albert, P. S (1988). Models for longitudinal data: a generalized estimating equation approach. *Biometrics* **44**, 1049–1060.
76. Zeng, D and Lin, D. Y (2006). Efficient estimation of semiparametric transformation models for counting processes. *Biometrika* **93**, 627–640.

About the Authors

Colin O. Wu is a Mathematical Statistician at the Office of Biostatistics Research, Division of Cardiovascular Sciences, National Heart, Lung and Blood Institute, National Institutes of Health (USA). He is also an Adjunct

Professor at the Department of Biostatistics, Bioinformatics, and Biomathematics, Lombardi Comprehensive Cancer Center, Georgetown University School of Medicine, and a Professorial Lecturer at the Department of Statistics, The George Washington University. He received his Ph.D. in statistics from the University of California, Berkeley, in 1990. His former positions include Visiting Assistant Professor at the University of Michigan, Ann Arbor, Assistant and Associate Professor at the Johns Hopkins University, and Guest Lecturer at University of Maryland, College Park. He has published over 90 research articles in statistics, biostatistics and medical journals. He has been a Guest Editor for Statistics in Medicine, and he is currently serving as an Associate Editor for Biometrics and a Data Monitoring Committee member for the United Sates Department of Veterans Affairs. He is an Elected Member of the International Statistical Institute, and a Fellow of the American Statistical Association.

Xin Tian is currently a Mathematical Statistician in the Office of Biostatistics Research, Division of Cardiovascular Sciences, National Heart, Lung and Blood Institute, National Institutes of Health. She obtained her PhD in Statistics (2003) from Rutgers, the State University of New Jersey. Her research interests include design and analysis of clinical trials, statistical genetics, and longitudinal data analysis with structural nonparametric models.

Kai Fun Yu is a Professor of Mathematical Sciences at Tsinghua University in the People's Republic of China. His former positions include Senior Investigator and Mathematical Statistician at the United States National Institutes of Health, Associate Professor of Statistics at the University of South Carolina and Assistant Professor of Statistics at Yale University. He was on the visiting faculty of some universities including Columbia University and Stanford University. He has published over 100 articles in scientific journals. He was a statistical consultant to the New Haven Legal Assistance Association, South Carolina State Re-organization Commission, South Carolina Water Resources Commission and South Carolina Department of Corrections. He performed many community services such as serving on the National Instituted of Health Institutional Review Board, the American Statistical Association Committee on Scientific Freedom and Human Rights, as the Biometric Section Chairman of the International Chinese Statistical Association et cetera. He is a fellow of American Statistical Association, an elected member of International Statistical Institute, and a member of Institute of Mathematical Statistics, International Chinese

Statistical Association and Hong Kong Statistical Society. He was educated at Saint Francis Xavier's College, Dartmouth College, Princeton University and Columbia University.

Mi Xia Wu is an Associate Professor of Applied Sciences at Beijing University of Technology in China. Her former positions include visiting researcher at Department of Applied Mathematics, The Hong Kong Polytechnic University and postdoctoral fellow at Eunice Kennedy Shriver National Institute of Child Health and Human Development, the United States National Institutes of Health. She received her Ph.D. in Statistics from Beijing University of Technology in 2004. She was awarded "Zhong Jiaqing" prize in 2004, Excellent PH.D thesis of Beijing University of Technology in 2004, Training Program Foundation for the Beijing Municipal Excellent Talents in 2010 and Project for Academic Human Resources Development in Institutions of Higher Learning Under the Jurisdiction of Beijing Municipality PHR in 2011. She has published over 20 research articles and 3 books in statistics. Her research interests include mixed effects model, multivariate analysis and longitudinal data analysis.

CHAPTER 30

LOCAL MODELING: DENSITY ESTIMATION AND NONPARAMETRIC REGRESSION

JIANQING FAN

Department of Operations Research and Financial Engineering, Princeton University, Princeton, NJ 08544, USA; jqfan@princeton.edu

RUNZE LI

Department of Statistics, Penn State University, University Park, PA 16802, USA; rzli@psu.edu

1. Introduction

Local modeling approaches are useful tools for exploring features of data without imposing a parametric model. These approaches have been received increasing attention in last two decades and successfully applied to various scientific disciplines, such as, economics, engineering, medicine, environmental science, health science and social science. There are a vast amount of literature on this topic.[29, 34] A comprehensive account of local modeling can be found in the books.[6, 28, 48, 72, 75, 76, 85] see also Fan and Gijbels[29] and Fan and Müller[34] for a brief overview on this topic. In this chapter, we will introduce fundamental ideas of local modeling and illustrate the ideas by real data examples. For ease of presentation, we will omit all technical parts.

This chapter basically consists of two parts: Kernel density estimation and local polynomial fitting. In Sec. 2, the kernel density estimation method will be introduced. Important issues, including bandwidth selection, will be addressed. Real data examples will be used to illustrate the ideas how to implement this type of method. Local polynomial regression will be introduced in Sec. 3. In this section, we also discuss how to decide the amount of smoothing, and extend the ideas of local polynomial regression to other contexts. The idea is further extended to the local likelihood and local partially likelihood in Sec. 4. Section 5 introduces the ideas of nonparametric smoothing tests. Section 6 summarizes some applications of local modeling, including estimation of conditional quantile functions, conditional variance functions and conditional densities, and change point detection.

2. Density Estimation

Suppose that $X_1, \ldots, X_n$ are an independent and identically distributed sample from a population with an unknown probability density $f(x)$. Of interest is to estimate the density f. In explanatory data analysis, we may construct a histogram for the data. If the resulting histogram has a bell shape, then we may assume that the samples were taken from a normal distribution. In this situation, one may just estimate the population mean and variance using the sample mean and sample variance because a normal distribution is completely determined by its mean and variance. In general, parametric approaches to estimation of a density function assume that the density belongs to a parametric family of distributions, such as normal, gamma or beta family. In order to fully specify the density function, one has to estimate the unknown parameters using, for example, maximum likelihood estimation. One may use prior knowledge or scientific reasons to determine a parametric distribution family. In explanatory data analysis, data analysts frequently construct a histogram based on the sample, and then draw reasonable conclusions on the population density.

2.1. *Histogram*

A histogram is usually formed by partitioning the range of data into equally length intervals, called bins, and then drawing a block over each interval with height being the proportion of the data falling in the bin divided by the width of the bin. Specifically, the histogram estimate at a point x is given by

$$\hat{f}(x,h) = \frac{\text{number of observations in the bin containing } x}{nh},$$

where h is the width of the bins, namely binwidth. For a fixed choice of bins, it can be shown that under some mild conditions, $\hat{f}(\cdot,h)$ is a maximum likelihood estimate of the unknown density f. It is worthwhile to note that the nonparametric maximum likelihood estimate of the unknown density f

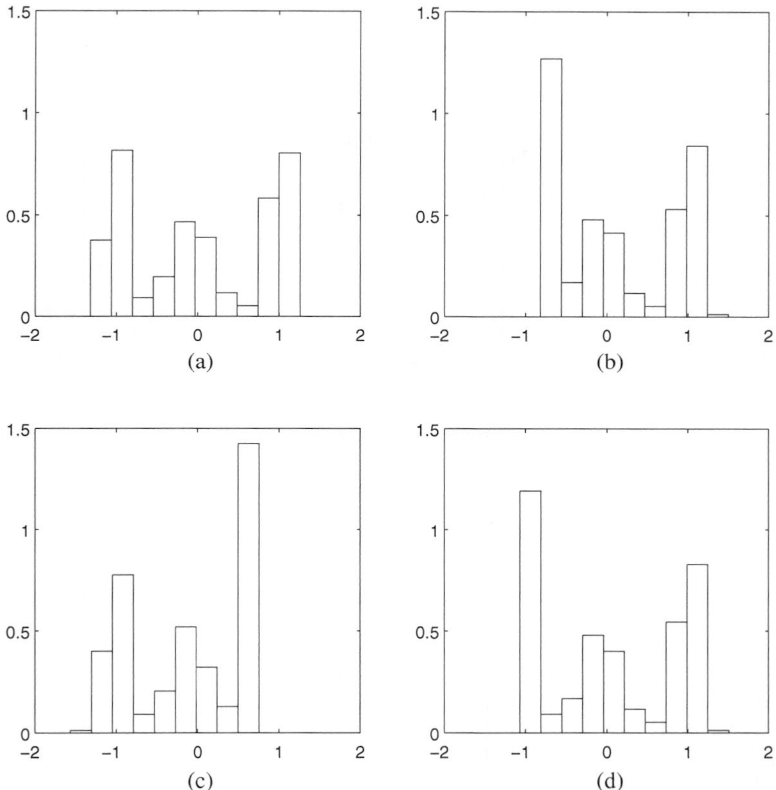

Fig. 1. Histograms of a sample of size 300 from a mixture of normal distribution $1/3N(-1, 0.1^2) + 1/3N(0, 0.25^2) + 1/3N(1, 0.1^2)$.

without any further restriction does not exist, since

$$\max_{\{f: f\geq 0, \int f = 1\}} \prod_{i=1}^{n} f(X_i) = \infty\,.$$

When one constructs a histogram, one has to choose the binwidth and the centers of bins. Figure 1 depicts four histograms based on the same data set and the same binwidth, but using different locations of bin centers. It can be seen from Fig. 1 that the shapes of the resulting histograms are quite different. This implies that the histogram suffers the "edge" effect. Figure 2 shows four histograms of the lengths of crabs, collected from 1973 to 1986, but with different binwidths. The crab data set is available from the website of statlib at Carnegie Mellon University at http://lib.stat.cmu.edu.

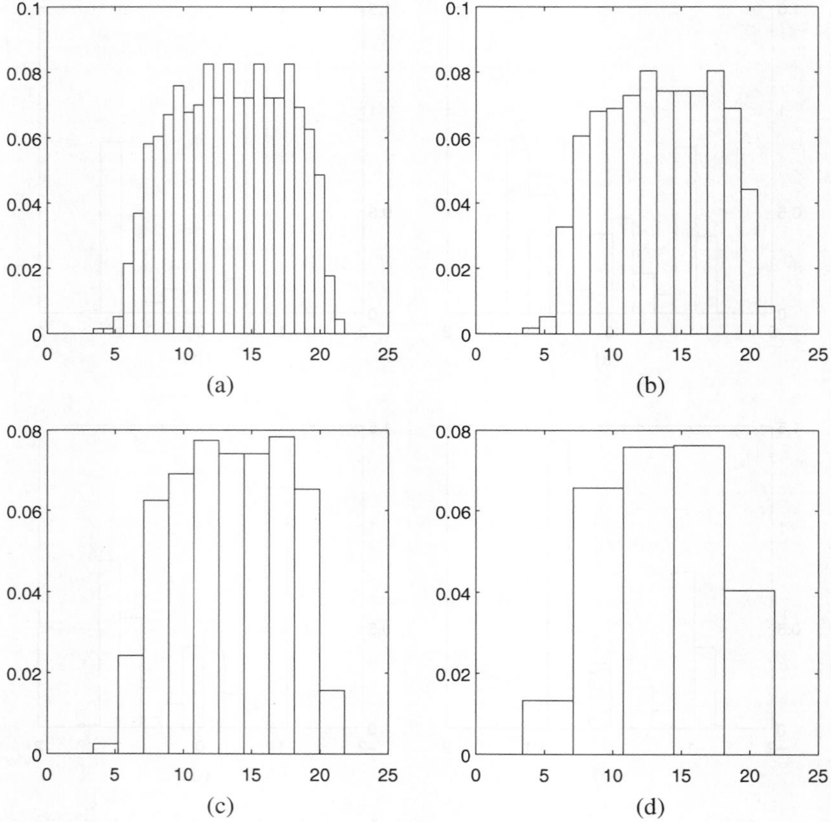

Fig. 2. Histograms for crab sizes. The data is the length of crab (cm).

From Fig. 2, if the binwidth h is too small, then the resulting histogram is rough, on the other hand, if the binwidth is too large, then the resulting histogram is too smooth. Thus constructing a histogram actually is not so simple! Usually one may start from an undersmoothed histogram, and then increase gradually the binwidth until getting a satisfactory result.

The histogram is the oldest and most widely used nonparametric estimate of density. The choice of binwidth is a smoothing problem. The edge effect of histograms can be repaired by the kernel density estimation introduced in next section. Furthermore, the kernel estimate will result in a smooth density curve rather than a step function as in histograms. It is an improved technique over the kernel density estimation.

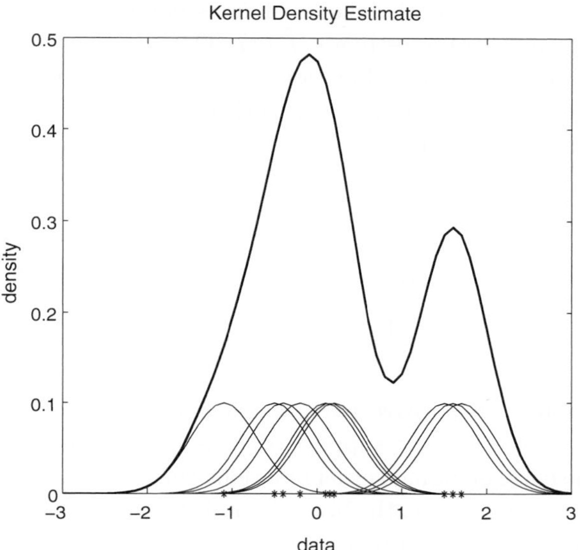

Fig. 3. Kernel density estimate for an hypothetical data set (thick curve). It smoothly redistributes the point mass at X_i by the function $(nh)^{-1}K\{(x - X_i)/h\}$. The small bumps show how point masses are redistributed.

2.2. *Kernel density estimation*

A kernel density estimate is defined as

$$\hat{f}_h = (nh)^{-1} \sum_{i=1}^{n} K\{(x - X_i)/h\},$$

where $K(\cdot)$ is a function satisfying $\int K(x)dx = 1$, called a *kernel function* and h is a positive number, called a *bandwidth* or a *smoothing parameter*. A density function such as the plot (thick curve) in Fig. 3 is usually obtained by evaluating the function $\hat{f}_h(x)$ over a few hundred of grid points. From the definition, indeed, the kernel estimate is the average of density functions $h^{-1}K\{(x - X_i)/h\}$, which smoothly redistribute the point mass at the point X_i. Figure 3 depicts the redistribution of point masses. To facilitate notation, let $K_h(t) = \frac{1}{h}K(t/h)$ be a rescaling function of K. This allows us to write

$$\hat{f}_h = n^{-1} \sum_{i=1}^{n} K_h(x - X_i). \tag{1}$$

It is well known that the choice of K is not very sensitive, scaled in a canonical form[64] to the estimate $\hat{f}_h(x)$. Thus it is assumed throughout this chapter that the kernel function is a symmetric probability density function. The most commonly used kernel function is the Gaussian density function given by

$$K(t) = \frac{1}{\sqrt{2\pi}} \exp(-t^2/2) . \tag{2}$$

Other popular kernel functions include the symmetric beta family

$$K(t) = \frac{1}{\beta(1/2, \gamma+1)} (1-t^2)_+^{\gamma} , \quad \gamma = 0, 1, \dots , \tag{3}$$

where + denotes the positive part, which is assumed to be taken before exponentiation, so that the support of K is $[-1, 1]$, and $\beta(\cdot, \cdot)$ is a beta function. The corresponding kernel functions when $\gamma = 0$, 1, 2 and 3 are the uniform, the Epanechnikov, the biweight and the triweight kernel functions. Figure 4 shows these kernel functions.

The smoothing parameter h controls the smoothness of density estimates, acting as the binwidth in histograms. The choice of the bandwidth is of crucial importance. If h is chosen too large, then the resulting estimate misses fine features of the data, while if h is selected too small then spurious

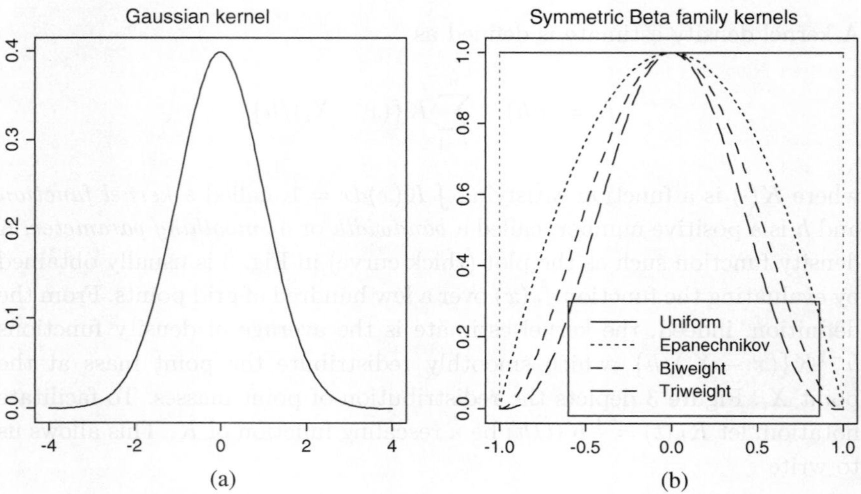

Fig. 4. Commonly-used kernels. (a) Gaussian kernel; (b) Symmetric Beta family of kernels that are renormalized to have maximum height 1.

sharp structure become visible. See Fig. 6 for example. In fact, it can be shown that under some mild conditions, when $n \to \infty$, $h \to 0$ and $nh \to \infty$,

$$E\hat{f}_h(x) - f(x) = \frac{f''(x)}{2}\mu(K)h^2 + o(h^2) \tag{4}$$

and

$$\text{var}\{\hat{f}_h(x)\} = \frac{R(K)f(x)}{nh}(1 + o(1)), \tag{5}$$

where $\mu(K) = \int t^2 K(t)dt$ and $R(K) = \int K^2(t)dt$. Thus, from (4) and (5), a large bandwidth h results in a large bias while a small bandwidth produces an estimate with a large variance. A good choice of bandwidth would balance the bias and variance trade-off. This is conveniently assessed by the *Asymptotic Mean Integrated Square Error* (AMISE) which is defined as

$$\text{AMISE}(h) = \frac{\mu^2(K)h^4}{4}\int \{f''(x)\}^2 dx + \frac{R(K)}{nh}. \tag{6}$$

Minimizing (6) with respect to h gives the ideal bandwidth

$$h_I = \left(\frac{R(K)}{\mu^2(K)\int\{f''(x)\}^2 dx}\right)^{1/5} n^{-1/5}, \tag{7}$$

which involves the unknown density function, and cannot be directly used in kernel smoothing. Since the choice of bandwidth is critical to kernel density estimation, there has a large literature on this topic. See Jones *et al.*[56,57] for a survey. In practice, we may take the Gaussian density with variance σ^2 as a reference density. In this situation, Eq. (7) becomes

$$h_I = \left(\frac{8\sqrt{\pi}R(K)}{3\mu^2(K)}\right)^{1/5} \sigma n^{-1/5}. \tag{8}$$

Here we focus on a rule of thumb.[75] The rule of thumb of bandwidth selection is to replace σ by the sample standard deviation s_n. Thus, for the Gaussian kernel,

$$\hat{h}_I = 1.06 s_n n^{-1/5},$$

and for the symmetric β family

$$\hat{h}_I = \left[\frac{8\sqrt{\pi}\beta(1/2, 2\gamma+1)}{\{\beta(3/2, \gamma+1)\}^2}\right]^{1/5} s_n n^{-1/5}.$$

Figure 5 depicts a kernel density estimate of the length of crab using the bandwidth $\hat{h}_I$ with the Gaussian kernel. From the shape of the estimated

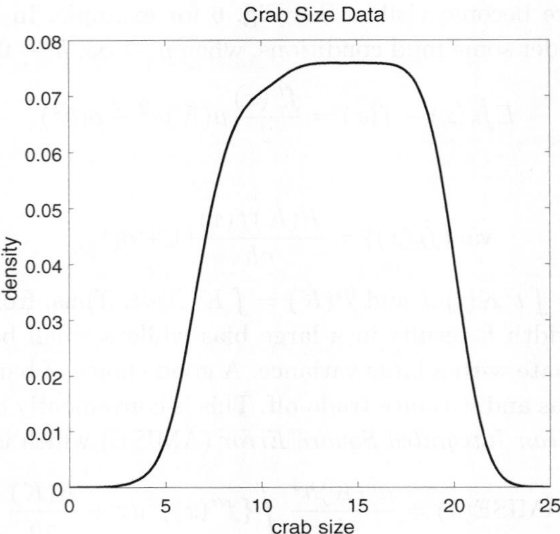

Fig. 5. Automatic kernel density estimates using the bandwidth according the rule of thumb. The data set is the crab size data collected from 1973 to 1986.

density curve, it seems that a normal distribution is not appropriate for modeling the crab size.

While the rule of thumb works well for many data sets, it tends to produce oversmooth estimates as the referenced density is a Gaussian density. Another method to avoid choosing a single optimal bandwidth is the family smoothing approach. This can be done by using a family of estimates

$$\{\hat{f}_h, h = 1.4^j \hat{h}_I, j = -3, -2, -1, 0, 1, 2\} \tag{9}$$

and then overlaying them in the same plot. The family smoothing approach allows us to explore possible patterns contained in data using different scale of bandwidths. This is closely related to scale space ideas in computer science. Choosing a smaller bandwidth acts as "zoom in", while selecting a larger bandwidth corresponds to "zoom out" in the scale space. These ideas have been further developed in a SiZer map.[13] The SiZer map can detect significant features in estimated curve with different scales. Figure 6 depicts a family smoothing plot for the crab size data.

The density estimation method is also a powerful graphic tool for comparing the results of two experiments. This is related to the classical two-sample mean problem. The advantage of the kernel smoothing approach over the traditional two sample tests is that the smoothing approach can show an overall pattern of the experiments, including the locations of

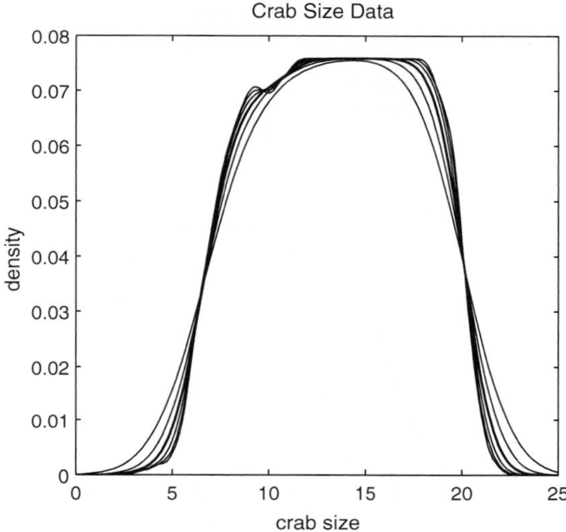

Fig. 6. A family of kernel estimates. The data set is the crab 5size data. The thick curve corresponds to $\hat{h}_I$.

centers and the dispersions of the data. Further, it gives us some ideas of two population distributions. To illustrate the idea, we applied the smoothing techniques for two subsets of the crab size data. One contains the 1976 data set and the other consists of the 1986 data set. The two estimated density curves are depicted in Fig. 7. They have different centers and dispersions.

In this section, the bandwidth remains constant, that is, it depends on neither the location x nor the datum point X_i. This kind of bandwidth is referred as a global bandwidth. From (7), it is desirable to use a larger bandwidth when changes of curvature is small and use a smaller bandwidth when curvature of underlying density dramatically changes. This leads to studying variable bandwidth selection, which suggests the use of different bandwidth at different location of x. Usually, a global bandwidth is easier to choose than the variable bandwidth. In order to use a constant bandwidth, one may first transform the data by

$$Y_i = g(X_i)\,, \quad i = 1, \ldots, n\,,$$

where g is a given monotone increasing function. The transformation g should be chosen so that the transformed data have a density with more homogeneous degree of smoothness so that a global bandwidth for the transformed data is more appropriate. Then apply the kernel density estimate

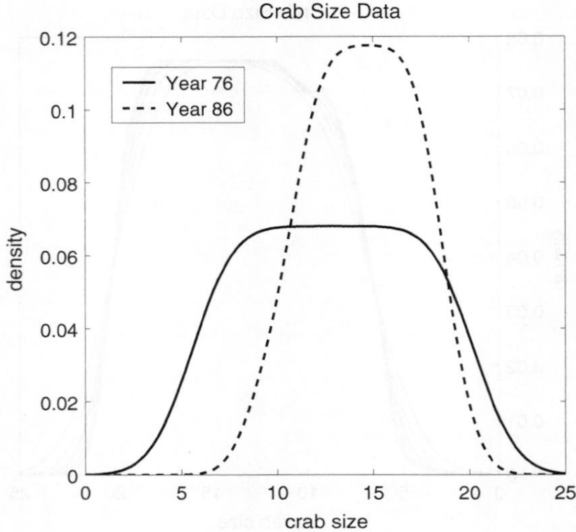

Fig. 7. Comparison of the length of crabs between 1976 and 1986. The sample mean and standard deviation for 1976 are 12.9020 and 4.2905, while the sample mean and standard deviation for 1986 are 14.4494 and 2.6257, respectively.

to the transformed data set and obtain the estimate $\hat{f}_Y(y)$. Finally apply the inverse transform to obtain the density of X:

$$\hat{f}_X(x) = g'(x)\hat{f}_Y(g(x)) = g'(x)n^{-1}\sum_{i=1}^{n} K_h(g(x) - g(X_i)).$$

The performance of this type estimate has been illustrated in Wand *et al.*[86] Marron and Yang (1999) proposed an approach to selecting a good transformation g.

3. Local Polynomial Fitting

Regression is one of the most useful techniques in statistics. Consider the $(d+1)$-dimensional data $(\mathbf{X}_1, Y_1), \ldots, (\mathbf{X}_n, Y_n)$, which form an independent and identically distributed sample from a population $(\mathbf{X}, Y)$, where $\mathbf{X}$ is a d-dimensional random vector and Y is a random variable. Of interest is to estimate the regression function $m(\mathbf{x}) = E(Y|\mathbf{X} = \mathbf{x})$. In other words, the data are regarded as realizations from the model:

$$Y = m(\mathbf{X}) + \varepsilon\,,$$

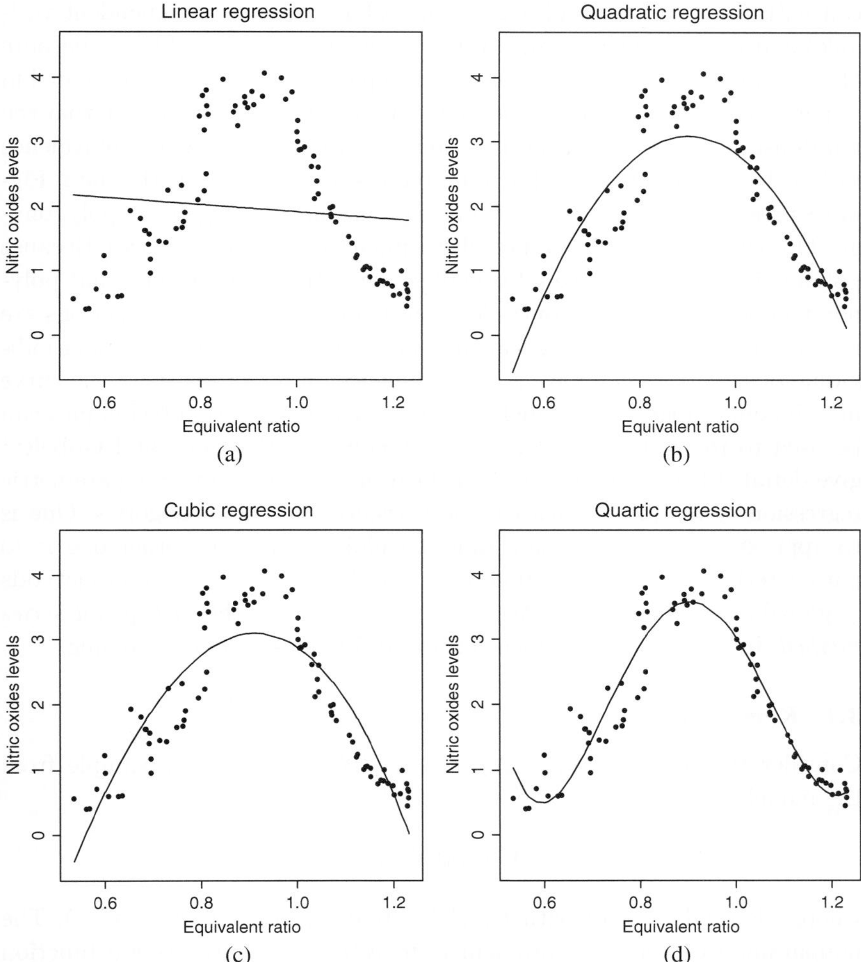

Fig. 8. Polynomial fits to the ethanol data. Presented are the scatter plots of the concentration of nitric oxides against the equivalence ratio along with the fitted polynomial regression functions. Adapted from Fan and Gijbels.[29]

where ε is a random error with zero mean. For a given data set, one may try to fit the data by using a linear regression model. If a nonlinear pattern appears in the scatter plot of Y against $\mathbf{X}$, one may employ polynomial regression to reduce the modeling bias of linear regression. Consider, for example, the data plotted in Fig. 8, where the relationship between the concentration of nitric oxides in engine exhaust (taken as dependent variable) and the equivalence ratio (taken as independent variable), a measure of the richness of the air/ethanol mix, is depicted for a burning of ethanol in a single-cylinder automobile test engine. From Fig. 8, it can be seen that the relationship between the concentration of nitric oxides and the equivalence ratio is highly nonlinear. Polynomial regression is used to fit the data. Figure 8 presents the resulting fits by using four different degrees of polynomials. One can easily see that all resulting fits have substantial biases. Because polynomial functions have all orders of derivatives everywhere, and polynomial degree cannot be controlled continuously, polynomial functions are not very flexible in modeling features encountered in practice. Further individual observations can have a large influence on remote parts of the curve in polynomial regression models. Nonparametric regression techniques can be used to repair the drawbacks of polynomial fitting. Fan and Gijbels[28] give detailed background and excellent overview on various nonparametric regression techniques, which can be classified into two categories. One is to approximate the regression function globally and the other one is to parameterize the regression function $m(\mathbf{x})$ locally. Two common methods of global approximation are the *spline approach* and the *orthogonal series method.* In this section, we focus on the techniques of local modeling.

3.1. *Kernel regression*

Consider the bivariate data $(X_1, Y_1), \ldots, (X_n, Y_n)$, an i.i.d. sample from the model:

$$Y = m(X) + \varepsilon\,,$$

where ε is random error with $E(\varepsilon|X) = 0$ and $\mathrm{var}(\varepsilon|X = x) = \sigma^2(x)$. The nonparametric regression problem is to estimate the regression function $m(\cdot)$ with imposing a form. Usually, a datum point closer to x carries more information about the value of $m(x)$. Therefore an intuitive estimator for the regression function $m(x)$ is the running local average. An improved version of this is the locally weighted average. That is

$$\hat{m}(x) = \sum_{i=1}^{n} w_i(x) Y_i \Big/ \sum_{i=1}^{n} w_i(x)\,.$$

An alternative interpretation of locally weighted average estimators is that the resulting estimator is the solution to the following weighted least-squares problem:

$$\min_{\theta} \sum_{i=1}^{n} (Y_i - \theta)^2 w_i(x) .$$

In other words, the kernel regression estimators are a weighted least squares estimate at the point x using a local constant approximation.

Setting the weights $w_i(x) = K_h(X_i - x)$ results in the NW kernel regression estimator, which is given by[68, 87]

$$\hat{m}_h(x) = \frac{\sum_{i=1}^{n} K_h(X_i - x) Y_i}{\sum_{i=1}^{n} K_h(X_i - x)} . \tag{10}$$

See Nadaraya[68] and Watson.[87]

Since the denominator in (10) is a random variable, it is inconvenient to take derivatives with respect to x and to derive the asymptotic properties of the estimator. Assume that the data have already been sorted according to the X-variable. Taking the local weights $w_i(x) = \int_{s_{i-1}}^{s_i} K_h(u - x) du$ with $s_i = (X_i + X_{i+1})/2$, $X_0 = -\infty$ and $X_{n+1} = +\infty$, we obtain the GM regression estimator given by

$$\hat{m}_h(x) = \sum_{i=1}^{n} \int_{s_{i-1}}^{s_i} K_h(u - x)\, du Y_i .$$

See Gasser and Müller.[41]

Just like the kernel density estimate, the choice of bandwidth is critical to the quality of the estimate. A too large bandwidth yields an over-smooth estimate, while a too small bandwidth gives a rough estimate. The basic asymptotic properties of the NW and GM regression estimators have been well established. The asymptotic biases and variances of these two estimators are depicted in Table 1.[23] The properties on the GM estimator were established in Mack and Müller[63] and Chu and Marron.[16]

3.2. *Local polynomial regression*

As indicated in the last section, both the NW estimator and the GM estimator are a local constant fit. It is natural to extend this to a local polynomial fit. The idea of local polynomial regression has been around for a long time. Since both a local constant and local polynomial fits use effectively datum points in a local neighborhood, this idea is referred as local modeling. It appeared in the statistical literature.[17, 79] Stone[80, 81] shows that local regression achieves optimal rates in a minimax sense. Müller[16]

Table 1. Leading terms in the asymptotic biases and variances.[25]

Method	Bias	Variance
NW Estimator	$\left\{m''(x) + \dfrac{2m'(x)f'(x)}{f(x)}\right\} b_n$	V_n
GM Estimator	$m''(x)b_n$	$1.5V_n$
Local Linear	$m''(x)b_n$	V_n

Here $b_n = \dfrac{1}{2}\displaystyle\int_{-\infty}^{+\infty} u^2K(u)du h^2$ and $V_n = \dfrac{\sigma^2(x)}{f(x)nh}\displaystyle\int_{-\infty}^{+\infty} K^2(u)du.$

establishes the equivalence between a local polynomial fit and a local constant fit under an equally-spaced design model. Fan[23,24] focus on local linear regression in the random design case and show that it has many advantages, such as simple expression for local bias and variance, spatial adaptation and high minimax efficiency. Fan and Gijbels[28] proved that theoretically the local linear regression estimator adapts automatically to the boundary. This was also empirically observed by Tibshirani and Hastie.[82] Ruppert and Wand[70] extended the results of Fan and Gijbels[28] to the case of local polynomial estimation. A thorough study of this topic can also be found in Chaps. 3 and 4 of Fan and Gijbels.[28]

Suppose that the regression function m is smooth. For z in a neighborhood of x, it follows from using Taylor's expansion that

$$m(z) \approx \sum_{j=1}^{p} \frac{m^{(j)}(x)}{j!}(z-x)^j \equiv \sum_{j=1}^{p} \beta_j (z-x)^j \,. \tag{11}$$

Thus, for X_i close enough to x,

$$m(X_i) \approx \sum_{j=0}^{p} \beta_j (X_i - x_0)^j \equiv \mathbf{X}_i^T \boldsymbol{\beta} \,,$$

where $\mathbf{X}_i = (1, (X_i - x_0), \ldots, (X_i - x_0)^p)^T$ and $\boldsymbol{\beta} = (\beta_0, \beta_1, \ldots, \beta_p)^T$. Intuitively datum points further from x have less information about $m(x)$. This suggests using a locally weighted polynomial regression

$$\sum_{i=1}^{n} (Y_i - \mathbf{X}_i^T \boldsymbol{\beta})^2 K_h(X_i - x) \,. \tag{12}$$

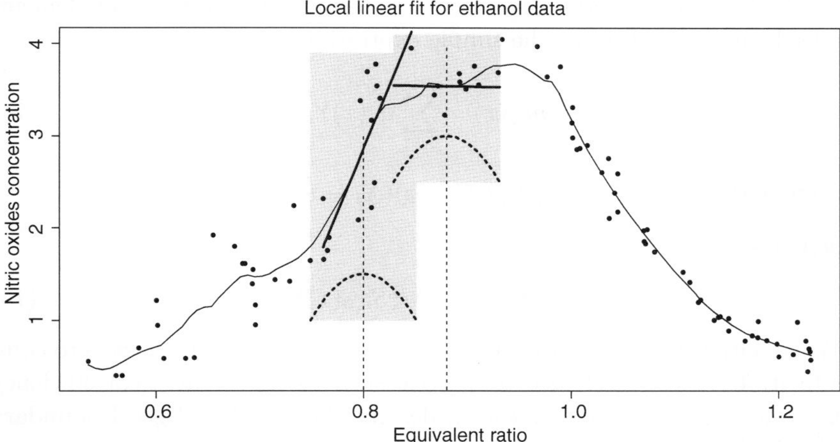

Fig. 9. Illustration of the local linear fit. For each given x_0, a linear regression is fitted through the data contained in the strip $x_0 \pm h$, using the weight function indicated at the bottom of the strip. The interactions of the fitted lines and the short dashed lines are the local linear fits. Adapted from Fan and Gijbels.[29]

Denote by $\hat{\beta}_j (j = 0, \ldots, p)$ the minimizer of (12). The above exposition suggests that an estimator for the regression function $m(x_0)$ is

$$\hat{m}(x_0) = \hat{\beta}_0(x_0) . \tag{13}$$

Furthermore, an estimator for the νth order derivative of $m(x_0)$ at x_0 is

$$\hat{m}_\nu(x_0) = \nu! \hat{\beta}_\nu(x_0) .$$

In general, local polynomial fitting has certain advantages over the NW and the GM estimators not only for estimating regression curves, but also for derivative estimation.

To better appreciate the above local polynomial regression, consider the ethanol data presented in Fig. 8. The window size h is taken to be 0.051 and the kernel is the Epanechnikov kernel. To estimate the regression function at the point $x_0 = 0.8$, we use the local data in the strip $x_0 \pm h$ to fit a regression line (c.f. Fig. 9). The local linear estimate at x_0 is simply the intersection of the fitted line and the line $x = x_0$. Suppose that we wish to estimate the regression function at another point $x_0 = 0.88$, another line is fitted using the data in the window 0.88 ± 0.051. The whole curve is obtained by estimating the regression function in a grid of points. Indeed, the curve in Fig. 9 was obtained by 101 local linear regressions, taking the 101 grid points from 0.0535 to 1.232.

The *local linear regression smoother* is particularly simple to implement. Indeed, the estimator has the simple expression

$$\hat{m}_L(x) = \sum_{i=1}^{n} w_i(x) Y_i \,, \tag{14}$$

where with $S_{n,j}(x) = \sum_{i=1}^n K_h(X_i - x)(X_i - x)^j$,

$$w_i(x) = K_h(X_i - x)$$
$$\{S_{n,2}(x) - (X_i - x)S_{n,1}(x)\}/(S_{n,0}(x)S_{n,2}(x) - S_{n,1}^2(x))\,. \tag{15}$$

We can either use the explicit formula (15) or a regression package to compute it. It has several nice properties such as high statistical efficiency (in an asymptotic minimax sense), design adaption[24] and good boundary behavior.[28, 70] The asymptotic bias and variance for this estimator is

$$E\{\hat{m}_L(x)|X_1,\ldots,X_n\} - m(x) = \mu(K)\frac{m''(x)}{2}h^2 + o(h^2) \tag{16}$$

and

$$\operatorname{var}\{\hat{m}_L(x)|X_1,\ldots,X_n\} = R(K)\frac{\sigma^2(x)}{f(x)nh} + o\left(\frac{1}{nh}\right), \tag{17}$$

provided that the bandwidth h tends to zero in such a manner that $nh \to \infty$, where f is the marginal density of X, namely, *the design density.*[29] Table 1 lists the leading term in the asymptotic bias and variance. By comparing the leading terms in the asymptotic variance, clearly the local linear fit uses locally one extra parameter without increasing its variability. But this extra parameter creates opportunities for significant bias reduction, particularly at the boundary regions and slope regions. This is evidenced by comparing their asymptotic biases.

Local linear fitting requires a choice for the smoothing parameter h and for the kernel function K. It is well known that the choice of the kernel function is of less importance in kernel smoothing. This holds truely for local polynomial regression. It has been shown that the Epanechnikov kernel is optimal in some sense. See Gasser, Müller, and Mamitzsch,[42] Granovsky and Müller[45] and Chap. 3 of Fan and Gijbels.[28]

The bandwidth selection is critical to all nonparametric estimators. A too-large bandwidth creates excessive biases in nonparametric estimates and a too small bandwidth results in a large variance in nonparametric estimate. There are two basic choices of bandwidth: subjective and data-driven.

In subjective choices, data analysts use different bandwidths to estimate the regression function and choose the one that visually balances the bias and variance trade-off. Trials-and-errors are needed in this endeavor. Alternatively, one can present the nonparametric estimates using a few different bandwidths (c.f. Fig. 6 for a similar idea). The data-driven bandwidth is to let data themselves choose a bandwidth that balances the bias and variance, via minimizing certain estimated *Mean Integrated Square Errors* (MISE).

We now briefly discuss some data-driven choices of the bandwidth. By (16) and (17), the weighted MISE of the local linear estimator is

$$\frac{\mu(K)^2h^4}{4}\int\{m''(x)\}^2w(x)dx+\frac{R(K)}{nh}\int\frac{\sigma^2(x)}{f(x)}w(x)dx\,.$$

The asymptotic optimal bandwidth, that minimizes the asymptotic weighted MISE of $\hat{m}_L(x)$, is given by

$$h_{\text{opt}}=\left(\frac{R(K)\int\sigma^2(x)f^{-1}(x)w(x)dx}{\mu^2(K)\int\{m''(x)\}^2w(x)dx}\right)^{1/5}n^{-1/5}\,, \tag{18}$$

where $w(x)$ is a weight function.

The optimal bandwidth involves the unknown regression function and the unknown density function of X. Hence it cannot be applied directly. There are many references on the topic of bandwidth selection. See Chap. 4 of Fan and Gijbels[28] and references therein. Here, we focus on the cross-validation method, which is conceptually simple, but needs intensive computation. Let $\hat{m}_{h,(-i)}(x)$ be the local linear regression estimator (12) without using the ith-observation (X_i, Y_i). We now analogously validate the "goodness-of-fit" by measuring the "prediction error" $Y_i-\hat{m}_{h,(-i)}(X_i)$. The cross-validation criterion measures the overall "prediction errors", which is defined by

$$CV(h)=n^{-1}\sum_{i=1}^{n}\{Y_i-\hat{m}_{h,(-i)}(X_i)\}^2\,. \tag{19}$$

The cross-validation bandwidth selector $\hat{h}_{CV}$ chooses the one that minimizes $CV(h)$.

In what follows, we illustrate the methodology of local linear regression in details by an environmental data set. This data set consists of 612 observations of 15 variables and has been analyzed by Rawlings and Spruill.[69] See Sec. 2 of Rawlings and Spruill[69] for a detailed description. Here, we are interested in how *depth to mottling* (DMOT) of soil affects the increment of diameter growth of some kinds of pine. Thus we take the increment of diameter as a response variable Y and the DMOT of soil as an independent variable X. After excluding the data points with missing values, we have 216 observations. The scatter plot of the data is depicted in Fig. 10.

The cross-validation method was used to search a bandwidth over 20 grid points $0.15 * 1.1^j$ multiplying the range of X variable, $j = 0, \ldots, 19$. With the smallest bandwidth 0.15 multiplying the range of X, we used 15% of data around x_0 to estimate $m(x_0)$, while with the largest bandwidth 0.15×1.1^{19} multiple the range of X, we used about 92% of data around x_0 to estimate $m(x_0)$. Here the Epanechnikov kernel was used. The plot of cross-validation scores against candidate bandwidths is depicted in Fig. 10(a). The corresponding $\hat{h}_{CV}$ is 12.776.

With the selected bandwidth, we are able to estimate the regression function. In nonparametric regression, one usually plots the curve of the estimated regression function. Thus one has to evaluate the regression function over a grid of points. Usually we take the grid of points evenly distributing over the range of X. A natural question arises here is how many grid points at which the estimate needed to be evaluated. Figure 10(c)–(e) depicts the resulting estimated curve with the number of grid points (Ngrid) being 100, 200 and 400, respectively. The plots shows nonlinear between the increment and the DMOT. From these plots, the estimated curves are almost the same, since the underline estimate is relatively smooth. In practice, we recommend using 100 or 200 grid points to evaluate estimated regression functions.

Now we take the natural logarithm of DMOT as the X-variable, and then use the cross-validation method to choose a bandwidth. The CV scores are depicted in Fig. 10(b). This yields $\hat{h}_{CV} = 1.3271$. The estimated curve is depicted in Fig. 10(h). Figure 10(h) shows that increment of diameter growth versus log(DMOT) is nearly linear. For such an implementation, it spent about 2 seconds (using MATLAB on PC Pentium II 450 MHz) to compute the estimated function over 200 grid points, including bandwidth selection using the cross-validation method.

Direct implementation of local polynomial regression for a large data set needs a considerable amount of computation. Fast computation algorithms have been proposed in Fan and Marron.[33] Many computer codes are available through internet. For example, S-plus codes can be downloaded from Matt Wand's homepage at

http://www.biostat.harvard.edu/ mwand/software.html,

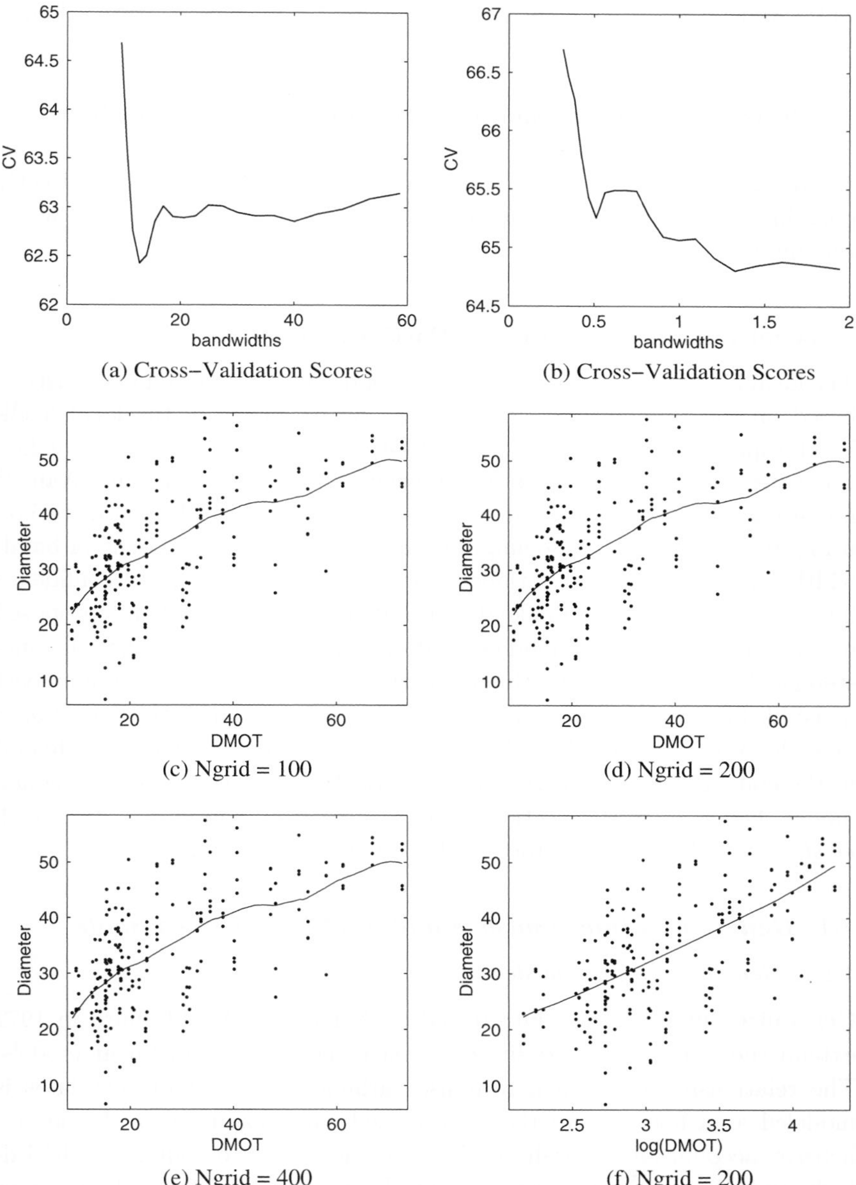

Fig. 10. Estimated regression functions. (a) and (b) are plots of cross-validation scores for increment of diameter versus depth of mottling (DMOT) and for versus log(DMOT), respectively. (c)–(e) are estimated regression function curves $E(\text{increment}|\text{DMOT})$ with scatter plot of data, corresponding to the number of grid points 100, 200 and 400, respectively. (h) is the estimated regression curve $E(\text{increment}|\log(\text{DMOT}))$.

while Matlab codes can be downloaded from James S. Marron's homepage at

http://www.stat.unc.edu/faculty/marron/marron_software.html

or through the authors. These codes can be easily implemented by directly plugging-in data. There is also a procedure of kernel smoothing in the latest version of SAS.

4. Local Likelihood and Local Partial Likelihood

The local likelihood approach was first proposed by Tibshirani and Hastie[82] based on the running line smoother. As an extension of the local likelihood approach, local quasi-likelihood estimation using local constant fits, was considered by Severini and Staniwalis.[74] Fan, Heckman and Wand[31] investigated the asymptotic properties of the local quasi-likelihood method using local polynomial modeling. Fan *et al.*[27] addressed the issue of bandwidth selection, bias and variance assessment and constructed confidence intervals in local maximum likelihood estimation. Fan and Chen[26] proposed one-step local quasi-likelihood estimation, and demonstrated that the one-step local quasi-likelihood estimator performs as well as the maximum local quasi-likelihood estimator using the ideal optimal bandwidth. Fan *et al.*[30] extended the idea of the local likelihood approach to local partial likelihood in the context of censored survival data analysis, such as Cox's regression model. The ideas in this section are motivated from Fan *et al.*[30, 31] Carroll *et al.*[11] extend the idea further to the likelihood equations.

4.1. *Generalized linear models and local likelihool estimate*

4.1.1. *Generalized linear models*

Generalized linear models introduced by Nelder and Wedderburn in 1972 extend the scope of the traditional least squares fitting of linear models. The relationship between a response variable and a set of covariates is modeled as a linear fit to the transformed conditional mean. A comprehensive account of generalized linear models can be found in McMullagh and Nelder.[65] Suppose that we have n independent observations $(\mathbf{X}_1, Y_1), \ldots, (\mathbf{X}_n, Y_n)$ of random vector $(\mathbf{X}, Y)$, where $\mathbf{X}$ is a d-dimensional real vector of covariates, and Y is a scalar response variable. The conditional density of Y given covariate $\mathbf{X} = \mathbf{x}$ belongs to the canonical exponential family:

$$f_{Y|\mathbf{X}}(y|\mathbf{x}) = \exp\{[\theta(\mathbf{x})y - b\{\theta(\mathbf{x})\}]/a(\phi) + c(y,\phi)\} \tag{20}$$

for known functions $a(\cdot)$, $b(\cdot)$ and $c(\cdot,\cdot)$. In parametric generalized linear models it is usual to model a transformation of the regression function $m(\mathbf{x}) = E(Y|\mathbf{X} = \mathbf{x})$ as linear, that is

$$\eta(\mathbf{x}) = g\{m(\mathbf{x})\} = \mathbf{x}^T\boldsymbol{\beta}\,,$$

and g is a known *link* function. If $g = (b')^{-1}$, then g is called the canonical link because it transform the regression function into the canonical parameter: $(b')^{-1}\{m(\mathbf{x})\} = \theta(\mathbf{x})$.

Here are a few examples that illustrate the model (20). The first example is that the conditional distribution of Y given $\mathbf{X} = \mathbf{x}$ has a normal distribution with mean $m(\mathbf{x})$ and variance σ^2. The normal density can be rewritten as

$$f_{Y|\mathbf{X}} = \exp\left\{\frac{m(\mathbf{x})y - m^2(\mathbf{x})/2}{\sigma^2} - \frac{y^2}{2\sigma^2} - \log(\sqrt{2\pi\sigma^2})\right\}.$$

It can be easily seen that

$$\phi = \sigma^2,\ a(\phi) = \phi,\ b(m) = m^2/2$$

and

$$c(y,\phi) = -y^2/(2\phi) - \log(\sqrt{2\pi\phi})\,.$$

The canonical link function is the identity link $g(t) = t$. This model is useful for a continuous response with homoscedastic errors.

Suppose that the conditional distributions of Y given $\mathbf{X} = \mathbf{x}$ is a Bernoulli distribution with the probability of success $p(\mathbf{x})$, in which case it can be seen that

$$f_{Y|\mathbf{X}}(y|\mathbf{x}) = \exp\left(y\log[p(\mathbf{x})/\{1 - p(\mathbf{x})\}] + \log\{1 - p(\mathbf{x})\}\right).$$

The canonical parameter in this example is $\theta(\mathbf{x}) = \text{logit}\{p(\mathbf{x})\}$, and the logit function is the canonical link.

Under model (20), it can be easily shown that the conditional mean and conditional variance are given respectively by $m(\mathbf{x}) = E(Y|\mathbf{X} = \mathbf{x}) = b'\{\theta(\mathbf{x})\}$, and $\text{var}(Y|\mathbf{X} = \mathbf{x}) = a(\phi)b''\{\theta(\mathbf{x})\}$. Hence,

$$\theta(\mathbf{x}) = (b')^{-1}\{m(\mathbf{x})\}\,.$$

Using the definition of $\eta(\cdot)$, we have

$$\theta(\mathbf{x}) = (b')^{-1}\{g^{-1}[\eta(\mathbf{x})]\}\,. \tag{21}$$

Since our primary interest is to estimate the mean function, without loss of generality, the factors related to the dispersion parameter ϕ are omitted.

This leads to the following conditional log-likelihood function

$$\ell\{\theta, y\} = \theta(\mathbf{x})y - b\{\theta(\mathbf{x})\}\,.$$

By (21), the above log-likelihood can be expressed as

$$\ell\{\theta, y\} = \left[y(b')^{-1} \circ g^{-1}(\eta(\mathbf{x})) - b\{(b')^{-1} \circ g^{-1}(\eta(\mathbf{x}))\}\right], \tag{22}$$

where $\circ$ denotes composition. In particular, when g is the canonical link,

$$\ell\{\theta, y\} = \eta(\mathbf{x})y - b\{\eta(\mathbf{x})\}\,.$$

4.1.2. *Local likelihood estimate*

It has been of interest to adapt these models to situations where the functional form for the dependence of $g(m(\mathbf{x}))$ on $\mathbf{x}$ is unknown. In what follows, the covariate $\mathbf{X}$ is assumed to be a scalar random variable. If $\eta(x)$ is a smooth function of x, then for X_i close enough to a given point x_0,

$$\eta(X_i) \approx \sum_{j=0}^{p} \beta_j (X_i - x_0)^j \equiv \mathbf{X}_i^T \boldsymbol{\beta}\,, \tag{23}$$

where $\mathbf{X}_i = (1, (X_i - x_0), \ldots, (X_i - x_0)^p)^T$ and $\boldsymbol{\beta} = (\beta_0, \beta_1, \ldots, \beta_p)^T$. Intuitively data points close to x_0 have more information about $\eta(x_0)$ than those away from x_0. Therefore, by (22), the local log-likelihood function based on the random sample $\{(X_i, Y_i)\}_{i=1}^n$ is

$$\ell(\boldsymbol{\beta}) = \sum_{i=1}^{n} [Y_i (b')^{-1} \circ g^{-1}(\mathbf{X}_i^T \boldsymbol{\beta}) - b\{(b')^{-1} \circ g^{-1}(\mathbf{X}_i \boldsymbol{\beta})\}] K_h(X_i - x_0)\,. \tag{24}$$

Define the local maximum likelihood estimator of $\boldsymbol{\beta}$ to be

$$\hat{\boldsymbol{\beta}} = \arg\max\nolimits_{\boldsymbol{\beta} \in R^{p+1}} \ell(\boldsymbol{\beta})\,.$$

Thus $\eta(x_0)$ and the νth derivative of $\eta(x_0)$ can be estimated by

$$\hat{\eta}(x_0) = \hat{\beta} \quad \text{and} \quad \hat{\eta}^{(\nu)} = \nu! \hat{\beta}_\nu$$

respectively, assuming that η has p derivatives. When the canonical like $g = (b')^{-1}$ is used, (24) becomes

$$\ell(\boldsymbol{\beta}) = \sum_{i=1}^{n} [Y_i (\mathbf{X}_i^T \boldsymbol{\beta}) - b(\mathbf{X}_i \boldsymbol{\beta})] K_h(X_i - x_0)\,.$$

The log-likelihood function (24) is really a weighted log-likelihood and hence can be computed by using the existing software. In fact, suppose that

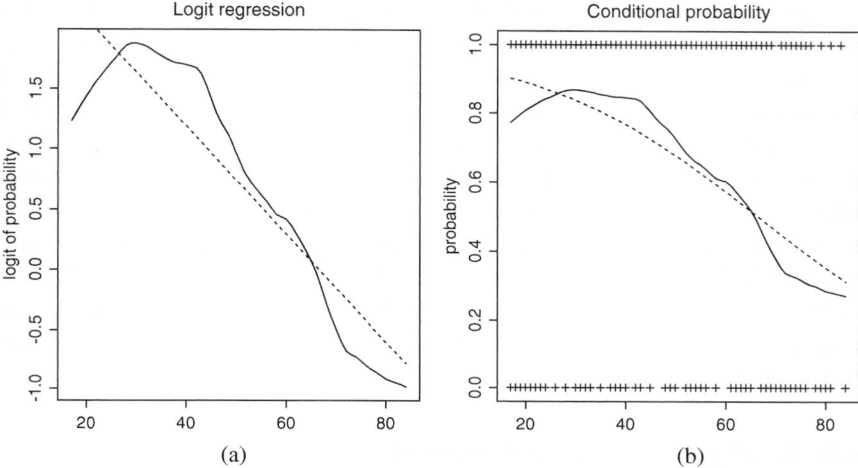

Fig. 11. Illustration of local likelihood approach for the burn data. (a) Estimated logit transform of the conditional probability. (b) Estimated conditional probability. Solid curve — local modeling with about 40% of the data points in each local neighborhood; dashed curve — global parametric logit linear model. Taken from Fan and Gijbels.[29]

we want to estimate $\hat{\eta}(\cdot)$ in a given interval. Take a grid of points (200, say) in that interval. For each given grid point x_0, model (24) can be maximized by using existing software packages such as SAS and Splus that contains the parametric Glim function. The whole estimated function is obtained by plotting the estimates obtained at grid points.

The choice of the link function g is not as crucial as for parametric generalized linear models, because the fitting is localized. Indeed it is conceivable to dispense with the link function and just estimate $m(x)$ directly. But there are several drawbacks to having the link equal to the identity. An identity link may yield a local likelihood that is not convex, allowing for the possibility of multiple maxima, inconsistency and computational problems. Use of the canonical link guarantees convexity. Furthermore the canonical link ensures that the final estimate has the correct range. For example, in the logistic regression context using the logit link leads to an estimate that is always a probability whereas using the identity link does not have. A final reason for preferring the canonical link is that the estimate of $m(x)$ approaches the usual parametric estimate as the bandwidth becomes large. This can be useful as a diagnostic tool.[31]

We now illustrate the local likelihood approach via analyzing the data set: *Burns data*, collected by General Hospital Burn Center at the University of South California. It is of interest to estimate the probability of surviving given the age of victims. Local likelihood estimate was computed over a grid of points with bandwidth 0.4 multiplying the range of X, and the estimated curves are depicted in Fig. 11. Note that the conditional probability function must be monotonic for the parametric linear model, whereas for the local linear model, the conditional probability function can be any curve. The former model can overstate the probability of survival for the younger group and for the senior group. The solid curves in Fig. 11 suggest that the conditional probability function is unimodal, which is reasonable in the current context.

4.2. *Local partial likelihood estimate*

In this section, we apply the local likelihood techniques to survival data analysis. Let T, C and X be respectively the survival time, the censoring time and their associated covariates. Correspondingly, let $Z = \min\{T, C\}$ be the observed time and $\delta = I(T \le C)$ be the censoring indicator. It is assumed that T and C are conditionally independent given X and that the censoring mechanism is noninformative. Suppose that $\{(X_i, Z_i, \delta_i) : i = 1, \ldots, n\}$ are an i.i.d. sample from the population (X, Z, δ). For a thorough introduction to survival analysis, see books by Fleming and Harrington[40] and Andersen *et al.*[2]

Let $h(t|x)$ be the conditional hazard rate function. The proportional hazards model assumes that

$$h(t|x) = h_0(t)\exp\{\theta(x)\}\,. \tag{25}$$

This model indicates that the covariate x inflates or deflates the hazard risk by a factor of $\exp\{\theta(x)\}$. The function $\theta(x)$ is called a hazard regression function, and characterizes the risk contribution of the covariate at value x. See Cox[19] for proportional hazard models with time-dependent covariates.

In the parametric model, a linear form $\theta(x) = \beta x$ is imposed on the hazard regression function. The local modeling methodology aims at removing this restriction and exploring possible nonlinearity, and is applicable to any smooth hazard regression function. For simplicity of discussion, we focus on the univariate cases. For multivariate settings, a dimensionality reduction technique such as additive models should be used.[52]

A commonly-used technique for estimating the hazard regression function is the *partial likelihood* technique introduced by Cox.[20] Let $t_1^o <$

$\cdots < t_N^o$ denote the ordered observed failure times. Let (j) provide the label for the item failing at t_j^o so that the covariates associated with the N failures are $X_{(1)}, \ldots, X_{(N)}$. Denote by $R_j = \{i : Z_i \geq t_j^o\}$, the risk set at time instantaneously before t_j^o. Then, the log-partial likelihood in our context is given by

$$\sum_{j=1}^{N} \left[\theta(X_{(j)}) - \log \left(\sum_{k \in R_j} \exp\{\theta(X_k)\} \right) \right]. \tag{26}$$

See Cox,[20] Fleming and Harriton[40] and Fan and Gijbels.[28] Substituting the parametric form of $\theta(\cdot)$ into (26) yields a maximum partial likelihood estimate of the hazard regression function.

We now apply the local modeling technique to estimate the hazard regression function $\theta(\cdot)$. For a given x_0, approximate $\theta(x)$ by

$$\theta(x) \approx \beta_0 + \cdots + \beta_p (x - x_0)^p \,, \tag{27}$$

for x in a neighborhood of x_0. Let

$$\beta = (\beta_1, \ldots, \beta_p)^T \quad \text{and} \quad \mathbf{X}_j = \{(X_j - x_0), \ldots, (X_j - x_0)^p\}^T \,.$$

Then the *local partial likelihood* is

$$\sum_{j=1}^{N} K_h(X_{(j)} - x_0) \left[\mathbf{X}_{(j)}^T \beta - \log \left\{ \sum_{k \in R_j} \exp(\mathbf{X}_k^T \beta) K_h(X_k - x_0) \right\} \right]. \tag{28}$$

See Fan *et al.*[30] for a derivation of the local partial likelihood (28). When the kernel function is uniform and the bandwidth is of the nearest neighbor type, the local likelihood (28) was introduced by Tibshirani and Hastie.[82] For a related approach based on the local likelihood, see Gentleman and Crowley.[43]

The function value $\theta(x_0)$ is not directly estimable since (28) does not depend on the intercept β_0. However, the derivative functions are directly estimable. Let $\hat{\beta}(x_0)$ be the maximum local log-partial likelihood estimate that maximizes (28). An estimate $\hat{\theta}_\nu(x_0)$ of $\theta^{(\nu)}(x_0)$ is given by $\nu! \hat{\beta}_\nu(x_0)$.

We impose the condition $\theta(0) = 0$ for identifiability. With this extra constraint, the function $\theta(x)$ can be estimated by

$$\hat{\theta}(x) = \int_0^x \hat{\theta}'(t) dt \,, \tag{29}$$

where $\hat{\theta}'(t) = \hat{\theta}_1(t)$ is the derivative estimator. In practice, the function $\hat{\theta}_1(x)$ is often evaluated at either grid points or the design points. Assume that $\hat{\theta}_1(x_j) = \hat{\beta}_1(x_j)$ are computed at points $\{x_0, \ldots, x_m\}$. Then, $\hat{\theta}(x_i)$ can be approximated by the trapezoidal rule

$$\hat{\theta}(x_i) = \sum_{j=1}^{i}(x_j - x_{j-1})(\hat{\beta}_{1,j} + \hat{\beta}_{1,j-1})/2\,,$$

where $\hat{\beta}_{1,j} = \hat{\beta}_1(x_j)$. The coefficients can simply be computed by using existing software packages for parametric Cox's proportional hazards model.

We conclude this section with an analysis of the Primary Biliary Cirrhosis (PBC) data set, which can be found in Fleming and Harrington.[40] PBC is a rare but fatal chronic liver disease of unknown cause. The analysis is here based on the data collected at Mayo Clinic between January 1974 and May 1984. Of 312 patients who participated in the randomized trial, 187 cases were censored. In our analysis, we take the time (in days) between registration and death, or liver transplantation or the time of the study analysis (July 1986) as response and the ages of the patients as a covariate. The observed data are presented in Fig. 12(a). The local partial likelihood method (28) with $p = 2$ was employed for three different bandwidths $h = 10$, 20 and 30. The estimated hazard regression function and its derivative function are respectively given in Figs. 12(b) and (c). Note that since the hazard regression function is only identifiable within a constant, the curves in Fig. 12(c) are normalized to have the same average height so that they can be better compared. Figure 12(c) reveals the fact that it is reasonable to model linearly the hazard regression function of covariate age.

5. Nonparametric Goodness of Fit Tests

Nonparametric goodness of fit test has received increasing attention recently. A motivating and simple example is to consider a simple nonparametric regression model. Suppose that $(X_1, Y_1), \ldots, (X_n, Y_n)$ are a random sample from the nonparametric regression model

$$Y_i = m(X_i) + \varepsilon_i$$

with $E(\varepsilon_i|X_i) = 0$ and $\text{var}(\varepsilon_i|X_i) = \sigma^2$. Of interest is to test the hypothesis

$$H_0 : m(x) = \alpha_0 + \alpha_1 x_1 + \cdots + \alpha_p x^p \text{ versus } H_1 : m(x) \neq \alpha_0 + \alpha_1 x_1 + \cdots + \alpha_p x^p\,.$$

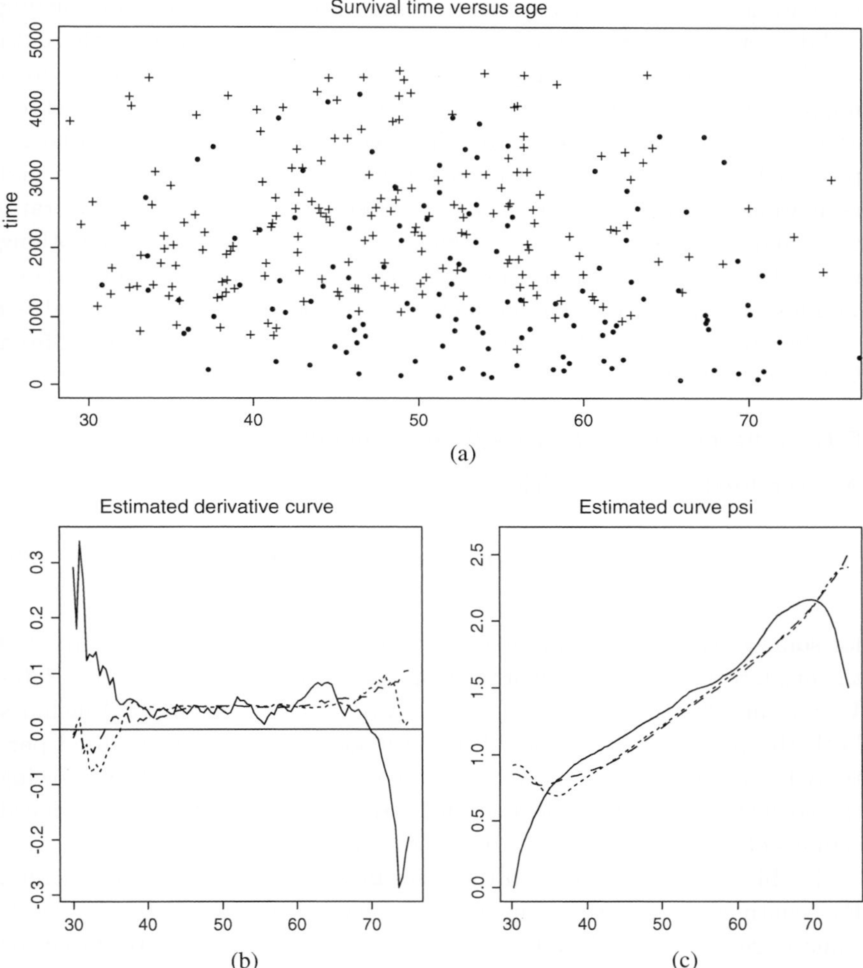

Fig. 12. Local partial likelihood estimation of the hazard regression function. (a) Observed time versus age with "+" indicating censored observations. (b) Estimated derivative function $\theta'(\cdot)$. (c) Estimated hazard regression function $\theta(\cdot)$; solid curve — bandwidth = 10; short-dashed curve — bandwidth = 20; long-dashed curve — bandwidth = 30. From Fan and Gijbels.[29]

This testing problem is well known as test of linearity in the context of model diagnostic where the question arises whether a family of parametric models fit adequately the data. It is natural to use the nonparametric model as an alternative hypothesis. On the other hand, it is known that nonparametric regression may yield a complicated model. Thus, after fitting a data set by a nonparametric model, we may check whether the data can be fitted by a less complicated parametric model. This leads to a nonparametric goodness of fit test. Hart[51] gives a comprehensive study and presents many examples on this topic. Fan[25] and Fan and Huang[32] proposed some goodness of fit tests for various parametric models and nonparametric models. Fan *et al.*[37] proposed generalized likelihood ratio tests and established a general framework for nonparametric smoothing tests. Many related literature, are available[1, 3, 4, 21, 22, 50, 55, 58] In this section, we illustrate the idea of nonparametric likelihood ratio test by generalized varying coefficient models. Some material of this section was extracted from Cai *et al.*,[8] referred as CFL.

5.1. *Generalized varying coefficient models*

A generalized varying-coefficient model has the form

$$\eta(\mathbf{u}, \mathbf{x}) = g\{m(\mathbf{u}, \mathbf{x})\} = \sum_{j=1}^{p} a_j(\mathbf{u}) x_j \tag{30}$$

for some given link function $g(\cdot)$, where $\mathbf{x} = (x_1, \ldots, x_p)^T$, and $m(\mathbf{u}, \mathbf{x})$ is the mean regression function of the response variable Y given the covariates $\mathbf{U} = \mathbf{u}$ and $\mathbf{X} = \mathbf{x}$ with $\mathbf{X} = (X_1, \ldots, X_p)^T$. Clearly, model (30) includes both the parametric generalized linear model[65] and the generalized partially linear model.[9, 14, 46, 77] An advantage of model (30) is that by allowing the coefficients $\{a_j(\cdot)\}$ to depend on $\mathbf{U}$, the modeling bias can be reduced significantly and the "curse of dimensionality" is avoided.

In this section, we focus on the cases in which the response is discrete. For continuous responses, many works have been done. In the least-squares setting, model (30) with the identity link was introduced by Cleveland *et al.*[18] and extended by Hastie and Tibshirani[53] to various aspects. Varying-coefficient models are a simple and useful extension of classical generalized linear models. They are particularly appealing in longitudinal studies where they allow one to explore the extent to which covariates affect responses changing over time. See Hoover *et al.*,[54] Brumback and Rice[7] and Fan and Zhang[38] for details on novel applications of the varying-coefficient models to longitudinal data. For nonlinear time series applications, see Chen and Tsay[15] and Cai *et al.*[9] for statistical inferences based on the functional-coefficient autoregressive models. Kauermann and Tutz[59] used varying coefficient models for model disgnostics.

5.2. *Estimation procedures*

For simplicity, we consider the important case that $\mathbf{u}$ is one-dimensional. Extension to multivariate $\mathbf{u}$ involves no fundamentally new ideas. However, implementations with $\mathbf{u}$ having more than two dimensions may have some difficulties due to the "curse of dimensionality".

In this section, it is assumed that the conditional log-likelihood function $\ell(v, y)$ is known and linear in y for fixed v. This assumption is satisfied for the canonical exponential family, which is the focus of this section. The methods, introduced in this section, are directly applicable to situations in which one cannot specify fully the conditional log-likelihood function $\ell(v, y)$, but can model the relationship between the mean and variance by $\text{var}(Y|\mathbf{U} = \mathbf{u}, \mathbf{X} = \mathbf{x}) = \sigma^2 V\{m(\mathbf{u}, \mathbf{x})\}$ for a known variance function $V(\cdot)$ and unknown σ. In this case, one needs only to replace the log-likelihood function $\ell(v, y)$ by the quasi-likelihood function $Q(\cdot, \cdot)$, defined by $\frac{\partial}{\partial \mu} Q(\mu, y) = \frac{y-\mu}{V(\mu)}$.

5.2.1. *Local MLE*

Local linear modeling will be used here, though general local polynomial methods are also applicable. Suppose that $a_j(\cdot)$ has a continuous second derivative. For each given point u_0, $a_j(u)$ can be approximated locally by a linear function $a_j(u) \approx a_j + b_j(u - u_0)$ for u in a neighborhood of u_0. Based on a random sample $\{(U_i, \mathbf{X}_i, Y_i)\}_{i=1}^n$, one may use the following local likelihood method to estimate the coefficient functions

$$\ell_n(\mathbf{a}, \mathbf{b}) = \frac{1}{n} \sum_{i=1}^{n} \ell \left[g^{-1} \left\{ \sum_{j=1}^{p} (a_j + b_j(U_i - u_0)) X_{ij} \right\}, Y_i \right] K_h(U_i - u_0), \tag{31}$$

where $\mathbf{a} = (a_1, \ldots, a_p)^T$ and $\mathbf{b} = (b_1, \ldots, b_p)^T$. Note that a_j and b_j depend on u_0, and so does $\ell_n(\cdot, \cdot)$. Maximizing the local likelihood function $\ell_n(\mathbf{a}, \mathbf{b})$ results in estimates $\hat{\mathbf{a}}(u_0)$ and $\hat{\mathbf{b}}(u_0)$. The components in $\hat{\mathbf{a}}(u_0)$ provide an estimate of $a_1(u_0), \ldots, a_p(u_0)$. For simplicity of notation, let $\boldsymbol{\beta} = \boldsymbol{\beta}(u_0) = (a_1, \ldots, a_p, b_1, \ldots, b_p)^T$, and write the local likelihood function (31) as $\ell_n(\boldsymbol{\beta})$. Likewise, the local MLE is denoted by $\hat{\boldsymbol{\beta}}_{\text{MLE}} = \hat{\boldsymbol{\beta}}_{\text{MLE}}(u_0)$. The sampling properties have been established in CFL.

5.2.2. *One-step local MLE*

Computation for the above local MLE is expensive. We have to maximize the local likelihood (31) for usually hundreds of distinct values of u_0, with each maximization requiring an iterative algorithm, in order to obtain the estimated functions $\{\hat{a}_j(\cdot)\}$. To alleviate this expense, we replace an iterative local MLE by the one-step estimator, which has been frequently used in parametric models.[5,61] The one-step local MLE does not lose any statistical efficiency provided that the initial estimator is good enough. See CFL for theoretic insights.

Let $\ell_n'(\boldsymbol{\beta})$ and $\ell_n''(\boldsymbol{\beta})$ be the gradient and Hessian matrix of the local log-likelihood $\ell_n(\boldsymbol{\beta})$. Given an initial estimator $\hat{\boldsymbol{\beta}}_0 = \hat{\boldsymbol{\beta}}_0(u_0) = (\hat{\mathbf{a}}(u_0)^T, \hat{\mathbf{b}}(u_0)^T)^T$, one-step of the Newton-Raphson algorithm updates its solution by

$$\hat{\boldsymbol{\beta}}_{\mathrm{OS}} = \hat{\boldsymbol{\beta}}_0 - \{\ell_n''(\hat{\boldsymbol{\beta}}_0)\}^{-1}\ell_n'(\hat{\boldsymbol{\beta}}_0)\,, \tag{32}$$

thus featuring the computational expediency of least-squares local polynomial fitting. Furthermore, the sandwich formula can be used as an estimate for standard errors of the resulting estimate

$$\widehat{\mathrm{cov}}(\hat{\boldsymbol{\beta}}_{\mathrm{OS}}) = \{\ell_n''(\hat{\boldsymbol{\beta}}_0)\}^{-1}\widehat{\mathrm{cov}}\{\ell_n'(\hat{\boldsymbol{\beta}}_0)\}\{\ell_n''(\hat{\boldsymbol{\beta}}_0)\}^{-1}\,.$$

This formula has been tested in CFL to be accuracy enough for most of practical purpose.

In univariate generalized linear models, Fan and Chen[26] carefully studied properties of the local one-step estimator. In that setting, the least-squares estimate serves a natural candidate as an initial estimator. However, in the multivariate setting, it is not clear how an initial estimator can be constructed. The following is proposed in CFL. Suppose that we wish to evaluate the functions $\hat{\mathbf{a}}(\cdot)$ at grid points $u_j, j = 1, \ldots, n_{\mathrm{grid}}$. Our idea of finding initial estimators is as follows. Take a point u_{i_0}, usually the center of the grid points. Compute the local MLE $\hat{\boldsymbol{\beta}}_{\mathrm{MLE}}(u_{i_0})$. Use this estimate as the initial estimate for the point u_{i_0+1} and apply (32) to obtain $\hat{\boldsymbol{\beta}}_{\mathrm{OS}}(u_{i_0+1})$. Now, use $\hat{\boldsymbol{\beta}}_{\mathrm{OS}}(u_{i_0+1})$ as the initial estimate at the point u_{i_0+2} and apply (32) to obtain $\hat{\boldsymbol{\beta}}_{\mathrm{OS}}(u_{i_0+2})$ and so on. Likewise, we can compute $\hat{\boldsymbol{\beta}}_{\mathrm{OS}}(u_{i_0-1})$, $\hat{\boldsymbol{\beta}}_{\mathrm{OS}}(u_{i_0-2})$, etc. In this way, we obtain our estimates at all grid points.

A refine alternative of the above proposal is to calculate a fresh local MLE as a new initial value after iterating along the grid points for a while. For example, if we wish to evaluate the functions at 200 grid points and are willing to compute the local maximum likelihood at five distinct points. A sensible placement of these points is $u_{20}, u_{60}, u_{100}, u_{140}$ and u_{180}. Use for example $\hat{\boldsymbol{\beta}}_{\mathrm{MLE}}(u_{60})$ along with the idea in the last paragraph to compute $\hat{\boldsymbol{\beta}}_{\mathrm{OS}}(u_i)$ for $i = 40, \ldots, 79$, and use $\hat{\boldsymbol{\beta}}_{\mathrm{MLE}}(u_{100})$ to compute $\hat{\boldsymbol{\beta}}_{\mathrm{OS}}(u_i)$ for $i = 80, \ldots, 119$, and so on.

Note that $\ell_n''(\hat{\boldsymbol{\beta}}_0)$ can be nearly singular for certain u_0, due to possible data sparsity in certain local regions. Seifert and Gasser[73] and Fan and Chen[26] explored the use of the ridge regression as an approach to handling such problems in the univariate setting. See CFL[8] for details.

5.3. *Hypothesis testing*

When fitting a varying-coefficient model, it is natural to ask whether the coefficient functions are actually varying or whether any particular covariate is significant in the model. For simplicity of description, we only consider the first hypothesis testing problem

$$H_0 : a_1(u) \equiv a_1, \ldots, a_p(u) \equiv a_p\,, \tag{33}$$

though the technique also applies to other testing problems. A useful procedure is based on the nonparametric likelihood ratio test statistic

$$T = 2\{\ell(H_1) - \ell(H_0)\}\,, \tag{34}$$

where $\ell(H_0)$ and $\ell(H_1)$ are respectively the log-likelihood functions computed under the null and alternative hypotheses. Note that the normalization constant in (34) does not change the testing procedure. However, in order for it to possess a χ^2 distribution, it needs to be normalized as in Ref. 37

$$T_K = r_K\{\ell(H_1) - \ell(H_0)\}\,, \tag{35}$$

where

$$r_K = \frac{K(0) - \frac{1}{2}\int K^2(t)dt}{\int (K(t) - \frac{1}{2}K * K(t))^2 dt}\,.$$

Table 2 gives the value of r_K for a few commonly used kernels.

For parametric models, it is well known that the likelihood ratio statistic follows asymptotically a χ^2-distribution. The asymptotic null distribution is independent of nuisance parameters under the null hypothesis. This is the Wilks type of phenomenon. Fan *et al.*[37] has shown the Wilks phenomenon still holds for the nonparametric likelihood ratio tests. Furthermore, they

Table 2. Normalization constant r_K.

Kernel	Uniform	Epanechnikov	Biweight	Triweight	Gaussian
r_K	1.2000	2.1153	2.3061	2.3797	2.5375

showed that the null distribution of the nonparametric likelihood ratio test is a χ^2-distribution in some sense and does not depend on the values of $a_1, \ldots, a_p$. Thus one may use the following *conditional bootstrap* to construct the null distribution of T_K and hence the P-value. Let $\{\hat{a}_j\}$ be the MLE under the null hypothesis. Given the covariates $(U_i, \mathbf{X}_i)$, generate a bootstrap sample Y_i^* from the given distribution of Y with the estimated linear predictor $\hat{\eta}(U_i, \mathbf{X}_i) = \sum_{j=1}^p \hat{a}_j X_{ij}$ and compute the test statistic T_K^* in (34). Use the distribution of T_K^* as an approximation to the distribution of T_K.

Note that the above conditional bootstrap method applies readily to setting without presence of dispersion parameter, such as the Poisson and Bernoulli distributions. It is really a simulation approximation to the conditional distribution of T_K given observed covariates under the particular null hypothesis: $H_0 : a_j(u) = \hat{a}_j$ $(j = 1, \ldots, p)$. As pointed out above, this approximation is valid under both H_0 and H_1 as the null distribution does not asymptotically depend on the values of $\{a_j\}$. In the case where model (30) involves a dispersion parameter (e.g. the Gaussian model), the dispersion parameter should be estimated based on the residuals from the *alternative* hypothesis.

It is also of interest to investigate whether some covariates are significant. For example, we want to check whether the covariate X_p can be excluded from the model. This is equivalent to testing the hypothesis $H_0 : a_p(\cdot) = 0$, the above conditional bootstrap idea can be employed to obtain the null distribution of T_K under the model (30) and the generalized likelihood ratio statistics continue to apply. In this case, the data should be generated from the mean function $g\{m(\mathbf{u}, \mathbf{x})\} = \sum_{j=1}^{p-1} \hat{a}_j(\mathbf{u}) x_j$, where $\hat{a}_j(\cdot)$ is an estimate under the alternative hypothesis.

5.4. *An application*

We conclude this section via illustrating the proposed methodology to analyze the *Burn Data* set. The binary response variable Y is 1 for those victims who survived their burns and 0 otherwise, and covariates $X_1 = age$, $X_2 = sex$, $X_3 = \log(\text{burn area} + 1)$ and binary variable $X_4 = Oxygen$ (0 if oxygen supply is normal, 1 otherwise) are considered. Of interest is to study how burn areas and the other variables affect the survival probabilities for victims at different age groups. This naturally leads to the following varying-coefficient model

$$\operatorname{logit}\{p(x_1, x_2, x_3, x_4)\} = a_1(x_1) + a_2(x_1)x_2 + a_3(x_1)x_3 + a_4(x_1)x_4. \tag{36}$$

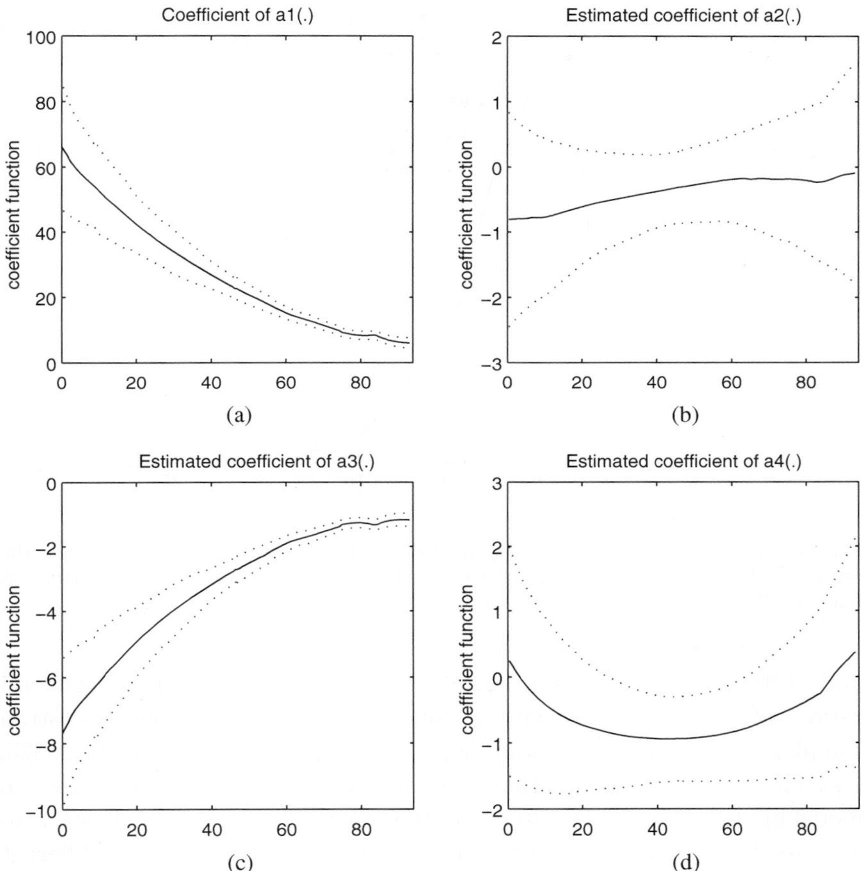

Fig. 13. The estimated coefficient functions (the solid curves) via the one-step approach with bandwidth chosen by the CV. The dot curves are the estimated functions plus/minus twice estimated standard errors. Adapted from Cai, Fan and Li.[8]

Figure 13 presents the estimated coefficients for model (36) via the one-step approach with bandwidth $h = 65.7882$, selected by a cross-validation method. See CFL[8] for details.

A natural question arises whether the coefficients in (36) are actually varying. To see this, we consider the parametric logistic regression model

$$\text{logit}\{p(x_1, x_2, x_3, x_4)\} = \beta_0 + \beta_1 x_1 + \beta_2 x_2 + \beta_3 x_3 + \beta_4 x_4 \qquad (37)$$

as the null model. As a result, the MLE of $(\beta_0, \ldots, \beta_4)$ in model (37) and its standard deviation are $(23.2213, -6.1485, -0.4661, -2.4496, -0.9683)$

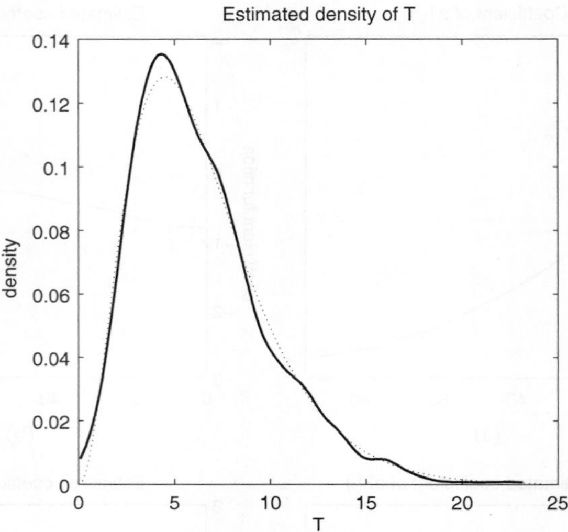

Fig. 14. The estimated density of T_K by Monte Carlo simulation. The solid curve is the estimated density, and the dashed curve stands for the density of chi-squared distribution (gamma distribution) with 6.5 degrees of freedom.

and (1.9180, 0.6647, 0.2825, 0.2206, 0.2900), respectively. The likelihood ratio test T_K is 58.1284 with p-value 0.000, based on 1000 bootstrap samples (the sample mean and variance of T_K^* are 6.3201 and 11.98023, respectively). This implies that the varying-coefficient logistic regression model fits the data much better than the parametric fit. It also allows us to examine the extent to which the regression coefficients vary over different ages. The estimated density of T_K^* is depicted in Fig. 14, from which we can seen that the null distribution is well approximated by a χ^2 distribution with 6.5 degrees of freedom (a gamma distribution).

To examine whether there is any gender gap for different age groups or if the variable X_4 affects the survival probabilities for different age of burn victims, we consider testing the null hypothesis H_0 : both $a_2(\cdot)$ and $a_4(\cdot)$ are constant under model (36). The corresponding test statistic T_K is 3.4567 with p-value 0.7050 based on 1000 bootstrap samples. This in turn suggests that the coefficient functions $a_2(\cdot)$ and $a_4(\cdot)$ are independent of age and indicates that there are no gender differences for different age groups.

Finally, we examine whether both covariates *sex* and *oxygen* are statistically significant in model (36). The likelihood ratio test for this problem is $T_K = 11.9256$ with p-value 0.0860, based on 1000 bootstrap samples (the sample mean and variance of T_K^* are 5.5915 and 10.9211, respectively). Both covariates *sex* and *oxygen* are not significant at level 0.05. This suggests that gender and oxygen do not play a significant role in determining the survival probability of a victim.

6. Other Applications

There are many other applications of local modeling methods. This section briefly introduces some of them and gives some relevant references for those who wish for more details. Suppose that $(X_1, Y_1), \ldots, (X_n, Y_n)$ are a random sample from a population (X, Y). We are interested in estimating a population parameter function θ. The function $\theta(\cdot)$ can be, for example, the conditional mean function $E(Y|X)$ and the conditional quantile function. In parametric settings, we model $\theta(x)$ using a parametric family $\theta(x) = g(x; \beta)$. To get an estimator of β, we optimize (either minimize or maximize) an objective function

$$L(\beta) = \sum_{i=1}^{n} \ell\{X_i, Y_i, g(X_i, \beta)\}\,. \tag{38}$$

Here ℓ is a discrepancy loss function or the log-likelihood function of an individual observation. For example, the L_2-loss function leads to a least squares estimate, while the L_1-loss function corresponds to a robust linear regression.

The local modeling method can be used to relax the global parametric model assumption and to significantly reduce the modeling bias. For a given point x_0, we replace the objective function by its local version

$$L\{\beta(x_0)\} = \sum_{i=1}^{n} \ell\{X_i, Y_i, g(X_i, \beta(x_0))\}K_h(X_i - x_0)\,. \tag{39}$$

Optimizing (39) yields an estimate $\hat\beta(x_0)$, just like the local likelihood estimate discussed in the last section. Thus, an estimate of the function $\theta(\cdot)$ by $\hat\theta(x_0) = g\{x_0; \hat\beta(x_0)\}$. Since the local estimate $\hat\beta(x_0)$ optimizes (39), the estimate $g\{x_0, \hat\beta(x_0)\}$ should converge to its population version. Therefore the estimate $\hat\theta(x_0)$ is a consistent estimator of the function $\theta(x_0)$ if $h \to 0$ in such a way that $nh \to \infty$.

For a given x_0, by Taylor's expansion, we can parametrize the function in a local neighborhood of x_0 as

$$g(x; \beta) = \beta_0(x_0) + \beta_1(x_0)(x - x_0) + \cdots + \beta_p(x_0)(x - x_0)^p\,. \tag{40}$$

With suppressing the dependence of β's on x_0, (39) can be rewritten as

$$L\{\beta(x_0)\} = \sum_{i=1}^{n} \ell\{X_i, Y_i, \beta_0 + \beta_1(X_i - x_0) + \cdots + \beta_p(X_i - x_0)^p\} \times K_h(X_i - x_0)\,. \tag{41}$$

Let $\hat{\beta}_j$ $(j = 0, 1, \ldots, p)$ optimize (41). Then as in last section,

$$\hat{\theta}(x_0) = \hat{\beta}_0$$

and

$$\hat{\theta}_\nu(x_0) = \nu!\hat{\beta}_\nu\,, \quad \nu = 1, \ldots, p$$

estimates the νth derivative of the function $\theta(x)$ at $x = x_0$.

It is clear that local polynomial regression and local likelihood approach are special cases hereof. An extension of the ideas for estimating bias and variance can be found in Fan *et al.*,[27] in which methods for selecting bandwidths and constructing confidence intervals are also proposed. A closely related framework is the local estimating equation method introduced by Carroll *et al.*[11] and the kernel generalized estimating equation (GEE) proposed by Lin and Carroll.[62]

6.1. *Estimation of conditonal quantiles and median*

In explanatory data analysis, quantiles provide us informative summary of a population. In regression analysis, conditional quantiles have important applications for constructing predictive intervals and detecting heteroscedasticity. When the error distribution is asymmetric, the conditional median regression function is more informative than the conditional mean regression.

Take the loss function in (38) to be $\ell(x, y, \theta) = \ell_\alpha(y - \theta)$ with

$$\ell_\alpha(t) = |t| + (2\alpha - 1)t\,. \tag{42}$$

The minimizer of $E\ell(X, Y, \theta)$ in this situation is the conditional α-quantile function $\xi_\alpha(x) = G^{-1}(\alpha|x)$, where $G^{-1}(y|x)$ is the conditional distribution of Y given $X = x$.

Now we apply the local modeling approach to estimate the conditional quantile function. Minimize

$$\sum_{i=1}^{n} \ell_\alpha\{Y_i - \beta_0 - \beta_1(X_i - x_0) - \cdots - \beta_p(X_i - x_0)^p\}K_h(X_i - x_0) \tag{43}$$

and the resulting estimator for $\xi_\alpha(x_0)$ is simply $\hat{\beta}_0$.

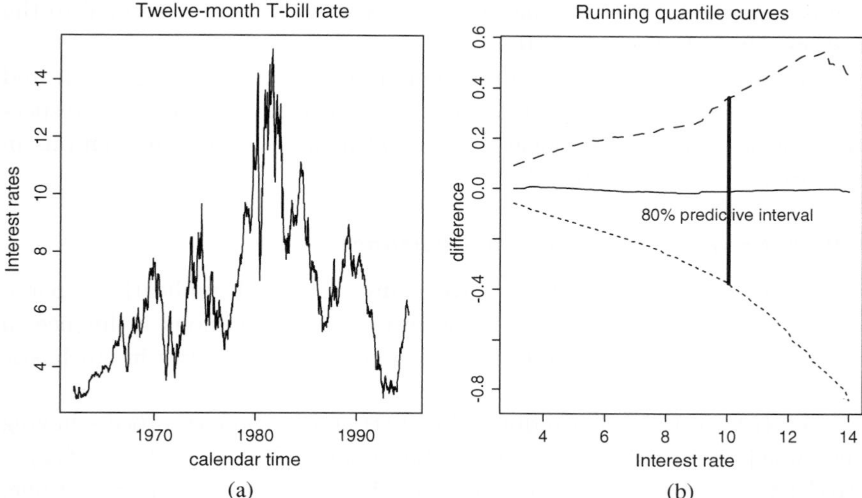

Fig. 15. Quantile regression. (a) The yields of 12-month Treasury bill. (b) Conditional quantiles - - - - - : $\alpha = 0.1$, solid curve — $\alpha = 0.5$, — — — — — : $\alpha = 0.9$. The vertical bar indicates the 80%-predictive interval at the point $x = 10$. Taken from Fan and Gijbels.[29]

Now we apply the proposed approach to the 12-month Treasury bill data presented in Fig. 15(a). Figure 15(b) depicts the estimated conditional median, the conditional 10th percentile and the conditional 90th percentile. The fan shape of the conditional quantiles shows that the variability gets larger as the interest rate gets higher. The intervals sandwiched by conditional 10th and 90th percentiles are 80%-predictive intervals. For example, given the current interest rate being 10%, with probability 80% the difference of the next week's rate and this week's rate falls in the interval $[-0.373\%, 0.363\%]$.

For robust estimation of the regression function, one can simply replace the loss function in (42) by an outlier-resistant loss function such as

$$\ell(t) = \begin{cases} t^2/2 & \text{when } |t| \le c \\ c|t| - c^2/2 & \text{when } |t| > c\,, \end{cases}$$

namely, taking the derivative of $\ell(t)$ to be Huber's ψ-function: $\psi_c(t) = \max\{-c, \min(c, t)\}$. When the conditional distribution of Y given $X = x$ is symmetric about the regression function $m(x)$, the resulting estimates are consistent for all $c \ge 0$. Another useful robust procedure is LOWESS, introduced by Cleveland,[17] which reduces the influence of outliers by an iterative reweighted least-squares scheme with weights proportional to the residuals from the previous iteration.

There is a large literature on nonparametric quantile regression and robust regression. Härdle and Gasser[49] and Tsybakov[84] considered respectively local constant and local polynomial fitting. Other contributions in this area are also available.[12, 28, 47, 60, 83]

6.2. *Estimation of conditional variance*

Conditional variance functions have many statistical applications, particularly in finance. Because of their important applications in finance in which data are often dependent, we formulate the problems in stochastic setup.

Let $\{(X_i, Y_i)\}$ be a two-dimensional strictly stationary process having the same joint distribution as (X, Y). Let $m(x) = E(Y|X = x)$ and $\sigma^2(x) = \text{var}(Y|X = x)$ be respectively the regression function and the conditional variance function. Our approach is based on the residuals of the local fit. Let $\hat{m}_{h_1,K}(\cdot)$ be the local fit of $m(\cdot)$ using a kernel K and a bandwidth h_1. Consider the squared residuals

$$\hat{r}_i = \{Y_i - \hat{m}_{h_1,K}(X_i)\}^2 . \tag{44}$$

Note that the conditional variance function can be expressed as

$$\sigma^2(x) = E[\{Y - m(X)\}^2 | X = x] ,$$

which is the regression function of the squared residuals. Therefore, a natural procedure is to run a local fit on the squared residuals. Let $\hat{\sigma}^2_{h_2,W}(x)$ be the local fit based on the data $\{(X_i, \hat{r}_i), i = 1, \ldots, n\}$, using a bandwidth h_2 and a kernel W. Then, it was shown by Fan and Yao,[35] Ruppert *et al.*[71] that the estimator $\hat{\sigma}^2_{h_2,W}(x)$ performs as well as the ideal estimator, which is a local linear fit to the true squared residuals

$$\{(X_i, \{Y_i - m(X_i)\}^2),\ i = 1, \ldots, n\}$$

using the same bandwidth h_2 and the same kernel W. They also obtained the order of bias and variance of the resulting estimators. Their results suggest that if the bandwidth h_1 is of order $n^{-1/5}$, then the residual-based *conditional variance estimator* performs asymptotically as well as the ideal one. In particular, the optimal bandwidth for estimating the mean regression function is permitted to be used for computing the residuals. Thus a data-driven procedure can be established.[35]

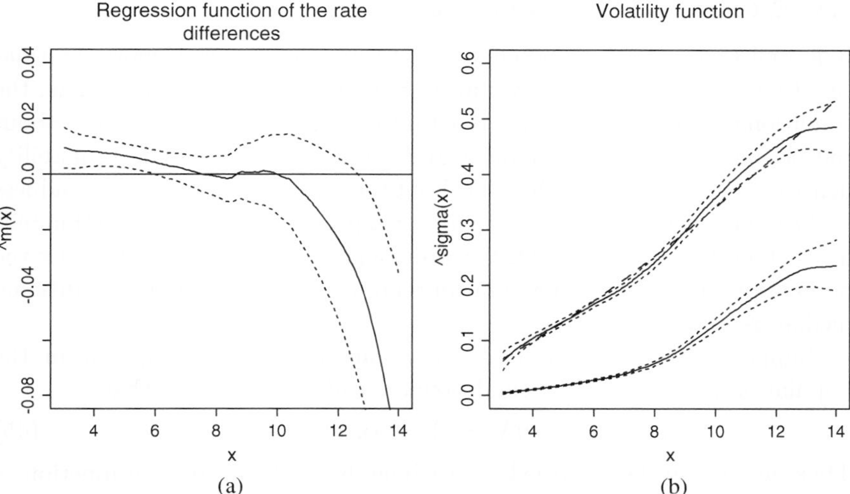

Fig. 16. The regression function and the volatility function for the 12-month Treasury bill data. (a) The estimated mean regression function and, (b) Estimated volatility function (thick curve) and the estimated conditional variance function (thin curve). The two dashed curves around a solid one indicate one standard error above and below the estimated mean regression function. From Fan and Gijbels.[29]

To illustrate the usefulness of the above automatic method, consider the yields of 12-month Treasury bill. The refined global bandwidth selector of Fan and Gijbels[28] and the Epanechnikov kernel. Figure 16(a) gives the estimated mean regression function. The bandwidth $\hat{h}_1 = 3.99$ was chosen by the software. Figure 16(b) depicts the estimated conditional standard deviation (the volatility function) and the conditional variance function. The bandwidth $\hat{h}_2 = 3.63$ was selected by the software. Visual inspection suggests that the volatility function should be a power function. Indeed, the correlation coefficient between $\{\log(x_j)\}$ and $\{\log(\hat{\sigma}(x_j))\}$ is 0.997!, where $x_j, (j = 1, \ldots, 201)$ are grid points in the interval [3, 14]. Fitting a line through the data $\{(\log(x_j), \log\{\hat{\sigma}(x_j)\}), j = 1, \ldots, 201\}$, we obtain the estimate

$$\hat{\sigma}(x) = 0.0154x^{1.3347}.$$

This estimate is presented as a thick-dashed curve in Fig. 16(b). This is an example where the nonparametric analyses yield a good parametric model $\sigma(x) = \alpha x^{\beta}$. Based on the linear regression on the data $(\log(X_i), \log(\hat{r}_i))$, one can also obtain directly an estimate of α and β.

6.3. *Estimation of conditional density*

It is well known that probability density function is much more informative than the mean and the variance. Similarly, in regression settings, the conditional probability density function provided more information about the population than the conditional regression function. The probability density function plots can show us about the center as well as the spreadness of the population. The shape of conditional probability density function tells us whether it is symmetric. This provides a guidance for us to summarize the population via the conditional mean regression function or the conditional median regression function.

Suppose that $(X_1, Y_1), \ldots, (X_n, Y_n)$ are a random sample from the population (X, Y) with the conditional density $g(y|x)$. Note that

$$E\{K_{h_2}(Y - y)|X = x\} \approx g(y|x)\,, \quad \text{as } h_2 \to 0\,. \tag{45}$$

Thus, $g(y|x)$ can be regarded approximately as the regression function of the variable $K_{h_2}(Y - y)$ on X. Considerations of this nature lead to the following local polynomial regression problem:

$$\sum_{i=1}^{n} \left\{ K_{h_2}(Y_i - y) - \sum_{j=0}^{p} \beta_j (X_i - x)^j \right\}^2 W_{h_1}(X_i - x)\,, \tag{46}$$

for a given bandwidth h_1 and a kernel function W. Let $\{\hat{\beta}_j(x, y), j = 0, \ldots, p\}$ be the solution of the least-squares problem. Then an estimator of $g^{(\nu)}(y|x) = \frac{\partial^\nu g(y|x)}{\partial x^\nu}$ is $\nu!\hat{\beta}_\nu(x, y)$. We write $\hat{g}(y|x) = \hat{\beta}_0(x, y)$ as the estimator of the conditional density.

To apply the proposed approach of conditional density estimation, we have to choose two bandwidths h_1 and h_2. The method for constructing a data-driven bandwidth for local polynomial regression can be used to compute a bandwidth for h_1, and the method for choosing a bandwidth for kernel density estimation can be employed to find a bandwidth h_2.[36]

With the estimated conditional density function, one can derive many statistical estimators. For example, the mean regression function can simply be estimated by

$$\hat{m}(x) = \int y\hat{g}(y|x)dy\,.$$

It can be shown that this estimator is the same as the local polynomial regression estimator when the kernel function K has mean zero. Similarly, one can derive estimates for the conditional variance and conditional quantile functions.

6.4. *Change point detection*

Change point detection is useful in medical monitoring and quality control. For example, when the treatment effects change suddenly without warning or planning, *jump points* arise. The statistical problem can be formulated as follows.

Let $(X_1, Y_1), \ldots, (X_n, Y_n)$ be a random sample from a population (X, Y) with conditional mean function m, which is smooth except for a few number of jump discontinuities. For simplicity, we assume that there is only one single discontinuity point, also called a *change point*.

One may regard the change point as the location where the derivative function $|m'(\cdot)|$ is maximized. Thus, a naive method is to first estimate the derivative curve and then find the maximizer of the absolute value of the estimated derivative function. Let $D(x, h)$ be a derivative estimator resulting from a local polynomial fit of order p with bandwidth h and kernel K. For simplicity, assume that the support of K is $[-1, 1]$. The above idea translates into the following estimating scheme: plot the function $|D(\cdot, h)|$ for a range of values of h and identify the jump as the point x in the vicinity of which $|D(x, h)|$ is consistently large for a *range of values of* h. More precisely, let $\tilde{x}(h)$ be the global maximum of the function $|D(\cdot, h)|$. Put

$$\tilde{x}_-(h) = \sup_{h_1 \in [h, \eta_n]} \{\tilde{x}(h_1) - 2h_1\}, \quad \tilde{x}_+(h) = \inf_{h_1 \in [h, \eta_n]} \{\tilde{x}(h_1) + 2h_1\}, \tag{47}$$

for $h \leq \eta_n$, where $\eta_n > 0$ is a prescribed number, tending to zero more slowly than $n^{-1} \log n$. Let $\tilde{h}$ denote the infimum of values h such that $\tilde{x}_-(h) \leq \tilde{x}_+(h)$. The proposed jump point estimator is $\hat{x}_0 = \tilde{x}(\tilde{h})$.[44]

Gijbels *et al.*[44] also propose a further refinement of the above idea. For a given bandwidth h, pretend the change point lies in the interval $\tilde{x}(h) \pm 2h$ and the regression function is a step function on this interval. Then, find the unknown location of the jump such that it minimizes the residual sum of squares, using only the data in the strip $\tilde{x}(h) \pm 2h$. The resulting estimator is a refinement of the estimator $\tilde{x}(h)$. In particular, we can take $h = \tilde{h}$ to yield a refinement of $\hat{x}_0$.

Müller[67] proposed an alternative method based on a one-sided kernel approach. The idea can be extended to the local polynomial setting as follows. Denote by K_- a kernel function supported on $[-1, 0]$ and $\hat{m}_-(x, h)$ a local polynomial fit using the bandwidth h and the kernel K_-. Note that the estimator $\hat{m}_-(x, h)$ uses only the local data on the left-hand side of the point x. Analogously, let K_+ be a kernel function supported on [0, 1] and

$\hat{m}_+(x, h)$ be a local polynomial fit using the bandwidth h and the kernel K_+. Then, $\hat{m}_+(x, h)$ uses only the data on the right-hand side of the point x. At the smooth locations, the estimates $\hat{m}_-(x, h)$ and $\hat{m}_+(x, h)$ are about the same, since both are consistent estimates of $m(x)$. At the discontinuity point, however, they estimate respectively the left-limit and the right-limit of the function m at the point x. Thus, a natural estimator is the location such that the difference function $|\hat{m}_+(x, h) - \hat{m}_-(x, h)|$ is maximized. The bandwidth for detecting the change point is typically much smaller than the optimal bandwidth for curve estimation. Müller[67] and Gijbels *et al.*[44] also gave some interesting examples.

References

1. Aerts, M., Claeskens, G. and Hart, J. D. (1999). Testing the fit of a parametric function. *Journal of the American Statistical Association* **94**: 869–879.
2. Andersen, P. K., Borgan, Ø., Gill, R. D. and Keiding, N. (1993). *Statistical Models Based on Counting Processes*, Springer-Verlag, New York.
3. Azzalini, A. and Bowman, A. N. (1993). On the use of nonparametric regression for checking linear relationships. *Journal of the Royal Statistical Society Series* **B55**: 549–557.
4. Azzalini, A., Bowman, A. N. and Härdle, W. (1989). On the use of nonparametric regression for model checking. *Biometrika* **76**: 1–11.
5. Bickel, P. J. (1975). One-step Huber estimates in linear models. *Journal of the American Statistical Association* **70**: 428–433.
6. Bowman, A. W. and Azzalini, A. (1997). *Applied Smoothing Techniques for Data Analysis, The Kernel Approach with S-Plus Illustrations*, Oxford Science Publications, Oxford.
7. Brumback, B. and Rice, J. (1998). Smoothing spline models for the analysis of nested and crossed samples of curves. *Journal of the American Statistical Association* **93**: 961–976.
8. Cai, Z., Fan, J. and Li, R. (2000). Efficient estimation and inferences for varying-coefficient models. *Journal of the American Statistical Association* **95**: 888–902.
9. Cai, Z., Fan, J. and Yao, Q. (2000). Functional-coefficient regression models for nonlinear time series. *Journal of the American Statistical Association* **95**: 941–956.
10. Carroll, R. J., Fan, J., Gijbels, I. and Wand, M. P. (1997). Generalized partially linear single-index models. *Journal of the American Statistical Association* **92**: 477–489.
11. Carroll, R. J., Ruppert, D. and Welsh, A. H. (1998). Local estimating equations. *Journal of the American Statistical Association* **93**: 214–227.
12. Chaudhuri, P. (1991). Nonparametric estimates of regression quantiles and their local Bahadur representation. *The Annals of Statistics* **19**: 760–777.

13. Chaudhuri, P. and Marron, J. S. (1999). SiZer for exploration of structures in curves. *Journal of the American Statistical Association* **94**: 807–822.
14. Chen, H. (1988). Convergence rates for parametric components in a partly linear model. *The Annals of Statistics* **16**: 136–146.
15. Chen, R. and Tsay, R. S. (1993). Functional-coefficient autoregressive models. *Journal of the American Statistical Association* **88**: 298–308.
16. Chu, C. K. and Marron, J. S. (1991). Choosing a kernel regression estimator (with discussions). *Statistical Sciences* **6**: 404–436.
17. Cleveland, W. S. (1979). Robust locally weighted regression and smoothing scatterplots. *Journal of the American Statistical Association* **74**: 829–836.
18. Cleveland, W. S., Grosse, E. and Shyu, W. M. (1992). Local regression models. In *Statistical Models in S*, eds. J. M. Chambers and T. J. Hastie, Wadsworth and Brooks, California, 309–376.
19. Cox, D. R. (1972). Regression models and life-tables (with discussion). *Journal of the Royal Statistical Society* **B34**: 187–220.
20. Cox, D. R. (1975). Partial likelihood. *Biometrika* **62**: 269–276.
21. Eubank, R. L. and Hart, J. D. (1992). Testing goodness-of-fit in regression via order selection criteria. *The Annals of Statistics* **20**: 1412–1425.
22. Eubank, R. L. and LaRiccia, V. M. (1992). Asymptotic comparison of Cramér-von Mises and nonparametric function estimation techniques for testing goodness-of-fit. *The Annals of Statistics* **20**: 2071–86.
23. Fan, J. (1992). Design-adaptive nonparametric regression. *Journal of the American Statistical Association* **87**: 998–1004.
24. Fan, J. (1993). Local linear regression smoothers and their minimax. *The Annals of Statistics* **21**: 196–216.
25. Fan, J. (1996). Test of significance based on wavelet thresholding and Neyman's truncation. *Journal of the American Statistical Association* **91**: 674–688.
26. Fan, J. and Chen, J. (1999). One-step local quasi-likelihood estimation. *Journal of the Royal Statistical Society* **B61**: 927–943.
27. Fan, J., Farmen, M. and Gijbels, I. (1998). A blueprint of local maximum likelihood estimation. *Journal of the Royal Statistical Society* **B60**: 591–608.
28. Fan, J. and Gijbels, I. (1996). *Local Polynomial Modelling and Its Applications*, Chapman and Hall, London.
29. Fan, J. and Gijbels, I. (2000). Local polynomial fitting, *Smoothing and Regression. Approaches, Computation and Application*, ed. M. G. Schimek, John Wiley and Sons, 228–275.
30. Fan, J., Gijbels, I. and King, M. (1997). Local likelihood and local partial likelihood in hazard regression. *The Annals of Statistics* **25**: 1661–1690.
31. Fan, J., Heckman, N. E. and Wand, M. P. (1995). Local polynomial kernel regression for generalized linear models and quasi-likelihood functions. *Journal of the American Statistical Association* **90**: 141–150.
32. Fan, J. and Huang, L. (2001). Goodness-of-fit test for parametric regression models. *Journal of the Americal Statistical Association*, to appear.
33. Fan, J. and Marron, J. S. (1994). Fast implementations of nonparametric curve estimators. *Journal of Computational and Graphical Statistics* **3**: 35–56.

34. Fan, J. and Müller, M. (1995). Density and regression smoothing. In *XploRe: An Interactive Statistical Computing Environment*, eds. W. Härdle, S. Klinke and B. A. Turlach, Springer, Berlin, 77–99.
35. Fan, J. and Yao, Q. (1998). Efficient estimation of conditional variance functions in stochastic regression. *Biometrika* **85**: 645–660.
36. Fan, J., Yao, Q. and Tong, H. (1996). Estimation of conditional densities and sensitivity measures in nonlinear dynamical systems. *Biometrika* **83**: 189–206.
37. Fan, J., Zhang, C. and Zhang, J. (2001). Generalized likelihood ratio statistics and Wilks phenomenon. *The Annals of Statistics* **29**, to appear.
38. Fan, J. and Zhang, J. (2000). Functional linear models for longitudinal data. *Journal of the Royal Statistical Society* **B62**: 303–332.
39. Fan, J. and Zhang, W. (1999). Statistical estimation in varying-coefficient models. *The Annals of Statistics* **27**: 1491–1518.
40. Fleming, T. R. and Harrington, D. P. (1991). *Counting Processes and Survival Analysis*, Wiley, New York.
41. Gasser, T. and Müller, H.-G. (1984). Estimating regression functions and their derivatives by the kernel method. *Scandinavian Journal of Statistics* **11**: 171–185.
42. Gasser, T., Müller, H.-G. and Mammitzsch, V. (1985). Kernels for nonparametric curve estimation. *Journal of the Royal Statistical Society* **B47**: 238–252.
43. Gentleman, R. and Crowley, J. (1991). Local full likelihood estimation for the proportional hazards model. *Biometrics* **47**: 1283–1296.
44. Gijbels, I., Hall, P. and Kneip, A. (1995). On the estimation of jump points in smooth curves. Discussion Paper #9515, Institute of Statistics, Catholic University of Louvain, Louvain-la-Neuve, Belgium.
45. Granovsky, B. L. and Müller, H.-G. (1991). Optimizing kernel methods: a unifying variational principle. *International Statistical Review* **59**: 373–388.
46. Green, P. J. and Silverman, B. W. (1994). *Nonparametric Regression and Generalized Linear Models: A Robust Penalty Approach*, Chapman and Hall, London.
47. Hall, P. and Jones, M. C. (1990). Adaptive M-estimation in nonparametric regression. *The Annals of Statistics* **18**: 1712–1728.
48. Härdle, W. (1990). *Applied Nonparametric Regression*, Cambridge University Press, Boston.
49. Härdle, W. and Gasser, T. (1984). Robust non-parametric function fitting. *Journal of the Royal Statistical Society* **B46**: 42–51.
50. Härdle, W. and Mammen, E. (1993). Comparing nonparametric versus parametric regression fits. *The Annals of Statistics* **21**: 1926–47.
51. Hart, J. D. (1997). *Nonparametric Smoothing and Lack-of-fit Tests*, Springer, New York.
52. Hastie, T. J. and Tibshirani, R. (1990). *Generalized Additive Models*. Chapman and Hall, London.
53. Hastie, T. J. and Tibshirani, R. J. (1993). Varying-coefficient models (with discussion). *Journal of the Royal Statistical Society* **B55**: 757–796.

54. Hoover, D. R., Rice, J. A., Wu, C. O. and Yang, L. P. (1998). Nonparametric smoothing estimates of time-varying coefficient models with longitudinal data. *Biometrika* **85**: 809–822.
55. Inglot, T., Kallenberg, W. C. M. and Ledwina, T. (1994). Power approximations to and power comparison of smooth goodness-of-fit tests. *Scandinavian Journal of Statistics* **21**: 131–45.
56. Jones, M. C., Marron, J. S. and Sheater, S. J. (1996a). A brief survey of bandwidth selection for density estimation. *Journal of the American Statistical Association* **91**: 401–407.
57. Jones, M. C., Marron, J. S. and Sheater, S. J. (1996b). Progress in data-based bandwidth selection for kernel density estimation. *Computational Statistics* **11**: 337–381.
58. Kallenberg, W. C. M. and Ledwina, T. (1997). Data-driven smooth tests when the hypothesis is composite. *Journal of the American Statistical Association* **92**: 1094–1104.
59. Kauermann, G. and Tutz, G. (1999). On model diagnostics using varying coefficient models. *Biometrika* **86**: 119–128.
60. Koenker, R., Portnoy, S. and Ng, P. (1992). Nonparametric estimation of conditional quantile function. In *Proceedings of the conference on L_1 — Statistical Analysis and Related Methods*, ed. Y. Dodge, Elsevier, 217–229.
61. Lehmann, E. L. (1983). *Theory of Point Estimation*, Pacific Grove, Wadsworth and Brooks/Cole, California.
62. Lin, X. and Carroll, R. J. (2000). Nonparametric function estimation for clustered data when the predictor is measured without/with error. *Journal of the American Statistical Association* **95**: 520–534.
63. Mack, Y. P. and Müller, H. G. (1989). Convolution type estimators for nonparametric regression estimation. *Statistics and Probability Letters* **7**: 229–239.
64. Marron, J. S. and Nolan, D. (1988). Canonical kernels for density estimation. *Statistics and Probability Letters* **7**: 195–199.
65. McCullagh, P. and Nelder, J. A. (1989). *Generalized Linear Models*. Chapman and Hall, London.
66. Müller, H.-G. (1987). Weighted local regression and kernel methods for nonparametric curve fitting. *Journal of the American Statistical Association* **82**: 231–238.
67. Müller, H.-G. (1992). Change-points in nonparametric regression analysis. *The Annals of Statistics* **20**: 737–761.
68. Nadaraya, E. A. (1964). On estimating regression. *Theory Probability Applied* **9**: 141–142.
69. Rawlings, J. O. and Spruill, S. E. (1994). Estimating pine seedling response to ozone and acidic rain. In *Case Studies in Biometry*, eds. N. Lange, L. Ryan, L. Billard, D. Brillinger, L. Conquest and J. Greenhouse, Wiley, New York, 81–106.
70. Ruppert, D. and Wand, M. P. (1994). Multivariate weighted least squares regression. *The Annals of Statistics* **22**: 1346–1370.

71. Ruppert, D., Wand, M. P., Holst, U. and Hössjer, O. (1997). Local polynomial variance function estimation. *Technometrics* **39**: 262–73.
72. Scott, D. W. (1992). *Multivariate Density Estimation: Theory, Practice, and Visualization*, John Wiley and Sons, New York.
73. Seifert, B. and Gasser, T. (1996). Finite-sample variance of local polynomials: analysis and solutions. *Journal of the American Statistical Association* **91**: 267–275.
74. Severini, T. A. and Staniswalis, J. (1994). Quasi-likelihood estimation in semiparametric models. *Journal of the American Statistical Association* **89**: 501–511.
75. Silverman, B. W. (1986). *Density Estimation for Statistics and Data Analysis,* Chapman and Hall, London.
76. Simonoff, J. S. (1996). *Smoothing Methods in Statistics.* Springer, New York.
77. Speckman, P. (1988). Kernel smoothing in partial linear models. *Journal of the Royal Statistical Society* **B50**: 413–436.
78. Spokoiny, V. G. (1996). Adaptive hypothesis testing using wavelets. *The Annals of Statistics* **24**: 2477–2498.
79. Stone, C. J. (1977). Consistent nonparametric regression. *The Annals of Statistics* **5**: 595–645.
80. Stone, C. J. (1980). Optimal rates of convergence for nonparametric estimators. *The Annals of Statistics* **8**: 1348–1360.
81. Stone, C. J. (1982). Optimal global rates of convergence for nonparametric regression. *The Annals of Statistics* **10**: 1040–1053.
82. Tibshirani, R. and Hastie, T. J. (1987). Local likelihood estimation. *Journal of the Americal Statistical Association* **82**: 559–567.
83. Truong, Y. K. (1989). Asymptotic properties of kernel estimators based on local medians. *The Annals of Statistics* **17**: 606–617.
84. Tsybakov, A. B. (1986). Robust reconstruction of functions by the local-approximation method. *Problems of Information Transmission* **22**: 133–146.
85. Wand, M. P. and Jones, M. C. (1995). *Kernel Smoothing,* Chapman and Hall, London.
86. Wand, M. P., Marron, J. S. and Ruppert, D. (1991). Transformations in density estimation, *Journal of the Americal Statistical Association* **86**: 343–361.
87. Watson, G. S. (1964). Smooth regression analysis. *Sankhyā Series* **A26**: 359–372.
88. Yang, L. and Marron, J. S. (1999). Iterated transformation — Kernel density estimation. *Journal of the American Statistical Association* **94**: 580–589.

About the Authors

Jianqing Fan is Frederick L. Moore Professor of Finance, Professor of Statistics, Chairman of Department of Operations Research and Financial

Engineering, and Director of Committee of Statistical Studies, Princeton University, where he directs both financial econometrics and statistics labs. He was the past president of the Institute of Mathematical Statistics and International Chinese Statistical Association, and was an invited speaker at the 2006 International Congress of Mathematicians. He is co-editing *Journal of Econometrics* and is an associate editor of *Econometrica* and *Journal of American Statistical Association*, and was the co-editor of *The Annals of Statistics*, *Probability Theory and Related Fields* and *Econometrics Journal.* After receiving his Ph.D. from the University of California at Berkeley, he has been appointed as assistant, associate, and full professor at the University of North Carolina at Chapel Hill (1989–2003), professor at the University of California at Los Angeles (1997–2000), Professor and Chairman at Chinese University of Hong Kong (2000–2003), and professor at Princeton University (2003–). His published work on statistics, computational biology, and finance has been recognized by the 2000 COPSS Presidents' Award, the Myrto Lefkopoulou distinguished lecture of Harvard School of Public Health, the 2007 Morningside Gold Medal of Applied Mathematics, Guggenheim Fellow in 2009, and election to Academician of Academia Sinica and fellow of American Associations for Advancement of Science, Institute of Mathematical Statistics, and American Statistical Association.

Runze Li is distinguished professor of statistics, The Pennsylvania State University. He received his Ph.D. in Statistics from University of North Carolina at Chapel Hill in 2000. He served as associate editor for Annals of Statistics, Journal of American Statistical Association and Statistica Sinica. He currently serves as co-editor of Annals of Statistics. Runze Li is interested in the development of statistical methods and theories as well as novel statistical applications to various scientific fields. He is an elected fellow of Institute of Mathematical Statistics and American Statistical Association. He won the United Nations' World Meteorological Organization Gerbier-Mumm International Award for 2012.

CHAPTER 31

STATISTICAL METHODS FOR DEPENDENT DATA

FENG CHEN

Department of Medical Statistics,
Nantong Medical College,
Nantong, Jiangsu 226001, PR China
Tel: 0086-513-5517191-2012;
chenfeng@public.nt.js.cn

1. Introduction

Most classical statistical methods require independent observations. The issue here is not independence of multiple variables, rather of the samples. There are many cases of dependent in medical research when requirement of independence cannot be hold, i.e. observations are correlated.

The existence of such correlation is not a coincident, but due to the design of the experiments. In some cases, this type of correlation can be eliminated by suitable procedure without losing any information. The simplest case is paired design where the observations within the same paired is correlated. For example, to investigate a new drug's effects on hypertension, a 2-by-2 crossover design can be used to measure the diastolic pressure before and after treatment for each subject. Although the pressures across subjects are independent, the observations of the same subject are correlated.

Unfortunately, we could not eliminate intra-unit correlations in most cases by traditional statistical methods. For example, in a toxicological study, 32 pregnant rats were randomly allocated into test and control groups. Rats in control group were fed with regular food, while rats in test group were fed with combinations of regular food and suspected teratogen. The proportion of malformation of pups of two groups was compared after rat delivery. In this study, the pregnant rats are independent with each other, but genetic factors, antepartum internal womb environments and metabolism conditions of teratogen have effects on the rat pups. Thus, the rat pups cannot be treated as independent observations because siblings are more likely to encounter the similar proportion of malformation than pups from different litters. The litter effect must be taken into account. Special procedure must be used to deal with this type of data.

The intra-unit correlation or intra-class correlation is a measure of similarity (or non-independence) among individuals that share some characteristics. The intra-unit correlation means that observations in the same unit are not dependent. There are overlaps between the information they present. It is inappropriate to ignore the intra-unit correlation. For example, in a clinical trail, many variables, i.e. vital signs, physiological index, effects and side effects, should be observed successively in different time for each subject during the trial period to show the efficacy and safety of the tested drug. Each subject should be observed several times. We refer to this type of study as repeated measurement study. There are two classical ways to deal with this sort of data. One is, to test the significance of the difference between the test group and the control group on each occasion respectively including test for the homogeneity of two groups before treatment and to compare the difference of changes (such as absolutely increase or decrease, relatively increase or decrease, etc.) between the two groups at each time. The alternative is to take k observations of each one of n subjects as one response variable, (the sample size will be nk) to fit a model (or generalized linear model) in which time is an explanatory variable. The former one will have low statistical power because it treats the observations of each occasion independently. The latter considers the correlations between the treatment effect and time. However, it ignores the intra-subject correlation of the observations and takes the data as independent data. Thus, it will increase the type I error which may result in the approval of the inefficiency drug to the market.

The set of observations taken from the same subject tend to be correlated. They provide rather less information than the same number independent observations taken from different subjects. The larger the intra-unit correlation is, the less information will be provided. Therefore, it will increase the type I error if we use nk observations to fit general linear model.

The statistical methods for dependent data are described and illustrated in this chapter. The methods cover estimation of intra-correlation coefficient, hypotheses test, estimation of sample size, etc.

2. Examples of Dependent Data

Dependent data is omnipresent in medical researches, such as, repeated measurement data, longitudinal data, data of cross-over design, data of multicenter clinical trial, cluster sampling survey data, and infective disease, inherited disease, etc. They share the same property, which is the dependence or intra-unit correlation of observations. We refer to this type of data as dependent data. In this section, we will illustrate some types of examples for dependent data, and discuss their common and distinguishing features.

2.1. *Example 1. Randomized block design*

To compare the effects on the clotting time of serum of four treatments, 8 volunteers were recruited. Four samples of serum from each subject were assigned to the four treatments in a random order. The results of the experiment were presented in Table 1.

The property of the data shown in Table 1 is that the observations of the same block are correlated, while the observations from different blocks are independent. Thus, the effects of 4 treatments of 4 serums from one person are correlated. That is to say the data from block design are dependent. Observations in the same block in split-plot design and in split-split-plot design have the same property.

2.2. *Example 2. Cluster sampling*[1]

A simple random sample of 30 households was drawn from a census taken in 1947. The question here is whether they had consulted a doctor in the

Table 1. Clotting time (min) of serum from 8 volunteers, treated by 4 methods.

	Treatment			
subject	A	B	C	D
1	8.4	9.4	9.8	12.2
2	12.8	15.2	12.9	14.4
3	9.6	9.1	11.2	9.8
4	9.8	8.8	9.9	12.0
5	8.4	8.2	8.5	8.5
6	8.6	9.9	9.8	10.9
7	8.9	9.0	9.2	10.4
8	7.9	8.1	8.2	10.0

last 12 months. Data are shown below. The denominator is the number of persons in a household, and the nominator is the number of persons who saw a doctor.

5/5, 0/5, 2/3, 3/3, 0/2, 0/3, 0/3, 0/3, 0/4, 0/4, 0/3, 0/2, 0/7, 4/4, 1/3, 2/5, 0/4, 0/4, 1/3, 3/3, 2/4, 0/3, 0/3, 0/1, 2/2, 2/4, 0/3, 2/4, 0/2, 1/4

The property of this data is that the members of the same family tend to be similar, while persons from different families are assumed to be independent. Our purpose is to estimate the proportion of people who consulted a doctor, and to measure the similarity of the members in the same family. Similar results would be obtained for any characteristic in which the members of the same family trend to act in the same way.

2.3. *Example 3. Toxicological study*[2]

In a toxicological study, 32 pregnant rats were randomly allocated into 2 groups: test group and control group. Rats in control group were fed with regular food, while rats in test group were fed with combination of regular food with suspected teratogen. The proportions of malformation of pups of two groups were compared after delivery. The results are shown as follows:

Control group	13/13	12/12	9/9	8/8	8/8	12/13	11/12	9/10	9/10	8/9
	11/13	4/5	5/7	7/10	7/10	9/9				
Test group	12/12	11/11	10/10	9/9	10/11	9/10	9/10	8/9	8/9	4/5
	7/9	4/7	5/10	3/6	3/10	0/7				

The denominator is the number of offspring in a litter, and the nominator is the number of offsprings that are malformation in the litter.

In this study, the pregnant rats are independent to each other, but genetic factors, antepartum internal womb environments and metabolism conditions of teratogen have effects on the rat pups. The rat pups cannot be treated as independent observations because siblings are more alike than pups from different litters. Data in Example 2 have similar property. Similar property would be obtained from genetics studies in which the members of the same family tend to be similar.

2.4. *Example 4. Crossover design*

For studying the bioequivalence of domestic and imported rosiglitazone maleate tablets (RMT), 24 volunteers were recruited in a 4 × 4 crossover study. Four sequence groups are formed by the randomized Latin square below

ADBC
BACD
CBDA
DCAB

Where A, B, C, D are imported RMT 2 mg, domestic RMT 2 mg, imported RMT 4 mg and domestic 4 mg, respectively.

Twenty-four volunteers were randomly allocated in 4 treatment groups with 6 in each sequence. Each subject received different treatment on different cycles. To minimize carryover effects, a 7-day wash-out period between the two treatment occasions was made. Plasma concentration of rosiglitazone maleate was detected within 24 hours after orally taking RMT. Data in Table 2 is the area under curve (AUC), maximum concentration ($C_{\max}$) and time to half maximum concentration (T_{50}). The aim is to test whether there is difference between domestic and imported RMT.

This is a four-by-four crossover design with 3 variables. In this data set, the observations in 4 periods and the variables (AUC, $C_{\max}$ and T_{50}) are correlated.

2.5. *Example 5. Repeated measurement, linear regression*

In a multicenter, randomized, double-blind, three doses (high, middle, and low = placebo) controlled clinical study, the researchers evaluated the efficacy and safety of urokinase (UK) in the treatment of acute cerebral infarctions within 6 hours from the onset of stroke. One interesting variable is the European stroke scale (ESS). Data are shown in Table 3.

Repeated measurement design, also known as within-subject design, is a quite common design in medical researches. The feature of this type of data set is that individuals are measured repeatedly through time. We are interested in both treatment and temporal effects. Figure 1 displays the data graphically. Each line connect the repeated observations at different times of a subject. This simple graph reveals apparent and important patterns. First, all of 30 subjects are getting better within 8 weeks as ESS is becoming larger. Second, patients with larger ESS at the beginning of the period tend to remain larger throughout. This phenomenon is called "tracking."

There are two ways to deal with this type of data by classical methods. First, we estimate the average of ESS for each week and fit a regression model of the means of ESS over time. In fact, we aggregate the data.

Table 2. Results of 4 × 4 cross-over trial for testing bioequivalence of domestic and imported rosiglitazone maleate tablets.

Id	sequence	Stage 1			Stage 2			Stage 3			Stage 4		
		AUC	$C_{\max}$	T_{50}	AUC	$C_{\max}$	T_{50}	AUC	$C_{\max}$	T_{50}	AUC	$C_{\max}$	T_{50}
1	DCAB	884.27	204.63	3.47	905.09	222.94	3.86	2330.77	455.14	5.50	1936.98	395.55	4.35
2	CBDA	919.50	178.27	3.92	2201.98	346.89	4.58	855.89	205.31	3.79	1939.36	327.12	4.01
3	ADBC	1738.12	326.72	3.95	901.70	130.61	4.56	1889.72	375.37	4.08	870.93	158.99	4.09
4	BACD	2000.29	382.25	3.51	2350.58	479.88	3.83	952.86	187.72	3.68	955.46	202.02	3.69
5	CBDA	823.39	158.72	3.86	1864.97	329.66	3.65	710.06	133.87	3.22	1372.77	309.07	2.99
6	ADBC	2102.11	360.38	4.47	946.33	155.29	4.68	2005.84	339.67	3.53	934.45	176.23	3.72
7	DCAB	907.86	170.88	3.95	991.65	197.54	4.06	2139.65	369.21	3.98	2408.84	368.93	4.62
8	BACD	2139.72	366.84	3.80	2012.09	411.87	3.99	1134.23	200.43	3.94	924.12	223.98	3.70
9	DCAB	787.80	163.07	2.73	905.52	172.22	3.23	1966.42	362.11	3.77	1640.15	331.95	3.15
10	BACD	1785.35	347.46	3.93	1934.66	373.82	4.38	892.89	163.78	3.78	826.27	151.87	3.78
11	ADBC	2031.55	320.43	3.39	975.70	165.38	3.56	1893.99	313.81	3.48	788.06	128.56	3.23
12	BACD	1524.61	381.50	3.12	2525.23	439.42	4.35	952.05	177.75	4.07	940.57	187.22	3.58
13	ADBC	2013.54	314.76	4.99	1005.49	168.16	4.39	2322.68	406.54	4.98	946.92	152.94	4.73
14	DCAB	990.04	163.73	4.63	1118.63	177.61	4.82	2300.18	334.58	4.51	2197.79	293.69	4.72
15	CBDA	839.94	136.99	4.02	1956.45	374.10	3.97	611.43	132.20	2.63	1707.48	273.61	4.03
16	CBDA	1159.85	167.43	4.57	2760.90	349.34	5.59	1007.45	178.00	4.59	2477.37	327.36	5.88
17	DCAB	1032.22	182.99	4.01	1039.21	173.00	3.96	2440.50	380.79	4.53	1860.15	353.41	3.77
18	BACD	1782.62	376.58	3.64	1917.01	426.42	3.44	1048.27	179.42	4.04	882.46	149.33	3.23
19	CBDA	852.84	150.20	3.87	2256.02	284.50	4.04	982.67	157.35	4.19	1924.09	360.50	3.96
20	ADBC	2178.77	436.64	4.09	1273.04	186.33	4.58	2074.44	296.02	4.08	1009.09	190.86	4.57
21	ADBC	2529.23	449.49	4.58	1365.57	190.35	5.21	1868.99	412.40	4.15	1064.39	208.41	4.95
22	CBDA	989.89	167.33	3.85	1936.16	334.66	4.03	904.53	175.76	4.10	2029.20	420.12	4.24
23	BACD	1579.55	328.00	3.72	1756.96	284.65	3.69	949.38	188.22	4.11	951.75	201.15	4.12
24	DCAB	889.20	186.69	3.95	757.79	196.20	3.10	1813.93	441.25	3.57	1523.54	327.47	3.33

Table 3. ESS of 30 acute cerebral infarctions.

Id	treat	Age	weeks								
			0	1	2	3	4	5	6	7	8
1	0	27	107	106	106	108	108	112	112	112	112
2	0	21	107	106	106	106	106	112	112	114	116
3	0	21	100	100	100	106	109	108	114	116	116
4	0	36	107	106	106	107	106	111	112	117	109
5	0	17	110	111	112	112	113	113	113	116	116
6	0	22	105	108	108	106	108	108	108	109	110
7	0	29	102	101	104	100	94	106	106	105	106
8	0	15	97	97	97	99	99	99	101	101	103
9	0	21	108	108	108	110	116	116	120	128	120
10	0	27	108	108	108	114	116	118	118	124	128
11	1	34	98	98	102	121	120	124	124	132	140
12	1	37	100	98	114	118	126	126	134	138	138
13	1	31	104	123	127	129	130	130	136	140	140
14	1	28	108	120	115	119	134	126	126	127	140
15	1	32	106	108	108	108	112	112	112	114	116
16	1	18	103	102	102	104	114	114	116	128	143
17	1	15	101	103	104	108	113	113	118	122	126
18	1	31	91	90	92	93	89	95	102	105	108
19	1	39	94	94	96	99	116	124	135	138	145
20	1	34	104	104	105	105	122	128	131	129	138
21	2	36	107	111	112	127	127	128	138	141	141
22	2	45	109	114	120	130	131	132	139	142	143
23	2	40	103	103	108	112	116	118	123	125	135
24	2	44	110	114	120	124	133	135	142	144	144
25	2	22	95	103	115	113	119	122	126	134	136
26	2	25	92	102	110	108	116	116	116	122	127
27	2	32	98	106	112	112	120	124	126	136	141
28	2	38	106	121	127	126	128	130	132	138	140
29	2	22	102	112	110	119	119	123	125	133	142
30	2	19	109	109	124	127	128	132	133	144	147

As a result, it increases the correlation and causes a spurious association between ESS and time. Second, we fit a regression model for all the data on time. These two models give the same regression coefficients but different standard errors. Both of them ignore the intra-subject correlation.

2.6. *Example 6. Pharmacokinetics study, repeated measurements, nonlinear regression*

A single oral dose Ciclosporin A Capsule was given to 10 healthy volunteers. Plasma concentration (ng/ml) was detected after medication. The results are shown in Table 4.

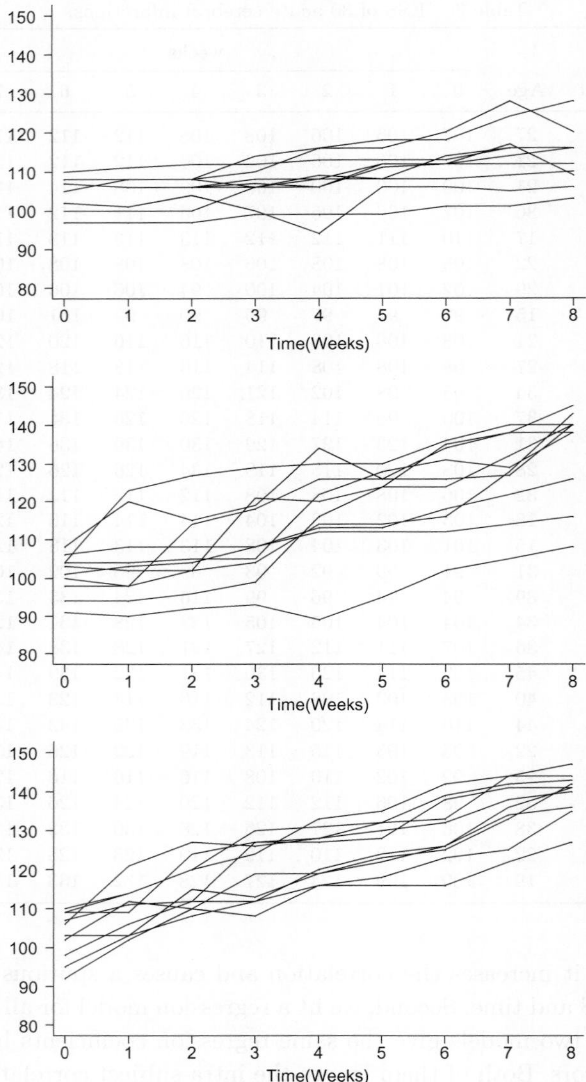

Fig. 1. ESS over time of 30 acute cerebral infarctions for three groups.

This is an example of repeated measurement with nonlinear trend, which are distinct from Example 5.

In experimental or pharmacokinetical study, the sample size is relatively small and the period is usually short. Dropout seldom occurs. Furthermore

Table 4. Plasma concentrations of Ciclosporin A Capsule after medication of 10 volunteers.

	Time (*hour*)									
Subject	0.5	1	2	3	4	5	6	8	12	16
1	343.3	783.6	443.1	426.8	267.0	155.5	125.0	98.3	75.2	23.8
2	86.6	501.1	817.9	542.7	273.9	226.4	195.7	114.0	79.9	26.6
3	256.1	534.8	486.8	420.1	370.6	316.7	250.6	192.6	124.5	75.9
4	300.2	849.7	846.0	521.1	373.2	269.4	258.1	182.7	93.0	68.0
5	344.6	826.4	631.0	485.0	389.7	257.7	204.7	172.4	124.5	44.2
6	230.0	780.7	912.3	551.2	299.8	219.3	148.7	75.1	55.9	27.6
7	116.5	943.4	848.2	747.3	410.4	345.5	171.4	129.5	63.0	17.5
8	66.7	239.2	814.6	526.9	426.6	213.5	152.5	118.5	73.1	38.1
9	67.7	789.1	551.6	520.2	463.0	295.7	191.8	154.4	108.4	32.5
10	216.2	599.9	1099.5	562.9	413.9	297.5	233.2	146.6	94.8	38.7

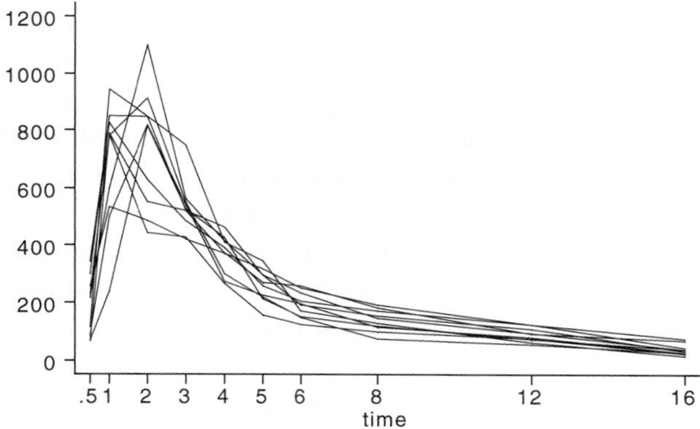

Fig. 2. Plasma concentration-time curve of Ciclosporin A capsule after a single oral dose in 10 volunteers.

both times of repeated measure and time intervals are similar to each other. However, it is not the case in clinical trial. The observed period is usually long. Compliance varies among patients and dropouts are routine. Last, but not least, the times and time intervals are different among patients.

2.7. *Example 7. Multi-center clinical study, ranked data*

To investigate the effect of nerve growth factor (NGF) for subjects of extraneuritis caused by chemical products, an random, double blind, placebo controlled clinical trial was developed.

One hundred two subjects were random allocated into treatment and placebo groups. The effectiveness was observed in 8 consecutive weeks for 102 subjects. The results are shown in Table 5, in which Id represents identification of subjects; Cnt represents the center; Trt represents groups (Trt = P for placebo, Trt = T for NGF); Com represents companies; Base represents the MDNS base level before treatment; and x1–x8 are effects at time from 1 to 8 weeks after treatment. Here, x = 0 stands for invalid or worse effect of treatment on the subject, 1 for improved, 2 for notable improved, 4 for recovery, and m for missing.

Except for the intra-subject correlation, the intra-center correlation of the subjects in the same hospital should be considered for this type of data.

2.8. *Example 8. Repeated measurement, count data*[3]

In order to understand whether the progabide reduces the rate of epileptic seizures, 59 patients of epileptics were recruited in a clinical trial. For each patient, the number of epileptic seizures was recorded during a baseline period of 8 weeks. Patients were then randomized to treatment with the anti-epileptic drug progabide, or placebo. In addition, all of the patients were treated with standard chemotherapy. The number of seizures was then recoded in 4 consecutive two-weeks for each epileptic.

Where, treatment variable is group (0 = placebo, 1 = progabide). What is different from Examples 5 and 7 is that the response variable is the seizure counts in unit time (two-week). Poisson regression would be used here for count data.

In this study, only recurrence episodes were included, not first episode. The reason of not including the first episode was that the factors associated with recurrence of a disease are usually different from those with that disease. For example, in a model of development of breast cancer, we should not include women who already had breast cancer, because family history and late childbearing have the strongest association with development of breast cancer, whereas stage of disease, hormone receptors, and histological grade are the strongest risk factors for recurrence of breast cancer.

For those diseases for which it is sensible to speak of a second distinct episode, the risk factors for a second episode may be similar to the risk factors for a first episode. Hooton and colleagues were interested in studying urinary track infections in young women.[4] With urinary track infections, patients can have a second (or third, etc.) episode after a "crude" first episode. Repeated episodes in the same person are not independent

Table 5. Effects of 102 subjects of extra-neuritis caused by chemical products.

Id	cnt	Trt	com	sex	age	base	x1	x2	x3	x4	x5	x6	x7	x8
1	1	T	A	0	21	13	1	2	2	2	2	2	2	3
2	1	P	A	0	27	12	1	2	2	2	2	2	2	2
3	1	T	A	0	27	13	1	2	2	2	2	2	2	2
4	1	P	B	0	21	13	1	2	2	2	2	2	2	2
5	1	T	B	0	34	7	0	1	1	2	2	2	2	2
6	1	T	B	0	45	13	1	2	2	2	2	2	2	3
7	1	T	B	0	37	13	1	2	2	2	2	2	2	
8	1	P	A	0	21	13	1	2	2	2	2	2	2	2
9	1	T	A	0	31	14	1	2	2	2	3	3	3	3
10	1	T	B	0	23	14	2	2	2	2	3	3	3	3
11	1	T	A	0	22	13	1	2	2	2	2	2	2	2
12	1	P	B	1	28	14	2	2	2	2	2	2	2	2
13	2	P	A	1	24	15	2	2	2	2	3	3	m	m
14	2	T	A	0	28	13	2	2	2	2	3	3	3	m
15	2	T	B	0	29	14	2	2	2	2	3	3	m	m
16	2	T	A	0	21	10	1	2	2	2	3	3	3	3
17	2	P	B	0	31	15	2	2	2	2	m	m	m	3
18	2	T	B	1	25	10	1	1	1	1	2	2	3	3
19	2	P	A	0	29	8	0	1	1	1	2	2	2	1
20	2	T	B	0	20	10	1	1	2	2	2	3	3	3
21	2	T	A	0	32	13	1	2	2	2	2	2	2	2
22	3	T	A	0	18	14	2	2	2	2	3	3	3	3
23	3	T	A	0	31	6	0	0	0	1	1	1	1	1
24	3	T	A	0	39	10	1	1	1	2	2	2	2	3
25	3	T	B	0	34	9	1	1	1	1	1	2	2	2
26	4	P	A	0	15	12	1	1	1	1	2	2	2	2
27	5	P	B	0	36	7	1	1	1	1	1	1	1	1
28	5	T	B	0	37	5	1	1	1	1	1	1	1	2
29	6	T	A	1	15	1	0	0	0	0	0	0	1	1
30	6	T	A	1	16	1	0	0	0	0	1	1	1	1
31	6	T	B	0	15	11	1	2	2	2	2	2	2	3
32	6	P	B	1	16	8	1	1	1	1	1	1	1	1
33	6	P	A	1	17	13	1	2	2	2	2	2	2	2
34	7	T	B	0	29	13	1	2	2	2	2	2	2	3
35	7	P	B	0	19	15	2	2	2	2	3	3	3	3
36	7	T	B	0	29	13	1	2	2	2	2	2	2	2
37	7	P	A	0	29	13	2	2	2	2	m	m	m	m
38	8	T	B	0	17	13	1	2	2	2	2	1	2	1
39	8	P	A	0	18	13	1	2	2	2	2	2	2	2
40	8	T	B	0	17	12	2	2	2	2	2	2	3	3
41	8	T	A	0	18	11	1	2	2	2	2	2	2	2
42	0	P	B	0	45	7	0	1	2	2	2	2	2	2
43	9	T	A	0	30	9	0	0	1	1	1	1	2	2
44	9	P	A	0	43	12	1	2	2	2	2	2	2	2
45	9	T	A	0	36	14	2	2	2	2	3	2	2	2

(*Continued*)

Table 5. (*Continued*)

Id	cnt	Trt	com	sex	age	base	x1	x2	x3	x4	x5	x6	x7	x8
46	9	T	B	0	45	14	2	2	2	2	3	3	3	3
47	9	P	B	0	32	14	2	2	2	2	3	3	3	3
48	9	T	A	0	40	11	1	1	2	2	2	2	2	2
49	1	P	A	0	36	13	1	2	2	2	2	2	2	2
50	1	T	A	0	44	13	1	2	2	2	2	3	3	3
51	10	P	B	0	35	13	1	2	2	2	2	2	2	2
52	10	T	B	0	38	13	1	2	2	2	2	2	2	2
53	10	T	A	0	33	13	1	2	2	2	2	3	3	3
54	10	T	B	0	41	13	1	2	2	2	2	2	2	3
55	11	T	A	0	22	13	2	2	2	2	2	3	m	m
56	11	P	B	0	22	14	1	1	1	1	2	2	2	2
57	11	T	B	0	28	8	1	1	1	1	1	2	2	2
58	11	P	A	0	31	14	2	2	2	2	3	3	3	3
59	11	T	A	0	37	15	2	2	2	2	3	3	3	3
60	11	T	B	0	21	14	2	2	2	2	2	3	3	3
61	11	P	B	1	24	12	1	2	2	2	2	2	2	2
62	11	T	B	0	25	7	1	1	1	2	2	2	2	2
63	11	T	A	0	32	12	1	1	2	2	2	2	2	2
64	11	T	A	0	21	15	2	2	2	2	3	3	3	3
65	11	P	A	0	20	13	2	2	2	2	3	3	3	3
66	11	T	B	1	30	14	2	2	2	2	3	m	m	m
67	11	T	A	1	38	13	1	2	2	2	2	3	3	3
68	11	T	A	0	19	16	2	2	2	2	3	3	3	3
69	11	T	B	0	21	14	2	2	2	2	2	3	3	3
70	11	P	B	0	25	11	1	m	2	2	m	m	m	m
71	11	T	B	1	22	15	2	2	2	2	m	3	m	3
72	11	P	A	1	23	10	1	1	1	1	1	1	m	m
73	11	T	A	0	21	14	2	2	2	2	3	3	3	3
74	11	T	A	0	26	14	2	m	2	m	3	m	3	m
75	11	T	B	0	20	15	2	2	2	2	3	3	3	3
76	11	P	B	0	18	13	2	2	2	m	m	m	m	m
77	11	P	A	1	23	8	1	1	1	1	1	1	1	2
78	11	T	B	0	24	15	m	2	m	2	m	3	m	3
79	11	P	B	0	26	10	1	1	1	1	1	2	2	m
80	11	T	A	0	20	15	2	2	2	2	3	3	3	3
81	11	P	A	0	18	13	2	2	m	m	m	m	m	m
82	11	T	B	0	22	14	2	2	2	2	m	m	3	m
83	11	T	B	0	25	15	2	2	2	2	3	3	3	3
84	11	T	A	0	19	15	2	2	2	2	3	3	3	3
85	11	T	B	0	20	15	2	2	2	2	3	3	m	m
86	11	T	A	0	29	15	2	2	2	2	3	3	m	m
87	11	P	A	0	25	8	m	m	1	m	m	1	m	m
88	11	T	A	0	24	15	2	2	2	m	m	3	m	m
89	11	P	B	0	21	11	m	1	1	m	m	m	m	m
90	11	T	B	0	19	15	2	2	2	2	3	3	3	m

(*Continued*)

Table 5. (*Continued*)

Id	cnt	Trt	com	sex	age	base	x1	x2	x3	x4	x5	x6	x7	x8
91	11	T	A	0	21	15	2	2	2	2	3	3	3	m
92	11	T	B	0	22	14	2	2	2	2	3	3	3	m
93	11	T	A	0	20	15	2	2	2	2	3	3	3	3
94	11	P	A	0	29	4	0	0	0	0	1	1	1	1
95	11	T	B	0	19	14	2	2	2	2	3	3	3	3
96	11	P	B	0	28	12	1	2	m	2	3	2	2	m
97	11	P	B	0	21	8	1	1	1	1	1	1	m	m
98	11	T	B	0	30	15	2	2	2	2	3	3	3	3
99	11	T	B	1	27	15	2	2	2	2	3	3	3	3
100	12	P	A	0	25	7	0	1	1	1	1	2	1	2
101	12	T	B	0	35	7	1	1	1	1	1	2	2	2
102	12	T	A	0	33	8	1	1	1	1	2	2	2	2

observations because the causes of urinary track infections are likely to be more similar in repeated episodes in the same person than in separate episodes in different people. Therefore, Hooton and colleagues included repeat episodes in their analysis, which increased the power of their study.

2.9. *Other examples*

Clinical researchers in the fields of ophthalmology, orthopedics, and dentistry have a distinct advantage over cardiologists, neurologists, and hepatologists. That is while humans have only one heart, one brain, and one liver, we have two eyes, thirty-two teeth or so, and most of our joints in duplicates. In those fields with duplicate organs, it is possible to follow (or assess) a single subject and have multiple observations. For the cases with outcomes that are observed more than once in a single subject, you must use special methods to deal with outcomes that can occur in more than one body part in the same person.

In a study of complications after breast implantation most women had bilateral implants.[5] Some had multiple implants in the same breast. The investigators therefore performed follow-up of each breast implant until a complication occurred, the implant was removed, or the end of follow-up occurred. The survival times of the implants for the same woman are dependent.

In a study of the relationship of vitamin D to development of osteoarthritis of knees, the investigators used the fact that their participants had two knees to their advantage.[6] Although the Framingham's study consists of

Table 6. Four successive two-week seizure counts for each 59 patients of epileptics.

ID	y1	y2	y3	Y4	treat	baseline	Age	ID	y1	y2	y3	y4	treat	baseline	Age
1	5	3	3	3	0	11	31	31	0	4	3	0	1	19	20
2	3	5	3	3	0	11	30	32	3	6	1	3	1	10	20
3	2	4	0	5	0	6	25	33	2	6	7	4	1	19	18
4	4	4	1	4	0	8	36	34	4	3	1	3	1	24	24
5	7	18	9	21	0	66	22	35	22	17	19	16	1	31	30
6	5	2	8	7	0	27	29	36	5	4	7	4	1	14	35
7	6	4	0	2	0	12	31	37	2	4	0	4	1	11	57
8	40	20	23	12	0	52	42	38	3	7	7	7	1	67	20
9	5	6	6	5	0	23	37	39	4	18	72	5	1	41	22
10	14	13	6	0	0	10	28	40	2	1	1	0	1	7	28
11	26	12	6	22	0	52	36	41	0	2	4	0	1	22	23
12	12	6	8	5	0	33	24	42	5	4	0	3	1	13	40
13	4	4	6	2	0	18	23	43	11	14	25	15	1	46	43
14	7	9	12	14	0	42	36	44	10	5	3	8	1	36	21
15	16	24	10	9	0	87	26	45	19	7	6	7	1	38	35
16	11	0	0	5	0	50	26	46	1	1	2	4	1	7	25
17	0	0	3	3	0	18	28	47	6	10	8	8	1	36	26
18	37	29	28	29	0	111	31	48	2	1	0	0	1	11	25
19	3	5	2	5	0	18	32	49	102	65	72	63	1	151	22
20	3	0	6	7	0	20	21	50	4	3	2	4	1	22	32
21	3	4	3	4	0	12	29	51	8	6	5	7	1	42	25
22	3	4	3	4	0	9	21	52	1	3	1	5	1	32	35
23	2	3	3	5	0	17	32	53	18	11	28	13	1	56	21
24	8	12	2	8	0	28	25	54	6	3	4	0	1	24	41
25	18	24	76	25	0	55	30	55	3	5	4	3	1	16	32
26	2	1	2	1	0	9	40	56	1	23	19	8	1	22	26
27	3	1	4	2	0	10	19	57	2	3	0	1	1	25	21
28	13	15	13	12	0	47	22	58	0	0	0	0	1	13	36
29	11	14	9	8	1	76	18	59	1	4	3	2	1	12	37
30	8	17	9	4	1	38	32								

over 5000 subjects, only 556 participants had X-rays of their knees and assessments of their vitamin D intake and serum levels. Therefore, they did this by looking at both knees to maximize their statistical power.

3. Common Structures of Intra-unit Correlation for Dependent Data

The feature of dependent data is that the variance-covariance matrix of response variable is not diagonal but block diagonal.

Because the dependent data do not meet the independent requirement that is essential in classical statistical methods, special methods are needed to deal with it. For example, random effects models and/or mixed effects models are used for repeated measurement or longitudinal data and meta-analysis is used for multicenter clinical trial.[3] Many systematic researches have been achieved in the field. In this section, we try to demonstrate the connotations of dependent data, how to judge the type of the data set, to construct reasonable covariance structure or intra-unit correlations structure, draw valid scientific inferences for the data set. In this section, we focus on the common structures of intra-unit correlation of dependent data.[7]

3.1. *A simple case*

We first consider the simplest case of a paired design. In this paired design, the subjects are independent, while two observations on the same subjects are correlated. If we assume the correlations of two observations of subjects are equal, say ρ, then the correlation matrix of $2m$ observations from m subjects could be

$$\boldsymbol{R}_Y = \begin{bmatrix} \boldsymbol{R} & \mathbf{0} & \cdots & \mathbf{0} \\ \mathbf{0} & \boldsymbol{R} & \cdots & \mathbf{0} \\ \vdots & \vdots & \ddots & \vdots \\ \mathbf{0} & \mathbf{0} & \cdots & \boldsymbol{R} \end{bmatrix} \quad (1)$$

where,

$$\boldsymbol{R} = \begin{bmatrix} 1 & \rho \\ \rho & 1 \end{bmatrix} \quad (2)$$

where $\mathbf{0}$ is 0 matrix with all elements being 0, $\boldsymbol{R}_Y$ is block diagonal matrix with $\boldsymbol{R}$ in diagonal.

For random block trial, we have a treatments and b blocks. While individuals from different blocks are independent, those from the same block tend to be similar and correlated. Because the individuals in the same block are in the same status, so we can assume that there is a positive correlation, ρ, between any two individuals from the same block. The intra-block correlation matrix is defined as

$$\boldsymbol{R}_2 = \begin{bmatrix} 1 & \rho & \cdots & \rho \\ \rho & 1 & \cdots & \rho \\ \vdots & \vdots & \ddots & \vdots \\ \rho & \rho & \vdots & 1 \end{bmatrix} \quad (3)$$

$a \times b$ observations form a correlation matrix which has the same structure as $\boldsymbol{R}_Y$ in (1). Matrices in diagonal block of $\boldsymbol{R}_Y$ have the same structure as $\boldsymbol{R}_2$. It is obviously that $\boldsymbol{R}$ in (1) is a special case of $\boldsymbol{R}_2$.

Now let's consider some types of correlation structure of longitudinal studies. The defining characteristic of a longitudinal study is that individuals are measured repeatedly through time in a follow-up study. Correlation structures vary from data set. The commonly used correlation matrices are equal correlation, neighbor correlation, autocorrelation and unstructured correlation, etc.

3.1.1. *Equal correlation*

It is similar to $\boldsymbol{R}_2$, We also refer to equal correlation as exchangeable or compound symmetry.

3.1.2. *Neighbor correlation*

Neighbor correlation is that only two closed observations are correlated, others are independent. For 5 times repeated measurement, the correlation matrix is given by

$$\boldsymbol{R}_3 = \begin{bmatrix} 1 & \rho_1 & 0 & 0 & 0 \\ \rho_1 & 1 & \rho_2 & 0 & 0 \\ 0 & \rho_2 & 1 & \rho_3 & 0 \\ 0 & 0 & \rho_3 & 1 & \rho_4 \\ 0 & 0 & 0 & \rho_4 & 0 \end{bmatrix} . \tag{4}$$

When the correlations of two closed observations are equal, the correlation is refered to as stationary 1-dependence), otherwise, nonstationary 1-dependence. Stationary 2-dependence has the structure as follows

$$\boldsymbol{R}_4 = \begin{bmatrix} 1 & \rho & \rho & 0 & 0 \\ \rho & 1 & \rho & \rho & 0 \\ \rho & \rho & 1 & \rho & \rho \\ 0 & \rho & \rho & 1 & \rho \\ 0 & 0 & \rho & \rho & 1 \end{bmatrix} . \tag{5}$$

It is not difficult to extend to stationary k-dependence. Obviously, stationary correlation is a special case of nonstationary, and exchangeable correlation is a special case of stationary.

3.1.3. *Autocorrelation*

Autocorrelation means that correlation depends on the spacing of two measurements. The correlation between a pair of measurements on the same subject decays towards 0 as the time separation between the measurements increases. If the correlation of two observations next to each other is ρ, the correlation of two separated observations is ρ's power of number of the observations separated. For 5 times repeated measurements, the correlation matrix is given by

$$\boldsymbol{R}_5 = \begin{bmatrix} 1 & \rho & \rho^2 & \rho^3 & \rho^4 \\ \rho & 1 & \rho & \rho^2 & \rho^3 \\ \rho^2 & \rho & 1 & \rho & \rho^2 \\ \rho^3 & \rho^2 & \rho & 1 & \rho \\ \rho^4 & \rho^3 & \rho^2 & \rho & 1 \end{bmatrix}. \tag{6}$$

We refer to (6) as the first order autocorrelation or the first order autoregressive process. A natural extension of (6) is given by (7), $\boldsymbol{R}_6$, the correlation is inversed to the time interval or spacing of two measurements.

$$\boldsymbol{R}_6 = \begin{bmatrix} 1 & \rho^{t_2-t_1} & \rho^{t_3-t_1} & \rho^{t_4-t_1} & \rho^{t_5-t_1} \\ \rho^{t_2-t_1} & 1 & \rho^{t_3-t_2} & \rho^{t_4-t_2} & \rho^{t_5-t_2} \\ \rho^{t_3-t_1} & \rho^{t_3-t_2} & 1 & \rho^{t_4-t_3} & \rho^{t_5-t_3} \\ \rho^{t_4-t_1} & \rho^{t_4-t_2} & \rho^{t_4-t_3} & 1 & \rho^{t_5-t_4} \\ \rho^{t_5-t_1} & \rho^{t_5-t_2} & \rho^{t_5-t_3} & \rho^{t_5-t_4} & 1 \end{bmatrix}. \tag{7}$$

3.1.4. *Unstructured or general structure*

In this case elements on nondiagonal of block matrix $\boldsymbol{R}$ are unequal.

3.1.5. *Independent, zero correlation*

Elements on nondiagonal of block matrix $\boldsymbol{R}$ are 0.

The relationships of the matrices mentioned above are as follow

$$\text{independent} \subset \text{exchangeable} \subset \text{autocorrelation} \subset \text{stationary}$$
$$\subset \text{nonstationary} \subset \text{unstructured}$$

where A $\subset$ B means A is a special case of B.

3.2. *Complicated cases*

In random cluster sample study, individuals in the same cluster (household, class in school, group in enterprise, etc.) tend to act in a similar way on healthy attitude, eating habit, and so on, and share the same environment, etc. If family is the unit in cluster sampling, genetic factor should be considered because the observations measured on the members from the same family are correlated. For example, in a cluster sampling, a simple random sample of 54 households was drawn.[8] The blood pressure observations of 209 subjects were detected. Let Y_{ij} represent a response variable, systolic pressure, for member j ($j = 1, 2, \ldots, n_i$) in household i ($i = 1, 2, \ldots, 54$). Where $j = 1$ stands for father, 2 for mother, 3 and more for children.

Generally speaking, if the interesting variable is affected by genetic factor or other family factors, the correlation between parents is lower than the correlations between father and children, mother and children, and children themselves. In this case, a special but common correlation structure could be defined as (for example, 4 persons in a family with parents and two children)

$$\begin{array}{c} \\ Y_{i1} \\ Y_{i2} \\ Y_{i3} \\ Y_{i4} \end{array} \begin{array}{c} \begin{array}{cccc} Y_{i1} & Y_{i2} & Y_{i3} & Y_{i4} \end{array} \\ \begin{pmatrix} 1 & r_1 & r_2 & r_2 \\ r_1 & 1 & r_3 & r_3 \\ r_2 & r_3 & 1 & r_4 \\ r_2 & r_3 & r_4 & 1 \end{pmatrix} \end{array} \begin{array}{l} \\ \text{father} \\ \text{mother} \\ \text{child 1} \\ \text{child 2} \end{array} . \tag{8}$$

In fact, the correlation structure matrix of 4 members (parents and two children) in one family in the example mentioned above is

$$\begin{pmatrix} 1.0000 & 0.2056 & 0.4212 & 0.4212 \\ 0.2056 & 1.0000 & 0.4292 & 0.4292 \\ 0.4212 & 0.4292 & 1.0000 & 0.5622 \\ 0.4212 & 0.4292 & 0.5622 & 1.0000 \end{pmatrix}.$$

For stratified cluster sampling and other data with hierarchical structure, the same strategy could be used to construct the intra-cluster correlation matrices.

In the crossover design, each subject is randomized to a sequence of two or more treatments and hence acts as his own control for treatment comparisons. In the simplest paired 2 × 2 crossover design, two subjects are paired, the first subject in the same paired receives either of two treatments in randomized order in two successive treatment periods which often separated by a washout period, while the other received two treatments in adverse order to the first one in two successive treatment periods. There are 3 possible correlations in this type of data: (1) correlation between two observations of the same subject in two periods; (2) correlation between two subjects in the same paired in the same period; and (3) correlation between two subjects in the same paired in different periods. The correlation structure, therefore, could be defined as:

		Subject 1		Subjects 2	
		Period 1	Period 2	Period 1	Period 2
Subject 1	Period 1	1	r_1	r_2	r_3
	Period 2	r_1	1	r_3	r_2
Subject 2	Period 1	r_2	r_3	1	r_1
	Period 2	r_3	r_2	r_1	1

In multicenter clinical trial, although the protocol and standard operating procedures are implemented similarly at all centers, the level and opinions of doctors and nurses, equipments, and medical conditions, etc., vary from the centers. This is so-called center-effects. Subjects in the same center are correlated. The repeated observations through time from the same subjects are also correlated. This is hierarchical structure data. If subjects from different centers are independent, the intra-center correlation structure could be defined as (3 visits for each subject):

		Subject 1			Subject 2			$\cdots$	Subject n		
		t_1	t_2	t_3	t_1	t_2	t_3	$\cdots$	t_1	t_2	t_3
Subject 1	t_1	1	r_1	r_1	r_2	r_2	r_2		r_2	r_2	r_2
	t_2	r_1	1	r_1	r_2	r_2	r_2	$\cdots$	r_2	r_2	r_2
	t_3	r_1	r_1	1	r_2	r_2	r_2	$\cdots$	r_2	r_2	r_2
Subject 2	t_1	r_2	r_1	r_2	r_2	1	r_1		r_2	r_2	r_2
	t_2	r_2	r_2	r_2	1	r_1	r_1	$\cdots$	r_2	r_2	r_2
	t_3	r_2	r_2	r_2	r_1	r_1	1		r_2	r_2	r_2
	$\cdots$		$\cdots$			$\cdots$				$\cdots$	
Subject n	t_1	r_2	r_2	r_2	r_2	r_2	r_2		1	r_1	r_1
	t_2	r_2	r_2	r_2	r_2	r_2	r_2	$\cdots$	r_1	1	r_1
	t_3	r_2	r_2	r_2	r_2	r_2	r_2		r_1	r_1	1

Although, for a real data set, the correlation structure could be defined and selected by statistical methods, the author suggests that the biological and medical backgrounds should be considered to get a reasonable and acceptable correlation matrix structure.

4. ANOVA Methods and Its Limitation

4.1. *Parameter estimations for dependent data*

4.1.1. *Estimation of means*

If there are n observations of variable X, denoted by $x_1, x_2, x_3, \ldots, x_n$ with mean $\bar{X}$ and variance σ^2. We assume the data are dependent.

(1) x_i is correlated with x_j with a correlate coefficient ρ

If x_i is correlated with x_j with a correlation coefficient ρ (ρ is assumed to be larger than 0 without losing general), thus the variance of $\bar{X}$ was

$$\begin{aligned} \operatorname{var}(\bar{X}) &= \frac{1}{n^2}\operatorname{cov}(x_1 + x_2 + \cdots + x_n,\, x_1 + x_2 + \cdots + x_n) \\ &= \frac{1}{n^2}[n\sigma^2 + n(n-1)\rho\sigma^2] \\ &= \frac{\sigma^2}{n}[1 + (n-1)\rho]. \end{aligned} \tag{9}$$

Formula (9) shows that standard error of mean is larger when the data are dependent than the case when the data are independent. Moreover, it is in proportion to correlation. In this case, the confidence interval of population mean is as follows

$$\bar{X} \pm t_{n-1,\nu}\frac{\sigma}{\sqrt{n}}\sqrt{1 + (n-1)\rho}. \tag{10}$$

It is wider than that when the data are independent. When intra-unit correlation is 0, the confidence interval given by (10) is similar to the confidence interval when data are independent.

(2) x_i is correlated with x_j with autocorrelation

If x_i is correlated with x_j with autocorrelation

$$\operatorname{cov}(x_i, x_j) = \sigma^2\rho^{|i-j|}. \tag{11}$$

The variance of

$$\operatorname{var}(\bar{X}) = \frac{1}{n^2}[n + 2(n-1)\rho + 2(n-2)\rho^2 + \cdots + 2\rho^{n-1}]\sigma^2. \tag{12}$$

(3) Correlation between x_i and x_j is unstructured

If the correlation between x_i and x_j is unstructured

$$\operatorname{cov}(x_i, x_j) = \lfloor \rho_{ij}\sigma^2 \rfloor_{n\times n}. \tag{13}$$

The variance of $\bar{X}$ is

$$\operatorname{var}(\bar{X}) = \frac{1}{n^2}\left[n + 2\left(\sum_{i\neq j}\rho_{ij}\right)\right]\sigma^2. \tag{14}$$

Thus, the standard error of mean in this case when the data are dependent is larger than the one when the data are independent from each other. The standard error is in proportion to the correlation as well. The confidence interval is wider than that of independent data.

4.1.2. *Estimation of rate*

The independent binary data should generally be handled by the methods based on binominal distribution. Let incidence rate be π and its variance be $\pi(1-\pi)$, then the standard error is $\sqrt{\pi(1-\pi)/n}$.

If the data are correlated with each other, the variance and the standard error of rate increase. For example, in Example 2, the total incident rate is $\pi = 30/104 = 0.2885$, the variance is 0.00197 and 95% CI is 0.2038–0.3855 if we apply the methods based on binominal distribution. And its 95% CI is 0.2014–0.3756 if we apply the methods based on normal approximation.

However, the actual variance of the incident rate in each family is 0.00520, much larger than that given by the pure binominal distribution. This is because that the incidence, "visiting doctors in the last year", has a family aggregation. As a result, we underestimated the variance of dependent incidences by applying methods based on binomial distribution.

The classic way of handling dichotomous data is firstly coding the incidence that happens as 1, otherwise, as 0, and then applying Eq. (9) to the data. When it comes to a dichotomous data with equal correlation, the standard error of rate is

$$\sigma_\pi = \sqrt{\frac{\pi(1-\pi)}{n}[1+(n-1)\rho]}. \tag{15}$$

Others can be handled in similar ways.

4.2. *ANOVA with random effect*

We begin with the repeated one-way testing designs, of which the block design is the simplest case. We may assume that there are a treatments and b blocks. The model of ANOVA can be represented as

$$y_{ij} = \mu + \tau_j + e_{ij}. \tag{16}$$

In the equation below, μ is the population's mean, τ_j is the effect of the jth treatment ($j = 1, 2, \ldots, a$), e_{ij} is the total residual error of observations receiving the jth treatment in the ith block.

When we apply a randomized block design, the units in the same block may have good homogeneity, while units in different blocks may have many differences. This is the characteristic of block design that makes the observations in every block to be homoplasy, which is called intra-block correlation. For this moment, the error term e_{ij} may be denoted as

$$e_{ij} = \nu_i + u_{ij}. \tag{17}$$

ν_i is the residual error of the ith block ($i = 1, \ldots, b$), u_{ij} is the residual error of observations receiving the jth treatment in the ith block. Therefore, the ANOVA model of block design should be

$$y_{ij} = \mu + \tau_j + \nu_i + u_{ij}. \tag{18}$$

In most cases, the treatment factors of a block design are fixed effects, while blocks are random effects. Namely, τ_j is fixed effect, μ_j is the mean of observations in the jth level, and ν_i is random effects with

$$\begin{gathered} \tau_j = \mu_j - \mu, \quad \Sigma\tau_j = 0 \\ \nu_i = \mu_i - \mu, \quad \Sigma\nu_i = 0, \\ \mathrm{var}(\nu_i) = \sigma_2^2, \quad \text{and } \mathrm{cov}(\nu_i, \nu_{i'}) = 0,\ i \neq i', \end{gathered} \tag{19}$$

where μ_i is the mean of the ith block. u_{ij} is the random effect, and

$$\begin{gathered} u_{ij} = y_{ij} - \mu - \tau_j - \nu_i, \quad \Sigma u_{ij} = 0, \\ \mathrm{var}(u_{ij}) = \sigma_1^2, \quad \text{and } \mathrm{cov}(u_{ij},\ u_{i'j'}) = 0,\ j \neq j' \\ \mathrm{cov}(u_{ij}, \nu_k) = 0 \quad \text{for all } i, j, k. \end{gathered} \tag{20}$$

In this way, the variance of y_{ij} is

$$\mathrm{var}(y_{ij}) = \sigma_2^2 + \sigma_1^2, \tag{21}$$

the covariance is

$$\mathrm{cov}(y_{ij}, y_{ij'}) = \mathrm{cov}(\nu_i + u_{ij}, \nu_i + u_{ij'}) = \sigma_2^2,\ j \neq j',$$

and others are 0.

Expressed by matrix, the variance and covariance of y_{ij} is

$$\mathrm{cov}(e_{ij}) = \sigma^2 \begin{pmatrix} \boldsymbol{R} & 0 & \cdots & 0 \\ 0 & \boldsymbol{R} & \cdots & 0 \\ \vdots & \vdots & \ddots & \vdots \\ 0 & 0 & \cdots & \boldsymbol{R} \end{pmatrix}_{ab\times ab}. \tag{22}$$

Here, $\sigma^2 = \sigma_1^2 + \sigma_2^2$,

$$\boldsymbol{R} = \begin{pmatrix} 1 & \rho & \cdots & \rho \\ \rho & 1 & \cdots & \rho \\ \vdots & \vdots & \ddots & \vdots \\ \rho & \rho & \cdots & 1 \end{pmatrix}_{a\times a}. \tag{23}$$

The intra-unit correlation coefficient is

$$\rho = \frac{\sigma_2^2}{\sigma_1^2 + \sigma_2^2}. \tag{24}$$

Based on the idea of ANOVA, it is obvious that

$$\begin{aligned} E(MS_{\text{treatment}}) &= b\sum_{i=1}^{a} \tau_1^2/(a-1) + \sigma_1^2, \\ E(MS_{\text{block}}) &= b\sigma_2^2 + \sigma_1^2, \\ E(MS_{\text{residual}}) &= \sigma_1^2. \end{aligned} \tag{25}$$

And the variance component σ_1^2 and σ_2^2 are

$$\begin{aligned} \sigma_1^2 &= E(MS_{\text{residual}}), \\ \sigma_2^2 &= \frac{MS_{\text{block}} - MS_{\text{residual}}}{b}. \end{aligned} \tag{26}$$

If we substitute σ_1^2 and σ_2^2 in Eq. (24) by equations above, the intra-correlation coefficient is

$$\rho = \frac{MS_{\text{block}} - MS_{\text{residual}}}{MS_{\text{block}} + (b-1)MS_{\text{residual}}}. \tag{27}$$

If every block has a different size (e.g. missing values), the intra-unit correlation of randomized block design data can be denoted as

$$\rho = \frac{MS_{\text{block}} - MS_{\text{residual}}}{MS_{\text{block}} + (m_0-1)MS_{\text{residual}}}, \tag{28}$$

Table 7. ANOVA of the serum coagulation time of four methods.

Source	SS	DF	MS	F	P
Total	105.7787	31	3.4122		
Between Groups	13.0163	3	4.3388	6.62	0.0025
In Groups	92.7624	28	3.3129		
Between Block	78.9888	7	11.2841	17.20	0.0000
Residual	13.7738	21	0.6559		

Table 8. ANOVA of log AUC.

Source	SS	DF	MS	F	P
Total	15.67277346	95			
ID(sequence)	0.96107428	20	0.04805371	4.71	<0.0001
Sequence	0.06927165	3	0.02309055	2.26	0.0892
Period	0.13519601	3	0.04506534	4.42	0.0068
Treat	13.83396718	3	4.61132239	452.05	<0.0001
Residual	0.67326434	66	0.01020097		

where

$$m_0 = \bar{m} - \frac{\sum(m_i - \bar{m})^2}{(a-1)\sum m_i}. \tag{29}$$

4.3. *Example 9. Analysis of randomized block design data*

The analysis of Example 1. We begin with the ANOVA Table 7.[9]

The variance component σ_1^2 and σ_2^2 are

$$\sigma_0^2 = MS_{\text{residual}} = 0.6559,$$

$$\sigma_1^2 = \frac{MS_{\text{block}} - MS_{\text{residual}}}{b} = \frac{11.2841 - 0.6559}{4} = 2.6571.$$

And the intra-correlation coefficient is

$$r = \frac{\sigma_1^2}{\sigma_0^2 + \sigma_1^2} = \frac{2.6571}{0.6599 + 2.6571} = 0.8020.$$

Though ANOVA of correlated data is similar to that of traditional randomized block design in process and result, ANOVA of correlated data not only answers the question, “whether there is a difference between treatment groups”, on which that of traditional randomized block design emphasizes, but also puts more emphasis on the further decomposition of variance and affords the intra-unit correlation. Thus, its model is more precise with richer information.

4.4. *Example* 10. 4 × 4 *cross-over design*

The analysis of log AUC data in Example 4. For this moment, the fixed effects that we should take into consideration is 4 treatments, A, B, C, D, 4 different periods and 4 different sequences. The 4 observations of the same subject are correlated.

And,

$$\sigma_0^2 = MS_{\text{Residual}} = 0.01020097,$$

$$\sigma_1^2 = \frac{MS_{ID(\text{Sequence})} - MS_{\text{Residual}}}{b} = \frac{0.04805371 - 0.01020097}{4}$$

$$= 0.009463185.$$

Accordingly,

$$\rho = \frac{MS_{ID(\text{Sequence})} - MS_{\text{Residual}}}{MS_{ID(\text{Sequence})} + (b-1)MS_{\text{Residual}}}$$

$$= \frac{0.04805371 - 0.01020097}{0.04805371 + (4-1) \times 0.01020097} = 0.4812.$$

4.5. *The condition of using ANOVA*

The ANOVA is limited to fairly balanced designs where there are tidy partitions of the total sum of squares. The model should be fairly simple so that a suitable covariance structure (symmetry) for the observations can be produced. For example, if $t = 4$ in repeated measurement data, the covariance matrix should be

$$\begin{pmatrix} \sigma_{11} & \sigma_{12} & \sigma_{13} & \sigma_{14} \\ \sigma_{21} & \sigma_{22} & \sigma_{23} & \sigma_{24} \\ \sigma_{31} & \sigma_{32} & \sigma_{33} & \sigma_{34} \\ \sigma_{41} & \sigma_{42} & \sigma_{43} & \sigma_{44} \end{pmatrix}.$$

So the symmetry means

(1) $\sigma_{ii} = \sigma_{jj} = \sigma^2$,
(2) $\sigma_{ij} = \rho\sigma^2$, $i \neq j$.

In other wards, symmetry means equal variance and equal intra-unit correlation.

When the data are not symmetry, the ANOVA would increase type I error. In 1958, Greenhouse and Geisse suggested a correction coefficient

$$\varepsilon = \frac{t^2(\bar{\sigma}_{ii} - \bar{\sigma}_{..})^2}{(t-1)(\sum \sigma_{ij}^2 + t^2\bar{\sigma}_{..}^2 - 2t\sum \bar{\sigma}_i^2)} \tag{30}$$

where t represents the times of repeated measurement, $\bar{\sigma}_{ii}$ is the average of variances in diagonal of covariance matrix, $\bar{\sigma}_{..}$ is the average of all elements in covariance matrix, and $\bar{\sigma}_i$ is the average of elements in ith row of covariance matrix.

Greenhouse and Geisse have shown that, $1/(t-1) \le \varepsilon \le 1$. If ε is not equal to 1, a modified $F = MS_{\text{Treatment}}/MS_{\text{Residual}}$ would not follow F distribution with degree of freedom $\nu_{\text{Treatment}}$ and ν_{Residual} but follow F distribution with degree of freedom $\varepsilon\nu_{\text{Treatment}}$ and $\varepsilon\nu_{\text{Residual}}$. Because of the cutting down of degree of freedom, the modified F test is conservative.

For the data in Example 1, the variance-covariance matrix is

$$\begin{pmatrix} 2.40286 & & & \\ 3.23143 & 5.26411 & & \\ 2.13857 & 3.00518 & 2.29125 & \\ 2.13143 & 3.41536 & 2.02036 & 3.29357 \end{pmatrix}.$$

Greenhouse–Geisser's $\varepsilon = 0.7996$. Thus, the degree of freedoms

$$\nu_{\text{Treatment}} = 0.7996 \times 3 = 2.4,$$

$$\nu_{\text{Residual}} = 0.7996 \times 21 = 16.8,$$

then $F = 6.62$, $P = 0.0056$, larger than $P = 0.0025$.

In 1970, Huynh and Feldt have proved that when $\varepsilon = 1$, the F test is valid. If covariance matrix is symmetry, then $\varepsilon = 1$ or otherwise $\varepsilon < 1$. On the other hand, $\varepsilon = 1$ does not necessary implies the covariance being symmetry. The exception is for 2×2 covariance matrix for twice repeated measurements, ε always equal to 1 even if the variances are unequal.

We should select a suitable method for dependent data according to the feature of the data set. Unfortunately, the suitable systematic methods for all types of dependent data have not been developed. Only several methods for special data set can be used now. For instance, the mixed models are employed for repeated measurements or data from randomized block design, crossover design, and some special procedures for longitudinal data, etc. The multilevel models analysis[7] would be used if the structure of variance-covariance matrix is block diagonal. For general structure of variance-covariance matrix, which is not block diagonal, generalized least square procedure with Newton–Raphson iterations may be useful. Further research is needed.

5. GEE for Dependent Data

Generalized estimating equations (GEE) was put forward by Liang Zeger[10] which is an extension of generalized linear models that provides a unified and flexible approach to analysis of data from a longitudinal study. Of particular relevance when the repeated measurements are binary variables or counts, and a number of time dependent covariates are also measured (Qiguang Chen,[11] Lingping Xiong *et al.*[12]). GEE plays an important rule in modeling the possible correlations among the repeated observations for a given subject.[13]

5.1. *Introduction of GEE*

The key ideas are presented in terms of repeated measurements with the simplest dependent structure. Let y_{ij} be the observation of jth measurement of the ith unit, where $i = 1, 2, \ldots, n$ and $j = 1, 2, \ldots, m_i$. $X_{ij} = (x_{1ij}, x_{2ij}, \ldots, x_{pij})$ represents the explanatory variables. The observations from the same unit are likely to be correlated, but the observations from different units are assumed in general to be independent.

If the marginal distribution of response variable y_{ij} is one of exponential family, then, by the theory of generalized linear models, the density functions would be

$$f(y_{ij}) = \exp[\{y_{ij}\mu_{ij} - a(\mu_{ij}) + b(y_{ij})\}\phi], \tag{31}$$

where ϕ is known as dispersion parameter or additional scale, $\mu_{ij} = h(\eta_{ij})$, $\eta_{ij} = \boldsymbol{X}_{ij}\boldsymbol{\beta}$. It can be proved that $E(y_{ij}) = a'(\mu_{ij})$, $\text{var}(y_{ij} = a''(\mu_{ij})/\phi$.

For random effects model, we have

$$\begin{cases} \hat{y}_{ij} = \mu_{ij} \\ g(\mu_{ij}) = \beta_0 + \beta_1 x_{1ij} + \cdots + \beta_p x_{pij} \end{cases}, \tag{32}$$

where $g(\cdot) = h^{-1}(\cdot)$ as a link function. If there is correlation between the repeated observations, the correlation between n_i observations in unit i can be described by working correlation matrix $\boldsymbol{R}_i(\alpha)$. The times of repeated measurement on subjects are different from each other, so the ranks of correlation matrices are also different from each other. $R_i(\alpha)$ depends on unknown parameter α, to which we refer as correlate parameter. For instance, for $\boldsymbol{R}_2$ in (3)

$$\rho_{st} = \begin{cases} 1 & \text{if } s = t, \\ \alpha & \text{if } s \neq t. \end{cases} \tag{33}$$

for $\boldsymbol{R}_4$ in (5)

$$\rho_{st} = \begin{cases} 1 & \text{if } s = t, \\ \alpha & \text{if } 0 < |s-t| \leq 2, \\ 0 & \text{if } |s-t| > 2. \end{cases} \tag{34}$$

for $\boldsymbol{R}_5$ in (6)

$$\rho_{st} = \begin{cases} 1 & \text{if } s = t, \\ \alpha^{|s-t|} & \text{if } s \neq t. \end{cases} \tag{35}$$

then the variance-covariance matrix of $\boldsymbol{y}_i = (y_{i1}, y_{i2}, \ldots, y_{im_i})'$ has the form

$$\boldsymbol{V}_i = \boldsymbol{A}_i^{1/2} \boldsymbol{R}(\alpha) \boldsymbol{A}_i^{1/2} / \phi, \tag{36}$$

where $\boldsymbol{A}_i$ is diagonal matrix with the elements $h(\mu_{ij}) = \nu_{ij}\phi$ in diagonal, which are the function of the variance ν and the mean μ of y. Liang and Zeger[10] defined the GEE as

$$\sum_{i=1}^{n} \boldsymbol{D}_i' \boldsymbol{V}_i^{-1} \boldsymbol{E}_i = 0, \tag{37}$$

where $\boldsymbol{D}_i = \frac{\partial \boldsymbol{\mu}_i}{\partial \boldsymbol{\beta}}$, $\boldsymbol{E}_i = \boldsymbol{y}_i - \boldsymbol{\mu}_i$, and $\boldsymbol{\mu}_i = (\mu_{i1}, \mu_{i2}, \ldots, \mu_{im_i})'$.

5.2. *Parameters estimations of GEE*

There are three types of parameters in GEE, covariate coefficients $\boldsymbol{\beta}$, the scale parameter ϕ, the correlation parameter α. But ϕ and α are functions of $\boldsymbol{\beta}$. We can get the estimation of $\boldsymbol{\beta}$ only if ϕ and α are known. Consequently, the estimation procedure of GEE is iterative.

The initial value of $\boldsymbol{\beta}$ will be the estimations from generalized linear model under the assumption that the observations are independent of one another, say $\boldsymbol{\beta}_i$.

The crude residuals of the model is

$$e_{ij} = y_{ij} - \mu_{ij} = y_{ij} - g^{-1}(\beta_0 + \beta_1 x_{1ij} + \cdots + \beta_p x_{pij}). \quad (38)$$

The Pearson residuals are

$$r_{ij} = \frac{\hat{y}_{ij} - \mu_{ij}}{\sqrt{\nu_{ij}}}. \quad (39)$$

Thus

$$\hat{\phi} = \sum_{i=1}^{n}\sum_{j=1}^{m_i} r_{ij}/(N-p). \quad (40)$$

The intra-unit correlation can be estimated from the current Pearson residuals. For exchangeable correlation, we have

$$\hat{\alpha} = \sum_{i=1}^{n}\left[\frac{\sum_{j=1}^{m_i}\sum_{l=1}^{m_i} r_{ij}r_{il} - \sum_{j=1}^{m_i} r_{ij}^2}{m_i(m_i-1)}\right] \Bigg/ \left[\sum_{i=1}^{n}\frac{\sum_{j=1}^{m_i} r_{ij}^2}{m_i}\right]. \quad (41)$$

For first order autocorrelation

$$\hat{\alpha} = \sum_{i=1}^{n}\frac{\sum_{j=1}^{m_i-1} r_{ij}r_{ij+1}}{m_i-1} \Bigg/ \left[\sum_{i=1}^{n}\frac{\sum_{j=1}^{m_i} r_{ij}^2}{m_i}\right]. \quad (42)$$

For stationary k-dependence

$$\hat{\alpha} = \sum_{i=1}^{n}\left[\frac{\sum_{j=1}^{m_i} r_{ij}^2}{m_i}, \frac{\sum_{j=1}^{m_i-1} r_{ij}r_{ij+1}}{m_i-1}, \ldots, \frac{\sum_{j=1}^{m_i-k} r_{ij}r_{i,j+k}}{m_i-k}\right] \Bigg/ \left[\sum_{i=1}^{n}\frac{\sum_{j=1}^{m_i} r_{ij}^2}{m_i}\right], \quad (43)$$

where the first element of α is 1 and the elements after k-order are 0.

At a given iteration, the scale parameter ϕ and correlation parameters α can be estimated from the current Pearson residuals. Given the estimated of ϕ and α, we can calculate an updated estimate of $\boldsymbol{\beta}$ by iteratively reweighed least squares (IRLS). These two steps are iterated until the procedure convergence.

5.3. *Analysis of examples*

5.3.1. *Example* 11. *Analyses of the data in Example* 1

The random effect model is

$$y_{ij} = \beta_0 + \beta_2 g_{2ij} + \beta_3 g_{3ij} + \beta_4 g_{4ij} + e_{ij},$$

where g_1, g_2, g_3 and g_4 are dummy variables of treatment groups. The correlations between the observations of different treatments for the same subjects are assumed equal. Results are shown in Table 9.

Table 9. Estimated results of data in Example 1 by GEE.

Variables	Coefficient	*SE*	*Z*	*P*
g_2	0.4125	0.378783	1.09	0.276
g_3	0.6375	0.378783	1.68	0.092
g_4	1.7250	0.378783	4.55	0.000
Constant	9.3000	0.601958	15.45	0.000

Table 10. The results of fitting two GEE models for data in Example 3.

	Logistic				Probit			
	Coefficient	Std.	*Z*	*P*	Coefficient	Std.	*Z*	*P*
Group	−1.0144	0.4985	−2.03	0.042	−0.5611	0.2702	−2.08	0.038
Constant	2.1484	0.4039	5.32	0.000	1.2564	0.2086	6.02	0.000

Intra-subject correlation $\rho = 0.8020$. We obtain the same results as in Example 9.

5.3.2. *Example* 12. *Analysis of data in Example* 3

We fit both logistic regression model and probit model as follows

$$y_{ij} = \frac{e^{\alpha+\beta \text{ treat}}}{1+e^{\alpha+\beta \text{ treat}}} + e_{ij},$$

$$y_{ij} = \Phi^{-1}(\alpha + \beta \text{ treat}) + e_{ij},$$

where the subscripts of *treat* are omitted. Table 10 shows the results.

Two intra-litter correlation coefficients are estimated based on logistic model and probit model and they are all equal to 0.1556.

5.3.3. *Example* 13. *Analysis of data in Example* 8

Example 8 has count data, with successive two-week seizure counts for each of 59 epileptics. Poisson regression model will be used. In contrast to the examples mentioned above, beside treatment effects, the covariables, such as *age*, *ln*(*base*), and *time* effects, should also be considered. The mixed effect Poisson regression model for the data is

$$\ln(\lambda) = \alpha + \beta_1 \, treat + \beta_2 \, time + \beta_3 \, age + \beta_4 \, ln(base).$$

For repeated measurement data, the intra-subject correlation structure may be exchangeable or first order auto-correlation.

Table 11. GEE estimators for data in Example 8.

Parameter	Coefficient	SE	Z	P
Constant	−1.7760	0.3692	−4.81	<0.0001
Treat	−0.2938	0.1445	−2.03	0.0420
Time	−0.0443	0.0353	−1.26	0.2092
Age	0.0231	0.0067	3.46	0.0005
ln(base)	0.9817	0.0796	12.33	<0.0001

For exchangeable structure, intra-subject correlation estimated from GEEs is 0.7690, and deviance = 3551.0. For autocorrelate structure the intra-subject correlation is 0.7990^t, where t is time interval between two observations (1 unit of t is 2 weeks) and deviance = 3554.79.

The working matrix of autocorrelation structure is

$$\begin{matrix} 1.0000 & 0.4533 & 0.2055 & 0.0931 \\ 0.4533 & 1.0000 & 0.4533 & 0.2055 \\ 0.2055 & 0.4533 & 1.0000 & 0.4533 \\ 0.0931 & 0.2055 & 0.4533 & 1.0000 \end{matrix}$$

The numbers of parameter of two models are equal. Therefore, the smaller the deviance is, the better the model will be. According to this, we conclude that exchangeable structure is suitable for the data. Estimated results are shown in Table 11.

The results show that the two-week seizure counts for those in test group are significantly smaller than those in placebo group. The counts are related to age and the baseline. No evidence shows that the counts change over time.

GEE can cope with data with missing values. For the numerical data in a paired design or randomized block design, the paired t-test and ANOVA require the data are balanced without missing, while the GEE does not. Furthermore, when the times of measurement are not common to all the experimental units, or when the numbers of the unit in clusters are not the same, the use of GEE will still be applicable. Liang[9] has proved that if there are not too many missing values and missing is random, the GEE estimation is robust.

GEE obtains the estimation of covariance matrix $\boldsymbol{V}$ or working correlation matrix $\boldsymbol{R}$ by using simple regression or "moment" procedures based upon functions of the actual calculated raw residuals. Theoretically, the structure of working correlation matrix can be specified arbitrarily. However, GEE focuses on modeling the fixed effects rather than exploring the structure of the random component of the model. It does not consider the case where the explanatory variables have an influence on covariance of response variable.

6. Multilevel Models for Dependent Data

Many kinds of dependent data collected in medical and biological sciences have a *hierarchical* or *clustered* structure. We refer to a hierarchy as consisting of *units* grouped at different *levels*. For example, in a clustered sampling survey where the sampling units are families, offsprings may be the level 1 units in a 2-level structure where the level 2 units are the families. Repeated measurements are the level 1 units in a 2-level structure where the level 2 units are the individuals. Repeated measurements are the level 1 unit in a 3-level structure where the level 3 units are the hospitals and level 2 units are the patients. The existence of such data hierarchies is created by experimental design. Low levels are nested in the high levels.

6.1. *Introduction of multilevel model*

Multilevel model was put forward by Harver Goldstein[14] for the data with hierarchical or clustered structure. The key ideals are to estimate variances on each level and to address how the explanatory variables affect the variances. The multilevel model, therefore, enables data analysis to obtain statistically efficient estimations of regression coefficients, and provides correct standard errors, confidence intervals and significance tests by using the clustering information.

We discuss a simple 2-level model, without lose of generalizibility, of one explanatory variable x_1.

$$y_{ij} = \beta_{0j} + \beta_{ij}x_1 + \varepsilon_{ij} \tag{44}$$

i stands for level 1 units, j for level 2 units. $i = 1, \ldots, n_j; j = 1, \ldots, m$, where, β_{0j} and β_{1j} are random variables with

$$\beta_{0j} = \beta_0 + u_{0j}, \quad \beta_{1j} = \beta_1 + u_{1j},$$

where β_0 and β_1 are fixed parameters, u_{0j}, u_{1j} are random variables in level 2 with parameters

$$E(u_{0j}) = E(u_{1j}) = 0$$

$$\mathrm{var}(u_{0j}) = \sigma_{u0}^2, \quad \mathrm{var}(u_{1j}) = \sigma_{u1}^2, \quad \mathrm{cov}(u_{0j}, u_{1j}) = \sigma_{u01}.$$

ε_{ij} are random variables in level 1 with parameter

$$E(\varepsilon_{1j}) = 0, \quad \text{var}(\varepsilon_{ij}) = \sigma_0^2.$$

We also assume that $\text{cov}(\varepsilon_{ij}, u_{0j}) = \text{cov}(\varepsilon_{ij}, u_{1j}) = 0$.

We can now write the level 2 model in the form

$$y_{ij} = \beta_0 + \beta_1 x + (u_{0j} + u_{1j}x + \varepsilon_{ij}). \tag{45}$$

The model consists of a fixed part and a random part. In contrast to a general mixed effect model (for example, variance component model, mixed linear model, GEE), explanatory variables can be included in random part of multilevel model with random coefficients u_{1j}. The multilevel model, therefore, is also refered to as random coefficient model.

The covariance matrices is block diagonal

$$\boldsymbol{V} = \begin{pmatrix} \boldsymbol{V}_{n_1} & & & \\ & \boldsymbol{V}_{n_2} & & \\ & & \ddots & \\ & & & \boldsymbol{V}_{n_m} \end{pmatrix}. \tag{46}$$

If no covariate is included in the random part of the model, $\sigma_{u1}^2 = 0$ and the model reduces to a general mixed effects model with

$$\boldsymbol{V}_{n_i} = \text{cov}(y_{ij}|\boldsymbol{X\beta}) = \begin{pmatrix} \sigma_{u0}^2 + \sigma_0^2 & \sigma_{u0}^2 & \cdots & \sigma_{u0}^2 \\ \sigma_{u0}^2 & \sigma_{u0}^2 + \sigma_0^2 & \cdots & \sigma_{u0}^2 \\ \vdots & \vdots & \cdots & \vdots \\ \sigma_{u0}^2 & \sigma_{u0}^2 & \cdots & \sigma_{u0}^2 + \sigma_0^2 \end{pmatrix}_{n_i \times n_i}. \tag{47}$$

Equation (47) can be denoted as $\sigma_{u0}^2 \boldsymbol{J}_{(n_i)} + \sigma_0^2 \boldsymbol{I}_{(n_i)}$. Where, $\boldsymbol{J}_{(n)}$ is $n \times 1$ vector with all elements 1, $\boldsymbol{I}_{(n)}$ is n dimension unit matrix with all elements in diagonal 1, others 0. Then the intra-unit correlation can be estimated by

$$\rho = \frac{\text{cov}(u_{0j} + \varepsilon_{i_1 j} + u_{0j} + \varepsilon_{i_2 j})}{\sqrt{\text{var}(u_{0j} + \varepsilon_{i_1 j}) \cdot \text{var}(u_{0j} + \varepsilon_{i_2 j})}} = \frac{\sigma_{u0}^2}{\sigma_{u0}^2 + \sigma_0^2}. \tag{48}$$

If covariate was considered, $\sigma_{u1}^2 \neq 0$ and

$$\boldsymbol{V}_{n_i} = (\sigma_{u0}^2 + 2\sigma_{u01}x + \sigma_{u1}^2 x^2)\boldsymbol{J}_{(n_i)} + \sigma_0^2 \boldsymbol{I}_{(n_i)}. \tag{49}$$

The intra-unit correlation can be estimated by

$$\rho = \frac{\sigma_{u0}^2 + 2\sigma_{u01}x + \sigma_{u1}^2 x^2}{\sigma_{u0}^2 + 2\sigma_{u01}x + \sigma_{u1}^2 x^2 + \sigma_0^2}. \tag{50}$$

It is thus clear that intra-unit correlation has relation to the explanatory variables.

6.2. *Estimation of parameters of multilevel model*

Parameters in multilevel model can be estimated by iterative generalized least squares (IGLS)[14] or Restricted Iterative Generalized Least Squares (RIGLS).[15]

Let $\mathrm{cov}(\boldsymbol{Y}|\boldsymbol{X\beta}) = \boldsymbol{V}$, if $\boldsymbol{V}$ is known, then according to the generalized least square estimation

$$\hat{\boldsymbol{\beta}} = (\boldsymbol{X}^T\boldsymbol{V}^{-1}\boldsymbol{X})^{-1}\boldsymbol{X}^T\boldsymbol{V}^{-1}\boldsymbol{Y}, \quad \mathrm{cov}(\hat{\boldsymbol{\beta}}) = (\boldsymbol{X}^T\boldsymbol{V}^{-1}\boldsymbol{X})^{-1}. \tag{51}$$

But in fact, $\boldsymbol{V}$ is usually unknown and expressed by random coefficients. For known $\boldsymbol{\beta}$ we form the residuals of y_{ij}

$$\tilde{\boldsymbol{Y}} = \{\tilde{y}_{ij}\} = \{y_{ij} - \boldsymbol{X}_{ij}\boldsymbol{\beta}\}. \tag{52}$$

If we form the cross-product matrix $\tilde{\boldsymbol{Y}}\tilde{\boldsymbol{Y}}^T$) we see that the expected value of this is simply $\boldsymbol{V}$. From the equation

$$\mathrm{vec}(\tilde{\boldsymbol{Y}}\tilde{\boldsymbol{Y}}^T) = \mathrm{vec}(\boldsymbol{V}) + \boldsymbol{R}, \tag{53}$$

we estimate parameters σ_{u0}^2, σ_{u1}^2, σ_{u01} and σ_0^2 by means of generalized least squares where $\mathrm{vec}(\cdot)$ is the vector operator.

The estimation procedure is iterative. We would usually start from "reasonable" estimates of the fixed parameters $\boldsymbol{\beta}$. Typically these will be those from an initial OLS estimation. From these we form the "raw" residuals (52), estimate random coefficients; and obtain an improved estimator of $\boldsymbol{V}$; then return to (51) to obtain new estimates of the fixed effects $\boldsymbol{\beta}$; and so on. Alternate between the random and fixed parameters estimation until the procedure convergence.

The IGLS procedure produces biased estimates in general and this can be important in small samples. Goldstein[15] shows how a simple modification leads to restricted iterative generalized least squares (RIGLS) by substituting $\boldsymbol{V} - \boldsymbol{X}(\boldsymbol{X}^T\boldsymbol{V}^{-1}\boldsymbol{X})\boldsymbol{X}^T$ for its corresponding term $\boldsymbol{V}$ in (53) to produce an unbiased estimate.

For multilevel generalized linear model, in order to work with a linearized model, we will use Taylor expansion. There are two produces to treat high-level residuals when forming Taylor expansion. One is to add current residuals to the linear component of the nonlinear function and the another does not add. The former is predictive quasi-likelihood (PQL), while the latter is marginal quasi-likelihood (MQL). In many applications, MQL procedure tends to underestimate the values of both the fixed and random parameters, especially where n_{ij} is small. So Goldstein[14] suggested that PQL be used in fitting generalized model rather than MQL. In addition, he also pointed out that greater accuracy is to be expected if the second-order approximation is used rather than first-order based upon the first term in the Taylor expansion.[16]

6.3. *Example* 14. *Analysis of data in Example* 1

This is the simplest case with 4 units in level 1 in a 2-level structure where the level 2 units are the subjects. The model has the form as

$$y_{ij} = \beta_0 + \beta_2 g_{2ij} + \beta_3 g_{3ij} + \beta_4 g_{4ij} + u_{0j} + e_{ij}.$$

To obtain IGLS estimation of the parameters, we use software *MLn*.[17] The results are shown in Table 12. The estimation of variance in level 1 is $\sigma_0^2 = 0.6559$, in level 2 $\sigma_{u_0}^2 = 2.6571$, with standard error $SE[\sigma_0^2] = 0.1893$, $SE[\sigma_{u_0}^2] = 1.411$, respectively.

Then

$$\rho = \frac{\sigma_{u0}^2}{\sigma_{u0}^2 + \sigma_0^2} = \frac{2.6571}{2.6571 + 0.6559} = 0.8020.$$

This results are similar to those from ANOVA and GEE.

6.4. *Example* 15. *Analysis of data in Example* 7

This is a 3-level model. Subjects are level 2 units clustered within centers that are level 3 units. Repeated measurements from the same subject are level 1 units nested within level 2 unit. The results are shown in Table 13.

Table 12. *MLn* estimation for data in Example 1.

Variable	Coefficient	*SE*	*Z*	*P*
g_2	0.4125	0.4049	1.0188	0.3083
g_3	0.6375	0.4049	1.5745	0.1154
g_4	1.7250	0.4049	4.2603	0.0000
Constant	9.3000	0.6435		

Table 13. *MLn* estimation of data in Example 7.

			Coefficient	*SE*
Fixed effect	CONS		1.7230	0.2545
	TREAT		0.3273	0.1135
	COMP		0.0384	0.0900
	AGE		−0.0090	0.0076
	SEX		−0.2285	0.1483
	TIME		0.1616	0.0056
Random effect	Level 3	$\sigma^2_{\nu 0}$	0.1190	0.0657
	Level 2	σ^2_{u0}	0.3151	0.0859
	Level 1	σ^2_0	0.1156	0.0065

The multilevel model decomposes the variance into 3 levels. 0.1156 for level 1, 0.3151 for level 2 and 0.1190 for level 3. Thus, intra-subject correlation can be estimated as

$$\frac{\sigma^2_{u0} + \sigma^2_{\nu 0}}{\sigma^2_0 + \sigma^2_{u0} + \sigma^2_{\nu 0}} = \frac{0.3151 + 0.1190}{0.1156 + 0.3151 + 0.1190} = 0.7897.$$

And, intra-center correlation can be estimated as

$$\frac{\sigma^2_{\nu 0}}{\sigma^2_0 + \sigma^2_{u0} + \sigma^2_{\nu 0}} = \frac{0.1190}{0.1156 + 0.3151 + 0.1190} = 0.2165.$$

Theoretically, multilevel model can fit for arbitrary levels. The most powerful software *MLwin* could fit models up to 7 levels. It is sufficient in practice.

6.5. *Multilevel logistic regression*

Multilevel model can be expanded to the case where the error term in the model is non-normal distribution.[18] In the rest of this section we will focus on the multilevel models with binomial distribution, or Poisson distribution.

To make matters concrete, consider the data in Example 3. Let y_{ij} be an observation of ith pup from jth pregnant rat. If the pup is normal then $y_{ij} = 0$, else $y_{ij} = 1$. Let f_{ij} be fixed part of the model, and r_j be the random part, and π_{ij} be the expected value of the response for the ijth level 1 unit. A 2-level logistic regression model would have the form

$$y_{ij} = \pi_{ij} + \varepsilon_{ij} = \frac{\exp(f_{ij} + r_j)}{1 + \exp(f_{ij} + r_j)} + \varepsilon_{ij} \tag{54}$$

$$f_{ij} = \alpha + \beta_1 x_{1ij} + \cdots + \beta_p x_{pij},$$

$$\varepsilon_{ij} = e_{ij}\sqrt{\pi_{ij}(1 - \pi_{ij})}.$$

In general, ε_{ij} follows a binomial distribution, but sometimes it is extra-binomial. The variance of ε_{ij} can be written in the form of $\sigma_0^2\pi_{ij}(1 - \pi_{ij})$. Here, σ_0^2 is refered to as extra-binomial variance (or over dispersion). When $\sigma_0^2 = 1$, it is purely binomial. We will assume $\sigma_0^2 = 1$, and $r_j \sim N(0, \sigma_0^2)$ in this section.

Let r_{ij} be the Pearson residual of the model

$$r_{ij} = \frac{y_{ij} - \pi r_{ij}}{\sqrt{\pi_{ij}(1 - \pi_{ij})/n_{ij}}}. \tag{55}$$

Then the intra-unit correlation can be defined as

$$\rho = \sum_{j=1}^{m} \left[\frac{\sum_{i=1}^{n_j} \sum_{k=1}^{n_j} r_{ij} r_{kj} - \sum_{i=1}^{n_j} r_{ij}^2}{n_j(n_j - 1)} \right] \Bigg/ \left[\sum_{j=1}^{m} \frac{\sum_{i=1}^{n_j} r_{ij}^2}{n_j} \right]. \tag{56}$$

In contrast to GEE, 2-level logistic model decompose the residuals into each level. The residuals in the level 1 are linear to the response, while the residues in level 2 are nonlinear.

The 2-level logistic model for Example 3 can be written as

$$y_{ij} = \frac{\exp(\alpha + \beta_{\text{Group}} + r_j)}{1 + \exp(\alpha + \beta_{\text{Group}} + r_j)} + e_{ij}\sqrt{\pi_{ij}(1 - \pi_{ij})}$$

where the subscripts of Group are omitted. The results are shown in Table 14.

Table 14. Results of fitting 3 2-level models for data in Example 3.

Parameter	Models		
	Logit	Probit	C log-log
α	1.127(0.3380)	0.6933(0.1929)	0.3463(0.1686)
β	1.028(0.5099)	0.5655(0.2824)	0.4692(0.2383)
σ_1^2	1.212(0.5061)	0.3822(0.1578)	0.2779(0.1131)
σ_0^2	1	1	1
intra-unit correlation ρ	0.1731	0.1734	0.1739
$-2\ln(L)$	210.686	211.610	213.084

6.6. *Multilevel Probit model and complementary log-log model*

The expected proportion π_{ij} in (55) is modeled using a logit link function. If we use probit link function, a 2-level probit model would have the form

$$y_{ij} = \pi_{ij} + \varepsilon_{ij} = \Phi(f_{ij} + r_j) + \varepsilon_{ij}. \tag{57}$$

If we use complementary log-log link function, then a 2-level complementary log-log model would have the form

$$y_{ij} = \pi_{ij} + \varepsilon_{ij} = 1 - \exp\{-\exp(f_{ij} + r_j)\} + \varepsilon_{ij}. \tag{58}$$

Other notations are similar to a level 2 logistic model in (54).

6.7. *Example* 16

We fitted 2-level logistic, probit, and complementary log-log models for data in Example 3 respectively. The results are shown in Table 14.

The results show that the intra-unit correlations estimated from 3 models are quite similar.

6.8. *Multilevel Poisson regression model*

For count data multilevel Poisson regression model would be fitted. For a 2-level model, it can be written as

$$\begin{aligned} y_{ij} &= m_{ij} + \varepsilon_{ij} = \exp(f_{ij} + r_j) + \varepsilon_{ij}, \\ f_{ij} &= \alpha + \beta_1 x_{1ij} + \cdots + \beta_p x_{pij}. \end{aligned} \tag{59}$$

We usually assume that ε_{ij} follows a Poisson distribution with $\text{var}(y_{ij}|m_{ij}) = m_{ij}$. But sometimes it is extra-Poisson with conditional variance of $\text{var}(y_{ij}|m_{ij}) = m_{ij} + km_{ij}^2$. When $k > 0$, it is negative binomial distribution. When $k = 0$, it is purely Poisson. Here we keep $k = 0, r_j \sim N(0, \sigma_1^2)$.

Let r_{ij} be Pearson residuals of the model as follow:

$$r_{ij} = \frac{y_{ij} - \mu_{ij}}{\sqrt{\mu_{ij}}}. \tag{60}$$

The definition of intra-unit correlation is similar to (55).

6.9. *Example* 17. *Fitting a 2-level Poisson regression model for data in Example* 8

The response is two-week seizure counts for epileptics and is a count data.

The Poisson model is sufficed here. The results are shown in Table 15.

Table 15. Estimated results of random effect model for Example 8.

Parameter	Coefficient	SE	Z	P
Treat	−0.07606	0.27020	−0.28150	0.7783
Trial	0.19900	0.05859	3.39648	0.0007
Time	−0.05743	0.02026	−2.83465	0.0046
Age	−0.01685	0.01788	−0.94239	0.3460
Constant	1.88100	0.55440		

The results show that the counts are correlated with age and time. No significance can be detected in test group and placebo group. But it is significantly different between the counts before and after medication. The intra-subject correlation estimated from the model is 0.7776.

6.10. *Multilevel logistic models for multiple response categories*

In this section we extend the multilevel logistic model for binomial response to the cases of multiple categories and ordinal categories. When the response is multiple categories without order, a multilevel polytomous logistic model will be fitted. And when the response is ordinal, a multilevel ordinal logistic model will be fitted.

For example, let's consider a 2-level model with one explanatory variable. The response is now multiple with k categories. A multilevel polytomous logistic model can be defined as

$$\pi_{ij}^{(s)} = \frac{\exp(\beta_0 + \beta_1 x_{1ij}^{(s)} + u_{0j}^{(s)})}{1 + \exp(\beta_0 + \beta_1 x_{1ij}^{(s)} + u_{0j}^{(s)})} + \varepsilon_{ij}, \tag{61}$$

$s = 1, 2, \ldots, k$. Under the standard assumption that the observed response proportions follow a multinomial distribution, the level 2 covariance matrix has the form

$$n_{ij}^{-1} \begin{pmatrix} \pi_{ij}^{(1)}(1-\pi_{ij}^{(1)}) & \cdots & & \\ -\pi_{ij}^{(1)}\pi_{ij}^{(2)} & \pi_{ij}^{(2)}(1-\pi_{ij}^{(2)}) & & \\ \vdots & \vdots & \ddots & \\ -\pi_{ij}^{(1)}\pi_{ij}^{(k)} & -\pi_{ij}^{(2)}\pi_{ij}^{(k)} & \cdots & \pi_{ij}^{(k)}(1-\pi_{ij}^{(k)}) \end{pmatrix}. \tag{62}$$

If k categories are ordered, we should base our model upon the cumulative response probabilities rather than the responses probabilities for each category. The multilevel ordinal logistic model can be defined as

$$\gamma_{ij}^{(s)} = \frac{\exp(\beta_0 + \beta_1 x_{1ij}^{(s)} + u_{0j}^{(s)})}{1 + \exp(\beta_0 + \beta_1 x_{1ij}^{(s)} + u_{0j}^{(s)})}, \tag{63}$$

where $\gamma_{ij}^{(s)}$ is cumulative probability for $s = 1, 2, \ldots, k$. If we assume an underlying multinomial distribution for the category probabilities, the cumulative proportions have a covariance matrix given by $\pi_{ij}^{(r)}(1 - \pi_{ij}^{(s)})/n_{ij}$, $(r < s)$.

6.11. *Example* 18. *Analysis of data in Example* 7

The effectiveness variable in Example 7 is an ordinal response, with 0 stands for invalid or worse effects of treatment on the subject, 1 for improved, 2 for notable improved, and 3 for recovery. A multilevel ordinal logistic model with cumulative odds was fitted. The results are shown in Table 16.

Where, the centers are level 3 units, the subjects are level 2 units and repeated observations are level 1 units.

6.12. *Relationship between intra-unit correlation and explanatory variable*

The key idea of multilevel model is to express the variance in each level by explanatory variables. In many applications, mean squared error is related to some explanatory variables. As a result, the intra-unit correlations are

Table 16. The results of a 3-level cumulative logistic model for data in Example 7.

Parameter	Estimation	*SE*
Fixed parameters		
Y1	−1.482	0.8162
Y2	0.9309	0.8089
Y3	4.299	0.8284
Comp	−0.03902	0.2977
Treat	−1.187	0.3245
Sex	0.5575	0.4685
Age	0.03687	0.02515
Time	−0.5268	0.03924
Random parameters		
Level 3	1.001	0.5818
Level 2	1.586	0.3197
Level 1	1	0

Table 17. The results of fitting a 2-level model for data in Example 5.

	Parameter	Estimate	SE
Fixed	Cons	98.19	4.175
	Time	1.283	0.1285
	Age	0.18	0.1531
	G1	−8.356	3.23
	G2	−2.972	3.255
	G1*Time	2.778	0.2771
	G2*Time	2.977	0.1902
Random			
Level 2	Cons/Cons	38.59	10.48
Level 1	Cons/Cons	9.914	1.44
Level 1	G1*Time/Cons	3.195	0.7093
Level 1	G2*Time/Cons	0.195	0.2165

related to them, too. This issue would be resolved by adding the explanatory variables to the random part of multilevel models.

6.13. *Example* 19. *Analysis of the data in Example* 5

The data show that the variance of ESS is changing over time. Let G1 and G2 be the dummy variables of groups. We fit a 2-level model for the data in which the time variable is added into random part at level 1 of the model. The results are shown in Table 17.

The results show that in the middle dose group ($treat = 1$) and the high dose group ($treat = 2$), the intra-subject correlation is 0.7956, which is independent on time. But in the low dose (placebo) group ($treat = 0$), the intra-subject correlation coefficient depends upon time. The correlation of observations at $Time_1$ and $Time_2$ would be estimated by

$$\frac{38.59}{\sqrt{(38.59 + 9.914 + 3.195 \times Time_1)(38.59 + 9.914 + 3.195 \times Time_2)}}.$$

6.14. *Multivariate multilevel models*

So far, we have only considered a single response variable. In many applications, we wish simultaneously to model several responses functions of explanatory variables. In Example 4, AUC, $C_{\max}$ and T_{50} will be considered together as responses to test the bioequivalence of domestic and imported

Table 18. The results fitting multivariate multilevel model for data in Example 4.

	Parameters	Coefficient	SE	Intra-subject correlation
Fixed effects	Cons_AUC	6.82577	0.02661	
	Cons_$C_{\max}$	5.13547	0.02550	
	Treat_AUC	0.03252	0.02198	
	Treat_$C_{\max}$	0.03563	0.02099	
	Drug_AUC	0.75844	0.02198	
	Drug_$C_{\max}$	0.73093	0.02099	
Random effects				
Subject level	Cons_AUC/Cons_AUC	0.008301	0.003274	1
	Cons_$C_{\max}$/Cons_AUC	0.003883	0.002426	0.486
	Cons_$C_{\max}$/Cons_$C_{\max}$	0.007678	0.003017	1
Period level	Cons_AUC/Cons_AUC	0.011595	0.001936	1
	Cons_$C_{\max}$/Cons_AUC	0.003444	0.001369	0.311
	Cons_$C_{\max}$/Cons_$C_{\max}$	0.010572	0.001765	1

rosiglitazone maleate tablets (RMT). This goal could be achieved by fitting a multivariate multilevel model.

For the sake of convenience, we consider the multivariate multilevel model with two response, the logarithmic values of AUC (also denoted AUC) and $C_{\max}$, and treat the subject as a subject-level unit and 4 treatment effects (observations repeated measured on subjects) as period-level units which are clustered in subject-level. Besides intra-subject correlation, other properties of this model should be considered: observations of AUC are correlated between different periods of trial, and so do $C_{\max}$; and AUC and $C_{\max}$ are correlated either in the same period or in different periods.

The results shown that: the intra-subject correlation of AUC is

$$0.008301/(0.008301 + 0.011595) = 0.4172.$$

The intra-subject correlations of $C_{\max}$ is

$$0.007678/(0.007678 + 0.010572) = 0.4207.$$

The Pearson correlation of AUC and $C_{\max}$ is 0.311 in level 1, and 0.486 in level 2.

7. Sampling Distribution and Confidence Interval of Intra-unit Correlation

7.1. *Confidence interval of intra-unit correlation*

The intra-unit correlation coefficient estimated by a generalized estimation equation or a multilevel model is a point estimation. But we did not estimate its estimation errors and had little ideas of its sampling distribution. The bootstrap may be applied to estimate the CI of intra-unit correlation.[19]

Bootstrap is a data-based simulation method for statistical inference, which can be used to study the variability of estimated characteristics of the probability distribution of a set of observations, and provide confidence intervals for parameters and hypothesis test in situations where these are difficult or impossible to derive closed form formulas. The basic idea of the procedure involves sampling with replacement to produce random samples of size n from original data, each of these is known as a bootstrap sample and each provides an estimate $\theta(b)$ of the interesting parameter, θ. Repeating the process a large number of times, say $\mathrm{B} = 500$ or more, provides the required information on the variability of the estimator. For example, the type of distribution, standard error of the bootstrap estimates. An approximate 95% confidence interval can be derived from mean ± 1.96 SD if the bootstrap estimates are normally distributed, and from the 2.5% and 97.5% quartiles of the replicate values if the bootstrap estimates is not normally distributed. The confidence interval derived from bootstrap sampling is known as bootstrap confidence interval.

If the population distribution is known, bootstrap samples can be randomly samped not from the original data, but from the population distribution. The former produce is known as non-parametric bootstrap, and the latter as parametric bootstrap.

Research shows that there are two particularities in applying the bootstrap estimation to data of dependent design.[20] First, it is not proper to adopt a parametric estimation because of the difficulty in making a judgment to the distribution of the data. So we suggest adopting a non-parametric estimation. Second, it is not proper to apply a random sample directly to observations because of the non-independence of observations. So we suggest that we sample high level units. And if some high level unit is sampled, all the observations in this unit will be sampled. As examples, data of Example 2 should be sampled by family; data of Example 3 should be sampled by litter; and data of Examples 1, 4 and 5 should be sampled by patient.

The estimator of intra-family correlation of Example 2 is 0.5674. If we sample the data on families, make 500 resamplings, and estimated by GEE, then the non-parametric 95% CI of intra-family correlation is 0.2875–0.8874. If we sample the data of Example 8 on patients and make the same analysis, we estimated the non-parametric 95% CI of correlation 0.5219–0.8874. Both of the two bootstrap sampling distributions of intra-unit correlation are skew. Because both of the two CIs do not include 0, we may accept that the intra-subject correlations exist.

7.2. *The sampling distribution of intra-unit correlation*

To estimate the type and characteristic of distribution of intra-unit correlation, we use the Monte Carlo method. One thousand simulations were generated from specific population with known ρ and corresponding assumed parameters. For each set of simulated data, we fit a 2-level model, estimate σ_0^2, σ_e^2, and then the intra-unit correlation. We then investigate the distribution of intra-unit correlation based on 1000 estimators of ρ.

We may assume that there are m individuals (two-level unit) and each individual have k repeatedly measured values (one-level unit), then we have $n = m \times k$ observations. In order to investigate the effect of units of level 1 and units of level 2 on the intra-unit correlation when overall sample size of observations are the same, we design the grids are $(k, m) = (4, 10)$, (4, 20), (4, 30), ...,(4, 100) and $(k, m) = (8, 5)$, (8, 10), (8, 15), ...,(8, 50) respectively, and the intra-unit correlation coefficients is 0.1–0.9 respectively.

Without losing generality, in analog investigation, we do not take fixed but random effect into account, because the intra-unit correlation is related only to random effect. Furthermore, we assume that the intra-unit correlation structure is exchangeable.

Now we may consider two situations. One is the simplest situation

$$y_{ij} = \mu_j + e_{ij}. \tag{64}$$

Only one random effect is considered both in levels 1 and level 2. Then the variance of y is $\sigma_0^2 + \sigma_e^2$; The variance-covariance matrix of y is $\boldsymbol{V} = \text{diag}(\boldsymbol{R}, \boldsymbol{R}, \ldots, \boldsymbol{R})$. If k is 4,

$$\boldsymbol{R} = \begin{pmatrix} \sigma_0^2 + \sigma_e^2 & & & \\ \sigma_0^2 & \sigma_0^2 + \sigma_e^2 & & \\ \sigma_0^2 & \sigma_0^2 & \sigma_0^2 + \sigma_e^2 & \\ \sigma_0^2 & \sigma_0^2 & \sigma_0^2 & \sigma_0^2 + \sigma_e^2 \end{pmatrix}, \tag{65}$$

the intra-unit correlation can be calculated by Eq. (48).

Another situation is more complex

$$y_{ij} = \mu_j + \nu_j x_{ij} + e_{ij}. \tag{66}$$

Level 1 has two random effect terms: one is random error. Another random effect term is related to independent variable, namely the variance of y, $\sigma_0^2 + \sigma_1^2(x_{ij})^2 + \sigma_e^2$, and is affected by explanatory variable. Let $x_{ij} = j - 1$, the variance-covariance matrix of y is $\boldsymbol{V} = \mathrm{diag}(\boldsymbol{R}, \boldsymbol{R}, \ldots, \boldsymbol{R})$, when $k = 4$,

$$\boldsymbol{R} = \begin{pmatrix} \sigma_0^2 + \sigma_e^2 & & & \\ \sigma_0^2 & \sigma_0^2 + \sigma_1^2 + \sigma_e^2 & & \\ \sigma_0^2 & \sigma_0^2 & \sigma_0^2 + 4\sigma_1^2 + \sigma_e^2 & \\ \sigma_0^2 & \sigma_0^2 & \sigma_0^2 & \sigma_0^2 + 9\sigma_1^2 + \sigma_e^2 \end{pmatrix}. \tag{67}$$

We may calculate intra-unit correlation by Eq. (48) after deducting the effect of explanatory variable to y.

The parameters of the model can be estimated by the Restricted Iterative Generalized Least Square (RIGLS) method. The simulation study is made by using specialized multilevel model software MLn.[17]

Table 19 lists the simulated results of six models. Models A–D are generated based on Eq. (64), and their amounts of units of levels 1 and 2 are model A with $(k, m) = (4, 10)$, model B with $(k, m) = (8, 5)$, model C with $(k, m) = (4, 100)$, model D with $(k, m) = (8, 50)$, respectively. The overall sample size of model A is equal to that of model B, while the overall sample size of model C is equal to that of model D. Models E and F are generated based on Eq. (66), and their amounts of units are respectively model E with $(k, m) = (4, 100)$ and model F with $(k, m) = (8, 50)$.

The result shows that the type of distribution is related to the value of intra-unit correlation. And the distribution of intra-unit correlation of these models indicates that when $\rho = 0.5$, its distribution is symmetrical and resembles the normal distribution; when $\rho > 0.5$, its distribution is positively skew; and when $\rho < 0.5$, negatively skew, just as Fig. 3 shows.

In one model, the estimated error is larger when ρ approaches 0.5, and becomes smaller gradually as ρ approaches 0.1 or 0.9.

The mean intra-unit correlation coefficients of model C is closer to the theoretical value than that of model A, and its standard error is smaller. Similarly, the mean intra-unit correlation coefficient of model D is closer to theoretical value than that of model B, and its standard error is also smaller. Therefore, the larger the sample size, the better the effect of estimation.

Table 19. 500 simulated results of intra-unit correlation of 6 populations.

Theoretical values	Model A $k = 4, m = 10$	Model B $k = 8, m = 5$	Model C $k = 4, m = 100$	Model D $k = 8, m = 50$	Model E $k = 4, m = 100$	Model F $k = 8, m = 50$
0.1	0.1235 ± 0.1279	0.1057 ± 0.1146	0.0980 ± 0.0471	0.0965 ± 0.0411	0.1150 ± 0.0933	0.1121 ± 0.1178
0.2	0.2017 ± 0.1485	0.1786 ± 0.1467	0.1987 ± 0.0540	0.1981 ± 0.0522	0.2019 ± 0.1067	0.2075 ± 0.1450
0.3	0.2855 ± 0.1633	0.2666 ± 0.1722	0.3026 ± 0.0534	0.2988 ± 0.0572	0.2978 ± 0.1081	0.2963 ± 0.1635
0.4	0.3787 ± 0.1725	0.3428 ± 0.1884	0.3973 ± 0.0560	0.3936 ± 0.0616	0.3995 ± 0.1123	0.3934 ± 0.1599
0.5	0.4595 ± 0.1749	0.4288 ± 0.2054	0.4971 ± 0.0534	0.4942 ± 0.0609	0.4995 ± 0.1078	0.4981 ± 0.1563
0.6	0.5635 ± 0.1608	0.5207 ± 0.2042	0.5964 ± 0.0463	0.5931 ± 0.0570	0.5965 ± 0.1018	0.5920 ± 0.1507
0.7	0.6663 ± 0.1379	0.6232 ± 0.1928	0.6967 ± 0.0389	0.6947 ± 0.0481	0.6974 ± 0.0957	0.6891 ± 0.1435
0.8	0.7647 ± 0.1146	0.7278 ± 0.1702	0.7974 ± 0.0287	0.7935 ± 0.0375	0.7986 ± 0.0865	0.8042 ± 0.1211
0.9	0.8786 ± 0.0734	0.8492 ± 0.1216	0.8985 ± 0.0153	0.8965 ± 0.0213	0.8912 ± 0.0727	0.8891 ± 0.0957

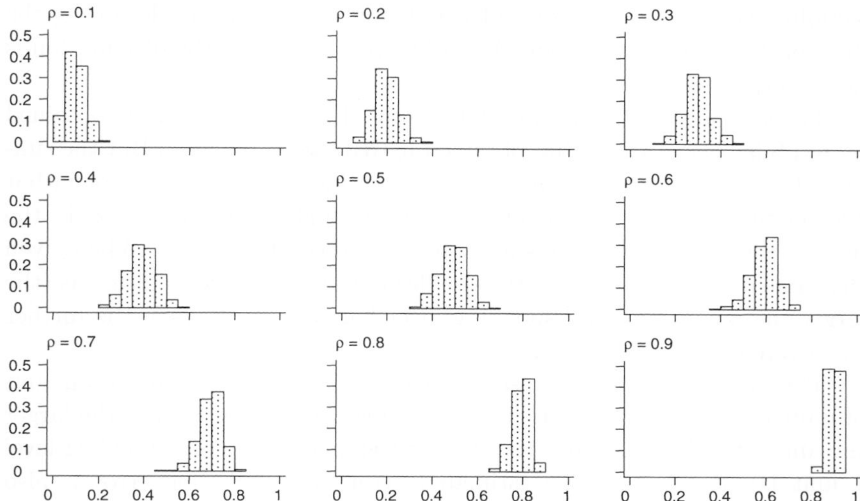

Fig. 3. Sampling distibution of the intra-unit correlations base on model C.

In comparisons of model A with B, model C with D and model E with F respectively, for which each pair has the same sample size, the estimation of model B is not as good as A, model D not as good as C and model F not as good as E except that $\rho = 0.1$ or 0.2. This is because the amount of two-level units is small while that of one-level units is large. In fact, because of the presence of intra-unit correlation, the amount of information is overlapped. As an example, the amount of information obtained by measuring k times repeatedly to the same individual is smaller than that obtained by measuring once to k individuals.

If we compare model E with C and model F with D respectively, their overall sample sizes, the amount of one-level units and two-level units are equal respectively. But models E and F have larger estimated error because the variance terms of models E and F are more complex.

The statistical simulation shows that the estimator of ρ is little smaller than the theoretical value. But the larger the sample size is, the closer the estimator is to its theoretical value. And when given the same overall sample size, the larger the amount of level 2 units is (the smaller the amount of corresponding level 1 unit is), the closer the estimated value is to the theoretical value.

If ρ is close to 0.5, the sampling distribution of intra-unit correlation is approximately normal distribution. As ρ approaches 0, or approaches 1, the sampling error is becoming smaller and smaller. When ρ is close to 0, the distribution is positively skew. And when ρ is close to 1, the distribution is negatively skew.

Theoretically, as Goldstein (1998) pointed out, the estimators obtained by IGLS is biased, while that obtained by RIGLS is unbiased. But the simulated results show that estimators of ρ obtained by RIGLS are somewhat smaller than the theoretical values. And the smaller the sample size is, the further the estimated value is away from its theoretical value. When given the same overall sample size, the smaller the amount of level 2 unit is (the larger the amount of corresponding level 1 unit is, of course), the further the estimated value is biased.

The sampling error of intra-unit correlation is also related to the amount of units of every level. When given the same overall sample size, the larger the amount of level 2 units (the smaller the amount of corresponding level 1 unit is), the smaller the estimated error. The sampling error is also related to how complex the variance of responding variable is: the larger the variance, the larger the sampling error.

This section focuses only on the situation when responding variable is numeric, that is to say that data should be distributed normally. Further investigation is needed, especially with regard to skew distributions, such as binominal and Poisson distributions.

8. Sample Size and the Cost-effect of Dependent Test

This section will take the repeated measurement (sampling) as an example to discuss sample size and power of hypothesis testing and cost-effect for dependent data. Because of the overlap of information, the dependent data tells us less than independent data given the same sample size, which leads to a low power. And the larger the relationship in groups is, the less information the data offers and the lower the power shows.

8.1. *Sample size and power of test*

Let Y_{ijg} represent the jth observation of the ith subject in the gth group ($i = 1, \ldots, m, j = 1, \ldots, k; g = 0, 1$). We also assume the individuals are independent to each other, and the intra-subject correlations are equal. If the type I error is α and the power is $1 - \beta$, the sample size of each group can be estimated by the equation below:

$$m = [1 + (k-1)\rho]\frac{\sigma^2(Z_\alpha + Z_\beta)^2}{k\delta^2}. \qquad (68)$$

Where δ is the difference of effects of the two groups ($g = 0$ and $g = 1$). It is oblivious that the number of observations m needed in this design is smaller, while the overall number of observations $n = mk$ is larger than those of the independent design. And when $\rho = 0$, it is equal to the sample size of independent design.

The table below is the result of a simulated experiment on the power of a group of repeated measurements. The intra-unit correlation is 0, 0.1, 0.2, ... ,0.9, respectively; the sample size m and the times of repeated measures k are (50, 4), (100, 2), (20, 4), (40, 2), respectively; And δ are 0, 0.2, 0.4, 0.6, 0.8, 1.0, respectively. All designs were balanced. Based on each grid, 1000 simulations were generated by using the MLn package.[17] For each set of simulated data, we fit a multilevel model. The power is then estimated by the proportion of times of the rejections of null hypothesis in 1000 simulations.

The results corresponding to $\delta = 0$ is type I error, while that to $\rho = 0$ is the power of the independent data. From the Table 20, we can conclude that the power decreases as the intra-unit correlation within group increases. And unless δ is large enough, the extent of the decrease is large. For example, when the repeated times are the same, the power of the design with $m = 50$, $k = 4$ and $\rho = 0.9$ is only half of that with $n = 200$ and $\rho = 0$. When the repeated times are equal, the power has a tendency to increase as m increases; And when $n = mk$ are equal, the power of the design with twice measured is larger than that with 4 repeated times.

8.2. *Cost-effect analysis*

The estimations of design efficiency and sample size are important considerations during the experiment design. Researchers always have to balance among design efficiency, sample size and cost-benefit before making a decision. For example, a physiological experiment uses several rats' liver cells. Researchers may sample only once (single sample test, independent) or several times (repeated sample test, dependent) on each rat. The latter needs fewer rats than the former, which means the latter costs less. But data from the latter are dependent while those of the former are independent. So, the problem researchers confront is that the test should not only cost litter, but also achieve enough power of test.

Table 20. Power of repeated measurement (times of the rejection to null hypothesis in 1000 simulations).

	$m = 50,\ k = 4$						$m = 100,\ k = 2$					
	δ						δ					
ρ	0	0.2	0.4	0.6	0.8	1.0	0	0.2	0.4	0.6	0.8	1.0
0	44	234	789	984	1000	1000	54	272	781	989	1000	1000
0.1	55	232	689	961	998	1000	43	268	757	986	999	1000
0.2	68	220	598	915	995	999	55	279	709	979	999	1000
0.3	57	169	557	854	975	999	52	226	692	963	999	1000
0.4	60	181	474	820	961	998	57	233	661	957	996	1000
0.5	56	157	447	756	936	990	43	205	645	942	999	999
0.6	66	143	393	718	931	983	62	119	600	916	989	1000
0.7	56	138	357	692	889	971	54	208	593	902	992	1000
0.8	62	151	331	647	860	970	62	190	564	883	981	999
0.9	58	117	342	595	829	952	58	168	519	875	988	1000
	$m = 20,\ k = 4$						$m = 40,\ k = 2$					
	δ						δ					
ρ	0	0.2	0.4	0.6	0.8	1.0	0	0.2	0.4	0.6	0.8	1.0
0	59	133	384	746	927	992	36	139	412	759	932	997
0.1	56	125	336	631	870	967	44	143	380	708	916	993
0.2	63	119	302	573	812	939	62	141	375	678	890	928
0.3	80	108	279	488	744	891	69	140	356	634	887	974
0.4	58	106	258	464	682	849	61	129	344	592	859	967
0.5	65	110	228	440	626	805	53	113	296	612	825	959
0.6	69	109	175	372	535	767	57	130	318	577	787	950
0.7	71	94	194	361	546	731	48	103	301	524	780	927
0.8	59	102	193	333	492	696	61	109	288	528	759	908
0.9	69	103	179	313	490	692	69	101	263	490	729	898

When we discussed the estimation of sample size in the last section, we did not consider the cost. But the funds are limited in practice. So it is related to cost-benefit problems. On one hand, given restricted funds (the cost is constant), we should consider whether to select single sample or repeated sample to make the effect as large as possible (the variance is minimum). On the other hand, when the benefit is constant (the variance is restricted), we should consider whether to sample independently or repeatedly to make the cost the least.

8.2.1. *When the cost is constant, how to evaluate the benefits of independently sampling design and repeated sampling design?*

In a repeated sampling design, individual is independent with each other. We can assume the average elemental cost of each individual is C_1, the average direct cost of sampling once to each individual is C_2, the variation among individualities and repeated sample measures is σ_2, and the intra-subject correlation of samples from the same subject is ρ.

Let the overall cost be C, the individual numbers (or pairs) needed for repeated sampling design is m, and the times of repeated sample to each individual is k, then

$$C = m(C_1 + kC_2). \tag{69}$$

It is not difficult to find:

$$\mathrm{var}(\bar{Y}) = \frac{\sigma^2}{mk}[1 + (k+1)\rho]. \tag{70}$$

When the restricted overall cost is C, to make $\mathrm{var}(\bar{Y})$ as little as possible (equivalent to making the power as large as possible), the optimal number of individuals m and the times of repeated sample k to each subject are the solutions of conditional minimum of function (70) restricted by Eq. (69).

Let $f(m,k) = \sigma^2[1+(k-1)\rho]/(mk) + \lambda(mC_1 + kmC_2 - C)$, then

$$\begin{cases} \dfrac{\partial f(m,k)}{\partial k} = \dfrac{-\sigma^2(1-\rho)}{mk^2} + \lambda m C_2 = 0 \\ \dfrac{\partial f(m,k)}{\partial m} = \dfrac{-\sigma^2[1+(k-1)\rho]}{mk^2} + \lambda(C_1 + kC_2) = 0. \end{cases} \tag{71}$$

That is

$$\begin{cases} m = \sqrt{\dfrac{\sigma^2\rho}{\lambda C_1}} \\ k = \sqrt{\dfrac{(1-\rho)C_1}{\rho C_2}}. \end{cases} \tag{72}$$

Substituting m and k in (72) for their corresponding terms in (69), because C is a specific value, the optimal number of individuals is

$$m = \frac{C\sqrt{C_1\rho}[\sqrt{C_1\rho} - \sqrt{C_2(1-\rho)}]}{C_1[C_1\rho - C_2(1-\rho)]}. \tag{73}$$

So the minimum variance is

$$\mathrm{var}(\bar{Y}) = \sigma^2(\sqrt{\rho C_1} + \sqrt{(1-\rho)C_2})^2/C. \tag{74}$$

If the sample size of independent sampling design is N, the overall cost and sample error are $C = NC_1$ and $\mathrm{var}(\bar{Y}) = \sigma^2/N$ respectively.

And if the restricted overall cost is C, to make $\mathrm{var}(\bar{Y})$ as little as possible (make the power as large as possible), the optimal number of subjects m is the solution of conditional minimum of function $\mathrm{var}(\bar{Y}) = \sigma^2/N$ restricted by equation $C = NC_1$.

Let $g(N) = \sigma^2/N + \lambda NC_1$, then

$$N = C/C_1. \tag{75}$$

And the minimum variance of independent sample is

$$\mathrm{var}(\bar{Y}) = \sigma^2 C_1/C. \tag{76}$$

So given restricted overall funds C, whether to sample independently or repeatedly depends on the value of sample error, which means to work out when Eqs. (76) and (74) will have minimum values, when

$$\rho < \left(\frac{C_1 - C_2}{C_1 + C_2}\right)^2. \tag{77}$$

The repeated sample design can result in a minimum sample error (the power is the largest and the effect is better). Otherwise, it would be better to choose independent sampling design.

8.2.2. *When the benefit is constant, how to compare the cost of independent sample with that of repeated sample?*

We should follow the method in the last section to make the overall cost C as little as possible when $\mathrm{var}(\bar{Y}) = V$ is constant.

The optimal individual number of repeated sampling design m and the optimal sample times of each subject k can be worked out by the equations below, respectively:

$$\begin{cases} m = \dfrac{\sigma^2\sqrt{C_1\rho}[\sqrt{C_1\rho} + \sqrt{C_2(1-\rho)}]}{C_1 V}, \\ k = \sqrt{\dfrac{C_1(1-\rho)}{C_2\rho}}. \end{cases} \tag{78}$$

The minimum overall cost of repeated sampling design is

$$C = m(C_1 + kC_2) = \sigma^2[\sqrt{C_1\rho} + \sqrt{C_2(1-\rho)}]^2/V, \tag{79}$$

The optimal individual number of independent sampling design is

$$N = \sigma^2/V. \tag{80}$$

And the minimum overall cost of independent sample is

$$C = NC_1 = \sigma^2 C_1/V. \tag{81}$$

So under the condition of restricted sample error (the same benefit), should we select the independent sampling design or the repeated sampling design? This depends on the overall cost of the sample. We should compare when Eqs. (79) and (82) will have their minimum values. And only if the intra-subject correlation ρ meets the need of Eq. (77) can repeated sampling design make the sample cost as little as possible. Otherwise we'd better use an independent sampling design.

8.3. *Example 20. The cost benefit problems of rat's test data*

Physiology Laboratory, Nantong Medical College, had finished a test that needed four rats. Four sets of single spleen T cells turbid liquid were prepared for each rat by normal methods. Then researcher mixed ConA with each liquid and measured OD. From pre-experiments or experiences, they estimated that

$$\sigma^2 = 0.00054844 \quad \text{and} \quad \rho = 0.52895.$$

Then if we restricted sampling overall cost C or sample error $\text{var}(\bar{Y})$, should we select an independently sampling design or a repeated sampling design? This is related to the average elemental cost of each rat C_1, the average direct cost of repeated sampling once to each rat C_2 and the intra-subject coefficient of repeated measurement. We assume that each rat costs $C_1 = 20$ yuan, each portion (1 ml) of medium and 0.1 ml calf serum costs $C_2 = 0.12$ yuan. Because

$$\rho = 0.52895 < \left(\frac{C_1 - C_2}{C_1 + C_2}\right)^2 = \left(\frac{20 - 0.12}{20 + 0.12}\right)^2 = 0.97629,$$

this case meets the need of Eq. (77). Thus, it is wise to do repeated sampling instead of an independent sampling. From Eq. (72), we known that the repeated sampling times of each rat k is 13.

If the restricted overall cost $C = 110$ yuan, the repeated sampling design needs 5 rats and the minimum sampling error is $\text{var}(\bar{Y}) = 0.000062$ from Eqs. (73) and (74).

If the restricted sampling error is $\text{var}(\bar{Y}) = 0.000052$, the repeated sampling design needs $m = 6$ rats and the minimum sampling cost is $C = 130$ yuan from Eqs. (78) and (82).

In this section we focus on the power of the repeated sample design in one group, the estimation of sample size and some problems about cost-effect. The principles of analysis can also be applied to repeated measurement data of grouped design and longitudinal data, etc.

When estimating the power and sample size of the repeated sampling, we should take full advantages of the prior information to specify the values of variation among individuals and repeated samples, the value of intra-subject correlation coefficient and the values of acceptable error because of the affection these values have on the estimation of sample size. If there is not enough prior information, it is better to obtain it through pilot studies. And the importance of types I and II errors should be determined according to damages caused by the respectively wrong decisions.

There are two other design methods similar to repeated sampling design. One of them is the multiple repeated measures, which can improve the precision of measurements, and reflect whether the measured results have stability, namely reliablity. And the degree of reliability can be represented by constructed validity. The intra-subject correlation among repeated measures of these data is always low and always has nothing to do with the covariates. The another one is the regular or irregular follow-up in a longitudinal study, such as the follow up studies of kid's growth and development and the metabolism of some kind of drug, etc., in which we are interested in the occurring, developing, or law of variation of an event. The intra-subject correlation of these data is always related with the interval of the follow up. However, repeated sampling is sampling from the same subject. These samples always have a low intra-subject correlation and are related to some covariates. Though in several literatures they are all refered to as repeated measurement and have similar methods of processing and analyzing, they have their own particular emphases. So the structures of covariances matrix of response variables are different. But to applied researchers, more emphases should be laid on the distinctions of different designs.

References

1. Cochran, W. G. (1977). Sampling Techniques. John Wiley and Son. Inc. New York.
2. Willams, D. A. (1975). The analysis of binary responses from toxicological experiments involving reproduction and teralogenicity. *Biometrics* **31**: 941–952.

3. Diggle, P. J., Liang, K. Y. and Zeger, S. T. (1995). Analysis of longitudinal data. Clarendon Press. Oxford.
4. Hooton, T. M., Scholes, D., Hughes, J. P. *et al.* (1996). A prospective study of risk factors for symptomatic urinary tract infection in young women. *NEJM* **335**: 468–474.
5. Gabriel, S. E., Woods, J. E. and O'Fallon, W. M. *et al.* (1997). Complications leads to surgery after breast implantation. *NEJM* **336**: 677–682.
6. McAlindon, T. E., Felson, D. T. and Zhang, Y. *et al.* (1996). Relation of dietary intake and serum levels of vitamin D to progression of osteoarthritis of the knee among participants in the Framingham study. *Ann. Int. Med.* **125**: 353–359.
7. Chen, F., Ren, S.-Q. and Lu, S. Z. (1998). On intra-correlations of dependent data. *Modern Prevent. Med.* **25**: 269–271.
8. Ren, S.-Q. and Chenfeng (1998). Expression for covariance structure for dependent data. *Chinese Health Statist.* **15**(4): 4–8.
9. Prescott, R. and Brown, H. (1995). *Mixed Models Analysis of Clinical Trials Using SAS*: *Proc Mixed and Beyond.* Course Presenters.
10. Liang, K. Y. and Zeger, S. T. (1986). Longitudinal data analysis using generalized linear models. *Biometrika* **73**(1): 13.
11. Chen, Q.-G. (1995). GEE analysis for repeated measurement in longitudinal study. *Chinese Health Statist.* **12**(1): 22.
12. Xiong, L.-P., Cao, X.-T. and Xu, Y.-Y. *et al.* (1999). Log linear model for longitudinal data. *Chinese Health Statist.* **16**(2): 68.
13. Chen, F., Ren, S.-Q. and Lu, S.-Z. (1999). Intra-unit correlation of dependent data and GEE. *Acta Academia Med. Nantong* **19**(6): 359–362.
14. Goldstein, H. (1986). Multilevel mixed linear model analysis using iterative generalized least square. *Biometrika* **73**: 43–56.
15. Goldstein, H. (1989). Restricted unbiased iterative generalised least squares estimation. *Biometrika* **76**: 622–623.
16. Goldstein, H. (1995) *Multilevel Statistics Models*, 2nd edn., Chapman, London.
17. Rasbash, J. and Woodhouse, G. (1995). *MLn Command Reference*, Institute of Education. London.
18. Goldstein, H. (1991). Nonlinear multilevel models with an application to discrete response data. *Biometrika* **78**: 45–51.
19. Chen, F., Lu, S.-Z. and Yang, M. (1997). Bootstrap estimation and its apolication. *Chinese Health Statist.* **14**(5): 5–8.
20. Ren, S.-Q. (1999). The statistics methods for non-independent data. PhD dissertation. West China University of Medical Sciences.

About the Author

Chen Feng, Ph.D, is currently professor at the School of Public Health, Nanjing Medical School, P.R. China. He received his B.S. in mathematics from Zhushan University, Guangzhou, China, in 1983 and a Ph.D in biostatistics from the Huaxi Medical University, Chengdu, China, in 1994. Dr. Chen is a senior member of the committee of the statistical theory and methodology of the association of the Chinese Medical Informatics. Dr. Chen is also the director of Chinese Clinical Trial Statistical group (CCTS). He was visiting scholar and London University and Harvard University. His research interest includes statistical methods in analyzing dependent data, high-dimensional data and clinical trial data.

CHAPTER 32

BAYESIAN METHODS

MING-HUI CHEN
Department of Statistics, University of Connecticut,
Stoors, CT 06269, USA
mhchen@stat.uconn.edu

KEYING YE
Department of Management Science and Statistics,
University of Texas at San Antonio,
San Antonio, TX 78249, USA

1. Introduction

In the practice of applied statistics and data analysis, summarizing data points, making inference to the unknowns, fitting probability models and predicting the future are all important elements to be considered. Many statistical methodologies have been developed in modern days to deal with different problems in the world full of randomness. Two schools of statistics are popular nowadays. One of them is called *classic* or *frequentist* statistics. The other one, which has progressed rapidly in the last decade and which has been more and more used in common practice, is called *Bayesian statistics*. Due to the current advances in computing technology and the development of efficient computational algorithms, Bayesian statistics are now becoming more popular in many applied fields such as agriculture, bioinformatics, medicine, biology, public health, and epidemiology. Chen *et al.* (2010) provide a nice review of current and future research frontiers in Bayesian inference and decision making.

The Bayesian paradigm is based on specifying a probability model for the observed data $D = (n, \boldsymbol{y}, X)$, where n is the sample size, $\boldsymbol{y}$ is the $n \times 1$ response vector, and X is the $n \times p$ matrix of covariates, given a vector of unknown parameters $\boldsymbol{\theta}$, leading to the likelihood function $L(\boldsymbol{\theta}|D)$. Then we assume that $\boldsymbol{\theta}$ is random and has a *prior* distribution denoted by $\pi(\boldsymbol{\theta})$.

Inference concerning $\boldsymbol{\theta}$ is then based on the *posterior* distribution, which is obtained by Bayes' theorem. The posterior distribution is given by

$$\pi(\boldsymbol{\theta}|D) = \frac{L(\boldsymbol{\theta}|D)\pi(\boldsymbol{\theta})}{\int_\Omega L(\boldsymbol{\theta}|D)\pi(\boldsymbol{\theta})\, d\boldsymbol{\theta}}, \tag{1}$$

where Ω denotes the parameter space of $\boldsymbol{\theta}$. From (1) it is clear that $\pi(\boldsymbol{\theta}|D)$ is *proportional* to the likelihood multiplied by the prior,

$$\pi(\boldsymbol{\theta}|D) \propto L(\boldsymbol{\theta}|D)\pi(\boldsymbol{\theta}),$$

and thus it involves a contribution from the observed data through $L(\boldsymbol{\theta}|D)$, and a contribution from prior information quantified through $\pi(\boldsymbol{\theta})$. The quantity $m(D) = \int_\Omega L(\boldsymbol{\theta}|D)\pi(\boldsymbol{\theta})\, d\boldsymbol{\theta}$ is the *normalizing constant* of $\pi(\boldsymbol{\theta}|D)$, and is often called the *marginal* distribution of the data or the prior predictive distribution.

Notice that other than the data D to be random, from a Bayesian point of view, the parameter $\boldsymbol{\theta}$ is also random. Foundationally speaking, to gain information of an unknown, say $\boldsymbol{\theta}$, it would be natural if the knowledge of $\boldsymbol{\theta}$ can be described by using a form of statistical distribution. The more of the information about the unknown through data is obtained, the better knowledge of the unknown is gained. The posterior in (1) can also be viewed as a prior distribution for future experimental observations, if any. Hence, Bayesian thinking requires a sequential learning process that leads to understanding unknowns in the scientifical world.

In this chapter, we are going to describe a few aspects of Bayesian statistics, including posterior inference (Section 2), prior elicitation (Section 3), Bayesian computations (Section 4), Bayesian design of non-inferiority clinical trials (Section 5), and applicational examples (Section 6).

2. Posterior Inference

2.1. *Summary of posterior distributions*

In Bayesian data analysis, many posterior quantities are of the form

$$E[h(\boldsymbol{\theta})|D] = \int_{R^p} h(\boldsymbol{\theta})\pi(\boldsymbol{\theta}|D)\, d\boldsymbol{\theta}, \tag{2}$$

where $h(\cdot)$ is a real-valued function of $\boldsymbol{\theta} = (\theta_1, \theta_2, \ldots, \theta_p)'$. We call (2) an integral-type posterior quantity, or the posterior expectation of $h(\boldsymbol{\theta})$. In

(2), we assume that

$$E(|h(\boldsymbol{\theta})| \mid D) = \int_{R^p} |h(\boldsymbol{\theta})|\pi(\boldsymbol{\theta}|D)\, d\boldsymbol{\theta} < \infty.$$

Integral-type posterior quantities include posterior means, posterior variances, covariances, higher-order moments, and probabilities of sets by taking appropriate functional forms of h. For example, (2) reduces to:

(a) the posterior mean of $\boldsymbol{\theta}$ when $h(\boldsymbol{\theta}) = \boldsymbol{\theta}$;
(b) the posterior covariance of θ_j and θ_{j^*} if $h(\boldsymbol{\theta}) = (\theta_j - E(\theta_j|D))(\theta_{j^*} - E(\theta_{j^*}|D))'$, where $E(\theta_j|D) = \int_{R^p} \theta_j \pi(\boldsymbol{\theta}|D)\, d\boldsymbol{\theta}$;
(c) the posterior predictive density when $h(\boldsymbol{\theta}) = f(z|\boldsymbol{\theta})$, where $f(z|\boldsymbol{\theta})$ is the predictive density given the parameter $\boldsymbol{\theta}$; and
(d) the posterior probability of a set A if $h(\boldsymbol{\theta}) = 1\{\boldsymbol{\theta} \in A\}$, where $1\{\boldsymbol{\theta} \in A\}$ denotes the indicator function.

In (d), the posterior probability leads to a Bayesian p-value (see Meng 1994) by taking an appropriate form of A.

Some other posterior quantities such as normalizing constants, Bayes factors, and posterior model probabilities, may not simply be written in the form of (2). However, they are actually functions of integral-type posterior quantities. Posterior quantiles, Bayesian credible intervals, and Bayesian Highest Posterior Density (HPD) intervals are often viewed as nonintegral-type posterior quantities. Even for these types of posterior quantities, we can express them as functions of integral-type posterior quantities under certain conditions. For example, let $\xi = h(\boldsymbol{\theta})$, and $\xi_{1-\alpha}$ be the $(1-\alpha)^{th}$ posterior quantile of ξ with respect to $\pi(\boldsymbol{\theta}|D)$, where $0 < \alpha < 1$ and $h(\cdot)$ is a real-valued function. Then, $\xi_{1-\alpha}$ is the solution of the following equation:

$$\int_{R^p} 1\{h(\boldsymbol{\theta}) \le t\}\pi(\boldsymbol{\theta}|D)\, d\boldsymbol{\theta} = 1 - \alpha.$$

Therefore, the posterior quantile is a function of the posterior expectation of $1\{h(\boldsymbol{\theta}) \le t\}$.

2.2. *Predictive distributions*

A major aspect of the Bayesian paradigm is prediction. Prediction is often an important goal in regression problems, and usually plays an important role in model selection problems. The *posterior predictive* distribution of a future observation vector z given the data D is defined as

$$\pi(z|D) = \int_{\Omega} f(z|\boldsymbol{\theta})\pi(\boldsymbol{\theta}|D)\, d\boldsymbol{\theta}, \tag{3}$$

where $f(z|\boldsymbol{\theta})$ denotes the sampling density of z, and $\pi(\boldsymbol{\theta}|D)$ is the posterior distribution of $\boldsymbol{\theta}$. We see that (3) is just the posterior expectation of $f(z|\boldsymbol{\theta})$, and thus sampling from (3) is easily accomplished via the Gibbs sampler (See Section 4 for detail) from $\pi(\boldsymbol{\theta}|D)$. This is a nice feature of the Bayesian paradigm since (3) shows that predictions and predictive distributions are easily computed once samples from $\pi(\boldsymbol{\theta}|D)$ are available.

Regarding the complementary roles of the predictive and posterior distributions in Bayesian data analysis, Box (1980) notes that the posterior distribution provides a basis for "estimation of parameters conditional on the adequacy of the entertained model" while the predictive distribution enables "criticism of the entertained model in light of current data." In this spirit, Gelfand, Dey, and Chang (1992) consider a cross-validation approach, in which the predictive distribution is used in various ways to assess model adequacy. The main idea of this cross-validation approach is to validate conditional predictive distributions arising from single observation deletion against observed responses.

Let $\boldsymbol{y} = (y_1, y_2, \ldots, y_n)'$ denote the $n \times 1$ vector of the observed responses. Let X denote the $n \times p$ matrix of covariates whose i^{th} row $\boldsymbol{x}_i'$ is associated with y_i. Then, the observed data can be written as $D = (n, \boldsymbol{y}, X)$. Also let $\boldsymbol{y}^{(-i)}$ denote the $(n-1)\times 1$ response vector with y_i deleted, let $X^{(-i)}$ denote the $(n-1) \times p$ matrix that is X with the ith row $\boldsymbol{x}_i'$ deleted, and the resulting observed data are written as $D^{(-i)} = ((n-1), \boldsymbol{y}^{(-i)}, X^{(-i)})$. In addition, let $\boldsymbol{\theta}$ be the vector of model parameters. We assume that $y_i \sim f(y_i|\boldsymbol{\theta}, \boldsymbol{x}_i)$ and we let $\pi(\theta)$ denote the prior distribution of θ. Then, the posterior distribution of $\boldsymbol{\theta}$ based on the data D is given by

$$\pi(\boldsymbol{\theta}|D) \propto \left[\prod_{i=1}^{n} f(y_i|\boldsymbol{\theta}, \boldsymbol{x}_i)\right] \pi(\theta), \tag{4}$$

and the posterior distribution of $\boldsymbol{\theta}$ based on the data $D^{(-i)}$ is given by

$$\pi(\boldsymbol{\theta}|D^{(-i)}) \propto \left[\prod_{j\neq i} f(y_j|\boldsymbol{\theta}, \boldsymbol{x}_j)\right] \pi(\theta). \tag{5}$$

Let $\boldsymbol{z} = (z_1, z_2, \ldots, z_n)'$ denote future values of a replicate experiment. Also let $\pi(z_i|\boldsymbol{x}_i, D^{(-i)})$ denote the conditional density of z_i given $\boldsymbol{x}_i$ and

$D^{(-i)}$ defined as

$$\pi(z_i|\boldsymbol{x}_i, D^{(-i)}) = \int f(z_i|\boldsymbol{\theta}, \boldsymbol{x}_i)\pi(\theta|D^{(-i)})\, d\boldsymbol{\theta}, \tag{6}$$

for $i = 1, 2, \ldots, n$. The conditional predictive density $\pi(z_i|\boldsymbol{x}_i, D^{(-i)})$ is also called the cross-validated predictive density. This density is to be checked against y_i, for $i = 1, 2, \ldots, n$ in the sense that, if the model holds, y_i may be viewed as a random observation from $\pi(z_i|\boldsymbol{x}_i, D^{(-i)})$. To do this, we take $z_i = y_i$ in (6) and then we obtain the Conditional Predictive Ordinate (CPO):

$$\mathrm{CPO}_i = \pi(y_i|\boldsymbol{x}_i, D^{(-i)}). \tag{7}$$

CPO_i, which was proposed by Geisser (1980) and further discussed in Gelfand, Dey, and Chang (1992), is a very useful quantity for model checking, since it describes how much the ith observation supports the model. Large CPO values indicate a good fit.

Another application of the predictive distribution to construct the Bayesian standardized residual. Similar to the Studentized residuals with the current observation deleted, the Bayesian standardized residual can be computed as

$$d_i = E[g(z_i, y_i)|\boldsymbol{x}_i, D^{(-i)}] = \frac{y_i - E(z_i|\boldsymbol{x}_i, D^{(-i)})}{\sqrt{\mathrm{Var}(z_i|\boldsymbol{x}_i, D^{(-i)})}}, \tag{8}$$

where $\mathrm{Var}(z_i|\boldsymbol{x}_i, D^{(-i)})$ is the variance of z_i with respect to the predictive distribution $\pi(z_i|\boldsymbol{x}_i, D^{(-i)})$ given by (6). Large $|d_i|$'s cast doubt upon the model but retaining the sign of d_i allows patterns of under or over fitting to be revealed.

Example 1. Chen and Deely (1996) consider the problem of estimating apple production y in New Zealand. Let β_j denote the average number of cartons per tree, conditional on the age of the tree, j, for $j = 1, 2, \ldots, 10$. These averages are combined using the linear model

$$y = \sum_{j=1}^{10} \beta_j x_j + \epsilon, \tag{9}$$

where x_j is the number of trees of age j and $\epsilon \sim N(0, \sigma^2)$. Younger trees are known to produce fewer apples on average, so the model is subject to the constraints

$$0 \le \beta_1 \le \beta_2 \le \cdots \le \beta_{10}. \tag{10}$$

Given data D on the number of trees and production by year and by orchard, Chen and Deely (1996) choose a noninformative prior for β_1, ...,

β_9, and σ^2 as well as a proper prior for β_{10}, which allow them to derive the full joint posterior density

$$\pi(\boldsymbol{\beta}, \sigma^2|D) = \frac{\exp\left\{-\frac{(\beta_{10}-\mu_{10})^2}{2\sigma_{10}^2}\right\}}{c(D)\sigma^{N+1}} \exp\left\{-\frac{1}{2\sigma^2}\sum_{i=1}^{N}\left(y_i - \sum_{j=1}^{10}\beta_j x_{ij}\right)^2\right\}, \tag{11}$$

where $\boldsymbol{\beta} = (\beta_1, \beta_2, \ldots, \beta_{10})'$, $c(D)$ is the normalizing constant, $0 \leq \beta_1 \leq \beta_2 \leq \cdots \leq \beta_{10}$, and $\sigma^2 > 0$. For the New Zealand apple data, $N = 207$, $\mu_{10} = 0.998$, and $\sigma_{10}^2 = 0.0891$, where μ_{10} and σ_{10}^2 are specified using method-of-moments estimates from the growers' data for trees of age 10.

For the model given in (9), we have

$$f(z_i|\boldsymbol{\beta}, \sigma^2, \boldsymbol{x}_i) = \frac{1}{\sqrt{2\pi}\sigma}\exp\left\{-\frac{(z_i - \boldsymbol{x}_i'\boldsymbol{\beta})^2}{2\sigma^2}\right\},$$

where $\boldsymbol{x}_i = (x_{i1}, x_{i2}, \ldots, x_{i,10})'$. Thus,

$$E(z_i|\boldsymbol{x}_i, D^{(-i)}) = \int (\boldsymbol{x}_i'\boldsymbol{\beta})\pi(\boldsymbol{\beta}, \sigma^2|D^{(-i)})\, d\boldsymbol{\beta}\, d\sigma^2 .$$

Note that CPO_i given by (7) can be rewritten as

$$\text{CPO}_i = f(y_i|\boldsymbol{x}_i, D^{(-i)}) = \left(\int \frac{1}{f(y_i|\boldsymbol{\beta}, \sigma^2, \boldsymbol{x}_i)}\pi(\boldsymbol{\beta}, \sigma^2|D)\, d\boldsymbol{\beta}\right)^{-1}.$$

Let $\{(\boldsymbol{\beta}_l, \sigma_l^2),\ l = 1, 2, \ldots, L\}$ denote a Gibbs sample from $\pi(\boldsymbol{\beta}, \sigma^2|D)$ using the Gibbs sampler given in Section 4. Then, the Monte Carlo estimate of CPO_i is given by

$$\widehat{\text{CPO}}_i = L\left[\sum_{l=1}^{L}\left(f(y_i|\boldsymbol{\beta}_l, \sigma_l^2, \boldsymbol{x}_i)\right)^{-1}\right]^{-1}, \tag{12}$$

and the Monte Carlo estimates of $E(z_i|\boldsymbol{x}_i, D^{(-i)})$ and $\text{Var}(z_i|\boldsymbol{x}_i, D^{(-i)})$ are given by

$$\hat{E}(z_i|\boldsymbol{x}_i, D^{(-i)})) = \widehat{\text{CPO}}_i L^{-1}\sum_{l=1}^{L}\frac{\boldsymbol{x}_i'\boldsymbol{\beta}_l}{f(y_i|\boldsymbol{\beta}_l, \sigma_l^2, \boldsymbol{x}_i)}, \tag{13}$$

and

$$\begin{aligned}\widehat{\text{Var}}(z_i|\boldsymbol{x}_i, D^{(-i)})) &= \hat{E}(z_i^2|\boldsymbol{x}_i, D^{(-i)}) - [\hat{E}(z_i|\boldsymbol{x}_i, D^{(-i)})]^2\\ &= \widehat{\text{CPO}}_i L^{-1}\sum_{l=1}^{L}\frac{\sigma_l^2 + (\boldsymbol{x}_i'\boldsymbol{\beta}_l)^2}{f(y_i|\boldsymbol{\beta}_l, \sigma_l^2, \boldsymbol{x}_i)} - [\hat{E}(z_i|\boldsymbol{x}_i, D^{(-i)})]^2,\end{aligned} \tag{14}$$

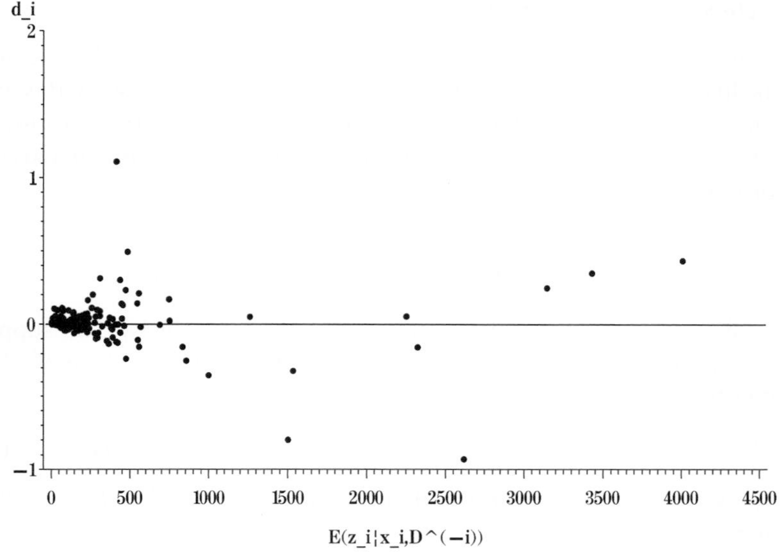

Fig. 1. The Bayesian standardized residual plot.

respectively. Using (13) and (14), the Monte Carlo estimate of the Bayesian standardized residual d_i is

$$\hat{d}_i = \frac{y_i - \hat{E}(z_i|\boldsymbol{x}_i, D^{(-i)})}{\sqrt{\widehat{\text{Var}}(z_i|\boldsymbol{x}_i, D^{(-i)})}}. \tag{15}$$

For the New Zealand apple data, Chen and Deely (1996) use 50,000 Gibbs iterations to obtain the $\hat{d}_i$'s, and the results are displayed in Figure 1.

From Figure 1, it can be seen that: (i) the $\hat{d}_i$'s are small when the $\hat{E}(z_i|\boldsymbol{x}_i, D^{(-i)})$'s are small; and (ii) the $\hat{d}_i$'s are roughly symmetric about zero, which implies that the model is neither over-fitted nor under-fitted. Chen and Deely (1996) also check the distribution of $\hat{d}_i$ and find that the $\hat{d}_i$'s roughly follow a Student t distribution. Noting that $f(y_i|\boldsymbol{\beta}, \sigma^2, \boldsymbol{x}_i)$ is a normal distribution and $\hat{f}(y_i|\boldsymbol{x}_i, D^{(-i)})$ in (12) is a finite mixture of normal distributions, it follows from a result of Johnson and Geisser (1983) that $f(y_i|\boldsymbol{x}_i, D^{(-i)})$ is approximately a Student t distribution. Hence the results obtained by Chen and Deely (1996) are consistent with the theoretical result of Johnson and Geisser (1983), and give further support that the normal assumption of the error terms in the constrained multiple linear regression model is appropriate.

2.3. *Marginal distributions*

In Bayesian inference, a joint posterior distribution is available through the likelihood function and a prior distribution. One purpose of Bayesian inference is to calculate and display marginal posterior densities because the marginal posterior densities provide complete information about parameters of interest.

Let

$$\boldsymbol{\theta}^{(j)} = (\theta_1, \dots, \theta_j)' \quad \text{and} \quad \boldsymbol{\theta}^{(-j)} = (\theta_{j+1}, \dots, \theta_p)'$$

be the first j and last $p - j$ components of $\boldsymbol{\theta}$, respectively. The support of the conditional joint marginal posterior density of $\boldsymbol{\theta}^{(j)}$ given $\boldsymbol{\theta}^{(-j)}$ is denoted by

$$\Omega_j(\boldsymbol{\theta}^{(-j)}) = \{(\theta_1, \dots, \theta_j)' : (\theta_1, \dots, \theta_j, \theta_{j+1}, \dots, \theta_p)' \in \Omega\}, \tag{16}$$

and the subspace of Ω, given the first j components $\boldsymbol{\theta}^{*(j)} = (\theta_1^*, \dots, \theta_j^*)'$, is denoted by

$$\Omega_{-j}(\boldsymbol{\theta}^{*(j)}) = \left\{(\theta_{j+1}, \dots, \theta_p)' : (\theta_1^*, \dots, \theta_j^*, \theta_{j+1}, \dots, \theta_p)' \in \Omega\right\}. \tag{17}$$

Then the marginal posterior density of $\boldsymbol{\theta}^{(j)}$ evaluated at $\boldsymbol{\theta}^{*(j)}$ has the form

$$\pi(\boldsymbol{\theta}^{*(j)}|D) = \int_{\Omega_{-j}(\boldsymbol{\theta}^{*(j)})} \pi(\boldsymbol{\theta}^{*(j)}, \boldsymbol{\theta}^{(-j)}|D)\, d\boldsymbol{\theta}^{(-j)}. \tag{18}$$

In general, the analytical evaluation of $\pi(\boldsymbol{\theta}^{*(j)}|D)$ is not available. Thus, a Monte Carlo method is much needed to estimate it. There are several Monte Carlo methods available. These include the kernel density estimation, the conditional density estimation, and the importance weighted marginal density estimation (IWMDE) of Chen (1994). Here, we briefly describe how IWMDE works, and we refer the interesting readers to Chen, Shao, and Ibrahim (2000) for detailed discussion of other methods.

Consider the following identity:

$$\pi(\boldsymbol{\theta}^{*(j)}|D) = \int_{\Omega} \frac{w(\boldsymbol{\theta}^{(j)}|\boldsymbol{\theta}^{(-j)})\pi(\boldsymbol{\theta}^{*(j)}, \boldsymbol{\theta}^{(-j)}|D)}{\pi(\boldsymbol{\theta}|D)} \pi(\boldsymbol{\theta}|D)\, d\boldsymbol{\theta}, \tag{19}$$

where $w(\boldsymbol{\theta}^{(j)}|\boldsymbol{\theta}^{(-j)})$ is a completely known conditional density whose support is contained in, or equal to, the support, $\Omega_j(\boldsymbol{\theta}^{(-j)})$, of the conditional density $\pi(\boldsymbol{\theta}^{(j)}|\boldsymbol{\theta}^{(-j)}, D)$. Here, "*completely* known" means that $w(\boldsymbol{\theta}^{(j)}|\boldsymbol{\theta}^{(-j)})$ can be evaluated at any point of $(\boldsymbol{\theta}^{(j)}, \boldsymbol{\theta}^{(-j)})$. In other words, the kernel *and* the normalizing constant of this conditional density are available in closed form. Using the identity (19), the IWMDE of $\pi(\boldsymbol{\theta}^{*(j)}|D)$ is defined by

$$\hat{\pi}(\boldsymbol{\theta}^{*(j)}|D) = \frac{1}{n}\sum_{i=1}^{n} w(\boldsymbol{\theta}_i^{(j)}|\boldsymbol{\theta}_i^{(-j)})\frac{\pi(\boldsymbol{\theta}^{*(j)},\boldsymbol{\theta}_i^{(-j)}|D)}{\pi(\boldsymbol{\theta}_i^{(j)},\boldsymbol{\theta}_i^{(-j)}|D)}, \tag{20}$$

where $\{\boldsymbol{\theta}_i = (\boldsymbol{\theta}_i^{(j)},\boldsymbol{\theta}_i^{(-j)}),\ i = 1,2,\ldots,n\}$ is an MCMC sample from $\pi(\boldsymbol{\theta}|D)$. In (20), w plays the role of a weight function. Further, $\hat{\pi}(\boldsymbol{\theta}^{*(j)}|D)$ does not depend on the unknown normalizing constant $c(D)$, since $c(D)$ cancels in the ratio $\pi(\boldsymbol{\theta}^{*(j)},\boldsymbol{\theta}_i^{(-j)}|D)/\pi(\boldsymbol{\theta}_i^{(j)},\boldsymbol{\theta}_i^{(-j)}|D)$. In fact, using (1), we can rewrite (20) as

$$\hat{\pi}(\boldsymbol{\theta}^{*(j)}|D) = \frac{1}{n}\sum_{i=1}^{n} w(\boldsymbol{\theta}_i^{(j)}|\boldsymbol{\theta}_i^{(-j)})\frac{L(\boldsymbol{\theta}^{*(j)},\boldsymbol{\theta}_i^{(-j)}|D)\pi(\boldsymbol{\theta}^{*(j)},\boldsymbol{\theta}_i^{(-j)})}{L(\boldsymbol{\theta}_i|D)\pi(\boldsymbol{\theta}_i)}.$$

The choice of w and the properties of $\hat{\pi}(\boldsymbol{\theta}^{*(j)}|D)$ can be found in Chen (1994). Thus, the detail is omitted here for brevity.

2.4. *Posterior model probabilities*

Suppose there are $\mathcal{K}$ models under consideration. Assume model m has a vector $\boldsymbol{\theta}^{(m)}$ of unknown parameters, with dimension p_m, which may vary from model to model, for $m = 1,2,\ldots,\mathcal{K}$. Under model m, the posterior distribution of $\boldsymbol{\theta}^{(m)}$ takes the form

$$\pi(\boldsymbol{\theta}^{(m)}|D,m) \propto \pi^*(\boldsymbol{\theta}^{(m)}|D,m) = L(\boldsymbol{\theta}^{(m)}|D,m)\pi(\boldsymbol{\theta}^{(m)}|m), \tag{21}$$

where $L(\boldsymbol{\theta}^{(m)}|D,m)$ is the likelihood function, D denotes the data, $\pi(\boldsymbol{\theta}^{(m)}|m)$ is the prior distribution, and $\pi^*(\boldsymbol{\theta}^{(m)}|D,m)$ is the unnormalized posterior density. Let $p(m)$ denote the prior probability of model m. Then, using Bayes' theorem, the posterior probability of model m can be written as

$$p(m|D) = \frac{p(D|m)p(m)}{\sum_{j=1}^{\mathcal{K}} p(D|j)p(j)}, \tag{22}$$

where

$$p(D|m) = \int L(\boldsymbol{\theta}^{(m)}|D,m)\ \pi(\boldsymbol{\theta}^{(m)}|m)\ d\boldsymbol{\theta}^{(m)} = \int \pi^*(\boldsymbol{\theta}^{(m)}|D,m)d\boldsymbol{\theta}^{(m)} \tag{23}$$

denotes the marginal distribution of the data D under model m. The marginal density $p(D|m)$ is precisely the normalizing constant of the joint posterior density of $\boldsymbol{\theta}^{(m)}$. We choose the model with the largest posterior model probability $p(m|D)$.

Model selection, in particular variable selection, is one of the most frequently encountered problems in statistical data analysis. In cancer or AIDS clinical trials, for example, one often wishes to assess the importance of certain prognostic factors such as treatment, age, gender, or race in predicting survival outcome. Bayesian approach to model selection is more attractive than a criterion-based classical method such as the Akaike Information Criterion (AIC) (Akaike 1973) or Bayesian Information Criterion (BIC) (Schwarz 1978), since available prior information can be incorporated into the posterior model probability via $p(m)$ and $\pi(\boldsymbol{\theta}^{(m)}|m)$ and thus more power can be achieved in order to identify the correct model. However, Bayesian model selection is often difficult to carry out because of the challenge in

(i) specifying prior distributions for the regression parameters for all possible models;
(ii) specifying a prior distribution on the model space; and
(iii) computations.

Other than focusing on a particular model selection using the largest posterior probability, one may also use the probability in (22) as a weight function to incorporate model uncertainty in a prediction. Such a criterion is called *Bayesian Model Averaging* or simply *BMA*. Suppose that one is interested in predicting certain quantity Δ such as predicting a future observation or a coefficient estimation for a regression problem. Instead of using just one model in prediction, one makes a prediction by average all feasible models through a weighted average whereas the weights are calculated from the posterior probabilities of the models. The posterior distribution given data D is

$$p(\Delta|D) = \sum_{\text{model } m} p(\Delta|m, D)p(m|D). \tag{24}$$

The models used in the above calculation are the ones with significant posterior probabilities. The purpose of this model averaging is to avoid any risk of believing that the data belongs to a particular model. Instead, it accounts for the model uncertainty in predictions.

The two elements of the model selection problem (model search and model selection criterion) are naturally integrated in model averaging.

Table 1. Regular model selection results for the body fat data.

Method	Variable names	R^2	s^2
Stepwise	Age, Weight, Neck, Abdomen, Thigh, Forearm, Wrist	0.7445	18.41
Adjusted R^2	Age, Weight, Neck, Abdomen, Hip, Thigh, Biceps, Forearm, Wrist	0.7447	18.32

This overcomes the inherent deficiency of the deterministic model selection approach by combining (averaging) information on all or a subset of models when estimating parameters, making inferences, or predicting new observations, instead of using a single model.

More details of *BMA* and some of its applications can be found in Hoeting, *et al.* (1999), Hoeting, Raftery, and Madigan (1996, 1999), Lipkovich, Smith and Ye (2008), Madigan and Raftery (1994), Raftery (1995) and Raftery, Madigan and Volinsky (1997) and the references therein. Assessment of the BMA performance, the performance of BIC in BMA computation, and using Bayes factor to account for model uncertainty can be found in Boone, Ye and Smith (2005), Lipkovich, Ye, and Smith (2010) and Raftery (1996). As an illustration, we look at the following example.

Example 2. A variety of popular health books suggest that the readers assess their health, at least in part, by estimating their percentage of body fat. A data set used in Penrose, Nelson and Fisher (1985) studied the predictive equations of human's body fat with other variables such as Age, Weight, Height, Neck circumference, Chest circumference, Abdomen 2 circumference, Hip circumference, Thigh circumference, Knee circumference, Ankle circumference, Biceps (extended) circumference, Forearm circumference and Wrist circumference. Apparently a multiple linear regression model can be used here. However, since there are a lot of independent variables, it is quite natural to use certain model selection techniques to obtain a "best" model. The two commonly used methods, namely stepwise regression and adjusted R^2 method come up with two different models as follows.

From Table 1, it seems both methods yielded quite comparative results in terms of variation explanation and regression accuracy. Suppose that we want to predict somebody's body fat at the values Age = 36, Weight = 226.75, Height = 71.75, Neck = 41.5, Chest = 115.3, Abdomen = 108.8, Hip = 114.4, Thigh = 69.2, Knee = 42.4, Ankle = 24, Biceps = 35.4, Forearm = 21 and Wrist = 20.1. The stepwise regression gave

Table 2. Posterior probabilities of models for the body fat data.

Model	Variable names	R^2	$p(m\|D)$
1	Weight,Abdomen,Forearm,Wrist	0.7350	0.47043
2	Weight, Abdomen, Wrist	0.7277	0.24656
3	Weight, Abdomen, Biceps, Wrist	0.7328	0.16415
4	Weight, Neck, Abdomen, Forearm, Wrist	0.7379	0.11885

an estimate of 21.39 with a prediction variance 22.73, while the adjusted R^2 resulted in an estimate of 21.73 with a prediction variance 22.81. Note that those variances are the variances of the predictions under given models. If the prediction model is not a correct one, then the variance in prediction would be very different.

On the other hand, we may use the method of *BMA* to deal with this data set. The models with significant posterior probabilities are given in Table 2.

In Table 2, it clearly shows that both models selected by classical sequential model selection methods are not with high posterior probabilities. To predict the person's body fat for the same values as above, the prediction is at 24.26 with a prediction variance of 26.82. However, this is the variance over all plausible models and it can be decomposed by two parts. The first part is 21.37 which is quite comparable to the variances we derived using sequential methods. This part is called pooled variances of all the models used in *BMA*. The second part, which is 5.45, is the part due to model uncertainty.

Bayesian approaches are now feasible due to recent advances in computing technology and the development of efficient computational algorithms. In particular, Chen, Ibrahim, and Yiannoutsos (1999) and Ibrahim, Chen, and Ryan (2000) propose informative prior distributions $\pi(\boldsymbol{\theta}^{(m)}|m)$ and $p(m)$ for the parameter $\boldsymbol{\theta}^{(m)}$ and model m, and develop novel methods for computing the marginal distribution of the data. In addition, the stochastic search variable selection of George and McCulloch (1993) and a novel reversible jump MCMC algorithm proposed by Green (1995) make the computation of posterior model probabilities possible when $\mathcal{K}$ is large. In Section 6 below, we present a real data example from a series of animal toxicological experiments performed in the Department of Biology at the University of Waterloo to illustrate Bayesian model selection using informative priors.

3. Prior Elicitation

Prior distribution is one of the most important elements in Bayesian methodology. As the matter of fact, it is the most challenging element to practitioners. Rather than having a large amount of data when people can use large sample theory, most of the experiments consist of small to moderate sample size data sets. Thus, prior distribution plays a very important role in Bayesian analysis. We insist that whenever a practitioner can summarize historical or subjective information on an unknown, an informative prior should be elicited. The difficulty of seeking an informative prior lies in how one can connect the known or subjective information to a prior distribution. Conjugate priors are most commonly sought before because of the simplicity of the distributional forms and computational reason. However, the recent development in Bayesian computation overcome much of the difficulty using non-conjugate priors. Hence, to a practitioner, it is important to summarize all the information about an unknown to an approximate distribution form and use such a distribution as a prior.

On the other hand, many times, either historical or subjective knowledge of the unknown is not available, or there are too many parameters whose prior distributions need to be specified, noninformative priors are constantly used as alternatives. However, as contrary to its name, all noninformative priors are actually informative. They are usually based on different criteria people use to generate prior distributions serving different purposes.

In subsequent subsections, we discuss in more details about informative and noninformative priors.

3.1. *Informative priors*

Informative priors are useful in applied research settings where the investigator has access to previous studies measuring the same response and covariates as the current study. For example, in many cancer and AIDS clinical trials, current studies often use treatments that are very similar or slight modifications of treatments used in previous studies. We refer to data arising from previous similar studies as *historical data*. In carcinogenicity studies, for example, large historical databases exist for the control animals from previous experiments. In all of these situations, it is natural to incorporate the historical data into the current study by quantifying it with a suitable prior distribution on the model parameters. The methodology discussed here can be applied to each of these situations as well as in other applications that involve historical data.

From a Bayesian perspective, historical data from past similar studies can be very helpful in interpreting the results of the current study. For example, historical control data can be very helpful in interpreting the results of a carcinogenicity study. According to Haseman, Huff and Boorman (1984), historical data can be useful when control tumor rates are low and when marginal significance levels are obtained in a test for dose effects. Suppose, for example, that 4 of 50 animals in an exposed group develop a specific tumor, compared with 0 of 50 in a control group. This difference is not statistically significant ($p = 0.12$, based on Fisher's exact test). However, the difference may be biologically significant if the observed tumor type is known to be extremely rare in the particular animal strain being studied. By specifying a suitable prior distribution on the control response rates that reflect the observed rates of a particular defect over a large series of past studies, one can derive a modified test statistic that incorporates historical information. If the defect is rare enough in the historical series, then even the difference of 4/50 versus 0/50 will be statistically significant based on a method that appropriately incorporates historical information.

To fix ideas, suppose we have historical data from a similar previous study, denoted by $D_0 = (n_0, y_0, X_0)$ where n_0 is the sample size of the historical data, y_0 is the $n_0 \times 1$ response vector, and X_0 is the $n_0 \times p$ matrix of covariates based on the historical data. Chen, Ibrahim, and Shao (2000) and Ibrahim and Chen (2000) proposed the power prior to incorporate historical information. The power prior is defined to be the likelihood function based on the historical data D_0, raised to a power a_0, where $0 \leq a_0 \leq 1$ is a scalar parameter that it controls the influence of the historical data on the current data. One of the most useful applications of the power prior is for model selection problems, since these priors inherently automate the informative prior specification for all possible models in the model space. They are quite attractive in this context, since specifying meaningful informative prior distributions for the parameters in each model is a difficult task requiring contextual interpretations of a large number of parameters. In variable subset selection, for example, the prior distributions for all possible subset models are automatically determined once the historical data D_0, and a_0 are specified. Berger and Mallows (1988) refer to such priors as "semi-automatic" in their discussion of Mitchell and Beauchamp (1988). Chen, Manatunga, and Williams (1998) use the power prior for heritability estimates from human twin data. Chen, Ibrahim, and Yiannoutsos (1999) demonstrate the use of the power prior in variable selection contexts for logistic regression. Ibrahim, Chen, and Ryan (1999) and Chen,

Ibrahim, Shao, and Weiss (2001) develop the power prior for the class of generalized linear mixed models. Ibrahim and Chen (1998), Ibrahim, Chen, and MacEachern (1999), Chen, Ibrahim, and Sinha (1999), Chen, Dey, and Sinha (2000) develop the power prior for various types of models for survival data, and Duan, Smith, Ye (2006), Duan, Ye, and Smith (2006), Neuenschwander, Branson, and Spiegelhalter (2009), Hobbs *et al.* (2011), and Hobbs, Sargent, and Carlin (2012) extend the power prior of Ibrahim and Chen (2000) to develop the normalized power prior and its variations.

Let $\pi_0(\boldsymbol{\theta})$ denote the prior distribution for $\boldsymbol{\theta}$ before the historical data D_0 is observed. We shall call $\pi_0(\boldsymbol{\theta})$ the *initial prior* distribution for θ. Given a_0, we define the *power prior* distribution of θ for the current study as

$$\pi(\boldsymbol{\theta}|D_0, a_0) \propto L(\boldsymbol{\theta}|D_0)^{a_0}\ \pi_0(\boldsymbol{\theta}), \tag{25}$$

where a_0 is a scalar prior parameter that weights the historical data relative to the likelihood of the current study. The parameter a_0 can be interpreted as a precision parameter for the historical data. It is reasonable to restrict the range of a_0 to be between 0 and 1, and thus we take $0 \leq a_0 \leq 1$. One of the main roles of a_0 is that it controls the heaviness of the tails of the prior for $\boldsymbol{\theta}$. As a_0 becomes smaller, the tails of (25) become heavier. Setting $a_0 = 1$, (25) corresponds to the update of $\pi_0(\boldsymbol{\theta}|c_0)$ using Bayes theorem. That is, with $a_0 = 1$, (25) corresponds to the posterior distribution of $\boldsymbol{\theta}$ from the previous study. When $a_0 = 0$, then the prior does not depend on the historical data, and in this case, $\pi(\boldsymbol{\theta}|D_0, a_0 = 0) \equiv \pi_0(\boldsymbol{\theta})$. Thus, $a_0 = 0$ is equivalent to prior specification with no incorporation of historical data. Therefore, (25) can be viewed as a generalization of the usual Bayesian update of $\pi_0(\boldsymbol{\theta})$. The parameter a_0 allows the investigator to control the influence of the historical data on the current study. Such control is important in cases where there is heterogeneity between the previous and current study, or when the sample sizes of the two studies are quite different.

The hierarchical power prior specification is completed by specifying a (proper) prior distribution for a_0. Thus we propose a joint power prior distribution for (θ, a_0) of the form

$$\pi(\boldsymbol{\theta}, a_0|D_0)\ \propto\ L(\boldsymbol{\theta}|D_0)^{a_0}\pi_0(\boldsymbol{\theta})\pi(a_0|\gamma_0), \tag{26}$$

where $\boldsymbol{\gamma}_0$ is a specified hyperparameter vector. A natural choice for $\pi(a_0|\gamma_0)$ is a beta prior. However, other choices, including a truncated gamma prior or a truncated normal prior can be used. These three priors for a_0 have similar theoretical properties, and our experience shows that they have similar computational properties. In practice, they yield similar results when the hyperparameters are appropriately chosen. Thus, for a clear focus and exposition, we will use a *beta* distribution for $\pi(a_0|\gamma_0)$, which takes the form

$$\pi(a_0|\gamma_0) \propto a_0^{\delta_0 - 1}(1-a_0)^{\lambda_0 - 1},$$

where $\gamma_0 = (\delta_0, \lambda_0)$. The beta prior for a_0 appears to be the most natural prior to use and leads to the most natural elicitation scheme. The prior in (26) does not have a closed form in general, but it has several attractive theoretical and computational properties for the classes of models considered here. One attractive feature of (26) is that it creates heavier tails for the marginal prior of $\boldsymbol{\theta}$ than the prior in (25), which assumes that a_0 is a fixed value. This is a desirable feature since it gives the investigator more flexibility in weighting the historical data. In addition, the construction of (26) is quite general, with various possibilities for $\pi_0(\boldsymbol{\theta})$. If $\pi_0(\boldsymbol{\theta})$ is proper, then (26) is guaranteed to be proper. Further, (26) can be proper even if $\pi_0(\boldsymbol{\theta})$ is an improper uniform prior. Specifically, Ibrahim, Ryan and Chen (1998) and Chen, Ibrahim, and Yiannoutsos (1999) characterize the propriety of (26) for generalized linear models, and also show that for fixed a_0, the prior converges to a multivariate normal distribution as $n_0 \to \infty$. For the class of generalized linear mixed models, Ibrahim, Chen, and Ryan (1999), Chen, Ibrahim, Shao, and Weiss (2001), and Chen, Dey, and Sinha (2000) characterize the propriety of (26) and derive various other theoretical properties of the power prior. Ibrahim, Chen, and MacEachern (1999), and Ibrahim and Chen (1998) characterize various properties of (26) for proportional hazards models, and Chen, Ibrahim, and Sinha (1999) examine various theoretical properties of (26) for a class of cure rate models.

Example 3. For illustrative purposes, we consider an analysis of the AIDS study ACTG036 using the data from ACTG019 as historical data.

The ACTG019 study was a double blind placebo-controlled clinical trial comparing zidovudine (AZT) to placebo in persons with CD4 counts less than 500. The results of this study were published in Volberding *et al.* (1990). The sample size for this study, excluding cases with missing data, was $n_0 = 823$. The response variable (y_0) for these data is binary with a 1 indicating death, development of AIDS, or AIDS related complex (ARC), and a 0 indicates otherwise. Several covariates were also measured. The ACTG036 study was also a placebo-controlled clinical trial comparing AZT to placebo in patients with hereditary coagulation disorders. The results of this study have been published by Merigen *et al.* (1991). The sample size in this study, excluding cases with missing data, was $n = 183$. The response variable (y) for these data is binary with a 1 indicating death, development of AIDS, or AIDS related complex (ARC), and a 0 indicates otherwise. Several covariates were measured for these data. A summary of both data sets can be found in Chen, Ibrahim, and Yiannoutsos (1999). Therefore, we let D_0 denote the data from the ACTG019 study and D denote the data from the ACTG036 study.

Chen, Ibrahim, and Yiannoutsos (1999) use the priors given by (26) and the logistic regression model to carry out variable subset selection, which yields the model containing an intercept, CD4 count (cell count per mm^3 of serum), age, and treatment as the best model. For this model, we use the power prior (26) to obtain posterior estimates of the regression coefficients for various choices of $(\mu_{a_0}, \sigma_{a_0})$, where $\mu_{a_0} = \frac{\delta_0}{\delta_0+\lambda_0}$ and $\sigma_{a_0}^2 = \mu_{a_0}(1 - \mu_{a_0})(\delta_0 + \lambda_0 + 1)^{-1}$. The results based on the standardized covariates and the logit model with an improper uniform prior for the regression coefficients are given in Table 3. The values of $(\mu_{a_0}, \sigma_{a_0})$ and the corresponding values of (δ_0, λ_0) are also reported in the table. We used 50,000 Gibbs iterations for all posterior computations and the Monte Carlo method of Chen and Shao (1999) to calculate 95% highest probability density (HPD) intervals for the parameters of interest. From Table 3, we see that as the weight for ACTG019 study increases, the posterior mean of a_0 (denoted $E(a_0|D, D_0)$) increases, the posterior standard deviations (Std Dev) for all parameters decrease, and the 95% HPD intervals get narrower. Most noticeably, when $(\delta_0, \lambda_0) = (100, 1)$, none of the HPD intervals for the regression coefficients contain 0. Table 3 also indicates that the HPD intervals are not too sensitive for moderate changes in $(\mu_{a_0}, \sigma_{a_0})$. This is a comforting feature, since it implies that the HPD intervals are fairly robust with respect to the hyperparameters of a_0. This same robustness feature is also exhibited in posterior model probability calculations (see Chen, Ibrahim, and Yiannoutsos, 1999).

3.2. *Conjugate priors*

Conjugate priors were quite popular before the powerful breakthrough of the Bayesian computational techniques. Suppose $\mathcal{F}$ is a class of prior distributions for $\boldsymbol{\theta}$, where $\boldsymbol{\theta}$ is the parameter, $\mathcal{P}$ a class of sampling distributions $f(y|\boldsymbol{\theta})$. The class $\mathcal{F}$ is conjugate for $\mathcal{P}$ for any $f(y|\boldsymbol{\theta})$ in $\mathcal{P}$ if the prior $\pi(\boldsymbol{\theta})$ and the posterior $\pi(\boldsymbol{\theta}|y)$ all from the same family $\mathcal{F}$. Since the posterior distributions have the same form as the prior, the closed form of the posteriors can be derived accordingly. Hence, it does not cause much trouble

Table 3. Posterior estimates for AIDS Data.

(δ_0, λ_0)	$(\mu_{a_0}, \sigma_{a_0})$	$E(a_0 \mid D, D_0)$	Variable	Posterior Mean	Posterior Std Dev	95% HPD Interval
(5, 5)	(0.50, 0.151)	0.02	Intercept	−4.389	0.725	(−5.836, −3.055)
			CD4 count	−1.437	0.394	(−2.238, −0.711)
			Age	0.135	0.221	(−0.314, 0.556)
			Treatment	−0.120	0.354	(−0.817, 0.570)
(20, 20)	(0.50, 0.078)	0.09	Intercept	−3.803	0.511	(−4.834, −2.868)
			CD4 count	−1.129	0.300	(−1.723, −0.559)
			Age	0.176	0.195	(−0.214, 0.552)
			Treatment	−0.223	0.300	(−0.821, 0.364)
(30, 30)	(0.50, 0.064)	0.13	Intercept	−3.621	0.436	(−4.489, −2.809)
			CD4 count	−1.028	0.265	(−1.551, −0.515)
			Age	0.194	0.185	(−0.170, 0.557)
			Treatment	−0.259	0.278	(−0.805, 0.288)
(50, 1)	(0.98, 0.019)	0.26	Intercept	−3.337	0.323	(−3.978, −2.715)
			CD4 count	−0.865	0.211	(−1.276, −0.448)
			Age	0.233	0.160	(−0.081, 0.548)
			Treatment	−0.314	0.230	(−0.766, 0.138)
(100, 1)	(0.99, 0.010)	0.53	Intercept	−3.144	0.231	(−3.601, −2.705)
			CD4 count	−0.746	0.161	(−1.058, −0.429)
			Age	0.271	0.135	(0.001, 0.529)
			Treatment	−0.356	0.181	(−0.717, −0.011)

in computing the posterior as described in Section 1. One simple example is given as follows.

Example 4. Suppose that a random variable Y follows a Poisson distribution with mean λ. The density function of Y given λ can be written as

$$f(y|\lambda) = e^{-\lambda}\frac{\lambda^y}{y!}, \quad \text{for } y = 0, 1, \ldots. \tag{27}$$

Further suppose that the prior distribution of λ is a Gamma distribution with parameters α and β, as follows

$$\pi(\lambda) \propto \lambda^{\alpha} e^{-\beta\lambda}, \quad \text{for } \lambda > 0. \tag{28}$$

The posterior distribution of λ thus can be calculated as

$$\pi(\lambda|y) \propto \pi(\lambda) f(y|\lambda) \propto \lambda^{\alpha} e^{-\beta\lambda} \lambda^{y} e^{-\lambda} \propto \lambda^{\alpha+y} e^{-(\beta+1)\lambda}, \tag{29}$$

which is another Gamma distribution. Clearly, the prior (28) and the posterior (29) all belong to the same Gamma distribution family for any Poisson family sampling distribution.

The practical advantage of the conjugate prior distributions is obvious. This is the reason why it is still popular when practitioners often use it if they believe that their priors may be specified as conjugate priors. Although, it is flexible to elicit a conjugate prior due to changing the hyper-parameter values, many times it is not accurate to decide a prior knowledge by only choosing one or two parameter values. On the other hand, sometimes a finite mixture of conjugate priors may be a good idea to overcome this difficulty since the mixture of conjugate priors is also a conjugate prior (see Berger 1985).

We have to note here that the conjugacy depends on the family $\mathcal{F}$ and $\mathcal{P}$ one chooses. Also, it depends on dimensions of the parameter space. For instance, normal priors on the mean of normal sampling distribution when the variance is known constitute a conjugate prior family, while inverse gamma priors on the variance of normal sampling distribution when the mean is assumed known constitute another conjugate prior family. However, normal priors on the mean and inverse gamma priors on the variance of the normal sampling distribution do not constitute a conjugate family since the marginal posteriors of the mean parameter is no longer normal. This suggests that people have to be careful when examining conjugacy for multi-dimensional parameter problems.

Another point about conjugacy we like to point out is that it is often quite useful to have conditionally conjugacy to parameters for a multi-dimensional parameter model. Conditional conjugacy or sometimes called semi-conjugacy means that the conditional posterior distributions of a set of parameters given others and the prior distribution of the same set of parameters belong to the same distributional family, for instance, to the example we just mentioned above about normal mean and normal variance. Although the marginal posterior distribution of the normal mean is no longer normal, the conditional posterior distribution of the normal mean given that the normal variance is still normal. Likewise, the conditional posterior distribution of the normal variance given the normal mean is still inverse Gamma. The advantage of this semi-conjugacy can be used in full conditional distributions in Gibbs sampling (see Section 4.1).

3.3. *Noninformative priors*

As described in the opening of this section, none of the noninformative priors are non-informative. The derivations of those so called noninformative priors all depend on certain informative criteria. One of the earliest methods of defining noninformative priors was based on the principle of insufficient reason. This method, sometimes referred to as *Laplace's rule*, prescribes a uniform prior on the parameter space $\boldsymbol{\Theta}$. By the way, Laplace used uniform priors on the probabilities of two binomial populations.

Laplace's rule, and the principle of insufficient reason, are intuitively appealing. The reasoning is that if no prior information is available that favors certain parameter values over others, then all parameter values should be considered equally likely. However, the immediate criticism of this uniform prior is that it does not follow probability law in the sense of invariance in parameter transformation. Here is an example:

Example 5. Suppose that Y follows a Binomial distribution with parameters n and p, while n is known. Using Laplace's argument, if there is no subjective prior information available for p, a uniform prior $\pi(p) = 1$, for $0 < p < 1$ should be used. Now assume that we are interested in the parameter $q = 1/(1+p)$. Since we still do not have information about q, we *have to* assume the prior distribution of q as uniform, i.e., $\pi(q) = 2$, for $1/2 < q < 1$. Since q is a variable transformation of p, with the Jacobian $1/q^2$, following the probability law it follows that $\pi(q) = \pi(p(q))/q^2 = 1/q^2$ for $1/2 < q < 1$. However, if both uniform distributions are used, the above equality cannot hold. This implies that the uniform prior is not invariant under transformation.

There is also another issue that has been discussed extensively in Bayesian school. Suppose we are going to use Laplace's rule and assign a uniform prior on the parameter. If the parameter space is finite, the uniform distribution is proper (that is, its integration over it's domain is finite). However, if the parameter space is infinite such as the mean of a normal distribution, a uniform prior is improper (not integrable). Such a phenomenon does not only happen for a uniform prior, it may happen to many other noninformative priors we will discuss later. As a matter of fact, many of the noninformative priors we use are improper.

Although an improper prior is not supported by Bayes' rule, it does not necessarily lead to problems in Bayesian analysis as long as the posterior distributions are proper. For more discussions of improper priors, readers are referred to Berger (1985), Bernardo and Smith (1995), and Kass and Wasserman (1996). Once a posterior distribution is integrable, after normalization to a probability distribution, the final posterior distribution still represents a post-knowledge of the unknowns. Therefore, if an improper noninformative prior is used in practice, it is important to verify that the posterior distribution is integrable before making posterior inferences. This is even more important if simulation methods (see Section 4) are used to draw posterior inference because even if the posterior distribution is improper, sometimes it cannot be detected by using simulation. Therefore, it may lead to inappropriate conclusion when the true posterior distribution is actually improper.

Since the pioneer work of Laplace to use Bayesian methodology into applied statistics, there have been a lot of attempts to seek *default* or *automatic* prior distributions. In the following subsections, we will discuss Jeffreys priors, the reference priors and the probability matching priors.

3.4. *Jeffreys priors*

To overcome the difficulty of the non-invariant uniform prior criterion, Jeffreys (1961) derived a prior using invariance of parameter transformations. Before we present the Jeffreys prior, one term called expected Fisher information needs to be defined. Suppose that a random vector $\boldsymbol{Y}$, given $\boldsymbol{\theta}$, has a probability density function $f(\boldsymbol{y}|\boldsymbol{\theta})$ which is twice differentiable with respect to $\boldsymbol{\theta}$. The expected Fisher information matrix, denoted by $I(\boldsymbol{\theta}) = \{I_{ij}(\boldsymbol{\theta})\}$, is defined as

$$I_{ij}(\boldsymbol{\theta}) = -E_{\boldsymbol{\theta}}\Big[\frac{\delta^2}{\delta\theta_i\delta\theta_j}\log(f(\boldsymbol{y}|\boldsymbol{\theta}))\Big]. \tag{30}$$

Once a sampling distribution is known with the density satisfying the existence of the Fisher information matrix, the Jeffreys prior is simply

$$\pi_J(\boldsymbol{\theta}) \propto \sqrt{\det(I(\boldsymbol{\theta}))}, \tag{31}$$

where det stands for a determinant. For any one-to-one transformation between two parameters $\boldsymbol{\theta}$ and $\boldsymbol{\eta}$, the two priors for $\boldsymbol{\theta}$ or $\boldsymbol{\eta}$ calculated using (31) will not cause any ambiguous results, i.e., the method used here is invariant through parameter transformation. On the other hand, like a uniform prior, Jeffreys prior may be improper. A couple of simple examples can be seen as follows.

Example 6. Suppose that Y follows a Binomial distribution with unknown parameter p and known n. The density function of this distribution is $f(y|p) \propto p^y(1-p)^{n-y}$. Taking second derivative to $-\log(f)$, with respect to p, yields $y/p^2 + (n-y)/(1-p)^2$. The expectation of this form becomes $n/p(1-p)$. Thus, the Jeffreys prior is proportional to $1/\sqrt{p(1-p)}$.

Example 7. Suppose $y_1, \ldots, y_n$ form a random sample from a normal population $N(\mu, \sigma^2)$. The density function is given as $f(y|\mu, \sigma) \propto e^{-(y-\mu)^2/2\sigma^2}/\sigma$. To calculate the Fisher information matrix, note that $I_{11}(\mu, \sigma) = E(1/\sigma^2) = 1/\sigma^2$, $I_{12} = I_{21} = 0$ and $I_{22} = 2/\sigma^2$. Hence the Jeffreys prior for (μ, σ) is $1/\sigma^2$.

Example 8. Suppose that $\{(\boldsymbol{x}_i, y_i, n_i),\ i = 1, 2, \ldots, n\}$ are independent observations, where y_i is a binomial response variable taking a value between 0 and n_i (≥ 1), and $\boldsymbol{x}_i = (x_{i0}, , x_{i1}, \ldots, x_{ik})'$ is a $(k+1) \times 1$ vector of (possibly random) covariates and $x_{i0} = 1$ for the intercept term. The binomial regression model assumes $f(y_i|\boldsymbol{x}_i, n_i, \boldsymbol{\beta}) = \binom{n_i}{y_i}[F(\boldsymbol{x}_i'\boldsymbol{\beta})]^{y_i}[1 - F(\boldsymbol{x}_i'\boldsymbol{\beta})]^{n_i - y_i}$, where $\boldsymbol{\beta} = (\beta_0, \beta_1, \ldots, \beta_k)'$ denotes a $(k+1)$ vector of regression coefficients, $F(\cdot)$ denotes a cumulative distribution function (cdf), and F^{-1} is called the link function. The likelihood function of $\boldsymbol{\beta}$ is $L(\boldsymbol{\beta}|X, \boldsymbol{y}) = \prod_{i=1}^n \binom{n_i}{y_i}\{F(\boldsymbol{x}_i'\boldsymbol{\beta})\}^{y_i}\{1 - F(\boldsymbol{x}_i'\boldsymbol{\beta})\}^{n_i - y_i}$, where $\boldsymbol{y} = (y_1, y_2, \ldots, y_n)'$ and $X = (\boldsymbol{x}_1, \boldsymbol{x}_2, \ldots, \boldsymbol{x}_n)'$ is the $n \times (k+1)$ design matrix. Assume that $F(\cdot)$ is twice differentiable and $f(z) = dF(z)/dz$ denotes the probability density function. Then, Jeffreys's prior for $\boldsymbol{\beta}$ under the binomial regression model is then given by $\pi(\boldsymbol{\beta}|X) \propto |X'W(\boldsymbol{\beta})X|^{1/2}$, where $|X'W(\boldsymbol{\beta})X|$ denotes the determinant of the matrix $X'W(\boldsymbol{\beta})X$, $W(\boldsymbol{\beta}) = \text{diag}(w_1(\boldsymbol{\beta}), w_2(\boldsymbol{\beta}), \ldots, w_n(\boldsymbol{\beta}))$, and $w_i(\boldsymbol{\beta}) = \frac{n_i\{f(\boldsymbol{x}_i'\boldsymbol{\beta})\}^2}{F(\boldsymbol{x}_i'\boldsymbol{\beta})\{1 - F(\boldsymbol{x}_i'\boldsymbol{\beta})\}}$ for $i = 1, 2, \ldots, n$. As shown in Ibrahim and Laud (1991), when X is of full rank, Jeffreys's prior $\pi(\boldsymbol{\beta}|X)$ is proper and the corresponding moment generating function of $\boldsymbol{\beta}$ exists. Chen, Ibrahim, and Kim (2008) show that for certain class of distribution functions F, Jeffreys's prior $\pi(\boldsymbol{\beta}|X)$ is unimodal and has lighter tails than a multivariate t-distribution with ν degrees of freedom for any $\nu > 0$ and heavier tails than a multivariate normal distribution. Chen, Ibrahim, and Kim (2008) also show that the prior and posterior normalizing constants under Jeffreys's prior are linear transformation invariant in the covariates and further establish an interesting theoretical connection between the BIC criterion and the induced dimension penalty term using Jeffreys's prior for binomial regression models with general links in variable selection problems.

Note that while the prior distributions in Examples 6 and 8 are proper, the prior in Example 7 is improper. Yet, in the later example, the posterior distributions are usually proper except in certain degenerate cases. Jeffreys priors are very commonly used for many different models. Even in many other developments of noninformative priors, one can always trace them back to Jeffreys priors in some sense. We will discuss more of those in the following subsections.

One property of the Jeffreys priors is the invariance under parameter transformations. However, the use of Jeffreys prior is not quite appealing in multi-dimensional situations. For instance, Jeffreys prior in Example 7, is $1/\sigma^2$. Of making inference about the mean variable, even Jeffreys himself pointed out that this prior does not yield satisfactory results. Instead, in this case a prior $1/\sigma$ is usually used for the parameterization (μ, σ) which is the product of the Jeffreys prior of μ alone (uniform) and that of σ alone $(1/\sigma)$. Here alone means that when the Jeffreys prior is calculated for one parameter, the other parameter is treated as fixed. In this case, both individual priors do not depend on the fixed parameter. When the product of the two priors is used, it means that "independence" of the prior knowledge of those two parameters is assumed. However, once the data is used, in the posterior analysis, those two parameters are rarely independent.

The above discussion raises a question that what kind of prior is good for multi-dimensional parameter problems. In most of the applied statistical problems, there are more than one parameters and some of them are treated as very important and the others are treated as nuisance. To find a noninformative prior for such kinds of models, Berger and Bernardo (1989) developed an iterative algorithm to calculate noninformative priors for multi-parameter problems. Such priors are called the reference prior which will be briefly described in the next subsection.

3.5. *The reference priors*

The reference prior method, introduced by Bernardo (1979) and further developed by Berger and Bernardo (1989, 1992), is motivated by the notion of maximizing the expected amount of information about the parameter $\boldsymbol{\theta}$ provided by the data $\mathbf{y}$. The amount of information provided by the experiment is quantified by the *Kullback-Liebler divergence*, which is defined by

$$D(g,h) = \int_{\Theta} g(\boldsymbol{\theta}) \log\left(\frac{g(\boldsymbol{\theta})}{h(\boldsymbol{\theta})}\right) d\boldsymbol{\theta},$$

for two densities g and h. The expected information about $\boldsymbol{\theta}$ provided by the data can be naturally defined as

$$E_{\mathbf{Y}}(D(\pi(\boldsymbol{\theta}|\boldsymbol{y}), \pi(\boldsymbol{\theta}))), \tag{32}$$

where $\pi(\boldsymbol{\theta})$ and $\pi(\boldsymbol{\theta}|\boldsymbol{y})$ are prior and posterior distributions, respectively. Theoretically, the reference prior approach is to find a prior such that the quantity (32) is maximized. However, the actual process of this maximization involves a modification of the form (32) and asymptotic process using infinitely many independent replications of the experiments would be used. Now we briefly mention the idea and procedure of the algorithm developed by Berger and Bernardo (1992).

To derive the reference priors for an experiment, one has to decompose the parameter space by ordered groups in the order of importance of the groups: $\boldsymbol{\theta}_{(1)}, \boldsymbol{\theta}_{(2)}, \ldots, \boldsymbol{\theta}_{(m)}$, where each group $\boldsymbol{\theta}_{(j)}$ contains one or more of the scalar parameter in $\boldsymbol{\theta}$. The reference prior is developed iteratively by first computing the marginal prior for $\boldsymbol{\theta}_{(m)}$, then the conditional prior for $\boldsymbol{\theta}_{(m-1)}$ given $\boldsymbol{\theta}_{(m)}$, then the conditional prior for $\boldsymbol{\theta}_{(m-2)}$ given $\boldsymbol{\theta}_{(m-1)}$ and $\boldsymbol{\theta}_{(m)}$, etc. Finally, a reference prior can be obtained by multiplying all the priors above together. In the derivation, the parameter spaces should be truncated to compact sets and certain limiting procedures may be used. The detailed algorithm can be found in Berger and Bernardo (1992).

Note that in addition to being divided into groups, the parameters in $\boldsymbol{\theta}$ are also ordered. The order of the importance of the groups may be different by different users, although the parameter of interests stay the same. Berger and Bernardo recommended single group ordering, which means that there is only one parameter in each group (see also Ye and Berger 1989 and Ye 1993). This recommendation is based on their experience in applying the reference prior method to various applied problem. Since different groupings may yield different reference priors (Berger and Bernardo 1992 and Ye 1994), it is possible that there exist different reference priors for the same model.

Berger and Bernardo also state, concerning the ordering of the parameters in terms of inferential importance, that "... beyond putting the 'parameters of interest' first, it is too vague to be of much use." They recommend that, if possible, all reference priors for which the parameters of interest are placed first in the ordering should be computed. This provides a set of prior distributions which can be compared, to assess the sensitivity of the resulting analyses to the choice of prior distribution.

Finally, we want to point it out that interestingly, under certain regular conditions, the reference prior is the same as the Jeffreys prior which means that using the Jeffreys prior, the expected information about the parameter coming from data only is maximized. More studies of the reference priors can be found in Datta and Ghosh (1996), Ghosh and Mukerjee (1992), Sun and Ye (1995) and Ye (1993). Many more references can also be found in

Kass and Wasserman (1996). In Section 6.3, we will discuss the reference priors for a statistical calibration model.

3.6. *Probability matching priors*

From inference point of view, confidence interval is quite frequently used in practice. Although, the concept of confidence interval creates a lot of confusing in interpretation, this interval however, gives quite important information in accuracy of an estimate. In the frequentist domain such that for many runs of experiments, the probability associated with a confidence interval provides coverage probability of the random intervals covering the true unknown. On the other hand, one can also derive a credible interval in Bayesian study. Such an interval is quite similar to a confidence interval, except that the probability of this credible interval implies the probability that the unknown parameter belonging to two fixed numbers. This is actually how people usually interpret a confidence interval. The advantage in this interpretation comes from the fact that the parameter in consideration is random and the posterior probability is calculated under the parameter domain, not in the frequentist domain anymore.

Getting an *automatic* prior is one purpose of developing a noninformative prior method. This means that the prior derived using this method can be applied to any data created from the statistical model in study. Obviously, not only a Bayesian credible interval is of interest, but also the confidence interval. Probability matching priors are those priors to have the property that posterior probabilities of the posterior quantiles from the resulting Bayesian analysis match frequentist coverage probabilities of the same quantiles, at least asymptotically.

Suppose that θ is a parameter of interest and an interval $(\phi(\boldsymbol{y}) \leq \theta)$ has the posterior probability $\alpha = P(\{\phi(\boldsymbol{y}) \leq \theta)|\boldsymbol{y})$ (α^{th} posterior quantile). On the other hand, if we treat θ as fixed, the frequentist coverage probability of this interval can also be calculated as $P(\phi(\boldsymbol{y}) \leq \theta|\theta)$. If a prior can be obtained such that

$$\alpha = P(\phi(\boldsymbol{y}) \leq \theta|\boldsymbol{y}) \approx P(\phi(\boldsymbol{y}) \leq \theta|\theta), \tag{33}$$

for all $\boldsymbol{y}$ and θ, asymptotically, we say the prior a probability matching prior.

Welch and Peers (1963) are the first ones to study such kind of priors. In one-dimensional case, they found that the Jeffreys priors satisfies this equality in the order of $O(1/\sqrt{n})$, which means that when n goes to infinity, the rate of the difference between the two probabilities in (33) goes to zero in the rate same as $1/\sqrt{n}$. This is called the first order matching. Stein (1985) and Tibshirani (1989) extended their work and used differential equations to obtain more first order matching priors.

The probability matching priors have played certain justification rules to many of the noninformative priors. For instance, in many models, the reference priors are matching priors. However, in a few occasions, they are not. Since there are usually many priors satisfying the differential equations in deriving the probability matching priors, only using this method does not lead to a single prior which may be satisfactory.

4. Bayesian Computation

There are two major challenges involved in advanced Bayesian computation. These are how to sample from posterior distributions and how to compute posterior quantities of interest using Markov chain Monte Carlo (MCMC) samples. Several books, including Tanner (1996), Gilks, Richardson, and Spiegelhalter (1996), Chen, Shao, and Ibrahim (2000), Robert and Casella (2004), Gamerman and Lopes (2006), and Liang, Liu, and Carroll (2010) cover the development of MCMC sampling and advanced Monte Carlo (MC) methods for computing posterior quantities using the samples from the posterior distribution.

4.1. *Sampling from posterior distribution*

During the last decade, Monte Carlo (MC) based sampling methods for evaluating high-dimensional posterior integrals have been rapidly developing. Those sampling methods include MC importance sampling (Hammersley and Handscomb 1964; Ripley 1987; Geweke 1989; and Wolpert 1991), Gibbs sampling (Geman and Geman 1984; Gelfand and Smith 1990), Metropolis–Hastings sampling (Metropolis *et al.* 1953; Hastings 1970; and Green 1995), and many other hybrid algorithms.

The Gibbs sampler may be one of the best known MCMC sampling algorithms in the Bayesian computational literature. As discussed in Besag and Green (1993), the Gibbs sampler is founded on the ideas of Grenander (1983), while the formal term is introduced by Geman and Geman (1984). The primary bibliographical landmark for Gibbs sampling in problems of Bayesian inference is Gelfand and Smith (1990). A similar idea termed as *data augmentation* is introduced by Tanner and Wong (1987). Casella and George (1992) provide an excellent tutorial on the Gibbs sampler.

Let $\boldsymbol{\theta} = (\theta_1, \theta_2, \ldots, \theta_p)'$ be a p-dimensional vector of parameters and let $\pi(\boldsymbol{\theta}|D)$ be its posterior distribution given the data D. Then, the basic scheme of the Gibbs sampler is given as follows:

Step 0. Choose an arbitrary starting point $\boldsymbol{\theta}_0 = (\theta_{1,0}, \theta_{2,0}, \ldots, \theta_{p,0})'$, and set $i = 0$.

Step 1. Generate $\boldsymbol{\theta}_{i+1} = (\theta_{1,i+1}, \theta_{2,i+1}, \ldots, = \theta_{p,i+1})'$ as follows:

- Generate $\theta_{1,i+1} \sim \pi(\theta_1|\theta_{2,i}, \ldots, \theta_{p,i}, D)$;
- Generate $\theta_{2,i+1} \sim \pi(\theta_2|\theta_{1,i+1}, \theta_{3,i}, \ldots, \theta_{p,i}, D)$;

  $\cdots \quad \cdots \quad \cdots$
- Generate $\theta_{p,i+1} \sim \pi(\theta_p|\theta_{1,i+1}, \theta_{2,i+1}, \ldots, \theta_{p-1,i+1}, D)$.

Step 2. Set $i = i + 1$, and go to Step 1.

Thus each component of $\boldsymbol{\theta}$ is visited in the natural order and a cycle in this scheme requires generation of p random variates. Gelfand and Smith (1990) show that under certain regularity conditions, the vector sequence $\{\boldsymbol{\theta}_i,\ i = 1, 2, \ldots\}$ has a stationary distribution $\pi(\boldsymbol{\theta}|D)$. Schervish and Carlin (1992) provide a sufficient condition that guarantees geometric convergence. Other properties regarding geometric convergence are discussed in Roberts and Polson (1994).

Example 9. For the constrained linear model considered in Example 1, the posterior distribution for $(\boldsymbol{\beta}, \sigma^2)$ based on the New Zealand apple data D is given by (11). The Gibbs sampler can be implemented by taking

$$\beta_j|\beta_1, \ldots, \beta_{j-1}, \beta_{j+1}, \ldots, \beta_{10}, \sigma^2, D \sim N(\theta_j, \delta_j^2) \tag{34}$$

subject to $\beta_{j-1} \leq \beta_j \leq \beta_{j+1}$ ($\beta_0 = 0$) for $j = 1, 2, \ldots, 9$,

$$\beta_{10}|\beta_1, \ldots, \beta_9, \sigma^2, D \sim N(\psi\theta_{10} + (1-\psi)\mu_{10}, (1-\psi)\sigma_{10}^2) \tag{35}$$

subject to $\beta_{10} \geq \beta_9$ and

$$\sigma^2|\boldsymbol{\beta}, D \sim \mathcal{IG}\left(\frac{n}{2}, \frac{1}{2}\sum_{i=1}^{n}(y_i - \sum_{j=1}^{10} x_{ij}\beta_j)^2\right), \tag{36}$$

where in (34) and (35), $\psi = \sigma_{10}^2/(\sigma_{10}^2 + \delta_{10}^2)$,

$$\theta_j = \left(\sum_{i=1}^{n} x_{ij}^2\right)^{-1} \left[\sum_{i=1}^{n} \left(y_i - \sum_{l \neq j} x_{il}\beta_l\right) x_{ij}\right], \tag{37}$$

and

$$\delta_j^2 = \left(\sum_{i=1}^{n} x_{ij}^2 \right)^{-1} \sigma^2 \tag{38}$$

for $j = 1, \ldots, 10$, and $\mathcal{IG}(\xi, \eta)$ denotes the inverse gamma distribution with parameters (ξ, η), whose density is given by

$$\pi(\sigma^2 | \xi, \eta) \propto (\sigma^2)^{-(\xi+1)} e^{-\eta/\sigma^2} .$$

The Metropolis–Hastings algorithm is developed by Metropolis *et al.* (1953) and subsequently generalized by Hastings (1970). Tierney (1994) gives a comprehensive theoretical exposition of this algorithm, and Chib and Greenberg (1995) provide an excellent tutorial on this topic.

Let $q(\boldsymbol{\theta}, \boldsymbol{\vartheta})$ be a proposal density, which is also termed as a *candidate-generating density* by Chib and Greenberg (1995), such that

$$\int q(\boldsymbol{\theta}, \boldsymbol{\vartheta}) \, d\boldsymbol{\vartheta} = 1.$$

Also let $U(0,1)$ denote the uniform distribution over $(0,1)$. Then, a general version of the Metropolis–Hastings algorithm for sampling from the posterior distribution $\pi(\boldsymbol{\theta}|D)$ can be described as follows:

Step 0. Choose an arbitrary starting point $\boldsymbol{\theta}_0$ and set $i = 0$.
Step 1. Generate a candidate point $\boldsymbol{\theta}^*$ from $q(\boldsymbol{\theta}_i, \cdot)$ and u from $U(0,1)$.
Step 2. Set $\boldsymbol{\theta}_{i+1} = \boldsymbol{\theta}^*$ if $u \le a(\boldsymbol{\theta}_i, \boldsymbol{\theta}^*)$ and $\boldsymbol{\theta}_{i+1} = \boldsymbol{\theta}_i$ otherwise, where the acceptance probability is given by

$$a(\boldsymbol{\theta}, \boldsymbol{\vartheta}) = \min \left\{ \frac{\pi(\boldsymbol{\vartheta}|D) q(\boldsymbol{\vartheta}, \boldsymbol{\theta})}{\pi(\boldsymbol{\theta}|D) q(\boldsymbol{\theta}, \boldsymbol{\vartheta})}, 1 \right\} . \tag{39}$$

Step 3. Set $i = i + 1$, and go to Step 1.

The performance of a Metropolis–Hastings algorithm depends on the choice of a proposal density q. In the context of the random walk proposal density, which is of the form $q(\boldsymbol{\theta}, \boldsymbol{\vartheta}) = q_1(\boldsymbol{\vartheta} - \boldsymbol{\theta})$, where $q_1(\cdot)$ is a multivariate density, Roberts, Gelman, and Gilks (1997) show that if the target and proposal densities are normal, then the scale of the latter should be tuned so that the acceptance rate is approximately 0.45 in one-dimensional problems and approximately 0.23 as the number of dimensions approaches infinity, with the optimal acceptance rate being around 0.25 in six dimensions. For the *independence chain*, in which we take $q(\boldsymbol{\theta}, \boldsymbol{\vartheta}) = q(\boldsymbol{\vartheta})$, it is important to ensure that the tails of the proposal density $q(\boldsymbol{\vartheta})$ dominate those of the target density $\pi(\boldsymbol{\theta}|D)$, which is similar to a requirement on the importance sampling function in Monte Carlo integration with importance sampling.

Example 10. Consider a Poisson mixed model:

$$y_i \sim \mathcal{P}(\mu_i),$$

where $\mu_i = \exp(\boldsymbol{x}_i'\boldsymbol{\beta}+\epsilon_i)$ for $i = 1, 2, \ldots, n$, $\boldsymbol{x}_i$ is a $p\times 1$ vector of covariates, and $\boldsymbol{\beta}$ is a $p \times 1$ vector of regression coefficients. We assume the random effects

$$\boldsymbol{\epsilon} = (\epsilon_1, \epsilon_2, \ldots, \epsilon_n)' \sim N(0, \Sigma),$$

where

$$\Sigma = \sigma^2 \begin{pmatrix} 1 & \rho & \rho^2 & \cdots & \rho^{n-1} \\ \rho & 1 & \rho & \cdots & \rho^{n-2} \\ \vdots & \vdots & \vdots & \ddots & \vdots \\ \rho^{n-1} & \rho^{n-2} & \rho^{n-3} & \cdots & 1 \end{pmatrix}.$$

Assume that a noninformative prior for $(\boldsymbol{\beta}, \sigma^2, \rho)$ has the form

$$\pi(\boldsymbol{\beta}, \sigma^2, \rho) \propto (\sigma^2)^{-(\delta_0+1)} \exp(-\sigma^{-2}\gamma_0),$$

where the hyperparameters $\delta_0 > 0$ and $\gamma_0 > 0$ are prespecified. Then, the joint posterior distribution for $(\boldsymbol{\beta}, \sigma^2, \rho, \boldsymbol{\epsilon})$ is given by

$$\pi(\boldsymbol{\beta}, \rho, \sigma^2, \boldsymbol{\epsilon}|D) \propto \exp\left\{y'(X\boldsymbol{\beta} + \boldsymbol{\epsilon}) - J_n'Q(\boldsymbol{\beta}, \epsilon) - \frac{1}{2}\boldsymbol{\epsilon}'\Sigma^{-1}\boldsymbol{\epsilon}\right\}$$
$$\times \frac{1}{\sigma^n(1-\rho^2)^{\frac{n-1}{2}}} \times (\sigma^2)^{-(\delta_0+1)} \exp(-\frac{\lambda_0}{\sigma^2}), \quad (40)$$

where $\boldsymbol{y} = (y_1, y_2, \ldots, y_n)'$, $J_n = (1, 1, \ldots, 1)'$, $Q(\boldsymbol{\beta}, \boldsymbol{\epsilon}) = (q_1, q_2, \ldots, q_n)'$, $q_i = \exp(\boldsymbol{x}_i\boldsymbol{\beta} + \epsilon_i) + \log(y_i!)$, X is the covariate matrix with the ith row equal to $\boldsymbol{x}_i'$, and $D = (n, \boldsymbol{y}, X)$.

To obtain a more efficient MCMC sampling algorithm, we consider a hierarchically centered reparameterization, which is given by

$$\boldsymbol{\eta} = X\boldsymbol{\beta} + \boldsymbol{\epsilon}.$$

Using (40), the reparameterized posterior for $(\boldsymbol{\beta}, \sigma^2, \rho, \boldsymbol{\eta})$ is written as

$$\pi(\boldsymbol{\beta}, \sigma^2, \rho, \boldsymbol{\eta}|D) \propto \exp\{\boldsymbol{y}'\boldsymbol{\eta} - J_n'Q(\boldsymbol{\eta}) - J_n'C(\boldsymbol{y})\}$$
$$\times (2\pi\sigma^2)^{-n/2}(1-\rho^2)^{-(n-1)/2}$$
$$\times \exp\left\{-\frac{1}{2\sigma^2}(\boldsymbol{\eta} - X\boldsymbol{\beta})'\Sigma^{-1}(\boldsymbol{\eta} - X\boldsymbol{\beta})\right\}, \quad (41)$$

where $\boldsymbol{\eta} = (\eta_1, \eta_2, \ldots, \eta_n)'$, and $Q(\boldsymbol{\eta})$ is an $n \times 1$ vector with the tth element equal to $q_i = \exp(\eta_i)$. We note that the hierarchical centering method of Gelfand, Sahu, and Carlin (1995, 1996) is a tool to improve convergence of MCMC sampling. As discussed in Chen, Shao, and Ibrahim (2000), this technique is particularly useful for the Poisson mixed model.

To sample from the reparameterized posterior $\pi(\boldsymbol{\beta}, \sigma^2, \rho, \boldsymbol{\eta}|D)$, the following steps are required:

Step 1. Draw $\boldsymbol{\eta}$ from its conditional posterior distribution

$$\pi(\boldsymbol{\eta}|\boldsymbol{\beta}, \sigma^2, \rho, D) \propto \exp\left\{\boldsymbol{y}'\boldsymbol{\eta} - J_n'Q(\boldsymbol{\eta}) - \frac{(\boldsymbol{\eta} - X\boldsymbol{\beta})'\Sigma^{-1}(\boldsymbol{\eta} - X\boldsymbol{\beta})}{2\sigma^2}\right\}. \tag{42}$$

Step 2. Draw $\boldsymbol{\beta}$ from

$$\boldsymbol{\beta}|\boldsymbol{\eta}, \sigma^2, \rho, D \sim N((X'\Sigma^{-1}X)^{-1}X'\Sigma^{-1}\boldsymbol{\eta}, \sigma^2(X'\Sigma^{-1}X)^{-1}).$$

Step 3. Draw σ^2 from its conditional posterior

$$\sigma^2|\boldsymbol{\beta}, \rho, \boldsymbol{\eta}, D \sim \mathcal{IG}(\delta^*, \gamma^*),$$

where $\delta^* = \delta_0 + n/2$, $\gamma^* = \gamma_0 + \frac{1}{2}(\boldsymbol{\eta} - X\boldsymbol{\beta})'\Sigma^{-1}(\boldsymbol{\eta} - X\boldsymbol{\beta})$, and $\mathcal{IG}$ (δ^*, γ^*) is an inverse gamma distribution.

Step 4. Draw ρ from its conditional posterior

$$\pi(\rho|\sigma^2, \boldsymbol{\beta}, \boldsymbol{\eta}, D) \propto (1 - \rho^2)^{-(n-1)/2} \times \exp\left\{-\frac{1}{2\sigma^2}(\boldsymbol{\eta} - X\boldsymbol{\beta})'\Sigma^{-1}(\boldsymbol{\eta} - X\boldsymbol{\beta})\right\}. \tag{43}$$

In Step 1, it can be shown that $\pi(\boldsymbol{\eta}|\boldsymbol{\beta}, \sigma^2, \rho, D)$ is log-concave in each component of $\boldsymbol{\eta}$. Thus $\boldsymbol{\eta}$ can be drawn using the adaptive rejection sampling algorithm of Gilks and Wild (1992). The implementation of Steps 2 and 3 is straightforward, which may be a bonus of hierarchical centering, since sampling $\boldsymbol{\beta}$ is much more expensive before the reparameterization. In Step 4, we use a so-called "*Localized Metropolis*" algorithm, which was introduced in Chen, Shao, and Ibrahim (2000).

The *Localized Metropolis* algorithm requires the following transformation:

$$\rho = \frac{-1 + e^{\xi}}{1 + e^{\xi}}, \ -\infty < \xi < \infty.$$

Using (43), we have

$$\pi(\xi|\sigma^2, \boldsymbol{\beta}, \boldsymbol{\eta}, D) = \pi(\rho|\sigma^2, \boldsymbol{\beta}, \boldsymbol{\eta}, D)\frac{2e^{\xi}}{(1+e^{\xi})^2}.$$

Now, we generate ξ by using a normal proposal $N(\hat{\xi}, \hat{\sigma}^2_{\hat{\xi}})$, where $\hat{\xi}$ is a maximizer of the logarithm of $\pi(\xi|\sigma^2, \boldsymbol{\beta}, \boldsymbol{\epsilon}, D)$, which can be obtained by, for example, the Newton-Raphson algorithm, and $\hat{\sigma}^2_{\hat{\xi}}$ is the minus of the inverse of the second derivative of $\log \pi(\xi|\sigma^2,\ \boldsymbol{\beta},\ \boldsymbol{\eta}, D)$ evaluated at $\xi = \hat{\xi}$, that is,

$$\hat{\sigma}^{-2}_{\hat{\xi}} = -\left.\frac{d^2 \log \pi(\xi|\sigma^2, \boldsymbol{\beta}, \boldsymbol{\eta}, D)}{d\xi^2}\right|_{\xi=\hat{\xi}}.$$

The algorithm to generate ξ operates as follows:

(a) Let ξ be the current value.
(b) Generate a proposal value ξ^* from $N(\hat{\xi}, \hat{\sigma}^2_{\hat{\xi}})$.
(c) A move from ξ to ξ^* is made with probability

$$\min\left\{\frac{\pi(\xi^*|\sigma^2, \boldsymbol{\beta}, \boldsymbol{\eta}, D)\phi\left(\frac{\xi-\hat{\xi}}{\hat{\sigma}_{\hat{\xi}}}\right)}{\pi(\xi|\sigma^2, \boldsymbol{\beta}, \boldsymbol{\eta}, D)\phi\left(\frac{\xi^*-\hat{\xi}}{\hat{\sigma}_{\hat{\xi}}}\right)}, 1\right\},$$

where ϕ is the $N(0,1)$ probability density function.

We note that the proposal $(\hat{\xi}, \hat{\sigma}^2_{\hat{\xi}})$ does not depend on the current value of ξ, which will typically produce a small autocorrelation among ξ's.

Recently, several Bayesian software packages have been developed. These include BUGS for analyzing general hierarchical models via MCMC (http://www.mrc-bsu.cam.ac.uk/bugs/), BATS for Bayesian time series analysis (http://www.stat.duke.edu/~mw/bats.html), Matlab and Minitab Bayesian computational algorithms for introductory Bayesian analysis (http://www-math.bgsu.edu/~albert/), SAS version 9.3, and many others. A more complete listing and description of pre-1990 Bayesian software can be found in Goel (1988). A listing of some of the Bayesian software developed since 1990 is given in Berger (1999).

4.2. *Computing posterior quantities*

In Bayesian inference, MC methods are often used to compute the posterior expectation $E(h(\boldsymbol{\theta})|D)$, since the analytical evaluation of $E(h(\boldsymbol{\theta})|D)$

is typically not available. Assuming that $\{\boldsymbol{\theta}_i,\ i=1,2,\ldots,n\}$ is an MCMC sample from $\pi(\boldsymbol{\theta}|D)$, the MC estimator of $E(h(\boldsymbol{\theta})|D)$ is given by

$$\hat{E}(h) = \frac{1}{n}\sum_{i=1}^{n} h(\boldsymbol{\theta}_i). \tag{44}$$

Asymptotic or small sample properties of $\hat{E}(h)$ depend on the algorithm used to generate the sample $\{\boldsymbol{\theta}_i,\ i=1,2,\ldots,n\}$. Under certain regularity conditions such as *ergodicity*, the MC estimator $\hat{E}(h)$ is consistent.

Since $\hat{E}(h)$ is a random quantity, it is important to compute the simulation standard error of $\hat{E}(h)$, as it provides the magnitude of the simulation accuracy of the estimator $\hat{E}(h)$. Let $\mathrm{Var}(\hat{E}(h))$ be the variance of $\hat{E}(h)$, and let $\widehat{\mathrm{Var}}(\hat{E}(h))$ be an estimate of $\mathrm{Var}(\hat{E}(h))$. Then, the simulation standard error of $\hat{E}(h)$ is defined as

$$\mathrm{se}(\hat{E}(h)) = [\widehat{\mathrm{Var}}(\hat{E}(h))]^{1/2}, \tag{45}$$

which is the square root of the estimated variance of the MC estimator $\hat{E}(h)$. Since the sample generated by an MCMC sampling algorithm is often dependent, a complication that arises from the autocorrelation is that $\mathrm{Var}(\hat{E}(h))$ is difficult to obtain. A variety of methods for obtaining a dependent sample based estimate of $\mathrm{Var}(\hat{E}(h))$ are discussed in system simulation textbooks, as, for example, in Bratley, Fox and Schrage (1987), Ripley (1987), or Law and Kelton (1991). In this subsection, we briefly discuss a general overlapping batch statistics (obs) method considered in Schmeiser, Avramidis, and Hashem (1990) for computing $\widehat{\mathrm{Var}}(\hat{E}(h))$.

Suppose that $\{\boldsymbol{\theta}_i,\ i=1,2,\ldots,n\}$ is a dependent sample, from which a point estimator $\hat{\xi}$ of the posterior quantity of interest is computed. (Here, $\hat{\xi}=\hat{E}(h)$.) The obs estimate of the variance of $\hat{\xi}$ is

$$\hat{V}(m) = \left[\frac{m}{n-m}\right]\frac{\sum_{j=1}^{n-m+1}(\hat{\xi}_j-\hat{\xi})^2}{(n-m+1)}, \tag{46}$$

where $\hat{\xi}_j$ is defined analogously to $\hat{\xi}$, but is a function of only $\boldsymbol{\theta}_j$, $\boldsymbol{\theta}_{j+1}$, ..., $\boldsymbol{\theta}_{j+m-1}$. Sufficient conditions for obs estimators to be unbiased and have variance inversely proportional to n are given in Schmeiser, Avramidis, and Hashem (1990). Using (46), the simulation standard error of $\hat{\xi}$ is $\mathrm{se}(\hat{\xi}) = \sqrt{\hat{V}(m)}$. The primary difficulty in using the obs estimator is the choice of the batch size m to balance bias and variance, since no optimal batch size formula is known for general obs estimators. Limiting behavior for $\hat{V}(m)$ for some special obs estimators is discussed by Goldsman and Meketon (1986) and Song and Schmeiser (1995). For many situations, choosing m so that $10 \leq n/m \leq 20$ is reasonable.

There are several other efficient Monte Carlo methods for computing posterior quantities other than $E(h(\boldsymbol{\theta})|D)$ in the literature. These include the bridge sampling method of Meng and Wong (1996), the path sampling method of Gelman and Meng (1998), and the ratio importance sampling method of Chen and Shao (1997) for computing normalizing constants and Bayes factors; and the MC methods of Chen and Shao (1999) for calculating HPD intervals. The detailed description and discussion of these methods can be found in Chen, Shao, and Ibrahim (2000).

5. Bayesian Design of Non-Inferiority Clinical Trials

In February, 2010, the US Food and Drug Administration (FDA) released "Guidance for the Use of Bayesian Statistics in Medical Device Clinical Trials" (www.fda.gov/MedicalDevices/DeviceRegulationandGuidance/GuidanceDocuments/ucm071072.htm). This document lays out detailed guidance on the determination of the sample size in a Bayesian clinical trial. It also provides guidance on the evaluation of the operating characteristics of a Bayesian clinical trial design, including type I error (probability of erroneously approving an ineffective or unsafe device), type II error (probability of erroneously disapproving a safe and effective device), and power (the probability of appropriately approving a safe and effective device).

Sample size determination (SSD) is an important aspect of clinical trial design. Our main focus of this section is on the design and analysis of non-inferiority trials. There is a rich literature on the frequentist methods of SSD in various non-inferiority trials, which includes, for example, D'Agostino Sr., Massaro, and Sullivan (2003), Hung *et al.* (2003), Rothmann *et al.* (2003), Wang and Hung (2003a,b), Hung, Wang, and O'Neill (2005, 2007), Kieser and Friede (2007), and Fleming (2008). The literature on Bayesian SSD has been growing recently due to recent advances in Bayesian computation and Markov chain Monte Carlo sampling. Joseph, Wolfson, and Du Berger (1995a,b), Lindley (1997), Rubin and Stern (1998), Katsis and Toman (1999), and Inoue, Berry, and Parmigiani (2005) are the Bayesian SSD articles cited in the FDA 2010 Guidance. An early review of Bayesian SSD is given in Adcock (1997). The recent work includes Rahme and Joseph (1998), Simon (1999), Wang and Gelfand (2002), De Santis (2007), and M'Lan, Joseph, and Wolfson (2006, 2008). The existing literature on Bayesian SSD primarily focuses on simple normal, one or two sample binomial problems, standard normal linear regression, and generalized linear models. Although the literature on Bayesian SSD discusses a variety of performance criteria, the widely used ones include the Bayes factor (Weiss, 1997), the average posterior variance criterion (APVC) (see, for example, Wang and Gelfand, 2002), the average coverage criterion (ACC), the average length criterion (ALC), and the worst outcome criterion (WOC) (e.g., Joseph, Wolfson, Du Berger, 1995a,b; Joseph and Bélisle, 1997), and the approach based on the range of equivalence (Spiegelhalter *et al.*, 2004) for superiority/non-inferiority trials. Lindley (1997), Pham-Gia (1997), and Lam and Lam (1997) provide SSD through a maximization of expected utility or a minimization of the Bayes risk. M'Lan, Joseph, and Wolfson (2006, 2008) extend ACC and ALC to ACC_k and ALC_k. Most recently, Chen *et al.* (2011) develop a very general Bayesian approach of sample size determination (SSD) for the design of non-inferiority clinical trials.

5.1. *Non-inferiority trials with two treatment arms*

Suppose that we have a randomized trial with two arms: treatment and control. Let $\boldsymbol{y}_1^{(n_1)} = (y_{11}, y_{12}, \ldots, y_{1n_1})'$ and $\boldsymbol{y}_2^{(n_2)} = (y_{21}, y_{22}, \ldots, y_{2n_2})'$ be the data corresponding to the treatment and control arms, respectively, from this trial. Let $n = n_1 + n_2$ denote the total sample size. Also, we write $\boldsymbol{y}^{(n)} = ((\boldsymbol{y}_1^{(n_1)})', (\boldsymbol{y}_2^{(n_2)})')'$. We assume that the ratio of two sample sizes, $r = \frac{n_2}{n_1}$, is fixed. Thus, we have

$$n_1 = \frac{n}{1+r} \text{ and } n_2 = \frac{rn}{1+r}.$$

The common choices of the ratio r are $r = 1/2$ and $r = 1/4$. When $r = 1/2$, $n_1 = n_2$ and when $r = 1/4$, $n_1 > n_2$. The goal of the trial is to show that the treatment is non-inferior to the control.

We assume that $\boldsymbol{y}_1^{(n_1)}$ and $\boldsymbol{y}_2^{(n_2)}$ are two independent random samples and y_{ji} has a density in the exponential class with the form

$$f(y_{ji}|\mu_j, \tau) = \exp\left\{a^{-1}(\tau)(y_{ji}\mu_j - b(\mu_j)) + c(y_{ji}, \tau)\right\}, \quad i = 1, \ldots, n_j,\ j = 1, 2, \tag{47}$$

indexed by the canonical parameter μ_j and scale parameter τ. The functions b and c determine a particular family in the class, such as the Bernoulli and normal distributions. The function $a(\tau)$ is commonly of the form $a(\tau) = \tau^{-1}w^{-1}$, where the w is a known weight. We consider two special cases of (47).

Bernoulli: $y_{ji}|p_j \sim \text{Bernoulli}(p_j)$, $\mu_j = \log\left(\frac{p_j}{1-p_j}\right)$, $\tau = 1$, $w = 1$, $b(\mu_j) = \log(1 + \exp(\mu_j))$, and $c(y_{ji}, \tau) = 0$.

Normal: $y_{ji}|\mu_j, \tau \sim N(\mu_j, \tau)$, where τ is the precision, i.e., $\text{Var}(y_{ji}) = \frac{1}{\tau}$. In this case, we take $b(\mu_j) = \mu_j$, $w = 1$, and $c(y_i, \tau) = -\frac{1}{2}\{\tau y_{ji}^2 + \log(2\pi) - \log(\tau)\}$.

Let $\boldsymbol{\theta} = (\mu_1, \mu_2, \tau)$. Then, the joint distribution of $\boldsymbol{y}^{(n)}$ is given by

$$f(\boldsymbol{y}^{(n)}|\boldsymbol{\theta}) = \prod_{j=1}^{2}\prod_{i=1}^{n_j} \exp\left\{a^{-1}(\tau)(y_{ji}\mu_j - b(\mu_j)) + c(y_{ji}, \tau)\right\}. \tag{48}$$

The design parameter $h(\boldsymbol{\theta})$ is the difference between μ_1 and μ_2, namely, $\mu_1 - \mu_2$. Let δ denote the non-inferiority margin. Similar to Hung *et al.* (2003), the hypotheses for non-inferiority testing are given by

$$H_0\colon \mu_1 - \mu_2 \geq \delta \quad \text{versus} \quad H_1\colon \mu_1 - \mu_2 < \delta. \tag{49}$$

The trial is successful if H_1 is accepted.

5.2. *Bayesian sample size determination*

Chen *et al.* (2011) propose a general method to determine Bayesian sample size for a non-inferiority trial. Let $\pi(\boldsymbol{\theta})$ denote the prior distribution of $\boldsymbol{\theta}$. Using (48), the joint distribution of $\boldsymbol{y}^{(n)}$ and $\boldsymbol{\theta}$ is given by $f(\boldsymbol{y}^{(n)}|\boldsymbol{\theta})\pi(\boldsymbol{\theta})$. Let $h(\boldsymbol{\theta})$ be a scalar function that measures the "true" size of the treatment effect. Then, the general hypotheses for non-inferiority testing can be formulated as follows:

$$H_0\colon h(\boldsymbol{\theta}) \geq \delta \quad \text{versus} \quad H_1\colon h(\boldsymbol{\theta}) < \delta. \tag{50}$$

Again, in (50), δ is the non-inferiority margin. Consequently, we let Θ_0 and Θ_1 denote the parameter spaces corresponding to H_0 and H_1. For the hypotheses given in (49), $h(\boldsymbol{\theta}) = \mu_1 - \mu_2$. For the model in (47), $\Theta_0 = \{\boldsymbol{\theta} = (\mu_1, \mu_2, \tau)\colon \mu_1 - \mu_2 \geq \delta, \tau > 0\}$ and $\Theta_1 = \{\boldsymbol{\theta}\colon \mu_1 - \mu_2 < \delta, \tau > 0\}$.

Following Wang and Gelfand (2002), we introduce two types of priors for $\boldsymbol{\theta}$, namely, the sampling prior and the fitting prior denoted by $\pi^{(s)}(\boldsymbol{\theta})$ and $\pi^{(f)}(\boldsymbol{\theta})$, respectively. The sampling prior captures a certain specified portion of the parameter space in achieving a certain level of performance in SSD, which is used to generate the data. The fitting prior is used to fit the model once the data is obtained. The sampling prior must be proper while the fitting prior may be improper as long as the resulting posterior,

$$\pi^{(f)}(\boldsymbol{\theta}|\boldsymbol{y}^{(n)}) \propto f(\boldsymbol{y}^{(n)}|\boldsymbol{\theta})\pi^{(f)}(\boldsymbol{\theta}),$$

is proper. In addition, we let $f^{(s)}(\boldsymbol{y}^{(n)})$ denote the marginal distribution that is induced from the sampling prior. The key quantity for Bayesian SSD introduced by Chen *et al.* (2011) is given by

$$\beta_s^{(n)} = E_s\Big[1\{P(h(\boldsymbol{\theta}) < \delta|\boldsymbol{y}^{(n)}, \pi^{(f)}) \geq \gamma\}\Big], \tag{51}$$

where the indicator function $1\{A\}$ is 1 if A is true and 0 otherwise, $\gamma > 0$ is a prespecified quantity, the probability is computed with respect to the posterior distribution given the data $\boldsymbol{y}^{(n)}$ and the fitting prior $\pi^{(f)}(\boldsymbol{\theta})$, and the expectation is taken with respect to the marginal distribution of $\boldsymbol{y}^{(n)}$ under the sampling prior $\pi^{(s)}(\boldsymbol{\theta})$.

Let $\overline{\Theta}_0$ and $\overline{\Theta}_1$ denote the closures of Θ_0 and Θ_1. Let $\pi_0^{(s)}(\boldsymbol{\theta})$ denote a "sampling prior" with support $\Theta_B = \overline{\Theta}_0 \cap \overline{\Theta}_1$. Also let $\pi_1^{(s)}(\boldsymbol{\theta})$ denote a "sampling prior" with support $\Theta_1^* \subset \Theta_1$. We further let $\beta_{s0}^{(n)}$ and $\beta_{s1}^{(n)}$ be the two special quantities of (51) corresponding to $\pi^{(s)} = \pi_0^{(s)}$ and $\pi^{(s)} = \pi_1^{(s)}$. Then, $\beta_{s0}^{(n)}$ is the Bayesian type I error while $\beta_{s1}^{(n)}$ is the Bayesian power. For given $\alpha_0 > 0$ and $\alpha_1 > 0$, we first compute

$$n_{\alpha_0} = \min\{n:\ \beta_{s0}^{(n)} \leq \alpha_0\} \text{ and } n_{\alpha_1} = \min\{n:\ \beta_{s1}^{(n)} \geq 1 - \alpha_1\}. \tag{52}$$

Then, the Bayesian sample size is given by

$$n_B = \max\{n_{\alpha_0}, n_{\alpha_1}\}. \tag{53}$$

In (51), we choose $\gamma \geq 0.95$. Common choices of α_0 and α_1 include $\alpha_0 = 0.05$ and $\alpha_1 = 0.20$ so that the Bayesian sample size n_B guarantees that the type I error rate is less than or equal to 0.05 and the power is at least 0.80. In addition, for a given sample size n_B, the operating characteristic curve can be constructed by varying Θ_1^* inside of Θ_1. If $h(\boldsymbol{\theta})$ is a monotonic function of the distance between Θ_1^* and Θ_B, then the further Θ_1^* is away from Θ_B, the higher the power will be.

Example 11. Suppose $\{y_i,\ \ i=1,2,\ldots,n\}$ is a random sample from $N(\theta, \tau^{-1})$, where τ is a known precision parameter. Suppose the hypotheses for non-inferiority testing are formulated as follows: H_0: $\theta \geq \delta$ versus H_1: $\theta < \delta$. We take $\pi^{(f)}(\theta) \propto 1$. In addition, we specify two point mass sampling priors for θ such that $\pi_0^{(s)}(\theta) = 1$ if $\theta = \delta$ and $\pi_1^{(s)}(\theta) = 1$ if $\theta = 0$. After some algebra, it is easy to show that a necessary condition for achieving a type I error rate of α_0 is $1-\gamma \leq \alpha_0$ and if $1-\gamma \leq \alpha_0$, the Bayesian sample size is the smallest integer n_B satisfying

$$n_B \geq \frac{1}{\tau\delta^2}\left[\Phi^{-1}(1-\alpha_1)+\Phi^{-1}(\gamma)\right]^2,$$

where Φ denotes the $N(0,1)$ cumulative distribution function. In this simple case, $\beta_0^{(n)} \leq \alpha_0$ always holds for all n as long as $1-\gamma \leq \alpha_0$ and the Bayesian sample size n_B is identical to the classical sample size formulation for a one-sided alternative hypothesis when $\alpha_0 = 1-\gamma$.

5.3. *Specification of fitting and sampling priors*

One of the advantages of the Bayesian SSD method compared to frequentist SSD methods is that Bayesian SSD allows the incorporation of historical data, which may potentially yield a substantial reduction of the sample size. Assume that historical data are available only for the control arm. Suppose that there are K historical datasets for the control arm, denoted by

$$\boldsymbol{y}_{0k} = (y_{0k1}, y_{0k2}, \ldots, y_{0kn_{0k}})'$$

for $k=1,2,\ldots,K$. Let $\boldsymbol{y}_0 = (\boldsymbol{y}_{01}', \ldots, \boldsymbol{y}_{0K}')'$ denote all K historical datasets. There are several approaches available in the Bayesian literature as discussed in Chen *et al.* (2011). Here, we discuss only the power prior (Section 3.1; Ibrahim and Chen, 2000; Duan, Smith, Ye (2006), Duan, Ye, and Smith, 2006; and Neuenschwander, Branson, and Spiegelhalter, 2009) to incorporate the historical data $\boldsymbol{y}_0$.

Under the exponential family model, we assume that y_{0ki} follows the same model given in (47) with density given by

$$f(y_{0ki}|\mu_2,\tau) = \exp\left\{a^{-1}(\tau)(y_{0ki}\mu_2 - b(\mu_2)) + c(y_{0ki},\tau)\right\}, \tag{54}$$

for $i = 1,2,\ldots,n_{0k}$ and $k = 1,2,\ldots,K$. Then, the power prior for μ_2 and τ given multiple historical data $\boldsymbol{y}_0$,

$$\pi(\mu_2,\tau|\boldsymbol{y}_0,\boldsymbol{a}_0) = \prod_{k=1}^{K}\prod_{i=1}^{n_{0k}} \exp\{a_{0k}a^{-1}(\tau)(y_{0ki}\mu_2 - b(\mu_2))\}, \tag{55}$$

where $\boldsymbol{a}_0 = (a_{01},\ldots,a_{0K})'$ and $0 \leq a_{0k} \leq 1$ is fixed for $k = 1,2,\ldots,K$. When $\boldsymbol{a}_0$ is random, (55) can be extended to the normalized power prior (Duan, Ye, Smith, 2006, Duan, Ye, and Smith, 2006 and Neuenschwander,

Branson, and Spiegelhalter, 2009) given by

$$\pi(\mu_2, \tau | \boldsymbol{y}_0, \boldsymbol{a}_0) = \frac{1}{C(\boldsymbol{a}_0)} \prod_{k=1}^{K} \prod_{i=1}^{n_{0k}} \exp\{a_{0k} a^{-1}(\tau)(y_{0ki}\mu_2 - b(\mu_2))\}, \quad (56)$$

where

$$C(\boldsymbol{a}_0) = \int_0^\infty \int_{-\infty}^{\infty} \Big[\prod_{k=1}^{K} \prod_{i=1}^{n_{0k}} \exp\{a_{0k} a^{-1}(\tau)(y_{0ki}\mu_2 - b(\mu_2))\} \Big] d\mu_2 d\tau.$$

In the random $\boldsymbol{a}_0$ case, we further assume that the a_{0k}'s are independent and distributed as

$$a_{0k} \sim \text{beta}(\alpha_0, \beta_0), \quad (57)$$

where $\alpha_0 > 0$ and $\beta_0 > 0$ are prespecified hyperparameters. Then, the joint prior for $\boldsymbol{a}_0$ is given by

$$\pi(\boldsymbol{a}_0) \propto \prod_{k=1}^{K} a_{0k}^{\alpha_0 - 1}(1 - a_{0k})^{\beta_0 - 1}.$$

Let $\pi(\mu_2, \tau | \boldsymbol{y}_0) = \pi(\mu_2, \tau | \boldsymbol{y}_0, \boldsymbol{a}_0)$ for fixed $\boldsymbol{a}_0$ and $\pi(\mu_2, \tau | \boldsymbol{y}_0) = \int \pi(\mu_2, \tau | \boldsymbol{y}_0, \boldsymbol{a}_0)\pi(\boldsymbol{a}_0) d\boldsymbol{a}_0$ for random $\boldsymbol{a}_0$. The fitting prior of $\boldsymbol{\theta}$ is of the form

$$\pi^{(f)}(\boldsymbol{\theta}) = \pi(\mu_1, \mu_2, \tau | \boldsymbol{y}_0) \propto \pi(\mu_2, \tau | \boldsymbol{y}_0)\pi_0(\mu_1, \mu_2, \tau), \quad (58)$$

where $\pi_0(\mu_1, \mu_2, \tau)$ is an initial prior which may be improper, for example, $\pi_0(\mu_1, \mu_2, \tau) \propto \frac{1}{\tau}$. To specify the sampling prior $\pi^{(s)}(\boldsymbol{\theta})$, we assume μ_1, μ_2, and τ are independent, then specify point mass priors for μ_1 and μ_2, and use the historical data to specify the sampling prior for τ. Specifically, we take

$$\pi^{(s)}(\boldsymbol{\theta}) = \pi^{(s)}(\mu_1)\pi^{(s)}(\mu_2)\pi^{(s)}(\tau), \quad (59)$$

where $\pi^{(s)}(\mu_1)$ and $\pi^{(s)}(\mu_2)$ are two prespecified point mass priors,

$$\pi^{(s)}(\tau) \propto \int \pi(\mu_2, \tau | \boldsymbol{y}_0)\pi_0^{(s)}(\tau) d\mu_2, \quad (60)$$

and $\pi_0^{(s)}(\tau)$ may be an improper initial prior such as $\pi_0^{(s)}(\tau) \propto 1/\tau$.

5.4. *Computational algorithm for Bayesian SSD*

The fitting posterior distribution of $\boldsymbol{\theta} = (\mu_1, \mu_2, \tau)$ is given by

$$\pi^{(f)}(\boldsymbol{\theta} | \boldsymbol{y}^{(n)}, \boldsymbol{y}_0) \propto f(\boldsymbol{y}^{(n)} | \boldsymbol{\theta})\pi^{(f)}(\boldsymbol{\theta}),$$

where $f(\boldsymbol{y}^{(n)}|\boldsymbol{\theta})$ is given by (48) and $\pi^{(f)}(\boldsymbol{\theta})$ is defined by (58). Instead of directly sampling from $\pi^{(f)}(\boldsymbol{\theta}|\boldsymbol{y}^{(n)}, \boldsymbol{y}_0)$, we consider the augmented fitting posterior distribution parameters $\boldsymbol{\theta}^*$, where $\boldsymbol{\theta}^* = (\mu_1, \mu_2, \tau, \boldsymbol{a}_0)$ for the normalized power prior. Then, the augmented fitting posterior distribution of $\boldsymbol{\theta}^*$ is given by

$$\pi(\boldsymbol{\theta}^*|\boldsymbol{y}_0) \propto \pi(\mu_2, \tau|\boldsymbol{y}_0, \boldsymbol{a}_0)\left[\prod_{k=1}^{K} a_{0k}^{\alpha_0-1}(1-a_{0k})^{\beta_0-1}\right]\pi_0(\mu_1, \mu_2, \tau)$$

with $\pi(\mu_2, \tau|\boldsymbol{y}_0, \boldsymbol{a}_0)$ defined in (56) under the normalized power prior. Although the posterior distribution $\pi^{(f)}(\boldsymbol{\theta}|\boldsymbol{y}^{(n)}, \boldsymbol{y}_0)$ is analytically intractable, sampling from this distribution via the Gibbs sampler is quite straightforward, because the conditional posterior distributions of the components of $\boldsymbol{\theta}$ (except for $\boldsymbol{a}_0$) are either known distributions or log-concave for exponential family models. For $\boldsymbol{a}_0$, we use the localized Metropolis algorithm discussed in Chen, Shao, and Ibrahim (2000) to sample from its conditional posterior distribution.

Let $\{\boldsymbol{\theta}^{*(m)},\ m = 1, 2, \ldots, M\}$ denote a Gibbs sample from the augmented fitting posterior distribution $\pi^{(f)}(\boldsymbol{\theta}^*|\boldsymbol{y}^{(n)}, \boldsymbol{y}_0)$. As $\boldsymbol{\theta}$ is a subvector of $\boldsymbol{\theta}^*$, let $\boldsymbol{\theta}^{(m)}$ denote the corresponding components of $\boldsymbol{\theta}^{*(m)}$ from the mth Gibbs iteration. Then, it is easy to show that $\{\boldsymbol{\theta}^{(m)},\ m = 1, 2, \ldots, M\}$ is a Gibbs sample from the fitting posterior distribution $\pi^{(f)}(\boldsymbol{\theta}|\boldsymbol{y}^{(n)}, \boldsymbol{y}_0)$. Using this Gibbs sample, a Monte Carlo estimate of $P(h(\boldsymbol{\theta}) < \delta|\boldsymbol{y}^{(n)}, \pi^{(f)})$ is given by

$$\hat{P}_f = \frac{1}{M}\sum_{m=1}^{M} 1\{h(\boldsymbol{\theta}^{(m)}) < \delta\}. \tag{61}$$

The following computational algorithm can be used to compute $\beta_s^{(n)}$ in (51).

Computational Algorithm:

Step 0: Specify n_1, n_2, δ, γ, and N;
Step 1: Generate $\boldsymbol{\theta} \sim \pi^{(s)}(\boldsymbol{\theta})$;
Step 2: Generate $\boldsymbol{y}^{(n)} \sim f(\boldsymbol{y}^{(n)}|\boldsymbol{\theta})$;
Step 3: Run the Gibbs sampler to generate a Gibbs sample $\{\boldsymbol{\theta}^{(m)}, m=1, 2, \ldots, M\}$ of size M from the fitting posterior distribution $\pi^{(f)}(\boldsymbol{\theta}|\boldsymbol{y}^{(n)}, \boldsymbol{y}_0)$;
Step 4: Compute $\hat{P}_f$ via (61);
Step 5: Check whether $\hat{P}_f \geq \gamma$; and

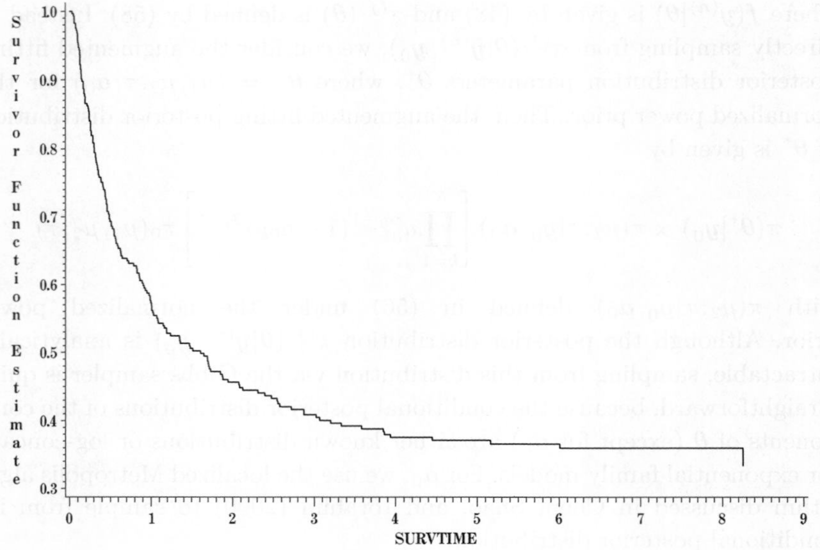

Fig. 2. Kaplan-Meier plot for E1684 data.

Step 6: Repeat Steps 1-5 N times.

Step 7: Compute the proportion of $\{\hat{P}_f \geq \gamma\}$ in these N runs, which gives an estimate of $\beta_s^{(n)}$.

6. Applications and Examples

6.1. *Bayesian analysis for survival data with a cure fraction*

The cure rate model is needed for modelling time-to-event data for various types of cancers, including breast cancer, non-Hodgkins lymphoma, leukemia, prostate cancer, melanoma, and head and neck cancer, where for these diseases, a significant proportion of patients are "cured". To demonstrate such a phenomenon, we consider a recent phase III clinical trial in malignant melanoma (E1684) undertaken by the Eastern Cooperative Oncology Group (ECOG). The graph in Figure 2 gives the Kaplan-Meier survival curve for 284 patients in E1684, with the survival time given in years. We see from Figure 2 that a plateau in the curve occurs at approximately 0.36, suggesting that 36% fraction of patients are "cured" after sufficient follow-up.

An important issue with cure rate modelling is model comparison. It will be of interest to compare various cure models to the Cox model. It will also be of interest to compare various semi-parametric models to obtain the most parsimonious and best fitting semi-parametric model. For model comparisons, Bayes factors require proper priors, and criterion based statistics such as the L measure (Ibrahim and Laud 1994) will not be well defined for cure rate models since the cure rate model does not have proper probability density. As a result, we need to turn to other measures to carry out model comparisons. Here, we use the Conditional Predictive Ordinate (CPO) as a goodness of fit statistic that is well defined for these models and will allow us to do formal model comparisons.

We compare three types of models for modelling time-to-event data.

6.1.1. *Cox model*

A proportional hazards model is defined by a hazard function of the form

$$h(t, \boldsymbol{x}) = h_0(t) \exp(\boldsymbol{x}'\boldsymbol{\beta}), \tag{62}$$

where $h_0(t)$ denotes the baseline hazard function at time t, $\boldsymbol{x}$ denotes the covariate vector for an arbitrary individual in the population, and $\boldsymbol{\beta}$ denotes a vector of regression coefficients. Suppose we have n subjects, and let $y_1, \ldots, y_n$ denote the observed failure times or censoring times for the individuals, and ν_i is the indicator variable taking on the value 1 if y_i is a failure time, and 0 if it is a censoring time. Our semi-parametric development for this model is based on a piece-wise constant hazard. We construct a finite partition of the time axis, $0 < s_1 < \cdots < s_J$, with $s_J > y_i$ for all $i = 1, 2, \ldots, n$. Thus, we have the J intervals $(0, s_1], (s_1, s_2], \ldots, (s_{J-1}, s_J]$. In the jth interval, we assume a constant hazard λ_j. Throughout, we let $D = (n, \boldsymbol{y}, X, \boldsymbol{\nu})$ denote the observed data for the current study, where $\boldsymbol{y} = (y_1, \ldots, y_n)'$, $\boldsymbol{\nu} = (\nu_1, \ldots, \nu_n)'$, and X is the $n \times p$ matrix of covariates with i^{th} row $\boldsymbol{x}_i'$. Letting $\boldsymbol{\lambda} = (\lambda_1, \ldots, \lambda_J)'$, we can write the likelihood function of $(\boldsymbol{\beta}, \boldsymbol{\lambda})$ for all n subjects as

$$\begin{aligned} L(\boldsymbol{\beta}, \boldsymbol{\lambda}|D) = \prod_{i=1}^{n}\prod_{j=1}^{J} &(\lambda_j \exp(\boldsymbol{x}_i'\boldsymbol{\beta}))^{\delta_{ij}\nu_i} \\ &\times \exp\left\{-\delta_{ij}\left[\lambda_j(y_i - s_{j-1}) + \sum_{g=1}^{j-1}\lambda_g(s_g - s_{g-1})\right]\exp(\boldsymbol{x}_i'\boldsymbol{\beta})\right\}, \end{aligned} \tag{63}$$

where $\delta_{ij} = 1$ if the ith subject failed or was censored in the jth interval, and 0 otherwise, $\boldsymbol{x}_i' = (x_{i1}, \ldots, x_{ip})$ denotes the $p \times 1$ vector of covariates for the ith subject, and $\boldsymbol{\beta} = (\beta_1, \ldots, \beta_p)'$ is the corresponding vector of regression coefficients. The indicator δ_{ij} is needed to properly define the likelihood over the J intervals for the semi-parametric models. The semi-parametric model in (63), sometimes referred to as a piecewise exponential model, is quite general and can accommodate various shapes of the baseline hazard over the intervals. Moreover, we note that if $J = 1$, then the model reduces to a parametric exponential model with failure rate parameter $\lambda \equiv \lambda_j$, $j = 1, 2, \ldots, J$. This semi-parametric proportional hazards model is a useful and simple model for modelling survival data. It serves as the benchmark for comparisons with other semi-parametric or fully parametric models for survival data.

6.1.2. *Parametric cure rate model*

We present a version of the cure rate model discussed by Yakovlev and Tsodikov (1996), and Chen, Ibrahim, and Sinha (1999). Suppose that for an individual in the population, we let N denote the number of *metastatic-competent* tumor cells for that individual left active after the initial treatment. A metastatic-competent tumor cell is a tumor cell which has the potential of metastasizing. Further, we assume that N has a Poisson distribution with mean θ. We let Z_i denote the random time for the ith metastatic-competent tumor cell to produce detectable metastatic disease. That is, Z_i can be viewed as an incubation time for the ith tumor cell. The variables Z_i, $i = 1, 2, \ldots$, are assumed to be independent and identically distributed with a common distribution function $F(t) = 1 - S(t)$ and are independent of N. The time to relapse of cancer can be defined by the random variable $T = \min\{Z_i, 0 \le i \le N\}$, where $P(Z_0 = \infty) = 1$ and N is independent of the sequence $Z_1, Z_2, \ldots$. The survival function for T, and hence the survival function for the population, is given by

$$\begin{aligned} S_p(t) &= P(\text{no metastatic cancer by time t}) \\ &= P(N = 0) + P(Z_1 > t, \ldots, Z_N > t, N \ge 1) \\ &= \exp(-\theta) + \sum_{k=1}^{\infty} S(t)^k \, \frac{\theta^k}{k!} \exp(-\theta) = \exp(-\theta + \theta S(t)) \\ &= \exp(-\theta F(t)). \end{aligned} \tag{64}$$

Since $S_p(\infty) = \exp(-\theta) > 0$, (64) is not a proper survival function. We see that (64) shows explicitly the contribution to the failure time of two distinct characteristics of tumor growth: the initial number of metastatic-competent cells and the rate of their progression. Thus the model incorporates parameters bearing clear biological meaning. The model in (64) is quite different from the standard mixture cure rate model proposed by Berkson and Gage (1952), and has several attractive properties. For a detailed discussion of the various properties of (64), we refer the reader to Yakovlev and Tsodikov (1996). Aside from the biological motivation, the model in (64) is suitable for any type of failure-time data with a surviving fraction. Thus, failure-time data which do not "fit" the biological definition given above can still certainly be modeled by (64) as long as the data has a surviving fraction and can be thought of as being generated by an unknown number N of latent independent competing risks (Z_i's). Yakovlev *et al.* (1993) discuss a similar modeling technique for tumor latency, but do not consider a Bayesian formulation of the model.

We also see from (64) that the cure fraction (i.e., cure rate) is given by

$$S_p(\infty) \equiv P(N = 0) = \exp(-\theta). \tag{65}$$

As $\theta \to \infty$, the cure fraction tends to 0, whereas as $\theta \to 0$, the cure fraction tends to 1. The sub-density corresponding to (64) is given by

$$f_p(t) = \theta f(t) \exp(-\theta F(t)), \tag{66}$$

where $f(t) = \frac{d}{dt}F(t)$ is a proper probability density function. The hazard function is given by

$$h_p(t) = \theta f(t). \tag{67}$$

We note that $h_p(t)$ is *not* a hazard function corresponding to a probability distribution since $S_p(t)$ is not a proper survival function.

Suppose we have n subjects and for the ith subject, let y_i denote the observed survival time, let ν_i be the censoring indicator that equals 1 if y_i is a failure time and 0 if it is right censored, and also let N_i denote the number of metastatic-competent tumor cells. Further, we assume that the N_i's are *i.i.d.* Poisson random variables with mean θ_i, which is related to the covariates by $\theta_i \equiv \theta(\boldsymbol{x}_i'\boldsymbol{\beta}) = \exp(\boldsymbol{x}_i'\boldsymbol{\beta})$. Letting $\boldsymbol{N} = (N_1, \ldots N_n)'$, the "complete data" is given by $D_{comp} = (n, \boldsymbol{y}, \boldsymbol{\nu}, \boldsymbol{N})$, where $\boldsymbol{N}$ is an unobserved vector of latent variables. Then, we can write the complete data likelihood of $(\boldsymbol{\beta}, \lambda)$ as

$$L(\boldsymbol{\beta}, \lambda|D_{comp}) = \left(\prod_{i=1}^{n} S(y_i \mid \lambda)^{N_i-\nu_i} \ (N_i f(y_i \mid \lambda))^{\nu_i}\right) \times \exp\left\{\sum_{i=1}^{n} [N_i x_i' \beta - \log(N_i!) - \exp(\boldsymbol{x}_i' \boldsymbol{\beta})]\right\}, \quad (68)$$

where $f(y_i|\lambda)$ is exponential density given above, and $S(y_i|\lambda) = 1 - F(y_i|\lambda) = \exp(-\lambda y_i)$. Since the latent vector $\boldsymbol{N}$ is not observed, the likelihood function based on the observed data $D = (n, \boldsymbol{y}, X, \boldsymbol{\nu})$ is obtained by summing (68) over $\boldsymbol{N}$, leading to

$$L(\boldsymbol{\beta}, \lambda|D) = \sum_{\boldsymbol{N}} L(\boldsymbol{\beta}, \lambda|D_{comp}). \quad (69)$$

6.1.3. *Semi-parametric cure rate model*

We consider a semi-parametric version of the parametric cure rate model in (68). We do this by considering a piecewise constant hazard model, and thus assume that the hazard is equal to λ_j for the jth interval, $j = 1, \ldots, J$. With this assumption, the complete data likelihood can be written as

$$\begin{aligned} L(\boldsymbol{\beta}, \boldsymbol{\lambda}|D_{comp}) &= \prod_{i=1}^{n}\prod_{j=1}^{J} \exp\left\{-(N_i - \nu_i)\delta_{ij}\left[\lambda_j(y_i - s_{j-1}) + \sum_{g=1}^{j-1} \lambda_g(s_g - s_{g-1})\right]\right\} \\ &\times \prod_{i=1}^{n}\prod_{j=1}^{J} (N_i \lambda_j)^{\delta_{ij}\nu_i} \\ &\times \exp\left\{-\nu_i \delta_{ij}\left[\lambda_j(y_i - s_{j-1}) + \sum_{g=1}^{j-1} \lambda_g(s_g - s_{g-1})\right]\right\} \\ &\times \exp\left\{\sum_{i=1}^{n} [N_i x_i' \beta - \log(N_i!) - \exp(\boldsymbol{x}_i' \boldsymbol{\beta})]\right\}, \end{aligned} \quad (70)$$

where $\boldsymbol{\lambda} = (\lambda_1, \ldots, \lambda_J)'$. The model in (70) is a semi-parametric version of (68). If we take $J = 1$ in (70), then the model reduces to the fully parametric model given in (68). There are several attractive features of the model in (70). First, we note the degree of the non-parametricity is controlled by J. The larger the J, the more non-parametric the model is.

However, by picking a small to moderate J, we get more of a parametric shape for the survival function. This is an important aspect for the cure rate model, since the estimation of the cure rate parameter θ could be highly affected by the non-parametric nature of the survival function. For this reason, it may be desirable to choose small to moderate values of J for cure rate modelling. In practice, we recommend doing analyses for several values of J to see the sensitivity of the posterior estimates of the regression coefficients. We recommend doing sensitivity analyses for small, moderate, and large values of J. Thus, the semi-parametric cure rate model (70) is quite flexible, as it allows us to model general shapes of the hazard function, as well as choose the degree of parametricity through suitable choices of J. Again, since $\boldsymbol{N}$ is not observed, the observed data likelihood, $L(\boldsymbol{\beta}, \boldsymbol{\lambda}|D)$ is obtained by summing out N from (70) as in (69).

6.1.4. *Prior distributions*

First, we consider a noninformative prior. We take

$$\pi(\boldsymbol{\beta}, \boldsymbol{\lambda}) \propto \prod_{j=1}^{J} \lambda_j^{\zeta_0 - 1} \exp(-\tau_0 \lambda_j), \tag{71}$$

where $\zeta_0 \geq 0$ and $\tau_0 \geq 0$, so that β has an improper uniform prior and $\lambda_j \sim \text{Gamma}(\zeta_0, \tau_0)$. The prior given in (71) includes two special cases: (i) Jeffreys's prior for λ when $\zeta_0 = \tau_0 = 0$, and (ii) uniform prior for λ when $\zeta_0 = 1$ and $\tau_0 = 0$.

Second, we consider an informative prior. We use the *power prior* to formally construct an informative prior distribution from *historical data* D_0. Let n_0 denote the sample size for the historical data, $\boldsymbol{y}_0 = (y_{01}, y_{02}, \ldots, y_{0n_0})'$ be an $n_0 \times 1$ vector of right censored failure times for the historical data with censoring indicators $\boldsymbol{\nu}_0 = (\nu_{01}, \nu_{02}, \ldots, \nu_{0n_0})'$, and X_0 is an $n_0 \times k$ matrix of covariates with i^{th} row $\boldsymbol{x}'_{0i}$. Let $D_0 = (n_0, \boldsymbol{y}_0, X_0, \boldsymbol{\nu}_0)$ denote the observed historical data. The power prior given by (26) has the form

$$\pi(\boldsymbol{\beta}, \boldsymbol{\lambda}, a_0|D_0) \propto L(\boldsymbol{\beta}, \boldsymbol{\lambda}|D_0)^{a_0} \pi_0(\boldsymbol{\beta}, \boldsymbol{\lambda}) a_0^{\alpha_0 - 1}(1 - a_0)^{\lambda_0 - 1}, \tag{72}$$

where $L(\beta, \lambda|D_0)$ is the likelihood function based on the observed historical data, and α_0 and λ_0 are prespecified hyperparameters. The quantity $\pi_0(\boldsymbol{\beta}, \lambda)$ is the initial prior for $(\boldsymbol{\beta}, \boldsymbol{\lambda})$, which is (71).

It is well known that with insufficient follow-up or with too few events, the estimate of the cure rate can be quite unreliable and unstable. In addition, the model itself may not be identifiable or nearly identifiable if there is insufficient follow-up and there are too few events. The use of informative prior distributions can help overcome such difficulties, which can provide better estimates of the cure rate and make the model identifiable.

6.1.5. *Model assessment*

We use a summary statistic of the CPO_i's given by (7), the logarithm of the *pseudo-Bayes factor*, for model assessment. The CPO_i given by (7) has the form

$$\text{CPO}_i = f(y_i|y_{(i)}) = \int f(y_i|\boldsymbol{\beta}, \boldsymbol{\lambda})\ \pi(\boldsymbol{\beta}, \boldsymbol{\lambda}|y_{(i)})\ d\boldsymbol{\beta}\ d\boldsymbol{\lambda}, \tag{73}$$

where y_i denotes the response variable for case i, and $y_{(i)}$ denotes the entire response vector with the ith case deleted. Then, the logarithm of the pseudo-Bayes factor is defined as

$$B = \sum_{i=1}^{n} \log(\text{CPO}_i). \tag{74}$$

In the context of survival data, the statistic B has been discussed by Gelfand and Mallick (1995), Sinha and Dey (1997), and Dey, Chen, and Chang (1997). In Ibrahim, Chen, and Sinha (2001), the B statistic is also called the logarithm of pseudo marginal likelihood (LPML).

We see from (73) that B is always well defined as long as the posterior predictive density is proper. Thus, B is well defined under improper priors, and in addition, it is very computationally stable. Therefore, B has a clear advantage over the Bayes factor as a model assessment tool, since it is well known that the Bayes factor is not well defined with improper priors, and is generally quite sensitive to vague proper priors. Thus, the Bayes factor is not applicable for many of our models here, since we consider several models involving improper priors. In addition, the B statistic also has clear advantages over other model selection criteria, such as the *L measure* proposed by Ibrahim and Laud (1994) and Laud and Ibrahim (1995). The L measure is a Bayesian criterion requiring finite second moments of the sampling distribution of y_i, whereas the B statistic does not require existence of any moments. Since the cure rate models in (68) and (70) have improper survival functions, no moments of the sampling distribution exist, and therefore the L measure is not well defined for these models. Thus, for the models considered here, the B statistic is well motivated.

6.1.6. *E1690 melanoma study*

To demonstrate the methodologies, we consider the second ECOG trial, E1690, in malignant melanoma. This study had $n = 427$ patients on the high dose interferon arm and observation arm combined. ECOG initiated this trial, right after the completion of E1684, to attempt to confirm the results of E1684 and to study the benefit of Interferon Alpha-2b (IFN) given at a lower dose. The E1690 trial accrued patients from 1991 until 1995, and was unblinded in 1998. The E1690 trial was designed for exactly the same patient population as E1684, and the high dose IFN arm in E1690 was identical to that of E1684. See Kirkwood *et al.* (1996, 1999) for detail.

We carry out a Bayesian analysis of E1690 using E1684 as historical data using relapse-free survival (RFS) as the response variable with the treatment as a covariate. Since E1684 has longer follow-up than E1684, the use of E1684 as a historical may help to improve the accuracy in the estimates of cure rates based on E1690. But, in this example, we solely focus on model comparisons. We consider Cox model, parametric cure rate (PCR) model, and semiparametric cure rate (SPCR) model with $J = 1$, $J = 5$, and $J = 10$ for noninformative and informative priors. Table 4 shows the results of Pseudo-Bayes Factors (B's) when $a_0 = 0$ with probability 1, $E(a_0|D) = 0.05$, 0.20, 0.30, and 0.60, and $a_0 = 1$ with probability 1. We note that $a_0 = 0$ implies the use of noninformative prior, which is equivalent to a prior specification with no incorporation of historical data, while with $a_0 = 1$, we simply combine D and D_0 together.

Table 4 is quite informative. First, for the degree of parametricity, $J = 5$ is better than $J = 1$ or $J = 10$. However, for SPCR $J = 1$ and $J = 5$ are fairly close. Second, for both $J = 1$ or $J = 5$, the cure rate model yields a better fit than the Cox model. Third, the incorporation of E1684 in the

Table 4. Pseudo-Bayes factors (B's).

Model		$a_0 = 0$	$E(a_0\|D) \simeq$ 0.05	0.20	0.30	0.60	$a_0 = 1$
Cox	$J = 1$	−575.60	−575.45	−575.23	−575.13	−574.95	−574.64
	$J = 5$	−522.30	−522.05	−521.67	−521.59	−521.61	−522.24
	$J = 10$	−523.62	−523.20	−522.39	−522.12	−522.02	−522.71
SPCR	$J = 1$	−519.75	−519.61	−519.39	−519.34	−519.40	−519.67
	$J = 5$	−520.24	−519.89	−519.43	−519.31	−519.67	−520.16
	$J = 10$	−524.42	−523.82	−522.83	−522.53	−522.56	−522.97

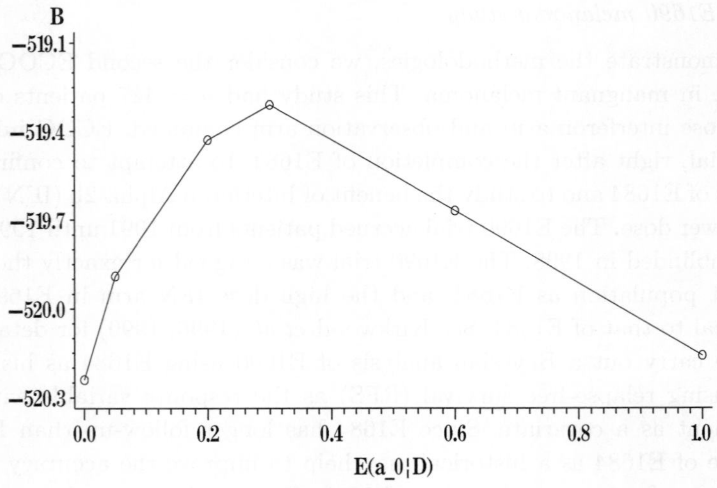

Fig. 3. Plot of Pseudo-Bayes Factors for SPCR with $J = 5$.

analysis improves the model fit over the exclusion of historical data. Fourth, for all the cases, B is a concave function of $E(a_0|D)$, see Figure 3 for an illustration. This is an interesting feature in B in that it demonstrates that there is an "optimal" weight for the historical data with respect to the statistic B, and thus this property is potentially very useful in selecting a model and the prior weight a_0.

6.2. *Bayesian model selection for multivariate mortality data with large families*

To illustrate Bayesian model selection, we consider an analysis of the multivariate mortality data with large families from a series of animal toxicological experiments performed in the Department of Biology at the University of Waterloo. One of these experiments to study the toxic effect of potassium thiocyanate (KSCN) on the mortality of trout fish eggs. In this experiment, each of the six levels of KSCN were added to different tanks each containing many trout fish eggs (61 to 179 eggs per vial). Half of the tanks were water hardened before the application of the KSCN ($x_1 = 1$) and other half were water hardened after the application of the KSCN ($x_1 = 0$). Another covariate is the continuous variable x_2, which is defined as the natural logarithm of the level of KSCN. Each experimental condition was replicated 4 times, so there were in total 48 tanks. Another similar experiment was conducted in the same laboratory with a different toxicant, sodium thiocyanate (NaSCN). For the KSCN data, mortality counts for each tank were taken at 5, 11, 19, 31 and 35 days after the application of KSCN, while for the NaSCN data mortality counts for each tank were taken at 1, 6, 13, 20, and 27 days after the application of the NaSCN. We refer the reader to O'Hara Hines (1989) and O'Hara Hines and Lawless (1993) for the more detailed description of these two experiments. Since NaSCN is a toxicant similar to KSCN and both experiments were similar in design and purpose, the data from the NaSCN experiment will be used to build an informative prior distribution for the KSCN study.

For the KSCN data, there are $K = 48$ tanks (families) of fishes (subjects). Suppose that the observation times for each tank are $t_0 = 0 < t_1 < \cdots < t_m$ $(m = 5)$. Moreover, it is given that $t_1 = 5, t_2 = 11, t_3 = 19, t_4 = 31$ and $t_5 = 35$. The cumulative mortality counts (the observed data) in each tank at these five days, can be summarized as $\{(d_{kj}, r_{kj}) : j = 1, \ldots, 5; k = 1, \ldots, 48\}$ where d_{kj} is the number of fishes dying and r_{kj} is the number of fishes at risk in the kth tank during the time interval $(t_{j-1}, t_j] = I_j$. Let h_{kj} be the mortality rate, which can be also interpreted as the discrete hazard rate, for a fish from the kth tank at the time interval I_j:

$$h_{kj} = P\Big(T_i \in \ I_j \mid i \in \ R_{kj}, \boldsymbol{x}_i\Big) \ ,$$

where T_i is the time of death for a fish from the kth tank, and R_{kj} is the set of fishes still 'at risk' (alive) in the kth tank at the beginning of the time interval $(t_{j-1}, t_j]$ (for $j = 1, 2, \ldots, 5$ and $k = 1, 2, \ldots, K$). There are two covariates x_{1k} and x_{2k} for each tank, where x_{2k} is the primary covariate, the natural logarithm of the KSCN level applied to the kth tank, and x_{1k} is the water hardening of the kth tank. Thus, the number of fishes dying in the kth tank during I_j is distributed as Binomial with success probability h_{kj} and the number of trials is equal to the number of fishes at risk during that interval in the kth tank, i.e., $d_{kj} \sim Binomial(r_{kj}; h_{kj})$.

Chen, Dey, and Sinha (2000) assume that for a logit link function,

$$\text{logit}(h_{kj}) = \log\Big(\frac{h_{kj}}{1 - h_{kj}}\Big) \ = \boldsymbol{x}_k'\boldsymbol{\beta} + g_\gamma(t_j) + e_{kj}, \tag{75}$$

where g_γ is a known function with unknown parameters γ, possibly vector valued, $\boldsymbol{x}_k = (1, x_{1k}, \ x_{2k})'$, $\boldsymbol{\beta} = (\beta_0, \beta_1, \beta_2)'$ is a 3×1 vector of the regression coefficients with respect to covariates $\boldsymbol{x}_k$. In (75), e_{kj}'s are the random effects for the hazard rate of the fishes in the kth tank during the time interval I_j. Let $\boldsymbol{e}_k = (e_{k1}, e_{k2}, \ldots, e_{k,m})'$ for $k = 1, 2, \ldots, K$. We assume that these random effects, e_{kj}'s, are dependent on each other within the same tank (family) but independent between any two different tanks. Also let $\boldsymbol{A} = diag(a_1, a_2, \ldots, a_m)$, where $a_j = (t_j - t_{j-1})^{1/2}$ is the square root of the length of consecutive time intervals for $j = 1, 2, \ldots, m$. We build the dependence structure using a m-dimensional multivariate normal distribution within each tank, so that

$$\boldsymbol{e}_k \sim N_m(0, \sigma^2 \boldsymbol{\Sigma}), \tag{76}$$

where $\boldsymbol{\Sigma}$ is a $m \times m$ matrix defined by

$$\boldsymbol{\Sigma} = \boldsymbol{A} \begin{pmatrix} 1 & \rho & \rho^2 & \cdots & \rho^{m-1} \\ \rho & 1 & \rho & \cdots & \rho^{m-2} \\ \vdots & \vdots & \vdots & \ddots & \vdots \\ \rho^{m-1} & \rho^{m-2} & \rho^{m-3} & \cdots & 1 \end{pmatrix} \boldsymbol{A}. \tag{77}$$

The function $g_\gamma(t)$ in (75) is a function of time known up to the unknown parameter γ. The choice of g_γ depends on the entertained response-time model of these kinds of mortality data. The most simple form of $g_\gamma(t)$ is linear, i.e., $g_\gamma(t) = \gamma_1 t$, the constant term is absent to preserve the identifiability of the model. There are many other possible choices for the function $g_\gamma(t)$ such as quadratic, $g_\gamma(t) = \gamma_1 t + \gamma_2 t^2$, and even more complex one such as a spline function of known order with a known number of knots but, with unknown knot positions. In this example, we use Bayesian variable selection approach to explore a suitable form for $g_\gamma(t)$ from the data. Here, we assume that $g_\gamma(t)$ takes the form

$$g_\gamma(t) = \gamma_1 g_1(t) + \gamma_2 g_2(t) + \cdots + \gamma_q g_q(t), \tag{78}$$

where the $g_j(t)$ are the known functions of t and $q \geq 0$. For the notational convenience, we denote $g_\gamma(t) \equiv 0$ when $q = 0$. We further denote $\gamma = (\gamma_1, \gamma_2, \ldots, \gamma_q)'$.

Let D denote the complete data, that is, $D = ((\mathbf{d}_k, \mathbf{r}_k, \boldsymbol{x}_k, g_1(t_{k1}), \ldots, g_q (t_{km})), k = 1, \ldots, 48)$, where $\mathbf{d}_k = (d_{kj}, j = 1, 2, \ldots, m)$ and $\mathbf{r}_k = (r_{kj}, j = 1, 2, \ldots, m)$. Also let $\phi_m(\mathbf{e}_k|\mu, \sigma^2\Sigma)$ denote the m-dimensional normal density of the random effect $\mathbf{e}_k$ with mean μ and covariance matrix $\sigma^2\Sigma$, i.e.,

$$\phi_m(\boldsymbol{e}_k|\mu, \sigma^2\Sigma) = \frac{|\boldsymbol{\Sigma}|^{-1/2}}{(2\pi\sigma^2)^{m/2}} \exp\left(-\frac{1}{2\sigma^2}(\mathbf{e}_k - \mu)'\boldsymbol{\Sigma}^{-1}(\mathbf{e}_k - \mu)\right). \tag{79}$$

Then, it can be shown that the likelihood function is given by

$$L(\boldsymbol{\beta}, \gamma, \sigma^2, \rho|D) = \prod_{k=1}^{K} \left\{ \int \left[\prod_{j=1}^{m} (h_{kj})^{d_{kj}} (1 - h_{kj})^{r_{kj} - d_{kj}} \right] \phi_m(\mathbf{e}_k | 0, \sigma^2 \Sigma) d\mathbf{e}_k \right\}, \quad (80)$$

where h_{kj} and e_{kj} are given in (75). Notice that from (77), we have

$$|\boldsymbol{\Sigma}| = (1 - \rho^2)^{m-1} \times \prod_{j=1}^{m} a_j.$$

We use the NaSCN added fish tank data (see O'Hara Hines, 1989) to build our prior distributions. Let D_0 denote the complete NaSCN data, that is, $D_0 = ((\mathbf{d}_{0k}, \mathbf{r}_{0k}, \boldsymbol{x}_{0k}, g_1(t_{01}), \ldots, g_q(t_{0m_0})), k = 1, 2, \ldots, K_0 = 36)$, where $\boldsymbol{x}_{0k} = (1, x_{01k}, x_{02k})'$, $\mathbf{d}_{0k} = (d_{0kj}, j = 1, 2, \ldots, m_0 = 5)$ and $\mathbf{r}_{0k} = (r_{0kj}, j = 1, 2, \ldots, m_0 = 5)$. In the NaSCN data, d_{0kj} is the number of fishes dying and r_{0kj} is the number of fishes at risk in the kth tank during the time interval $I_{0j} = (t_{0,j-1}, t_{0j})$ for $j = 1, 2, \ldots, m_0 = 5$, where $t_{01} = 1$, $t_{02} = 6$, $t_{03} = 13$, $t_{04} = 20$, $t_{05} = 27$, and $m_0 = 5$ for $k = 1, 2, \ldots, K_0$ ($K_0 = 36$).

To determine the form of g_γ, let $\mathcal{M}$ denote the model space with each model containing $\boldsymbol{\beta}$ and a specific choice of covariates $g_l(t_j)$. The full model is defined here as the model containing all of the available covariates in the toxicity experiment. Also, let $\boldsymbol{\theta}^{(\mathcal{Q})} = (\boldsymbol{\beta}', \gamma_1, \gamma_2, \ldots, \gamma_q)'$ and let $\boldsymbol{\theta}^{(m)}$ denote a $q_m \times 1$ vector of regression coefficients for model m with $\boldsymbol{\beta}$, and a specific choice of $q_m - 3$ covariates $g_l(t_j)$. We write $\boldsymbol{\theta}^{(\mathcal{Q})} = (\boldsymbol{\theta}^{(m)'}, \boldsymbol{\theta}^{(-m)'})'$, where $\boldsymbol{\theta}^{(-m)}$ is $\boldsymbol{\theta}^{(\mathcal{Q})}$ with $\boldsymbol{\theta}^{(m)}$ deleted.

Using the power prior given by (26), we construct the prior distribution for $(\boldsymbol{\theta}^{(m)}, \sigma^2, \rho)$ under model m as

$$\begin{aligned} \pi(\boldsymbol{\theta}^{(m)}, \sigma^2, \rho|m) &\propto \pi_0^*(\boldsymbol{\theta}^{(m)}, \sigma^2, \rho|D_0, m) \\ &= \int_0^1 \prod_{k=1}^{K_0} \left\{ \prod_{j=1}^{m_0} \int \frac{\exp\left\{a_0 d_{0kj} \left((\boldsymbol{x}_{0kj}^{*(m)})' \boldsymbol{\theta}^{(m)} + e_{0kj} \right) \right\}}{\left[1 + \exp\left\{ (\boldsymbol{x}_{0kj}^{*(m)})' \boldsymbol{\theta}^{(m)} + e_{0kj} \right\}\right]^{a_0 r_{0kj}}} \right. \\ &\qquad \left. \phi_{m_0}(\mathbf{e}_{0k} | 0, \sigma^2 \boldsymbol{\Sigma}_0) d\mathbf{e}_{0k} \right\} \\ &\qquad \times \pi_1(\sigma^2)\ \pi_2(\rho)\ \pi_3(a_0) da_0, \end{aligned} \quad (81)$$

where $\mathbf{e}_{0k}$ is a $m_0 \times 1$ vector of random effects, and $\boldsymbol{x}_{0kj}^{*(m)}$ is a $q_m \times 1$ vector of covariates corresponding to $\boldsymbol{\theta}^{(m)}$. Note that under the full model, $\boldsymbol{x}_{0kj}^* = (1, x_{01k}, x_{02k}, g_1(t_{0kj}), \ldots, g_q(t_{0kj}))'$. In (81), we specify an inverse gamma prior for σ^2 given as $\pi_1(\sigma^2) \propto (\sigma^2)^{-(\delta_0+1)} \exp(-\sigma^{-2}\zeta_0)$, a scaled beta prior for ρ given as $\pi_2(\rho) \propto (1+\rho)^{\nu_0-1}(1-\rho)^{\psi_0-1}$, and independent beta priors for each a_0 given as $\pi_3(a_0) \propto a_0^{\alpha_0-1}(1-a_0)^{\lambda_0-1}$. Let $L(\boldsymbol{\theta}^{(m)}, \sigma^2, \rho|D, m)$ denote the likelihood function given by (80) under model m. Then, the marginal likelihood given in (23) has the following expression:

$$p(D|m) = \int L(\boldsymbol{\theta}^{(m)}, \sigma^2, \rho|D, m)\pi(\boldsymbol{\theta}^{(m)}, \sigma^2, \rho|m) d\boldsymbol{\theta}^{(m)} d\sigma^2 d\rho. \qquad (82)$$

To completely determine the posterior probability of model m given by (22), we elicit the prior model probability $p(m)$ as:

$$p(m) = \frac{\int \pi_0^*(\boldsymbol{\theta}^{(m)}, \sigma^2, \rho|D_0, m)\ d\boldsymbol{\theta}^{(m)} d\sigma^2 d\rho}{\sum_{j=1}^{\mathcal{Q}} \int \pi_0^*(\boldsymbol{\theta}^{(j)}, \sigma^2, \rho|D_0, j)\ d\boldsymbol{\theta}^{(j)} d\sigma^2 d\rho}. \qquad (83)$$

The choice for $p(m)$ in (83) is a natural one since the numerator is just the normalizing constant of the joint prior of $(\boldsymbol{\theta}^{(m)}, \sigma^2, \rho)$ under model m. The prior model probabilities in (83) are based on coherent Bayesian updating. It can be shown that $p(m)$ in (83) corresponds to the posterior probability of model m based on the data D_0 using a uniform prior on the model space for the previous study, $p_0(m) = 2^{-q}$ for $m \in \mathcal{M}$ as $\alpha_0 \to \infty$. That is, $p(m) \propto p(m \mid D_0^{(m)})$, and thus $p(m)$ corresponds to the usual Bayesian update of $p_0(m)$ using D_0 as the data.

Next, we briefly discuss how to compute the posterior model probability $p(m|D)$. From (82) and (83), it can be seen that $p(m|D)$ is a function of the ratios of analytically intractable prior and posterior normalizing constants, which are expensive to compute. However, the following result can greatly ease such computational burden. Using (22), (82), and (83) along with the Savage-Dicky ratio (see, for example, Verdinelli and Wasserman 1995), it directly follows from Ibrahim, Chen, and Ryan (2000) that the posterior probability $p(m|D)$ in (22) of model m reduces to

$$p(m|D) = \frac{\pi(\boldsymbol{\theta}^{(-m)} = 0|D, \mathcal{Q})}{\sum_{j=1}^{\mathcal{Q}} \pi(\boldsymbol{\theta}^{(-j)} = 0|D, \mathcal{Q})}, \qquad (84)$$

$m = 1, \ldots, \mathcal{Q}$, where $\pi(\boldsymbol{\theta}^{(-m)} = 0|D, \mathcal{Q})$ is the marginal posterior density of $\boldsymbol{\theta}^{(-m)}$ evaluated at $\boldsymbol{\theta}^{(-m)} = 0$ under the full model. In (84), for notational convenience we assume that $\pi(\boldsymbol{\theta}^{(-\mathcal{Q})} = 0|D, \mathcal{Q}) = 1$. Note that the joint posterior distribution of $\boldsymbol{\theta}$ is given by

$$\pi(\boldsymbol{\theta}|D, \mathcal{Q}) \propto \int L(\boldsymbol{\theta}, \sigma^2, \rho|D)\pi(\boldsymbol{\theta}, \sigma^2, \rho|\mathcal{Q})d\sigma^2 d\rho.$$

The result in (84) is attractive since it shows that the posterior model probability $p(m|D)$ is simply a function of the marginal posterior density functions of $\boldsymbol{\theta}^{(-m)}$ for the full model evaluated at $\boldsymbol{\theta}^{(-m)} = 0$. This formula does not algebraically depend on the prior model probability $p(m)$ since it cancels out in the derivation due to the structure of $p(m)$. This is an important feature since it allows us to compute the posterior model probabilities directly *without* numerically computing the prior model probabilities. This has a clear computational advantage and as a result, allows us to compute posterior model probabilities efficiently. Although the analytical evaluation of $\pi(\boldsymbol{\theta}^{(-m)} = 0|D, \mathcal{Q})$ does not appear possible due to the complexity of our model, it can be easily computed by using the IWMDE method discussed in Section 2.3.

We implement the above Bayesian variable subset selection to determine the form of g_γ. The terms $t, t^2, log(t)$ were previously used in the toxicological mortality estimation literature by authors such as O'Hara Hines (1989), O'Hara Hines and Lawless (1993) and others to model the effect of time. We do not know which form of $g(t)$ fits the data best before our analysis, and therefore, we use the formal Bayesian model selection procedure allowing the possibility of including all of these coefficients in the selected model. So, we consider that the full model for $g_\gamma(t_j)$ contains t_j, t_j^2, and $\ln t_j$, that is, $g_\gamma(t_j) = \gamma_1 t_j + \gamma_2 t_j^2 + \gamma_3 \ln t_j$. Thus, the model space $\mathcal{M}$ has a dimension of $\mathcal{Q} = 2^3 = 8$. We specify noninformative priors for ρ and σ^2. Specifically, we take a uniform prior for ρ on $[-1, 1]$ (i.e., $\nu_0 = \psi_0 = 1$) and take an inverse gamma prior for σ^2 given as $\pi_1(\sigma^2) \propto (\sigma^2)^{-(\delta_0+1)} \exp(-\sigma^{-2}\zeta_0)$ with $\delta_0 = \zeta_0 = 0.005$. Then, we consider several choices of hyperparameters (α_0, λ_0) for a_0 to perform a small scale sensitivity study. Similar to Example 3, we let $\mu_{a_0} = \alpha_0/(\alpha_0 + \lambda_0)$, and $\sigma_{a_0} = \left(\mu_0(1 - \mu_0)(\alpha_0 + \lambda_0 + 1)^{-1}\right)^{1/2}$. We generate 50,000 Gibbs iterations from the posterior distribution under the full model to obtain IWMDE. Table 5 gives results for the top three models based on several values of $(\mu_{a_0}, \sigma_{a_0})$. In Table 5, we let T, T^2, and $\ln T$ denote time, time square, and the natural logarithm of time. From Table 5, it can be seen that (i) for all choices of $(\mu_{a_0}, \sigma_{a_0})$, the order of the top three models does not change while model (x_1, x_2, T) is clearly the top model, and (ii) the posterior model probabilities for all top three models

Table 5. Posterior model probabilities for the fish tank data.

(μ_0, σ_0)	Model	$p(m \mid D)$
(0.50, 0.109)	(x_1, x_2, T)	0.486
	(x_1, x_2, T^2)	0.352
	$(x_1, x_2, \ln T)$	0.153
(0.50, 0.050)	(x_1, x_2, T)	0.484
	(x_1, x_2, T^2)	0.351
	$(x_1, x_2, \ln T)$	0.153
(0.91, 0.027)	(x_1, x_2, T)	0.484
	(x_1, x_2, T^2)	0.350
	$(x_1, x_2, \ln T)$	0.153
(0.98, 0.006)	(x_1, x_2, T)	0.483
	(x_1, x_2, T^2)	0.350
	$(x_1, x_2, \ln T)$	0.154

are almost the same for all choices of $(\mu_{a_0}, \sigma_{a_0})$ despite the one with a strong prior on a_0 (see $(\mu_{a_0}, \sigma_{a_0}) = (0.98, 0.006)$). Therefore, model choice is reasonably robust to the choice of $(\mu_{a_0}, \sigma_{a_0})$. In addition, the total sum of the posterior model probabilities for the top three models is close to 1, for example, this sum equals 0.988 for $(\mu_{a_0}, \sigma_{a_0}) = (0.50, 0.050)$. This result implies that for the purpose of posterior prediction, it suffices to use these three models to apply model averaging techniques (Raftery 1996) to incorporate model uncertainty in posterior densities for parameters. Also, from the principle of parsimony and from the result of Bayesian variable selection, the best model to use is $g(t) = \gamma_1 + \gamma_2 t$.

6.3. *Reference prior analysis to a statistical calibration model*

A statistical calibration problem (or, more precisely, an *absolute* statistical calibration problem), bears a resemblance to a regression problem. It is still assumed that the variables x and y are related through a function of specified form. However, in calibration, interest centers on the estimation of an unknown value of x, corresponding to an observed value of y. Inferences are based on two samples of data. At a first stage of data collection, n pairs (x_i, y_i) are observed, with the x values fixed at known levels. At a second stage, c replications of the response variable y are observed, corresponding to an unknown value of the regressor x_0; estimation of this regressor value is of primary interest. A review of statistical calibration is given by Osbourne (1991).

Noninformative priors for the linear calibration problem have been presented by several authors, including Kubokawa and Robert (1994), du Plessis, van der Merwe and Groenewald (1995), Philippe and Robert (1998) and Ghosh, Carlin and Srivastava (1995). Also, Eno and Ye (2000) studied the reference priors for the polynomial calibration models, as well as the probability matching prior for an extended calibration problem (Eno and Ye 2001). In here we present an example of polynomial calibration model.

6.3.1. *An example of polynomial calibration*

The data set was presented by Aitchison and Dunsmore (1975). These data resulted from an assay of an antibiotic, based on the "clearance circle" technique. The goal of such an experiment is to estimate the concentration of the active constituent in a particular test preparation of the antibiotic.

In a clearance circle assay, the regressor variable x is a precise measure of the concentration of active constituent in a preparation of antibiotic. This concentration is controlled in a laboratory experiment, where it is set at several different values by diluting a known full-strength antibiotic preparation to varying degrees. Each response y_i is obtained by placing a drop of antibiotic solution (of a specified volume) on a petri dish which is uniformly infected with bacteria. The actual response variable y_i is the measured diameter of the circle which has been disinfected by the antibiotic preparation after a specified period of time. It is expected that the diameter of this clearance circle depends on the concentration of the active constituent in an antibiotic solution. Based on the known dilutions of the standard preparation, this regression relationship can be estimated.

At the same time that the clearance circles corresponding to the known antibiotic concentrations are measured, clearance circles are also measured for the test preparation whose unknown antibiotic concentration is of interest. What we want to do here is to use the reference prior Bayesian analysis to estimate this unknown antibiotic concentration. The data are plotted in Figure 4.

In the plot (Figure 4), the response is transformed via the square root transformation and the regressor is transformed via the log transformation. The plot really fits a quadratic model well.

6.3.2. *The model and the reference priors*

The polynomial calibration problem can be formally stated as follows. Data in the form of n pairs (x_i, y_i) are collected. In addition to these n data pairs,

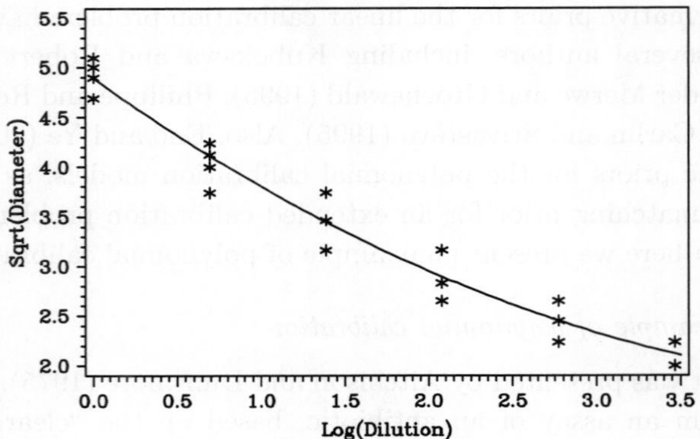

Fig. 4. Scatterplot of the transformed data in clearance circle assay.

we observe c values of the response, $y_{n+1}, y_{n+2}, \ldots, y_{n+c}$, which correspond to a single unknown value of the regressor x_0. The response variable y is assumed to be related to the regressor x via a polynomial function of order p:

$$y_i = \alpha + \beta_1 x_i + \beta_2 x_i^2 + \cdots + \beta_p x_i^p + \epsilon_i, \quad \text{for } i = 1, 2, \ldots, n+c.$$

For convenience, we have written x_i in place of x_0, for $i = n+1, n+2, \ldots, n+c$. We assume that the errors ϵ_i are independent and identically distributed normal deviates, with mean 0 and standard deviation σ.

Of primary interest in this problem is the estimation of the unknown regressor value x_0. A feature that distinguishes the polynomial calibration problem from the linear calibration problem is that, since a polynomial function need not be monotonic, more than one value of x_0 may give rise to a particular mean response $\bar{y}_0$. This issue in the context of the clearance circle assay described above has been discussed and addressed in Eno and Ye (2000).

Reference priors for the univariate polynomial calibration problem, as described above, are given as follows.

$$\begin{aligned}\pi_k(x_0, \alpha, \beta, \sigma) &\propto \sigma^{-k}\left(\frac{\zeta_0'\zeta_0}{1 + c\xi_0'(\mathbf{X}_{\alpha,1}'\mathbf{X}_{\alpha,1})^{-1}\xi_0}\right)^{\frac{1}{2}} \\ &= \sigma^{-k}(\zeta_0'\zeta_0)^{\frac{1}{2}}\left(1 + \frac{cn}{n+c}(\mathbf{x}_0 - \bar{\mathbf{x}})'(\mathbf{X}_1'\mathbf{X}_1)^{-1}(\mathbf{x}_0 - \bar{\mathbf{x}})\right)^{-\frac{1}{2}},\end{aligned} \tag{85}$$

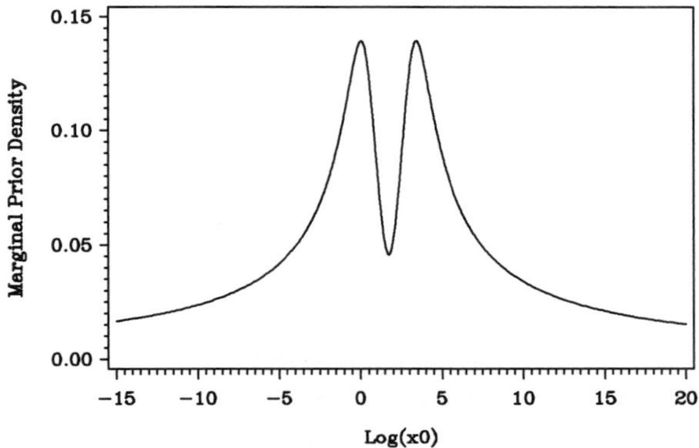

Fig. 5. Reference prior for the quadratic model, for the clearance circle assay example.

where, $\mathbf{X}_1$ is the $n \times p$ matrix whose i^{th} row is $\mathbf{x}_i'$, the vector of regressor at i^{th} observation, $\mathbf{X}_{\alpha,1}$ is the $n \times (s+1)$ matrix whose i^{th} row is $(1, \mathbf{x}_i')$, $\zeta_0' = (1, 2x_0, 3x_0^2, \ldots, px_0^{p-1})$ is a vector of derivative terms of $\mathbf{x}_0$, and k is the number of parameters in the group involving σ in the implementation of the reference prior algorithm.

Clearly the prior in (85) is improper. As we noted in Section 3.3, it is necessary to check the propriety of the posteriors once an improper prior is used. In Eno and Ye (2000), integrability of the reference prior in form (85) was proven. The prior function is shown in Figure 5 for the clearance circle assay problem.

6.3.3. *Posterior results*

Applying the reference prior (85) to the clearance circle assay problem, we are ready to estimate the antibiotic concentration level for the observed responses. The marginal posterior distribution of the log (*concentration*) is shown in Figure 6. It is quite clear to see the bi-modal properties of both the prior and the posterior since the model considered here is quadratic. Furthermore, it can be easily seen that the small bump in the posterior distribution reflects to x_0 value may beyond the region of original regressor. It is conceivable that this local mode does not belong to this data set.

Since the model is not likely to be reliable outside the range of the controlled regressor values, we truncate the range of the posterior density and transform the logarithm back to the original scale. Figure 7 shows the marginal posterior distribution of x_0.

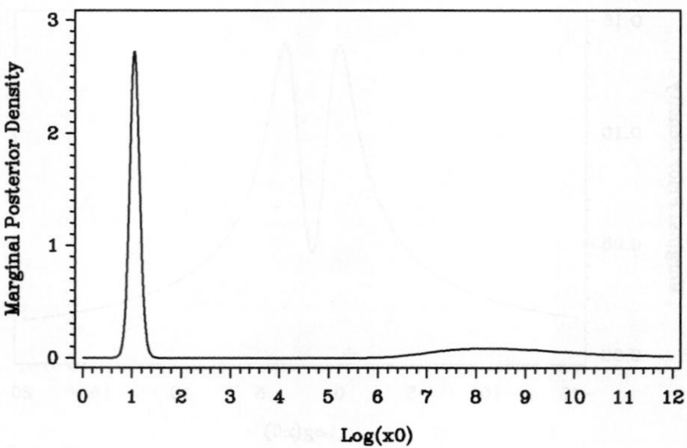

Fig. 6. Marginal reference posterior for $\log(x_0)$.

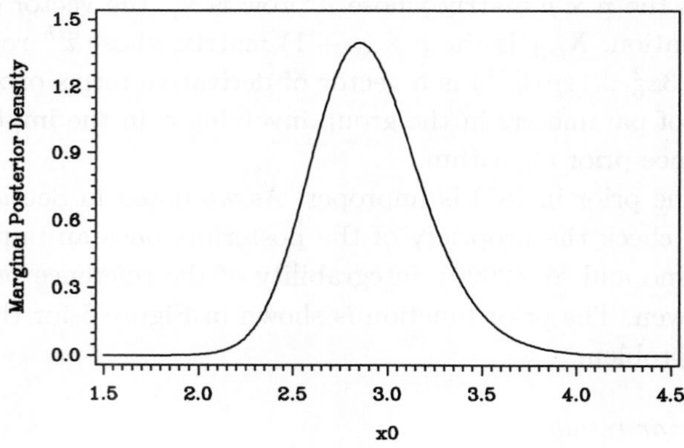

Fig. 7. Marginal reference posterior for x_0.

6.4. *Bayesian design of a non-inferiority trial for medical devices using historical data*

We apply the Bayesian SSD discussed in Section 5 for designing a clinical trial to evaluate the performance of a new generation of drug-eluting stent (DES) ("treatment") with a non-inferiority comparison to the first generation of DES ("control"). We consider only the primary endpoint, which is the 12-month Target Lesion Failure (TLF) (binary) composite endpoint. TLF is an ischemia-driven revascularization of the target lesion (TLR), myocardial infarction (MI) (Q-wave and non-Q-wave) related to the target vessel, or (cardiac) death related to the target vessel.

As discussed in Chen *et al.* (2011), historical data are available from two previous trials on the first generation of DES. The first trial conducted in 2002 evaluated the safety and effectiveness of the slow release paclitaxel-eluting stent for treatment of de novo coronary artery lesions. The second trial conducted in 2004 expanded on the first trial, studied more complex de novo lesions, and involved multiple overlapping stents and smaller and larger diameter stents. Our historical data based on lesion size matched criteria are subsets of the data published in Stone *et al.* (2004, 2005). The sample sizes for these two historical trials were 535 and 304. A summary of the historical data can be found in Chen *et al.* (2011). We use these historical datasets to construct our priors in Bayesian SSD.

For the primary endpoint, we assume that y_{1i} (y_{2i}) follows a Bernoulli distribution $\text{Ber}(p_1)$ ($\text{Ber}(p_2)$). In this case, $\mu_j = \text{logit} = \log\left(\frac{p_j}{1-p_j}\right)$ for $j = 1, 2$ and the joint distribution of $\boldsymbol{y}^{(n)}$ is given by

$$f(\boldsymbol{y}^{(n)}|\boldsymbol{\theta}) = \prod_{j=1}^{2}\prod_{i=1}^{n_j} \frac{\exp(y_{ji}\mu_j)}{1+\exp(\mu_j)}.$$

Under the Bernoulli model, $\tau = 1$ and the normalized power prior (56) for μ_2 reduces to

$$\pi(\mu_2|\boldsymbol{y}_0, \boldsymbol{a}_0) = \frac{\exp\left\{\mu_2 \sum_{k=1}^{K} a_{0k} n_{0k} \bar{y}_{0k}\right\}}{B\left(\sum_{k=1}^{K} a_{0k} n_{0k} \bar{y}_{0k}, \sum_{k=1}^{K} a_{0k} n_{0k}(1-\bar{y}_{0k})\right)[1+\exp(\mu_2)]^{n_0(\boldsymbol{a}_0)}},$$

where $B(.,.)$ denotes the complete beta function, $\bar{y}_{0k} = \frac{1}{n_{0k}} \sum_{i=1}^{n_{0k}} y_{0ki}$, and $n_0(\boldsymbol{a}_0) = \sum_{k=1}^{K} a_{0k} n_{0k}$.

The margin was set to be $\delta = \text{logit}(4.1\%) = \log\left\{\frac{0.041}{1-0.041}\right\}$. We took $\pi_0(\mu_2) \propto 1$ and $b_{01} = b_{02} = 1$ for the initial priors of μ_1 and a_{0k} in (58). We computed the powers at $\mu_1 = \mu_2$ and the type I error at $\frac{\exp(\mu_1)}{1+\exp(\mu_1)} = \frac{\exp(\mu_2)}{1+\exp(\mu_2)} + \frac{\exp(\delta)}{1+\exp(\delta)}$. In the sampling prior given by (59), we assume a point mass prior at $\mu_2 = \text{logit}(9.2\%)$ for $\pi^{(s)}(\mu_2)$, where 9.2% is the pooled proportion for the two historical control datasets, and a point mass prior at $\mu_1 = \mu_2$ or $\mu_1 = \text{logit}\left[\frac{\exp(\mu_2)}{1+\exp(\mu_2)} + \frac{\exp(\delta)}{1+\exp(\delta)}\right]$ for $\pi^{(s)}(\mu_1)$. In all of the computations, In all calculations, a 3:1 sample size ratio, $N = 10,000$ and $M = 20,000$ were used.

Table 6. Powers and type I errors for the 12-month TLF with $\gamma = 0.95$.

Total Sample Size (n_1, n_2)		1000 (750, 250)	1080 (810, 270)	1200 (900, 300)	1280 (960, 320)	1480 (1110, 370)
Score Test	Power	0.672	0.699	0.736	0.758	0.807
No Borrowing	Power	0.648	0.676	0.718	0.738	0.800
$\boldsymbol{a}_0 = (0, 0)$	Type I Error	0.049	0.048	0.048	0.050	0.044
Power Prior	Power	0.840	0.856	0.884	0.892	0.923
Fixed $\boldsymbol{a}_0 = (0.3, 0.3)$	Type I Error	0.030	0.027	0.028	0.030	0.032
Power Prior	Power	0.843	0.878	0.897	0.902	0.914
Random $\boldsymbol{a}_0$	Type I Error	0.038	0.031	0.029	0.036	0.039

We first computed the powers and the type I errors for various sample sizes without the incorporation of historical data. Table 6 shows the results. Table 6 also presents the power of the frequentist method, namely, the score test (Farrington and Manning, 1990) for non-inferiority trials. PASS 2008 (Hintze, 2008) was used for computing the powers for the frequentist SSD method. We see from Table 6 that the Bayesian SSD without incorporation of historical data gives very similar powers compared to the frequentist SSD method, while the type I errors of the Bayesian SSD are controlled at or below 5%. Table 6 also shows the powers and the type I errors of the Bayesian SSD procedure with fixed and random $\boldsymbol{a}_0$. The powers based on the power prior with $\boldsymbol{a}_0$ random are comparable to those based on the power prior with $\boldsymbol{a}_0$ fixed at $\boldsymbol{a}_0 = (0.3, 0.3)$. These results imply that the power prior with random $\boldsymbol{a}_0$ borrow approximately 30% of the historical data. With incorporation of the historical data, a sample size of $(n_1, n_2) = (810, 270)$ achieves 80% power. However, based on the frequentist SSD or the Bayesian SSD without incorporation of historical data, a sample size of 1480 with $n_1 = 1110$ and $n_2 = 370$ is required to achieve 80% power. Thus, the Bayesian SSD with incorporation of historical data yields a substantial reduction in the sample size.

The Bayesian SSD works best if the historical data from the control device are compatible to the data from the current trial. However, the targeted type I error and power may not be well maintained when the data from the historical and current trials are not compatible. For illustrative purposes, we consider $n = 1200$ with $n_1 = 900$ and $n_2 = 300$. If a point mass sampling prior at $\mu_2 = \text{logit}(8.0\%)$ is assumed, the type I error and power

Table 7. Powers and type I errors under three sampling priors with $\gamma = 0.96$.

	Point mass sampling prior at $\mu_c = \text{logit}(p_c^*)$					
	$p_c^* = 8.0\%$		$p_c^* = 9.2\%$		$p_c^* = 10.0\%$	
$\boldsymbol{a}_0$	Power	Type I Error	Power	Type I Error	Power	Type I Error
$(0, 0)$	0.740	0.039	0.685	0.038	0.649	0.035
$(0.1, 0.1)$	0.860	0.039	0.762	0.029	0.694	0.022
$(0.2, 0.2)$	0.920	0.041	0.819	0.024	0.731	0.017
$(0.3, 0.3)$	0.953	0.049	0.856	0.021	0.750	0.013
$(0.4, 0.4)$	0.973	0.058	0.887	0.022	0.776	0.010
$(0.5, 0.5)$	0.980	0.069	0.906	0.017	0.799	0.009

were 0.07 and 0.945 for the power prior with $a_{0k} \sim \text{beta}(1, 1)$ and $\gamma = 0.95$. Chen *et al.* (2011) proposed two approaches for resolving this type I error problem. One approach is to change the initial prior $\text{beta}(b_{01}, b_{02})$ for a_{0k} in (58) to down-weight the historical control data. Another approach is to increase the value of γ, which is recommended in the FDA 2010 Guidance. Chen *et al.* (2011) empirically showed that each of these two approaches and a combination of these two approaches work quite effectively in controlling the type I error while maintaining good power at the same time. To further illustrate how the second approach works, we consider $(n_1, n_2) = (900, 300)$, $\gamma = 0.96$ and fixed $\boldsymbol{a}_0$ under three sampling priors for μ_2. Table 7 shows the type I errors and powers under various choices of $\boldsymbol{a}_0$. From this table, we see that when $\gamma = 0.96$ and $\boldsymbol{a}_0 = (0, 0)$, the type I error is well controlled below 5%. The type I error increases when more historical data are incorporated. When $\boldsymbol{a}_0 = (0.3, 0.3)$, the type I error is exactly controlled at around 5%. This illustration demonstrates that fixed $\boldsymbol{a}_0$ indeed provides us additional flexibility in controlling the type I error.

References

1. Adcock, C.J. (1997). Sample size determination: a review. *The Statistician*, **46**, 261–283.
2. Aitchison, J. and Dunsmore, I.R. (1975). *Statistical Prediction Analysis.* Cambridge University Press.
3. Akaike, H. (1973). Information theory and an extension of the maximum likelihood principle. In *International Symposium on Information Theory* (Eds. B.N. Petrov and F. Csaki). Budapest: Akademia Kiado, 267–281.
4. Berkson, J. and Gage, R.P. (1952). Survival curve for cancer patients following treatment. *Journal of the American Statistical Association*, **47**, 501–515.
5. Berger, J.O. (1999). Bayesian analysis today and tomorrow. *Technical Report 99-30.* Institute of Statistics and Decision Sciences, Duke University.

6. Berger, J.O. (1985). *Statistical Decision Theory and Bayesian Analysis.* Second Edition. New York: Wiley.
7. Berger, J.O. and Bernardo, J. (1989). Estimating a product of normal means: Bayesian analysis with reference priors. *Journal of the American Statistical Association*, **84**, 200–207.
8. Berger, J.O. and Bernardo, J. (1992). On the development of the reference prior method. In *Bayesian Statistics 4,* (eds.) Bernardo, J.M., Berger, J.O., Dawid, A.P. and Smith, A.F.M., Oxford University Press: London, pp. 35–60.
9. Berger, J.O. and Mallows, C.L. (1988). Discussion of Bayesian variable selection in linear regression. *Journal of the American Statistical Association*, **83**, 1033–1034.
10. Bernardo, J. (1979). Reference posterior distributions for Bayesian inference (with discussion). *J. Royal Statistical Society*, **B 41**, 113–147.
11. Bernardo, J.M. and Smith, A.F.M. (1995). *Bayesian Theory.* John Wiley and Sons, New York.
12. Besag, J. and Green, P.J. (1993). Spatial statistics and Bayesian computation. *Journal of the Royal Statistical Society, Series B*, **55**, 25–37.
13. Boone, E.L., Ye, K., and Smith, E. P. (2005), Assessment of two approximation methods for computing posterior model probabilities. *Computational Statistics and Data Analysis*, **48**, 221–234.
14. Box, G.E.P. (1980). Sampling and Bayes' inference in scientific modelling and robustness (with discussion). *Journal of the Royal Statistical Society, Series A*, **143**, 383–430.
15. Bratley, P., Fox, B.L., and Schrage, L.E. (1987). *A Guide to Simulation.* Second Edition. Springer-Verlag, New York.
16. Carlin, B.P. and Louis, T.A. (2000). *Bayes and Empirical Bayes Methods for Data Analysis.* Second Edition, Chapman & Hall, New York.
17. Casella, G. and George, E.I. (1992). Explaining the Gibbs sampler. *The American Statistician*, **46**, 167–174.
18. Chen, M.-H. (1994). Importance weighted marginal Bayesian posterior density estimation. *Journal of the American Statistical Association*, **89**, 818–824.
19. Chen, M.-H. and Deely, J.J. (1996). Bayesian analysis for a constrained linear multiple regression problem for predicting the new crop of apples. *Journal of Agricultural, Biological and Environmental Statistics*, **1**, 467–89.
20. Chen, M.-H., Dey, D.K., Müller, P., Sun, D., Ye, K. (Eds.) (2010). *Frontiers of Statistical Decision Making and Bayesian Analysis — In Honor of James O. Berger.* Springer-Verlag, New York.
21. Chen, M.-H., Dey, D.K., and Sinha, D. (2000). Bayesian analysis of multivariate mortality data with large families. *Applied Statistics*, **49**, 129–144.
22. Chen, M.-H., Ibrahim, J.G., and Kim, S. (2008). Properties and implementation of Jeffreys's prior in binomial regression models. *Journal of the American Statistical Association*, **103**, 1659–1664.

23. Chen, M.-H., Ibrahim, J.G., Lam, P., Yu, A., and Zhang, Y. (2011). Bayesian design of non-inferiority trials for medical devices using historical data. *Biometrics* **67**, 1163–1170.
24. Chen, M.-H., Ibrahim, J.G., and Shao, Q.-M. (2000). Power prior distributions for generalized linear models. *Journal of Statistical Planning and Inference*, **41**, 121–137.
25. Chen, M.-H., Ibrahim, J.G., Shao, Q.-M., and Weiss, R.E. (2001) Prior elicitation for model selection and estimation in generalized linear mixed models. *Journal of Statistical Planning and Inference*, to appear.
26. Chen, M.-H., Ibrahim, J.G., and Sinha, D. (1999). A new Bayesian model For survival data with a surviving fraction. *Journal of the American Statistical Association*, **94**, 909–919.
27. Chen, M.-H., Ibrahim, J.G., and Yiannoutsos, C. (1999). Prior elicitation and Bayesian computation for logistic regression models with applications to variable selection. *Journal of the Royal Statistical Society, Series B*, **61**, 223–242.
28. Chen, M.-H., Manatunga, A.K., and Williams, C.J. (1998). Heritability estimates from human twin data by incorporating historical prior information. *Biometrics*, **54**, 1348–1362.
29. Chen, M.-H. and Shao, Q.-M. (1999). Monte Carlo estimation of Bayesian credible and HPD intervals. *Journal of Computational and Graphical Statistics*, **8**, 69–92.
30. Chen, M.-H. and Shao, Q.-M. (1997). On Monte Carlo methods for estimating ratios of normalizing constants. *The Annals of Statistics*, **25**, 1563–1594.
31. Chen, M.-H., Shao, Q.-M., and Ibrahim, J.G. (2000). *Monte Carlo Methods in Bayesian Computation*. Springer-Verlag, New York.
32. Chib, S. and Greenberg, E. (1995). Understanding the Metropolis–Hastings algorithm. *The American Statistician*, **49**, 327–335.
33. Cox, D.R. and Reid, N. (1987). Parameter orthogonality and approximate conditional inference (with discussion). *Journal of the Royal Statistical Society*, **49**, 1–39.
34. Datta, G.S. and Ghosh, M. (1996). On the invariance of noninformative priors. *Technical Report 94-20*, Department of Statistics, University of Georgia.
35. D'Agostino Sr., R.B., Massaro, J.M., and Sullivan, L.M. (2003). Non-inferiority trials: design concepts and issues — the encounters of academic consultants in statistics. *Statistics in Medicine*, **22**, 169–186.
36. De Santis, F. (2007). Using historical data for Bayesian sample size determination. *Journal of the Royal Statistical Society, Series A*, **170**, 95–113.
37. Dey, D.K., Chen, M.-H., and Chang, H. (1997). Bayesian approach for nonlinear random effects models. *Biometrics*, **53**, 1239–1252.
38. Duan, Y., Smith E.P., and Ye, K. (2006), Using power priors to improve the binomial test in water quality, *Journal of Ag., Biol. and Envir. Stat.*, **11**, 151–168.
39. Duan, Y., Ye, K., and Smith, E.P. (2006). Evaluating water quality using power priors to incorporate historical information. *Environmetrics* **17**, 95–106.

40. du Plessis, J.L., van der Merwe, A.J., and Groenewald, P.C.N. (1995). Reference priors for the multivariate calibration problem. *South African Statistical Journal*, **29**, 155–168.
41. Eno, D.R. and Ye, K. (2000). Bayesian reference prior analysis for polynomial calibration models. *Test*, **9**, 191–208.
42. Eno, D.R. and Ye, K. (2001). Probability matching priors for an extended statistical calibration model. *Canadian Journal of Statistics*, to appear.
43. Farrington, C.P. and Manning, G. (1990). Test statistics and sample size formulae for comparative binomial trials with null hypothesis of non-zero risk difference or non-unity relative risk. *Statistics in Medicine*, **9**, 1447–1454.
44. Fleming, T.R. (2008). Current issues in non-inferiority trials. *Statistics in Medicine*, **27**, 317–332.
45. Gamerman, D. and Lopes, H.F. (2006). *Markov Chain Monte Carlo: Stochastic Simulation for Bayesian Inference*. Second Edition. Chapman & Hall, London.
46. Geisser, S. (1993). *Predictive Inference: An Introduction*. Chapman & Hall, London.
47. Geisser, S (1980). In discussion of G.E.P. Box. *Journal of the Royal Statistical Society, Series A*, **143**, 416–417.
48. Gelfand, A.E., Dey, D.K., and Chang, H. (1992). Model determinating using predictive distributions with implementation via sampling-based methods (with discussion). In *Bayesian Statistics* **4** (Eds. J.M. Bernado, J.O. Berger, A.P. Dawid, and A.F.M. Smith). Oxford: Oxford University Press, 147–167.
49. Gelfand, A.E. and Mallick, B. (1995). Bayesian analysis of proportional hazards models built from monotone functions. *Biometrics*, **51**, 843–852.
50. Gelfand, A.E., Sahu, S.K., and Carlin, B.P. (1996). Efficient parametrisations for generalized linear mixed models (with discussion). In *Bayesian Statistics* **5** (Eds. J.M. Bernardo, J.O. Berger, A.P. Dawid, and A.F.M. Smith). Oxford: Oxford University Press, 165–180.
51. Gelfand, A.E., Sahu, S.K., and Carlin, B.P. (1995). Efficient parametrisations for normal linear mixed models. *Biometrika*, **82**, 479–488.
52. Gelfand, A.E. and Smith, A.F.M. (1990). Sampling-based approaches to calculating marginal densities. *Journal of the American Statistical Association*, **85**, 398–409.
53. Gelman, A. and Meng, X.-L. (1998). Simulating normalizing constants: from importance sampling to bridge sampling to path sampling. *Statistical Science*, **13**, 163–185.
54. Geman, S. and Geman, D. (1984). Stochastic relaxation, Gibbs distributions and the Bayesian restoration of images. *IEEE Transactions on Pattern Analysis and Machine Intelligence*, **6**, 721–741.
55. Geweke, J. (1989). Bayesian inference in econometrics models using Monte Carlo integration. *Econometrica*, **57**, 1317–1340.
56. George, E.I. and McCulloch, R.E. (1993). Variable selection via Gibbs sampling. *Journal of the American Statistical Association*, **88**, 881–889.

57. Ghosh, J.K. and Mukerjee, R. (1992). Noninformative priors. In *Bayesian Statistic 4*, (eds.) Bernardo, J.M., Berger, J.O., Dawid, A.P. and Smith, A.F.M., Oxford University Press, London, 195–210.
58. Ghosh, M., Carlin, B.P., and Srivastava, M.S. (1998). Probability matching priors for linear calibration. *Test*, **4**, 333–357.
59. Gilks, W.R., Richardson, S., and Spiegelhalter, D.J. (1996). *Markov Chain Monte Carlo in Practice*. Chapman & Hall, London.
60. Gilks, W.R. and Wild, P. (1992). Adaptive rejection sampling for Gibbs sampling. *Applied Statistics*, **41**, 337–348.
61. Goel, P.K. (1988). Software for Bayesian analysis: current status and additional needs. In *Bayesian Statistics 3* (Eds. J.M. Bernardo, M.H. DeGroot, D.V. Lindley, and A.F.M. Smith). Oxford: Oxford University Press, 173–188.
62. Goldsman, D. and Meketon, M.S. (1986). A comparison of several variance estimators. *Technical Report J-85-12*. School of Industrial and Systems Engineering, Georgia Institute of Technology.
63. Green, P.J. (1995). Reversible jump Markov chain Monte Carlo computation and Bayesian model determination. *Biometrika*, **82**, 711–732.
64. Grenander, U. (1983). Tutorial in pattern theorey. *Technical Report*. Providence, R.I.: Division of Applied Mathematics, Brown University.
65. Hammersley, J.M. and Handscomb, D.C. (1964). *Monte Carlo Methods*. Methuen, London.
66. Haseman, J.K., Huff, J., and Boorman, G.A. (1984). Use of historical control data in carcinogenicity studies in rodents. *Toxocologic Pathology*, **12**, 126–135.
67. Hastings, W.K. (1970). Monte Carlo sampling methods using Markov chains and their applications. *Biometrika*, **57**, 97–109.
68. Hintze, J. (2008). PASS 2008. NCSS, LLC. Kaysville, Utah, USA. www.ncss.com.
69. Hobbs, B.P., Carlin, B.P., Mandekar, S.J., and Sargent, D.J. (2011). Hierarchical commensurate and power prior models for adaptive incorporation of historical information in clinical trials. *Biometrics*, **67**, 1047–1056.
70. Hobbs, B.P., Sargent, D.J., and Carlin, B.P. (2012). Commensurate priors for incorporating historical information in clinical trials using general and generalized linear models. *Bayesian Analysis*, **7**, 1–36.
71. Hoeting, J.A., Madigan, D., Raftery, A.E., and Volinsky, C.T. (1999). Bayesian model averaging: a tutorial. *Statistical Science*, **14**, 382–417.
72. Hoeting, J.A., Raftery, A.E., and Madigan, D. (1996). A method for simultaneous variable selection and outlier identification in linear regression. *Computational Statistics and Data Analysis*, **22**, 251–270.
73. Hung, H.M.J., Wang, S.-J., and O'Neill, R.T. (2007). Issues with statistical risks for testing methods in noninferiority trial without a placebo arm. *Journal of Biopharmaceutical Statistics*, **17**, 201–213.
74. Hung, H.M.J., Wang, S.-J., and O'Neill, R.T. (2005). A regulatory perspective on choice of margin and statistical inference issue in non-inferiority trials. *Biometrical Journal*, **47**, 28–36

75. Hung, H.M.J., Wang, S.-J., Tsong, Y., Lawrence, J., and O'Neill, R.T. (2003). Some fundamental issues with non-inferiority testing in active controlled trials. *Statistics in Medicine*, **22**, 213–225.
76. Ibrahim, J.G. and Chen, M.-H. (2000). Power prior distributions for regression models. *Statistical Sciences*, **15**, 46–60.
77. Ibrahim, J.G. and Chen, M.-H. (1998). Prior distributions and Bayesian computation for proportional hazards models. *Sankhyā, Series B*, **60**, 48–64.
78. Ibrahim, J.G., Chen, M.-H., and MacEachern, S.N. (1999). Bayesian variable selection for proportional hazards models. *The Canadian Journal of Statistics*, **27**, 701–717.
79. Ibrahim, J.G., Chen, M.-H., and Ryan, L.-M. (2000). Bayesian variable selection for time series count data. *Statistica Sinica*, **10**, 971–987.
80. Ibrahim, J.G., Chen, M.-H., and Sinha, D. (2001). *Bayesian Survival Analysis*. Springer-Verlag, New York.
81. Ibrahim, J.G. and Laud, P.W. (1994). A predictive approach to the analysis of designed experiments. *Journal of the American Statistical Association*, **89**, 309–319.
82. Ibrahim, J.G. and Laud, P.W. (1991). On Bayesian analysis of generalized linear models using Jeffreys's prior. *Journal of the American Statistical Association*, **86**, 981–986.
83. Ibrahim, J.G., Ryan, L.-M., and Chen, M.-H. (1998). Use of historical controls to adjust for covariates in trend tests for binary data. *Journal of the American Statistical Association*, **93**, 1282–1293.
84. Inoue, L.Y.T., Berry, D.A., and Parmigiani, G. (2005). Relationship between Bayesian and frequentist sample size determination. *The American Statistician*, **59**, 79–87.
85. Jeffreys, H. (1961). *Theory of Probability*. Oxford University Press.
86. Johnson, W. and Geisser, S. (1983). A predictive view of the detection and characterization of influential observations in regression analysis. *Journal of American Statistical Association*, **78**, 137–144.
87. Joseph, L. and Bélisle, P. (1997). Bayesian sample size determination for normal means and differences between normal means. *The Statistician*, **46**, 209–226.
88. Joseph, L., Wolfson, D.B., and Du Berger, R. (1995a). Sample size calculations for binomial proportions via highest posterior density intervals. *The Statistician: Journal of the Institute of Statisticians* **44**, 143–154.
89. Joseph, L., Wolfson, D.B., and Du Berger, R. (1995b). Some comments on Bayesian sample size determination. *The Statistician: Journal of the Institute of Statisticians* **44**, 167–171.
90. Kass, R.E. and Wasserman, L.A. (1996). Formal rules for selecting prior distributions. *Journal of the American Statistical Association,* **91**, 1343–1370.
91. Katsis, A. and Toman, B. (1999). Bayesian sample size calculations for binomial experiments. *Journal of Statistical Planning and Inference*, **81**, 349–362.

92. Kieser, M. and Friede, T. (2007). Planning and analysis of three-arm non-inferiority trials with binary endpoints. *Statistics in Medicine*, **26**, 253–273.
93. Kirkwood, J.M., Ibrahim, J.G., Sondak, V.K., Richards, J., Flaherty, L.E., Ernstoff, M.S., Smith, T.J., Rao, U., Steele, M., and Blum, R.H. (1999). The role of high- and low-dose interferon Alfa-2b in high-risk melanoma: first analysis of intergroup trial E1690/S9111/C9190. *Journal of Clinical Oncology*, **18**, 2444–2458.
94. Kirkwood, J.M., Strawderman, M.H., Ernstoff, M.S., Smith, T.J., Borden, E.C., Blum, R.H. (1996). Interferon alfa-2b adjuvant therapy of high-risk resected cutaneous melanoma: The Eastern Cooperative Oncology Group trial EST 1684. *Journal of Clinical Oncology*, **14**, 7–17.
95. Kubokawa, T. and Robert, C.P. (1994). New perspectives on linear calibration. *Journal of Multivariate Analysis*, **51**, 178–200.
96. Lam, Y. and Lam, C.V. (1997). Bayesian double-sampling plans with normal distributions. *The Statistician*, **46**, 193–207.
97. Laud, P.W. and Ibrahim, J.G. (1995). Predictive model selection. *Journal of the Royal Statistical Society, Series B*, **57**, 247–262.
98. Law, A.M. and Kelton, W.D. (1991). *Simulation Modeling and Analysis*. Second Edition. McGraw-Hill, New York.
99. Liang, F., Liu, C., and Carroll, R.J. (2010). *Advanced Markov Chain Monte Carlo Methods: Learning from Past Samples*. Wiley, New York.
100. Lindley, D.V. (1997). The choice of sample size. *The Statistician*, **46**, 129–138.
101. Lipkovich, I., Smith, E.P. and Ye, K. (2008). Detecting pattern in biological stressor response relationships using model based cluster analysis. *Environmental and Ecological Statistics*, **15**, 71–78.
102. Lipkovich, I., Ye, K. and Smith, E. (2010), An assessment of the performance of Bayesian model averaging in the linear model. In *Frontiers of Statistical Decision Making and Bayesian Analysis*, (eds.) Chen, M.H., Dey, D., Mueller, P., Sun, D., and Ye K., 146-155, Springer.
103. Madigan, D. and Raftery, A.E. (1994). Model selection and accounting for model uncertainty in graphical models using Occams window. *Journal of Amer. Stat. Assoc.*, **89**, 1535–1546.
104. Meng, X.-L. (1994). Posterior predictive p-values. *The Annals of Statistics*, **22**, 1142–1160.
105. Meng, X.-L. and Wong, W.H. (1996). Simulating ratios of normalizing constants via a simple identity: a theoretical exploration. *Statistica Sinica*, **6**, 831–860.
106. Merigan, T.C., Amato, D.A., Balsley, J., Power, M., Price, W.A., Benoit, S., Perez-Michael, A., Brownstein, A., Kramer, A.S., Brettler, D., Aledort, L., Ragni, M.V., Andes, A.W., Gill, J.C., Goldsmith, J., Stabler, S., Sanders, N., Gjerset, G., Lusher, J., and the NHF-ACTG036 Study Group (1991). Placebo-controlled trial to evaluate zidovudine in treatment of human immunodeficiency virus infection in asymptomatic patients with hemophilia. *Blood*, **78**, 900–906.

107. Metropolis, N., Rosenbluth, A.W., Rosenbluth, M.N., Teller, A.H., and Teller, E. (1953). Equations of state calculations by fast computing machines. *Journal of Chemical Physics*, **21**, 1087–1092.
108. Mitchell, T.J. and Beauchamp, J.J. (1988). Bayesian variable selection in linear regression (with discussion). *Journal of the American Statistical Association*, **83**, 1023–1036.
109. M'Lan, C.E., Joseph, L., and Wolfson, D.B. (2008). Bayesian sample size determination for bionomial proportions. *Bayesian Analysis*, **3**, 269–296.
110. M'Lan, C.E., Joseph, L., and Wolfson, D.B. (2006). Bayesian sample size determination for case-control studies. *Journal of the American Statistical Association*, **101**, 760–772.
111. Neuenschwander, B., Branson, M. and Spiegelhalter, D.J. (2009). A note on the power prior. *Statistics in Medicine* **28**, 3562–3566.
112. O'Hara Hines, R.J. (1989). Some methods for the analysis of toxicological mortality data grouped over time. *Unpublished PhD Thesis*, Department of Statistics and Actuarial Science, University of Waterloo, Canada.
113. O'Hara Hines, R.J. and Lawless, J.F. (1993), Modelling overdispersion in toxicological mortality data grouped over time. *Biometrics*, **49**, 107–122.
114. Osbourne, C. (1991). Statistical calibration: a review. *Journal of Statistical Review*, **59**, 309–336.
115. Penrose, K., Nelson, A., and Fisher, A. (1985). Generalized body composition prediction equation for men using simple measurement techniques" (abstract). *Medicine and Science in Sports and Exercise*, **17**, 189.
116. Pham-Gia, T. (1997). On Bayesian analysis, Bayesian decision theory and the sample size problem. *The Statistician*, **46**, 139–144.
117. Philippe, A. and Robert, C.P. (1998). A note on the confidence properties of reference priors for the calibration model. *Test*, **7**, 147–160.
118. Raftery, A.E. (1995). Bayesian model selection in social research (with discussion). In *Sociological Methodology*, Marsden, P.V., editor, 111–195. Blackwells Publishers, Cambridge, Mass.
119. Raftery, A.E. (1996). Approximate Bayes factors and accounting for model uncertainty in generalized linear models. *Biometrika*, **83**, 251–266.
120. Raftery, A.E., Madigan, D.M., and Hoeting, J. (1997). Model selection and accounting for model uncertainty in linear regression models. *Journal of the American Statistical Association*, **92**, 179–191.
121. Rahme, E., and Joseph, L. (1998). Exact sample size determination for binomial experiments. *Journal of Statistical Planning and Inference*, **66**, 83–93.
122. Ripley, B.D. (1987). *Stochastic Simulation.* Wiley, New York.
123. Robert, C.P. and Casella, G. (2004). *Monte Carlo Statistical Methods.* Second Edition. Springer-Verlag, New York.
124. Roberts, G.O., Gelman, A., and Gilks, W.R. (1997). Weak convergence and optimal scaling of random walk Metropolis algorithms. *Annals of Applied Probability*, **7**, 110–120.
125. Roberts, G.O. and Polson, N.G. (1994). On the geometric convergence of the Gibbs sampler. *Journal of the Royal Statistical Society, Series B*, **56**, 377–384.

126. Rothmann, M., Li, N., Chen, G., Chi, G.Y.H., Temple, R., and Tsou, H.-H. (2003). Design and analysis of non-inferiority mortality trials in oncology. *Statistics in Medicine*, **22**, 239–264.
127. Rubin, D.B., and Stern, H.S. (1998). Sample size determination using posterior predictive distributions. *Sankhyā, Series B* **60**, 161–175.
128. Schervish, M.J. and Carlin, B.P. (1992). On the convergence of successive substitution sampling. *Journal of Computational and Graphical Statistics*, **1**.
129. Schmeiser, B.W., Avramidis, A.N., and Hashem, S. (1990). Overlapping batch statistics. In *Proceedings of the 1990 Winter Simulation Conference*, 395–398.
130. Schwarz, G. (1978). Estimating the dimension of a model. *The Annals of Statistics*, **6**, 461–464.
131. Simon, R. (1999). Bayesian design and analysis of active control clinical trials. *Biometrics*, **55**, 484–487.
132. Sinha, D., and Dey, D.K. (1997). Semiparametric Bayesian analysis of survival data. *Journal of the American Statistical Association*, **92**, 1195–1212.
133. Song, W.-M.T. and Schmeiser, B.W. (1995). Optimal mean-squared-error batch sizes. *Management Science*, **41**, 110–123.
134. Spiegelhalter, D.J., Abrams, K.R., and Myles, J.P. (2004). *Bayesian Approaches to Clinical Trials and Health-Care Evaluation.* Wiley, New York.
135. Stein, C. (1985). On the coverage probability of confidence sets based on a prior distribution. In *Sequential Methods in Statistics,* (Ed. R. Zielinski), Warsaw: PWN-Polish Scientific Publishers, 485–514.
136. Stone, G.W., Ellis, S.G., Cannon, L., *et al.* (2005). Comparison of a polymer-based paclitaxel-eluting stent with a bare metal stent in patients with complex coronary artery disease: a randomized controlled trial. *Journal of the American Medical Association*, **294**, 1215–1223.
137. Stone, G.W., Ellis, S.G., Cox, D.A., *et al.* (2004). A polymer-based, paclitaxel-eluting stent in patients with coronary artery disease. *The New England Journal of Medicine*, **350**, 221–231.
138. Sun, D. and Ye, K. (1995). Reference prior Bayesian analysis for normal mean products. *Journal of American Statistical Association*, **90**, 589–597.
139. Tanner, M.A. (1996). *Tools for Statistical Inference.* Third Edition. Springer-Verlag, New York.
140. Tanner, M.A. and Wong, W.H. (1987). The calculation of posterior distributions by data augmentation. *Journal of the American Statistical Association*, **82**, 528–549.
141. Tibshirani, R. (1989). Noninformative priors for one parameter of many. *Biometrika,* **76**, 604–608.
142. Tierney, L. (1994). Markov chains for exploring posterior distributions (with discussions). *The Annals of Statistics*, **22**, 1701–1762.
143. Verdinelli, I. and Wasserman, L. (1995). Computing Bayes factors using a generalization of the Savage-Dickey density ratio. *Journal of the American Statistical Association*, **90**, 614–618.
144. Volberding, P.A., Lagakos, S.W., Koch, M.A., Pettinelli, C., Myers, M.W., Booth, D.K., Balfour, H.H., Reichman, R.C., Bartlett, J.A., Hirsch, M.S., Murphy, R.L., Hardy, D., Soeiro, R., Fischl, M.A., Bartlett, J.G., Merigan,

T.C., Hylsop, N.E., Richman, D.D., Valentine, F.T., Corey, L., and the AIDS Clinical Trials Group of the National Institute of Allergy and Infectious Diseases (1990). Zidovudine in asymptomatic human immunodeficiency virus infection. *New England Journal of Medicine*, **322**, 941–949.
145. Wang, F., and Gelfand, A.E. (2002). A simulation-based approach to Bayesian sample size determination for performance under a given model and for separating models. *Statistical Science*, **17**, 193–208.
146. Wang, S.-J. and Hung, H.M.J. (2003a). Assessing treatment efficacy in non-inferiority trials. *Controlled Clinical Trials*, **24**, 147–155.
147. Wang, S.-J. and Hung, H.M.J. (2003b). TACT method for non-inferiority testing in active controlled trials. *Statistics in Medicine*, **22**, 227–238.
148. Weiss, R. (1997). Bayesian sample size calculations for hypothesis testing. *The Statistician*, **46**, 185–191.
149. Welch, B.L. and Peers, H.W. (1963). On formulae for confidence points based on integrals of weighted likelihoods. *Journal of the Royal Statistical Society*, **25**, 318–329.
150. Wolpert, R.L. (1991). Monte Carlo importance sampling in Bayesian statistics. In *Statistical Multiple Integration* (Eds. N. Flournoy and R. Tsutakawa). *Contemporary Mathematics*, **116**, 101–115.
151. Yakovlev, A.Y., Asselain, B., Bardou V.J., Fourquet, A., Hoang, T. Rochefediere, A., and Tsodikov, A.D. (1993). A simple stochastic model of tumor recurrence and its applications to data on premenopausal breast cancer. In *Biometrie et Analyse de Donnees Spatio-Temporelles*, # 12, (eds.) B. Asselain, M. Boniface, C. Duby, C. Lopez, J. P. Masson, and J. Tranchefort , Rennes: France, 66–82.
152. Yakovlev, A.Y. and Tsodikov, A.D. (1996). *Stochastic Models of Tumor Latency and Their Biostatistical Applications*. World Scientific, New Jersey.
153. Ye, K. (1993). Reference priors when the stopping rule depends on the parameter of interest. *Journal of American Statistical Association*, **88**, 360–363.
154. Ye, K. (1994). Bayesian reference prior analysis on the ratio of variances for the balanced one-way random effect model. *Journal of Statistical Planning and Inference*, **41**, 267–280.
155. Ye, K. and Berger, J.O. (1989). Noninformative priors for inferences in exponential regression models. *Biometrika*, **78**, 645–656.

About the Authors

Ming-Hui Chen, Ph.D. is currently a full professor at Department of Statistics, University of Connecticut, USA. He obtained B.S. in Mathematics from Hangzhou University, M.S. in Applied Probability from Shanghai Jiao Tong University, and M.S. in Applied Statistics and Ph.D. in Statistics from Purdue University. He has coauthored the books, "Applied Statistics for Engineers" (Prentice-Hall, INC., 1999), "Monte Carlo Methods in Bayesian Computation" (Springer-Verlag, 2000), and "Bayesian Survival Analysis" (Springer-Verlag, 2001). He is also a co-editor of the book "Frontiers of Statistical Decision Making and Bayesian Analysis — In Honor of James O. Berger" (Springer-Verlag, 2010). His current research interests include Bayesian statistical methodology, Bayesian computation, Bayesian phylogenetics, categorical data Analysis, design of Bayesian clinical trials, DNA microarray data analysis, meta-analysis, missing data analysis (EM, MCEM, and Bayesian), Monte Carlo methodology, prior elicitation, statistical methodology and analysis for prostate cancer data, statistical modeling, and survival data analysis.

Keying Ye, Ph.D., currently a full professor at Department of Management Science and Statistics at the University of Texas at San Antonio, USA. Dr. Ye received his BS in Mathematics, Fudan University, MS in Mathematics, Institute of Applied Mathematics, Academia Sinica, in the People's Republic of China, and Ph.D. in Statistics from Purdue University, USA. He is a co-editor of the book "Frontiers of Statistical Decision Making and Bayesian Analysis — In Honor of James O. Berger" (Springer-Verlag, 2010). His research interests are in Bayesian methodology developments and statistical applications. His recent works involve financial predictive models, clinical trials, computational biology, cyber security, environmental and ecological sciences, experimental design, and meta analysis.

CHAPTER 33

VALID PRIOR-FREE PROBABILISTIC INFERENCE AND ITS APPLICATIONS IN MEDICAL STATISTICS

DUNCAN ERMINI LEAF, HYOKUN YUN, and CHUANHAI LIU*

Department of Statistics, Purdue University,
150 N. University Street, West Lafayette, IN 47907, USA
**chuanhai@purdue.edu*

Valid, prior-free, and situation-specific probabilistic inference is desirable for serious uncertain inference, especially in bio-medical statistics. This chapter introduces such an inferential system, called the Inferential Model (IM) framework, proposed recently. IMs do not require a prior to be specified, yet they produce probabilistic inferential results that have desireable frequency properties. This chapter illustrates the IM framework and demonstrates its potential applications in bio-medical statistics with a collection of benchmark examples, including (i) classification, (ii) inference with subgroup selection, (iii) 2×2 tables, and (v) a many-normal-means problem in meta-analysis. It concludes with a few remarks on further applications of IMs to modern, large-scale, and challenging statistical problems, such as Stein's paradox, the Behrens-Fisher problem, multiple hypothesis testing, and variable selection in linear regression.

1. Introduction

1.1. *Statistical inference: a brief historical review*

For serious statistical applications, such as bio-medical statistics, producing prior-free, frequency-calibrated (or valid), data-dependent (or situation-specific) probabilistic inference has been a longstanding dream of statisticians. Probabilistic inference is attractive as an easy-to-interpret quantitative assessment of uncertainty. It has a long history that can be traced back to Bayes (1763); see also Liang, Liu, and Carroll (2010). Bayes is clearly the most sensible approach when the statistician has a valid prior distribution for unknown quantities. Philosophically, there is nothing wrong and it probably should always be attempted in practice so long as the statistician and his or her clients are willing to accept the consequences of any decision made accordingly. Nevertheless, we shall not discuss philosophical differences here, such as those concerning the different meanings or interpretations of probability. In any case, when a prior is taken for everything, the inference problem is reduced to an exercise of usual probability calculus. Following, *e.g.*, Fraser (2011), for conceptual clarity we simply refer to such models as probability models. This chapter is concerned with statistical inference when there is no known prior for some unknown quantity.

For Bayesian approaches to statistical inference, it is a fair comment that not all Bayesian statisticians really put meaning on prior distributions for everything. Most often in practice, part of the prior is used for simplicity to produce inference that matches or beats the best possible frequentist results. This is supported, for example, by the use of Bayes factors and so-called conjugate and invariance priors, among many others. An agreed way of specifying priors, especially in modern, challenging, and large-scale problems, is yet to emerge.

When priors are unknown, it is perhaps due to the fact that Bayesian inferential results are generally not frequency-calibrated that most statisticians have fallen into what is known as the frequentist school. However, frequentist procedures are often created via what can be thought of as a *guess-and-check* process. A proposed procedure is often checked according to the criteria set forth by Fisher (1922), namely, sufficiency, efficiency, and consistency. Due to the limitations of Bayesian and frequentist schools of thought, around 1930 R. A. Fisher started developing an ideal inferential system, which he called fiducial. He spent the rest of his life, about 30 years, working on this. Although, some of the ideas in fiducial inference were reinterpreted by J. Neyman to create confidence intervals that have been central to frequentist statisticians, Fisher's fiducial has been perceived as his *"one great failure"* (Zabell, 1992).

While acknowledging the limited success of his efforts, R. A. Fisher apparently recognized that there was something valuable in fiducial. He wrote (see Savage (1964) p. 926): *"I don't understand yet what fiducial probability does. We shall have to live with it a long time before we know what it's doing for us. But it should not be ignored just because we don't yet have a clear interpretation."* Efforts continuing along this direction can be found in further developments of Fisher's fiducial inference and its variants: Fraser's structural inference (Fraser, 1966, 1968) and Dempster-Shafer theory (Dempster, 2008; Shafer, 1976); see Hannig (2009) for a recent discussion.

What is fiducial? A brief but good answer was given by Savage (1976), who wrote: "*The expressions 'fiducial probability' and 'fiducial argument' are Fisher's. Nobody knows just what they mean, because Fisher repudiated his most explicit, but definitely faulty, definition and ultimately replaced it with a few examples.*" When referring to the fiducial argument, we shall adopt the interpretation of Dempster (1963), namely, *continuing to believe that the pivotal quantity introduced in fiducial has the same distribution after seeing the observed data.* For example, consider inference about θ from an observation x that is assumed to have come from the normal distribution $N(\theta, 1)$ with unknown mean $\theta \in \mathbb{R} = (-\infty, \infty)$ and unit variance. We refer to this problem the one-normal-mean example. To obtain a fiducial probability, one writes

$$x = \theta + Z \qquad (Z \sim N(0,1)), \tag{1}$$

where the introduced random variable Z is called a pivotal variable. The connection between (1) and the familiar sampling distribution $x \sim N(\theta, 1)$ is made by assuming that $Z \sim N(0, 1)$ holds *a priori*, *i.e.*, before seeing x. After seeing x, *i.e.*, conditional on x, with the fiducial argument one continues to believe that $Z \sim N(0, 1)$. Since (1) implies that $\theta = x - Z$, the distribution on Z defines a distribution on θ when x is fixed at its observed value. That distribution is $\theta \sim N(x, 1)$ conditional on x, which is the same as the Bayesian posterior of θ obtained by putting the flat prior on θ; see Lindley (1958) and Fraser (2011). When used for inference, this posterior distribution has nice frequency properties for certain assertions or hypotheses on the unknown quantity θ. In general, however, it is questionable to manipulate it as a distribution using the usual probability calculus; see Ermini Leaf *et al.* (2009).

While not as popular as Bayesian inference nowadays, fiducial inference can provide better results than Bayesian methods for certain models; see Section 2. This observation is partially consistent with what Efron (1998) wrote: "*. . . but here is a safe prediction for the 21st century: statisticians will be asked to solve bigger and more complicated problems. I believe there is a good chance ... that something like fiducial inference will play an important role in this development. Maybe Fisher's biggest blunder will become a big hit in the 21st century!*" While this "something" remains to be discovered, we and our collaborators recently proposed a new promising inferential framework, called the inferential model (IM) framework, that produces prior-free, frequency-calibrated, and data-dependent probabilities for assessing uncertainty. Although it is both philosophically and technically different from fiducial, the IM framework was motivated by fiducial and its extension, the Dempster-Shafer theory of belief functions. As a matter of fact, the original but fundamental idea of IMs was explored in Martin, Zhang, and Liu (2010), Zhang and Liu (2011) and, Zhang (2010) in the context of Dempster-Shafer theory. In the sequel, we present the IM framework reformulated and extended most recently in Martin and Liu (2011); see also Martin and Liu (2013a,b), and Ermini Leaf and Liu (2012).

1.2. *Outline*

The key starting point for IMs is to consider reasoning with uncertainty toward predictive or probabilistic inference. Section 2.1 reviews the idea that probabilistic inference requires an unobserved but predictable quantity, called an auxiliary (a)-variable, to be introduced as an integral part of a full statistical model. Given a full statistical model that allows for probabilistic inference, Section 2.2 uses the one-normal-mean to summarize and illustrate a simple but general three-step procedure for constructing IMs. Section 3 reviews conditional and marginal IMs that are necessary for efficient inference.

The second part of this chapter, Sections 4–7, presents a sequence of potential applications of IMs in bio-medical statistics, including classification, constrained parameter problems, selective inference, 2×2 tables, and the many-normal-means problem in meta-analysis. We hope readers will agree with us that prior-free, valid, and data-dependent probabilistic inference is within reach rather than impossible, as might have been mistakenly perceived from the failure of Fisher's efforts in fiducial inference; see Zabell (1992). Serious statistical applications and challenging large-scale problems demand exact probabilistic inference such as that provided by IMs (see Martin and Liu (2013b)), or similar inferential methods yet to be developed. We also hope that readers share our vision that this line of thinking has a great future for many, many years to come.

2. Inferential Models

For the sake of simplicity, the one-normal-mean example, *i.e.*, inference about $N(\theta, 1)$ from a single observation x,

$$x \sim N(\theta, 1) \qquad (\theta \in \Theta \equiv \mathbb{R}), \tag{2}$$

serves as a running example in this section. Probabilistic inference about the unknown quantity θ from the observed data x is of interest. Any hypothesis about θ corresponds to a subset of Θ called an assertion. In this section, we consider inference about the truth and falsity of the assertion

$$\mathcal{A}_{\theta_0} = \{\theta_0\} \subseteq \Theta \tag{3}$$

where θ_0 is some specific value of interest, *e.g.*, $\theta_0 = 0$. For clarity, we note that the subset $\mathcal{A}_{\theta_0}$ of Θ is said to be *true* if the true value of the unknown θ belongs to $\mathcal{A}_{\theta_0}$. Otherwise, $\mathcal{A}_{\theta_0}$ is said to be *false* when the true value of θ is contained in $\mathcal{A}^c_{\theta_0}$, the complement or negation of $\mathcal{A}_{\theta_0}$.

2.1. *Association models for probabilistic inference*

The postulated model (2), known as a sampling model for the observed data x, is a familiar way of starting statistical inference. Perhaps, it is relatively less familiar (see, e.g., Dempster, 1964) that the sampling model (2) doesn't allow for desired predictive or probabilistic inference. This is because (i) the sampling model specifies a class of different probability measures indexed by θ, and (ii) the probability measure in the sampling model (2) only allows the evaluation of event probabilities to confirm or compare different explanations of observed data in different probability spaces. Since no *missing but predictable quantity* is present, no probabilistic inference is possible. To emphasize this observation, Martin and Liu (2011) introduced the following principle.

Principle 1. *The sampling model alone is insufficient for probabilistic inference about unknown parameters. Only if unobserved but predictable quantities are associated with the observed data and unknown parameters can predictive probabilistic inference be achieved.*

According to this principle, something that is missing but predictable, called an *auxiliary (a)-variable*, must be introduced as an integral part of modeling for statistical inference. Following this principle, IMs require the specification of an *association model* by introducing a-variables. The probability distribution of the a-variables determines the postulated sampling model for the observed data. For the running example of the one-normal-mean problem, an association model can be specified as in fiducial inference, *i.e.*,

$$x = \theta + z \qquad (z \sim N(0, 1)), \tag{4}$$

where the a-variable z is missing, but *a priori* assumed to follow the standard normal distribution, $N(0,1)$. Given x and the true value of z, the true value of the unknown quantity θ is then given by $\theta = x - z$. In the general setting, x denotes both the observable and the observed data. An association-model determines the mapping from (x, z) to θ, which in general can be set-valued and thus written as

$$\Theta_x(z) \subseteq \Theta. \tag{5}$$

Given an association model, predictive or probabilistic inference about θ amounts to predicting the unobserved realization of the a-variable, z. Motivated by the concepts of Bayesian credible intervals, frequentist confidence intervals that produce inferential results with desirable certainty (i.e., with probabilities close to one or zero), and frequentist rejection regions for hypothesis testing, predicting z can be made simple to create user-friendly inferential outputs. This explains, at least partially, the following use of *predictive random sets* (PRSs). The IM framework, built around this simple idea, is briefly reviewed next.

2.2. *The three-step representation of IMs*

The IM framework can be represented as a three-step procedure for inference about $\mathcal{A} \subseteq \Theta$, an assertion on θ. This three-step procedure consists of an Association (A) step, a Prediction (P) step, and a Combination (C) step as follows.

Inferential Model 1 (The three-step procedure for IMs). *An IM is built using three steps:*

A-STEP. *Associate the observable x and unknown θ with an a-variable z to obtain a set-valued mapping $\Theta_x(z)$ $(\subseteq \Theta)$, which consists of the candidate values of θ given z and x.*

P-STEP. *Predict z by specifying a credible (PRS) $\mathcal{S}_\theta$, possibly depending on θ; and*

C-STEP. *Combine $\Theta_x(z)$ and $\mathcal{S}_\theta$ to obtain the PRS $\Theta_x(\mathcal{S}_\theta) = \cup_{z \in \mathcal{S}_\theta} \Theta_x(z)$ for θ, and compute the probabilities*

$$\underline{\mathsf{e}}_x(\mathcal{A}) \equiv Pr(\Theta_x(\mathcal{S}_\theta) \subseteq \mathcal{A})$$

and

$$\overline{\mathsf{e}}_x(\mathcal{A}) \equiv 1 - Pr(\Theta_x(\mathcal{S}_\theta) \subseteq \mathcal{A}^c) = Pr(\Theta_x(\mathcal{S}_\theta) \cap \mathcal{A} \neq \emptyset)$$

as the lower evidence and upper evidence for $\mathcal{A}$.

Random variables represent uncertainty in the postulated sampling model. The A-step emphasizes the modeling of data using a-variables for probabilistic inference. For the one-normal-mean example, this step is formally written as

A-STEP. This is given by (4), which gives the singleton set-valued mapping

$$\Theta_x(z) = \{\theta : \ \theta = x - z\}. \tag{6}$$

A PRS is a random set $\mathcal{S}_\theta$ that takes values in the power set of the space of the a-variables. A realization of the PRS $\mathcal{S}_\theta$ can be interpreted as a set that is believed to include the unobserved value of the a-variable. The strength of this belief is defined by the probability distribution for $\mathcal{S}_\theta$. As mentioned previously, this set of possibilities can depend on the true value of θ. The use of a so-called credible PRS is intended to be user-friendly in the sense that the resulting probabilistic outputs can be interpreted and used for uncertain inference in a practical and straightforward manner; see Liu and Martin (2014) for more discussion on interpreting the evidence functions as belief probability in the context of scientific inference. Roughly speaking, a PRS in the P-step is said to be credible if it produces probabilities that have numerical values consistent with those of frequency or additive probabilities. Formally, the credibility of PRSs is defined as follows.

Definition 1 (Credibility). *Let Π_z be the probability distribution of the a-variable z. The PRS S for predicting z is said to be credible if it satisfies*

$$Pr(\mathcal{S} \not\ni z) \overset{Stochastically}{\leq} U \sim Unif(0,1) \qquad (z \sim \Pi_z), \tag{7}$$

where $Pr(\mathcal{S} \not\ni z)$ is computed with respect to the distribution of $\mathcal{S}$ for fixed z.

Note that (7) can be equivalently expressed as

$$\Pr\left(\Pr\left(\mathcal{S} \not\ni z\right) \geq 1 - \alpha\right) \leq \alpha,$$

for each $\alpha \in (0,1)$, where $\Pr(\mathcal{S} \not\ni z)$ is a function of the random a-variable, z. This can be interpreted as follows: for any fixed z, we can compute $\Pr(\mathcal{S} \not\ni z)$ as a measure of belief that z is *not* a realization from Π_z. If we use a threshold $1-\alpha$ to make a decision that z is not the unobserved a-variable realization from Π_z in a particular experiment of interest, then we would make wrong decision at most $100\alpha\%$ of the time for z realizations from Π_z over repeated experiements. For example, the PRS

$$\mathcal{S}_\theta = \{z : |z| \leq |Z|\} = [-|Z|, |Z|] \qquad (Z \sim N(0,1)) \tag{8}$$

is credible for predicting an unobserved z taken from $N(0,1)$ due to the fact that

$$\Pr(\mathcal{S}_\theta \not\ni z) = \Pr(|Z| < |z|) = F_{|Z|}(|z|) \sim \text{Unif}(0,1) \qquad (z \sim N(0,1)).$$

where $F_{|Z|}(.)$ stands for the cdf of $|Z|$. Using this PRS, we have the following P-step for the one-normal-mean problem.

P-STEP. Predict z using the PRS in (8).

This credibility requirement for PRSs is essential as it guarantees the validity of inference about θ. This is discussed below along with the explanation of the C-step.

The operations of the C-step should be self-explanatory. Here, we assume that $\Theta_x(\mathcal{S}_\theta) \neq \emptyset$ holds with probability one. For cases where $\Pr(\Theta_x(\mathcal{S}_\theta) = \emptyset) > 0$, Ermini Leaf and Liu (2012) replace the credible PRS with what they call a credible Elastic PRS (EPRS); see Section 4. Most important is that the resulting $\underline{\mathsf{e}}_x(\mathcal{A})$ and $\bar{\mathsf{e}}_x(\mathcal{A})$ probabilities are meaningful in the sense that their numerical values are consistent with a frequency interpretation of probabilities. To be more precise, we need the formal definition of what is called validity.

Definition 2 (Validity). *Suppose that $x \sim f(x|\theta)$ and $\mathcal{A} \subseteq \Theta$. An inferential framework is said to be valid for inference about $\mathcal{A} \subseteq \Theta$ if and only if it produces probabilities $\underline{\mathsf{e}}_x(\mathcal{A})$ and $\bar{\mathsf{e}}_x(\mathcal{A})$ for $\mathcal{A}$, as functions of the random variable x, that satisfy*

$$\underline{\mathsf{e}}_x(\mathcal{A}) \overset{stochastically}{\leq} U \sim \mathit{Unif}(0,1)$$

for $\theta \in \mathcal{A}^c$ and

$$\bar{\mathsf{e}}_x(\mathcal{A}) \overset{stochastically}{\geq} V \sim \mathit{Unif}(0,1)$$

for $\theta \in \mathcal{A}$. An inferential framework is said to be valid if and only if it is valid for all assertions $\mathcal{A} \subseteq \Theta$.

The validity theorem (see, *e.g.*, Martin and Liu, 2011) says that *an IM is valid as long as the PRS of the P-step is credible.* The implication can be explained by making analogy with frequentist procedures as follows. The values of $\underline{\mathsf{e}}_x(\mathcal{A})$ and $\bar{\mathsf{e}}_x(\mathcal{A})$ can be interpreted in practice as: *a very large value of the lower evidence $\underline{\mathsf{e}}_x(\mathcal{A})$ practically "confirms" the truth of $\mathcal{A}$, and a very small value of the upper evidence $\bar{\mathsf{e}}_x(\mathcal{A})$ practically "confirms" the falsity of $\mathcal{A}$.* The use of the word "confirm" is in the sense of the Cournot principle (see, e.g., Shafer, 2011): *an event of very small probability will not happen.* This interpretation will not lead to a contradiction because $\underline{\mathsf{e}}_x(\mathcal{A}) \leq \bar{\mathsf{e}}_x(\mathcal{A})$ always holds. For example, given $\alpha = 0.01$ as threshhold for small probabilities, corresponding to the common type-I level of Neyman's test, we have three cases to consider:

(1) The case $\underline{e}_x(A) > 1 - .01 = 0.99$: confirms the truth of $\mathcal{A}$;
(2) The case $\bar{e}_x(A) < 0.01$: confirms the falsity of $\mathcal{A}$ (or the truth of $\mathcal{A}^c$); and
(3) The other case: neither the truth of $\mathcal{A}$ nor the truth of $\mathcal{A}^c$ can be confirmed. In this case, there is not enough evidence to make a decision for the given threshold, or we fail to take a decisive action.

To complete the IM for the one-normal-mean example, we give the following C-step.

C-step. Combine $\Theta_x(z)$ and $\mathcal{S}_\theta$ to obtain $\Theta_x(\mathcal{S}) = [x-|Z|, x+|Z|]$, and compute probabilities

$$\underline{\mathsf{e}}_x(\mathcal{A}_{\theta_0}) = 0 \text{ and } \bar{\mathsf{e}}_x(\mathcal{A}_{\theta_0}) = 2[1 - \Phi(|x - \theta_0|)].$$

for the assertion A_{θ_0}, where $\Phi(.)$ stands for the cdf of the standard normal distribution, $N(0,1)$.

The evidence $\underline{\mathsf{e}}_x(\mathcal{A}_{\theta_0})$ and $\bar{\mathsf{e}}_x(\mathcal{A}_{\theta_0})$ in the C-step can be derived as follows:

$$\begin{aligned}
\underline{\mathsf{e}}_x(\mathcal{A}_{\theta_0}) &= \Pr(\Theta_x(\mathcal{S}) \subseteq \mathcal{A}_{\theta_0}) \\
&= \Pr(\{\theta : |x - z| \leq |Z|\} \subseteq \{\theta_0\}) \\
&= \Pr(\{\theta : |x - z| > |Z|\} \supseteq \{\theta_0\}^c) \\
&= \Pr(|Z| < |x - \theta| \text{ for all } \theta \neq \theta_0) \\
&= \Pr\left(|Z| < \min_{\theta \neq \theta_0} |x - \theta|\right) \\
&= 0
\end{aligned}$$

and

$$\begin{aligned}
\bar{\mathsf{e}}_x(\mathcal{A}_{\theta_0}) &= 1 - \Pr(\Theta_x(\mathcal{S}) \subseteq \mathcal{A}_{\theta_0}^c) \\
&= 1 - \Pr(\{\theta : |x - z| \leq |Z|\} \subseteq \{\theta_0\}^c) \\
&= 1 - \Pr(\{\theta : |x - z| > |Z|\} \supseteq \{\theta_0\}) \\
&= 1 - \Pr(|Z| < |x - \theta_0|) \\
&= 2[1 - \Phi(|x - \theta_0|)].
\end{aligned}$$

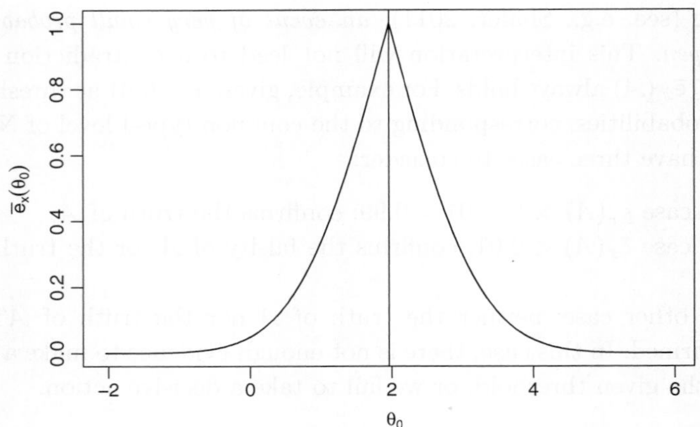

Fig. 1. The most evidence for $\mathcal{A}_{\theta_0} = \{\theta : \theta = \theta_0\}$ given the observed $x = 1.96$, indicated by the vertical line, in the one-normal-mean example in Section 2.

The logic in these algebraic operations is typical in computing evidence functions. In the sequel, we shall omit detailed calculations of evidence functions to save space.

For a simple numerical example, take $x = 1.96$ and $\mathcal{A}_0 = \{\theta = 0\}$. We have $\underline{\mathrm{e}}_x(\mathcal{A}_0) = 0$ and $\bar{\mathrm{e}}_x(\mathcal{A}_0) = 2[1 - \Phi(1.96)] = 0.05$. Unlike Fisher's p-value, our probability $\bar{\mathrm{e}}_x(\mathcal{A}_0)$ is predictive and therefore provides truly probabilistic inference. This probability has a meaningful probability interpretation for *situation-specific* inference, *i.e.*, it does not need repeated experiments, as in the frequentist school of thought, to help validate its meaningfulness. The results for a sequence of values of θ_0 are displayed in Figure 1. The region with small values of $\bar{\mathrm{e}}_x(\mathcal{A}_0)$ contains the least likely values of the unknown quantity θ. In other words, the evidence *against* $\mathcal{A}_{\theta_0}$ increases as θ_0 deviates away from the observed x. When θ_0 is close to the observed data point x, our uncertainty about the truth or falsity of $\mathcal{A}_{\theta_0}$ is large.

The preceding discussion shows how IMs can be used for hypothesis testing after translating a hypothesis into an assertion, $\mathcal{A}$. The upper evidence, $\bar{\mathrm{e}}_x(\mathcal{A})$ can be used in a similar manner to a p-value, although the interpretation is different. When $\bar{\mathrm{e}}_x(\mathcal{A})$ is small, the assertion $\mathcal{A}$ can be rejected. However, large $\bar{\mathrm{e}}_x(\mathcal{A})$ values do not mean that the assertion should be accepted. Only large values of $\underline{\mathrm{e}}_x(\mathcal{A})$ serve to confirm that $\mathcal{A}$ is true. As shown in the preceding example, $\underline{\mathrm{e}}_x(\mathcal{A})$ may be zero for any point assertions of the form $\mathcal{A}_{\theta_0}$. In these cases, the hypothesis that $\theta = \theta_0$ can never be confirmed. However, $\bar{\mathsf{e}}_x(\mathcal{A}_{\theta_0})$ can used for estimation. Simply choose the value of θ_0 that maximizes $\bar{\mathsf{e}}_x(\mathcal{A}_{\theta_0})$. This is the most plausible value of θ given the observed x. In the preceding example, the most plausible value of θ_0 is x (1.96). For an interval estimate, we can find

$$\Gamma_x(\alpha) = \{\theta_0 : \bar{\mathsf{e}}_x(\mathcal{A}_{\theta_0}) > \alpha\}.$$

This is known as a *plausibility interval.* Like a confidence interval, $\Gamma_x(\alpha)$ has $1-\alpha$ probability of covering a fixed θ value over repeated experiments.

2.3. *PRSs and efficiency considerations*

Efficiency of IMs is an important issue that is determined by the PRS specified in the P-step. First, it is easy to see that the PRS for predicting a-variables can be made stochastically as small as possible, provided that it is credible (and that the space of the a-variable is metric). For continuous a-variables, it is possible to construct a PRS such that the credibility condition (7) is replaced with

$$\Pr(\mathcal{S} \not\ni z) \sim \text{Unif}(0,1) \qquad (z \sim \Pi_z). \tag{9}$$

Such a PRS is called an *efficient* PRS. For example, for continuous a-variables, let $b(z)$ be an arbitrary continuous function defined on the a-space, the space of the a-variable. It is easy to show that the random set defined by the boundary function $b(z)$,

$$\mathcal{S} = \{z : b(z) \geq b(Z)\} \qquad (Z \sim \Pi_z), \tag{10}$$

is credible and efficient.

It should be noted that an efficient PRS doesn't necessarily mean that the resulting inference for any assertion $\mathcal{A}$ is efficient in the sense of maximizing the distribution of $\underline{\mathsf{e}}_{x,\mathcal{S}}(\mathcal{A})$ and minimizing the distribution of $\bar{\mathsf{e}}_{x,\mathcal{S}}(\mathcal{A})$ over all efficient and credible PRSs for predicting z. In some sense, the concept of efficient PRSs is meant to emphasize that PRSs do not need to be stochastically larger than necessary for credibility. Among a few topics that can be investigated based on this observation is the construction of assertion-specific PRSs. The shapes of PRSs can be specified according to assertions of interest. This is particularly useful for multiple-parameter inference problems. For single-parameter problems efficiency is less an issue because the inferential results for precise single-parameter assertions, such as those in the one-normal-mean example, based on different credible and efficient PRSs are not very different. Two important classes of methods for making efficient IM inference are discussed next.

3. Conditional and Marginal IMs

Although valid, IMs constructed by predicting a high-dimensional a-variable can be inefficient. Here we review two types of dimensionality reduction for efficient inference. One is to predict only a minimum number of a-variables, typically of the same dimension as the unknown quantity θ. The other is to predict an assertion-specific low dimensional quantity. These two types of dimension reduction of a-variables are considered in Sections 3.1 and 3.2. Inference about the Gaussian model $N(\mu, \sigma^2)$ with unknown μ and known or unknown variance σ^2 from an observed sample $x_1, \ldots, x_n$, a standard textbook example, is used in this section for both motivation and illustration.

3.1. *Combining information via dimension reduction: conditional IMs*

Suppose that the observed data $x_1, \ldots, x_n$ are considered as a sample from the Gaussian model $N(\mu, \sigma^2)$ with unknown mean $\mu \in \mathbb{R}$ and known variance σ^2. Without loss of generality, take $\sigma = 1$. It is natural to extend the discussion of the $n = 1$ case, the one-normal-mean example, to the present $n > 1$ case by writing the baseline association model

$$x_i = \mu + Z_i \qquad (Z_i \overset{iid}{\sim} N(0,1)), \tag{11}$$

where the a-variable is the random vector $Z = (Z_1, \ldots, Z_n)'$. One can predict the n-dimensional a-variable Z for making probabilistic inference about the unknown quantity μ. It is immediately clear that predicting one component of Z, say Z_1, would be sufficient for such a purpose. However, with a closer look at the association model (11) we would find that some functions, for example,

$$Z_i - Z_1 = x_i - x_1 \qquad (i = 2, \ldots, n) \tag{12}$$

are fully observed. These observed a-variables can help predict Z_1 more accurately. This motivates the idea of (i) associating x_1 and μ with an unobserved but predictable quantity Z_1

$$x_1 = \mu + Z_1; \tag{13}$$

(ii) predicting Z_1 using a credible PRS based on its conditional distribution given (12); and (iii) combining the PRS constructed in (ii) and the association model (13) to evaluate evidence functions for assertions about μ.

Care must be taken to check that when conditioning on (12) there are a-variables available to be predicted for inference about μ, *i.e.*, the fundamental principle of Section 2 is not violated. This is not a problem in this motivating example. For general cases, to preserve the fundamental principle of Section 2, assume that the baseline association model $x = a(U, \theta)$ can be represented by a conditional association model

$$h_1(x) = a_1(V_1, \theta) \tag{14}$$

and a conditioning equation

$$h_2(x) = a_2(V_2), \tag{15}$$

where $V_1 = \psi_1(U)$ and $V_2 = \psi_2(U)$ form a one-to-one mapping between $V = (V_1, V_2)'$ and U from the the space of a-variable U to that of the new a-variable V. When such a representation exists, a regular conditional IM can be constructed, as suggested by the motivating example above, in the same way as constructing the IM in Section 2. That is

Inferential Model 2 (Conditional IM). *The regular conditional IM (CIM) based on (14) and (15) has the following three steps.*

A-STEP. *Associate $h_1(x)$ and θ through the a-variable V_1, which gives the candidates of θ, $\Theta_{h_1(x)}(V_1) = \{\theta : h_1(x) = a_1(V_1, \theta)\}$, when $h_1(x)$ and V_1 become available, either observed or predicted.*

P-STEP. *Predict V_1 using a credible PRS $\mathcal{S}_\theta$ based on its conditional distribution given (15).*

C-STEP. *Combine $\mathcal{S}_\theta$ and $\Theta_{h_1(x)}(V_1)$ to obtain*

$$\Theta_{h_1(x)}(\mathcal{S}_\theta) = \{\theta : \theta \in \Theta_{h_1(x)}(v_1) \text{ for some } v_1 \in \mathcal{S}_\theta\}.$$

Then, evaluate evidence functions in exactly the same way as in IM 1.

Under mild conditions, mainly that (14) is a valid association model that is consistent with the fundamental principle, the CIM is valid; see Martin and Liu (2013a). Here we illustrate the CIM by completing the above motivating example. The A-step gives the candidate set $\{\mu : \mu = x_1 - Z_1\}$. The conditional distribution of Z_1 given $(Z_2 - Z_1, \ldots, Z_n - Z_1)$ is

$$N\left(-\frac{1}{n}\sum_{i=2}^{n}(x_i - x_1), \frac{1}{n}\right). \tag{16}$$

In the P-step, we define a PRS for predicting Z_1 by predicting the residuals from (16). The resulting PRS for Z_1 is given by

$$\mathcal{S} = \left\{ z_1 : z_1 = -\frac{1}{n}\sum_{i=2}^{n}(x_i - x_1) + z/\sqrt{n} \text{ for some } z \in (-|V|, |V|) \right\}$$
$$(V \sim N(0,1)).$$

The P-step generates the PRS for μ

$$\{\mu : |\bar{x} - \mu| \le |V|/\sqrt{n}\} \qquad (V \sim N(0,1)),$$

where $\bar{x}$ denotes the sample mean, i.e., $\bar{x} = n^{-1}\sum_{i=1}^{n} x_i$. In other words, the CIM is equivalent to the IM based on the sufficient statistic $\bar{x}$ alone. We note that this CIM can be easily derived by considering the conditional association model

$$\bar{x} = \mu + \frac{1}{\sqrt{n}} V$$

and the conditioning equation

$$x_i - \bar{x} = Z_i - \bar{Z} \qquad (i = 1, \ldots, n).$$

However, it should be verified that this system of conditioning equations requires only a $(n-1)$ dimensional observed characteristics to be given, leaving a one-dimensional observed quantity for preserving the fundamental principle.

Remark 1. *There are cases where regular CIMs may not exist. A many-normal-means problem in meta-analysis in Section 7 provides such an example. In such cases, the generalized CIM of Martin and Liu (2013a) can be used and illustrated in 7.*

Remark 2. *It should be noted that there is difference between conditional IM and Fisher's conditional inference. The latter is frequentist and, thereby, works with the sampling distribution of sufficient statistics conditional an ancillary statistics. That is, it requires other experiments for interpreting inferential results. IM conditional inference is data-dependent or situation-specific and doesn't need other experiments for interpretation.*

3.2. *Efficient inference via dimensional reduction: marginal IMs*

Suppose that the observed data $x_1, \ldots, x_n$ are considered as a sample from the Gaussian model $N(\mu, \sigma^2)$ with unknown $\mu \in \mathbb{R}$ and unknown $\sigma \in \mathbb{R}_+ =$

$(0, \infty)$. The natural baseline association model is

$$x_i = \mu + \sigma Z_i \qquad (Z_i \overset{iid}{\sim} N(0,1); i = 1, \ldots, n).$$

Let s_x^2 be the sample variance of $x_1, \ldots, x_n$ and let s_Z^2 be the sample variance of the unobserved sample $Z_1, \ldots, Z_n$ from a known population. Then it is straightforward to show that the CIM obtained by using the conditional association model

$$\bar{x} = \mu + \sigma \bar{Z} \quad \text{and} \quad s_x^2 = \sigma^2 s_Z^2 \tag{17}$$

and the conditioning equation

$$(Z - \mathbf{1}\bar{Z})/s_Z = (x - \mathbf{1}\bar{x})/s_x,$$

i.e., the observed direction of the centered Z, is given by the IM with (17) as the baseline association-model. That is, we can make inference about $\theta = (\mu, \sigma^2)$ based on the IM with the association model (17). The two a-variables $\bar{Z}$ and s_Z^2 are independent with

$$\bar{Z} \sim N(0, n^{-1}) \quad \text{and} \quad (n-1)s_Z^2 \sim \chi_{n-1}^2.$$

Now suppose that we are interested in inference about σ alone. In this case, we see that inference can be made by predicting s_Z^2 alone. In other words, we can consider a PRS predicting $(\bar{Z}, s_Z^2)$ but focus more on the accuracy of predicting s_Z^2. This suggests that we construct a credible PRS in such a way that when projected down to space of s_Z^2, it is minimized. Such a PRS is given by a product of a credible PRS for predicting s_Z^2 and a largest possible PRS, i.e., $\mathbb{R}$, for predicting $\bar{Z}$. For example, using a centered (marginal) PRS

$$\{s_Z^2 : |F(s_Z^2) - .5| \leq F(M^2) - .5|\} \qquad ((n-1)M^2 \sim \chi_{n-1}^2)$$

for s_Z^2 yields the PRS

$$\mathcal{S} = \mathbb{R} \times \{s_Z^2 : |F(s_Z^2) - .5| \leq F(M^2) - .5|\}$$

for predicting $(\bar{Z}, s_Z^2)$. This approach effectively "integrates" out $\bar{Z}$ or the so-called nuisance parameter μ and results in a marginal IM for inference about σ^2.

Before we discuss inference about μ alone with σ^2 viewed as a "nuisance" parameter, we consider the general case of inferring $\phi = \phi(\theta)$ alone. In what follows, we use a class of nuisance parameters. To be specific, let $(\phi, \xi) = (\phi(\theta), \xi(\theta))$ be a one-to-one mapping from the space Θ to the space of (ϕ, ξ). The approach in the above example of inferring σ^2 is generalized in Martin and Liu (2013b) as follows. Suppose that the baseline association model can be written as a (regular) system of two equations: a marginal association model

$$h(x, \phi) = m(\psi(U), \phi) \tag{18}$$

and a nuisance association model

$$c(U, x, \xi) = 0, \tag{19}$$

where U is the a-variable. Under the assumption that for any x and U, there exists ξ such that $c(U, x, \xi) = 0$ holds, then the baseline association model is equivalent to the marginal association model (18) for inference about ϕ. Thus, under mild conditions a valid IM for inference about ϕ, called a marginal IM (MIM), is obtained.

Inferential Model 3 (Marginal IM). *The marginal IM for inference about ϕ has the following three steps.*

A-STEP. *Obtain the candidate set of ϕ from (18),*

$$\Phi_x(\psi(U)) = \{\phi : h(x, \phi) = m(\psi(U), \phi)\}.$$

P-STEP. *Construct a credible PRS $\mathcal{S}_\phi$ to predict $\psi(U)$.*

C-STEP. *Compute for any assertion of interest $\mathcal{A}$ on ϕ the evidence functions*

$$\underline{\mathsf{e}}_x(\mathcal{A}) = Pr(\Phi_x(\mathcal{S}) \subseteq \mathcal{A})$$

and

$$\bar{\mathsf{e}}_x(\mathcal{A}) = 1 - Pr(\Phi_x(\mathcal{S}) \subseteq \mathcal{A}^c),$$

where $\Phi_x(\mathcal{S}) = \{\phi : h(x, \phi) = a_1(\psi(U), \phi), \psi(U) \in \mathcal{S}_\phi\}$.

It is easy to see that the above example of inferring σ^2 is an instance of MIM. For another illustrative example, consider marginal inference about μ. Write the baseline association model (17) as a regular system of a marginal association model

$$\frac{\sqrt{n}(\bar{x} - \mu)}{s_x} = \frac{\sqrt{n}\bar{Z}}{s_Z} \tag{20}$$

and a nuisance association model

$$s_x^2 - \sigma^2 s_Z^2 = 0.$$

Thus, the MIM for μ has the A-step obtained from (20), the P-step predicting

$$T = \frac{\sqrt{n}\bar{Z}}{s_Z} \sim t(0, 1, n-1),$$

and the standard C-step, where $t(0, 1, n-1)$ stands for the standard Student-t distribution with $n-1$ degrees of freedom. The marginal association model

$$\frac{\sqrt{n}(\bar{x}-\mu)}{s_x} = T$$

with the a-variable following $t(0, 1, n-1)$ gives IM results that are similar to familiar frequentist results, except that IM results have the desired interpretation for situation-specific uncertainty assessment.

Remark 3. *There are cases where regular MIMs may not exist. The Behrens-Fisher problem, a popular statistical problem in bio-medical statistics and elsewhere for inference about the difference of two normal population means with unknown variances, provides such an example. While more research is expected to be done on this interesting topic, Martin and Liu (2013b) proposed a parameter-expansion approach that leads to what they call weak marginal inferential models (WMIMs). With parameter-expansion, they gave an satisfactory IM solution to the Behrens-Fisher problem, a famous benchmark example in statistical inference.*

Remark 4. *To help understand Remark 2, it is interesting to note that from a frequentist point of view, marginal IM inference can also be considered as Fisherian conditional inference. For example, IM inference about* μ *gives similar frequentist results obtained by conditioning on* s_x^2 *(and direction of the residual vector). For IM inference, all observed data are considered as fixed and the efforts are made in predicting the unobserved a-variables in the particular experiment where the observed data were collected.*

4. Constrained Inferential Models

Here we discuss an important issue that occurs when the combination of the PRS $\mathcal{S}$ and the candidate set $\Theta_x(z)$ in the C-step of IMs is empty. We call this problem the constrained inferential model problem. It contains constrained-parameter problems as special cases, but appears to be more general from a constrained inferential model perspective.

As is often the case in IM applications, realizations of $\mathcal{S}$ are here assumed to be *monotone* in the sense that any two realizations S_1 and S_2 of $\mathcal{S}$ satisfy either $S_1 \subseteq S_2$ or $S_1 \supseteq S_2$. A simple way of dealing with the constrained inferential model problem is to discard realizations of $\mathcal{S}$ that do not intersect with $\Theta_x = \cup_z \Theta_x(z)$. Ermini Leaf and Liu (2012) show that the resulting IMs are indeed valid. This idea can be understood as that the discarded realizations are effectively replaced with larger realizations. Computationally, this approach can be implemented using an acceptance-rejection sampling scheme that rejects draws of $\mathcal{S}$ that are too small to intersect with Θ_x. Intuitively, replacing small realizations of $\mathcal{S}$ with large ones maintains the validity, but results in loss of efficiency. To overcome this problem, Ermini Leaf and Liu (2012) proposed what they call the elastic PRS. The basic idea is to replace an overly small realization with one that is large enough rather than throwing it away.

Loosely speaking, the elastic version of a regular PRS $\mathcal{S}$ is a collection of random sets each containing $\mathcal{S}$ as a subset. More precisely, let $\mathbb{S}$ be the sample space of a regular $\mathcal{S}$. Then the elastic PRS can be defined by

$$\mathsf{w}(\mathcal{S}) = \{W : \mathcal{S} \subseteq W \in \mathbb{S}\} \qquad (\mathcal{S} \in \mathbb{S}). \tag{21}$$

The constrained IM is obtained by replacing the intersection $\Theta_x(\mathcal{S})$ of the C-step of an IM with

$$\Theta_x(\mathcal{S}) = \cup_{z \in \mathcal{S}^*} \Theta_x(z), \tag{22}$$

where $\mathcal{S}^*$ is the "smallest" element in $\mathsf{w}(\mathcal{S})$ that intersects with $\Theta_x = \cup_z \Theta_x(z)$, i.e.,

$$\mathcal{S}^* = \cap_{W \in \mathcal{W}^*} W \qquad \text{with } \mathcal{W}^* = \{W : W \in \mathsf{w}(\mathcal{S}), W \cap \Theta_x \neq \emptyset\}.$$

The use of constrained IMs is illustrated below by its application in classification. More applications can be found in Ermini Leaf and Liu (2012); see also Ermini Leaf (2011) and Section 7.

4.1. *A classification problem*

Here we consider the simple problem of classifying an observation to one of two univariate Gaussian subpopulations. For conceptual clarity, we discuss the case with known populations in Section 4.1.1. The more practical version, with unknown populations, is considered in Section 4.1.2.

4.1.1. *Classification with known populations*

Suppose that an observation $z \in \mathbb{R}$ is known to have come from either $N(\mu_1, \sigma_1^2)$ or $N(\mu_2, \sigma_2^2)$. It is assumed that there is no prior knowledge about which of the two subpopulations this observation z belongs to, but μ_1, σ_1, μ_2, and σ_2 are all known. Thus we consider the association model

$$z = \mu_i + \sigma_i U \qquad (U \sim N(0,1); i = 1, 2), \tag{23}$$

where U is the a-variable and i is the unknown quantity. This association model gives the A-step with

$$\Theta_z(u) = \{i : z = \mu_i + \sigma_i U\}.$$

We use the centered PRS

$$\mathcal{S} = \{u : |u| \leq |U|\} \qquad (U \sim N(0,1))$$

to predict $u^\star$, the unobserved realization of U associated with the observed data z. It is easy to see that the PRS $\mathcal{S}$ and the candidate set Θ_z may have an empty intersection. Equipping the PRS with elasticity, we have the constrained IM that, computationally, acts like a regular IM with the (conditionally enlarged) PRS

$$\mathcal{S} = \left\{u : |u| \leq \max\left(|U|, \min_{i=1,2} \frac{|z - \mu_i|}{\sigma_i}\right)\right\} \qquad (U \sim N(0,1)).$$

The assertions of interest regarding the classification problem are $\mathcal{A}_1 = \{i = 1\}$ and $\mathcal{A}_2 = \{i = 2\}$. Let $k = \arg\min_{i=1,2} |z - \mu_i|/\sigma_i$. Then routine algebraic operations give for $i = 1, 2$

$$\underline{\mathsf{e}}_z(\mathcal{A}_i) = \begin{cases} 1 - 2\Phi\left(-\frac{|z-\mu_k|}{\sigma_k}\right), & \text{if } i = k; \\ 0, & \text{otherwise,} \end{cases}$$

and

$$\bar{\mathsf{e}}_z(\mathcal{A}_i) = \begin{cases} 1, & \text{if } i = k; \\ 2\Phi\left(-\frac{|z-\mu_i|}{\sigma_i}\right), & \text{otherwise.} \end{cases}$$

4.1.2. *Classification with unknown populations*

Consider the classification problem of Section 4.1.1 but with unknown parameters μ_1, σ_1^2, μ_2, and σ_2^2. Instead, it is assumed that two samples, $x_1, \ldots, x_{n_1}$, from $N(\mu_1, \sigma_1^2)$ and $y_1, \ldots, y_{n_2}$ from $N(\mu_2, \sigma_2^2)$, are available. The problem of inference remains the same, i.e., inferring about the unknown quantities regarding which subpopulation an observation z belongs to.

The discussion of Section 4.1.1 motivates us to consider inference about $(z - \mu_i)/\sigma_i$ for classification. The baseline association model is given by

$$z = \mu_i + \sigma_i U \qquad (U \sim N(0,1)),$$

$$x_i = \mu_1 + \sigma_1 V_i^{(x)} \qquad (V_i^{(x)} \overset{iid}{\sim} N(0,1); i = 1, \ldots, n_1),$$

and

$$y_i = \mu_2 + \sigma_2 V_i^{(y)} \qquad (V_i^{(y)} \overset{iid}{\sim} N(0,1); i = 1, \ldots, n_2),$$

where $U, (V_1^{(x)}, \ldots, V_{n_1}^{(x)})$ and $(V_1^{(y)}, \ldots, V_{n_2}^{(y)})$ are independent of each other. Applying the standard conditioning approach yields the reduced association model

$$\bar{x} = \mu_1 + \sigma_1 \bar{V}_x \quad \text{and } s_x = \sigma_1 M_1 \tag{24}$$

and

$$\bar{y} = \mu_2 + \sigma_2 \bar{V}_y \quad \text{and } s_y = \sigma_2 M_2, \tag{25}$$

where $\bar{x}$ and s_x are the sample mean and standard deviation of $x_1, \ldots, x_{n_1}$, $\bar{V}_x$ and M_1 are the "sample" mean and standard deviation of $U_1, \ldots, U_{n_1}$. The quantities $\bar{y}$, s_y, $\bar{V}_y$, and M_2 are introduced similarly but for $y_1, \ldots, y_{n_2}$ and the associated a-variables $V_1^{(y)}, \ldots, V_{n_2}^{(y)}$. The four a-variables $\bar{V}_x$, $\bar{V}_y$, M_1, and M_2 are independent with

$$\bar{V}_x \sim N(0, 1/n_1),\ \bar{V}_y \sim N(0, 1/n_2),\ (n_1 - 1)M_1^2 \sim \chi^2_{n_1-1}, \quad \text{and} \quad (n_2 - 1)M_2^2 \sim \chi^2_{n_2-1}.$$

For inference about $\delta_i \equiv (z - \mu_i)/\sigma_i$ for $i = 1, 2$, write (24) as

$$\frac{z - \bar{x}}{s_x} = \frac{\delta_1 + \bar{V}_x}{M_1} \quad \text{and } s_x = \sigma_1 M_1 \tag{26}$$

and (25) as

$$\frac{z - \bar{y}}{s_y} = \frac{\delta_2 + \bar{V}_y}{M_2} \quad \text{and } s_y = \sigma_2 M_2. \tag{27}$$

For efficient inference, marginalizing out σ_1 and σ_2 and noticing that $\delta_i = U$ leave the dimension-reduced association model for classification

$$\frac{z - \bar{x}}{s_x\sqrt{1 + \frac{1}{n_1}}} = \frac{U + \bar{V}_x}{M_1\sqrt{1 + \frac{1}{n_1}}} \quad \text{or} \quad \frac{z - \bar{y}}{s_y\sqrt{1 + \frac{1}{n_2}}} = \frac{U + \bar{V}}{M_2\sqrt{1 + \frac{1}{n_2}}}.$$

Let $F_1(.)$ denote the cdf of $(U+\bar{V}_x)/(M_1\sqrt{1+1/n_1})$, the standard Student-t with n_1-1 degrees of freedom, and, likewise, let $F_2(.)$ denote the cdf of $(U+\bar{V}_y)/(M_2\sqrt{1+1/n_2})$, the Student-t with n_2-1 degrees of freedom. Thus, via a change-of-variable we can write the reduced association model as

$$\frac{z-\bar{x}}{s_x\sqrt{1+\frac{1}{n_1}}} = F_1^{-1}(U) \quad \text{or} \quad \frac{z-\bar{y}}{s_y\sqrt{1+\frac{1}{n_2}}} = F_2^{-1}(U) \qquad (U \sim \text{Unif}\,(0,1)) \tag{28}$$

with U playing the role of the a-variable.

Technically, classification based on the reduced association model (28) with the uniform a-variable U is the same as that with known subpopulations discussed in Section 4.1.1. Let $k = \arg\min_{i=1,2}|F_i - .5|$, where $F_1 = F_1\left((z-\bar{x})/(s_x\sqrt{1+\frac{1}{n_1}})\right)$ and $F_2 = F_2\left((z-\bar{y})/(s_y\sqrt{1+\frac{1}{n_2}})\right)$. Take the centered PRS for predicting U and equip it with elasticity. The evidence functions for the assertions $\mathcal{A}_i = \{i\}$ in classification are given by

$$\underline{\mathsf{e}}_{z,x,y}(\mathcal{A}_i) = \begin{cases} 1 - 2F_k\left(-\frac{|z-\mu_k|}{\sigma_k\sqrt{1+\frac{1}{n_k}}}\right), & \text{if } i = k; \\ 0, & \text{otherwise,} \end{cases}$$

and

$$\bar{\mathsf{e}}_{z,x,y}(\mathcal{A}_i) = \begin{cases} 1, & \text{if } i = k; \\ 2F_i\left(-\frac{|z-\mu_i|}{\sigma_i\sqrt{1+\frac{1}{n_i}}}\right), & \text{otherwise} \end{cases}$$

for $i = 1, 2$.

5. Selective Inference

In this section, we consider a situation where the hypothesis of interest is not determined until after observing the data; see Ermini Leaf (2011) for more details. Suppose that a population has two subgroups: female and male. A treatment is administered to a sample of size n from each group. Without considering subgroups, the entire sample might not have significant evidence for a positive treatment effect in the entire population. However, when looking separately at each subgroup mean, there might be evidence for a positive treatment effect within one subgroup. Let $\bar{y}_{\text{F}}$ and $\bar{y}_{\text{M}}$ be the mean observed treatment effects for each group. Suppose further that

$\overline{y}_{\mathrm{F}}$ comes from a $\mathrm{N}(\mu_{\mathrm{F}}, \sigma^2/n)$ distribution and, similarly, $\overline{y}_{\mathrm{M}}$ comes from a $\mathrm{N}(\mu_{\mathrm{M}}, \sigma^2/n)$. The standard deviation, $\sigma > 0$ is assumed to be known. Suppose it is observed that

$$\overline{y}_{\mathrm{F}} > \overline{y}_{\mathrm{M}}. \tag{29}$$

This suggests there might be evidence for the hypothesis that $\mu_{\mathrm{F}} > 0$. An IM for this hypothesis is preseneted in this section.

Bias can occur when a hypothesis is tested after observing data that suggests it is true. From a frequentist perspective, if the hypothesis is actually false, *i.e.*, $\mu_{\mathrm{F}} \leq 0$, and we only test it when $\overline{y}_{\mathrm{F}} > \overline{y}_{\mathrm{M}}$ is observed, then we would decide that the hypothesis is true too often over repeated experiments. The inference would not be valid. The way to overcome this bias is to condition the inference procedure on the event that led to the choice of hypothesis. In this case, the event (29) will be incorporated into the IM.

The association model can be built using the conditional cdf of each sample mean. Let

$$u_{\mathrm{M}} = \frac{\int_{-\infty}^{\overline{y}_{\mathrm{M}}} \frac{\sqrt{n}}{\sigma}\phi(\frac{t-\mu_{\mathrm{M}}}{\sigma/\sqrt{n}})\left(1 - \Phi(\frac{t-\mu_{\mathrm{F}}}{\sigma/\sqrt{n}})\right) dt}{\Phi\left(\frac{\mu_{\mathrm{F}}-\mu_{\mathrm{M}}}{\sqrt{2\sigma^2/n}}\right)} \tag{30}$$

and

$$u_{\mathrm{F}} = \frac{\Phi(\frac{\overline{y}_{\mathrm{F}}-\mu_{\mathrm{F}}}{\sigma/\sqrt{n}}) - \Phi(\frac{\overline{y}_{\mathrm{M}}-\mu_{\mathrm{F}}}{\sigma/\sqrt{n}})}{1 - \Phi(\frac{\overline{y}_{\mathrm{M}}-\mu_{\mathrm{F}}}{\sigma/\sqrt{n}})} \tag{31}$$

for $\overline{y}_{\mathrm{F}} > \overline{y}_{\mathrm{M}}$. The a-variables, u_{M} and u_{F}, each have a $\mathrm{Unif}(0,1)$ distribution. However, the association model does not have a closed form expression.

The mean treatment effect in the male population subgroup, μ_{M}, is a nuisance parameter. It plays no role in the assertion of interest: $\mathcal{A} = \{\mu_{\mathrm{F}} : \mu_{\mathrm{F}} > 0\}$. A marginal IM (see Section 3.2) can be created by predicting u_{M} with the largest possible PRS, $[0,1]$. Since $\mathcal{A}$ is one-sided, the PRS for u_{F} can also be one-sided. The PRS for $(u_{\mathrm{F}}, u_{\mathrm{M}})$ is:

$$\mathcal{S} = \{u : u \geq U\} \times [0,1], \quad (U \sim \mathrm{Unif}(0,1))$$

The C-step requires the mapping (31) to be inverted with respect to μ_{F} for fixed u_{F}. This can be done numerically using a bracketing method (see, *e.g.*, chapter 2 of Givens and Hoeting, 2005), but technical details are omitted here.

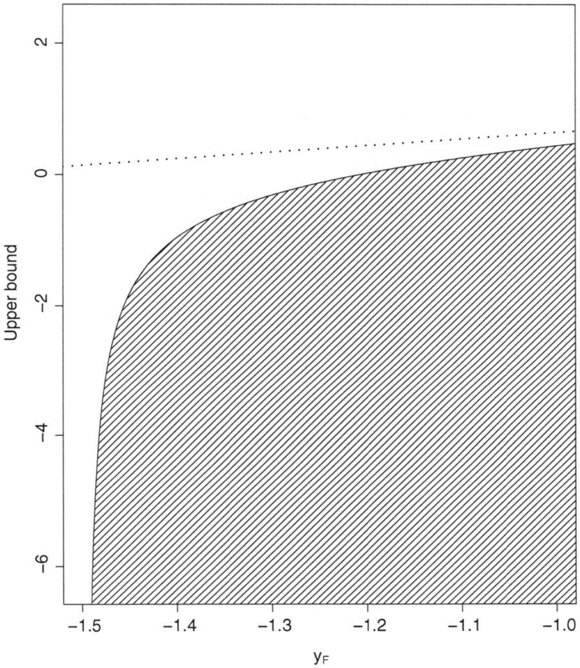

Fig. 2. Lower level-0.95 plausibility interval (shaded) for μ_{F} when $y_{\mathrm{M}} = -1.5$ and $\sigma/\sqrt{n} = 1$. The dotted line is the upper bound of the usual one-sided confidence interval.

Figure 2 shows the one-sided 95% plausibility interval for μ_{F} with different values of $\overline{y}_{\mathrm{F}}$ when $\overline{y}_{\mathrm{M}} = -1.5$. The upper bound of the usual one-sided confidence interval,

$$\overline{y}_{\mathrm{F}} + 1.645\sigma/\sqrt{n},$$

is also shown. When $\overline{y}_{\mathrm{F}} \gg \overline{y}_{\mathrm{M}}$, the plausibility interval bound approaches the confidence interval bound. However, as $\overline{y}_{\mathrm{F}}$ approaches $\overline{y}_{\mathrm{M}}$ the plausibility interval bound drops to $-\infty$. The plausibility interval has exact 0.95 coverage probability for fixed θ over repeated experiments with $\overline{y}_{\mathrm{F}} > \overline{y}_{\mathrm{M}}$. The confidence interval is too wide.

6. Inference for Binomial Data

This section considers inference about the parameters of a binomial distribution, $Bin(n, \theta)$, based on an observed binomial count, x. First, we simply consider inference about the success probability, θ. This idea is then extended to inference about the odds ratio in a 2×2 contingency table.

6.1. *Inference about a binomial proportion*

Following Martin and Liu (2013a), suppose that the observed data x follows binomial distribution $Bin(n, \theta)$ with known size n and unknown parameter θ. We are interested in inference about θ. In the A-step, we associate x and the unknown θ with an a-variable u as follows:

$$x = \min\{k : 1 - u < F_{n,\theta}(k)\} \quad (u \sim Unif(0, 1)), \tag{32}$$

where $F_{n,\theta}(\cdot)$ is the distribution function for the binomial distribution $Bin(n, \theta)$.

To complete the A-step, we derive $\Theta_x(u)$. From (32), we have

$$F_{n,\theta}(x - 1) \leq 1 - u < F_{n,\theta}(x). \tag{33}$$

Let $G_{a,b}(\cdot)$ be the distribution function of beta distribution with parameters a and b. The distribution function of the binomial distribution is related to that of beta distribution by the following equation

$$F_{n,\theta}(x) = G_{n-x,x+1}(1 - \theta) = 1 - G_{x+1,n-x}(\theta), \tag{34}$$

which can be shown using integration by parts. Therefore, (33) can be rewritten as

$$G^{-1}_{x,n-x+1}(u) \leq \theta < G^{-1}_{x+1,n-x}(u). \tag{35}$$

Therefore,

$$\Theta_x(u) = \{\theta : G^{-1}_{x,n-x+1}(u) \leq \theta < G^{-1}_{x+1,n-x}(u)\}. \tag{36}$$

Note that unlike previous examples, $\Theta_x(u)$ is *not* single-valued due to the discrete nature of the sampling distribution.

For the P-step, u can be predicted by the PRS

$$\mathcal{S}_\theta = \{u : |u - 0.5| \leq |U - 0.5|\} \quad (U \sim Unif(0, 1)). \tag{37}$$

Finally, in the C-Step $\Theta_x(u)$ and $\mathcal{S}_\theta$ are combined to obtain

$$\Theta_x(\mathcal{S}_\theta) = [G^{-1}_{x,n-x+1}(0.5 - |U - 0.5|), G^{-1}_{x+1,n-x}(0.5 + |U - 0.5|)), \tag{38}$$

with $U \sim Unif(0, 1)$.

6.2. *2 by 2 Contingency Table*

Now let us consider the more complicated case of observing counts from two independent binomial distributions,

$$x_1 \sim Bin(n_1, \phi_1) \quad \text{and} \quad x_2 \sim Bin(n_2, \phi_2), \tag{39}$$

when we are interested in inference about the odds ratio: $\theta = \frac{\phi_1}{1-\phi_1} / \frac{\phi_2}{1-\phi_2}$. Assume the sizes, n_1 and n_2, are known but parameters ϕ_1 and ϕ_2 are not known. When we are particularly interested in whether $\theta = 1$, it becomes the classical problem of testing association between two kinds of classification.

For the A-step, let $F_{n_1,\phi_1,n_2,\phi_2}(\cdot)$ be the distribution function of the sum of x_1 and x_2 so that

$$F_{n_1,\phi_1,n_2,\phi_2}(k) = \sum_{x_1+x_2 \le k} \binom{n_1}{x_1} \phi_1^{x_1}(1-\phi_1)^{n_1-x_1} \binom{n_2}{x_2} \phi_2^{x_2}(1-\phi_2)^{n_2-x_2}. \tag{40}$$

A CIM can be built using an a-equation for $z = x_1 + x_2$:

$$z = \min\{k : v_2 < F_{n_1,\phi_1,n_2,\phi_2}(k)\} \quad (v_2 \sim Unif(0,1)). \tag{41}$$

Given z from the a-equation (41), x_1 follows Fisher's noncentral hypergeometric distribution. Thus, letting $H_{n_1,n_2,z,\theta}(\cdot)$ be the distribution function of x_1,

$$x_{\min} = \max(0, z - n_2), \tag{42}$$

$$x_{\max} = \min(z, n_1), \tag{43}$$

$$H_{n_1,n_2,z,\theta}(k) = \frac{\sum_{x_{\min} \le x_1 \le k} \binom{n_1}{x_1}\binom{n_2}{z-x_1}\theta^{x_1}}{\sum_{x_{\min} \le x_1 \le x_{\max}} \binom{n_1}{x_1}\binom{n_2}{z-x_1}\theta^{x_1}}, \tag{44}$$

the conditional association model can be derived as:

$$x_1 = \min\{k : v_1 < H_{n_1,n_2,z,\theta}(k)\} \quad (v_1 \sim Unif(0,1)). \tag{45}$$

Note that unlike (15), the conditioning equation is not free of parameters ϕ_1 and ϕ_2. However, we can still conduct a conditional inference based on (45) using generalized conditional IM approach (Martin and Liu, 2013a). Thus, the conditional association model can be simplified as:

$$\Theta_{x_1}(v_1) = \{\theta : H_{n_1,n_2,z,\theta}(x_1 - 1) < v_1 \le H_{n_1,n_2,z,\theta}(x_1)\}. \tag{46}$$

For the P-step, we can predict v_1 by the marginal PRS

$$\mathcal{S}_\theta = \{v_1 : |v_1 - 0.5| \leq |V_1 - 0.5|\} \ (V_1 \sim Unif(0,1)). \tag{47}$$

In the C-step, although $\Theta_{x_1}(v_1)$ cannot be described as simply as in (38), for the assertion $\mathcal{A}_{\theta_0} = \{\theta_0\}$, it is possible to derive a simple expression for $\underline{e}(\mathcal{A}_{\theta_0})$ and $\overline{e}(\mathcal{A}_{\theta_0})$. Trivially, $\underline{e}(\mathcal{A}_{\theta_0}) = 0$ for any point assertion $\mathcal{A}_{\theta_0}$, since (46) is multiple-valued almost surely, thus $\Theta_{x_1}(v_1) \not\subseteq \mathcal{A}_{\theta_0}$ almost surely. Also, from (46) we have

$$\Theta_{x_1}^{-1}(\theta_0) = [a_{x_1}(\theta_0), b_{x_1}(\theta_0)). \tag{48}$$

where

$$a_{x_1}(\theta_0) = \frac{\binom{n_1}{x_1-1}\binom{n_2}{z-(x_1-1)}\theta^{x_1-1}}{\sum_{x_{\min}\leq t\leq x_{\max}}\binom{n_1}{t}\binom{n_2}{z-t}\theta^t},$$

and

$$b_{x_1}(\theta_0) = \frac{\binom{n_1}{x_1}\binom{n_2}{z-x_1}\theta^{x_1}}{\sum_{x_{\min}\leq t\leq x_{\max}}\binom{n_1}{t}\binom{n_2}{z-t}\theta^t}.$$

Therefore, when PRS in (47) is used,

$$\bar{\mathsf{e}}_x\left(\mathcal{A}_{\theta_0}\right) = \begin{cases} 1 & \text{if } a_{x_1}(\theta_0) \leq 0.5 \leq b_{x_1}(\theta_0); \\ 2(0.5 - b_{x_1}(\theta_0)) & \text{if } b_{x_1}(\theta_0) < 0.5; \\ 2(a_{x_1}(\theta_0) - 0.5) & \text{if } a_{x_1}(\theta_0) > 0.5. \end{cases}$$

For a concrete example, let us consider the case of Kidney stone treatment from Julious and Mullee (1994). Table 1 describes the result of applying treatment A to patients with small stones (n_1) and large stones (n_2), where x_1 and x_2 are the number of successful treatments for each group respectively. Fig. 3 plots the log of $\bar{\mathsf{e}}_x\left(\mathcal{A}_{\theta_0}\right)$ versus the log of θ_0. One can find a level $1-\alpha$ plausibility interval, by locating α on the vertical axis and choosing all the θ_0 values for which $\bar{\mathsf{e}}_x\left(\mathcal{A}_{\theta_0}\right) > \alpha$.

Note that conducting conditional inference based on (46) is similar to Fisher's exact test. In this respect, the IM approach provides another way of viewing and validating Fisher's exact test and conditional likelihood methods.

Table 1. Kidney stone experiment data.

$x_1 = 81$	$n_1 - x_1 = 6$	$n_1 = 87$
$x_2 = 192$	$n_2 - x_2 = 71$	$n_2 = 263$
$x_1 + x_2 = 273$	$n_1 + n_2 - x_1 - x_2 = 77$	$n_1 + n_2 = 350.$

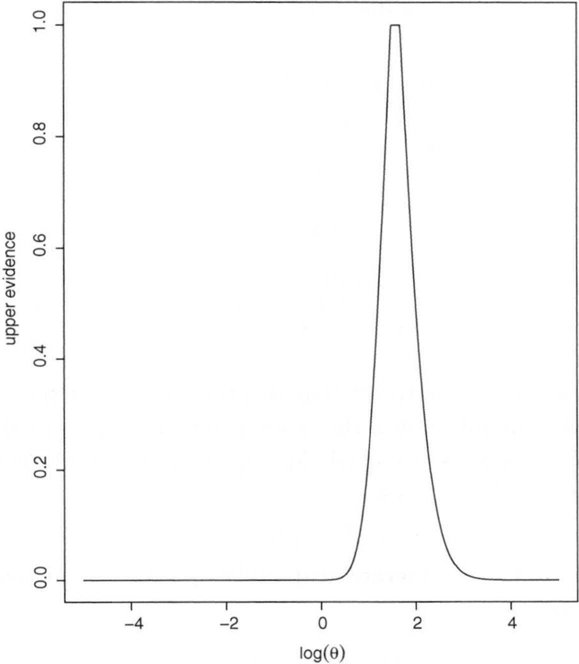

Fig. 3. Plot of upper evidence function for each point assertion $\mathcal{A}_{\theta_0}$.

7. Meta-Analysis: Many-Normal-Means Problems

We refer to Zhou *et al.* (2003) for a comprehensive review of meta-analysis. Here we focus on a popular statistical model for meta-analysis, namely, the many-normal-means model

$$y_i \overset{ind}{\sim} N(\theta_i, s_i^2) \qquad (i = 1, \ldots, n), \tag{49}$$

where y_i is the estimated or observed treatment effect in the i-th study. The mean, θ_i, is the unknown treatment effect to be inferred. The associated standard deviation s_i^2 is taken to be known, assuming that the sample sizes in all the studies are not too small.

For a numerical example of our exposition, we take the real-data example of Rubin (1981), which has the same data structure and inference problems. Rubin (1981) considers assessing effects of SAT coaching programs based on parallel randomized experiments in $n = 8$ schools. The estimated individual effects and the associated standard deviations are tabulated in Table 2. An argument for the use of the sampling model (49) is that each

Table 2. The data of Rubin (1981) on SAT coaching experiments.

School (i)	Estimated Treatment-Effects (y_i)	Associated Standard-Error (s_i)
1	28.39	14.9
2	7.94	10.2
3	−2.75	16.3
4	6.82	11.0
5	−0.64	9.4
6	0.63	11.4
7	18.01	10.4
8	12.16	17.6

y_i was obtained from a data set that is large enough for the acceptance of the normality assumption and the assumption that s_i^2's are known.

Section 7.1 discusses a formal IM approach to uncertainty assessment of the assertion or hypothesis

$$\mathcal{A}_0 = \{\theta : \theta_1 = \ldots = \theta_n\}. \tag{50}$$

Section 7.2 considers the hierarchical model specified by imposing a second stage structure

$$\theta_i \overset{iid}{\sim} N(\mu, \sigma^2) \qquad (i = 1, \ldots, n) \tag{51}$$

with unknown $\mu \in \mathbb{R}$ and unknown variance σ^2. The resulting model is also known as a random-effects model. Inference with unknown σ^2 has been challenging. For example, the method of maximum likelihood is problematic. Bayesian inference requires sensible operational priors to be carefully chosen for (μ, σ^2). This serves as a good example for the argument that practical Bayesian methods are approximating frequentist methods with resulting inference not necessarily valid in the sense of Section 2. After a brief discussion on an IM method for checking the postulated hierarchical model specified by (49) and (51), an IM approach to inference with the hierarchical model without requiring priors for (μ, σ^2) is presented in Section 7.2.

7.1. *Inference about equal means or homogeneity*

The sampling model (49) can be expanded for probabilistic inference as

$$y_i = \theta_i + s_i Z_i \qquad (Z_i \overset{iid}{\sim} N(0, 1);\ i = 1, \ldots, n), \tag{52}$$

where $Z_1, \ldots, Z_n$ are the a-variables. The problem here is to assess the truth and falsity of the assertion $\mathcal{A}_0$ given in (50).

Note that the assertion $\mathcal{A}_0$ is a point assertion in an $(n-1)$-dimensional space. That is, the common value of θ_i under the truth of $\mathcal{A}_0$ can be located anywhere on the real line $\mathcal{R}$. This means that no precise inference is needed for this unknown common mean. Thus, we consider an MIM that effectively integrates out a nuisance parameter representing this common value. We simply take the MIM consisting of the nuisance association model

$$y_1 = \theta_1 + s_1 Z_1$$

and the marginal association model

$$y_i - y_1 = \phi_i + U_i \qquad (i = 2, \ldots, n), \tag{53}$$

where $\phi_i = \theta_i - \theta_1$ and $U_i = s_i Z_i - s_1 Z_1$ for $i = 2, \ldots, n$. Since for any y and Z, there is a θ_1 such that the nuisance association model holds, we proceed with the marginal association model (53) alone.

Write $D = (y_2 - y_1, \ldots, y_n - y_1)'$, $\phi = (\phi_2, \ldots, \phi_n)'$, and $U = (U_2, \ldots, U_n)'$. Then (53) can be written in a vector form as

$$D = \phi + U \qquad (U \sim N_{n-1}(0, W)), \tag{54}$$

where the covariance matrix of U is

$$W = \text{diag}(s_2^2, \ldots, s_n^2) + s_1^2 \mathbf{1}\mathbf{1}'$$

with $\mathbf{1} = (1, \ldots, 1)'$, denoting the vector of $(n-1)$ ones. In terms of ϕ, the assertion of interest $\mathcal{A}_0$ is given by

$$\mathcal{A}_0 = \{\phi : \phi_2 = \ldots = \phi_n = 0\}.$$

For this precise or point assertion, we consider a credible PRS in the $n-1$ dimensional space of U. It is seen from (54) that the propagation of uncertainty from U to ϕ is subject to only a translation operation (i.e., additive transformation). To create an efficient PRS for predicting U, we construct smallest possible subsets with fixed coverage probabilities, that is, the highest-density regions

$$\mathcal{S} = \{u : u'W^{-1}u \leq U'W^{-1}U\} \qquad (U \sim N_{n-1}(0, W))$$

or, equivalently,

$$\mathcal{S} = \{u : u'W^{-1}u \leq R^2\} \qquad (R^2 \sim \chi^2_{n-1}). \tag{55}$$

It should be noted that the projected one-dimensional predictive random intervals in any one-dimensional space have the same coverage probabilities. This observation, together with the use of high-density sets and the translation operation from U to ϕ, explains intuitively the efficiency of the PRS (55).

Routine operations, using, for example, familiar matrix identities that can be easily established with the sweep operator, give the following evidence functions

$$\underline{\mathsf{e}}_y\left(\mathcal{A}_0\right) = 0 \tag{56}$$

and

$$\bar{\mathsf{e}}_y\left(\mathcal{A}_0\right) = 1 - F_{n-1}\left(\sum_{i=1}^{n} w_i (y_i - \bar{y})^2\right), \tag{57}$$

where $w_i = 1/s_i^2$ for $i = 1, \ldots, n$, $\bar{y} = \sum_{i=1}^n w_i y_i / \sum_{i=1}^n w_i$, and $F_{n-1}(.)$ denotes the cdf of the chi-square distribution with $n-1$ degrees of freedom. The evidence for $\mathcal{A}_0$ from the data in Table 2 are

$$\underline{\mathsf{e}}_y\left(\mathcal{A}_0\right) = 0 \quad \text{and} \quad \bar{\mathsf{e}}_y\left(\mathcal{A}_0\right) = 0.7131,$$

indicating no strong evidence is available for inference about the homogeneity of θ_i's.

We note that the results do not depend on the choice of $y_1 = \theta_1 + s_1 Z_1$ for the marginal inference. These results agree with the familiar classic results, but have the desirable interpretation for situation-specific inference.

7.2. *A hierarchical model*

Although there is no strong evidence *against* the assertion that the effects of all the coaching programs are the same, the evidence *for* this assertion is not strong either. Most importantly, it can be argued that these effects cannot be precisely the same. One purpose of the study is to evaluate how much difference there is among coaching programs, that is, the individual θ_i effects are viewed as random. A simple model for characterizing such an estimand is the hierarchical model given by (49) and (51):

$$y_i|\theta \overset{ind}{\sim} N(\theta_i, s_i^2) \quad \text{and} \quad \theta_i \overset{iid}{\sim} N(\mu, \sigma^2).$$

Integrating out the random θ_i effects yields the sampling model for the observed data given by the association model

$$y_i = \mu + \sqrt{s_i^2 + \sigma^2}\, Z_i \qquad (Z_i \overset{iid}{\sim} N(0,1); i = 1, \ldots, n). \tag{58}$$

7.2.1. *Model checking*

In practice, it is necessary to check if this postulated model fits the observed data. A simple IM approach can be carried out by producing evidence for the assertion that *there exists some value of* (μ, σ^2) *such that*

$$\frac{y_i - \mu}{\sqrt{s_i^2 + \sigma^2}} \qquad (i = 1, \ldots, n)$$

is a sample from the standard normal distribution. The IM proposed for such an assertion in Liu and Xie (2013) can be applied here with a simple modification obtained by including the corresponding optimization over (μ, σ^2). We refer to Liu and Xie (2010) for the technical details regarding the essential part of this IM method. For the present example, we applied this IM method to the data in Table 2. The pair of lower and upper evidence for this model-checking assertion is $(0, 0.95)$, indicating that the model fits the data well. In what follows, we consider inference about σ^2 based on the association model (58) with the observed data $y_1, \ldots, y_n$.

7.2.2. *A simple IM for inference about* σ^2

Inference about σ^2 appears to be a challenging problem. It is easy to see that the $n = 2$ case and the $s_1 = \ldots = s_n$ case are simple constrained parameter problems. In the $n = 2$ case, marginalizing out μ gives the association model

$$y_2 - y_2 = \sqrt{s_1^2 + s_2^2 + 2\sigma^2}\, Z \qquad (Z \sim N(0, 1))$$

with the unobserved a-variable Z to be predicted. This is effectively a constrained parameter problem because the unknown quantity $s_1^2 + s_2^2 + 2\sigma^2$ is subject to the constraint that $s_1^2 + s_2^2 + 2\sigma^2 \geq s_1^2 + s_2^2$. Inference about σ^2 in this case can be done using the method in Section 4. IM inference can also be carried out easily for the case where $s \equiv s_1 = \ldots = s_n$ by making inference about $\phi^2 = s^2 + \sigma^2$ subject to the constraint $\phi^2 \geq s^2$. For the general case, we present a simple IM approach below and discuss its efficiency; see Remark 5.

A simple IM approach is obtained by noticing the fact that

$$\sum_{i=1}^{n} \frac{(y_i - \bar{y}(\sigma^2))^2}{s_i^2 + \sigma^2} = S^2 \qquad (S^2 \sim \chi^2_{n-1}) \tag{59}$$

where S^2 is the a-variable and $\bar{y}(\sigma^2) = \sum_{i=1}^{n} w_i(\sigma^2) y_i / \sum_{i=1}^{n} w_i(\sigma^2)$ with $w_i(\sigma^2) = 1/(s_i^2 + \sigma^2)$ for $i = 1, \ldots, n$. Using a PRS to predict S^2 alone results in valid inference about σ^2; see Remark 5 for more discussion.

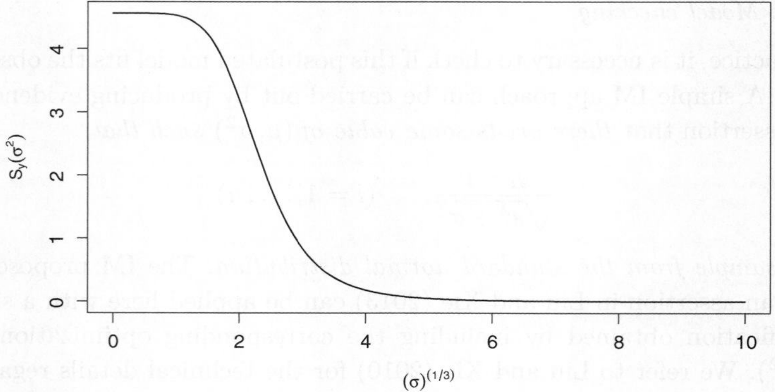

Fig. 4. The function $S_y(\sigma^2)$ for the SAT coaching example.

Let

$$S_y(\sigma^2) = \sum_{i=1}^{n} \frac{(y_i - \bar{y}(\sigma^2))^2}{s_i^2 + \sigma^2}.$$

The function $S_y(\sigma^2)$ for the SAT data is displayed in Figure 4, which shows that $S_y(\sigma^2)$ is bounded from above. Thus the EPRS $\mathcal{S}$ for predicting S^2 is used to ensure that $\mathcal{S}$ has non-empty intersection with the interval $[0, \max_{\sigma^2} S_y(\sigma^2)]$. We use, for example, the equal-tails/two-sided PRS to build an EPRS $\mathcal{S}$. In this example, the median of χ^2_7 is 6.3458 and $\max_{\sigma^2} S_y(\sigma^2) = 4.5632$. Thus, EPRS $\mathcal{S}$ has a point mass of 0.4262 at $\mathcal{S} = [4.5632, 8.5460]$. The resulting upper evidence function for the sequence of point assertions

$$\mathcal{A}_{\sigma_0^2} = \{\sigma_0^2\}$$

is shown in Figure 5, where the 95% plausibility interval for σ is $[0, 16.50]$.

Remark 5. *Write*

$$V(y, \sigma^2) \equiv \left(\frac{y_1 - \bar{y}(\sigma^2)}{\sqrt{s_1^2 + \sigma^2}}, \ldots, \frac{y_n - \bar{y}(\sigma^2)}{\sqrt{s_n^2 + \sigma^2}} \right)'$$

and

$$U(Z, \sigma^2) \equiv \left(Z_1 - \frac{\tilde{Z}(\sigma^2)}{\sqrt{s_1^2 + \sigma^2}}, \ldots, Z_n - \frac{\tilde{Z}(\sigma^2)}{\sqrt{s_n^2 + \sigma^2}} \right)',$$

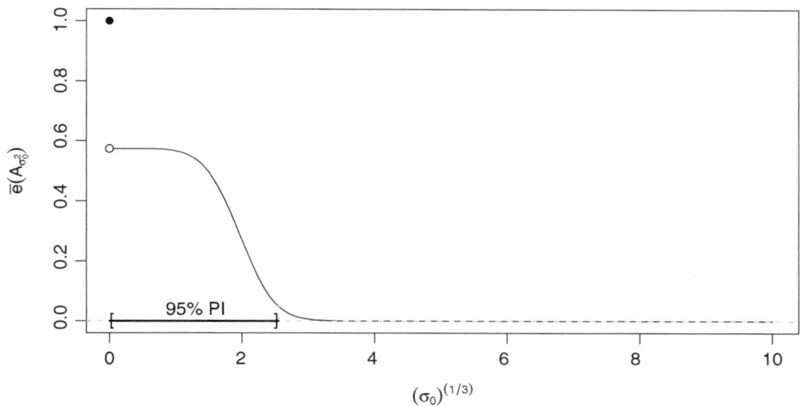

Fig. 5. The upper evidence function for the point assertion $\mathcal{A}_{\sigma_0^2} = \{\sigma_0^2\}$ and the 95% plausibility interval for σ, $[0, 16.50]$.

where

$$\tilde{Z}(\sigma^2) = \frac{\sum_{i=1}^{n} \frac{Z_i}{\sqrt{s_i^2+\sigma^2}}}{\sum_{i=1}^{n} \frac{1}{s_i^2+\sigma^2}}.$$

A formal argument for the validity of the simple approach in the last section can be made by writing the association model (58), after integrating out μ, as a system of equations consisting of (59), i.e.,

$$\|V(y, \sigma^2)\| = \|U(Z, \sigma^2)\|, \tag{60}$$

representing the length of the vector, and

$$\|V(y, \sigma^2)\|^{-1} V(y, \sigma^2) = \|U(Z, \sigma^2)\|^{-1} U(Z, \sigma^2), \tag{61}$$

for the direction of $V(y, \sigma^2)$. For the case of $s = s_1 = \ldots = s_n$, the unknown parameter σ^2 disappears from (61). This results in a simple conditional IM, from which we infer σ^2 based on the association (60) with $\|U(Z, \sigma^2)\|$ conditioned on the observed direction of $U(Z, \sigma^2)$ in (61). Since the length and direction of $U(Z, \sigma^2)$ are independent of each other, the simple approach is in fact based on a CIM and, thereby, is efficient. When the length and direction are not independent, one can ignore (61) or, equivalently, predict the direction of $U(Z, \sigma^2)$ with a (projected) vacuous PRS. This implies that although valid, efficiency may be gained by making use of (61). Research on developing general IM approaches for such problems, under the umbrella of the so-called generalized CIM (GCIM) approach, is on-going. Nevertheless,

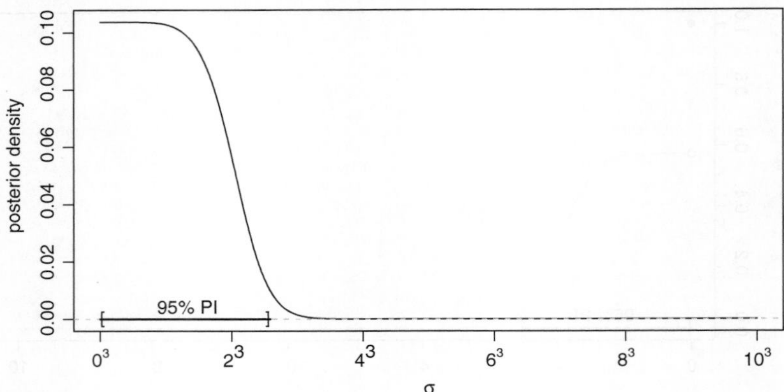

Fig. 6. The (marginal) Bayesian posterior density and 95% credible interval (CI), $[0, 17.27]$, for σ, obtained with the prior $\pi(\mu, \sigma) \propto 1$.

a Bayesian analysis is given below for indirectly verifying the efficiency of the above IM approach.

For a comparison, consider the Bayesian inference using the (flat) prior distribution (see, e.g., Rubin (1981) and Gelman *et al.* (2005)):

$$\pi(\mu, \sigma) \propto \text{const.}$$

The posterior density of σ and the 95% Bayesian credible inference (CI) are shown in Figure 6. Note that the Bayesian CI, $[0, 17.27]$, is slightly longer than IM plausibility interval (PI), $[0, 16.50]$. It should also be noted that the posterior can be very sensitive to the specification of the prior for σ. For example, different results will be produced if the alternative prior $\pi(\mu, \sigma^2) \propto 1/(\sigma^2 + \min_{1\leq i\leq n} s_i^2)$ is used.

References

1. Bayes, T. (1763). An essay towards solving a problem in the doctrine of chances. By the late Rev. Mr. Bayes, FRS communicated by Mr. Price, in a letter to John Canton, AMFRS. *Phil. Trans.*, **53**, 370–418.
2. Dempster, A. P. (1963). Further examples of inconsistencies in the fiducial argument. *Ann. Math. Statist.*, **34**, 884–891.
3. Dempster, A. P. (1964). On the difficulties inherent in Fisher's fiducial argument. *American Statistical Ass. J.*, **59**, 56–66.
4. Dempster, A. P. (2008). Dempster-Shafer calculus for statisticians. *Internat. J. of Approx. Reason.*, **48**, 265–277.
5. Efron, Bradley. (1998). R. A. Fisher in the 21st Century. *Statistical Science* **13**, 95–122.

6. Ermini Leaf, D. (2011). *Inferential Models and Restricted Spaces.* PhD thesis. Purdue University.
7. Ermini Leaf, D., Hui, J., and Liu, C. (2009). Statistical inference with a single observation of $N(\theta, 1)$. *Pakistan J. Statist.* **25**(4), 571–586.
8. Ermini Leaf, D., and Liu, C. (2012). Inference about constrained parameters using the elastic belief method, *International Journal of Approximate Reasoning*, **53**, 709–727.
9. Fisher, R. A. (1922). On the Mathematical Foundations of Theoretical Statistics. *Philosophical Transactions of the Royal Society*, A, **222** 309–368.
10. Fraser, D. A. S. (1966). On the definition of fiducial probability. *Bull. Int. Statist. Inst.*, **40**, 842–856.
11. Fraser, D. A. S. (1968). *The Structure of Inference.* Krieger, Huntington, New York.
12. Fraser, D. A. S. (2011). Is Bayes posterior just quick and dirty confidence? (with discussion). to appear in *Statistical Science.*
13. Gelman, A., Carlin, J. B., Stern, H. S., Rubin, D. B. (1995). *Bayesian Data Analysis.* Chapman and Hall, London.
14. Givens, G. H. and Hoeting, J. A. (2005). *Computational statistics.* Wiley Series in Probability and Statistics. Wiley-Interscience. Hoboken, NJ.
15. Hannig, J. (2009). On generalized fiducial inference. *Statist. Sinica* **19**, 491–544.
16. Liang, F., Liu, C. and Carroll, R.J. (2010). *Advanced Markov chain Monte Carlo: Learning from Past Samples*, Wiley.
17. Lindley, D. V. (1958). Fiducial distributions and Bayes theorem. *J. Roy. Statist. Soc. Ser.* B **20** 102–107.
18. Julious, S. A. and Mullee, M. A. (1994). Confounding and Simpson's paradox. *BMJ*, **309**, 1480–1481.
19. Lindley, D. V. (1958). Fiducial distributions and Bayes' theorem. *J. Roy. Statist. Soc. Ser. B.* **20**, 102–107
20. Liu, C. and Martin. R. (2014). *Inferential Models: reasoning with uncertainty*, monograph in preparation.
21. Liu, C. and Xie, J. (2013). Probabilistic Inference for Multiple Testing. *International Journal of Approximate Reasoning*, to appear.
22. Martin, R. and Liu, C. (2011). Inferential models. This is an early version of Martin, R. and Liu, C. (2013). Inferential models: a framework for prior-free posterior probabilistic inference, *Journal of the American Statistical Association*, **108**, 301–313.
23. Martin, R. and Liu, C. (2013a). Conditional inferential models: combining information for prior-free probabilistic inference, unpublished manuscript, arXiv:1211.1530.
24. Martin, R. and Liu, C. (2013b). Marginal inferential models: prior-free probabilistic inference on interest parameters, unpublished manuscript, arXiv:1306.3092.
25. Martin, R., Zhang, J. and Liu, C. (2010). Dempster-Shafer theory and statistical inference with weak beliefs. *Statist. Sci.* **25**, 72–87.

26. Rubin, D. B. (1981). Estimation in Parallel Randomized Experiments. *Journal of Educational Statistics* **6**, 377–401.
27. Savage, L. J. (1964). Discussion. *Bull. Inst. Internat. Statist.* **40**, 925–927.
28. Savage, L. J. (1976). On Rereading R. A. Fisher, *The Annals of Statistics*, **4**, 441–500.
29. Shafer, G. (1976). *A mathematical theory of evidence.* Princeton University Press, Princeton, N.J.
30. Shafer, G. (2011). A betting interpretation for probabilities and Dempster–Shafer degrees of belief. *Journal International Journal of Approximate Reasoning*, **52**, 127–136.
31. Zabell, S. L. (1992) R. A. Fisher and the fiducial argument. *Statist. Sci.*, **7**(3), 369-387.
32. Zhang, J. and Liu, C. (2011). Dempster-Shafer inference with weak beliefs. *Statist. Sinica* **21**, 475–494.
33. Zhang, Z., Xu, H., Martin, R., and Liu, C. (2011). Inferential models for linear regression. *Pakistan Journal of Statistics and Operation Research*, **7**, 413–432.
34. Zhang, J. (2010). Statistical inference with weak beliefs. Ph.D thesis, Purdue University.
35. Zhou X, Fang J, Yu C, Xu Z, and Lu Y. (2003). Meta analysis method, in *Advanced Medical Statistics*, 1st edition, eds. Lu Y, Fang J., River Edge, NJ; World Scientific.

About the Authors

Duncan Ermini Leaf is a Research Programmer at the University of Southern California Leonard D. Schaeffer Center for Health Policy and Economics. He received his Ph.D. degree from the Department of Statistics at Purdue University in 2011. His research interests include the foundations of statistical inference and computational methods for inference and forecasting.

Hyokun Yun is a Ph.D candidate of Statistics at Purdue University. Before joining Purdue, he got his dual BS in Mathematics and Industrial Engineering at POSTECH, and worked as a software engineer in Cyram(c). His main research interests are statistical machine learning and large scale distributed optimization.

Chuanhai Liu is Professor of Statistics at Purdue University. He received his MS degree in Probability and Statistics in 1987 from Wuhan University and Ph.D. degree in Statistics in 1994 from Harvard University. Before joining Purdue in 2005, he worked at Bell Laboratories as a technical staff for ten years. His research interests include modeling, statistical computing, and reasoning with uncertainty (or foundations of statistical inference).

CHAPTER 34

STOCHASTIC PROCESSES AND THEIR APPLICATIONS IN MEDICAL SCIENCE

CAIXIA LI

Department of Statistics,
School of Mathematics and Computational Science,
Sun Yat-Sen University, Guangzhou 510275, P.R. China
sysu_licx@hotmail.com

JIQIAN FANG

Department of Medical Statistics and Epidemiology,
School of Public Health, Sun Yat-Sen University,
Guangzhou 510080, P.R. China

A stochastic process $X = \{X(t), t \in T\}$ is a t-indexed collection of random variables. That is to say, for any $t \in T$, $X(t)$ is a random variable. t is a parameter. We often interpret t as time. If the set T is a countable set, we call the process a discrete-time stochastic process, usually denoted by $\{X_n, n = 1, 2, \ldots\}$. If T is continuum, we call it a continuous-time stochastic process, usually denoted by $\{X(t), t \geq 0\}$. $X(t)$ is called the state of process at time t. The collection of possible values of $X(t)$ is called state space. If the state space is a countable set, we call the process a discrete-state process, and if the space is a continuum, we call the process a continuous-state process.

Stochastic processes have always been applied in many fields. Now we introduce some important stochastic processes and their applications in medical science.

1. Markov Chains

1.1. *Discrete-time Markov chains*

Suppose that we roll a six-sided dice. The probability of rolling 1 is denoted p_1 ($0 < p_1 < 1$). Now consider a sequence of consecutive rolls. Suppose that they are all independent. If we let X_n denote the accumulative number of rolling 1 after n consecutive rolls, it's easy to see that the variables

$\{X_n, n = 1, 2, \ldots\}$ are not independent. However, if the value of X_n is given, for example $X_n = i$, we can see X_{n+1} either takes the value i (with probability $1-p_1$) or the value $i+1$ (with probability p_1). That is to say, the process $\{X_n, n = 1, 2, \ldots\}$ shows the property that conditional distribution of the future state X_{n+1}, given the present state X_n, depends only on the present state and is independent of the past states of $X_1, X_2, \ldots X_{n-1}$. This property is called Markovian property. Markov chains are discrete-state stochastic processes with Markovian property.

Definition.[2,19,21] Consider a stochastic process $\{X_n, n = 0, 1, 2, \ldots\}$ that takes on a finite or countable values. $\{X_n, n = 0, 1, 2, \ldots\}$ is said to be Markov chain if

$$\begin{aligned} P\{X_{n+1} = j \mid X_n = i, X_{n-1} = i_{n-1}, \ldots, X_1 = i_1, X_0 = i_0\} \\ = P\{X_{n+1} = j \mid X_n = i\} \end{aligned} \tag{1}$$

For all states $i_0, i_1, \ldots, i_{n-1}, i, j$ and all $n \geq 0$.

$P\{X_{n+1} = j \mid X_n = i\}$ in the equation (1) is associated with a transition taking place in one step, so it is called (one-step) transition probability and is denoted as $p_{i,j}(n, n+1)$. A Markov chain is said to be homogeneous if $p_{i,j}(n, n+1)$ is independent of n. Then $p_{i,j}(n, n+1)$ can be denoted as p_{ij}. Let P denote the matrix of transition probability p_{ij}, so that

$$P \hat{=} (p_{ij}) = \begin{pmatrix} p_{00} & p_{01} & p_{02} & \cdots \\ p_{10} & p_{11} & p_{12} & \cdots \\ \cdots & \cdots & \cdots & \cdots \end{pmatrix}.$$

It is obvious that $\sum_j p_{ij} = 1$ for any i.

1.1.1. *A simple example — simple random walk*

A particle makes a random walk on the integer points. Wherever it is, it will either go up one step (with probability p) or down one step (with probability $1-p$). Let X_n denote the site of the particle after n steps.

It is easy to see the simple random walk is a Markov chain. Its transition probability

$$p_{ij} = \begin{cases} p & j = i+1 \\ 1-p & j = i-1 \quad\quad i = 0, \pm 1, \ldots \\ 0 & \text{else} \end{cases}$$

As similar as one-step transition probability p_{ij}, m-step ($m > 1$) transition probability is

$$p_{ij}^{(m)} \hat{=} P\{X_{n+m} = j \mid X_n = i\}.$$

Let $P^{(m)}$ denote the matrix of $p_{ij}^{(m)}$, i.e. $\boldsymbol{P^{(m)}} = (\boldsymbol{p_{ij}^{(m)}})$.

1.1.2. *Chapman-Kolmogorov equation (C-K equation)*

For any m, n,

$$p_{ij}^{(m+n)} = \sum_k p_{ik}^{(m)} p_{kj}^{(n)}, \tag{2}$$

or, in terms of the transition probability matrices:

$$P^{(m+n)} = P^{(m)} \cdot P^{(n)}, \tag{3}$$

especially,

$$P^{(n)} = [P^{(1)}]^n.$$

So C-K equation can be used to derive higher order transition probability from one-step transition probability. Chiang C. L.[11] pointed out that

$$p_{ij}^{(n)} = \sum_{l=1}^{s} \frac{A'_{ij}(\lambda_l)\lambda_l^n}{\prod_{\substack{m=1 \\ m\neq l}}^{s} (\lambda_l - \lambda_m)}, \quad i, j = 1, 2, \ldots, s \tag{4}$$

where the $s \times s$ transition probability matrix P has s distinct eigenvalues $\lambda_1, \lambda_2, \ldots, \lambda_s$, and the matrix $A'(\lambda_l) = (\lambda_l I - P)'$.

The probability distribution of X_n

$$\begin{aligned} p_j^{(n)} \hat{=} P\{X_n = j\} &= \sum_i P\{X_0 = i\} P\{X_n = j \mid X_0 = i\} \\ &= \sum_i P\{X_0 = i\} p_{ij}^{(n)}. \end{aligned}$$

And in terms of the matrices,

$$P_{X_n} = (p_j^{(n)}) = P_{X_0} \cdot P^{(n)}. \tag{5}$$

So, the probability distribution of a Markov chain can be derived from transition probability matrix and initial distribution.

1.1.3. *Example: Hardy-Weinberg law of equilibrium in genetics)*[2,11]

Consider a biological population. Each individual in the population is assumed to have a genotype AA or Aa or aa, where A and a are two alleles. Suppose that the initial genotype frequency composition (AA, Aa, aa) equals to (d, $2h$, r), where $d + 2h + r = 1$. Then the gene frequencies of A and a are p and q, where $p = d + h, q = r + h$ and $p + q = 1$. We can use Markov chain to describe the heredity process. We number the three genotypes AA, Aa and aa by 1, 2, 3 and denote by p_{ij} the probability that an offspring has genotype j given that a specified parent has genotype i. For example,

$$\begin{aligned} p_{12} &= P\{\text{a child has genotype } Aa| \text{ his mother has genotype } AA\} \\ &= P\{\text{his father has gene } a| \text{ his mother has genotype } AA\}. \end{aligned}$$

Under random mating assumption,

$$\begin{aligned} &P\{\text{his father has gene } a \,|\, \text{his mother has genotype } AA\} \\ &\quad = P\{\text{his father has gene } a\}. \end{aligned}$$

So $p_{12} = q$. Similar computations yield the other transition probabilities. The one-step transition probability matrix is

$$P = \begin{pmatrix} p_{11} & p_{12} & p_{13} \\ p_{21} & p_{22} & p_{23} \\ p_{31} & p_{32} & p_{33} \end{pmatrix} = \begin{pmatrix} p & q & 0 \\ \frac{1}{2}p & \frac{1}{2} & \frac{1}{2}q \\ 0 & p & q \end{pmatrix}.$$

Let $p_i^{(k)}$ denote the probability that the k-th generation has genotype i. The initial genotype distribution of the 0-th generation

$$(p_1^{(0)}, p_2^{(0)}, p_3^{(0)}) = (d, 2h, r).$$

And then the genotype distribution of the first generation

$$\begin{aligned} (p_1^{(1)}, p_2^{(1)}, p_3^{(1)}) &= (p_1^{(0)}, p_2^{(0)}, p_3^{(0)})P \\ &= (d, 2h, r) \begin{pmatrix} p & q & 0 \\ \frac{1}{2}p & \frac{1}{2} & \frac{1}{2}q \\ 0 & p & q \end{pmatrix} \\ &= ((d + h)p, dq + h + rp, (h + r)q) \\ &= (p^2, 2pq, q^2) \end{aligned}$$

The genotype distribution of the second generation

$$
\begin{aligned}
(p_1^{(2)}, p_2^{(2)}, p_3^{(2)}) &= (p_1^{(1)}, p_2^{(1)}, p_3^{(1)})P \\
&= (p^2, 2pq, q^2)\begin{pmatrix} p & q & 0 \\ \frac{1}{2}p & \frac{1}{2} & \frac{1}{2}q \\ 0 & p & q \end{pmatrix} \\
&= (p^2(p+q), pq(p+q+1), q^2(p+q)) \\
&= (p^2, 2pq, q^2).
\end{aligned}
$$

and has the same distribution as that of the first generation. Similar computations show the distributions of the 3rd, 4th, ...are all same and still are $(p^2, 2pq, q^2)$. This is Hardy-Weinberg law of equilibrium. That is, whatever the parent genotype frequency compositions (*d, 2h, r*) may be, under random mating assumption, the first generation progenies will have the genotype composition $(p^2, 2pq, q^2)$ and this composition will remain in equilibrium forever.

1.2. *Stationary distribution and limiting distribution*

State j is said to be accessible[2] from state i if for some $n \geq 0$, $p_{ij}^{(n)} > 0$. Two states accessible to each other are said to communicate.[2] We say that the Markov chain is irreducible[2] if all states communicate with each other.

State i is said to have period d if $p_{ii}^{(n)} = 0$ whenever n is not divisible by d and d is the greatest integer with the property. A state with period 1 is called aperiodic.[20]

A probability distribution $\{\pi_j\}$ related to a Markov chain is called stationary if it satisfied the relation

$$\pi_j = \sum_i \pi_i p_{ij}. \tag{6}$$

If the initial distribution $\{P(X_0 = i)\}$ is stationary distribution, then

$$P\{X_1 = j\} = \sum_i P\{X_0 = i\}P\{X_1 = j \,|\, X_0 = i\} = \sum_i \pi_i p_{ij} = \pi_j$$

and, by induction, the probability $P\{X_n = j\} = \pi_j$. Therefore the distribution of X_n is independent of n (time) and the corresponding process is in a statistical equilibrium. In the example of Hardy-Weinberg Law of Equilibrium, the stationary distribution of the Markov chain is $(p^2, 2pq, q^2)$.

A Markov chain is called finite[2] if the chain has finite states. There must exist unique stationary distribution $\{\pi_j\}$ in a finite and irreducible Markov chain.[2] The $\pi_j, j \geq 0$, satisfying $\sum_j \pi_j = 1$, are the unique solution of equation (6).

If there is a distribution $\{\pi_j\}$ such that

$$\lim_{n\to\infty} \sum_i \pi_i p_{ij}^{(n)} = \pi_j \quad \text{for any } i, j, \tag{7}$$

$\{\pi_j\}$ is called long-run distribution (or limiting distribution)

If a Markov chain has long-run distribution $\{\pi_j\}$, the chain has asymptotic distribution $\{\pi_j\}$ no matter what the initial distribution is. A long-run distribution must be a stationary distribution. If a finite Markov chain is aperiodic, its stationary distribution is long-run distribution.[2,18,20]

1.2.1. *Example: Social status change*[2,18]

In sociology, there is a question about how much effect a father's social status has on a son's social status. We take it that one's occupation indicates his social status. Now consider the conditional probability distribution for son's occupation. In a research report about social status change, probability distribution is provided in Table 1.

We consider social status change as transition between states. If Markovian property is satisfied in the states, we can use a finite (three states) Markov chain to describe the social status change. This chain is irreducible and periodic, and there must be long-run distribution (π_1, π_2, π_3) satisfied

$$(\pi_1, \pi_2, \pi_3) \quad P = (\pi_1, \pi_2, \pi_3).$$

So we can get

$$\begin{pmatrix} \pi_1 \\ \pi_2 \\ \pi_3 \end{pmatrix} = \begin{pmatrix} 0.067 \\ 0.624 \\ 0.309 \end{pmatrix}.$$

Table 1. Change in the social status.

	Son's occupation		
Father's occupation	good	median	bad
good	0.448	0.484	0.068
median	0.054	0.699	0.247
bad	0.011	0.503	0.486

We can say, if social status change is a Markov chain with above transition probability, the social status takes asymptotically the proportions: 6.7% for good, 62.4% for median, 30.9% for bad.

1.3. *Continuous-time Markov chain*

Definition. For all states i, j, x_u and all $s, t \geq 0$, if the equation

$$P\{X_{t+s} = j \mid X_s = i, X_u = x_u,\ 0 \leq u < s\} = P\{X_{t+s} = j \mid X_s = i\} \quad (8)$$

is satisfied, the discrete process $\{X_t, t \geq 0\}$ is called continuous-time Markov chain. $P\{X_{t+s} = j \mid X_s = i\}$ in the equation is also called transition probability, denoted by $p_{i,j}(s, s+t)$. A continuous-time Markov chain is said to be homogeneous if $p_{i,j}(s, s+t)$ is independent of s (denoted by $p_{ij}(t)$ here).

If the state is i at time t, the chain transforms into state j with the probability

$$p_{ij}(\Delta t) = P\{X(t + \Delta t) = j \mid X(t) = i\}$$

after Δt. Let

$$\delta_{ij} = \begin{cases} 0 & j \neq i \\ 1 & j = i \end{cases}.$$

$q_{ij} \hat{=} \lim\limits_{\Delta t \to 0+} \frac{p_{ij}(\Delta t) - \delta_{ij}}{\Delta t}$ is said to be transition intensity.[20] The matrix $Q \hat{=} (q_{ij})$ is called transition intensity matrix.

$$\begin{array}{l} q_{ij}dt = P\{X(t+dt) = j \mid X(t) = i\} \quad (j \neq i) \\ q_{ii}dt = P\{X(t+dt) = i \mid X(t) = i\} - 1 = -P\{X(t+dt) \neq i \mid X(t) = i\} \end{array}.$$

So

$$\sum_j q_{ij} = 0.$$

For the continuous-time Markov chain with intensity matrix $Q = (q_{ij})$,

(1) the sojourn time of state i follows an exponential distribution with the mean $-q_{ii}$, and
(2) the chain step into state $j (j \neq i)$ with a probability $p_{ij} = -\frac{q_{ij}}{q_{ii}}$ after leaving state i.

The transition probability satisfies the Chapman-Kolmogorov equation

$$p_{ij}(t+s) = \sum_k p_{ik}(t)p_{kj}(s)$$

and two Chapman-Kolmogorov differential equations, i.e. Chapman-Kolmogorov forward equation

$$p'_{ij}(t) = \sum_k p_{ik}(t)q_{kj}, \quad \text{i.e. } P'(t) = P(t)Q \tag{9}$$

and Chapman-Kolmogorov backward equation

$$p'_{ij}(t) = \sum_k q_{ik}p_{kj}(t), \quad \text{i.e. } P'(t) = QP(t) \tag{10}$$

for all i, j and $t \geq 0$.

We can obtain transition probabilities from the differential equations.

Example. Now consider a two-state continuous-time Markov chain. The sojourn time of state 0 has an exponential distribution with rate λ and the sojourn time of state 1 has an exponential distribution with rate μ. Therefore the intensity matrix is

$$\begin{pmatrix} -\lambda & \lambda \\ \mu & -\mu \end{pmatrix}.$$

From forward equation

$$p'_{00}(t) = -\lambda p_{00}(t) + \mu p_{01}(t) = -\lambda p_{00}(t) + \mu(1 - p_{00}(t)) = -(\lambda+\mu)p_{00}(t) + \mu$$

we have

$$p_{00}(t) = \frac{\mu}{\lambda+\mu} + \frac{\lambda}{\lambda+\mu}\exp(-(\lambda+\mu)t).$$

Similarly,

$$p_{11}(t) = \frac{\lambda}{\lambda+\mu} + \frac{\mu}{\lambda+\mu}\exp(-(\lambda+\mu)t).$$

Hence, transition probability matrix

$$P(t) = \begin{pmatrix} \dfrac{\mu}{\lambda+\mu} + \dfrac{\lambda}{\lambda+\mu}\exp(-(\lambda+\mu)t) & \dfrac{\lambda}{\lambda+\mu} - \dfrac{\lambda}{\lambda+\mu}\exp(-(\lambda+\mu)t) \\ \dfrac{\mu}{\lambda+\mu} - \dfrac{\mu}{\lambda+\mu}\exp(-(\lambda+\mu)t) & \dfrac{\lambda}{\lambda+\mu} + \dfrac{\mu}{\lambda+\mu}\exp(-(\lambda+\mu)t) \end{pmatrix}.$$

Generally, for s-state chain, when the intensity matrix has distinct eigenvalues $\lambda_1, \lambda_2, \ldots, \lambda_s$, Chiang C.L.[11] presented the solution of

Chapman-Kolmogorov differential equations

$$P_{ij}(t) = \sum_{l=1}^{s} \frac{A'_{ij}(\lambda_l)\exp(\lambda_l t)}{\prod\limits_{\substack{m=1\\ m\neq l}}^{s} (\lambda_l - \lambda_m)}, i, j = 1, 2, \ldots, s \tag{11}$$

where $A'(\lambda_l) = (\lambda_l I - Q)'$.

2. Applications of Markov Chains

Markov chain is usually used to describe the systems with Markovian property. For example, we usually divide a certain disease into several states in medical science. Under Markovian property assumption, we can get the transition information among states.

2.1. *Example 1: Predict the structure of future system*

In the paper of Chen Jianzhong *et al.*,[1] to analyse the data which is investigated in 964 areas of NanPing in 1983 and 1988, a Markov model is built to predict forest resources with tree species. The tree species include *Cunninghamia lanceolata* (state 1), *Pinus massoniana* (state 2), broad-leaved trees (state 3), *Phyllostachys pubescens* (state 4), economic trees (state 5) and others (state 6). The data from two investigations (see Table 2).

The one step (five years) transition probability matrix P is estimated as follows,

$$P = \begin{pmatrix} 79.81 & 7.69 & 0 & 0 & 0.96 & 11.54 \\ 7.48 & 75.70 & 0 & 0 & 0 & 16.82 \\ 8.63 & 1.44 & 83.45 & 1.44 & 0.72 & 4.32 \\ 2.38 & 0 & 7.14 & 89.29 & 0 & 1.19 \\ 14.29 & 0 & 6.12 & 0 & 71.43 & 8.16 \\ 8.11 & 5.61 & 9.15 & 1.04 & 0.83 & 75.26 \end{pmatrix}$$

The chain with transition matrix P has stationary distribution. According to the initial distribution in 1988 and transition matrix P, the distributions of trees from 1993 to 2023 are computed in Table 3.

The stationary distribution shows the structure at present is not reasonable and needs to be adjusted. The transition probability matrix after

Table 2. Frequencies of tree species in 1983 and 1988.

1983	1988: 1	2	3	4	5	6	Total
1	83	8	0	0	1	12	104
2	8	81	0	0	0	18	107
3	12	2	116	2	1	6	139
4	2	0	6	75	0	1	84
5	7	0	3	0	35	4	49
6	39	27	44	5	4	362	481
Sum	151	118	169	82	41	403	964

Table 3. Prediction for occupied % of tree species in different years.

Year	1	2	3	4	5	6
1983	0.1079	0.1111	0.1442	0.0871	0.0508	0.4990
1988	0.1566	0.1224	0.1753	0.0851	0.0425	0.4180
1993	0.1913	0.1307	0.1932	0.0828	0.0366	0.3653
1998	0.2159	0.1369	0.2028	0.0805	0.0324	0.3318
2003	0.2335	0.1418	0.2073	0.0783	0.0295	0.3097
2008	0.2460	0.1457	0.2087	0.0761	0.02.73	0.2961
2013	0.2550	0.1488	0.2084	0.0740	0.0259	0.2879
2018	0.2614	0.1514	0.2071	0.0721	0.0248	0.2831
2023	0.2661	0.1536	0.2054	0.0703	0.0241	0.2805
⋮	⋮	⋮	⋮	⋮	⋮	⋮
Stationary	0.2805	0.1663	0.1901	0.0534	0.0226	0.2871

adjustment becomes

$$P = \begin{pmatrix} 79.81 & 7.69 & 0 & 0 & 0.96 & 11.54 \\ 7.48 & 75.70 & 0 & 0 & 0 & 16.82 \\ 2.88 & 1.44 & 89.21 & 1.44 & 0.72 & 4.32 \\ 2.38 & 0 & 7.14 & 89.29 & 0 & 1.19 \\ 14.29 & 0 & 6.12 & 0 & 71.43 & 8.16 \\ 3.95 & 5.61 & 7.28 & 3.12 & 4.78 & 75.26 \end{pmatrix}$$

The distributions of trees from 1993 to 2023 are computed similarly in Table 4.

Table 4. Prediction for occupied % of tree species in different years after adjustment.

Year	1	2	3	4	5	6
1983	0.1079	0.1111	0.1442	0.0871	0.0508	0.4990
1988	0.1276	0.1224	0.1743	0.0954	0.0622	0.4180
1993	0.1437	0.1285	0.1965	0.1008	0.0669	0.3637
1998	0.1562	0.1315	0.2131	0.1041	0.0680	0.3270
2003	0.1658	0.1330	0.2255	0.1062	0.0672	0.3023
2008	0.1728	0.1337	0.2348	0.1075	0.0657	0.2855
2013	0.1779	0.1339	0.2420	0.1083	0.0639	0.2741
2018	0.1815	0.1339	0.2474	0.1087	0.0622	0.2663
2023	0.1840	0.1338	0.2572	0.1089	0.0607	0.2609
⋮	⋮	⋮	⋮	⋮	⋮	⋮
Stationary	0.1872	0.1324	0.2698	0.1084	0.0545	0.2477

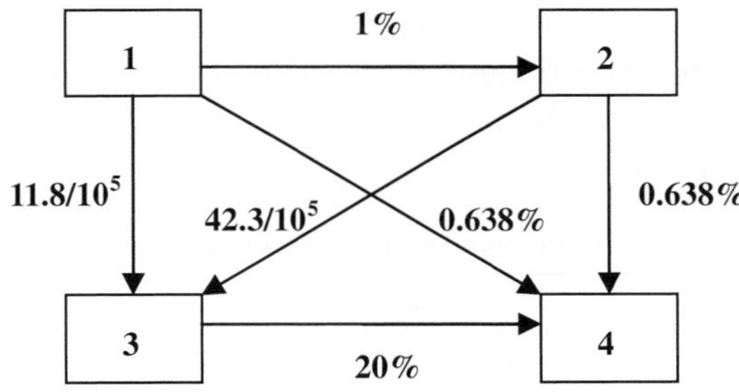

Fig. 1. Transition probabilities for HP infection model.

2.2. *Example 2: Decision analysis and cost-effectiveness analysis*

Helicobacter pylori (HP) infection is a factor for tummy cancer. A markov model is provided for cost analysis in the paper of Wang Qian *et al.*[9] Four states in the chain are without HP infection (state 1), HP infection (state 2), cancer (state 3) and death (state 4). The transition probabilities are given in Fig. 1.

Suppose that is 50% individuals in the population are HP infectious and the cancer incidence is $27/10^5$. For cost analysis, suppose that the heath values of four states are 1, 0.95, 0.3, 0 respectively. The cost of a cancer case is $\$10^4$ per year. The transitions and costs for the population are given in Table 5.

Table 5. The cost in the population (10,000 individuals) without screening.

	States				Communication value					
T	1	2	3	4	S	Q	Cost	S	Q	Cost
0	0.5	0.5	0	0	0	0	0	0	0	0
1	0.4918	0.5016	0.0003	0.0064	9936	9684	27050	9936	9684	27050
2	0.4836	0.5031	0.0005	0.0128	9872	9617	48660	19808	19301	75710
3	0.4757	0.5045	0.0007	0.0192	9808	9551	65916	29617	28852	141627
4	0.4678	0.5058	0.0008	0.0256	9745	9486	79687	39361	38338	221314
5	0.4601	0.5071	0.0009	0.0319	9681	9421	90667	49042	47759	311981
⋮	⋮	⋮	⋮	⋮	⋮	⋮	⋮	⋮	⋮	⋮
28	0.3138	0.5153	0.0013	0.1696	8304	8038	129002	254820	247422	3181863
29	0.3086	0.5150	0.0013	0.1751	8249	7982	128703	263069	255404	3310566
30	0.3036	0.5145	0.0013	0.1806	8194	7927	128387	271263	263332	3438953

T = time S = survival time Q = quality survival time

Suppose that the sensitivity and specificity are both 90% in the screening test and the cost of the screening test is $25 per individual. The cure rate of HP infection is 80% and the cost for cure is $300. Similarly, the transitions and costs for the population with screening can be computed. They are given in Table 6.

Table 6. The cost in the population (10,000 individuals) with screening.

	States				Communication value					
T	1	2	3	4	S	Q	Cost	S	Q	Cost
1	0.8458	0.1476	0.0002	0.0064	9936	9861	16070	9936	9816	1766070
2	0.8319	0.1551	0.0003	0.0128	9873	9793	29082	19809	19654	1795152
3	0.8181	0.1624	0.0004	0.0191	9809	9725	39642	29618	29379	1834794
4	0.8046	0.1694	0.0005	0.0254	9746	9658	48236	39363	39037	1883030
5	0.7914	0.1763	0.0006	0.0318	9682	9590	55251	49046	48627	1938281
⋮	⋮	⋮	⋮	⋮	⋮	⋮	⋮	⋮	⋮	⋮
28	0.5398	0.2916	0.0009	0.1677	8323	8171	91973	255075	251730	3848064
29	0.5309	0.2950	0.0009	0.1732	8268	8114	92283	263343	259844	3940347
30	0.5221	0.2983	0.0009	0.1786	8214	8085	92571	271557	267902	4032918

There is a contrast between them (see Table 7).

2.3. *Example 3: Using the transition dependent on covariates to analyse the factors for illness*

In the paper of Fang J.Q. *et al.*[3], two non-homogeneous Markov chains were used to study a two-stage model with time-dependent covariates for latent

Table 7. The costs between two populations.

	Screening	Non-Screening	Difference
S (year)	271557	271263	294
Q (year)	267902	263332	4570
Cancer frequency	55	82	−27
Summary cost ($)	4032918	3438953	593965
Screening cost ($)	1750000	—	1750000
Cost for cancer ($)	2282918	3438953	−1156035

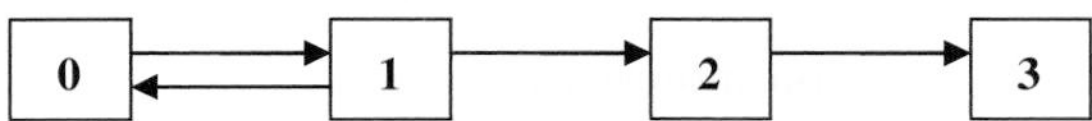

Fig. 2. The transitions between four states.

period of cancer. There are four states in the chains, which are inapparent illness (state 0), soakage stage (state 1), non-soakage stage (state 2) and observable clinic state (state 3). The transitions between the states are given as following Fig. 2.

2.3.1. *Model 1. A non-homogeneous discrete-time Markov model*

Let

$$p_{ij}(t) = P\{X(t+1) = j \mid X(t) = i\} \quad \text{and} \quad Z(t) = (Z_1(t), Z_2(t), \ldots, Z_p(t))',$$

where $Z_1(t), Z_2(t), \ldots, Z_p(t)$ are p covariates. The transition probability matrix is

$$P(t) = \begin{pmatrix} p_{00}(t) & p_{01}(t) & 0 & 0 \\ p_{10}(t) & p_{11}(t) & p_{12}(t) & 0 \\ 0 & 0 & p_{22}(t) & p_{23}(t) \\ 0 & 0 & 0 & 1 \end{pmatrix},$$

where

$$\begin{aligned} p_{01}(t) &= a_{01} \cdot \theta(t), & p_{00}(t) &= 1 - p_{01}(t), \\ p_{10}(t) &= a_{10} \cdot (1 - \theta(t)), & p_{12}(t) &= a_{12} \cdot \theta(t), \\ & & p_{11}(t) &= 1 - p_{10}(t) - p_{12}(t), \\ p_{23}(t) &= a_{23} \cdot \theta(t), & p_{22}(t) &= 1 - p_{23}(t), \\ \theta(t) &= 1 - \exp(-C'Z(t)), & C &= (r_1, r_1, \ldots, r_p)'. \end{aligned}$$

The model was applied to analyze a set of 12-year and 6-run screening data of cervical cancer in Jingan county, Jiangxi Province, China. The covariates are sex disorder, sex health, age, age-square and cervicitis. The estimation of parameters $C = (r_1, r_1, \dots, r_p)'$ is

$$\hat{r}_1 = 0.7095, \quad \hat{r}_2 = 0.0189, \quad \hat{r}_3 = 0.0152, \quad \hat{r}_4 = 2.23\times 10^{-4}, \quad \hat{r}_5 = 0.631,$$

i.e. $\hat{C} = (0.7095, 0.0189, 0.0152, 2.23 \times 10^{-4}, 0.631)$.

In the likelihood ratio tests for the hypothesis $r_i = 0$, the χ^2 statistics are 58.65, 59.62, 22.97, 39.72 and 77.38 respectively, with $P < 0.01$ for all. The results show the 5 covariates have effect on the transition.

2.3.2. *Model 2. A non-homogeneous continuous-time Markov model*

In the model, the transition intensities

$$\lambda_{ij}(t)dt = P\{X(t+dt) = j \mid X(t) = i\}$$

Let

$$\begin{aligned}\lambda_{01}(t) &= A_0 + A_1 Z_1(t) + \cdots + A_p Z_p(t)\\ \lambda_{10}(t) &= B_0 + B_1 Z_1(t) + \cdots + B_p Z_p(t)\\ \lambda_{12}(t) &= C_0 + C_1 Z_1(t) + \cdots + C_p Z_p(t)\\ \lambda_{23}(t) &= D_0 + D_1 Z_1(t) + \cdots + D_p Z_p(t)\end{aligned}.$$

A special model with $C_i = 0, D_i = 0$ $(i = 1, 2, 3, 4, 5)$ was also applied to analyze a set of 12-year and 6-run screening data of cervical cancer in Jingan county, Jiangxi Province, China. The covariates are sex disorder, sex health, age, age-square and cervicitis. The estimations of other parameters are

$$\begin{aligned}&\hat{A}_0 = 2.81 \times 10^{-5}, && \hat{A}_1 = 0.765, && \hat{A}_2 = 0.963,\\ &\hat{A}_3 = 4.16 \times 10^{-4}, && \hat{A}_4 = 7.61 \times 10^{-4}, && \hat{A}_5 = 1.333\\ &\hat{B}_0 = 8.25 \times 10^{-3}, && \hat{B}_1 = 0.019, && \hat{B}_2 = 0.116,\\ &\hat{B}_3 = 2.32 \times 10^{-3}, && \hat{B}_4 = 3.12 \times 10^{-3}, && \hat{B}_5 = 0.109\\ &\hat{C}_0 = 7.03 \times 10^{-4}, && \hat{D}_0 = 0.0279\end{aligned}$$

After hypothesis tests, except the age and age-square, all the other covariates have significant effect on the transition intensities.

2.4. *Modeling for sequence with short-term memory*

In a sequence $\{X_t\}$, the value of X_s usually has effect on the value of X_{s+t}, i.e. $Cov(X_s, X_{s+t}) \neq 0$. The effect attenuates gradually when the time length t gets longer. The sequence is said to have short-term memory if the attenuation is fast and to have long-term memory if the attenuation is slow. Markov chain is a sequence with short-term.

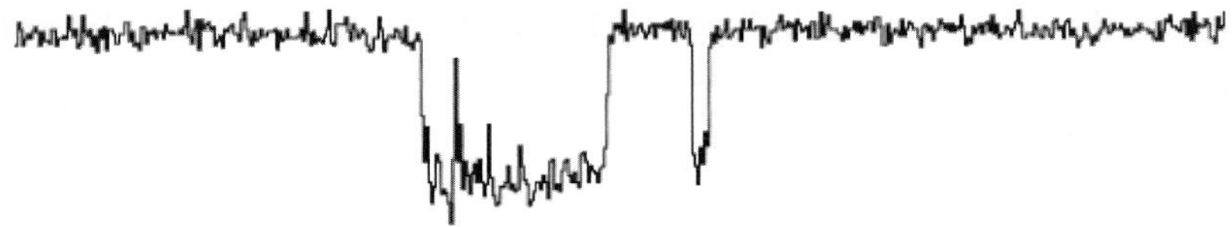

Fig. 3. Single ion-channel patch-clamp recordings.

Ion-channels are sometimes open and sometimes closed. The single ion-channel patch-clamp recordings recorded by patch-clamp are shown in Fig. 3.

Fang *et al.*[15] proposed two-state Markov model to study quantitatively memory existing in ion-channels. A two-state Markov process with constant transition intensities well fitted the short-term memory and a two-state Markov process within a kind of random environment well fitted the long-term memory. In the short-term memory model, the auto-correlation function is $\exp[-(\lambda+\mu)t]$.

3. Some Special Markov Chains

3.1. *Branching processes*

Branching Processes were studied by Galton and Watson in 1874. Consider a population, in which the individuals can produce offspring. Each individual can produce k new offspring with probability p_k, $k = 0, 1, 2, \ldots$, independently of the others' producing. That is to say, all individuals' producings have independent identical distribution (i.i.d.). Suppose that the number of initial individuals is X_0, which is called the size of the 0-th generation. The size of the first generation, which consists of all offspring of the 0-th generate, is denoted by $X_1, \ldots$. Let $Z_j^{(n)}$ denote the number of the offspring produced by the j-th individual in the n-th Generation. Then

$$X_n = Z_1^{(n-1)} + Z_2^{(n-1)} + \cdots + Z_{X_{n-1}}^{(n-1)} = \sum_{j=1}^{X_{n-1}} Z_j^{(n-1)}.$$

It shows that X_n is a sum of X_{n-1} random variables with i.i.d. $\{p_k, k = 0, 1, 2, \ldots\}$. The process $\{X_n\}$ is called Branching Processes.[18]

The Branching Processes is a Markov Chain,and its transition probability is

$$p_{ij} = P\{X_{n+1} = j \mid X_n = i\} = P\left(\sum_{\mathrm{k}=1}^{\mathrm{i}} \mathrm{Z}_{\mathrm{k}}^{(\mathrm{n})} = j\right).$$

Suppose that there are x_0 individuals in the 0-th generation, i.e. $X_0 = x_0$. Let $E(Z_j^{(n)}) = \sum_{k=0}^{\infty} kp_k = \mu$ and $Var(Z_j^{(n)}) = \sum_{k=0}^{\infty} (k-\mu)^2 p_k = \sigma^2$. Then it is easy to see

$$E(X_n) = x_0 \mu^n.$$

$$Var(X_n) = \begin{cases} x_0^2 \mu^{n-1} \sigma^2 \frac{\mu^{n-1}}{\mu-1} & \mu \neq 1 \\ n x_0^2 \sigma^2 & \mu = 1 \end{cases}$$

Now we can see that the expectation and variance of the size will increase when $\mu > 1$ and will decrease when $\mu < 1$.

In Branching Processes, the probability π_0 that the population dies out is shown in the following theorem.

Theorem. Suppose that $p_0 > 0$ and $p_0 + p_1 < 1$. Then
(1) $\pi_0 = q^{x_0}$ if $\mu > 1$, where q is the smallest positive number satisfying the equation

$$x = \sum_{k=0}^{\infty} p_k x^k \tag{12}$$

(2) $\pi_0 = 1$ if $\mu \leq 1$.

Example. Suppose that each individual in a population can produce 0, 1, 2, and 3 offspring with probabilities 1/8, 3/8, 3/8 and 1/8 respectively. Then the mean number of offspring per individual is

$$\mu = 0 \times \frac{1}{8} + 1 \times \frac{3}{8} + 2 \times \frac{3}{8} + 3 \times \frac{1}{8} = 1.5 > 1$$

If the size of 0-th generation is 1, i.e. $x_0 = 1$, the probability π_0 that the population dies out satisfies

$$x = x^0 \times \frac{1}{8} + x^1 \times \frac{3}{8} + x^2 \times \frac{3}{8} + x^3 \times \frac{1}{8}$$

i.e. $x^3 + 3x^2 - 5x + 1 = 0$

This equation has 3 roots, $1, -\sqrt{5} - 2$ and $\sqrt{5} - 2$. So $q = \sqrt{5} - 2$.

Lotka[2,18] proposed a branching process model to study the white American family. Suppose that a white generates k sons ($k = 0, 1, 2, \ldots$) with probability

$$p_k = \begin{cases} bc^{k-1} & k \neq 0 \\ 1 - \sum_{k=1}^{\infty} bc^{k-1} & k = 0 \end{cases},$$

where b, c are positive numbers with $b + c < 1$.

In this branching process,

$$\mu = \sum_{k=0}^{\infty} kp_k = \frac{b}{1-c^2}.$$

The equation

$$x = \sum_{k=0}^{\infty} p_k x^k$$

has two roots, 1 and $q = \frac{1-(b+c)}{c(1-c)}$. Lotka got $b = 0.2126, c = 0.5893$ according to a data collected in 1920. So we'll get

$$\mu = 1.26 > 1, q = 0.819.$$

That is to say, given $x_0 = 1$, the probability that the population will eventually die out is 0.819.

Suppose that survival times of each individual in simple branching processes have independent identical distribution F. Before dying, each individual will have produced k new offspring with probability p_k. Let $N(t)$ denote the number of living individuals at time t. For the process $\{N(t), t \geq 0\}$, when t is large enough,

$$E(N(t)) \approx \frac{(\mu-1)e^{\alpha t}}{\mu^2 \alpha \int_0^{\infty} xe^{-\alpha x} dF(x)},$$

where $\mu = \sum\limits_{k=0}^{\infty} kp_k$ is expectation of each individual's offspring. α is the positive number which satisfies the following equation

$$\int_0^{\infty} e^{-\alpha x} dF(x) = \frac{1}{\mu}.$$

Branching processes introduced above are in very simple cases.

(1) Each individual in certain generation produces offspring with the identical probability distribution.
(2) The probability distribution above is independent of generation.
(3) Any two individuals' producing is independent of each other.
(4) Each individual will not die before it produces offspring.
(5) The population is closed.

In this simple case, the size of the population will eventually become 0 or infinity. In fact, the above assumptions usually are violated before the size becomes infinity. There are some cases to generalize simple branching processes.

(i) Suppose that each individual survives with probability r before producing.
(ii) The distribution $\{p_k, k = 0, 1, 2, \ldots\}$ is dependent on generation n.
(iii) The population is not closed.

Lucas[17] used generalized branching processes to study plasmodia's producing. After a plasmodium comes into the cell in the liver, it propagates rapidly. When the number of plasmodia is large enough, the cell will be broken and plasmodia will go into red cells in blood. And with the number of plasmodia produced increasing, the red cell is broken and go into other red cells. The red cell's broken is periodical. Every period is about 48–72 hours. A branching process is used there. The initial plasmodia which go into red cells constitute 0-th generation. The offspring of 0th generation is called 1st generation, and so on. In the model, the individual may die before producing. The survival probability before producing is also dependent on generation n.

In addition, branching processes has ever used in genes mutation, genetics and epidemiology.

3.2. *Birth-death process*

Birth-death processes $\{N(t), t \geq 0\}$ were discussed in the processes that a population grows and declines. Birth-death processes are Markov chains with transition intensities satisfying $q_{ij} = 0$ if $|\, i - j \,| \geq 2$ (Fig. 4). Let

$$\lambda_i = q_{i,i+1}, \quad \mu_i = q_{i,i-1}.$$

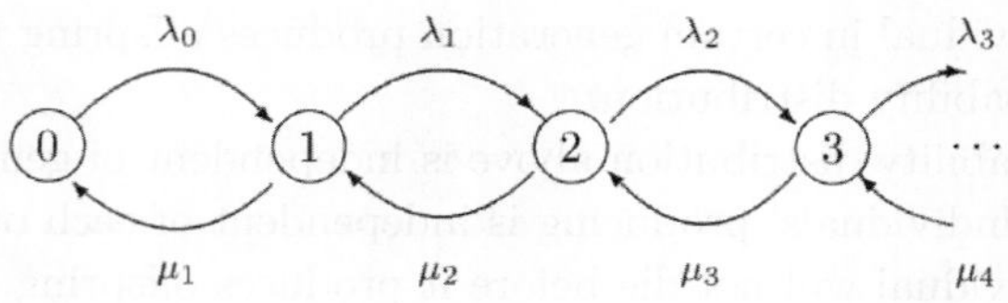

Fig. 4. The transitions in birth-death process.

The transition intensity matrix for Birth-death processes is

$$Q = \begin{pmatrix} -\lambda_0 & \lambda_0 & 0 & 0 & \cdots \\ \mu_1 & -(\lambda_1+\mu_1) & \lambda_1 & 0 & \cdots \\ 0 & \mu_2 & -(\lambda_2+\mu_2) & \lambda_2 & \cdots \\ \vdots & \vdots & \vdots & \vdots & \vdots \end{pmatrix}$$

Let $N(t)$ denote the size of a population at time t. We say that 1 birth (or 1 death) occurs in the population when the size increases by 1 (decreases by 1, respectively). λ_i and μ_i are called birth rate and death rate respectively.

According to the C-K forward equation, the distribution $p_k(t) \hat{=} P\{N(t) = k\}$ satisfies the equation

$$\begin{aligned} p_0'(t) &= -(\lambda_0 + \mu_0)p_0(t) + \mu_1 p_1(t), \\ p_k'(t) &= -(\lambda_k + \mu_k)p_k(t) + \lambda_{k-1}p_{k-1}(t) + \mu_{k+1}p_{k+1}(t), \quad k \geq 1, \end{aligned}$$

when $N(0) = 0$.

Example.[20] There are M mice in a cage, and there is infinite food provided for them to eat. A mouse will stop eating at time $t+h$ with probability $\mu h + o(h)$ if it is eating at time t and will have been eating before time $t+h$ with probability $\lambda h + o(h)$ if it is not eating at time t. Each mouse's eating is independent of others' eating. Let $N(t)$ denote the number of mice which are eating at time t. $\{N(t)\}$ is a birth-death process , and

$$\begin{aligned} P\{N(t+h) = i+1 \mid N(t) = i\} &= (M-i)\lambda h + o(h), \\ P\{N(t+h) = i-1 \mid N(t) = i\} &= i\mu h + o(h), \end{aligned}$$

Therefore the birth rate is $\lambda_i = (M-i)\lambda$, the death rate is $\mu_i = i\mu$.

The processes discussed above are homogeneous. A birth-death process is called homogeneous when the birth rate and death rate don't depend on time.

3.2.1. *Pure birth process*

A birth-death process is called pure birth process if $\mu_i = 0$ for all i. Therefore, the distribution $\{p_k(t)\}$ of pure birth process satisfies

$$\begin{aligned} p_0'(t) &= -\lambda_0 p_0(t), \\ p_k'(t) &= -\lambda_k p_k(t) + \lambda_{k-1}p_{k-1}(t), \quad k \geq 1. \end{aligned}$$

Poisson process and Yule[18] process are special cases of pure birth process with $\lambda_i = \lambda$ and $\lambda_i = i\lambda$, respectively.

3.2.2. *Example: Mckendrick model*[20]

There is one population which is constituted by 1 infected and $N-1$ susceptible individuals. The infected state is an absorbing state. Suppose that any given infected individual will cause, with probability $\beta h + o(h)$, any given susceptible individual infected in time interval $(t, t+h)$, where β is called infection rate. Let $X(t)$ denote the number of the infected individuals at time t. Then $\{X(t)\}$ is a pure birth process with birth rate

$$\lambda_n(t) = (N-n)n\beta.$$

This epidemic model was proposed by A. M. Mckendrick in 1926.

Let T denote the time until all individuals in the population are infected and T_i denote the time from i infective to $i+1$ infective. Then T_i has exponential distribution with mean $\frac{1}{\lambda_i} = \frac{1}{(N-i)i\beta}$. Therefore

$$\begin{aligned} ET &= E\left(\sum_{i=1}^{N-1} T_i\right) = \frac{1}{\beta}\sum_{i=1}^{N-1}\frac{1}{i(N-i)} \\ &= \frac{1}{\beta N}\left[\sum_{i=1}^{N-1}\frac{1}{i} + \sum_{i=1}^{N-1}\frac{1}{N-i}\right] = \frac{2}{\beta N}\sum_{i=1}^{N-1}\frac{1}{i}. \end{aligned}$$

3.2.3. *Example: M.J. Faddy and J.S. Fenlon*[13]

Some stochastic models based on pure birth processes are constructed to describe the invasion process of nematodes in fly larvae. Let $X(t)$ denote the number of nematodes which have invaded the host at time t. Then $\{X(t)\}$ is a pure birth process with birth rate λ_n, i.e.

$$\begin{aligned} &P\{X(t+\Delta t) = n+1 \mid X(t) = n\} = \lambda_n \Delta t + o(\Delta t) \\ &\lambda_n = (N-n)a_n \end{aligned}$$

where N is the number of nematodes outside the host at time 0 and $X(0) = 0$.

Five models in which appropriate forms for λ_n are given constructed as follows.

Let $\lambda_n = (N-n)a_n$.

Model 1. Let $a_n = a$, where a is a constant. From the differential equations, we can know that $X(t)$ has binomial distribution

$$P\{X(t) = n\} = \binom{N}{n} (1 - \exp(-at))^n \exp(-at)^{N-n}.$$

However, in practice, such a model is unlikely to be adequate.

Model 2. Let $a_n = \begin{cases} a_0 & n = 0 \\ a_1 & n \geq 1 \end{cases}$, where $a_1 > a_0$

Model 3. Let $a_n = \exp(a + bn)$, where $b > 0$

Model 4. Let $a_n = \frac{a}{1+\exp(b+cn)}$, where $c < 0$

Model 5. Let $a_n = \frac{a\exp(-dN)}{1+\exp(b+cn)}$, where $c < 0, d > 0$

The solution of the four differential equations for the latter 4 models can be calculated numerically using MATLAB software. Three data sets are given in Tables 8, 9 and 10 respectively.

Three data sets are analyzed. All models fitted to these data resulted in a log-likelihood. Let L_i denote the log-likelihood value for model i.

Table 8. Numbers of invading nematodes for various N.

	Number of larvae with the following numbers of invading nematodes										
N	0	1	2	3	4	5	6	7	8	9	10
10	1	8	12	11	11	6	9	6	6	2	0
7	9	14	27	15	6	3	1	0			
4	28	18	17	7	3						
2	44	26	6								
1	158	60									

Table 9. Numbers of invading nematodes for various N.

	Number of larvae with the following numbers of invading nematodes										
N	0	1	2	3	4	5	6	7	8	9	10
10	4	11	15	10	10	11	8	3	0	0	0
7	12	21	17	12	7	5	0	0			
4	32	22	15	6	0						
2	35	17	2								
1	165	59									

Table 10. Numbers of invading nematodes for various N.

	Number of larvae with the following numbers of invading nematodes										
N	0	1	2	3	4	5	6	7	8	9	10
10	21	13	11	11	9	4	2	2	1	0	0
7	34	15	13	1	2	3	1	1			
4	35	19	12	3	2						
2	45	26	3								
1	186	40									

For Table 8, $L_1 = -626.80$, $L_2 = -602.57$, $L_3 = -588.88$, $L_4 = -588.46$ and $L_5 = -588.21$. Model 3 is good enough. In model 3, $\hat{a} = -1.17(0.05), \hat{b} = 0.25(0.03)$ where the values in parentheses are standard errors. After combining some of the entries in Table 8 with low counts, a χ^2 goodness-of-fit statistic is calculated. $\chi^2 = 17.42$, degree of freedom $df = 16$ and p-value $p \approx 0.36$.

For Table 9, $L_1 = -559.28$, $L_2 = -545.04$, $L_3 = -542.12$, $L_4 = -540.041$ and $L_5 = -540.039$. Model 4 is better. In model 4, the estimators of parameters are $\hat{a} = 0.72(0.20), \hat{b} = 0.60(0.42), \hat{c} = -0.61(0.25)$. After combining some of the entries in Table 9 with low counts, $\chi^2 = 7.75$, $df = 13$ and $p \approx 0.86$.

For Table 10, $L_1 = -554.81$, $L_2 = -517.60$, $L_3 = -512.39$, $L_4 = -509.58$ and $L_5 = -503.71$. Model 5 is the best. In model 5, the estimators of parameters are $\hat{a} = 1.94(0.78), \hat{b} = 2.07(0.41), \hat{c} = -0.87(0.19)$, $\hat{d} = 0.062(0.018)$. After combining some of the entries in Table 10 with low counts, $\chi^2 = 19.22$, $df = 13$ and $p \approx 0.12$.

There are special processes, when the birth rate λ_i in homogeneous process or $\lambda_i(t)$ in non-homogeneous process takes appropriate forms.

3.3. *Pure death process*

A birth-death process $\{N(t)\}$ is said to be a pure death process if birth rates $\lambda_i = 0$ for all i. The pure death process is exactly analogous to the pure birth process.

In the usual applications, $N(t)$ is the number of individuals alive at time t and time t is interpreted as age. Let $\mu(t)$ denote the intensity that an individual alive at time t will die in the interval $(t, t + \Delta t)$. $\mu(t)$ is known as force of mortality, intensity of risk of dying, or failure rate. When $N(t) = i$, one death event occurs in the interval $(t, t + \Delta t)$ with probability

$i\mu(t)\Delta t + o(\Delta t)$. So you can see, $\{N(t)\}$ is a pure death process with death rates $i\mu(t)$. And $N(t)$ has binomial distribution

$$p_{ni}(t) \hat{=} P\{N(t) = i \mid N(0) = n\}$$
$$= \binom{n}{i} \exp\left(-\int_0^t \mu(\tau)d\tau\right)^i \left(1 - \exp\left(-\int_0^t \mu(\tau)d\tau\right)\right)^{n-i},$$
$$i = 0, 1, \ldots, n.$$

Suppose that i individuals are independent and have the same force of mortality. Let T denote the individual's survival time. The survival function is defined by

$$S(t) \hat{=} P\{T > t\} = 1 - F(t),$$

where $F(t)$ is distribution of T. It is easy to show

$$S(t) = \exp\left(-\int_0^t \mu(\tau)d\tau\right)$$

$$f(t) = \mu(t)\exp\left(-\int_0^t \mu(\tau)d\tau\right)$$

$$\mu(t) = \frac{f(t)}{S(t)} = \frac{f(t)}{\int_t^{+\infty} f(s)ds}.$$

For example, when T has a Weibull distribution

$$f(t) = \mu\gamma t^{\gamma-1}\exp(-\mu t^{\gamma-1}).$$

Then we can calculate

$$\mu(t) = \mu\gamma t^{\gamma-1},$$

and

$$S(t) = \exp(-\mu t^{\gamma-1}).$$

4. Applications in Statistic Computation

4.1. *MCMC*

In statistic computation, we usually compute the expectation of a function $f(x)$

$$E_\pi f = \int f(x)\pi(x)dx,$$

where $x = (x_1, x_2, \ldots, x_k)$ is k-dimensional vector and $\pi(x)$ is a density function. Markov chain Monte Carlo (MCMC)[8] methods are applied for this computation.

At present, there are two different definitions of Markov chain. In MCMC, the Markov chain is a discrete-state Markov process. There are transition probabilities for discrete-time chain and transition intensities for continuous-time chain. The transition probabilities and transition intensities are called transition kernel for discrete-state Markov process.

In MCMC, an aperiodic irreducible Markov chain $\{X^{(0)}, X^{(1)}, X^{(2)}, \ldots\}$ with stationary distribution $\pi(x)$ was built. If the initial state $X^{(0)}$ has a distribution $\pi(x)$, $X^{(t)}$ will have the same distribution $\pi(x)$. An aperiodic irreducible Markov chain with stationary distribution $\pi(x)$ has limiting distribution which is also $\pi(x)$. The distribution of $X^{(m)}$ bears little effect from the initial state$X^{(0)}$ and gets close to $\pi(x)$ when m is large enough. Therefore, the $n-m$ state, $X^{(m+1)}, X^{(m+2)}, \ldots X^{(n)}$, is used for computation.

The steps in MCMC methods are as follows.

Step 1. Building a Markov chain with stationary distribution $\pi(x)$.

Step 2. Getting a sample $X^{(0)}$, $X^{(1)}, X^{(2)}, \ldots, X^{(n)}$;

Step 3. Taking $m, n(m < n)$ and estimating of $E_\pi f$ by

$$\hat{E}_\pi f = \frac{1}{n-m} \sum_{t=m+1}^{n} f(X^{(t)}) \tag{13}$$

In MCMC methods, the transition kernel $p(x, x')$ is very important, where $x' = (x'_1, x'_2, \ldots, x'_k)$. In the different MCMC methods, the kernel is different.

In MCMC methods, the full conditional distribution $\pi(x_T \,|\, x_{-T})$ are often used, where $T \subset \{1, 2, \ldots, k\}$, $x_T = \{x_i, i \in T\}, x_{-T} = \{x_i, i \notin T\}$.

$$\pi(x_T \,|\, x_{-T}) = \frac{\pi(x_T)}{\int \pi(x) dx_T} \propto \pi(x)$$

Example. Suppose the joint distribution of X_1, X_2 is

$$\pi(x_1, x_2) \propto \exp\left\{-\frac{1}{2}(x_1-1)^2(x_2-1)^2\right\}.$$

Then the full conditional distribution

$$\begin{aligned}
\pi(x_1 \,|\, x_2) &\propto \pi(x_1, x_2) \propto \exp\left\{-\frac{1}{2}(x_1-1)^2(x_2-1)^2\right\} \\
&= N(1, (x_2-1)^{-2}) \\
\pi(x_2 \,|\, x_1) &\propto \pi(x_1, x_2) \propto \exp\left\{-\frac{1}{2}(x_1-1)^2(x_2-1)^2\right\} \\
&= N(1, (x_1-1)^{-2})
\end{aligned}$$

In the following, two important MCMC methods, Gibbs method and Metropolis-Hastings method, are introduced respectively.

4.1.1. *Gibbs sampling method*

Gibbs sampling method is proposed by Geman S. and Geman D (1984).[21]

Let $x'_{-T} = x_{-T}$. Consider the conditional distribution of $X_T \mid X_{-T}$. Let the transition kernel $p(x_T, x'_T \mid x_{-T}) \hat{=} \pi(x'_T \mid x_{-T})$. So x'_T can be gotten from the distribution $\pi(\cdot \mid x_{-T})$. It can be proved that $X' = (X'_T, X'_{-T})$ has distribution $\pi(x')$.

The simple Gibbs method is called if only one element is in T. Sampling from full conditional distribution becomes simple. The steps are given as follows.

Suppose that initial value $x^{(0)} = (x_1^{(0)}, x_2^{(0)}, \ldots, x_k^{(0)})$ is given and the $(t-1)$-th iterative value is $x^{(t-1)}$. The t-th iterative value $x^{(t)}$ is gotten as following k steps.

Step 1. Sample $x_1^{(t)}$ from the full conditional distribution $\pi(x_1 \mid x_2^{(t-1)}, \ldots, x_k^{(t-1)})$;

....

Step *i*. Sample $x_i^{(t)}$ from the full conditional distribution $\pi(x_i \mid x_1^{(t)}, \ldots, x_{i-1}^{(t)}, x_{i+1}^{(t-1)}, \ldots, x_k^{(t-1)})$;

....

Step k**.** Sample $x_k^{(t)}$ from the full conditional distribution $\pi(x_k \mid x_1^{(t)}, \ldots, x_{k-1}^{(t)})$.

Let $x^{(t)} = (x_1^{(t)}, x_2^{(t)}, \ldots, x_k^{(t)})$.

4.1.2. *Metropolis-Hastings sampling method*

Metropolis-Hastings sampling method is proposed by Metropolis (1953)[22] and Hastings (1970).[23] The transition kernel $p(x, x')$ is built as follows.

Suppose that $q(x, x')$ is an irreducible transition kernel. Let

$$p(x, x') = q(x, x')\alpha(x, x'), \quad x \neq x'$$

where $\alpha(x, x')$ is a function and $0 < \alpha(x, x') \leq 1$.

When the current state is x, i.e. $X^{(t)} = x$. We propose a transition $x \to x'$ with intensity $q(x, x')$. The proposal is not automatically accepted. The probability of acceptance is $\alpha(x, x')$. Therefore, the successive state will be changed as x' with probability $\alpha(x, x')$ and not changed with probability $1 - \alpha(x, x')$. That is to say,

$$x^{(t+1)} = \begin{cases} x' & u \leq \alpha(x, x') \\ x & u > \alpha(x, x') \end{cases}.$$

Where u is a random number from the $[0, 1]$ uniform distribution.

$q(x, \cdot)$ is a probability function or density function. It is called proposal distribution in Metropolis-Hastings sampling. $\alpha(x, x')$ is called acceptance probability. An expression for $\alpha(x, x')$ is derived to ensure the chain with stationary distribution $\pi(x)$.

$$\alpha(x, x') = \min\left\{1, \frac{\pi(x')q(x', x)}{\pi(x)q(x, x')}\right\}. \tag{14}$$

For full conditional distribution, let $x'_{-T} = x_{-T}$. The proposal distribution is $q(x_T, x'_T \,|\, x_{-T})$ and acceptance probability

$$\alpha(x, x') = \min\left\{1, \frac{\pi(x'_T \,|\, x_{-T})q(x'_T, x_T \,|\, x_{-T})}{\pi(x_T \,|\, x_{-T})q(x_T, x'_T \,|\, x_{-T})}\right\}. \tag{15}$$

Gibbs sampling is a special Metropolis-Hastings sampling, where proposal distribution is $\pi(x'_T \,|\, x_{-T})$ and acceptance probability is constant 1.

In the dissertation of Gao K.M. about Bayesian analysis of capture-recapture data, an application for MCMC is provided. In the capture-recapture model, the size of a closed population is N. N is unknown and needs to be estimated by k samples from the population. Suppose that the size of the i-th sample is n_i and n $(n < N)$ individuals are observed in all k samples. Suppose that every individual was captured with probability p_i in the i-th sample. When $k = 3$, the capture-recapture data can be summarized as in Table 11.

Table 11. The Capture-recapture Data when $k = 3$.

		3rd sample			
		Observed		Non-observed	
		2nd sample		2nd sample	
		Observed	Non-bserved	Observed	Non-observed
1st sample	Observed	x_{123}	$x_{1\bar{2}3}$	$x_{12\bar{3}}$	$x_{1\bar{2}\bar{3}}$
	Non-observed	$x_{\bar{1}23}$	$x_{\bar{1}\bar{2}3}$	$x_{\bar{1}2\bar{3}}$	$x_{\bar{1}\bar{2}\bar{3}}$

Where $x_{\bar{1}\bar{2}\bar{3}}$ is unknown. Let $u = x_{\bar{1}\bar{2}\bar{3}}$. Then $N = n + u$.

Let $\{\omega\} = \{123, 1\bar{2}3, 12\bar{3}, 1\bar{2}\bar{3}, \bar{1}23, \bar{1}\bar{2}3, \bar{1}2\bar{3}\}$ and $\{\omega'\} = \{\omega\} + \{\bar{1}\bar{2}\bar{3}\}$. When the three samples are independent, the likelihood function is

$$p(\{x_\omega\} \mid N, \{p_i\}) = \frac{N!}{(N-n)! \prod_\omega x_\omega!} \prod_1^3 p_i^{n_i} (1-p_i)^{N-n_i}.$$

The posterior distribution (N,$\{p_i\}$) is

$$p(N, \{p_i\} \mid x_{\omega'}) \propto \frac{N!}{(N-n)! \prod_\omega x_\omega!} \prod_\omega (p_i)^{x_\omega} (1-p_i)^{N-n_i} \pi(N, \{p_i\})$$

where $\pi(N, \{p_i\})$ is prior distribution of $(N, \{p_i\})$. If $\pi(N, \{p_i\})$ is uniform distribution, the full conditional distribution of $(N, \{p_i\})$ is

$$p(p_i \mid u, p_{-i}, \{x_\omega\}) \propto p_i^{n_i} (1-p_i)^{u+n-n_i} \sim \mathrm{Be}(n_i + 1, u + n - n_i + 1),$$

where $\mathrm{Be}(n_i + 1, u + n - n_i + 1)$ is Beta distribution, and

$$p(u|\{p_i\}, \{x_\omega\}) = \binom{u+n}{u} (p^*)^u (1-p^*)^n = b(n+u, p^*)$$

where $p^* = \prod_1^3 (1-p_i)$.

4.2. *Reversible jump MCMC computation*

In above MCMC methods, the dimension k of vector x is known and fixed. They are not available when k is not fixed. Green (1995)[16] proposed reversible jump MCMC samplers with jump between parameter subspaces of differing dimensionality.

4.2.1. *The general case*

Suppose that we have a countable collection of candidates model $\{M_k, k \in K\}$. Model M_k has a vector $\theta^{(k)}$of unknown parameters, where $\theta^{(k)} \in R^{n_k}$ and is a n_k dimensional vector. Let $x = (k, \theta^{(k)})$, $\Omega_k = \{k\} \times R^{n_k}$ and $\Omega = \bigcup_k \Omega_k, x \in \Omega_k$. For a given k, $\pi(x)$ is the joint posterior distribution of k and $\theta^{(k)}$, i.e.

$$\pi(x) = p(k, \theta^{(k)} \mid y) = p(k \mid y) p(\theta^{(k)} \mid k, y),$$

where y is an observed sample.

When the current state is x, we propose a move $x \to dx'$ of type m with probability $q_m(x, dx')$. Thus the successive state is not changed with the probability $1 - \sum\limits_m q_m(x, \Omega)$, where $\sum\limits_m q_m(x, \Omega) \leq 1$. Let $\alpha_m(x, x')$ is the acceptance probability of the move of type m. The dx', i.e., transition kernel is

$$P(x,B) = \sum_m \int_B q_m(x,dx')\alpha_m(x,x') + s(x)I(x\in B),$$

where $B \subset \Omega$, $I(\cdot)$ is indicator function and

$$s(x) = \sum_m \int_B q_m(x,dx')\{1-\alpha_m(x,x')\} + 1 - \sum_m q_m(x,\Omega)$$

is the probability of not moving from x.

$\alpha_m(x,x')$ given by Green[16] is

$$\alpha_m(x,x') = \min\left\{1, \frac{\pi(dx')q_m(x',dx)}{\pi(dx)q_m(x,dx')}\right\}. \tag{16}$$

Suppose that $\pi(dx)q_m(x,dx')$ has a finite density $f_m(x,x')$. Then

$$\alpha_m(x,x') = \min\left\{1, \frac{f_m(x',x)}{f_m(x,x')}\right\}. \tag{17}$$

4.2.2. *Switching between two simple subspaces*

We first give a simple example. Let two subspaces $\Omega_1 = \{1\}\times R, \Omega_2 = \{2\}\times R^2$. $x = (1,\theta) \in \Omega_1$ when $k=1$ and $x = (2,\theta_1,\theta_2)\in\Omega_2$ when $k=2$. Consider a move between Ω_1 and Ω_2. A move from Ω_1 to Ω_2 is defined as $(1,\theta)\to(2,\theta+u,\theta-u)$, where u and θ are independent random variables. Then the reversible move from Ω_2 to Ω_1 is $(2,\theta_1,\theta_2)\to(1,\frac{1}{2}(\theta_1+\theta_2))$. For dimensional matching of (θ,u) and (θ_1,θ_2), there is a bijection between (θ,u) and (θ_1,θ_2).

In general, $\Omega_1 = \{1\}\times R^{n_1}$, $\Omega_2 = \{2\}\times R^{n_2}$, $\Omega = \bigcup_k \Omega_k$, $x = (k,\theta^{(k)})$. For a given k, $x\in\Omega_k$ $(k=1,2)$. Consider just one move type between Ω_1 and Ω_2. The proposal distribution is $q(x,dx')$ and this move is chosen with probability $j(x)$. From Ω_1 to Ω_2, a m_1 dimension random vector $u^{(1)}$ independent with $\theta^{(1)}$ is generated. Set $\theta^{(2)}$ to be some function of $\theta^{(1)}$ and $u^{(1)}$. Then the move $(1,\theta^{(1)})\to(2,\theta^{(2)})$ is defined. Similarly, to switch back, a m_2 dimension random vector $u^{(2)}$ independent with $\theta^{(2)}$ is generated and set $\theta^{(1)}$ to be some function of $\theta^{(2)}$ and $u^{(2)}$. Then there is a bijection between $(\theta^{(1)},u^{(1)})$ and $(\theta^{(2)},u^{(2)})$. For dimensional matching, m_1 and m_2 must satisfy $n_1+m_1 = n_2+m_2$. Suppose that the densities of $u^{(1)}$ and $u^{(2)}$

are $q_1(u^{(1)})$ and $q_2(u^{(2)})$ respectively. Let $x = (1, \theta^{(1)}) \in \Omega_1, x' = (2, \theta^{(2)}) \in \Omega_2$, and

$$f(x, x') = p(1, \theta^{(1)} \mid y) j(1, \theta^{(1)}) q_1(u^{(1)}),$$
$$f(x', x) = p(2, \theta^{(2)} \mid y) j(2, \theta^{(2)}) q_2(u^{(2)}) \left| \frac{\partial(\theta^{(2)}, u^{(2)})}{\partial(\theta^{(1)}, u^{(1)})} \right| .$$

Then the acceptance probability

$$\alpha(x, x') = \min\left\{1, \frac{p(2, \theta^{(2)} \mid y) j(2, \theta^{(2)}) q_2(u^{(2)})}{p(1, \theta^{(1)} \mid y) j(1, \theta^{(1)}) q_1(u^{(1)})} \left| \frac{\partial(\theta^{(2)}, u^{(2)})}{\partial(\theta^{(1)}, u^{(1)})} \right| \right\} \tag{18}$$

Sometimes, m_1 or m_2 is 0. For example, when m_2 is 0, (18) becomes

$$\alpha(x, x') = \min\left\{1, \frac{p(2, \theta^{(2)} \mid y) j(2, \theta^{(2)})}{p(1, \theta^{(1)} \mid y) j(1, \theta^{(1)}) q_1(u^{(1)})} \left| \frac{\partial(\theta^{(2)})}{\partial(\theta^{(1)}, u^{(1)})} \right| \right\} .$$

5. Markov Models of Epidemics

5.1. *SIS model*

An epidemic model is a tool used to study the mechanisms by which diseases spread, to predict the future course of an outbreak and to evaluate strategies to control an epidemic.[24]

The simplest epidemic model is SIS model. The SIS epidemic model has been applied to sexually transmitted diseases.[25] In the SIS epidemic model, the population is divided into two compartments, those who are susceptible to the disease (denoted by S), and those who are infected (denoted by I). After a successful contact with an infectious individual, a susceptible individual becomes infected, but does not confer any long-lasting immunity. Therefore, the infected individuals become susceptible again after recovery. The flow of this model is shown in Fig. 5.

Let $S(t)$ and $I(t)$ denote the number of susceptible individuals and the number of infected individuals, respectively, at time t. Like the previous Mckendrick model, suppose that any given infected individual will cause, with probability $\beta h + o(h)$, any given susceptible individual infected in time interval $(t, t+h)$, where β is called infection rate. In addition, any given infected individual will recover and be susceptible again with probability

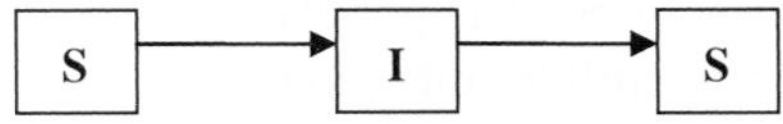

Fig. 5. The SIS model.

$\gamma h + o(h)$, where γ is called recovery rate. Using a fixed population, $N = S(t) + I(t)$, $\{I(t)\}$ is a birth and death process, a special Markov process, with

$$\lambda_i(t) = \beta i(N-i), \quad \mu_i(t) = \gamma i,$$

since

$$\begin{cases} P\{I(t+h) = i+1 \mid I(t) = i\} = \beta i(N-i)h + o(h), \\ P\{I(t+h) = i-1 \mid I(t) = i\} = i\gamma h + o(h), \\ P\{I(t+h) = i \mid I(t) = i\} = 1 - \beta i(N-i)h - i\gamma h + o(h). \\ P\{I(t+h) = j \mid I(t) = i\} = o(h), \mid j - i \mid \geq 2. \end{cases}$$

According to the C-K forward equation, the distribution of $I(t)$, $p_j(t) \hat{=} P\{I(t) = j\}$ satisfies the equation

$$\begin{aligned} p_0'(t) &= \gamma p_1(t), \\ p_j'(t) &= -[\beta j(N-j) + \gamma j]p_j(t) + \beta(j-1)(N-j+1)p_{j-1}(t) \\ &\qquad + \gamma(j+1)p_{j+1}(t), \quad j \geq 1, \end{aligned}$$

when $P\{I(0) = i\} = 1$.

The process $I(t)$ is a Markov chain with an absorbing state at $I(t) = 0$. When the parameter $R_0 = N\beta/\gamma$ is small, the infection will die out in the long run. When the parameter R_0 is large, the time to extinction may be extremely long and the infection will be able to spread in a population. This useful metric is called basic reproductive rate. The expected time to extinction of the basic SIS model is considered in Norden (1982).[26]

5.2. *SIR model*

For most common diseases that confer long-lasting immunity, the population is divided into three compartments: susceptible $S(t)$, infected $I(t)$, and recovered $R(t)$. The recovered individuals are no longer spreading the disease when they are removed from the infection process. This SIR model is an extension of the SIS model and the SIS model can be easily derived from the SIR model by simply considering that the individuals recover with no immunity to the disease. So, the population in SIR model is broken into three compartments: susceptible, infectious, and recovered (Fig. 6).

Suppose the total population size N is fixed constant, then the transition probabilities $p_{(s,i),(k,j)}(h) = P\{S(t+h) = k, I(t+h) = j \mid S(t) = s, I(t) = i\}$

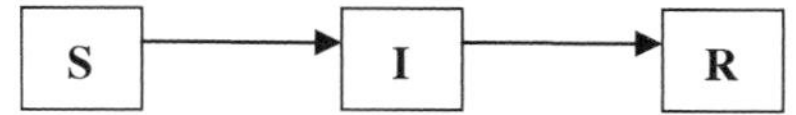

Fig. 6. The SIR model.

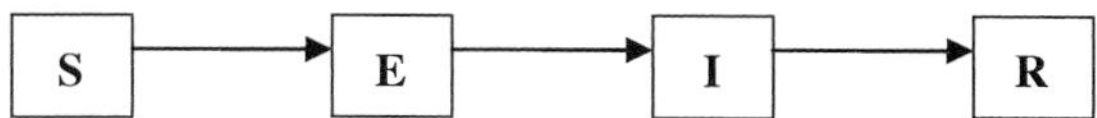

Fig. 7. The SEIR model.

for the bivariate Markov process $\{S(t), I(t)\}$ can be derived similarly:

$$p_{(s,i),(k,j)}(h) = \begin{cases} \beta i(N-i)h + o(h), & (k,j) = (s-1, i+1) \\ i\gamma h + o(h), & (k,j) = (s, i-1) \\ 1 - \beta i(N-i)h - i\gamma h + o(h), & (k,j) = (s,i) \\ o(h), & otherwise \end{cases} .$$

5.3. *SEIR model*

The SIR model discussed above takes into account only those diseases which cause an individual to be able to infect others immediately upon their infection. Many diseases have what is termed a latent or exposed phase, during which the individual is said to be infected but not infectious. The SEIR model takes into consideration the exposed or latent period of the disease. Hence, in this model the population is broken into four compartments: susceptible, exposed, infectious, and recovered (Fig. 7).

Maximum likelihood method can used to estimate parameter values for the basic SIS, SIR and SEIR models based on fully observed epidemic data. O'Neill *et al.* (1999, 2001)[27,28] also demonstrated how to use Bayesian methods via MCMC algorithm to fit SEIR general epidemic model based on partially observed data.

Severe acute respiratory syndrome (SARS) is a viral respiratory disease in humans. In early 2003, SARS spread from Hong Kong to 37 countries within weeks. Figure 8 plots the epidemic curve of 06/09/2003 showing the dates of onset of 1729 patients.[29] Several epidemic models on SARS data from the 2003 outbreak in Hong Kong have been published.[30,31,32] They adopted the stochastic SEIR models which contain susceptible, exposed (latent), infectious, and recovered individuals. They used the available data for SARS on latent and infectious periods and parametric distributions,

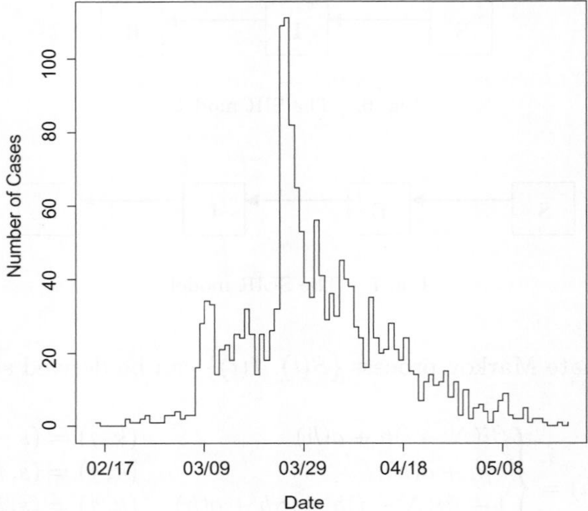

Fig. 8. Dates of onset of 1729 SARS patients.

such as Weibull or Gamma distributions, were assumed. The data were fitted by maximum likelihood estimation methods.

6. Counting Processes and Regression Models for Survival Data

6.1. *Life table*

There are two kinds of life tables, current life table and cohort life table, working for two different kinds of studies, cross-sectional study and follow-up study. For current life table, Chiang C.L. proposed a method to calculate the probability of death.

$$q_i = \frac{n_i M_i}{1 + (1 - a_i) n_i M_i},$$

where q_i is age specific probability of death, the probability in $(x_i, x_i + n_i)$, and M_i is age specific death rate.

Based on stage processes, a new life table is constructed by Chiang.[12] In this new table, probability of death is not only dependent on age, but also on stage of disease. The stage process is usually used to describe the development of chronic diseases. Generally, chronic diseases advance with time from mild through intermediate stages to death. The process often is irreversible but a patient may die while being in any one of the stages. For example, Evolution of cancer is always a stage process. There are many staging phenomena in many other areas, birth order and child spacing, engagement-marriage-divorce in demography, and so on.

6.2. *Counting process*

A process $\{N(t), t \geq 0\}$ is called a counting process if $N(t)$ represents the total number of events that occurred in $(0, t)$. A counting process must be a non-negative integer valued process. Let τ_i denote the time of the i-th event and it is said to be the arrival time of the i-th event. $\tau_1, \tau_2, \ldots$ are random variables and $0 < \tau_1 < \tau_2 < \cdots$. Let

$$T_1 = \tau_1, T_2 = \tau_2 - \tau_1, \ldots, T_n = \tau_n - \tau_{n-1}, \ldots.$$

$\{T_i, i = 1, 2, \ldots\}$ is called the sequence of interarrival times.

A counting process is called a renewal process if the inter-arrival times have independent and identical distribution. Especial, Poisson Process is called if the distribution is exponential distribution.

Now consider k different kinds of events may occur. Let $N_i(t)$ denote the total number of the i-th kind of events that occurred in $(0, t)$. $N(t) = (N_1(t), N_2(t), \ldots N_k(t))$ is called multiple counting process with k dimensions.

Let $X_1, X_2, \ldots, X_n$ denote survival times of n individuals. They are independent and have the same survival function $S(t)$. Let

$$N(t) = \#(i : X_i \leq t) = \sum_{i=1}^{n} I(X_i \leq t),$$

where $\#(\cdot)$ is a counting function and $I(\cdot)$ is a indicator function. Then $N(t)$ is the total number of deaths that occur in $(0, t]$ and $\{N(t), t \geq 0\}$ is a counting process.

In survival analysis problems, complete data is not possible. We can observe $(\tilde{X}_i, D_i), i = 1, 2, \ldots, n$, where D_i is a censoring indicator. Then

$$\begin{aligned} X_i &= \tilde{X}_i, \quad if\ D_i = 1, \\ X_i &> \tilde{X}_i, \quad if\ D_i = 0, \end{aligned}$$

Let

$$N(t) = \#\{i : \tilde{X}_i \leq t, D_i = 1\}.$$

6.3. *Kaplan-Meier estimator*

Kaplan-Meier estimator is a non-parametric estimator for survival function. It is also called product-limit estimator. It is

$$\hat{S}(t) = \prod_{s \leq t} \left(1 - \frac{\Delta N(s)}{Y(s)}\right),$$

where $\Delta N(s) = N(s) - N(s-)$, $Y(s) = \#\{i : \tilde{X}_i \geq s\}$ is the number at risk just before time s.

6.4. *Cox regression*

In above assumption, survival times of n individuals have identical distribution. However, survival time usually depends on some covariates. If the values of covariates are different for individuals, survival times of individuals have different distributions. That is to say, survival function depends on the covariates. Regression model can be used here. When the distribution is known to follow a certain distribution, for example, exponential distribution, a parametric regression model can be used. However, the distribution usually is unknown. Some semiparametric models are considered. Cox regression model is a semiparametric model. In Cox regression model, the intensity of hazard is

$$\mu_i(t, z) = \mu_0(t) \exp(\beta' Z_i),$$

where $Z_i = (z_{i1}, z_{i2}, \ldots z_{ip})'$ is the covariates vector, β is the regression coefficient vector and $\mu_0(t)$ is an intensity of risk independent of individuals. This model is also called proportional hazard model.

Because $\mu_0(t)$ is unknown, the estimators of parameters are based on partial likelihood function. Suppose that we observed d individuals, denoted by (1),(2),...,(d), dead. Let $X_{(i)}$ denote the survival time of individual (i). And $X_{(1)} < X_{(2)} < \ldots < X_{(\mathrm{d})}$. Let $R_{(i)} = \{j : \tilde{X}_j \geq X_{(i)}\}$, the number at risk just before the time $X_{(i.)}$. Then the partial likelihood function is

$$\begin{aligned} L &= \prod_{i=1}^{d} P\{\text{individual } (i) \text{ die at time } X_{(i)} \mid \text{one individual in } R_{(i)} \\ &\qquad \text{die at time } X_{(i)}\} \\ &= \prod_{i=1}^{d} \frac{\exp(\beta' Z_{(i)})}{\sum\limits_{j \in R_{(i)}} \exp(\beta' Z_{(j)})} \end{aligned}$$

Then logarithm partial likelihood function is

$$\ln L = \sum_{i=1}^{d} \left\{ \beta' Z_{(i)} - \ln \left[\sum_{j \in R_{(i)}} \exp(\beta' Z_{(j)}) \right] \right\}.$$

Therefore the maximal partial likelihood estimator of β can be calculated. It is also called Cox estimator.

Cox estimator is consistent. That is to say, the estimator $\to \beta$ in probability when the sample size $n \to \infty$.

Sometimes, the covariates are time-dependent. Some counting process models with time-dependent covariates are given as follows.

6.5. *Multiple renewal process model*

A multiple renewal process with time-dependent covariates is used as a model for acute respiratory infections (ARI) in the paper of Fang (1990).[13] Consider a marked renewal process with g marks $D_1, \ldots, D_g$ corresponding to g classes of diseases. Let $\mu_{si}(t)$, $s = 1, 2, \ldots, g$, $i = 1, 2, \ldots, n$ to denote the intensity that disease D_s for individual i happens at time t. Let $Z_i(t) = (z_i'(t), (t-t_{ri}), (t-t_{ri})^2, \ldots (t-t_{ri})^q)'$. It contains a set of p time dependent covariates $z_i(t)$ and quasi-covariates, $(t-t_{ri}), (t-t_{ri})^2, \ldots (t-t_{ri})^q$, representing the effect of time, where t_{ri} is the latest renewal time of individual i before time t. And let

$$\mu_{si}(t) = \exp(C_s' Z_i(t) + \theta_s),$$

where $C_s = (c_{s1}, c_{s2}, \ldots, c_{s,p+q})'$ is a $p+q$ dimensional column vector and θ_s are parameters related to the occurrence of D_s and expected to be estimated from the data.

For individual i, the records in the data include the beginning and the end of observed time, t_{0i} and t_{ei}, the occurrence times $t_{1i}, t_{2i}, \ldots t_{k_i i}$, and the corresponding states $d_{1i}, d_{2i}, \ldots d_{k_i i}$, where k_i is the number of transitions happening. The full log-likelihood function for n individuals can be written as

$$\ln L = \sum_{\substack{i=1 \\ k_i \neq 0}}^{n} \sum_{j=1}^{k_i} \ln \mu_{d_{ji} i}(t_{ji}) - \sum_{i=1}^{n} \int_{t_{0i}}^{t_{ei}} \left[\sum_{s=1}^{g} \mu_{si}(t) \right] dt.$$

As a especial case, if the parameter vectors C_s are assumed to be equal to C for all $s = 1, 2, \ldots, g$, the parameters are fewer. To estimate the vector C, a numerical method such as the Newton-Raphson algorithm is used.

The child survey data on ARI was analyzed. Eighteen covariates were included, of which nine were indices of health, seven were weather indices, and the last two were $(t - t_r)$ which was length of time since the latest illness (TEF), and $(t - t_r)^2$ which was the square of TEF (TEF^2), respectively, serving to explore the effect of time. The nine indices of health include hemochrome (HEM), history of tracheitis (HTR), rickets (RIC), age (AGE), history of tuberculosis (HTB), dental caries (CAR), sex (SEX), ratio of height and weight (RHW), family history of tracheitis (FHT). The seven indices of weather included low temperature for days (LTM), range of temperature for days (RTM), relative humidity for days (RHU), difference of minimal temperatures for two days (DLT), maximal wind velocity for days (MWV), atmospheric pressure for days (ATP).

By means of the likelihood ratio test, we find that one index of health HEM, three weather indices LTM, RTM, and RHU, and the effect of time, TEF and TEF^2 were significant on the risk of occurrence of disease D. The estimates of parameter θ_s corresponding to the six types of ARI were -2.0759, -3.9243, -7.6897, -4.4043, -2.0402 and -6.4517.

6.6. *Markov counting process model*

In the paper of Fang J.Q. *et al.*,[4] a Markov counting process with time-dependent covariates is used to build a model. Let N_{ij} denote the numbers of transitions $i \to j (i \neq j)$ that occur in $(0, t]$. Let $\mu_{ijh}(t)$ denote the intensity that the transition $i \to j$ for individual h happens at time t. We assume

$$\mu_{ijh}(t, z) = \mu_{ij0}(t) \exp(\beta'_{ij} Z_{ijh}(t)).$$

Then the partial likelihood function is

$$L = \prod_t \prod_{i,j,h} \left(\frac{\exp(\beta'_{ij} Z_{ijh}(t))}{\sum_{h=1}^{n} \exp(\beta'_{ij} Z_{si}(t)) Y_{ih}(t)} \right)^{\Delta N_{ijh}(t)},$$

where $N_{ijh}(t)$ is the number of transitions $i \to j (i \neq j)$ that occur in $(0, t]$ for the individual h, $\Delta N_{ijh}(t) = N_{si}(t) - N_{si}(t-)$ and Y_{ih} is the binary of the individual h at risk with respect to state i. That is to say,

$$Y_{ih}(t) = \begin{cases} 1 & \text{if individual } h \text{ at risk at time } t\text{, corresponding state } i \\ 0 & \text{else} \end{cases}.$$

Using this model, Fang analyzed a set of 12-year and 6-run screening data of cervical cancer in Jingan county, Jiangxi Province, China. The covariates are sex disorder, sex health, age, age-square and cervicitis. There are four states and five covariates dealt with. To obtain maximal partial likelihood estimator of parameter vector β, Marquardt modification algorithm was used. The estimators are solved as

$$\begin{aligned}\beta'_{01} &= (0.1348^*,\ -0.6567,\ 0.1088^*,\ -0.0012^*,\ 0.1838^*)\\ \beta'_{10} &= (-0.0450,\ -0.8642, 0.0542^*,\ -0.0010^*,\ -0.0173)\\ \beta'_{12} &= (-0.2087,\ -0.7219, 0.0691^*,\ -0.0008^*,\ 0.5787^*)\ ,\\ \beta'_{23} &= (1.7469^*,\ 0.0000,\ 0.0544,\ 0.0014^*,\ 0.6952)\end{aligned}$$

where * means that the covariate is significantly different from zero.

6.7. *General multiple counting process model*

Andersen, Borgan and Gill (1990)[10] proposed a statistical model based on multiple counting process. Now consider k types of event. Let $\mu_{si}(t,z)$ denote the occurrence intensity of type s event for individual i with time-dependent covariate vector z. We assume

$$\mu_{si}(t,z) = \mu_{s0}(t,\theta)f(\beta' Z_{si}(t)), \quad s = 1, 2, \ldots, k,$$

where $Z_{si}(t) = (z_{si1}(t), z_{si2}(t), \ldots z_{sip}(t))'$ is covariate vector, β is a regression coefficient vector and θ is a parameter.

The partial likelihood function is given as

$$L = \prod_t \prod_{s,i} \left(\frac{f(\beta' Z_{si}(t))}{\sum\limits_{i=1}^{n} f(\beta' Z_{si}(t)) Y_{si}(t)} \right)^{\Delta N_{si}(t)},$$

where $N_{si}(t)$ is the occurrence number of type s event by time t for the individual i, $\Delta N_{si}(t) = N_{si}(t) - N_{si}(t-)$, and Y_{si} is the binary indicator of the individual i at risk, corresponding type s event.

References

1. Cheng, J.Z., Zhou, S.Y., Xu, H.Y. (1994). Application of Markov process in structural dynamic forecasting of forest resources with tree species structure in Nanping region of Fujian province as an example. *Chinese Journal of Applied Ecology*, **5**(3): 232–236 (in Chinese).
2. Deng, Y.L. (1994). *Stochastic models and their applications.* Advanced Education Press.
3. Fang, J.Q. Mao, J.H., Zhou, W.Q. *et al.* (1995). Two-stage models, nonhomogeneous Markov chains, for cancer latent period. *Chinese Journal of Applied Probability and Statistics*, **11**(2). (in Chinese)

4. Fang, J.Q., Wu C.B. (1995). Two-stage model, counting process, and Bootstrap for cancer latent period. *Chinese Journal of Applied Probability and Statistics*, **11**(2). (in Chinese)
5. Fudan university (1981). *Stochastic processes.* Advanced Education Press. (in Chinese)
6. Gao, G.M. (2000). Probability models and Bayesian Analysis of capture-recapture data via Markov chain Monte Carlo simulation. *The Ph.D dissertation in Sun Yat-sen University.* (in Chinese)
7. Huang, Z.N. (1995). *Multiple Analysis in Medical.* Hunan Science and Technology Press. (in Chinese)
8. Mao, S.S., Wang, J.L., Pu X.L. (1998). *Advanced Statistics.* Advanced Education Press. (in Chinese)
9. Wang, Q., Jin P.H. (2000). Applications in economic hygiene for Markov model. *Chinese Journal of Health Statistics.* **17**(2): 86–88. (in Chinese)
10. Anderson, P. K., Borgan, ϕ, Gill, R.D. *et al* (1993). *Statistical Models Based on Counting Processes.* Springer-Verlag New York.
11. Chiang, C.L. (1980). *An Introduction to Stochastic Processes and their Application.* Robert E. Krieger Publishing Company, New York. (The Chinese version is translated by Fang J.Q. Shanghai translation press, 1986)
12. Chiang, C.L. (1983), *The Life Table and its Application.* (The Chinese version is translated by Fang J.Q. Shanghai translation press, 1984)
13. Faddy, M.J. and Fenlon, J.S. (1999). Stochastic modeling of the invasion process of nematodes in fly larvae. *Appl. Statist*, **48**, Part 1: 31–37.
14. Fang, Ji-Qian, Shi, Zhong-Lu, Wang, Yi *et al.* (1990). Parametric inference in a renewal process with time-dependent Covariates. *Biometrics*, **46**(3): 849–854.
15. Fang, J.Q., Ni, T.Y. Fan, Q. *et al.* (1996). Two-state stochastic models for memory in ion channels. *Acta Pharmacologica Sinica*, **17**(1): 13–18.
16. Green, P.J. (1995). Reversible jump Markov chain Monto Carlo computation and Bayesian model determination. *Biometrika* **82**(4): 711–732.
17. Lucas, W.F. (1983). *Modules in Applied Mathematics.* Vol. 4: Life Science Models. Springer-Verlag New York.
18. Parzen, E. (1962). *Stochastic Processes.* Holden-Day, San Francisco. (The Chinese version is translated by Deng Y.L., Yang Z.M., 1987).
19. Richard, J. B., Daniel, A. H. and Darren J.W. (2000). Detecting homogeneous segments in DNA sequences by hidden Markov models, *Appl. Statist.*, **49**, Part 2: 269–285.
20. Ross, S.M. (1983). *Stochastic Processes*, John Wiley & Sons Inc.
21. Geman, S. and Geman, D. (1984). Stochastic relaxation, Gibbs distributions and the Bayesian restoration of images. *IEER Trans. Pat. Anal. Mach. Intel.* **6**: 721–741.
22. Metropolis, N., Rosenbluth, A.W., Rosenbluth, M.N. *et al.* (1953). Equations of state calculations by fast computing machines. *J. Chem. Phys.* **21**: 1087–1091.

23. Hastings, W. K. (1970). Monte Carlo sampling methods using Markov chains and their applications.*Biometrika* **57**: 97–109.
24. Daley, D. J. and Gani, J. (2005). *Epidemic Modeling: An Introduction.* NY: Cambridge University Press.
25. Linda J.S. Allen. (2003). *An Introduction to Stochastic Processes with Biology Applications.* Prentice Hall.
26. Norden, R. (1982). On the distribution of the time to extinction in the stochastic logistic population model. *Adv. Appl. Probab.* **14**: 687–708.
27. O'Neill, P. D. and Roberts, G. O. (1999). Bayesian inference for partially observed stochastic epidemics. *J.R. Statist. Soc. A.* **162**: 121–129.
28. O'Neill, P. D. and Becker, N.G. (2001). Inference for an epidemic when susceptibility varies. *Biostatistics* **2**: 99–108.
29. Sars bulletin. *Technical report, Health, Welfare and Food Bureau,* Government of the Hong Kong Special Administrative Region, 10 June 2003. Available as http://www.info.gov.hk/info/sars/bulletin/bulletin0610e.pdf
30. Donelly, C. A., Ghani, A. C., Leung, G. M., *et al.* (2003). Epidemiological determinants of spread of causal agent of severe acute respiratory syndrome in Hong Kong. *The Lancet,* **361**: 1761–1766.
31. Riley, S., Fraser, C., Donnelly, C. A. *et al.* (2003). Transmission dynamics of the etiological agent of SARS in Hong Kong: Impact of Public Health Interventions, *Science,* **300**: 1961–1966. (deleted)
32. Lipsitch, M., Cohen, T., Cooper, B. *et al.* (2003). Transmission dynamics and control of severe acute respiratory syndrome, *Science,* **300**: 1966–1970.

About the Authors

Dr. Caixia Li is presently employed as Associate Professor at Sun Yat-Sen University in China. She received Master degree in Probability & Mathematical Statistics in 1996, and earned PhD degree in Medical Statistics & Epidemiology in 2002 from Sun Yat-Sen University. In 2006, she joined the post-doctoral program in Biostatistics at the University of California at San Francisco. In 2009, she returned to work at the Department of Statistics in Sun Yat-Sen University.

Ji-Qian Fang has been awarded "National Teaching Master" in 2009, and "Outstanding Contribution to Preventive Medicine" in 2010 by the Chinese Central Government. He is the leading professor in research and education of Medical statistics in China. Ji-Qian Fang was born in Shanghai 1939, earned his BS in 1961 from the Department of Mathematics, Fu Dan University and Ph.D in 1985 from the Program of Biostatistics, University of California at Berkeley. His Ph.D thesis studied multi-state survival analysis for life phenomena under the guidance of Professor Chin-Long Chiang. During 1985–1990, Dr. Fang was a Professor and Director, Department of Biostatistics and Biomathematics, Beijing Medical University. Since 1991, he has been the Director and Chair Professor, Department of Medical Statistics, Sun Yat-Sen University. Professor Fang was a visiting professor of University of Kent, UK in 1987 and Australian National University in 1990, as well as an adjunct professor of Chinese University of Hong Kong since 1993. He is the secretary for the Group China of International Biometric Society and vice president of Chinese Association of Health Informatics. Professor Fang has supervised many post graduate students and post-doctor fellows in medical statistics. His research projects widely covers various fields, including "Stochastic Models of Life Phenomena", "Gating Dynamics of Ion Channels", "Statistical Methods for Data on Quality of Life", "Health and Air Pollution", "Analysis of DNA Finger Printing", and "Linkage Analysis between Complex Trait and Multiple Genes" etc. These projects were sponsored by either the National Foundation of China or by International organizations, such as World Health Organization and European Commission. He is the chief editor of the textbook *Health Statistics* in Chinese (5, 6, 7-th ed.), and the co-editor of the monograph *Advanced Medical Statistics* in Chinese and English respectively (1st and 2nd Ed.).

CHAPTER 35

INTERPOLATION OF MISSING VALUES AND ADJUSTMENT OF MOVING HOLIDAY EFFECT IN TIME SERIES

ZHANG JIN-XIN*, ZHANG XI, XUE YUN-LIAN,
LI JI-BIN and HUANG BO

School of Public Health,
Sun Yat-Sen University, P.R. China
**zhjinx@mail.sysu.edu.cn*

In this chapter, we focus on two key issues: dealing with missing values and adjusting moving holiday effect in time series. For missing values, an interpolation method based on periodicity is introduced and then simulation study is applied in evaluating the interpolation effects in the first part of this chapter. The second part will explain how to adjust moving holiday effect in time series, which is commonly found in the dynamic data related to holidays corresponding with a lunar calendar.

1. Interpolation of Missing Values in Time Series Based on Statistically Significant Periodicity

1.1. *Background*

A relatively short sequence may reduce the stability of parameter estimation when fitting time series models. Therefore, a longer sequence is preferred in order to ensure the reliability of the model. In practice, the more historical observations the sequence covers, the more difficult data collection will become and the more likely missing values will occur.[1] If we ignore the missing values and fit the time series model directly based on the data, the model we get eventually will not reflect the true relations. For example, Fig. 1 shows a time series plot without missing values. Suppose there are three consecutive missing values (X_{35}, X_{36}, X_{37}) after observation X_{34}, we will get another plot (see Fig. 2) if we ignore the missing values and connect the two "break" sequences hastily. The ARIMA model is like the following

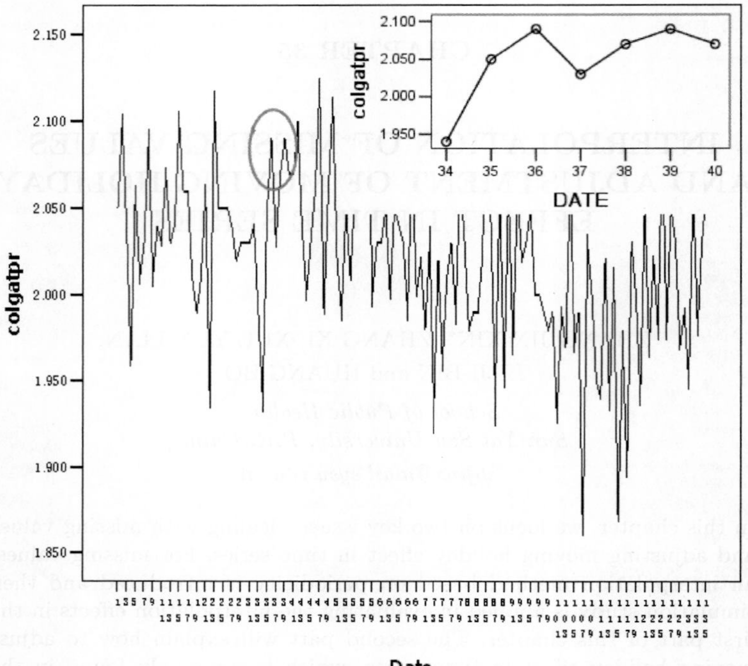

Fig. 1. Time series plot without missing values.

equation:

$$y_t = \varphi_1 y_{t-1} + \varphi_2 y_{t-2} + \cdots + \varphi_p y_{t-p} + a_t - \theta_1 a_{t-1} - \theta_2 a_{t-2} - \cdots - \theta_q a_{t-q} \quad (1)$$

There are 3 observations X_{35}–X_{37} between X_{34} and X_{38}, which can exert an influence on the estimation of parameter ϕ_4 in equation (1). If we delete them, X_{34} is next to X_{38} directly and then they will have an impact on the estimation of φ_2 ($\varphi_1, \varphi_2, \ldots, \varphi_p$ and $\theta_1, \theta_2, \ldots, \theta$ are autoregressive and moving average coefficients).

Generally there are two steps in processing data with missing values. Firstly, test the type of the missing values. Secondly, deal with the missing values with the appropriate operations. Classification criterion is based on Little and Rubin's missing mechanism theory.[2] Different treatments are required for different types. However, since any observation for different time points cannot be replaced in time series analysis, the genuine

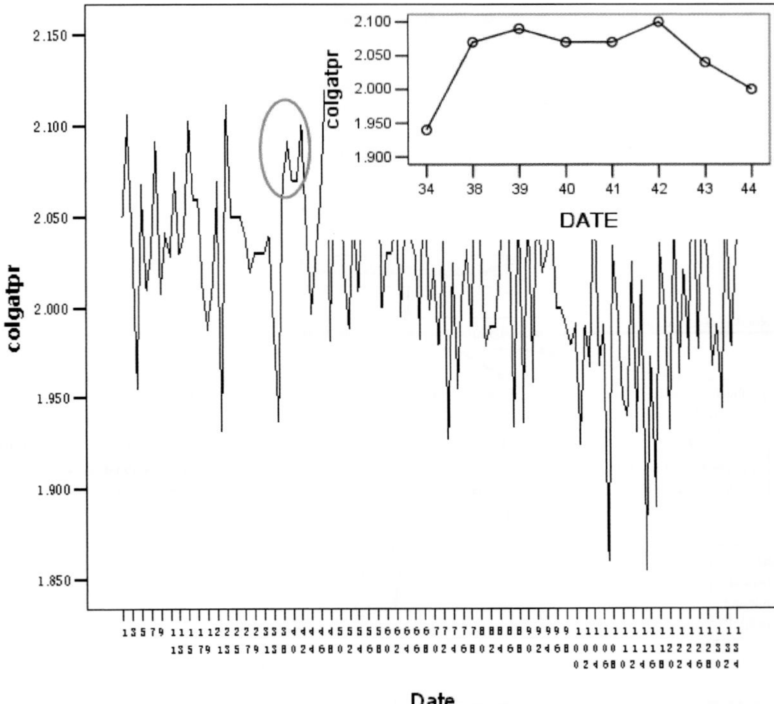

Fig. 2. Time series plot without missing values $X_{35} - X_{37}$.

correlation of real sequence will be misrepresented if the deletion operation is applied directly.

Several methods are used to deal with missing values but few are suitable for time series data. Time series data are "tall" and "thin": the data cover a long time and have only one single variable. So the general multiple interpolation and many other modern interpolation methods do not work in time series. Periodicity is an important frequency domain characteristic of the time-series. But many methods, such as ARIMA model estimation method, resample method, multiple imputations and so on, only use time domain information. These methods may be superior but cannot use frequency domain information sufficiently. Our research provides a new method to estimate the missing values of time series based on periodicity characteristic. Time-domain techniques and frequency domain techniques are both applied in this new method.

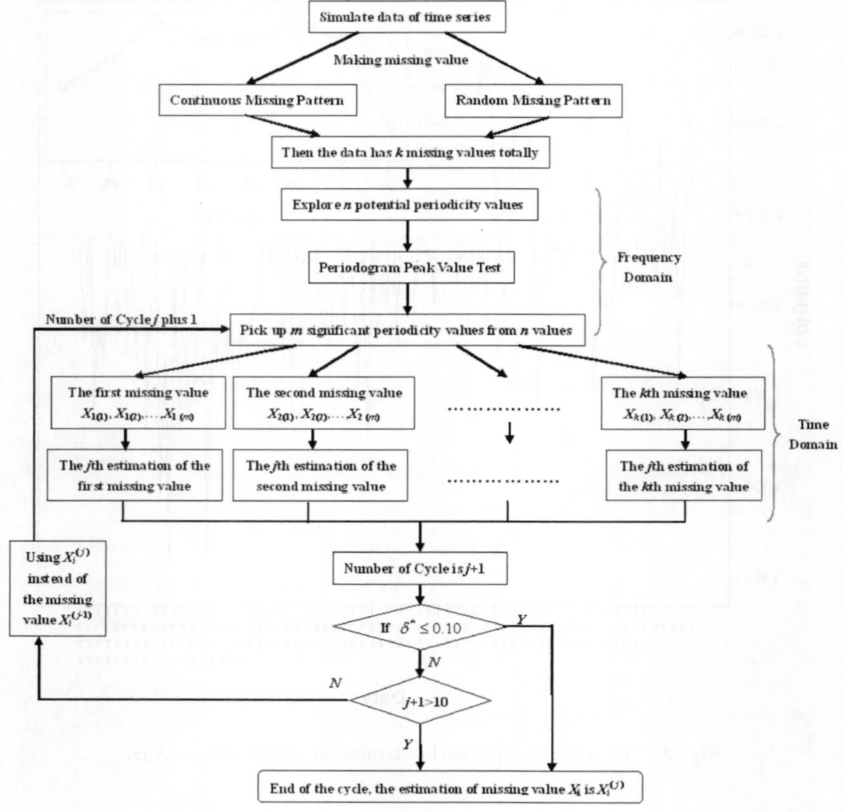

Fig. 3. Technology flow diagram of periodicity method.*

*δ can be computed by the formula as follows: $\delta = \max \left| \frac{X_i^{(j)} - X_i^{(j-1)}}{X_i^{(j-1)}} \right|$

1.2. *Methods*

1.2.1. *Research scheme*

Research scheme can be seen clearly from the technology flow diagram of this study (see Fig. 3).

ARMA model is a classical model in time series analysis.

j stands for the frequency of iteration, k represents the number of missing values, m indicates the number of period value;
T_m means the mth period value;

$X_{i(m)}$ means the estimation of ith missing value based on the mth significant statistical period value;
$X_i^{(j)}$ stands for the last estimation of ith missing value.

1.2.2. *Periodic test*

In this study, maximum periodogram method proposed by Fisher is used to explore the periodicity of time series. The statistics of this research are proposed by Priestley (1981)[3] and Chiu (1989)[4] and are calculated as follows:

$$U(r) = \frac{I_{n-r+1}}{\sum_{i=1}^{n} I_i}, \quad V(r) = \frac{I_{n-r+1}}{\sum_{i=1}^{n-r} I_i} \tag{2}$$

$$Z_1(r) = nU(r) - \ln(n - r + 1) \tag{3}$$

$$Z_2(r) = c(n - r)V(r) - \ln(n - r + 1) \tag{4}$$

$$c = 1 + \frac{r[\ln(\frac{r}{n})]}{n - r} \tag{5}$$

The probability distribution function of statistics is as follows:

$$P_i(r) = \exp\{-\exp[-Z_i(r)]\} \sum_{j=0}^{r-1} \exp\{-jZ_i(r)/j!\} \quad i = 1, 2 \tag{6}$$

The null hypothesis is "zero harmonics in X_t". Significant level is α. If $P_i(r) > (1 - \alpha), i = 1, 2$, then we accept H_1 and reject H_0. We arrange $n = \frac{T}{2}$ (T is the periodicity value) periodogram ordinates in ascending order as $I_1 < I_2 < \cdots < I_n$. Suppose r peak values are indicated by the statistics $U(r)$ or $V(r)$, then the estimation of the frequencies are taken to be the frequencies associated with the r periodogram ordinates $I_{n-r+1}, \ldots, I_n$. However, this test is only used to test the periodicity when (x_t) has exactly r hidden cycles. Actually, the test cannot be used directly as the number of hidden periods is unknown. So our study aims to determine the number of implicit initial value r by searching the periodogram for the number of peak values. Then test the peak values one by one in descending order. After that, determine the number of period values $k(k < r)$ which are statistically significant peak values. In the end, test whether the corresponding k period values are peak values through smoothing periodogram. If the value is significant, it will be ultimate period value of the sequence.

1.2.3. *Filling the missing values*

The fundamental steps of interpolation methods based on periodicity are as follows. First of all, search for hidden period values through periodic test. Suppose there are k values. Generally, we have $k > 3$. Secondly, divide the initial sequence into m sections. m is computed through the number of sequence over the period value. If there are f periodic values, then we will get f kinds of sequence division. Every section has many time points which can be called **period point**. The number of period points for each section is equal to the number of period values, so different sections with the same period can have the same number of period points. Then we can compute the proportion of missing values in every position which is exactly the means of missing values over the sum of observed values (exactly the sum of observed means) in the same section of one period, which means each missing value will have k proportions. After that, we can acquire the first estimation of missing value by actual sum of observed value timing means sum of observed in the section of missing value. The next step is to calculate the weighted means of k original estimations, weighted by the corresponding peak value of the periodogram. Finally, replace the missing values by the estimations and a complete sequence is acquired; then retest the new complete sequence, find new period values and repeat the previous steps till relative error of the value does not exceed 0.10. We will acquire the final estimation of the missing values. See Fig. 3.

1.2.4. *Evaluation of missing value estimation*

1.2.4.1. Comparison methods

Comparison method chosen in this research is cubic spline interpolation which is a common method of estimating missing values in time series. Time-series data is only a single variable sequence in many cases, so there is no auxiliary information provided by other related variables. That is partly why we chose the cubic spline as the contrast method.

1.2.4.2. Indicators of evaluation

Different indicators are applied in order to analyze the error (compare the errors between the two methods) and stability (examine the tolerance of missing proportional of the new method) of interpolation methods and explore application missing style of methods.

Evaluation of filling missing values is based on measuring the closeness of filling values and true values. The closer the filling value is with the true value, the better the filling method is. Generally, four evaluation indicators are applied[54]: Mean Error(*ME*), Absolute Mean Error(*AE*), Root Mean Square Error(*RMSE*) and Normalized Root Mean Square Error (*NRMSE*). Calculation formulas are as follows:

$$ME(\xi_i) = \sum_{n=1}^{N} (\hat{\xi}_{in} - \xi_i)/N \tag{7}$$

$$AE(\xi_i) = \sum_{n=1}^{N} \left|\hat{\xi}_{in} - \xi_i\right|/N \tag{8}$$

$$RMSE(\xi_i) = \sqrt{\sum_{n=1}^{N} (\hat{\xi}_{in} - \xi_i)^2/N} \tag{9}$$

$$NRMSE = \sqrt{\frac{\text{mean}[(\hat{\xi}_{in} - \xi_i)^2]}{\text{variance}(\xi_i)}} \tag{10}$$

$\hat{\xi}_{in}$ indicates the ith missing value estimation of nth times simulation, and ξ_i indicates the true value of missing observation of nth times simulation. N is the times of simulation, and $N = 100$ in this research. *NRMSE* value will change along with the change of the filling value. The smaller the *NRMSE* value is, the more precise the estimation $\hat{\xi}_{in}$ is. When $\hat{\xi}_{in}$ is extremely precise, *NRMSE* is almost equal to 0. In other words, the estimation of missing value is equal to the actual value as *NRMSE* is close to 0. Likewise, *RMSE* value states the same meaning as *NRMSE* value. The smaller *RMSE* value is, the more precise the filling value is.[6,7]

The significance of the three indicators is as follows. *RMSE* is a common indicator used to examine the degree of closeness of true value and corresponding missing estimation. This value can be used to discuss the distribution or gradual distribution of filling values. The sign and size of *ME* can show the system bias of missing estimation. *AE* does not have the above-mentioned advantages, but it is robust. *NRMSE* value can avoid the impacts of variations of different variables, which is the chosen indicator of this research.

1.3. *Results*

1.3.1. *Filling results of random missing pattern*

In simulation research, two kinds of missing styles, including random pattern and continuous pattern, are involved. Missing proportion and sequence

Table 1. *NRMSE* values of different missing proportions.

Missing proportion (%)	Mean difference$^{\triangle}$	SD	95% CI for mean difference *L*	*U*	*T*	*P*
10	−0.21	0.49	−0.31	−0.12	−4.41	<0.001*
20	−0.16	0.34	−0.23	−0.09	−4.62	<0.001*
30	−0.24	0.59	−0.36	−0.12	−4.06	<0.001*
40	−0.18	0.35	−0.24	−0.11	−5.06	<0.001*
50	−0.20	0.50	−0.30	−0.10	−4.03	<0.001*

$^{\triangle}$ Mean Difference: *NRMSE* value of periodicity method minus *NRMSE* value of spline;
$*P < 0.05$, the difference is statistically significant.

Table 2. *NRMSE* values of different sequence length.

Sequence length	Mean difference$^{\triangle}$	SD	95% CI for mean difference *L*	*U*	*T*	*P*
30	−0.37	2.12	−0.79	0.05	−1.77	0.080
50	−0.10	0.98	−0.29	0.10	−0.99	0.325
100	−0.14	0.67	−0.27	−0.01	−2.13	0.036*
200	−0.22	0.53	−0.32	−0.11	−4.12	<0.001*
250	−0.20	0.36	−0.27	−0.13	−5.56	<0.001*

$^{\triangle}$ Mean Difference: *NRMSE* value of periodicity method minus *NRMSE* value of spline;
$*P < 0.05$, the difference is statistically significant.

length are considered to be two key parameters in simulation of random pattern since they may affect the filling effectiveness. Considering missing proportion, we set 5 groups which have different proportions of missing observations, respectively. The proportions increase from 10% to 50% by 10%. Every group has 250 observations. In terms of sequence length, we set 6 groups with sequence length of 30, 50, 100, 150, 200 and 250, respectively.

Tables 1 and 2 show the filling results of two methods. In this study the missing style was random pattern and the sample size was 250, missing rates were from 10% to 50%.

For different missing proportions, the differences of *NRMSE* values between periodicity method and spline method are all statistically significant after testing by paired samples t test ($P < 0.01$). Therefore, we can conclude that two methods have different capability of filling missing values. Meanwhile, Fig. 4 shows the vertical variable NRMSE value varies along

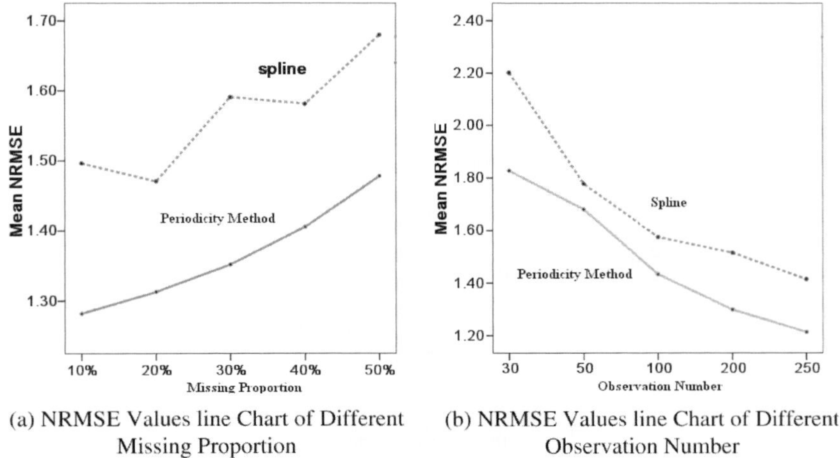

(a) NRMSE Values line Chart of Different Missing Proportion

(b) NRMSE Values line Chart of Different Observation Number

Fig. 4. *NRMSE* value line chart of different missing proportions and sequence length.

with the horizontal variable. The real line represents the result of spline method and the dashed line represents the result of periodicity method. In Fig. 4(a), X axis variable indicates missing proportion. The real line is always below the dashed line, which means the periodicity method is better than the spline method. The smaller *NRMSE* value is, the more precise the estimation of missing value is. Therefore, the periodicity method is a more precise method than spline method. Besides, *NRMSE* value increases as the missing proportion increases, which means the precision of two methods decreases when missing proportion rises. However, no matter what thesize of missing proportion is, periodicity method is always more precise than spline method. Another important phenomenon which can be seen clearly from Fig. 4(a) is the distances of the two lines stay at the same level with the increase of missing proportion, which indicates the two methods have the same variation tendency. X axis variable represents sequence length of missing values in Fig. 4(b). It can be seen that the dashed line is always over the real line. The difference is statistically significant (see Table 2). As the observation number ascends, the *NRMSE* value descends. We can conclude that periodicity method is more precise than spline method.

1.3.2. *Filling results of continuous missing pattern*

In continuous pattern, the number of missing values is considered in simulation. We set 6 groups with different numbers of missing values. The number rises from 5 to 30 by 5.

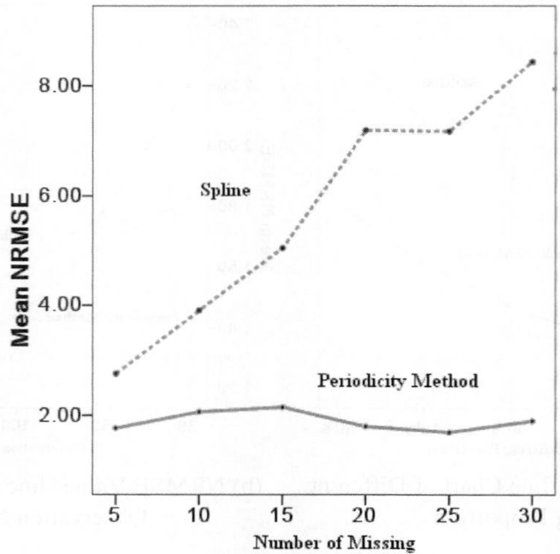

Fig. 5. *NRMSE* value line chart of different numbers of missing values.

Table 3. *NRMSE* values of different numbers of missing values.

Missing number	Mean difference$^{\triangle}$	SD	95% CI for mean difference L	95% CI for mean difference U	T	P
5	−0.99	1.70	−1.33	−0.65	−5.8	<0.001*
10	−1.84	5.54	−2.94	−0.74	−3.32	0.001*
15	−2.90	3.17	−3.53	−2.27	−9.13	<0.001*
20	−5.41	9.83	−7.37	−3.45	−5.47	<0.001*
25	−5.48	4.80	−6.43	−4.53	−11.42	<0.001*
30	−6.54	5.39	−7.60	−5.47	−12.13	<0.001*

$^{\triangle}$ Mean Difference: *NRMSE* value of periodicity method minus *NRMSE* value of spline;
$*P < 0.05$, the difference is statistically significant.

Figure 5 shows the *NRMSE* value of two methods changes along with the number of continuous missing values. The first thing that should be mentioned is that the dashed line is always over the real line, which means the *NRMSE* value of periodicity method is smaller than that of spline method. So the estimation of missing value based on periodicity is more precise than that of spline method. Also, the test shows the difference between the periodicity and the spline method is statistically significant ($P < 0.01$, see Table 3). Secondly, *NRMSE* value of spline method increases linearly

Table 4. *NRMSE* value of different missing proportions.

Missing proportion (%)	Mean difference$^{\triangle}$	SD	95% CI for Mean difference *L*	*U*	*T*	*P*
10	2.27	19.66	−1.63	6.17	1.16	0.25
20	−0.04	0.39	−0.12	0.03	−1.15	0.25
30	0.28	1.88	−0.10	0.65	1.47	0.14
40	0.71	2.59	0.20	1.23	2.76	0.01*
50	3.34	19.42	−0.51	7.19	1.72	0.09
60	13.93	49.07	4.19	23.67	2.84	0.01*

$^{\triangle}$ Mean Difference: *NRMSE* value of periodicity method minus *NRMSE* value of spline;
$*P < 0.05$, the difference is statistically significant.

while *NRMSE* value of periodicity method is nearly horizontal, which indicates that the periodicity method is more robust than spline method. In conclusion, the periodicity method is more precise and robust than spline method.

1.3.3. *Application results*

The data which comes from reference[8] is Northwest Pacific sea surface temperature field time series. There are 210 observations, and the sequence is from June 1, 1967 to December 1, 1984. The data is divided into 6 groups, which is the same as the simulated experiment.

1. Application results of random missing pattern

Table 4 is the test result of comparison between periodicity method and spline method. The difference of the *NRMSE* value for every missing proportion was tested.

Figure 6 represents the *NRMSE* value line chart. The y axis variable is means of *NRMSE* value in Fig. 6(a) while the y axis variable is the median of *NRMSE* value in Fig. 6(b). When missing proportion is from 10% to 30%, the mean differences of *NRMSE* values between the two methods are not statistically significant. The differences are statistically significant when missing proportion is 40% or 50%. When the missing proportion is lower than 30%, the *NRMSE* value of periodicity method is slightly larger than that of spline method. But the difference is not statistically significant ($P > 0.05$), which means the estimations of two methods are both suitable. When missing proportion is higher than 40%, the spline method seems more precise than the periodicity method. Another thing we can find is

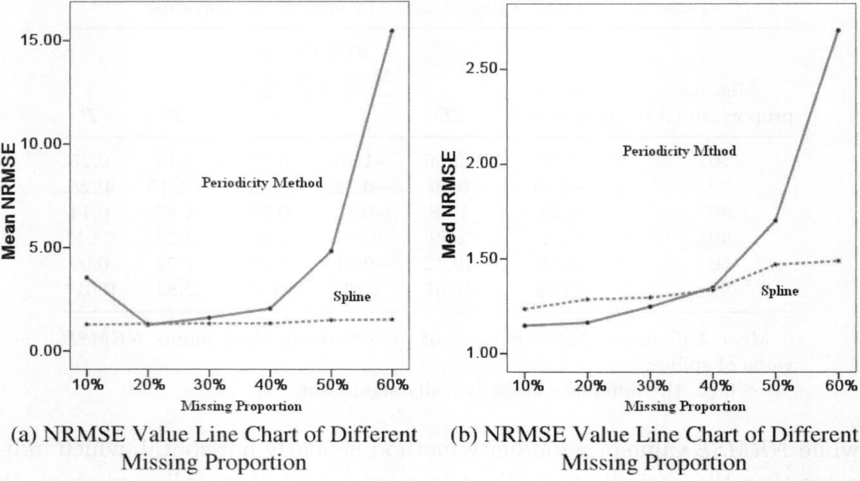

(a) NRMSE Value Line Chart of Different Missing Proportion

(b) NRMSE Value Line Chart of Different Missing Proportion

Fig. 6. *NRMSE* value line chart of different missing proportions.

that *NRMSE* value of periodicity method is changing quickly while *NRMSE* value of spline method is changing slowly. That means spline method is more robust than periodicity method. This result is different from the simulation result. We elaborate on the reason in theconclusion and discussion.

2. Application results of continuous missing pattern

Figure 7 and Table 5 are the results of factual application. We can conclude that the periodicity method is more precise and robust, which is the same as the simulation results.

1.4. *Conclusion and discussion*

A new method based on periodicity of time series is proposed to fill the missing values in the study. In order to evaluate the interpolation effects of periodicity method we compared the method with the spline method. There are two different types of missing values: random missing pattern and continuous missing pattern.

The results show that the interpolation effectiveness of periodicity method depends on the missing pattern. When dealing with random missing data, the periodicity method is no worse than spline method. In simulation study, the periodicity method showed better results than spline method. However, it is not the case in the actual application. Although the results of random missing are not perfect, periodicity method is always robust

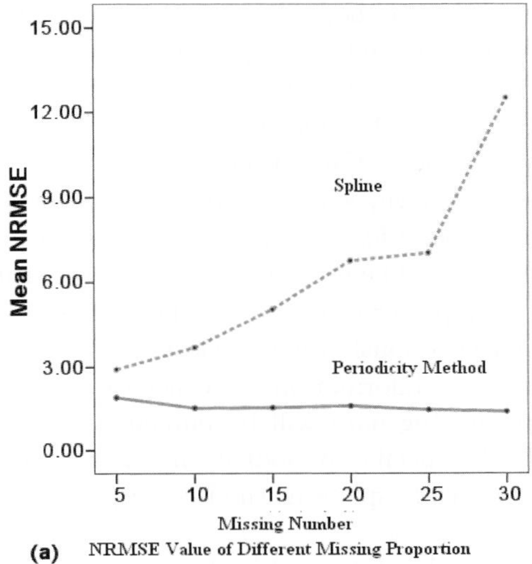

Fig. 7. *NRMSE* value line chart of different continuous missing number.

Table 5. *NRMSE* value of different numbers of missing values.

Missing number	Mean difference$^{\Delta}$	SD	95% CI for mean difference L	95% CI for mean difference U	T	P
5	−0.99	2.51	−1.49	−0.49	−3.93	<0.001*
10	−2.15	2.69	−2.68	−1.61	−7.98	<0.001*
15	−3.48	3.58	−4.19	−2.77	−9.71	<0.001*
20	−5.14	5.89	−6.31	−3.97	−8.72	<0.001*
25	−5.55	4.95	−6.53	−4.56	−11.20	<0.001*
30	−11.09	47.93	−20.60	−1.58	−2.31	0.023*

$^{\Delta}$ Mean Difference: *NRMSE* value of periodicity method minus *NRMSE* value of spline;
$^*P < 0.05$, the difference is statistically significant.

because *NRMSE* value remains almost the same as the missing proportion increases vigorously, while the spline method is quite the reverse. For random missing data, periodicity method displays satisfactory results no matter how tremendous the number of missing values is. For continuous missing pattern, periodicity method is more appropriate because it is more precise and robust in both simulation study and actual application.

Why does periodicity method perform well in continuous missing pattern but not so well in random missing pattern? The reason is that different methods rely on different information. The periodicity method is mainly based on the information of global time series while the spline method mainly depends on the local information of time series with missing values. For random missing pattern, when the missing proportion of time series data increases, the global information will decrease sharply while the local information of data can still be preserved. However, the situation is different for continuous missing pattern. As the missing number increases, the local information will be lost seriously while the loss of global information may be less compared with local information. So whichever method that is chosen when dealing with missing data will be influenced by the characteristics of missing data. To be specific, periodicity method corresponds to continuous missing pattern while spline method corresponds to random missing pattern.

The study has some limitations. Firstly, only two types of missing values (random pattern and continuous pattern) are considered. According to the results, periodicity method performs satisfactorily. The next step is to consider a more complicated situation, which is close to missing pattern of actual data. Besides, the periodicity can be used in dealing with irregular time series data. In addition, only a single variable time series data is considered, without considering multi-variable situation. The auxiliary information contained in other variables would help get better results.

2. Adjustment of Moving Holiday Effect for Daily Observation Sequence

In China, dates of some major festivals are determined by the lunar calendar. Hence, these holidays do not occur at a fixed date according to the Gregorian calendar but move from period to period over years. When these holidays take place, they tend to influence normal activities such as sales, production, service activity, inpatients, incidence rate of disease etc. Such effect is known as "moving holiday effect". Major moving holidays in the United States are Easter, Labor Day and Thanksgiving Day. In China, holidays tied to a lunar calendar are the Chinese New Year, Lantern Festival, Mid-Autumn Festival and Dragon-Boat Festival.

When the date of a holiday shifts from year to year, it can affect time series two or more months in a way that depends on the date. This will violate the comparability for the same month between different years.

Alper(2004)[9] pointed out that moving holidays could reduce the forecasting ability of a model fitting for time series. Specially, in the context of a regression problem, if such seasonal fluctuations affect the dependent and independent variables differently, the precision of estimation to coefficients will decrease. Thury(2005)[10] pointed out that calendar effects in monthly time series can sometimes cause considerable distortions in analytical tools such as the correlogram. By removing the moving holiday effect, the important features of economic series such as direction, turning points and consistency between several economic indicators could be easily identified (Ashley, 2001).[21] Shuja(2007)[11] stated that with consideration to the movement of holiday interval in seasonal adjustment process can avoid biased seasonally adjustment and trend estimation.

2.1. *Daylength-based proportional model*

X-12-ARIMA program which was designed by the American Census Bureau can be used to adjust moving holiday effects mentioned above. Holiday effects for one or several holidays can be estimated with built-in or user-defined regressors by means of a *reg*-ARIMA model (regression models with ARIMA errors), which can be denoted by formula (11)

$$\phi(B)\Phi(B^s)(1-B)^d(1-B^s)^D\left(Y_t-\sum_i \beta_i X_{it}\right)=\theta(B)\Theta(B^s)\varepsilon_t \tag{11}$$

Where B is the backshift operator ($BY_t = Y_{t-1}$); s is the seasonal period; $p(P)$, $d(D)$, and $q(Q)$ are integers greater than or equal to zero and respectively refer to the order of the autoregressive, integrated, and moving average of non-seasonal (seasonal) parts of the model; ε_t is independent identically distributed (*iid*), with mean zero and variance σ^2 (white noise); Y_t is dependent time series; X_{it} are regression variables observed concurrently with Y_t (such as trading day effect, leap year and seasonal effect); β_i are regression parameters; $Z_t = Y_t - \sum_i \beta_i X_{it}$ are time series of regression errors, which is assumed to follow the SARIMA(Seasonal ARIMA) model.

Moving holidays can be included in X-12-ARIMA program as regression variables. Bell and Hillmer(1983)[12] used a simple type of regressor to model effects of a variety of moving holidays that was proven to be versatile. With τ_t denoting the number of days in month t that belong to holiday interval, τ is the number of days in holiday interval. The value in month t of the holiday regressor $H(\tau,t) = \frac{\tau_t}{\tau}$ associated with this interval is defined to be the proportion of the interval contained within the month. It takes on the value zero for a particular month if the interval does not overlap with that month.

Although one single regressor is sufficient for modeling some moving holidays, such as Easter in the U.S and Chinese New Year, most series indicate changing activities around the holiday. Typically, the economic activity surges before the holiday, stops during the holiday and slowly accelerates after the holiday. Therefore, more researchers suggest using two or three regressors to adjust moving holiday effects. Those regression variables can be computed by the following formulas: $H_i(\tau_i, t) = \frac{\tau_{it}}{\tau_i}$. $H_1(\tau_1, t) = \frac{\tau_{1t}}{\tau_1}$, $H_2(\tau_2, t) = \frac{\tau_{2t}}{\tau_2}$, $H_3(\tau_3, t) = \frac{\tau_{3t}}{\tau_3}$, which respectively stand for effects of before, around and after the holiday.

Although X-12 ARIMA software explicitly includes a correction factor for the Easter effect, the correction is based on a North American Easter holiday interval. Findley and Soukup (2000)[13] noted that the X-12 ARIMA is only able to remove the holiday effect as experienced in the United States i.e. Easter, Labor Day and Thanksgiving, and has limitations in removing moving holiday effect that is tied to a lunar calendar, such as Chinese New Year. The software X-12-ARIMA was just used for American moving holidays, so Chinese moving holidays should be manually computed and included as user-defined variables.

The above methods of computing regression variables are all based on the length of the holiday intervals and premise the effects are the same for each day. In this chapter, we call them daylength-based proportional models. But they may fail to match the actual situation. In the following part of this chapter, we propose a method called observation-based proportional model, which is based on daily observations and considers unstable changes of observations among holiday intervals.

2.2. *Intervals of moving holiday effect*

One major question in adjustment of moving holiday is determination of the length of τ, since it is unknown in advance. Models with different τ are non-nested, hence a typical likelihood ratio test for model comparison is not appropriate. Findley and Soukup (2000) suggested two alternative approaches to address this model selection problem. One is using the AICC criterion proposed by Hurvich and Tsai (1989),[14] which is a modification of Akaike's AIC criterion. The other is comparison of out-of-sample forecast errors. As to two models with different number of intervals or lengths of intervals, the model with smallest AICC and out-of-sample forecast errors is preferred.

However, one must have a priori knowledge of the holiday effect and its length of intervals first and then can determine several models with different τ. That is to say, without prior knowledge, all the optional models with different holiday variables can be far away from the actuality. Besides, this method needs one to do the adjustment of moving holiday first, and it seems to be a too hard job for those inexperienced people to fulfill. It is very important to identify intervals of moving holiday effect properly and easily.

In addition to this introduction, section 2.3 illustrates those adverse effects of moving holidays using an inpatients sequence as an example. Section 2.4 expounds several methods to determine τ. Section 2.5 puts forward a new method called observation-based proportional model to determine $H(\tau, t)$ and provides the comparison of simulation results between observation-based proportional model and daylength-based proportional model. Conclusions are derived in section 2.6.

2.3. *Adverse effects of moving holidays*

In this section, we illustrate the adverse effects of moving holiday effect by comparing the period-to-period growth rate, sequence chart, periodogram and predicted values of the actual series and the adjusted series. The practical example is inpatients sequence from January 2002 to December 2007 in Foshan City of Guangdong province, China. We use observation-based proportional model to determine regressors of the moving holiday, which will be introduced in section 2.5.

Table 6 shows that there is no comparability of growth rate for actual series. For example, the period-to-period growth rate of Jan and Feb in 2004 is 0.9407 and 1.5421, but in 2005 is 1.3625 and 0.7899. However, for the adjustment series, the growth rates of Jan and Feb during the six years are comparable, which indicates that the inpatients sequence is affected by the moving Chinese New Year, and the adjustment method is necessary. It can also be found that the adjusted series eliminated the annual decline around the Chinese New Year which appeared before from the sequence chart (Fig. 8).

It can be seen from Fig. 9 that peak heights of the adjusted and pre-adjusted series are inconsistent. After periodic test (Fisher g test) of the adjusted and pre-adjust series, we found that the 12-month and 6-month periodicity was removed and the real 7-month periodicity was discovered in the adjusted series. Also, the adjusted series retained other statistical

Table 6. Observations and period-to-period growth rate of the actual and adjusted series.

	Actual series				Adjusted series			
	observations		growth rate		observations		growth rate	
Year	Jan	Feb	Jan	Feb	Jan	Feb	Jan	Feb
2002	7259	4601			7203.37	6499.21		
2003	7957	5348	1.0962	1.1624	7935.59	7174.04	1.1589	1.2177
2004	7485	8247	0.9407	1.5421	9196.44	8735.94	1.1234	1.1465
2005	10198	6514	1.3625	0.7899	10331.74	10015.66	1.1230	1.1049
2006	9723	8352	0.9534	1.2822	11602.78	11066.08	1.1889	1.1690
2007	13795	8805	1.4188	1.0542	13795.00	12936.42	1.1016	1.1038

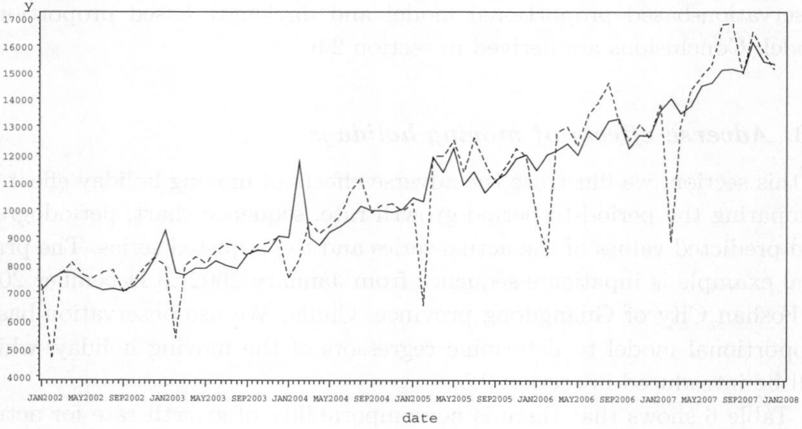

Fig. 8. Sequence chart of pre- and adjusted- series.
Notes: Dotted line represents pre-adjust series. Solid line represents adjusted series.

significance periodicities of the sequence, which considered better adjusted effects(Cleveland,1980; Soukup,1999).[15,16]

Table 7 provides the results of the paired Wilcoxon rank sum test about 1–3 step ahead absolute forecast errors. We use a 5-year length sequence (60 monthly observations point) as a fixed forecast period; then move the sequence from the beginning to the end of the series by one unit each time till the last forecasting value meets with the last real observation. According to this method, the sample size N is 10, from the 60th observation to the 69th observation. We would get ten 1–3 step ahead forecasts;

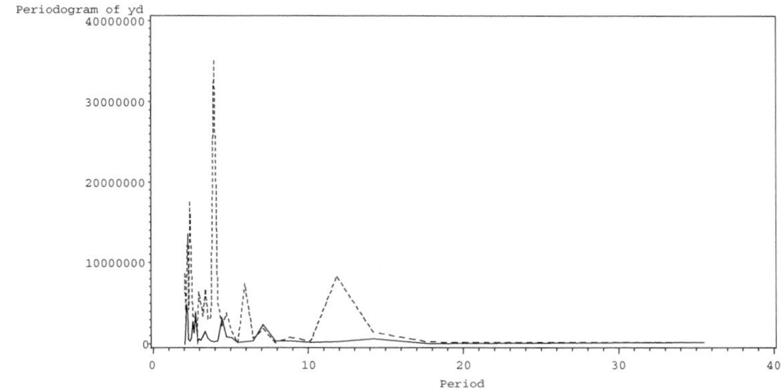

Fig. 9. Periodogram of pre- and adjusted-series.

Notes: Dotted line represents pre-adjust series. Solid line represents adjusted series.

Table 7. 1–3 step ahead absolute forecast errors of adjusted and pre-adjust series.*

Forecast	Series	$\overline{\chi}$ (1)	S (2)	M (3)	d_P_{25} (4)	d_P_{50} (5)	d_P_{75} (6)	d_S (7)	d_P (8)
1	Adjusted	520.608	408.178	427.581	353.611	551.093	874.601	24.5	0.01
	Pre-adjust	1170.087	680.272	1249.116					
2	Adjusted	598.916	377.888	518.626	181.178	440.317	1058.493	24.5	0.01
	Pre-adjust	1139.818	645.663	1340.966					
3	Adjusted	564.446	441.313	452.799	182.427	372.368	1070.326	27.5	0.002
	Pre-adjust	1071.358	666.118	847.345					

**Note*: (1)$\overline{\chi}$: mean of forecast error; (2) S: standard error of forecast error; (3) M: median of forecast error; (4) d_P_{25}: lower quartile of difference for forecast error of adjusted and pre-adjust series; (5) d_P_{50}: median of difference for forecast error of adjusted and pre-adjust series; (6) d_P_{75}: upper quartile of difference for forecast error of adjusted and pre-adjust series; (7) d_S: standard error of difference for forecast error of adjusted and pre-adjust series; (8) d_P: probability of difference for forecast error of adjusted and pre-adjust series.

then compute corresponding forecasting errors for 1–3 step ahead forecasts, respectively. We can see from Table 7 that the absolute forecast errors of adjusted series are significantly less than the pre-adjusted errors, indicating that the adjustment of Chinese New Year effect is successful.

2.4. *Methods of determining the moving holiday effects*

The length of moving holiday intervals is directly related to the adjustment effect of moving holidays and the predictive efficiency of adjusted series. Although statisticians use AICC and out-of-sample forecast errors

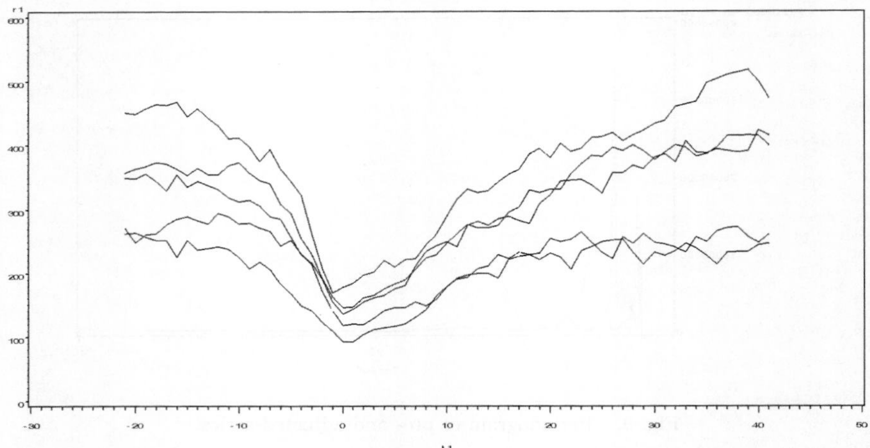

Fig. 10. Year-by-year sequence chart using daily observations in 1–4 month with Chinese New Year as mid-point.

to determine numbers of holiday intervals and length of each one (τ), they must have prior knowledge of the sequence and influence of the moving holidays. However, not all the people are good at the fields.

We propose some new methods based on literature review to identify numbers of holiday intervals and length of each one. The following four methods are proven to be effective.

2.4.1. *Year-by-year sequence chart*

We draw a year-by-year sequence chart (see Fig. 10, taking Chinese New Year for example) using daily observations in months (it refers to 1–4 month) that could be affected by moving holidays with holiday date as mid-point. If the sequence shows the same abnormal changes, we can conclude that it is affected by moving holiday effects. Furthermore, we can identify its pattern and determine its initial length.

2.4.2. *Paired t test*

Paired t test is applied to check which days are affected by the moving holiday. Theoretically, there are unstable changes for observations in moving holiday interval. Therefore, whether the observations fall into moving holiday interval can be determined by comparing observations in certain dates with the mean of yearly totals. The Chinese New Year for example, can mainly affect Jan, Feb and Mar. So paired t test is used to compare daily observations in the three months and the mean of yearly totals except observations in these three months. For those days with $P < 0.05$, we take them as moving holiday intervals. Also, the sign and size of their mean differences should also be considered in order to determine the number of segments and the start-stop points of the moving holiday interval.

2.4.3. *Selection criteria*

The former two methods are used to determine several possible models with different moving holiday intervals. Although these methods are simple and intuitive, they are not likely to have a uniform standard for the choice of a model. Findley (2005)[17] pointed that there is no standard statistical test to determine proper moving holiday interval. He proposed two criteria for model selection: AICC criterion and out-of-sample forecast errors. Firstly, the adjustment is necessary by taking each model that contains different moving holiday intervals into X-12-ARIMA software. After that, the two criteria are used to select the model. The moving holiday interval of the model with smallest AICC or forecasting error is the terminal one of the series (Lin 2002).[18]

Although out-of-sample forecast error can be used to compare models with different holiday intervals in terms of forecasting aspect, it can only compare two models at a time. Besides, it cannot indicate which model is better if the graph fluctuates markedly or remains horizontal. Therefore, AICC is preferred to do comparisons.

AICC (F-adjusted Akaike's information criterion) is a correction of Akaike's AIC criterion after considering the factor of sample size, which was proposed by Hurvich and Tsai (1989).[13] AICC is defined as below:

$$AICC = -2\log likelihood + 2p\frac{1}{1-(p+1)/(T-12D-d)} \tag{12}$$

Where p is the number of estimated parameters, D is the order of seasonal difference, and d is the order of regular difference. The model with the smallest AICC value is preferred. AICC can be applied when there are models with the same values of d and D and the same outlier regressors.

2.4.4. *Forecast error*

Although AICC is preferred for many statisticians, it is a parameter for retrospective fitting. We prefer perspective forecasting aspect to compare models with different holiday intervals. In this chapter, a stepwise forecast error is proposed to compare two models with different moving holiday intervals using daily observation series. We can not only compute each step ahead forecast error but also can obtain the testing P values of two models. The calculation steps are as follows:

For sequence with length N, take n as fixed forecast period (for monthly data, $60 \leq n \leq N - p$), move it from the beginning to the end of the sequence by one unit each time till the last forecasting value meet with the last real observation. Moving times can be considered as the sample size. In order to compare two models, we calculate their forecast errors separately and use paired Wilcoxon rank sum test. If $P \leq 0.05$, their forecast errors are statistically different. Then we need to compare medians of absolute forecast errors of the two sequences to determine which model is better. Of course, the one with smaller absolute forecast error is better from the point of prediction.

2.5. *Comparison of two proportional models*

2.5.1. *Introduction of two proportional models*

This chapter is aimed at introducing adjustment method of moving holiday effect for daily series. Currently, most articles use the same identification method of moving holiday intervals, which is based on the length of the holiday intervals and need to premise that effects are the same for each day. We call it "daylength-based proportional model". When using this model, only monthly observations of the sequence are required to do adjustment of moving holidays. In order to determine different intervals of length τ and patterns of the moving holiday effect, one should have a prior knowledge of the sequence. The set of interval length τ for daylength-based proportional model (represented by model one) can be seen in part 2-section 2.1.

Considering the disadvantages of daylength-based proportional model, we propose an observation-based proportional model (represented by model two), which uses daily observations to identify interval length τ which can be seen in Section 2.3. For observation-based proportional model, observations falling into month t each moving holiday interval are used to determine regressors of the moving holiday effect. Specifically, τ is the sum of observations in holiday interval, with τ_t denoting the sum of observations in month t that belong to holiday interval. If the value of the holiday regressor $H(\tau, t) = \frac{\tau_t}{\tau}$ in month t is associated with holiday interval, we can define it as the proportion of sum of observations contained within the month

t that belong to interval. The value can be zero for a particular month if the interval does not correspond to that month.

2.5.2. *Simulation*

In order to compare these two proportional models, Sine function $Y = abs(\sin(\omega x))$ and normal distribution function $X = M + sqrt(SQ) \times rannor(seed)$ are used to simulate 50 series which start from 1988.01.01 to 2007.12.31 with different random fluctuation levels of $\mu = 0$, $\sigma^2 = 6$ and $\mu = 100$, $\sigma^2 = 400$, respectively. Periods of the sequence are 3 and 12 months.

Based on these series, we add three common patterns of moving holiday (refers to Chinese New Year) effect. Three patterns can be explained through three examples. For instance, inpatients sequence declines before the holiday, stops during the holiday and slowly increases after the holiday (Fig. 11, named pattern one, graphic symbol is D); train capacity sequence increases before the holiday, decreases during the holiday and slowly increases after the holiday (Fig. 12, named pattern two, graphic symbol is T); energy production sequence increases before the holiday, stops during the holiday and slowly declines after the holiday (Fig. 13, named pattern three, graphic symbol is U). For each pattern, we add two different lengths of holiday effect intervals: short intervals and long intervals. To be specific, short intervals last for 13 days, including 5 days before holiday, 3 days during holiday and 5 days after holiday; long intervals last for 48 days, including 14 days before holiday, 3 days during holiday and 31 days after holiday. Accordingly, graphic symbols of series with different moving holiday effect in this study are D13, D48, T13, T48, U13 and U48.

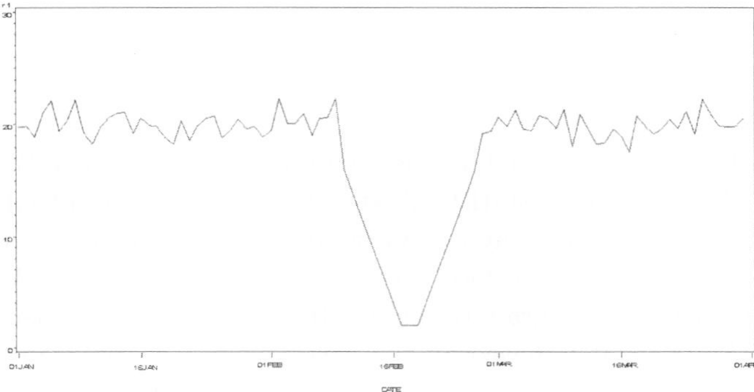

Fig. 11. Sequence chart of pattern one.

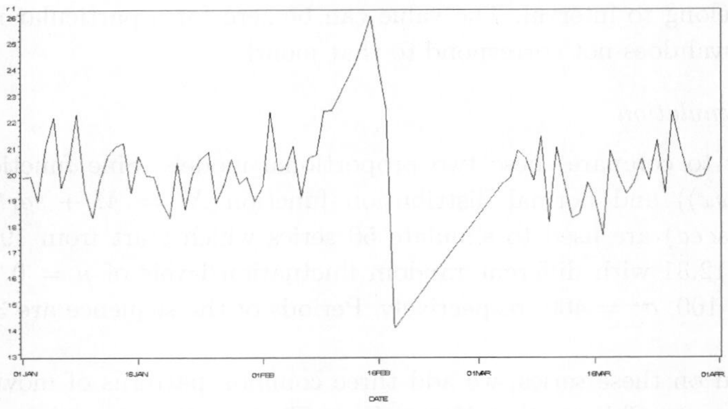

Fig. 12. Sequence chart of pattern two.

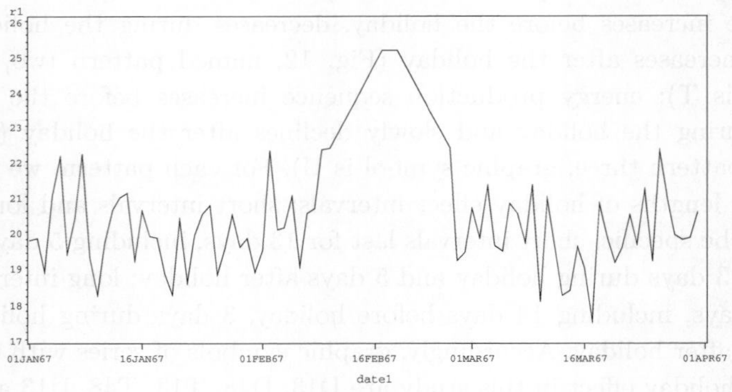

Fig. 13. Sequence chart of pattern three.

2.5.3. *Statistical packages*

The statistical packages used in this study are SAS 8.2 and X-12-ARIMA. SAS, the abbreviation of Statistical Analysis System, is used to do simulation work, set moving holiday regressors, draw basic sequence charts, compute forecast errors and perform hypothesis tests. X-12-ARIMA is a new seasonal adjustment program developed by the Bureau of Census, United States of America. It is based on the well-known X-11 program (Shiskin, 1967)[19] and Statistics Canada's X-11-ARIMA and X-11-ARIMA/88 (Dagum, 1988).[20] It uses regressors to adjust moving holiday effect and obtain AICC indicator. X-12-ARIMA package is available from the website http://www.census.gov/srd/www/x12a/x12down_pc.html#x12other, See also U.S. Bureau of the Census (2000).

2.5.4. *Comparison indicators*

AICC and forecast errors, which are introduced in Sections 2.4.3 and 2.4.4 of this chapter, are two key comparison indicators of the adjustment of moving holiday effects between two models.

Different conditions are set to compare adjustment effects of two proportional models. In this study, we propose the strength of moving holiday effect to do comparison. Strength of moving holiday effect is a measurement of influence from moving holidays to observations, indicated by the area of observations higher or lower than average years (except months affected by moving holidays).

2.5.5. *Results*

Two proportional models are applied to adjust the moving holiday effects, respectively (see Table 8. Average level sequence is made up by mean value in each time point of 50 sequences. From Table 8, we can see that from the point of average level sequence, AICC of model 2 is smaller than model 1 except D13. From the point of 50 sequences, the differences of AICC are of no statistical significance when $\mu = 0$; when $\mu = 400$, the differences of AICC are statistically significant for all six kinds of series.

We compute absolute forecast errors of two proportional models to compare their forecast results (see Figs. 14 and 15). When fluctuation level is low, the median curve of forecast errors fluctuates around zero reference line, which indicates that the absolute forecast errors of two proportional models are of small difference. When increasing fluctuation level of the sequence, the median curve of forecast errors fluctuates away from the zero reference line for most sequences, which means the absolute forecast errors of two proportional models may be different.

In order to further compare the absolute forecast errors of two proportional models, we separately compute 1–12 step ahead forecast errors of the adjusted series, and do paired Wilcoxon rank sum test. Here we only give comparison results of 1,6,12 steps ahead forecast errors (see Table 9). We use 5-year length (60 monthly observations point) as a fixed forecast period, move it from beginning to the end of the series by one unit each time till the last forecasting value meet with the last real observation. Accordingly,

Table 8. AICC of 6 kinds of series on two random fluctuation levels for mean and 50 sequences.*

Fluctuation level	Series	Average level Sequence				50 Sequences						
		Area	Model 2	Model 1	d	$n(d>0)$	$n(d<0)$	$n(d=0)$	$\overline{\chi}$	S	t	P
$\mu = 0$	D13	9.114	1110.302	1109.962	0.339	22	28	0	−2.461	17.720	−0.980	0.331
$\sigma^2 = 6$	D48	25.823	1167.871	1169.667	−1.796	28	22	0	0.761	4.641	1.160	0.252
	T13	7.791	1111.820	1117.314	−5.494	21	29	0	1.181	36.398	0.230	0.819
	T48	14.072	1140.784	1155.963	−15.179	21	29	0	−1.096	7.082	−1.090	0.279
	U13	15.190	1114.873	1116.305	−1.432	22	28	0	1.583	8.503	1.320	0.194
	U48	23.886	1213.392	1221.637	−8.245	18	31	1	−2.845	18.208	−1.110	0.275
$\mu = 400$	D13	2888.97	2519.016	2526.198	−7.182	0	50	0	−11.464	5.861	−13.83	<0.001
$\sigma^2 = 100$	D48	8185.43	2641.843	2940.146	−298.302	0	50	0	−211.174	42.076	−32.53	<0.001
	T13	2527.10	2269.822	2522.030	−252.208	14	36	0	−7.851	12.719	−4.36	<0.001
	T48	4766.81	2328.134	2666.328	−338.194	0	50	0	−143.278	36.537	−27.45	<0.001
	U13	4814.96	2578.642	2624.263	−45.622	0	50	0	−36.831	9.993	−26.06	<0.001
	U48	7571.52	2541.306	2705.914	−164.608	0	50	0	−212.115	59.835	−24.81	<0.001

* *Note*: Difference of AICC = AICC of model 2- AICC of model 1;
Model 1 is daylength-based proportional model; Model 2 is observation-based proportional model

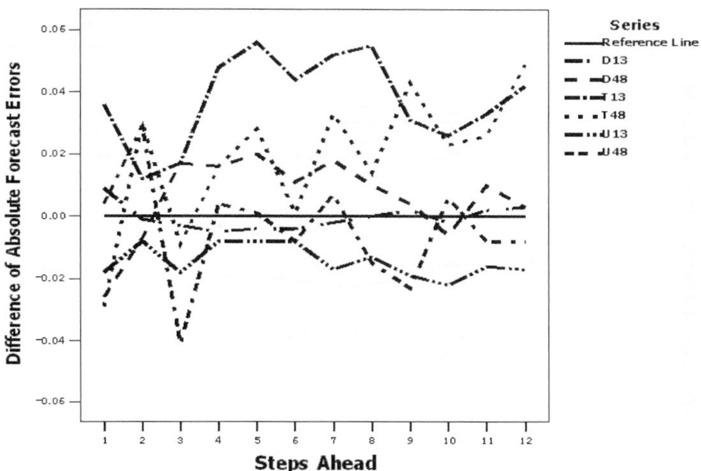

Fig. 14. Sequence chart of medians of absolute forecast errors for average level sequence with $\mu = 0$, $\sigma^2 = 6$.

Note: Difference of absolute forecast error = absolute forecast error of model 2- absolute forecast error of model 1.
Model 1 is daylength-based proportional model; Model 2 is observation-based proportional model.

we do 1–12 step ahead forecast with sample size $N = 109$, and compute corresponding forecast errors. From Table 9 we can see that when $\mu = 0$, although the absolute forecast errors of two proportional models are different, there is no statistical significance. When $\mu = 400$, the absolute forecast errors of two proportional models are statistically significant except for D13 and U13.

To sum up, when strength of moving holiday effect is small, fitting and forecasting results of observation-based proportional model and daylength-based proportional model are considerable. When increasing fluctuation level of the sequence and the strength of the moving holiday effect, observation-based proportional model has better fitting and forecasting results for four out of six series(except D13 and U13).

Also, we can see that different kinds of patterns have different sensitivity to the strength of moving holiday effect. Judging from the fitting and forecasting results of two proportional models, T pattern is more sensitive. However, D and U patterns show low sensitivity because only if the effect is long enough, will the forecast results of observation-based proportional model be better.

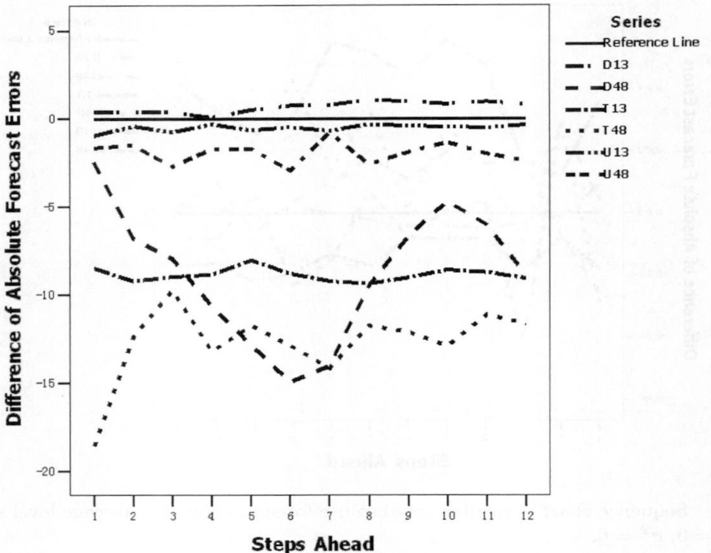

Fig. 15. Sequence chart of medians of absolute forecast errors for average level sequence with $\mu = 400$, $\sigma^2 = 100$.

Note: Difference of absolute forecast error = absolute forecast error of model 2- absolute forecast error of model 1.

Model 1 is daylength-based proportional model; Model 2 is observation-based proportional model.

After checking the regressors of two proportional models, we found that daylength-based proportional model only uses day length information which falls into each month among each holiday interval and assumes that observations in each holiday interval are level. However, observation-based proportional model uses daily observation in moving holiday interval to determine regressor and concludes abnormal changes in each interval. Therefore, when the strength of moving holiday effect is small, the fluctuation level of sequence is low, which means the amplitude of fluctuations is as small as level changes to sequence, so fitting and forecasting results of two proportional models are of no difference. When the intensity of moving holiday effect increases, fluctuation level of sequence is high, which means amplitude of fluctuations is big enough from level changes, so observation-based proportional model has better fitting and forecasting results.

Therefore, when fluctuation level of the sequence is high and intensity of moving holiday effect is large, the observation-based proportional model is strongly recommended.

Table 9. Test results of absolute forecast errors (d) of two proportional models ($N = 109$).*

Series	Steps ahead	fluctuation level with $\mu = 0$, $\sigma^2 = 6$					fluctuation level with $\mu = 400$, $\sigma^2 = 100$				
		P_{25}	P_{50}	P_{75}	S	P	P_{25}	P_{50}	P_{75}	S	P
D13	1	−0.072	0.009	0.070	92.500	0.781	−2.709	0.414	3.125	0.682	0.497
	6	−0.034	−0.004	0.036	−124.500	0.709	−2.017	0.758	3.517	0.910	0.365
	12	−0.012	0.003	0.029	434.500	0.190	−2.188	0.824	3.747	1.215	0.227
D48	1	−0.135	−0.026	0.113	−193.500	0.561	−74.885	−2.422	3.485	−1167.500	<0.001
	6	−0.074	0.011	0.115	310.500	0.350	−181.110	−14.943	−0.206	−1950.500	<0.001
	12	−0.072	0.003	0.103	274.500	0.409	−49.360	−8.906	1.260	−1765.500	<0.001
T13	1	−0.239	0.036	0.268	106.500	0.749	−21.112	−8.481	−0.950	−5.525	<0.001
	6	−0.121	0.044	0.147	344.500	0.300	−17.219	−8.801	−0.240	−5.318	<0.001
	12	−0.081	0.042	0.143	477.500	0.150	−17.348	−9.081	1.018	−5.168	<0.001
T48	1	−0.269	−0.029	0.333	6.500	0.984	−35.800	−18.584	−4.881	−6.072	<0.001
	6	−0.129	0.001	0.255	372.500	0.262	−29.117	−12.894	−1.529	−5.353	<0.001
	12	−0.119	0.049	0.257	721.500	0.029	−30.471	−11.649	−2.317	−5.174	<0.001
U13	1	−0.099	−0.018	0.070	−391.500	0.238	−4.015	−0.925	3.374	−1.870	0.064
	6	−0.058	−0.008	0.036	−437.500	0.187	−3.460	−0.470	2.123	−1.948	0.054
	12	−0.043	−0.017	0.039	−458.500	0.167	−3.812	−0.353	2.058	−2.078	0.040
U48	1	−0.343	0.004	0.330	−56.500	0.865	−8.346	−1.633	4.825	−2.869	0.005
	6	−0.172	−0.008	0.149	−136.500	0.682	−8.545	−2.918	4.260	−2.696	0.008
	12	−0.155	−0.008	0.189	31.500	0.925	−8.854	−2.389	3.384	−3.160	0.002

* *Note*: Difference of absolute forecast error = absolute forecast error of model 2- absolute forecast error of model 1; Model 1 is daylength-based proportional model; Model 2 is observation-based proportional model.

2.6. *Conclusion*

In this study, we have illustrated the impacts of moving holiday effect to observations by taking inpatients sequence as an example. Also, we proposed an improved adjustment method of moving holiday effect which is based on size of daily observations, called observation-based proportional model. The improvements of this model mainly can be reflected in two aspects. Firstly, the model that can determine the numbers and lengths of moving holiday intervals is more reasonable and accurate. Secondly, the model can take the abnormal changes of observations among moving holiday into account fully.

The observation-based proportional model we have introduced here can only be used for daily observation sequence and cannot be used to deal with monthly or yearly observation sequence. According to the simulation results of the two proportional models, we can see that when intensity of moving holiday effect is small, the adjustment effects of two proportional models are similar; when the intensity of moving holiday effect increases, observation-based proportional model has better fitting and forecasting effects. In conclusion, observation-based proportional model is worthy of strong recommendation to deal with daily observation sequence for the adjustment of moving holiday effects.

Acknowledgments

We are very grateful to Demetra P. Lytras and David F. Findley for their help in giving us software and theoretical support with X-12-ARIMA. We also gratefully thank for Yuewei Liu of Huazhong University of Science and Technology in PR China for his kindly help in programming.

References

1. Pascal, B. (2005). Influence of missing values on the prediction of a stationary time series. *Journal of time series analysis* **26**(4): 519–525.
2. Little, R. J. A., Rubin, D. B. (1987). *Statistical Analysis with Missing Data.* Wiley and Sons, Inc., New York..
3. Priestley, M. (1981). *Spectral Analysis and Time Series*, Academic Press, London.
4. Chiu, S. (1989). Detecting periodic components in a white Gaussian time series. *J. R. Statistic. Soc. B* **51**: 249–259.

5. Junninena, H., Niskaa, H., Tuppurainenc, K., *et al.* (2004). Methods for imputation of missing values in air quality data sets. *Atmospheric Environment* **38**(18): 2895–2907.
6. Xingyi, L., Nong, G. (2007). Comparing Several Popular Missing Data Imputation Methods. *Journal of Nanning Teachers College* **24**(3): 148–150. (In Chinese).
7. Zhang, X., Wang, H., Song, X. (2007). A non-parametric imputation method for microarray missing values. *Computers and Applied Chemistry* **24**(12): 1611–1616. (In Chinese)
8. Jia, X. (2005). Analysis of Time Series of Sea Surface Temperature in Northwest Pacific. *Master's work thesis*, Capital Normal University, Beijing (In Chinese).
9. Alper, C. E., Aruoba, S. B. (2004). Moving Holidays and Seasonal Adjustment: The Case of Turkey. *Review of Middle East Economics and Finance* **2**(3): 203–209.
10. Thury, G., Zhou, M. (2005) Calendar effects in monthly time series models. *Journal of Systems Science and Systems Engineering* **14**(2): 218–230.
11. Shuja, N., Lazim, M. A., Wah, Y. B. (2007). Moving Holiday Effects Adjustment for Malaysian Economic Time Series. *Journal of the Department of Statistics* **1**(1): 35–50.
12. Bell, W. R., Hillmer, S. C. (1983). Modeling Time Series with Calendar Variation. *Journal of the American Statistical Association* **78**(383): 526–534.
13. Findley, D. F., Soukup, R. J. (2000). Modeling and Model Selection for Moving Holidays. *Proceeding of the American Statistical Association Business and Economic Statistics Section*: 102–107.
14. Hurvich, C. M., Tsai, C. L. (1989). Regression and time series model selection in small samples. *Biometrika* **76**(2): 297–307.
15. Cleveland, W. S., Devlin, S. J. (1980). Calendar Effects in Monthly Time Series: Detection by Spectrum Analysis and Graphical Methods. *Journal of the American Statistical Association* **75**(371): 487–496.
16. Soukup, R. J., Findley, D.F. (1999). On the Spectrum Diagnostics Used by X-12-ARIMA to Indicate the Presence of Trading Day Effects after Modeling or Adjustment. *Journal of the American Statistical Association*: 144–149.
17. Findley, D. F., Wills, K., Monsell, B.C. (2005). Issues in Estimating Easter Regressions Using RegARIMA Models with X-12-ARIMA. http://www.census.gov/ts/papers/jem2005bcm.pdf.
18. Lin, J. L., Liu, T. S. (2002). Modeling lunar calendar holiday effects in Taiwan. *Taiwan Forecasting and Economic Policy Journal* **33**(2): 1–37.
19. Shiskin, J., Young, A. H., Musgrave, J. C. (1967). The X-11 Variant of the Census Method II Seasonal Adjustment Program. U.S.: *Department of Commerce, Bureau of the Census.*
20. Dagum, E. B. (1988). The X-11-ARIMA/88 Seasonal Adjustment Method: Foundations and User's Manual. *Statistics Canada*, Ottawa.
21. Ashley, J. D. (2001). Why Seasonal Adjustment. *U.S. Census Bureau.*

About the Authors

Zhang Jinxin, Associate Professor, obtained his doctoral degree of Epidemiology and Biostatistics in the Fourth Military Medical University in 2000. Since 2003, Dr. Zhang has worked in School of Public Health, Sun Yat-Sen University. He is the chair of the Department of Medical Statistics and Epidemiology in the school. Dr. Zhang's major research interests lie in developing statistical methods and its medical applications. He is particularly interested in developing statistical methods for design and data analysis of medical study and time series analysis in medicine. Dr. Zhang has hosted many research projects including the project from the Natural Science Foundation of China. He published more than 100 academic papers either in Chinese or English journals. Meanwhile, he is a reviewer of several journals such as *Chinese Journal of Preventive Medicine, Chinese Journal of Health Statistics, et al.*

Zhang Xi, Ph.D, Post doctor, Peking University Health Science Center, Beijing, China. Xi received her Bachelor of Medicine degree in 2006 from Shanxi Medical University. In 2006, Xi entered Sun Yat-Sen University for a Master of epidemiology and hygienic statistics degree in School of Public Health and involved research of the statistical methods of missing values. After obtaining the Master degree, she shifted to Fudan University for a doctoral degree of statistics in School of Public Health and continueed research on missing values in causal effect estimation. She works as a post-doctoral fellow in Peking University Health Science Center in Beijing now. Her research focuses on the statistical methods of missing values in casual inference, and methods when there are non-compliances in randomized controlled clinical trials.

Xue Yunlian, was born in Linyi, Shandong province. She works on hospital statistics as an assistant statistician in Sun Yat-Sen Memorial Hospital, Sun Yat-Sen Sniversity. She hasparticipated in the writing of the books, *Course of statistical analysis in SAS language*, *Correctly carrying out scientific research and statistical analysis*', *Medical statistics: using three forms theory to do modern regression analysis* and published 29 papers, 10 for which she was the first author in the last five years.

Li Ji-bin, had research interest in interpolation of missing values when he was a candidate for master degree in Sun Yat-Sen University. He is now a candidate for doctorate degree in the Chinese University of Hong Kong.

Huang Bo, has research interest in sample size estimation for multilevel data. She has published several papers on the application of mixed linear model.

CHAPTER 36

TREE-BASED METHODS

HEPING ZHANG
Department of Epidemiology and Public Health,
Yale University School of Medicine,
New Haven, CT 06520-8034, USA
heping.zhang@yale.edu

1. Introduction

In this chapter, I describe the developments and applications of tree-based methods. The thrust of these methods is the *recursive partitioning* technique that facilitates a process to divide an initially heterogeneous sample of observations into smaller subgroups within each of which the outcome of interest is relatively homogeneous.

The book by Breiman *et al.*[2] on classification and regression trees (CART^{TM}) is the milestone of the tree-based methodology. It provides much historical background and describes the methods and applications systematically. The associated CART program has become a commercial software. Since 1984, there has been a great deal of methodological developments as well as applications of tree-based methods, particularly in the area of survival trees. As in CART, the idea of recursive partitioning is still the heart and soul of the more recently developed methods. Please refer to Zhang and Singer[28] for a detailed introduction to those methods.

The rest of this chapter is organized as follows. First, the basic ingredients in CART is introduced. Then, survival trees is described. Finally, tree-based methods for analyzing multiple correlated responses is discussed.

2. The Basics of CART

One of the important and original applications of CART was to develop expert systems that can assist physicians in diagnosing patients potentially suffering heart attacks. Traditionally, the physicians made diagnoses in a

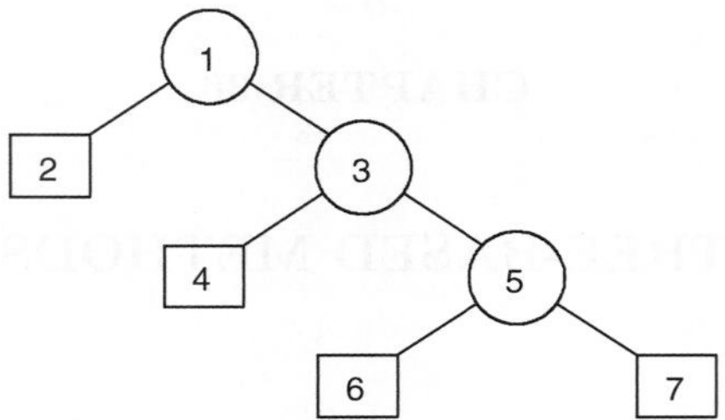

Fig. 1. A sample tree structure.

subjective, intuitive, idiosyncratic manner. A data-driven classification tree would enable the physician to interpret a patient's conditions by taking advantage of the empirical information from a large number of patients with similar conditions.[20] Now, the applications of the tree-based methods are far reaching.[1,3,4,8,11,12,14,24,27]

CART is arguably the most popular method among classification trees. All of tree-based approaches have in common the successive partitioning of a "feature space" of predictors into subsets. The partitioning is done on the basis of a *learning sample*, and it is sometimes validated by a *test sample*. Some of classification trees make use of a multi-level partition of a non-terminal node (a sub-group of the learning sample that is subject to a further division). However, only binary trees will be presented, i.e. a non-terminal node has exactly two daughter nodes. It is noteworthy that a tree that is constructed in a binary manner is not confined to be presented in the same manner as illustrated in Figure 1 of Zhang and Bracken[27] for the sake of an easier interpretation. In other words, a multi-level partition can be derived in principle by repeated binary partitions on the same variable.

Suppose that we have collected p covariates $\mathbf{x}$ and a response y from n subjects. For the ith subject, the measurements are

$$\mathbf{x}_i = (x_{i1}, \ldots, x_{ip})' \quad \text{and} \quad y_i, i = 1, \ldots, n.$$

The objective is to model the probability distribution of $P(y \mid \mathbf{x})$ or sometimes a function of this probability. The covariates $\mathbf{x}$ can be an array of mixed categorical (nominal or ordinal) and continuous variables, and they may have missing values for some subjects. In this section, we consider a single response y of either a categorical or continuous form. Later sections will deal with censored response or multiple responses. The characteristics of y mandate the choice of methodology.

Let us begin with an arbitrary tree as depicted in Figure 1. This tree has four layers of nodes. In general, the number of layers varies from case to case. At the top is the unique root node. Including the root node, there are three non-terminal, or internal nodes. They are represented by the circles and labeled as $1, 3$, and 5. The tree has four terminal nodes, represented by boxes and labeled as 2, 4, 6, and 7. The root and the internal nodes are connected to two nodes in the next layer that are called left and right daughter nodes, whereas the terminal nodes do not have "offspring." Moreover, the tree is not necessarily symmetric in that one of the two daughter nodes can be an internal node and the other a terminal one; for instance, nodes 2 and 3 are both the daughter nodes of node 1, and node 2 is terminal whereas node 3 is internal. The connection from a parent node to the two daughter nodes is determined by a splitting rule that I will elaborate in detail shortly.

Although the details and the implementation are complex, the nutshell of tree construction is really a few key questions: (a) How are the nodes determined from the data? (b) How do we split a node? (c) When does a node become terminal? I divide the answers to these questions in two steps: tree growing and tree pruning. After a tree is constructed, we need to interpret the tree structure and make statistical inferences to reveal the relationships among the predictors and the response. This issue is important and may determine the final tree, but it belongs to the use and interpretation of trees and does not have a clear-cut answer.

2.1. *Tree growing through node splitting*

Node is the most basic element of a tree. A node is simply a collection of observations. For example, the root node contains the learning sample, namely, all of the observations that are used during a tree construction. All nodes except the root node are subsets of the learning sample. When an internal node is divided into its daughter nodes, it means that a subset of the sample is further divided into sub-groups. Because the node division is exclusive, the terminal nodes are disjoint subgroups of the learning sample and the union of all terminal nodes is the root node.

The tree growing procedure begins with the split of the root node into its two daughter nodes. Once this is done, the resulting two daughters can be split recursively in the same way. This is why the procedure is called recursive partitioning. Obviously, the fundamental step is to partition one parent node (e.g. the root node) to the two daughter nodes. How do we split a node? The division of the root node is carried out through a predictor.

The purpose of splitting is to generate two daughter nodes within which the distributions of the response are more homogeneous than that in the parent node. Every predictor in $\mathbf{x}$ competes against another to achieve a combined maximum homogeneities in the two daughters. If x_j is an ordered covariate such as age, two subgroups result from the question of the form "Is $x_j > c$?" Here the cutoff point c is in the range of the observed values of x_j. The ith subject goes to the right or left node according to whether or not $x_{ij} > c$. The number of such distinct questions that can be asked upon an ordered covariate is one fewer than the number of the distinctly observed value of x_j. On the other hand, if x_j is nominal such as nationality, we can send a subject to the left or right node by asking questions such as "is the subject an Asian?" and "is the subject a Hispanic or an African?" If x_j has k levels, we can ask $2^{k-1} - 1$ meaningfully different questions, considering that the designation of left and right daughter nodes is arbitrary. For example, if x_j has four levels, A, B, C, and D, we can make seven distinct cut as follows: $\{A\}, \{B\}, \{C\}, \{D\}, \{A, B\}, \{A, C\}$, and $\{A, D\}$. We do not list $\{B, C\}$ and others, because its compliment $\{A, D\}$ is listed and asking "$x_{ij} \in \{B, C\}$?" or "$x_{ij} \in \{A, D\}$?" has the same effect. Considering p covariates and the number of possible cutoff points from each of them, we see that there are usually many possibilities to split a parent node into two daughter nodes. Therefore, we need a criterion to decide which split is preferable over the rest. This leads to the concept of impurity.

Let us use age as a predictor and cancer status as the response to explain how to evaluate the splits for a node (t) based on this age predictor. Suppose that we consider an age cutoff at c, e.g. 35. As a result of the question "Is x_j (age) $> c$ (35)?", we have the following table:

		Normal	Cancer	
Left Node (t_L)	$x_j \leq c$	n_{11}	n_{12}	$n_{1\cdot}$
Right Node (t_R)	$x_j > c$	n_{21}	n_{22}	$n_{2\cdot}$
		$n_{\cdot 1}$	$n_{\cdot 2}$	

What do we like to see? As stated earlier, we want a split such that the distributions of y in the daughter nodes are homogeneous. In other words, we would like to push as many observations as possible either along the diagonal n_{11}, n_{22} or along the off-diagonal n_{12}, n_{21}. A perfect example is $n_{11} = n_{22} = 0$. In this case, the two nodes are pure (or completely homogeneous) because each of them contains either the cancer patients only or the normal subjects only. In contrast, their parent node includes a mixture of n_{21} normal subjects and n_{12} cancer patients. Thus, the two daughter nodes are "more desirable" than their parent node. However, in most applications, whether the daughter nodes are more desirable than their parent node is not so clear cut and it generally requires a mathematical criterion to make the comparison.

One commonly used measure of node impurity for a categorical response is defined through the entropy function as follows:

$$i(t_L) = -\frac{n_{11}}{n_{1\cdot}} \log\left(\frac{n_{11}}{n_{1\cdot}}\right) - \frac{n_{12}}{n_{1\cdot}} \log\left(\frac{n_{12}}{n_{1\cdot}}\right). \tag{1}$$

Likewise, $i(t_R)$ and $i(t)$ can be defined. Then, we select a split that minimizes the weighted node impurity:

$$\frac{n_{\cdot 1}}{n} i(t_L) + \frac{n_{\cdot 2}}{n} i(t_R), \tag{2}$$

which can be regarded as the node splitting criterion.

For the later discussions, it is useful to note that $-i(t_L)$ is simply the maximum log likelihood of y by assuming that it follows a binomial distribution in node t_L. Minimizing criterion (2) is amount to maximizing the likelihood or homogeneity in this case.

When y is a continuous response, a node is pure when the responses within the node equal to the same constant. However, when the within-node responses are not constant, commonly used node impurity measures are the within-node variance and the absolute distance toward the median.

So far, I have described the splitting procedure based on completely observed ages from all subjects. In the presence of missing ages for some subjects, two strategies are available to deal with the splitting. One makes use of surrogate splits. The idea is this. If we cannot use age to decide how to send a subject to the left or right daughter node due to missing information, we try to find a split based on another predictor that hopefully resembles the age split sufficiently. The other strategy is much easier. We simply create another level for missing values. Then, all subjects with missing information will be sent to the same daughter node.

2.2. *Tree pruning by determining terminal nodes*

Applying the node splitting procedure described above to the root node, then to the resulting daughter nodes, and so on, we usually end up with a tree of excessive nodes. We do not need to worry about when to stop the recursive partitioning process because it stops by itself when further splitting is not possible or meaningless. In an extreme case, for example, we cannot split a node with one observation. And, the number of study subjects is always finite. What we need to be concerned with is how to deal with a tree of excessive size. In usual practice, such a tree is too large to be useful and trustworthy. This is why we need the tree pruning step to trim off some over-fitting nodes. Let us pretend that the tree in Figure 1 is large and subject to pruning. We need to address the question: "can we prune away some of the nodes?" If we have a general answer for this question, then we can prune any tree.

Tree pruning starts at the bottom of a tree, and the pruned tree is a subtree of the original one. Thus, pruning the tree in Figure 1 is equivalent to selecting one of its subtrees. The latter requires a measure of tree quality, reflecting our objective of extracting homogeneous subgroups of the study sample. Whether we construct trees for classification or prediction purpose, we make our decision based on the distributions of the response in the terminal nodes. All internal nodes play an intermediate role ultimately to lead to relatively homogeneous terminal nodes. Therefore, the quality of a tree depends on the quality of its terminal nodes. Let $Q(T)$ denote a certain quality measure of tree T, and we have

$$Q(T) = \sum_{t \in \tilde{T}} p(t)q(t), \tag{3}$$

where $\tilde{T}$ is the set of terminal nodes of tree T, $q(t)$ summarizes the quality of node t, and $p(t)$ is the proportion of subjects falling into node t.

For binary outcomes, $q(t)$ is usually replaced with the within-node misclassification cost $r(t)$, and $Q(T)$ with a tree misclassification cost $R(T)$. In other words, a tree is assessed by

$$R(T) = \sum_{t \in \tilde{T}} p(t)r(t).$$

There are two types of misclassifications, each of which is associated with a certain misclassification cost. The misclassification cost should reflect the severity of the error, for instance, when a cancer patient is classified to be cancer free or vice versa. Let $C(i|j)$ be the misclassification cost that a class j patient is classified as a class i patient. Here, we there are two classes of subjects: 0 for normal and 1 for cancer patients. For medical reasons, it is natural to choose $C(0|1) > C(1|0)$ because the consequence is potentially more severe when a patient with disease is wrongly diagnosed than when a normal person is classified to have the disease. Without loss of generality, we can set $C(1|0) = 1$ as the cost unit and let $C(0|1) = c$, which means that the a false positive diagnosis costs as many as c false negative ones. In addition, there is no cost when the classification is correct, namely, $C(i|i) = 0$. Unless a node is pure, we make mistakes one way or another. The within-node misclassification cost is the minimum of the two possible misclassification costs.

Although defining the measure in Eq. (3) is easy, using it is not straightforward unless there is an independent set of sample–the so-called test sample. When a test sample is available, we can estimate $p(t)$ and $r(t)$ from it, leading to an estimate of $R(T)$. Then, we can select a subtree that has the lowest estimated cost $\widehat{R}(T)$. However, in many applications, such a second sample is not feasible or too costly. Sample re-use methods are used as an alternative. For these methods, the size of a tree is another important aspect, indicating the tree complexity. Note that the total number of nodes in a tree, T, is $2|\tilde{T}| - 1$, where $|\tilde{T}|$ is the number of the terminal nodes of T. Hence, the complexity of T can be defined directly as $|\tilde{T}|$. Usually, a unit penalty, called a complexity parameter, is assigned to each terminal node, and the sum of these penalties becomes the penalty for the tree complexity. Therefore, the final quality measure of a tree is the following cost-complexity:

$$R_\alpha(T) = R(T) + \alpha|\tilde{T}|, \tag{4}$$

where $\alpha(>0)$ is the complexity parameter.

For a given complexity parameter and an initial tree such as the one in Figure 1, there is a unique smallest subtree of the initial tree that minimizes the cost-complexity measure Eq. (4). Importantly, if $\alpha_1 > \alpha_2$ the optimally pruned subtree corresponding to α_1 turns out to be a subtree of the one corresponding to α_2. So, as we increase the complexity parameter, we have a sequence of nested optimally pruned subtrees. The fact that the successive optimally pruned subtrees are nested can entail important savings in computation.[2] This nested sequence of subtrees has a finite length, because the number of subtrees is finite, and the last one is the root node. On the other hand, the complexity parameter takes a continuous value, which implies that an interval of the complexity parameter must correspond to the same subtree. Let T_0 be the initial tree. To prune off some nodes from T_0, we need to find the smallest α, denote by α_1, to allow some of the terminal nodes to be removed such that $R_{\alpha_1}(T_1)$ for the pruned T_1 is better than $R_{\alpha_1}(T_0)$ of the initial tree. It turns out

$$\alpha_1 = \min_{t \in \tilde{T}_0} \frac{r(t)p(t) - R(T(t))}{|\tilde{T}(t)| - 1},$$

where $T(t)$ represents a tree rooted at node t. Likewise, we proceed to find the next smallest α, denote by α_2, to allow some of the terminal nodes to be removed from T_1 such that $R_{\alpha_2}(T_2)$ for the pruned T_2 is better than $R_{\alpha_2}(T_1)$. As we continue this process until we reach the tree with the single root node, we end up with a sequence of increasing complexity parameters $\{\alpha_i\}_0^m$ (here $\alpha_0 = 0$) and a sequence of nested and shrinking subtrees $\{T_i\}_0^m$ (here T_m is the single root node tree).

The next step is to select a subtree from the nested sequence, and a cross-validation procedure is usually recommended. For example, we can randomly divide the study sample into several, say 5, sub-samples of about the same size. We use 4 of the 5 sub-samples to grow a large tree and prune it using the sequence $\{\alpha_i\}_0^m$ that leads to a new sequence of subtrees. Then, we compute $R(T)$ for each of those subtrees based on the left-over subsample, giving us one set of estimates for $\{R(T_i)\}_0^m$. We can do this 5 times and the average will be the final estimates for $\{R(T_i)\}_0^m$. With this sequence of estimates, we can select the subtree with the smallest or near the smallest $\hat{R}(T)$. Please refer to Breiman *et al.*[2] and Zhang and Singer[28] for details. Once the subtree is selected, the pruning step is accomplished.

3. Survival Trees

Although CART is a well-known brand name, the most frequently used tree-based method in biomedical research is survival trees, partly because survival analysis per se is a major topic in the health sciences. In this section, how to adapt the ideas expressed above for censored survival data will be explained. We face the same basic issues. One is to define a splitting criterion to divide a node into two, and the other is to choose a "right-sized" tree for subsequent use. Many criteria have been proposed in the literature, but they differ primarily in the way of declaring what daughter nodes are desirable. A few major ideas have emerged. First, as in CART, we can split a node to achieve better impurities in its daughter nodes. The concept of impurity is very intuitive in CART; however, for survival trees, we have to decide what we mean by node impurity. The second idea is to maximize the distributional difference between the two daughter nodes. In classical ANOVA, reducing within-group variances increases the between-group variances. But, for survival trees, it is not clear that reducing node impurity increases the distributional difference between the two daughter nodes. Finally, as hinted earlier, there is a connection between node impurity and maximum likelihood in CART. Although this connection may not hold in survival trees, we can nonetheless base our splitting decision on likelihood. In the following, the focus will be on presenting the approaches that have been implemented in the author's STREE program. Also see Zhang and Singer[28] and Zhang *et al.*[25]

3.1. *Use of the difference*

I begin the introduction of splitting rules with the use of Wasserstein metrics to measure the between-nodes distributional difference as proposed by Gordon and Olshen.[13] The within-node survival distribution is estimated by the Kaplan–Meier curve.[17] A desirable split can be characterized as one that results in two very different survival functions in the daughter nodes. Gordon and Olshen[13] used the so-called L^p Wasserstein metrics, $d_p(\cdot, \cdot)$, as the measure of discrepancy between the two survival functions. Specifically, for $p = 1$, the Wasserstein distance, $d_1(S_L, S_R)$, between two Kaplan–Meier curves, S_L and S_R, is the area sandwiched by the two Kaplan–Meier curves. Suppose that S_L and S_R are respectively the Kaplan–Meier curves for the left and right daughter nodes. We choose the split that maximizes the distance, $d_1(S_L, S_R)$. As before, we employ the recursive partitioning process to produce an initially large tree that will be pruned later.

A standard approach for comparing the survival times of two groups is the log-rank test. Thus, it is no surprise in the literature that the log-rank test is also used to separate the left and right daughter nodes. Indeed, Ciampi *et al.*[6] and Segal[18] adopted the log-rank test statistic as the splitting criterion.

3.2. *Use of likelihood functions*

One very flexible way of forming a splitting criterion is to use likelihood functions. Not only is this true for survival trees, but it is also the case for analyzing more complex responses. This approach is useful and convenient because we can assume a simple within-node distribution when we assess a split or node. In fact, a few likelihood based splitting and pruning criteria have been proposed. Davis and Anderson[9] assume that the survival function within any given node is an exponential function with a constant hazard. LeBlanc and Crowley[15] and Ciampi *et al.*[7] assume the proportional hazard models in two daughter nodes, but the hazard functions are unknown, but they respectively used the full and partial likelihoods for maximization.

3.3. *Use of impurity*

Note that we observe a binary death indicator and the (failure or censored) time. If we take these two outcomes for the separately for the momently, we can compute the within-node impurity, i_δ, of the death indicator and the within-node variation, i_y, of the time toward the median. By considering both of them together, we have the within-node impurity for both the death indicator and the time using a weighted combination, $w_\delta i_\delta + w_y i_y$. Zhang[21] examined a similar approach and recommended some choices of weights w_δ and w_y. Even though this approach does not fully incorporate the relationship between the censoring and observed time variables, existing evidence suggests that this simple extension outperforms the more sophisticated ones in discovering the underlying structures of data.

3.4. *Pruning survival trees*

I explained various ways of growing a survival tree. There is also a variety of options to prune a survival tree. We need the same recipes as before: a quality measure and a cost-complexity of a tree. They enable us use the cross validation procedure again to finish the pruning step.

Gordon and Olshen[13] suggested using the deviation of survival times toward their median as a measure of node quality $q(t)$ for a node t and (4) as the cost-complexity where $R(T)$ is taken as $Q(T)$.

In addition, a variety of tree cost-complexities has also been proposed by using the likelihood ratio statistic that compares the survival times in a parent node with those in its daughter nodes. A related method due to Therneau *et al.*[19] makes use of what are termed martingale residuals from the Cox model as the input to a cost-complexity scheme using least squares as the cost.

LeBlanc and Crowley[16] introduced the notion of "goodness-of-split" complexity as a substitute for cost-complexity in pruning the tree. Now, let $q(t)$ be the value of the log-rank test at node t. Then the split-complexity measure is

$$Q(T) = \sum_{t \in \tilde{T}} q(t) - \alpha(|\tilde{T}| - 1),$$

where the summation above is over the set of internal (non-terminal) nodes rather than the terminal nodes as in Eq. (4). The negative sign in front of the complexity part is a reflection of the fact that Q is to be maximized here, whereas the cost-complexity R is minimized there. In CART, cross validation is used to determine an optimal complexity parameter value, while here LeBlanc and Crowley[16] recommend choosing α between 2 and 4. I refer to their work for the justification of this choice.

Although the tree pruning procedures as described above are statistically elegant, they are rather sophisticated for researchers outside of the statistical society to comprehend. Even within the statistical community, we do not necessarily agree upon the correct use of these procedures. Thus, a practical and intuitive approach is appealing. Segal[18] recommended the following alternative for pruning survival trees. For each internal node (including the root node) of an initial tree, we assign it a value that equals the maximum of the log-rank statistics over all splits starting from the internal node of interest. Then, plot the values for all internal nodes in an increasing order and decide a threshold from the graph. If an internal node corresponds to a smaller value than the threshold, we prune all of its offspring. Although this usually works out fine, the choice of threshold could be arbitrary. In the author's RTEE program, pruning a tree (not necessarily a survival tree) at a different significance level is chosen. Analyzing genetic data, Zhang and Bonney[23] demonstrated how to decide a final tree based on both the scientific implication and computer output.

It is clear that there are plenty of choices to construct survival trees, which is good and bad. More choices give the data analysts the opportunity to select the ones that make a better scientific sense. Sometimes, however, too many choices can also lead the data analysts to wonder what to do. The state of the art is still to construct survival trees using a number of approaches and discuss them with experts to come up one or more trees that are as simple, informative, and interpretable as possible.

4. Classification Trees for Multiple Binary Responses

In this section, I introduce a tree-based approach for analyzing multiple correlated binary outcomes. Such outcomes are sometimes referred to as clustered outcomes. Correlated discrete responses can be generated from a single endpoint by repeatedly measuring it on individuals in a temporal or spatial domain. They are called longitudinal discrete responses. The correlated responses may also consist of distinct endpoints, which are actually the focus of this section.

Suppose that $\mathbf{Y}_i = (Y_{i1}, \ldots, Y_{iq_i})'$ is a vector of binary responses for subject i, $i = 1, \ldots, n$. The index length q_i may vary from individual to individual. This is particularly useful when some responses are missing for some individuals. Multiple correlated outcomes arise from many applications. For example, (Y_1, Y_2) may indicate the blindness of the left and right eyes or cancer status for a sib pair.

We have seen in both classification and survival trees that some of the simple parametric distributions form the foundations for tree constructions. For multiple correlated responses, the following distribution from an exponential family is proven useful:

$$P\{\mathbf{Y}_i = \mathbf{y}_i\} = \exp\left[\sum_{j=1}^{q_i} \theta_{ij} y_{ij} + \sum_{j_1<j_2} \theta_{ij_1 j_2} y_{ij_1} y_{ij_2} + \cdots \right.$$
$$\left. + \theta_{i1\cdots q_i} y_{i1} \cdots y_{iq_i} + A_i(\theta_i)\right], \tag{5}$$

where

$$\theta_i = (\theta_{i1}, \ldots, \theta_{iq_i}, \theta_{i12} \cdots \theta_{i,q_i-1,q_i}, \ldots, \theta_{1\cdots q_i})$$

is the $(2^{q_i-1} - 1)$-vector of canonical parameters and $\exp[A_i(\theta_i)]$ is the normalizing constant. The above model is commonly referred to as log-linear model.

In lieu of extensive search of node splitting, it is important that a distribution used to form the splitting criterion is as simple as possible. Even in more traditional, parametric data analyses, a much simplified version of model (5) is generally used by setting the canonical parameters with respect to the terms with the third- or higher-orders to zero.[10,29] Thus, Zhang[22] considered the following quadratic exponential model:

$$P\{\mathbf{Y} = \mathbf{y}\} = \exp\left[\sum_{j=1}^{q} \theta_j y_j + \sum_{j<k} \theta_{jk} y_j y_k + A(\Psi, \theta)\right], \tag{6}$$

where

$$\Psi = (\theta_1, \ldots, \theta_q)', \quad \theta = (\theta_{12} \cdots \theta_{q-1,q}).$$

He defined the generalized entropy criterion of node t as the maximum of the log-likelihood derived from this distribution, which equals

$$h(t) = \sum_{\{\text{subject } i \in t\}} (\hat{\Psi}' \mathbf{y}_i + \hat{\theta} w_i - A(\hat{\Psi}, \hat{\theta})), \tag{7}$$

where $\hat{\Psi}$ and $\hat{\theta}$ are the maximum likelihood estimates of Ψ and θ, respectively. Then, he chose a split to maximize $h(t_L) + h(t_R)$.

To determine the terminal nodes, Zhang[22] defined the tree quality measure as:

$$R(T) = -\sum_{t \in \tilde{T}} h(t). \tag{8}$$

To illustrate the use of this classification tree approach, Zhang[22] analyzed a subset of the data from a 1989 survey of 6,800 employees of the Library of Congress and the headquarters of the Environmental Protection Agency in the United States. The response variables are six cluster indicators for building-related occupant complaint syndrome, which is a nonspecific set of related symptoms of discomfort reported by occupants of buildings. The six clusters are: central nerve system, upper airway, pain, flu-like, eyes, and lower airway. Zhang[22] considered 22 predictors including those used in Figure 2 as the risk factors. Please refer to Zhang[22] for more details.

Figure 2 reveals that terminal nodes 7 and 17 have the highest incidences of symptoms. The table below the figure gives the number of symptoms reported in each terminal node and for each cluster. The respondents in terminal nodes 7 and 17 experienced more problems in nearly all clusters than others. The figure shows that it is because the air quality in their working area was poor, namely, often too stuffy or sometimes dusty. On the other hand, respondents in terminal node 14 had the least discomfort because they had the best air quality.

The subjects in terminal nodes 16 and 17 were allergic to dust whereas those in terminal node 11 were not. Due to this personal difference, many more symptoms in the central nervous system, upper airway, pain, and flu-like were reported among the allergic subgroups than among the non-allergic ones. Overall, the incidence rate of the eye symptoms is very low, and it appears to be mostly related to air stuffiness as shown in Figure 2. In fact, this figure reveals a lot more information about the symptom incidents than what is mentioned here. Please refer to Zhang[22] for a detailed analysis.

5. Final Remarks

The tree-based methods have become increasingly popular in medical research.[1,3–5,8,14,26,27] In addition, they have proven very useful in machine learning, marketing, finance, etc. The tree-based methods may become one of the standard analytic choices, but they likely complement rather than replace the classic statistical methods such as logistic regression models

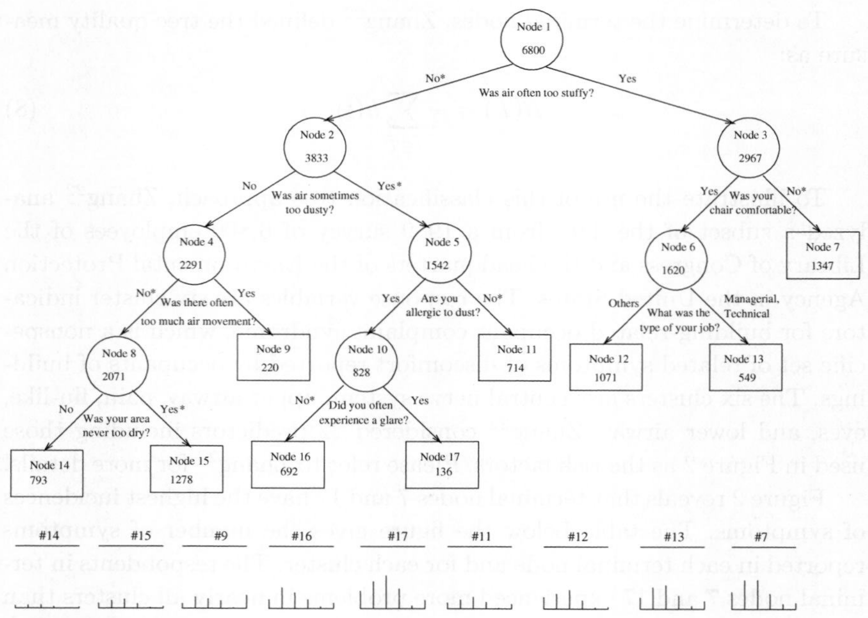

Terminal	Node	Cluster of symptoms					
node No.	Size	CNS	UA	Pain	Flu	Eyes	LA
7	1347	377	637	642	340	114	143
9	220	18	42	35	28	3	48
11	714	72	106	139	79	10	57
12	1071	206	267	333	152	27	35
13	549	103	194	214	120	27	71
14	793	36	41	45	26	2	16
15	1278	113	166	197	101	22	43
16	692	103	238	182	103	22	64
17	136	39	60	73	44	7	19

Fig. 2. Tree structure for the risk of symptoms.[22] Inside each node (○ or a □) are the node number and the number of subjects. The splitting question is given under the node. The asterisks indicate where the subjects with missing information are assigned. The nine diagrams under the tree show the incidence rates of the six clusters (CNS, upper airway, pain, flu-like, eyes, and lower airway) in the nine terminal nodes. The top and bottom lines in each diagram define the unit of 1.

and Cox proportional hazard models. The tree-based methods enable us to produce intuitive and interpretable tree structures without making restrictive parametric assumptions as in the classic models. For the same reason, however, it is more difficult to make statistical inference based on tree structures.

References

1. Bacchetti, P. and Segal, M. R. (1995). Survival trees with time-dependent covariates: Application to estimating changes in the incubation period of aids. *Lifetime Data Anal.* **1**: 35–47.
2. Breiman, L., Friedman, J. H., Olshen, R. A. and Stone, C. J. (1984). *Classification and Regression Trees.* Wadsworth, Belmont, California. Since 1993 this book has been published by Chapman and Hall, New York.
3. Carmelli, D., Halpern, J., Swan, G. E. *et al.* (1991). 27-year mortality in the western collaborative group study: Construction of risk groups by recursive partitioning. *Journal of Clinical Epidemiology* **44**: 1341–1351.
4. Carmelli, D., Zhang, H. P. and Swan, G. E. (1997). Obesity and 33 years of coronary heart disease and cancer mortality in the western collaborative group study. *Epidemiology.*
5. Chou, P. A., Lookabaugh, T. and Gray, R. M. (1989). Optimal pruning with applications to tree-structured source coding and modeling. *IEEE Transaction Information Theory* **35**: 299–315.
6. Ciampi, A., Thiffault, J., Nakache J.-P. and Asselain B. (1986). Stratification by stepwise regression, correspondence analysis and recursive partition: A comparison of three methods of analysis for survival data with covariates. *Computational Statistics and Data Analysis* **4**: 185–204.
7. Ciampi, A., Hogg, S., McKinney, S. and Thiffault, J. (1988). A computer program for recursive partition and amalgamation for censored survival data. *Computer Methods and Programs in Biomedicine* **26**: 239–256.
8. Curran, W. J. Jr., Scott, C. B., Horton, J. *et al.* (1993). Recursive partitioning analysis of prognostic factors in three radiation therapy oncology group malignant glioma trials. *Journal of the National Cancer Institute* **85**: 704–710.
9. Davis, R. and Anderson, J. *et al.* (1989). Exponential survival trees. *Statistics in Medicine* **8**: 947–962.
10. Fitzmaurice, G. and Laird, N. M. (1995). Regression Models for a bivariate discrete and continuous outcome with clustering. *Journal of the American Statistical Association* **90**: 845–852.
11. Goldman, L., Cook, F., Johnson, P., Brand, D., Rouan, G. and Lee, T. (1996). Prediction of the need for intensive care in patients who come to emergency departments with acute chest pain. *NEJM* **334**: 1498–504.
12. Goldman, L., Weinberg, M., Olshen, R. A., Cook, F., Sargent, R. *et al.* (1982). A computer protocol to predict myocardial infarction in emergency department patients with chest pain. *NEJM* **307**: 588–597.

13. Gordon, L. and Olshen, R. A. (1985). Tree-structured survival analysis. *Cancer Treatment Reports* **69**: 1065–1069.
14. Kwak, L. W., Halpern, J., Olshen, R. A. and Horning, S. J. (1990). Prognostic significance of actual dose intensity in diffuse large-cell lymphoma: Results of a tree-structured survival analysis. *Journal of Clinical Oncology* **8**: 963–977.
15. LeBlanc, M. and Crowley, J. (1992). Relative risk trees for censored survival data. *Biometrics* **48**: 411–425.
16. LeBlanc, M. and Crowley, J. (1993). Survival trees by goodness-of-split. *Journal of the American Statistical Association* **88**: 457–467.
17. Miller, R. G. (1981). *Survival Analysis*, Wiley, New York.
18. Segal, M. R. (1988). Regression trees for censored data. *Biometrics* **44**: 35–48.
19. Therneau, T. M., Grambsch, P. M. and Fleming, T. R. (1990). Martingale-based residuals for survival models. *Biometrika* **77**: 147–160.
20. Wasson, J. H., Sox, H. C., Neff, R. K., Goldman, L. (1985). Clinical prediction rules: Applications and methodologic standards. *The New England Journal of Medicine* **313**: 793–799.
21. Zhang, H. P. (1995). Splitting criteria in survival trees. In *Statistical Modelling: Proceedings of the 10th International Workshop on Statistical Modelling*, Innsbruck, Austria, July 1995, Springer-Verlag, pp. 305–314.
22. Zhang, H. P. (1988). Classification trees for multiple binary responses. *Journal of the American Statistical Association* **93**: 180–193.
23. Zhang, H. P. and Bonney, G. (2000). Use of classification trees for association studies. *Genetic Epidemiology.*
24. Zhang, H. P. and Bracken, M. B. (1995). Tree-based risk factor analysis of preterm delivery and small-for-gestational-age birth. *American Journal of Epidemiology* **141**: 70–78.
25. Zhang, H. P., Crowley, J., Sox, H. and Olshen, R. A. (1998). Tree structured statistical methods. *Encyclopedia of Biostatistics* **6**: 4561–4573, Wiley, Chichester, England.
26. Zhang, H. P., Holford, T. and Bracken, M. B. (1996). A tree-based methods of analysis for prospective studies. *Statistics in Medicine* **15**: 37–49.
27. Zhang, H. P. and Bracken, M. B. (1996). Tree-based, two-stage risk factor analysis for spontaneous abortion. *American Journal of Epidemiology* **144**: 989–996.
28. Zhang, H. P. and Singer, B. (1999). *Recursive Partitioning in the Health Sciences*, Springer, New York.
29. Zhao, L. P. and Prentice, R. L. (1990). Correlated binary regression using a quadratic exponential model. *Biometrika* 77: 642–648.

About the Author

Heping Zhang, Ph.D., is Susan Dwight Bliss Professor of Biostatistics, Professor of Statistics, and Professor in the Child Study Center at Yale University. He is also an honorary professor of the University of Hong Kong, a 1000-plan scholar appointed by Chinese Ministry of Logistics, and was a Chang-Jinang scholar at Sun Yat-Sen University appointed by Chinese Ministry of Education. He received his B.S in Mathematics from Jiangxi Normal University in 1982 and his Ph.D in Statistics from Stanford University in 1991. He is a fellow of the American Statistical Association and the Institute of Mathematical Statistics (IMS). He is the founding Editor-in-Chief of Statistics and Its Interface. He currently serves on the editorial boards of the Journal of the American Statistical Association (JASA), Genetic Epidemiology, and Fertility and Sterility. He was 2008 Myrto Lefkopoulou Distinguished Lecturer of Harvard School of Public Health, and 2011 IMS Medallion Lecturer. His research interests include nonparametric methods, longitudinal data, statistical genetics and bioinformatics, clinical trials, statistical modeling of epidemiological data, brain imaging analysis, statistical computation, and statistical methods in behavioral sciences. He is an author of a book on Recursive Partitioning and Its Applications published by Springer, and has also published extensively in statistical, genetic, epidemiological, and psychiatric journals from the Annals of Statistics, JASA to Science.

CHAPTER 37

INTRODUCTION TO ARTIFICIAL NEURAL NETWORKS

XIA JIELAI and JIANG HONGWEI

Department of Health Statistics,
The Fourth Military Medical University,
Xi'an, Shanxi 710033, PR China
Tel: (86) 29-3376979; jielaixia@yahoo.com

TANG QIYI

Institute of Insect Sciences, Zhejiang University,
866 Yuhang tang Road, HangZhon 310058, PR China
qytang@Zju.edu.cn

1. Introduction

While recent progress in neurology has led to the rapid development of artificial neural networks (ANN), the growing requirement of digital computer and artificial intelligence (AI) also promotes ANN. Today, in all problems that involve AI, human intelligence is still performed over AI. To develop a new generation of intelligent computers, we must fully understand the human intelligent processes; in particular, the mechanisms of dealing with information by the neural network systems in human brains. On the other hand, although the initial intention of ANN was merely to explore and simulate informational processing of humans, its superior capability has been demonstrated in problems that traditional digital computer systems and artificial intelligence encountered. Indeed, ANNs can be viewed as a major new break-through to various fields such as computational methodology and AI, etc.

Artificial neural networks (ANN) is an engineering method that simulates the structures and operating principles in the information processing systems possessed by human brain. It was a milestone that psychologist McCulloch and mathematician Pitts had originally proposed in the first mathematical model of ANNs in 1940s. Since then ANN has made rapid progress, and various perceptron models have been brought forth subsequently by many researchers such as F. Rosenblatt, Widrow, Hopf and J. J. Hopfield, etc.

In many ANN studies, simulated annealing (SA)[1,2,4] and Genetic Algorithm (GA)[3,4] are two popular stochastic optimization algorithms. The former was proposed by Metropolis to simulate the annealing process of metal heating, and the latter was proposed by Holland to simulate the natural evolutional process of living beings. Although the stimulated objectives are all different, both algorithms are extremely similar to each other in formulation of algebraic structures. SA holds for the ergodicity of state spaces by generation functions and ensures the directions of iteration processes by acceptation operator. GA holds for the ergodicity of state spaces by crossover operator and mutation operator, and ensures the directions of iteration processes by selection operator.

The traditional statistics, especially parametric statistics, usually assume a population distribution with unknown parameter. It is most perplexing to assure the validity of the assumptions that samples indeed come from the population specified before using statistical techniques such as t test, ANOVA, regression and so on. However, in accordance to directly learning from data sets, ANN dynamically modulates the "weight" of neurons, and sequentially is able to perceive newly resembled data. Because of its favorable resilience against distortions, ANN has unique advantages to processing imperfect data sets and to problems of complex nonlinear systems. Statistically ANN can be described as the nonparametric nonlinear models. Its applications include predictions, cluster analysis, pattern recognition engines, time series analysis and wick relationship gauge among complex systems. Depending on the nonlinear linkage of numerous simple rule sets (neurons), ANN, especially multilayer perceptron networks, is different in essence from normal expert systems, which is some enumerative procedures based on comprehensive rule systems. As knowledge of experts is collected and represented using some traditional measurements, the establishment of expert systems is more difficult than ANN.

2. Back Propagation (BP) Neural Networks

There are many different types of ANN, including the popular Hopfield model,[5] the connection networks by Feldmann,[6] the Baltzmann machine model by Hinton,[7] the multilayer perceptron model by Rumelhart[8] and

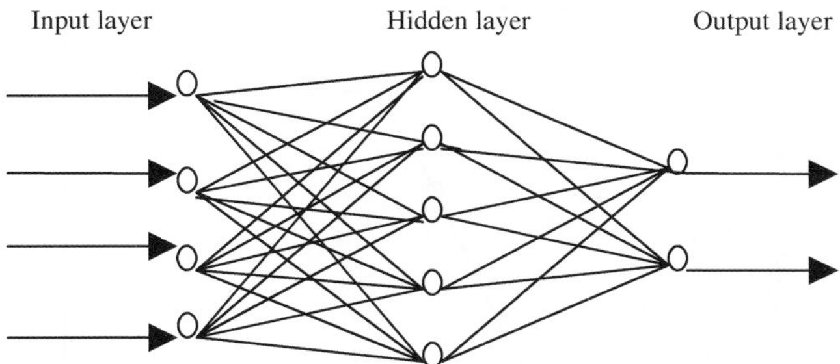

Fig. 1. A BP neural network model.

the self-organization networks models by Kohonen,[9] etc. Multilayer perceptron model is the most general among these ANN models. Although ANN had been around since the late 1940's, no major progress was made until the mid-1980's when the multilayer forward-propagation perceptron model was proposed by Minsky[10] and became sophisticated enough for general applications through combination with back-propagation (BP) algorithm by Rumelhart and simulated annealing (SA) algorithms. A manifold of three-layer BP neural network is shown in Fig. 1.

The BP neural networks (BPNN) systems with the hierarchical structure, include one input layer, several hidden layers and one output layer. Each layer consists of various neutrons taking on two phases: Activity and inactivity. Figure 1 illustrates a typical network with one input layer, one hidden layer and one output layer.

Typically in BPNN, after having processed the signals received from the input layer, the neutrons of the hidden layers propagate it forward to the output layer that completes the finial procedure to export the results. A conventional stimuli function of every neutron usually is a S-shaped curve function such as the logistic function.

$$f(x) = \frac{1}{1 + e^{-x/Q}}\,.$$

Here, Q is the threshold parameter to adjust the formulation of stimuli function. The learning procedure of this algorithm is made up of forward-propagation and backward-propagation. The special characteristic of this type of network is its simple dynamics: when a signal is inputted into the BPNN, it is propagated to the next layer by the interconnections between the neurons. The sign is processed by the neurons of one layer and then be

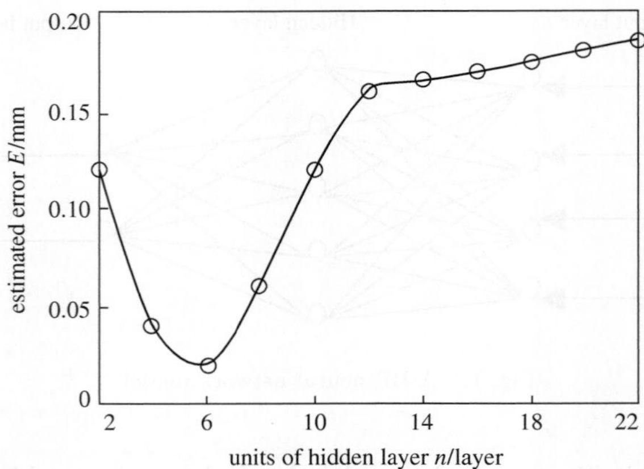

Fig. 2. Relationships between units of the hidden layer and estimated error.

propagated onto the next layer. It means that the state of each layer locally influence the next layer. This procedure will not stop until the signal reaches the output layer sending out the processed signal. In order to upgrade the precision of the system, signal errors feedback across the same pathways. Through modifications of the weights for all units of each layer, the differences between the expected and observed outcome are minimized.

At present, there is no mature theory on how to select the number of units and hidden layers. In general, the more units of hidden layers neural networks possess, the more complexity they reflect and higher precision of learning. Nevertheless, with the increment of units in hidden layers, overfitting to the learning data comes into being easily. If an ANN model is trained on a learning data set very well, its ability to predict subsequently future data set will be enhanced.

Figure 2 shows a special example in which the lowest error achieved when the system has 6 units in the hidden layer.

For simplicity, we assume that there are n sigmoid type units in a neural network which possesses only one unit x in the input layer and one unit y in the output layer. Let (x_k, y_k) $(k = 1, 2, 3, \ldots, N)$ be observations in which x_k is the input signal and y_k is the output signal for the kth sample. Also, let the output of any unit i as O_{ik} and the input of unit j is

$$\text{net}_{jk} = \sum_i W_{ij} O_{ik} \,.$$

And the error function is

$$E = \frac{1}{N}\sum_{k=1}^{N}(y_k - \hat{y}_k)^2 \,.$$

In this function $\hat{y}_k$ is the predicted value of the network output. If $E_k = (y_k - \hat{y}_k)^2$, $\delta_{jk} = \frac{\partial E_k}{\partial \mathrm{net}_{jk}}$ and $O_{jk} = f(\mathrm{net}_{jk})$, then

$$\frac{\partial E_k}{\partial W_{ij}} = \frac{\partial E_k}{\partial \mathrm{net}_{jk}}\frac{\partial \mathrm{net}_{jk}}{\partial W_{ij}} = \frac{\partial E_k}{\partial \mathrm{net}_{jk}} O_{ik} = \delta_{jk} O_{ik} \,.$$

If the unit j is in the output layer, $O_{jk} = \hat{y}_k$

$$\delta_{jk} = \frac{\partial E_k}{\partial \hat{y}_k}\frac{\partial \hat{y}_k}{\partial \mathrm{net}_{jk}} = -(y_k - \hat{y}_k) f'(\mathrm{net}_{jk}) \,. \tag{1}$$

If unit j is not in the output layer, then

$$\delta_{jk} = \frac{\partial E_k}{\partial \mathrm{net}_{jk}} = \frac{\partial E_k}{\partial O_{jk}}\frac{\partial O_{jk}}{\partial \mathrm{net}_{jk}} = \frac{\partial E_k}{\partial O_{jk}} f'(\mathrm{net}_{jk})$$

$$\begin{aligned}\frac{\partial E_k}{\partial O_{jk}} &= \sum_m \frac{\partial E_k}{\partial \mathrm{net}_{mk}}\frac{\partial \mathrm{net}_{mk}}{\partial O_{jk}} \\ &= \sum_m \frac{\partial E_k}{\partial \mathrm{net}_{mk}}\frac{\partial}{\partial O_{jk}}\sum_i W_{mi} O_{ik} \\ &= \sum_m \frac{\partial E_k}{\partial \mathrm{net}_{mk}}\sum_i W_{mj} = \sum_m \delta_{mk} W_{mj} \,.\end{aligned}$$

Thus,

$$\begin{cases} \delta_{jk} = f'(\mathrm{net}_{jk})\sum_m \delta_{mk} W_{mj} \\ \dfrac{\partial E_k}{\partial W_{ij}} = \delta_{mk} O_{ik} \,. \end{cases} \tag{2}$$

If a neural network has M layers in which the Mth only owns the output units and the first layer only possesses the input units, then BP algorithms are

(i) Select the initial weights W.
(ii) Repeat following procedures until converging:
   a. For K from 1 to N
      (a) Calculate O_{ik}, net_{jk} and $\hat{y}_k$ (in the procedure of forward-propagation)

(b) Implement the reversed calculation of layers from M to 2 (in the procedure of backward-propagation)

b. For the same unit $j \in M$, calculated δ_{jk} by (1) and (2).

(iii) Modulate weights, $W_{ij} = W_{ij} - \delta \frac{\partial E}{\partial W_{ij}}$, $\delta > 0$, for $\frac{\partial E}{\partial W_{ij}} = \sum_{k}^{N} \frac{\partial E_k}{\partial W_{ij}}$

From BP algorithms, it concludes that BP models transform input-to-output patterns of sampling data sets into the optimization of nonlinear models. Its optimization is totally different from the traditional gradient descend method. So neural networks are the absolutely nonlinear mapping projects between input and output.

The focal design of a neural network lies in how to estimate the structure of models and the selection of learning algorithms. To establish appropriate learning algorithms and model structure, we must rely on current theoretical developments of ANN and train these systems with enormous datasets. By dynamically adjusting the parameters of networks in the continuous procedures of learning, ANN can reach the precision required.

3. Introduction to Operation of DPS Data Process System

ANN packages have been embedded in statistical software packages, such as SPSS, MATLAB and so forth. They can be browsed in those statistical software websites. DPS, Data Processing System, programmed by Qiyi Tang, will be showed below in this section. The basic data structure is that each row is a single case (observation), each column is a single variable and the left is the data of input units (independent variables), the right is the data of output units (dependent variables). All values of cases are entered one by one. There is no need to enter the outputs (dependent variables) for the individuals to be recognized (predicted).

After the data-entering step has finished, press CTRL and right button of mouse to define the predicted data as the second block.

Before the learning procedure of neural networks, an optional dialogue, showed in Fig. 3 below, will appear to require entry of some parameters of neural network. The principles of setting parameters are:

(1) *Number of units*: The number of units of the input layer equals to the number of characteristic factors (independent variables), and the units of the output layer just amount to the number of system targets. Generally the number of units in hidden layers, greatly varies according to individual experiences, is 75% units of input layer. For example, if

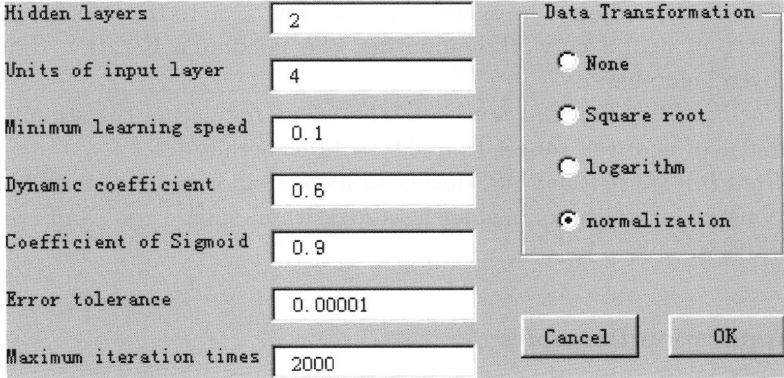

Fig. 3. Optional dialogue of parameters in neural network.

there are 7 units in an input layer and 1 unit in an output layer, the number of units in a hidden layer will be 5 to constitute a 7-5-1 model of neural network. In practice, due to comparing the output consequences of various units in a hidden layer, the most reasonable structure is established conclusively after the learning procedure of neural network.

(2) *Initial weights*: All initial weights must not be exactly equal to each other. For the fact that it has been verified that once the initial weights are identical, even if there exists a set of diverse weights so as to the minimum error of neural network, the weights of units will remain to be equal. Thus, in our software, a random generator is programmed to yield a set of random numbers ranged from -0.5 to $+0.5$ as the initial weight of neural network.

(3) *Optimum learning speed*: As a typical BP algorithm, the larger the learning speed is, the greater the change of the weights is, and the faster the convergence is. However when learning speed is beyond a certain limitation, the neural network will oscillate. Consequently learning speed is larger with the guarantee against system oscillation. So, in DPS, learning speed is optimized automatically, though user can specify a certain value, say 0.9.

(4) *Dynamic coefficient*: It is chosen empirically too, just as the range from 0.6 to 0.8.

(5) *Error tolerance*: Generally ranges from 0.001 to 0.00001. If the error between the results of two successive iterations is below the tolerance, computing stops systematically to provide the results.

(6) *Times of iteration*: The default value is 1000. Due to the possible divergence of neural network computing, the maximum iteration times is given beforehand.
(7) *Coefficient of Sigmoid function*: The value, regulating the stimuli formulas of neutron, ranges from 0.9 to 1.0 generally.
(8) *Data transformation*: DPS has advantage of allowing data transformations in several functions, such as logarithm, square root and normalization.

4. Application Examples

Example 1 is an illustration to use our software. Physicians under randomization collect the dataset. The influencing factors set of body surface area consists of 4 physical factors: Sex, age, weight and height. Figure 4 shows the nonlinear relationships between predictor variables and response variable.

Before establishing BP neural network, we split the data set into two segments: From No. 1 to No. 70 as learning sample and from No. 71 to No. 90 severally as predicted sample. The data structure is defined as the following blocks in Table 1.

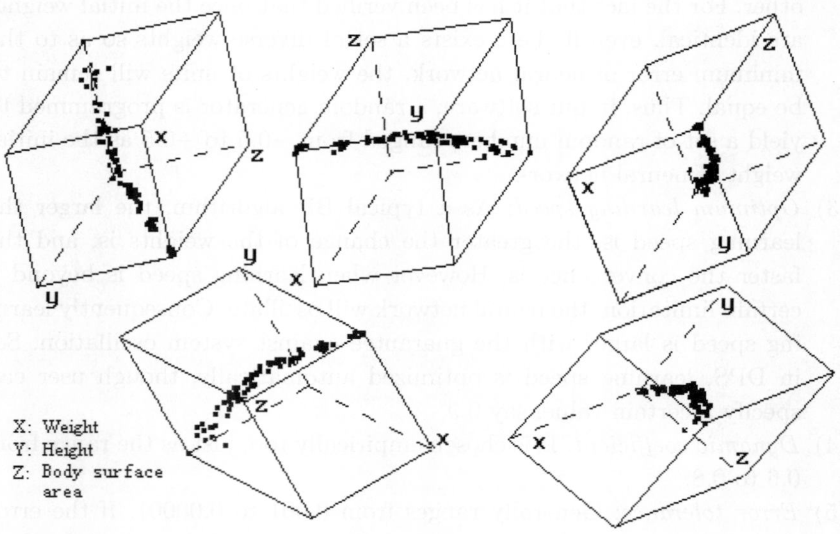

Fig. 4. 3-D Scatter of weight, height and body surface area.

Table 1. Random allotment of 90 persons' physical measurements.

No.	Sex	Age (year)	Weight (kg)	Height (cm)	Body Surface Area (cm^2)	No.	Sex	Age (year)	Weight (kg)	Height (cm)	Body Surface Area (cm^2)
1	1	13	30.5	138.5	10072.9	46	0	15	43	152	12998.7
2	0	5	15	101	6189	47	0	13	27.5	139	9569.1
3	0	0	2.5	51.5	1906.2	48	0	3	12	91	5358.4
4	1	11	30	141	10290.6	49	0	15	40.5	153	12627.4
5	1	15	40.5	154	13221.6	50	1	5	15	100	6364.5
6	0	11	27	136	9654.5	51	1	1	9	80	4380.8
7	0	5	15	106	6768.2	52	1	5	16.5	112	7256.4
8	1	5	15	103	6194.1	53	0	3	12.5	91	5291.5
9	1	3	13.5	96	5830.2	54	1	0	3.5	56.5	2506.7
10	0	13	36	150	11759	55	0	1	10	77	4180.4
11	0	3	12	92	5299.4	56	1	9	25	126	8813.7
12	1	0	2.5	51	2094.5	57	1	9	33	138	11055.4
13	0	7	19	121	7490.8	58	1	5	16	108	6988
14	1	13	28	130.5	9521.7	59	0	11	29	127	9969.8
15	1	0	3	54	2446.2	60	0	7	20	114	7432.8
16	0	0	3	51	1632.5	61	0	1	7.5	77	3934
17	0	7	21	123	7958.8	62	1	11	29.5	134.5	9970.5
18	1	11	31	139	10580.8	63	0	5	15	101	6225.7
19	1	7	24.5	122.5	8756.1	64	0	3	13	91	5601.7
20	1	11	26	133	9573	65	0	5	15	98	6163.7
21	0	9	24.5	130	9028	66	1	15	45	157	13426.7
22	1	9	25	124	8854.5	67	1	7	21	120	8249.2
23	1	0	2.25	50.5	1928.4	68	0	9	23	127	8875.8
24	0	11	27	129	9203.1	69	0	7	17	104	6873.5
25	0	0	2.25	53	2200.2	70	1	15	43.5	150	13082.8
26	0	5	16	105	6785.1	71*	1	15	50	168	14832
27	0	9	30	133	10120.8	72*	0	7	18	114	7071.8
28	0	13	34	148	11397.3	73*	1	3	14	97	6013.6
29	1	3	16	99	6410.6	74*	1	7	20	119	7876.4
30	1	3	11	92	5283.3	75*	0	0	3	54	2117.3
31	0	9	23	126	8693.5	76*	1	1	9.5	74	4314.2
32	1	13	30	138	9626.1	77*	0	15	44	163	13480.9
33	1	9	29	138	10178.7	78*	0	11	32	140	10583.8
34	1	1	8	76	4134.5	79*	1	0	3	52	2121
35	0	15	42	165	13019.5	80*	0	11	29	141	10135.3
36	1	15	40	151	12297.1	81*	0	3	15	94	6074.9
37	1	1	9	80	4078.4	82*	0	13	44	140	13020.3
38	1	7	22	123	8651.1	83*	1	5	15.5	105	6406.5
39	0	1	9.5	77	4246.1	84*	1	9	22	126	8267
40	1	7	25	125	8754.4	85*	0	15	40	159.5	12769.7

(*Continued*)

Table 1. (*Continued*)

No.	Sex	Age (year)	Weight (kg)	Height (cm)	Body Surface Area (cm^2)	No.	Sex	Age (year)	Weight (kg)	Height (cm)	Body Surface Area (cm^2)
41	1	13	36	143	11282.4	86*	1	1	9.5	76	3845.9
42	1	3	15	94	6101.6	87*	0	13	32	144	10822.1
43	0	0	3	51	1850.3	88*	1	13	40	151	12519.9
44	0	1	9	74	3358.5	89*	0	9	22	124	8586.1
45	0	1	7.5	73	3809.7	90*	1	11	31	135	10120.6

Note: The sign * denote predicted sample.

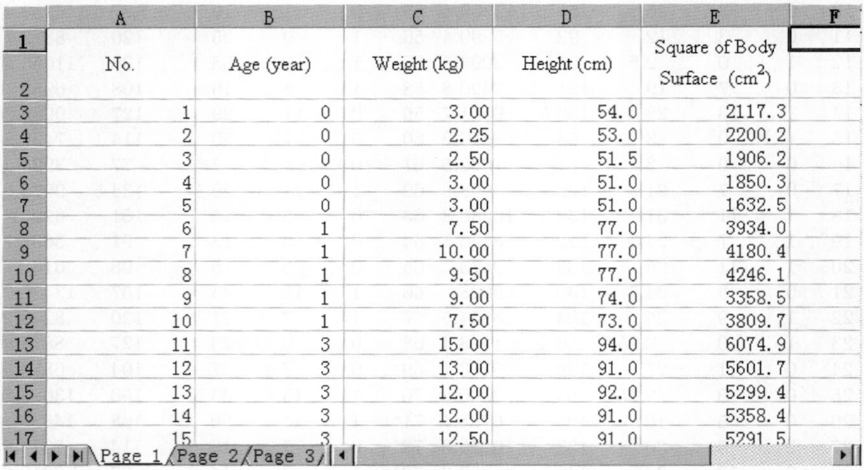

	A	B	C	D	E	F
1	No.	Age (year)	Weight (kg)	Height (cm)	Square of Body Surface (cm^2)	
2						
3	1	0	3.00	54.0	2117.3	
4	2	0	2.25	53.0	2200.2	
5	3	0	2.50	51.5	1906.2	
6	4	0	3.00	51.0	1850.3	
7	5	0	3.00	51.0	1632.5	
8	6	1	7.50	77.0	3934.0	
9	7	1	10.00	77.0	4180.4	
10	8	1	9.50	77.0	4246.1	
11	9	1	9.00	74.0	3358.5	
12	10	1	7.50	73.0	3809.7	
13	11	3	15.00	94.0	6074.9	
14	12	3	13.00	91.0	5601.7	
15	13	3	12.00	92.0	5299.4	
16	14	3	12.00	91.0	5358.4	
17	15	3	12.50	91.0	5291.5	

Page 1 / Page 2 / Page 3

Fig. 5. Diagram of the data editor window for BP neural network.

Figure 5 is an editor window of DPS system. The format of data is inputted as the following.

After launching the learning procedure of neural network, a window similar to Fig. 5 will be displayed. And then assign the parameter of network: Units in input layer is 4, hidden layer has 2 layers, optimum learning speed is 0.1, dynamic coefficient is 0.6, the coefficient of Sigmoid function is 0.9, error tolerance is 0.00001, maximum times of iteration are 2000, and the selection of data transformation is normalization.

Then press the "OK" button. Then we set 5 to the units of the first hidden layer and set 3 to the units of second hidden layer. After 2000 iterations, the error is 0.00000170. The weights of neutron in output layer is shown below:

Weights matrix of units in the first hidden layer

0.597230	−0.824710	0.566580	−1.065810	0.051900
0.750700	−0.151260	0.172180	−0.369140	−0.139280
−0.715220	2.044800	0.194420	−0.869060	−2.243410
−2.33773	−0.07406	1.46518	−0.12269	1.168

Weights matrix of units in the second hidden layer

−0.507940	−4.616450	3.675080
−0.928980	1.937520	−1.824980
−0.268910	0.21253	−3.046950
−0.708560	−4.81552	2.276470
−0.08934	−4.92864	−0.5283

Weights matrix of units in the output layer

1.12130
7.20956
−5.5911

Table 2 compared the predicted values with the observed values of the body surface area. And these predicted values from No. 71 to No. 90, used as predicted sample, are very close to the observed values. So the facts illustrate that the neural network has favorable abilities in model fitting and predicting.

Table 2. The predicted values and the observed values of neural network.

No.	Predicted Value	Observed Value	No.	Predicted Value	Observed Value	No.	Predicted Value	Observed Value
1	10226.87	10072.9	31	8511.77	8693.5	61	3793.63	3934
2	6370.82	6189	32	10085.21	9626.1	62	10024.22	9970.5
3	2076.073	1906.2	33	10138.25	10178.7	63	6370.82	6225.7
4	10320.32	10290.6	34	3896.33	4134.5	64	5528.03	5601.7
5	12589.19	13221.6	35	12830.50	13019.5	65	6183.77	6163.7
6	9544.59	9654.5	36	12484.89	12297.1	66	13052.96	13426.7
7	6651.57	6768.2	37	4353.68	4078.4	67	8072.70	8249.2
8	6510.22	6194.1	38	8353.89	8651.1	68	8536.07	8875.8
9	6034.13	5830.2	39	4053.10	4246.1	69	6733.68	6873.5
10	11881.13	11759	40	8993.87	8754.4	70	12893.16	13082.8
11	5461.66	5299.4	41	11713.91	11282.4	71*	13282.39	14832
12	2166.992	2094.5	42	6090.36	6101.6	72*	7358.28	7071.8
13	7748.67	7490.8	43	2082.186	1850.3	73*	6173.54	6013.6
14	9342.00	9521.7	44	3746.90	3358.5	74*	7875.99	7876.4
15	2275.284	2446.2	45	3485.76	3809.7	75*	2163.63	2117.3
16	2082.186	1632.5	46	12914.47	12998.7	76*	3909.322	4314.2
17	8109.89	7958.8	47	9703.54	9569.1	77*	13002.22	13480.9
18	10528.90	10580.8	48	5387.18	5358.4	78*	10854.05	10583.8
19	8803.51	8756.1	49	12658.19	12627.4	79*	2213.59	2121
20	9157.74	9573	50	6306.22	6364.5	80*	10094.41	10135.3
21	8894.74	9028	51	4353.68	4380.8	81*	6026.73	6074.9
22	8797.66	8854.5	52	7228.11	7256.4	82*	12950.38	13020.3
23	2145.221	1928.4	53	5457.31	5291.5	83*	6703.66	6406.5
24	9414.36	9203.1	54	2386.589	2506.7	84*	8315.04	8267
25	2104.641	2200.2	55	4120.19	4180.4	85*	12601.92	12769.7
26	6732.92	6785.1	56	8871.79	8813.7	86*	4075.91	3845.9
27	10243.62	10120.8	57	11159.89	11055.4	87*	10903.51	10822.1
28	11424.97	11397.3	58	6947.78	6988	88*	12564.37	12519.9
29	6584.85	6410.6	59	9869.52	9969.8	89*	8277.76	8586.1
30	5395.49	5283.3	60	7658.39	7432.8	90*	10423.74	10120.6

Note: The sign * denote predicted sample.

5. ANNs Based on Genetic Algorithm

Genetic Algorithm (GA), first proposed in 1975 by Holland in Michigan University, USA, is inspired by natural selection of Darwinism and the genetics machine. As a brand-new global optimization technique, the algorithm uses the population evolution principles to continuously optimize the prediction weights and eventually finds the optimal or nearly optimal solutions. Because it is simple, universal, robust and applicable to parallel computing, this method is effectively used in a wide variety of fields, such

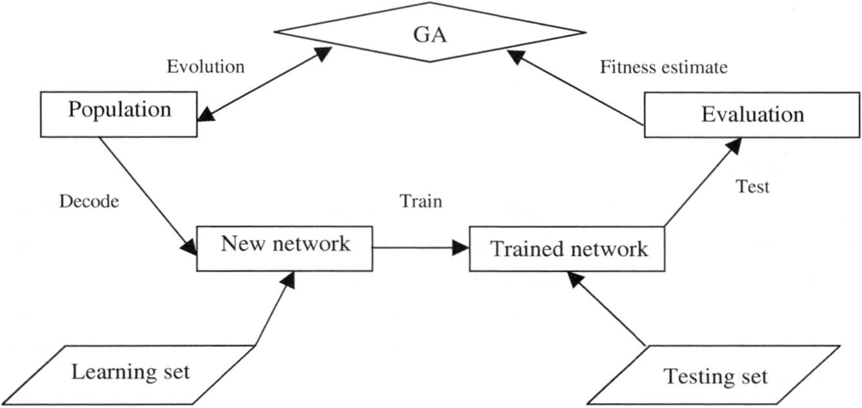

Fig. 6. The conjunction of GA and ANN.

as computer, dispatch optimization, transport problems and constitution optimizations etc.

GA, instead of many traditional methods, has been increasingly applied in ANNs design in the learning steps. The conjunction of GA and ANNs, showed below in Fig. 6, will be applied to the evaluation of crops in current research.

5.1. *Value encoding GA oriented to learning of weights in ANN*

5.1.1. *Encoding*

The procedure of weight learning in neural network is a continuously complicated optimization problem of parameters. Binary encoding gives too many possible chromosomes even with a small numbers of alleles. On the other hand, this encoding is often not natural for many problems and sometimes corrections must be made after crossover and/or mutation. By this method, the change of weights will step forward so as to influence the precision of learning in neural network. Therefore value encoding is adopted in the current study.

5.1.2. *Fitness function*

The weights of chromosomes are allocated to ANN, and the learning data sets are served as input/output. Then inverse mean squared error, coming out after ANN computing, is defined as fitness function:

$$f = 1 \Big/ \sum_{i=1}^{n} e_i^2 .$$

5.1.3. *Weights initialization*

Against that in ordinary BP algorithms performing with the uniform distribution from 0.0 to 1.0, the initial weights of neural network are obtained in accordance with the distribution of $e^{-|\gamma|}$, supported by enormous known trials, because all possible solution can be run around. As a result, the absolute values of weights are relatively small after neural network converges.

5.1.4. *Genetic operator*

Although genetic operators are different from various application circumstances, the weight crossover and weight mutation are two most important operators.

5.1.5. *Selection*

The selection probability of each individual is determined not by means of proportion, but by an elite ratio S, a measure of the surviving ratio of offspring. This can be written as:

$$P_2 = P_1 \cdot S$$

$$P_3 = P_2 \cdot S$$

$$\vdots$$

where P_1, P_2, P_3, ... represent the individual probabilities of various fitness functions: First-rate, second-rate, third-rate and so on.

5.2. *The conjunction of GA and ANN*

There is a 3-layer BP neural network with one input layer, one output layer and one hidden layer. Now first, using training sample A_k and expected output $C_k (k = 1, 2, \ldots, m)$, we calculate the stimuli values from the input layer to the hidden layer by formula

$$b_i = f\left(\sum_{h=1}^{n} a_h V_{hi} + \theta_i\right),$$

where $i = 1, 2, \ldots, p$, the units in output layer are a_h, the connection weights from input layer to hidden layer are V_{hi}, the thresholds of units in hidden layer are θ_i. The values of a_h, V_{hi}, θ_i are determined by the probability distributions, $e^{-|\gamma|}$. The stimuli algorithm is a logistic function:

$$f(x) = 1/(1 + e^{-x}). \tag{3}$$

And then using formula (3) and (4), we compute the stimuli values of units in the output layer:

$$C_j = f\left(\sum_{i=1}^{p} W_{ij} b_i + \gamma_j\right).$$

where $j = 1, 2, \ldots, q$, the connection weights from hidden layer to output layer are W_{ij}, the thresholds of units in the output layer are γ_j. And also the values of W_{ij}, γ_j are determined by the probability distribution, $e^{-|\gamma|}$. The method for calculating normalized error of output layer is given in (4):

$$d_j C_j (1 - C_j)(C_j^k - C_j), \tag{4}$$

where the expected value of unit j in output layer is C_j^k.

Finally, compute the error of units in hidden layer compared with each d_j

$$e_i = b_i (1 - b_i) \sum_{j=1}^{q} W_{ij} d_j.$$

On the basis of abiding on the above-mentioned steps and recombining crossover and mutation, we modulate the hidden-layer-to-output-layer connection weights and the thresholds of units in the output layer following the adjustment of the input-layer-to-hidden-layer connection weights and the thresholds of units in hidden layer. When the error between expected and observed outcomes converge to the pre-determined error tolerance, the learning of neural network stops.

6. Future Research Trends

Because the intelligent computing techniques, such as ANN, succeed in many applications, they attract considerable attention and play an important role in many research fields. As a popular utility, should become more matured in the future. But in terms of intelligent computing itself and statistics, several outstanding obstacles, which be urgently solved in this field are:

(1) It is known that AI still does not possess many inherent characteristics of brain, such as tolerance and robustness. Although ANNs have solved some problems in AI, their theories are not perfect and are still in their infancy. Moreover, AI and ANN may be completely different realizations of the natural principles on which the brain is based. So a number of mathematical principles should be developed right now. But this is ignored in lots of standard textbooks and reviews. Researchers should pay more attention to studying existing theories and to establishing mathematical foundations. To avoid getting lost in the "forest" of biological mechanisms, the nature of AI and ANN theories should be figured out. As there have been a multitude of materials and experiences, it is time to replace many seemingly faultless algorithms, which are full of analogues and metaphors, with the specifically objective methods and theories of quantification.

(2) It will take a longer time to reveal and understand the intelligent mechanisms of human beings. These biological discoveries are increasingly considered as a way to open up the scopes of AI and ANN. Once biology, neurology, genetics make break-throughs, AI and ANN can simulate high-level intelligent mechanisms to solve some unsolvable problems encountered today. Furthermore, they also urge biologic researchers to unveil more sealed puzzle in intelligence. Although AI and ANN are gray-box algorithms and approximately correspond to intelligence of human beings, they can provide some useful clues and foundations for further research. While verifying rationality of previous models, the methodology of AI and ANN, how to construct more sophisticated models, become more individualistic and explicit.

(3) Although AI and ANN have developed for near 50 years, their terminology has not standardized by any cases. Especially as to random system, most networks completely conceal or rigidly utilize the statistics. In the words of Anderson, Pellionisz and Rosenfeld:[22] Neural networks are statistics for amateurs. Most statisticians still soberly stand by the development of ANNs and will not to accept it in a short time because ANNs are quite imperfect compared with statistics. They, especially in statistical applications, are reluctant to waste valuable data and time in automatic processing of computer. However, along with maturity of MCMC theory and Gibbs sampling and the increasing Interactions between Frequency School and Bayesian School, the ANN based on Bayesian theory is growing rapidly. All the advantages of ANN are evaluated empirically based on practical applications rather

than in theoretical comparisons with statistic methods. The impact of ANNs on the theory and application of statistics is rather obscure at this stage. At present, as a system method between gray-box and black-box, we cannot evaluate ANNs advantages in generalized range. So how to combine ANN with statistics may be a feasible approach to get out of current dilemma. Statistician should pay more attention to the aspects of AI and ANN.

References

1. Metropolis, N., Rosenbluth, A. W., Rosenbluth, M. N., Teller, A. H. and Teller, E. (1953). Equation of state calculations by fast computing machines. *Journal of Chemical Physics* **21**: 1087–1092.
2. Rumelhart D. E., Hinton G. E. and Williams R. J. (1986). Learning representation by back propagation errors. *Nature* **323**(6188): 533–536
3. Holland J. H. (1992). *Adaptation in Natural and Artificial Systems.* MIT Press, Cambridge, Massachusetss.
4. Dong, C., Li, Z. N., Xia, R. W. and He, Q. Z. (1995). Advance and some problems on multilayer perceptron neural network. *Mechanics advance* **25**(2): 186–196.
5. Hopfield, J. J. (1982). Neural networks and physical systems with emergent collective computational abilities. *Proceedings of National Academic Sciences USA* **79**: 2445–2458.
6. Feldmann, R., Monien, B. and Mysliwietz, P. (1990). Distributed game tree search. In *Parallel Algorithms for Machine Intelligence and Vision*, eds. Kumar, Kanal and Gopalakrishan, Springer-Verlag, New York.
7. Hinton, G. E., Van Camp, D. (1993). Keeping neural networks simple by minimizing the description length of the weights. *Proceedings of the 6th Annual ACM Conference on Computational Learning Theory*, Santa Cruz, 5–13.
8. Rumbelhart, D. E., Hinton, G. E., Willians, R. J. (1986a). Learning representations by back-propagating errors. *Nature* **323**: 533–536.
9. Kohonen, T. (1984). *Associative Memory and Self-Organization*, Springer-Verlag, New York.
10. Minsky, M. L. and Papert, S. A. (1988). *Perceptrons. Expanded Edition*, MIT Press, Cambridge, Massachusetss. (First edn 1969.)
11. Lai, Y. X. and Lu, Y. S. (1999). BP neural network application in the distribution study of fluid diversity. *Journal of Beijing Chemistry University* **26**(2).
12. Radford, M. J. (1996). *Bayeian Learning for Neural Networks*, Springer, New York.
13. Watt, R. (1991). *Understanding Vision*, Academic Press, London.
14. Barndorff-Nielsen, O. E. and Jensen, J. L. (1993). *Networks and Chaos Statistical and Probabilistic Aspects*, Chapman and Hall, London.

15. Zhang, S. Q., Chen, C. and Wan, E. P. (1998). Gray system application in production evaluation. *Geography* **18**(6): 581–585.
16. Hechi Nielsen, R. (1989). Theory of the back propagation neural network. *International Journal of Conference Neural Network* **1**: 593–605.
17. Bornholdt, A. (1992). General asymmetric neural network and structure design by genetic algorithms. *Neural Network* **5**(2): 327–334.
18. Li, M. Q., Xu, B. Y. and Kou, J. S. (1999). The combination of GA and ANN. *Theory and Practice of System Engineering* **21**(2): 65–69.
19. Jin, L., Luo, Y., Mou, Q. L. *et al.* (1998). Study on ANN prediction model of the humidity in the soil of cornfield. *Agrology* **35**(1): 25–35.
20. Li, Z. and Zhang, J. T. (2000). The study on evaluation of mealie based on the combination of GA and ANN. *Natural Resource Journal* **15**(3).
21. Deng J. N. (1992). *The Basic Methods of Gray System*, Center China Sci. Tech. Univ. Press, 304–312.
22. Anderson, J. A., Pellionisz, A. and Rosenfeld, E. (1990). *Neuro-computing 2: Directions for Research*, MIT Press, Cambridge, Massachusetts.

About the Authors

Dr. Xia Jielai, is Professor of the Fourth Military Medical University. He earned his bachelor in applied mathematics from the Anhui University and master and Ph.D in healthy statistics from the Fourth Military Medical University. He taught in the bio-statistics department of the university as an assistant professor (1983–1988), lecturer (1988–1995), associate professor (1995–1998) and professor (1988-present). He visited clinical and epidemiological research center of Prince of Wales Hospital, the Chinese University of Hongkong (January–February 1994), and the Department of Genetics and Biometry, Louisiana State University Medical Center (March–October 1994). He serves as the Director of the Committee of Statistical Theory and Methodology, Chinese Medical Statistical Association. His research fields are biostatistics and data processing, including theory and methods of statistical modeling and soft development of NoSA (Non-typical data statistical analysis system). He has published numerous articles in various scientific journals.

Dr. Qiyi Tang, is Professor and senior scientist at the Insect Research Institute, Zhejiang University. Dr. Tang is a member of the Design Committee of Chinese Mathematical Association, fellow of the Chinese Association of Plant Protection and committee member of Pest Forecasting. Since 1981, Dr. Tang has been engaged in plant protection, pest forecasting, mathematical modeling of insect ecology, statistical analysis and software development. Dr. Tang was the winner of the National Science and Technology award and has published more than 50 articles and two monographs, *Applied statistical analysis and its computer platform* and *Applied statistical analysis and DPS data processing system.* The senior science has also developed a user-friendly statistical analysis software "DPBS Data Processing System", which has been widely used in various research areas. Dr. Tang has also participated in the software development of "Green Cross Doctor of Forecasting", "Rice Pests Zoning Management System", "Pest Forecasting Mapping System" and other plant protection software.

INDEX

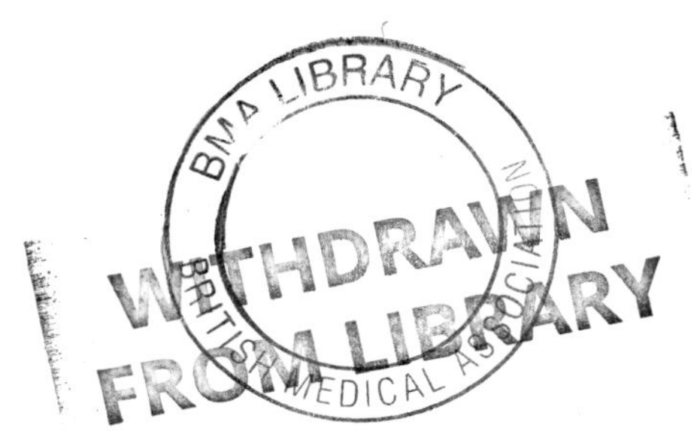